OKU

4

Orthopaedic Knowledge Update:
Trauma

AAOS
AMERICAN ACADEMY OF
ORTHOPAEDIC SURGEONS

OKU

4

Orthopaedic
Knowledge
Update:
Trauma

EDITORS:
Andrew H. Schmidt, MD
Professor, University of Minnesota
Faculty, Hennepin County Medical Center
Minneapolis, Minnesota

David C. Teague, MD
Professor and Don H. O'Donoghue Chair
Department of Orthopedic Surgery
University of Oklahoma
Oklahoma City, Oklahoma

DEVELOPED BY THE
ORTHOPAEDIC TRAUMA ASSOCIATION

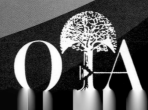

AAOS
AMERICAN ACADEMY OF
ORTHOPAEDIC SURGEONS

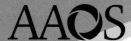

AMERICAN ACADEMY OF ORTHOPAEDIC SURGEONS

Published 2010 by the
American Academy of Orthopaedic Surgeons
6300 North River Road
Rosemont, IL 60018

Fourth Edition
Copyright 2010
by the American Academy of Orthopaedic Surgeons

ISBN 978-0-89203-692-9
Printed in the USA
Library of Congress Cataloging-in-Publication Data

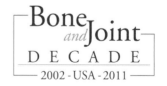

Bone *and* Joint
DECADE
2002 - USA - 2011

Acknowledgments

Editorial Board, Orthopaedic Knowledge Update: Trauma 4

Andrew H. Schmidt, MD
Professor, University of Minnesota
Faculty, Hennepin County Medical Center
Minneapolis, Minnesota

David C. Teague, MD
Professor and Don H. O' Donoghue Chair
Department of Orthopedic Surgery
University of Oklahoma
Oklahoma City, Oklahoma

Carlo Bellabarba, MD
Associate Professor
Director of Orthopaedic Spine Service
Department of Orthopaedics and Sports
  Medicine
University of Washington/Harborview Medical
  Center
Seattle, Washington

John T. Capo, MD
Associate Professor and Chief
Division of Hand and Microsurgery
Department of Orthopaedics
New Jersey Medical School
Newark, New Jersey

John T. Gorczyca, MD
Professor of Orthopaedic Surgery
Chief, Division of Orthopaedic Trauma
Department of Orthopaedics and Rehabilitation
University of Rochester Medical
Rochester, New York

Kenneth J. Koval, MD
Orthopaedic Surgeon
Wilmot, New Hampshire

Berton R. Moed, MD
Professor and Chairman
Department of Orthopaedic Surgery
Saint Louis University School of Medicine
St. Louis, Missouri

Kevin J. Pugh, MD
Director, Limb Reconstruction
Orthopaedic Trauma and Reconstructive
  Surgery
Grant Medical Center
Columbus, Ohio

Adam J. Starr, MD
Associate Professor
Department of Orthopaedic Surgery
UT Southwestern Medical Center
Dallas, Texas

Michael D. Stover, MD
Orthopaedic Surgery and Rehabilitation
Loyola University Medical Center
Maywood, Illinois

Orthopaedic Trauma Association Executive Committee

Timothy J. Bray, MD
President

Andrew N. Pollak, MD
President-Elect

Robert A. Probe, MD
2nd President-Elect

James P. Stannard, MD
Secretary

Alan L. Jones, MD
Chief Financial Officer
Finance and Audit Committee

David C. Templeman, MD
Immediate Past President
Nominating Committee

J. Tracy Watson, MD
2nd Past President
Strategic Plan Chairman

Brendan M. Patterson, MD
David J. Stephen, MD
Christopher T. Born, MD
Members-at-Large

William M. Ricci, MD
Annual Program Chair

Contributors

Animesh Agarwal, MD
Associate Professor
Chief, Division of Orthopaedic Trauma
Department of Orthopaedics
University of Texas Health Science Center at
San Antonio
San Antonio, Texas

Julie Agel, MA, ATC
Department of Orthopaedics
Harborview Medical Center
Seattle, Washington

Sam Agnew, MD
Partner, Senior Consultant
Orthopaedic Trauma Practice Consultants
Tampa, Florida

Jaimo Ahn, MD, PhD
Assistant Professor
Penn Orthopaedic Trauma and Fracture Service
Hospital of the University of Pennsylvania
Philadelphia, Pennsylvania

Peter Althausen, MD
Orthopaedic Surgeon
Reno Orthopaedic Clinic
Reno, Nevada

Daniel T. Altman, MD
Associate Professor
Director, Orthopaedic Spine Trauma
Allegheny Orthopaedic Associates
Allegheny General Hospital
Pittsburgh, Pennsylvania

Mark J. Anders, MD
Associate Professor, Orthopaedic Surgery
Director, Orthopaedic Trauma
Orthopaedic Surgery
State University of New York at Buffalo
Buffalo, New York

Romney C. Andersen, MD
Chief, Orthopaedic Surgery
Department of Orthopaedics and Rehabilitation
Walter Reed National Military Medical Center
Bethesda, MD; Washington, DC

Reto H. Babst, MD
Professor of Surgery
Chairman, Department of Surgery
Clinic of Trauma Surgery
Luzerner Kantonsspital
Lucerne, Switzerland

David P. Barei, MD
Associate Professor
Orthopaedics
Harborview Medical Center
Seattle, Washington

Murray J. Beuerlein, MD, MSC, FRCS(C)
Orthopaedic Surgeon
Department of Surgery
Red Deer Regional Hospital
Red Deer, Alberta, Canada

Earl R. Bogoch, MD, FRCSC
Professor
Department of Surgery
University of Toronto
Toronto, Ontario, Canada

Brett R. Bolhofner, MD
Director, Orthopedic Trauma Service
All Florida Orthopedic Associates
Bay Front Medical Center
St. Petersburg, Florida

Lawrence B. Bone, MD
Professor and Chairman
Department of Orthopaedics
State University of New York at Buffalo
Buffalo, New York

Christopher T. Born, MD, FACS
Professor of Orthopaedic Surgery
The Alpert School of Medicine
Brown University
Chief of Orthopaedic Trauma
Rhode Island Hospital
Providence, Rhode Island

Richard J. Bransford, MD
Assistant Professor
Department of Orthopaedics and Sports
  Medicine
University of Washington
Seattle, Washington

Timothy Bray, MD
Clinical Professor
University of California, Davis
Associate
Reno Orthopaedic Clinic
Reno, Nevada

Lisa K. Cannada, MD
Associate Professor
Orthopaedic Surgery
St. Louis University
St. Louis, Missouri

David B. Carmack, MD
Medical Director
Orthopedic Trauma Surgery
Surgery and Trauma Specialists of Maine
Eastern Maine Medical Center
Bangor, Maine

John T. Capo, MD
Associate Professor and Chief
Division of Hand and Microsurgery
Department of Orthopaedics
New Jersey Medical School
Newark, New Jersey

Troy Caron, DO
Assistant Professor
Department of Orthopaedic Sugery
University of Texas Southwestern
Dallas, Texas

MAJ Michael T. Charlton, MD
Chief of Orthopaedic Trauma
Department of Orthopaedic Surgery
Wilford Hall Air Force Medical Center
San Antonio, Texas

Peter A. Cole, MD
Professor
University of Minnesota
Chief of Orthopaedic Surgery
Regions Hospital
St. Paul, Minnesota

Cory A. Collinge, MD
Director of Orthopedic Trauma
Department of Orthopedics
Texas Health Harris Methodist Hospital
  Fort Worth
Fort Worth, Texas

Brett D. Crist, MD, FACS
Orthopaedic Surgery Department
University of Missouri
Columbia, Missouri

David Dalstrom, MD
Wright State University
Department of Orthopedics and Sports
  Medicine
Miami Valley Hospital
Dayton, Ohio

Thomas A. DeCoster, MD
Professor
Chief, Division of Trauma
Vice Chair
Department of Orthopaedics and Rehabilitation
University of New Mexico
Albuquerque, New Mexico

Gergory J. Della Rocca, MD, PhD, FACS
Assistant Professor
Co-Director, Orthopaedic Trauma Service
Department of Orthopaedic Surgery
University of Missouri
Columbia, Missouri

Paul J. Dougherty, MD
Associate Professor
Program Director
Orthopaedic Surgery
University of Michigan
Ann Arbor, Michigan

Kenneth A. Egol, MD
Professor and Vice Chairman
Orthopaedic Surgery
NYU Hospital for Joint Diseases
New York, New York

Thomas A. Einhorn, MD
Professor and Chairman
Department of Orthopaedic Surgery
Boston University Medical Center
Boston, Massachusetts

Hossein Elgafy, MD, MCh, FRCS Ed, FRCSC
Assistant Professor
Department of Orthopaedics
University of Toledo
Toledo, Ohio

Thomas J. Ellis, MD
Department of Orthopaedics
The Ohio State University
Columbus, Ohio

William J. J. Ertl, MD
Associate Professor
Department of Orthopedic Surgery
Health Sciences Center
University of Oklahoma
Oklahoma City, Oklahoma

Alun Evans, MSc, FRCS (Tr and Orth)
Consultant Orthopaedic Trauma Surgeon
Department of Orthopaedic Surgery
Morrison Hospital
Swansea, United Kingdom

COL James R. Ficke, MD
Chairman, Department of Orthopaedics and
*   Rehabilitation*
Orthopaedic Consultant, US Army Surgeon
*   General*
San Antonio Military Medical Center
Fort Sam Houston, Texas

Maureen Finnegan, MD
Associate Professor
Department of Orthopaedic Surgery
University of Texas Southwestern
Dallas, Texas

John C. France, MD
Professor
Orthopaedic Surgery
West Virginia University
Morgantown, West Virginia

Steven L. Frick, MD
Residency Program Director
Department of Orthopaedic Surgery
Carolinas Medical Center
Charlotte, North Carolina

David A. Fuller, MD
Assistant Professor of Surgery
Cooper University Hospital
Camden, New Jersey

Michael J. Gardner, MD
Assistant Professor
Orthopaedic Surgery
Washington University School of Medicine
St. Louis, Missouri

Peter Giannoudis, MD, FRCS
Professor in Trauma and Orthopaedic Surgery
Academic Unit of Trauma and Orthopaedics
Leeds General Infirmary
Leeds, United Kingdom

Paul J. Girard, MD
Assistant Clinical Professor
Department of Orthopaedic Surgery
University of California, San Diego
San Diego, California

Matt Graves, MD
Assistant Professor
Division of Trauma
Department of Orthopaedic Surgery and
*   Rehabilitation*
University of Mississippi Medical Center
Jackson, Mississippi

Andrew Green, MD
Associate Professor
Orthopaedic Surgery
Warren Alpert Medical School
Brown University
Providence, Rhode Island

Robert M. Greenleaf, MD
Department of Orthopaedics
Allegheny Orthopaedic Associates
Allegheny General Hospital
Pittsburgh, Pennsylvania

Jonatham M. Gross, MD, MPH
Assistant Professor
Orthopedic Surgery
University of Rochester
Rochester, New York

Gary S. Gruen, MD
Professor
Department of Orthopaedic Surgery
University of Pittsburgh
Pittsburgh, Pennsylvania

Pierre Guy, MD, MBA, FRCS(C)
Assistant Professor
Division of Orthopedic Trauma
University of British Columbia
Vancouver, British Columbia

George J. Haidukewych, MD
Professor
University of Central Florida
Co-Director of Orthopedic Trauma
Chief, Complex Adult Reconstruction
Orlando Health
Orlando, Florida

David J. Hak, MD, MBA
Associate Professor
Department of Orthopaedic Surgery
Denver Health
University of Colorado
Denver, Colorado

Mitchel Harris, MD, FACS
Associate Professor, Department of
  Orthopaedic Surgery
Chief, Orthopaedic Trauma Service
Harvard Medical Center
Brigham and Women's Hospital
Boston, Massachusetts

Edward J. Harvey, MD, MSc, FRCSC
Chief of Orthopaedic Trauma
Division of Orthopaedic Surgery
McGill University
Montreal, Canada

Roman A. Hayda, MD
Associate Professor, Orthopedic Surgery
Brown University
Warren Alpert School of Medicine
Department of Orthopedic Surgery
Rhode Island Hospital
Providence, Rhode Island

David L. Helfet, MD
Director
Orthopaedic Trauma Service
Hospital for Special Surgery
New York Presbyterian Hospital/Weill Cornell
  Medical Center
New York, New York

Thomas F. Higgins, MD
Associate Professor
Orthopaedic Trauma
Department of Orthopaedics
University of Utah School of Medicine
Salt Lake City, Utah

Matthew L. Jimenez, MD, FACS
Clinical Assistant Professor
Department of Orthopaedic Surgery
University of Illinois at Chicago
Illinois Bone and Joint Institute
Chicago, Illinois

Clifford B. Jones, MD, FACS
Clinical Professor, Michigan State University
Director of Orthopaedic Research, Spectrum
  Medical Center
Orthopaedic Associates of Michigan
Michigan State University
Grand Rapids, Michigan

David Kahler, MD
Associate Professor
Orthopaedic Surgery
University of Virginia
Charlottesville, Virginia

Steven M. Kane, MD
Chairman, Orthopedic Surgery Residency
Department of Orthopedic Surgery
Atlanta Medical Center
Atlanta, Georgia

Stephen A. Kottmeier, MD
Director of Orthopaedic Trauma
Associate Professor, Sports Medicine
Stony Brook University and Medical Center
Stony Brook, New York

James C. Krieg, MD
Associate Professor
Orthopaedics and Sports Medicine
Harborview Medical Center
University of Washington
Seattle, Washington

Paul R. Kuzyk, MD, MSc, FRCSC
Orthopaedic Lower Extremity Reconstruction
*   and Trauma Fellow*
Division of Orthopaedic Surgery
Department of Surgery
University of Toronto
St. Michael's Hospital
Toronto, Ontario, Canada

Matthew D. Layman, MD
Adjunct Assistant Professor of Anesthesiology
University of Minnesota Medical School
Intensivist and Anesthesiologist
Medical Director of Perioperative Services
Regions Hospital
St. Paul, Minnesota

Jackson Lee, MD
Associate Professor, Orthopedic Surgery
Director, Orthopedic Trauma Service
Service Chief, Orthopedic Surgery
Los Angeles County University of Southern
*   California Medical Center*
Department of Orthopedic Surgery
Keck School of Medicine
University of Southern California
Los Angeles, California

Mark A. Lee, MD
Associate Professor
Orthopaedic Surgery
University of California, Davis Medical Center
Sacramento, California

Kelly Lefaivre, MD, MSc, FRCSC
Assistant Professor
Department of Orthopaedic Surgery
University of British Columbia
Vancouver, British Columbia, Canada

Ross Leighton, MD, FRCS(C), FACS
Professor of Surgery
Division of Orthopedics
Dalhousie University
Halifax, Nova Scotia, Canada

Bruce A. Levy, MD
Assistant Professor
Department of Orthopaedic Surgery
Mayo Clinic
Rochester, Minnesota

David W. Lhowe, MD
Department of Orthopaedic Surgery
Massachusetts General Hospital
Boston, Massachusetts

Dean G. Lorich, MD
Associate Director
Orthopaedic Trauma Service
Hospital for Special Surgery
New York Presbyterian Hospital/Weill Cornell
*   Medical Center*
New York, New York

Douglas W. Lundy, MD, FACS
Orthopaedic Trauma Surgeon
Resurgens Orthopaedics
Kennestone Hospital
Atlanta, Georgia

Thuan V. Ly, MD
Assistant Professor
Department of Orthopaedic Surgery
Regions Hospital
St. Paul, Minnesota

Meir Marmor, MD
Orthopaedic Trauma Fellow
Department of Orthopaedic Surgery
University of California San Francisco
San Francisco, California

Amir Matityahu, MD
Assistant Clinical Professor of Orthopaedic
*   Surgery*
Director of Pelvic and Acetabular Trauma and
*   Reconstruction*
Department of Orthopaedic Surgery
University of California, San Francisco
San Francisco General Hospital
San Francisco, California

Michael T. Mazurek, MD
Residency Program Director
Orthopaedic Trauma
Department of Orthopaedic Surgery
Naval Medical Center San Diego
San Diego, California

Eric G. Meinberg, MD
Assistant Clinical Professor
Department of Orthopaedic Surgery
University of California, San Francisco
San Francisco General Hospital
San Francisco, California

Theodore Miclau, MD
Professor and Vice Chairman
Director, Orthopaedic Trauma Institute
Department of Orthopaedic Surgery
University of California, San Francisco
San Francisco, California

Keith O. Monchik, MD
Clinical Instructor of Orthopaedics
Alpert Medical School
Brown University
Department of Orthopaedic Surgery
Rhode Island Hospital
Providence, Rhode Island

Robert A. Morgan, MD
Director of Spine Trauma
Assistant Professor
Orthopaedic Surgery
Regions Hospital
University of Minnesota
St. Paul, Minnesota

Christopher E. Mutty, MD
Assistant Clinical Professor
Department of Orthopaedic Surgery
State University of New York at Buffalo
Buffalo, New York

Aaron Nauth, MD, FRCSC
Orthopaedic Trauma Fellow
Division of Orthopaedic Surgery
Department of Surgery
University of Toronto
St. Michael's Hospital
Toronto, Ontario, Canada

Sean E. Nork, MD
Associate Professor
Department of Orthopaedics and Sports
  Medicine
Harborview Medical Center
Seattle, Washington

Timothy O'Mara, MD
Orthopaedic Surgery
Reno Orthopaedic Clinic
Reno, Nevada

Michael J. Prayson, MD
Professor
Orthopaedic Surgery
Wright State University
Dayton, Ohio

Kevin J. Pugh, MD
Director, Limb Reconstruction
Orthopaedic Trauma and Reconstructive
  Surgery
Grant Medical Center
Columbus, Ohio

Mark Cameron Reilly, MD
Associate Professor
Co-Chief, Orthopaedic Trauma Service
New Jersey Medical School
Newark, New Jersey

William M. Ricci, MD
Professor
Chief, Orthopaedic Trauma Service
Department of Orthopaedic Surgery
Washington University School of Medicine
St. Louis, Missouri

Craig S. Roberts, MD, MBA
Professor
Residency Program Director
Department of Orthopaedic Surgery
University of Louisville School of Medicine
Louisville, Kentucky

Melvin Rosenwasser, MD
Robert E. Carroll Professor of Orthopaedic
  Surgery
Orthopaedic Surgery
Columbia University Medical Center
New York, New York

Milton L. Routt Jr, MD
Professor
Orthopaedics and Sports Medicine
Harborview Medical Center
Seattle, Washington

H. Claude Sagi, MD
Director of Fellowship Training and Research
Associate Clinical Professor
Orthopaedic Trauma Service
Tampa General Hospital
University of South Florida
Tampa, Florida

Emil H. Schemitsch, MD, FRCSC
Professor of Surgery
Division of Orthopaedic Surgery
Department of Surgery
University of Toronto
St. Michael's Hospital
Toronto, Ontario, Canada

Andrew J. Schoenfeld, MD
Assistant Professor
Department of Orthopaedic Surgery
Texas Tech University Health Sciences Center
William Beaumont Army Medical Center
El Paso, Texas

Alexandra K. Schwartz, MD
Associate Professor
Department of Orthopedic Surgery
University of California, San Diego
San Diego, California

Erik Paul Severson, MD
Department of Orthopaedics
Cuyuna Regional Medical Center
Crosby, Minnesota

Michael Sirkin, MD
Associate Professor
Vice Chairman
Department of Orthopaedics
New Jersey Medical School
Newark, New Jersey

Peter A. Siska, MD
Assistant Professor
Department of Orthopaedic Surgery
Division of Orthopaedic Traumatology
University of Pittsburgh Medical Center
Pittsburgh, Pennsylvania

Jeffrey M. Smith, MD
Orthopaedic Traumatologist
Orthopaedic Trauma and Fracture Specialists
  Medical Corporation
San Diego, California

Wade R. Smith, MD
Vice Chairman
Department of Orthopaedic Surgery
Geisinger Medical Center
Danville, Pennsylvania

Philip F. Stahel, MD
Department of Orthopaedics
Department of Neurosurgery
Denver Health Medical Center
Denver, Colorado

Michael D. Stover, MD
Orthopaedic Surgery and Rehabilitation
Loyola University Medical Center
Maywood, Illinois

Michael J. Stuart, MD
Professor
Department of Orthopaedic Surgery
Mayo Clinic
Rochester, Minnesota

Hobie Summers, MD
Assistant Professor
Department of Orthopaedic Surgery and
  Rehabilitation
Loyola University Medical Center
Maywood, Illinois

Takashi Suzuki, MD
Fellow
Department of Orthopaedic Surgery
Denver Health Medical Center
Denver, Colorado

Eric Swart, MD
Clinical Research Fellow
Orthopaedic Surgery
Columbia University Medical Center
New York, New York

Marc F. Swiontkowski, MD
Professor
Department of Orthopaedic Surgery
University of Minnesota
Minneapolis, Minnesota

Julie A. Switzer, MD
Assistant Professor
University of Minnesota
Director of Geriatric Trauma
Regions Hospital
St. Paul, Minnesota

Nirmal C. Tejwani, MD
Associate Professor
Department of Orthopaedic Surgery
NYU Hospital for Joint Diseases
New York, New York

Paul Tornetta III, MD
Professor, Program Director, Vice Chairman
Department of Orthopaedic Surgery
Boston University School of Medicine
Director, Orthopaedic Trauma
Boston Medical Center
Boston, Massachusetts

Heather A. Vallier, MD
Clyde L. Nash Professor of Orthopaedic
    Education
Case Western Reserve University
Department of Orthopaedic Surgery
The MetroHealth System
Cleveland, Ohio

David S. Weisman, MD
Clinical Assistant Professor
Department of Orthopedic Surgery
Robert Wood Johnson Medical School
New Brunswick, New Jersey

Brock T. Wentz, MD
Clinical Instructor
Department of Orthopaedic Surgery
University of California, San Francisco
Orthopaedic Trauma Institute
San Francisco General Hospital
San Francisco, California

Neil J. White, MD, FRCSC
Hand Surgery Fellow
Orthopaedic Surgeon
Hand Surgery
Columbia University
New York, New York

Raymond R. White, MD
Chief of Orthopaedic Trauma
Maine Medical Center
Portland, Maine

Philip R. Wolinsky, MD
Professor, Department of Orthopaedic Surgery
Chief, Division of Orthopaedic Trauma
University of California, Davis
Sacramento, California

Bruce H. Ziran, MD
Director of Orthopaedic Trauma
Orthopaedic Surgery
Atlanta Medical Center
Atlanta, Georgia

Preface

The American Academy of Orthopaedic Surgeons launched the Orthopaedic Knowledge Update series in 1984, followed by the launch of specialty OKU volumes in 1994. The goal of this ongoing endeavor is to provide practicing orthopaedic surgeons with a useful, comprehensive, yet concise update of new information available from the latest peer-reviewed orthopaedic literature, placed in context by expert authors. This volume represents the fourth in the series of *OKU Trauma*; the first three editions were published in 1996, 2000, and 2005.

The specialty of orthopaedic trauma continues to evolve rapidly, with dramatic changes in biotechnology, implants, and imaging. Tremendous advances have been made in the basic sciences, changing our understanding of the biology of fracture healing, muscle and tendon injury, and microbiology. Improved knowledge of clinical outcomes, along with an ever-expanding array of implant options, has led to many paradigm shifts in treatment during the past several years, as witnessed by the widespread adoption of volar plating for distal radius fractures or cephalomedullary nailing of the femur. As previous editors have done, we have added new chapters while generally maintaining the familiar organization of previous editions. *OKU Trauma 4* begins with a General Topics and New Technology section, with new chapters on practice management, new technology, and disaster and mass casualty preparedness. The second section addresses the polytrauma patient and fracture healing, with a new chapter on damage control orthopaedics. The remaining sections cover the upper extremity, axial skeleton, lower extremity, and the special problems of pediatric and geriatric trauma. Finally, following OKU tradition, each fully-referenced chapter provides annotations to the most current, peer-reviewed literature discussed by authors.

OKU Trauma 4 has been written by more than 100 volunteer authors from the Orthopaedic Trauma Association, and we are grateful to each of the expert contributors. Compiling this volume required much work by a large team of people, and we are especially indebted to our section editors for their important contributions and expertise: Kenneth J. Koval, MD; Adam J. Starr, MD; John T. Capo, MD; Berton R. Moed, MD; Carlo Bellabarba, MD; Kevin J. Pugh, MD; Michael D. Stover, MD; and John T. Gorczyca, MD; as well as the tremendous contributions of the Academy staff led by Lisa Claxton Moore. We trust that this fourth edition of *OKU Trauma* will provide you with valuable "pearls" and other information to help you care for your trauma patients, assist with board certification / maintenance of certification, or whatever your particular needs are.

Finally, we would like to dedicate this volume to the memory of Michael Mazurek, MD, Commander, Medical Corps, United States Navy, and to the honor of his military orthopaedic colleagues, many of whom contributed important new information to this volume. Dr. Mazurek wrote significant portions of the Infections chapter prior to his untimely death. His dedication to trauma care and orthopaedic education leaves a lasting and meaningful legacy. Many of his military orthopaedic colleagues continue to perform active duty tours in two war zones and care for wounded warriors abroad and at home, yet still find time to share their new knowledge with the orthopaedic community. We remember Dr. Mazurek, and we sincerely thank our military orthopaedic colleagues for their service.

Andrew H. Schmidt, MD
David C. Teague, MD

Tribute

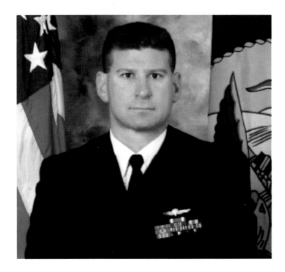

Tribute to Michael Mazurek, MD, Commander, Medical Corps, United States Navy, from all of his colleagues in Navy Medicine

On November 7, 2009, Navy Medicine and the orthopaedic trauma community lost a valued friend and colleague. Commander Michael Todd "Maz" Mazurek was a decorated battlefield veteran, a skilled surgeon, a trusted mentor, and a loving husband and father. His passion for orthopaedic trauma was surpassed only by that for his family – wife Lisa, and sons Adam, Dylan, and Spencer. He sought perfection in all that he did, and inspired those around him to do the same. Perhaps his greatest gift was his ability to teach, which he did as a residency program director, an AO instructor, and as author of numerous publications, including a chapter in this book. Maz routinely made us laugh, his passing made us cry, and his memory continues to make us better. Navy Medicine and the fighting men and women of the Unites States Marine Corps salute Commander Mazurek for battles well fought and a life well lived.

Table of Contents

Section 1

General Topics and New Technology

SECTION EDITOR:
KENNETH J. KOVAL, MD

Chapter 1
Outcomes of Musculoskeletal Trauma

Thuan V. Ly, MD   Julie Agel, MA, ATC   Marc F. Swiontkowski, MD   Thomas A. DeCoster, MD

Introduction

Outcomes of musculoskeletal trauma are increasingly reported in the literature, which requires the use of validated functional outcome instruments.[1-3] Outcome is defined as the end result of a treatment or disease.[4] Reported end results can be categorized into three general types: surgeon-based, patient-based, and mixed surgeon- and patient-based. Surgeon-based outcomes are associated with clinical measures performed by the surgeon or clinician. These clinical outcomes may include range of motion, infection, complications, strength, radiographic union, or implant failure. This information is documented in the surgeon's physical examination and clinical notes. Patient-based outcomes are those provided from the perspective of the patient on how the injury or treatment affects his or her life. This information is obtained from the patient via questionnaires. Mixed outcomes (for example,

Harris Hip Score) are measures that use a combination of both surgeon-based and patient-based outcomes to provide a final score or grade (such as poor, good, or excellent). There is significant interobserver variability with this method, and often these instruments are not validated for outcome assessment.[3,5,6] It is important to review why outcomes are assessed, the common types of patient-based functional outcome instruments currently in use, and which outcome measures to use.

Why Assess Outcomes?

There are internal and external factors that persuade orthopaedic surgeons to assess outcomes.[5,7,8] It is the orthopaedic surgeon's responsibility to understand how recommended nonsurgical or surgical treatment choices affect patients. With increasing numbers of novel treatments introduced and marketed, it becomes crucial to be aware of anticipated outcomes to provide patients with adequate information on treatment options and to assess and improve their care. The demands of the public and third-party payers encourage orthopaedic surgeons to collect outcomes data. With easy access to the Internet and the concern about costs, patients and health care systems expect information regarding individual surgeon outcomes or the effectiveness of a treatment before deciding on surgical intervention.

Outcomes are traditionally considered to be the clinical results of treatment. However, these clinical parameters often represent the surgeon's subjective or objective opinion of the patient's outcome and do not always equal a good or excellent outcome from the patient's perspective. The health-related quality of life (HRQOL) or the functional outcomes perceived by the patient are just as important, or more important, than the clinical results that have heretofore been collected by the surgeons and reported in the literature.[1,2,7,9] As with any effort to improve quality of care, there are multiple impediments to collecting outcomes, including time, cost, clinical relevance, and choice of the appropriate outcome instrument.[3,10]

Dr. Ly or an immediate family member is a member of a speakers' bureau or has made paid presentations on behalf of AO; and has received research or institutional support from Synthes and DePuy. Julie Agel or an immediate family member has received research or institutional support from National Institutes of Health (NIAMS and NICHD), Medtronic, Synthes, and AO. Dr. Swiontkowski or an immediate family member serves as a board member, owner, officer, or committee member of American Orthopaedic Association, American Board of Medical Specialties, and TRIA Orthopedic Center; serves as a paid consultant to or is an employee of Eli Lilly, Wyeth, Baxter Healthcare; serves as an unpaid consultant to Medtronic Sofamor Danek, National Institutes of Health (NIAMS and NICHD), Shriners Hospital for Children Clinical Outcomes Studies Advisory Board, and Synthes. Dr. DeCoster or an immediate family member serves as a board member, owner, officer, or committee member of Orthopaedic Trauma Association; has received royalties from Innomed; is a member of a speakers' bureau or has made paid presentations on behalf of AO, Biomet, EBI, Orthofix, Smith & Nephew, Stryker, and Synthes; serves as a paid consultant to or is an employee of Zimmer; serves as an unpaid consultant to EBI; has received research or institutional support from Biomet, EBI, Orthofix, Smith & Nephew, Stryker, and Zimmer; has stock or stock options held in Merck and Wyeth; and has received nonincome support (such as equipment or services), commercially derived honoraria, or other non–research-related funding (such as paid travel) from Smith & Nephew.

Orthopaedic Outcome Instruments

Patient-based functional outcomes are obtained directly from the patient through questionnaires. Depending on the type of outcome instrument, this assessment of patient function can cover physical, psychological, and social aspects, pain, health status, work activity, and activities of daily living. At the broadest level, outcome instruments are categorized into generic and specific measures.[2,5] Specific outcome instruments may be disease specific, region specific, or joint and injury specific. Most of these questionnaires are developed and established using psychometric principles. Appropriate outcome instruments are developed using the following steps: item development, item reduction, format selec-

tion, pretesting, reproducibility, responsiveness, and validity. The format of these questionnaires can be endorsable (yes or no), scaled (for example, a 3- or 5-point Likert scale with end point statements) or a visual analog scale (the patient makes a mark on a line of set length).[3,5-7,10,11]

The scientific development of these outcome instruments is complex, time consuming, and expensive. There are few reasons to consider developing new instruments; the exception would be condition-specific instruments for very common and/or expensive musculoskeletal conditions. Therefore, the use of existing instruments is recommended to accompany clinical outcome measures. Commonly used outcome instruments are described in **Tables 1** through **4**.

Table 1

Short Form-36 (SF-36)

What it is designed to assess	General health status
How to obtain instrument	http://www.sf-36.org/
Method of administration	Self-administered
Format and number of questions	Likert scale, 8 functional subscales, 36 questions
Time to complete	5 to 10 minutes
How results interpreted?	There is no total score. Range 0 to 100 points, high score = better function
Strength	Feasible in clinical setting
Weakness	Assessing upper extremity function
Miscellaneous	Shorter version available (SF-12); requires annual licensing fee. SF-36v2: more than 120 language translations available

Generic Instruments

Generic outcome instruments are synonymous with assessment of HRQOL. They are designed to evaluate the general health status of the patient, specifically looking at physical, mental, and social aspects of perceived well-being. Such measures assess overall patient function at the individual level and allow for comparison of patient's HRQOL among different injuries or diseases, although they may not be sensitive enough to discern changes among specific injuries or diseases.

The 36-Item Short Form (SF-36) is the most widely used outcome instrument for assessing general health status of the patient.[2,6,12] It is validated, reliable, and reproducible. The SF-36 consists of 36 multiple-choice questions with 8 subscale health concepts: physical functioning, role limitations due to physical problems, social functioning, bodily pain, general mental health, role limitations due to emotional problems, vitality, and general health perceptions. These subscales can be scored separately (range from 0 to 100 points, with high score indicating better function) and can be com-

Table 2

Sickness Impact Profile (SIP)

What it is designed to assess	General health status measure designed to evaluate the burden of disease on physical and psychosocial health
How to obtain instrument	http;//www.outcomes-trust.org/instruments.htm#SIP
Method of administration	Self-administered
Format and number of questions	Endorsable (yes/no). Two scales: Physical and Psychosocial, 136 questions
Time to complete	30 minutes
How are results interpreted?	Score of 0 to 3 indicates no disability, 4 to 9 indicates mild disability, 10 to 19 indicates moderate disability, and 20 or higher indicates severe disability
Strength	Long history of use in the literature
Weakness	Takes considerable time to complete, scale is unbalanced, with severe disability from 20 to 100 points
Miscellaneous	Scoring is complex. Other languages: none currently

Table 3	
Musculoskeletal Function Assessment (MFA)	
What it is designed to assess	Musculoskeletal function
How to obtain instrument	http://www.ortho.umn.edu/research/clinicaloutcomes.htm
Method of administration	Self-administered
Format and number of questions	Endorsable (yes/no), 100 questions, 10 domains
Time to complete	20 minutes
How results interpreted?	Total scores range from 0 to 100 points; high score = greater dysfunction
Strength	Provide general health status with emphasis on musculoskeletal injuries
Weakness	Time
Miscellaneous	Shorter version (SMFA): 46 questions. Other languages: German, Portuguese

Table 4	
Short Musculoskeletal Function Assessment (SMFA)	
What it is designed to assess	Musculoskeletal function
How to obtain instrument	http://www.ortho.umn.edu/research/clinicaloutcomes.htm
Method of administration	Self-administered
Format and number of questions	1 to 5 Likert scale, 46 questions, 4 domains
Time to complete	10 minutes
How results interpreted?	Total scores range from 0 to 100 points; high score = greater dysfunction
Strength	Feasible in clinical setting. Provide general health status with emphasis on musculoskeletal injuries
Weakness	May not provide sufficient discrimination between some diseases or treatments
Miscellaneous	Other languages: German, Portuguese

bined to create two summary scores—the physical component score and the mental component score. However, the SF-36 does not allow for a total score calculation. The method of administration can be self-administration or by a trained interviewer in person or by telephone. The SF-36 takes about 5 to 10 minutes to complete. In a busy clinical practice this instrument would be feasible, although scoring is not simple.[13]

The Sickness Impact Profile (SIP) is another commonly used generic outcome instrument for evaluating patients with musculoskeletal disorders.[14-16] The SIP is a validated and widely used self-reported health status of the patient. It contains 136 endorsable statements detailing functional status in five independent domains, four psychosocial domains, and three physical domains. The five independent domains are sleep and rest, eating, work, home management, and recreation and pastimes. The psychosocial domains consist of social interaction, alertness behavior, emotional behavior, and communication. The three physical domains are ambulation, mobility, and body care and movement. The overall SIP scores can range from 0 to 100 points. A score from 0 to 3 indicates no disability, 4 to 9 indicates mild disability, 10 to 19 indicates moderate disability, and a score of 20 or greater indicates severe disability. The SIP takes approximately 30 minutes to complete and is best administered with a trained interviewer. The SIP is cumbersome to use in the clinical setting because of the length of time required to administer. It is more commonly used in outcomes research in an academic setting.[13-16]

The Musculoskeletal Function Assessment (MFA) is a generic health status questionnaire that emphasizes

musculoskeletal function and can be used in the assessment of fractures, soft-tissue injuries, arthritis, and overuse injuries.[17] The MFA consists of 101 endorsable questions that assess patients' function in 10 domains: self-care; sleep and rest; hand and fine motor skills; mobility; housework; employment and work; leisure and recreational activities; family relationships; cognition and thinking; and emotional adjustment, coping, and adaptation. The MFA is comparable to the SF-36 and the SIP in terms of reliability, validity, and responsiveness. The overall MFA scores can range from 0 to 100 points, with a high score indicating poor function. The questionnaire can be completed in 15 to 20 minutes and can be self-administered or interviewer administered. Similar to the SIP, the MFA is often used in outcomes research and not routinely used in a busy clinical setting.[13,17-20]

The Short Musculoskeletal Function Assessment (SMFA) is a shortened version of the MFA.[21] The SMFA was developed to be used in community-based practice where time is limited. It consists of 46 Likert-scale items that provide two main scores: a Dysfunction index and a Bother index. The Dysfunction index has 34 items that assess patients' perceptions of their functional status. These questions cover daily activities; emotional status; function of the arm and head; and mobility. The Bother index has 12 questions that assess how patients are affected by their functional problems, such as the effect on recreation and leisure, sleep and rest, and work and family. The SMFA has been evalu-

1: General Topics and New Technology

ated for validity, reliability, and responsiveness. The total score can range from 0 to 100, with a higher score indicating poorer function. The SMFA can be completed by the patient or with a trained interviewer in about 5 to 10 minutes. Whereas the MFA is mainly useful in an academic setting, the SMFA is useful for clinical settings as well as academic settings.

A 2007 study described the current utilization and interpretation of the MFA and SMFA since their development.[1] Despite their increasing use as generic musculoskeletal outcome tools, the MFA and SMFA are not used to their potential. The authors recommended that major journals encourage consistent reporting of outcome data to allow for collection of large databases and comparison of data. Inhibiting factors are inconsistent reporting styles, confounding injuries, and determination of clinically relevant differences. It is recommended that variables such as diagnosis, age, gender, time frame, MFA domains, comorbidities, and treatment method be consistently collected and reported. This consistent format will allow comparison of data and provide better understanding of the impact of musculoskeletal diseases and injuries on patients.

Specific Measure Instruments

Specific outcome instruments are designed to assess problems related to a specific disease or injury process and/or body region. These questionnaires are more sensitive to change and able to detect small but clinically important differences in the outcome parameter of interest.

There are increasing numbers of specific measure instruments available. Some are well validated and some are not. A guide to outcome instruments for musculoskeletal trauma research was recently published in the *Journal of Orthopaedic Trauma*.[13] This supplement provides commonly used instruments that were found in the abstracts from the Orthopaedic Trauma Association (OTA) and the American Academy of Orthopaedic Surgeons trauma section meetings from 1997 to 2002. This supplement was designed as a reference for clinicians trying to determine the most appropriate instrument to use for their purpose and uses a table format to display the currently available tools for measuring outcomes in patients with musculoskeletal disease related to trauma. Information for each instrument includes a brief description and where to obtain the instrument, and it allows for comparison purposes.

Which Outcome Measure to Use

With many HRQOL and functional outcome instruments available, it can be difficult to determine the appropriate outcome tools to use. What may be appropriate for the researcher in an academic setting may not be feasible for the clinician in community practice. Several

review articles provide a logical way for researchers and clinicians to determine the correct outcome instrument.[2,5,6,9-11] The three components that are important when assessing which outcome tool to choose are content, methodology, and clinical utility.[6] Content is defined as the purpose of the instrument and is further categorized into type (clinician- or patient-derived outcome), scale (format and how questions are scored), and interpretation (what the score means). Methodology evaluates the validity, reliability, and responsiveness of the outcome instrument. Clinical utility is an assessment of whether the instrument would be practical for the patient and the clinician or researcher.

Another algorithm for assessing which outcome tool to choose starts with understanding and knowing the purpose of the study or the research question, followed by choosing the outcome instrument that will best answer the objective of the study.[5] Consultation with an experienced clinical researcher and performing a literature search are recommended. The outcome instrument of interest should be assessed for quality criteria such as validity, reliability, and responsiveness. The choice of the appropriate outcome instrument should depend on the question to be answered, what the outcome instrument is designed to assess, the availability of resources, and the feasibility of the instrument to be implemented (Figure 1). A multicenter, well-funded study with a well-defined injury and objectives of interest (for example, the Lower Extremity Assessment Project [LEAP] study of severe lower extremity injuries) can afford to use a longer questionnaire such as the SIP. However, a clinician in a community-based practice trying to improve care of a specific injury would be better advised to use a shorter and less intense questionnaire such as the SMFA. The general recommendation would be to use a generic HRQOL outcome instrument in conjunction with a region- or joint-specific outcome instrument. The generic instruments take into account other confounding factors, injuries, and preexisting conditions, and how they affect overall functional outcome. Adding a region- or joint-specific instrument increases sensitivity and allows the ability to distinguish the effect of a specific musculoskeletal injury from other confounding factors or conditions on the patient's long-term outcome. The use of existing validated outcome instruments for conditions they were designed to assess is suggested. Any attempt at modifying the scoring system or partially using the outcome tool should be avoided. Modification of the instrument will change the validity and reliability of the instrument and make it useless for comparison with other studies.[3,10,11]

Fracture Classification

The appropriate classification of fractures serves to guide treatment and help in the understanding of prognosis, and it is fundamental to the management of orthopaedic trauma. Since the publication of *Orthopaedic Knowledge Update: Trauma 3*, there has been

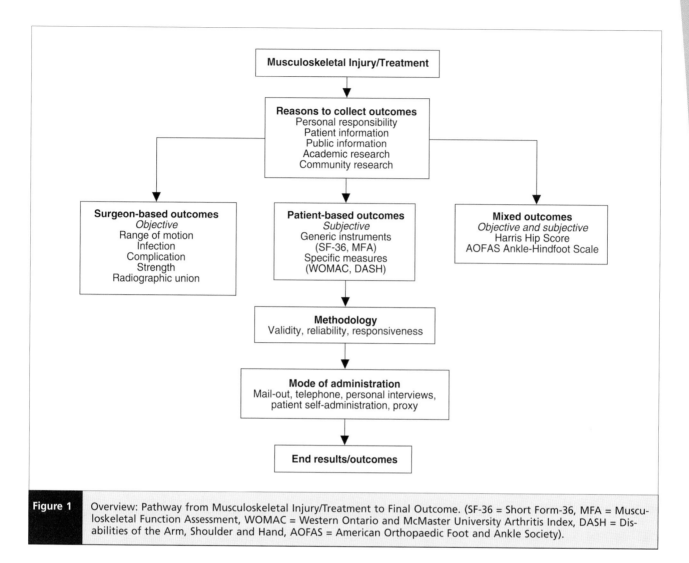

Figure 1 Overview: Pathway from Musculoskeletal Injury/Treatment to Final Outcome. (SF-36 = Short Form-36, MFA = Musculoskeletal Function Assessment, WOMAC = Western Ontario and McMaster University Arthritis Index, DASH = Disabilities of the Arm, Shoulder and Hand, AOFAS = American Orthopaedic Foot and Ankle Society).

significant advancement in fracture classification with the publication of new classifications, revision of previously described classifications, and most important, new information that helps the clinician understand the limitations of specific classifications as well as classifications in general. In addition, the OTA Fracture and Dislocation Classification Compendium 2007 was published in the *Journal of Orthopaedic Trauma* in November 2007.[22]

General Issues With Fracture Classification

Fractures are classified to accomplish several goals: first, to assist with choosing treatment options; second, to indicate the likelihood of complications; and third, to assign prognosis. An ideal classification would be simple and easy to understand, assign patients into groups based on straightforward criteria on which different observers can perfectly agree, correctly stratify among potential treatments without overlap, alert clinicians to specific risks, and provide immediate information about a given injury's prognosis. Obviously, such a classification does not exist for any injury. In fact, many "classic" classifications have become the lan-

guage for describing a given injury and continue to be used even though they may lack many of these characteristics and/or have been shown to have poor interobserver reliability.

For a given classification to be considered reliable, it must have reasonable intraobserver and interobserver reliability, content validity, and accuracy.[23] A recurrent problem with fracture classification is the issue of intraobserver and interobserver variability. An ideal classification requires different surgeons to classify a given patient the same way and the same surgeon evaluating a given injury at different times to assign the same classification. Interrater agreement is studied statistically by computing the so-called kappa statistic. Many fracture classifications were developed without attention to this matter and have been subsequently shown to have poor interobserver reliability, with kappa statistics that indicated only poor to fair agreement. Content validity means that different fracture classification categories are associated with relevant patient outcomes in the context of specific fracture management plans. Accuracy means that the classification categories fit the patterns of injuries that are actually seen in clinical

1: General Topics and New Technology

practice. Surgeons treating fractures and evaluating the medical literature should be aware of these limitations of existing fracture classifications, and those interested in developing new classifications should follow specific methodologic guidelines.[23]

The difficulty in assigning a specific fracture as either high energy or low energy is a problem that all fracture classifications have in common. The mechanism of injury is an important prognostic factor that is only indirectly assessed by descriptions of fracture pattern. Researchers from the University of Iowa have developed a CT-based algorithm to objectively and quantitatively measure fracture energy that incorporates measurement of fracture fragment surface area, displacement, and soft-tissue swelling. In a study of 20 distal tibial plafond fractures, fracture energy as determined by this imaging algorithm correlated well with a rank-order assessment of fracture severity as determined by three experienced traumatologists.[24] Such methods may well be incorporated into future classification schemes.

OTA Fracture and Dislocation Classification Compendium 2007

The OTA classification was originally published in 1996 and was an adaptation of The Comprehensive Classification of Fractures of the Long Bones, developed by Müller and the AO group. The general organization of the classification has remained the same.[22] The OTA Fracture Classification is comprehensive and all-inclusive in that it applies to all fractures treated by orthopaedic surgeons. The classification is also consistent in that the same concepts are applied throughout the body, facilitating recollection and ease of application and communication. It is an anatomically based classification that uses information available on plain radiographs, and each category is mutually exclusive, meaning that each individual fracture fits only one category. The classification is flexibly hierarchical, with the level of specificity varying from the general to very specific depending on the needs of the user. The most general category is the name of the fractured bone (1-9), followed by bone segment (1-3), type (A, B, C), group (1, 2, 3), subgroup (1.1, 1.2, 1.3), and specialized category (a, b, c). A supplementary alphanumeric designation of various categories assists in shorthand notation. The classification also provides a standard terminology for fracture categories that is particularly important at the bone segment level.

As an example, the humerus is designated with a 1 and the distal humerus bone segment (13) is distinguished from the humerus shaft (12) and proximal humerus (11) by the rule of squares. The rule of squares is used to distinguish the shaft from the proximal and distal segments of the long bones. The widest portion of the epiphysis on an AP radiograph defines the length of the side of the square. That distance from the articular surface toward the diaphysis defines the zone that comprises the distal or proximal segment. If the center of the fracture is contained within the square, the fracture is placed in the proximal or distal bone segment category. There are three types of distal humerus fracture patterns, namely extra-articular (13A), partial articular (13B), and total articular (13C). The type designations are letters A, B, and C for each bone segment throughout the body. Each of these types is subclassified into three groups based on anatomic location and pattern of comminution (13-A1, 13-A2, 13-A3, 13-B1, and so on) for a total of nine groups. For example, the partial articular types of distal humerus (bone segment) fractures are classified as group B1 (capitellum or lateral sagittal), B2 (trochlea or medial sagittal), or B3 (coronal or frontal plane fractures). A coronal plane (group B3) partial articular (B type) distal humerus (13 bone segment) is further classified into subgroups (B3.1 = capitellum only, B3.2 = trochlea only, B3.3 = capitellum and trochlea). The correct hierarchical terminology to describe an isolated coronal plane fracture of the capitellum is "distal humerus fracture, partial articular isolated coronal plane capitellum" = 13B3.1 for shorthand notation by code. Although slightly cumbersome, this terminology enhances effective communication by its clearness, logic, and consistency. If extremely detailed categories are required, then there are 3 subgroups for each group for a total of 27 categories. The changes to the 2007 classification include a unification of the OTA and AO classification, an expansion of the classification for short bones, an expansion of the dislocation section, and the introduction of a classification of skeletally immature bone fractures.

The dislocation section has been expanded to be more comprehensive. The alphanumeric shorthand and overall designation of categories have been revised. The first digit is the same body region as for fractures and the second digit is 0 for dislocation. The type level (A-E) is the specific joint within the region. For example, the shoulder is designated 10 with glenohumeral dislocation 10-A. Acromion-clavicular dislocations are 10-B, sternoclavicular 10-C, and scapulothoracic 10-D. The group level describes anatomic direction of dislocation, with an anterior glenohumeral dislocation a specific category with shorthand notation 10-A1. An overview of the overall approach was provided in 2007.[22]

As a general guideline, the bone segment level of fracture designation is appropriate for chapters in textbooks (for example, Proximal Tibia Fractures). The type level of designation may be appropriate for titles of articles in journals (for example, Treatment of Total Articular Distal Femur Fractures With Plating). The group level of designation may be appropriate for tables within an article; for example, reporting range of motion for patients with articular comminution, metaphyseal comminution, or no comminution. Alphanumeric shorthand (33-C3, 33-C2, 33-C1) could supplement the language in the legend. A paper might conclude that a specific modification of the technique was required for a specific subgroup; for example, comminuted intra-articular fractures of the distal femur with extension into the diaphysis (33-C3.3). In those subgroups a long plate with a lateral bow to accommodate the anatomic bow of the femur might be recommended. These examples illustrate how the hierarchical levels of the OTA Fracture Classification can be used to promote consistent and effective communication.

The OTA Classification for Children was developed by the AO Pediatric Classification Group. The classification was developed by an expert panel and then scientifically tested for applicability, consistency, and clinical relevance. This classification uses the same overall algorithm as the adult fracture classification and a very similar alphanumeric shorthand code. The growth plate is used to distinguish fracture location relative to bone segments including epiphyseal (E), metaphyseal (M), and diaphyseal (D) segments. Further categorization of types and groups is based on common patterns of injury and the relationship of the fracture lines and fragments to the growth plate. A discussion of the overall logic of the pediatric fracture classification was provided in 2007.[25]

The 2007 OTA Fracture and Dislocation Classification is now recommended for use by orthopaedic surgeons in publications, databases, and clinical care. It is required for articles submitted to the *Journal of Orthopaedic Trauma* and encouraged for other musculoskeletal journals. It has been adopted by many organizations and encouraged by many others. This classification, with its consistent clearly defined categories, is slowly replacing the haphazard array of fracture classifications in the literature.

Summary

Outcome instruments can be used to assess the end results of an injury or treatment in clinical practice or academic research. It is important to have a basic understanding of why outcomes are assessed, the different types of outcome instruments, and how to select them. Understanding these concepts will improve orthopaedic research and patient care. Consistency and use of available validated outcome instruments will allow for comparison across different studies and treatments. The 2007 OTA Fracture Classification is recommended for use in all orthopaedic communications and publications. The hierarchical level of specificity can be used to match the requirements of the author, ranging from the general (bones and bone segments) to very specific (groups and subgroups). Alphanumeric codes can be used when shorthand notation is needed.

Annotated References

1. Barei DP, Agel J, Swiontkowski MF: Current utilization, interpretation, and recommendations: The Musculoskeletal Function Assessments (MFA/SMFA). *J Orthop Trauma* 2007;21(10):738-742.

This special-interest article reported on the underutilization of the musculoskeletal function assessment MFA/SMFA for musculoskeletal diseases and injuries. The authors provided recommendations for improving the use of these instruments in clinical and research studies.

2. Beaton DE, Schemitsch E: Measures of health-related quality of life and physical function. *Clin Orthop* 2003; 413:90-105.

3. Swiontkowski MF: Outcomes measurement in orthopaedic trauma surgery. *Injury* 1995;26(10):653-657.

4. Codman E: The product of a hospital. *Surg Gynecol Obstet* 1944;18:491-496.

5. Poolman RW, Swiontkowski MF, Fairbank JC, Schemitsch EH, Sprague S, de Vet HC: Outcome instruments: Rationale for their use. *J Bone Joint Surg Am* 2009;91(Suppl 3):41-49.

A detailed explanation of the quality criteria for assessing outcome instruments is described. The authors provide guidelines for selecting an outcome instrument for research purposes.

6. Suk M, Norvell DC, Hanson B, Dettori JR, Helfet D: Evidence-based orthopaedic surgery: What is evidence without the outcomes? *J Am Acad Orthop Surg* 2008; 16(3):123-129.

This article depicts an algorithm of three important components (content, methodology, and clinical utility) to consider when assessing which outcome measure to use. The differences between clinician-based versus patient-reported outcomes are described. Available measurement instruments are provided.

7. Obremskey W, Swiontkowski M: Evaluation of outcomes for musculoskeletal injury, in Browner BD, Jupiter JB, Levine AM, et al, eds: *Skeletal Trauma*, ed 3. Philadelphia, PA, WB Saunders, 2003, pp 670-681.

8. Swiontkowski M: Why we should collect outcomes data. *J Bone Joint Surg Am* 2003;85 (Suppl 1):14-15.

9. Jackowski D, Guyatt G: Part III. Outcomes analysis in orthopaedic surgery. *Clin Orthop Relat Res* 2003;413: 80-89.

10. Swiontkowski MF, Buckwalter JA, Keller RB, Haralson R: The outcomes movement in orthopaedic surgery: Where we are and where we should go. *J Bone Joint Surg Am* 1999;81(5):732-740.

11. Pynsent PB: Choosing an outcome measure. *J Bone Joint Surg Br* 2001;83(6):792-794.

12. Ware JE Jr, Sherbourne CD: The MOS 36-item short-form health survey (SF-36): I. Conceptual framework and item selection. *Med Care* 1992;30(6):473-483.

13. Agel J, Swiontkowski MF: Guide to outcomes instruments for musculoskeletal trauma research. *J Orthop Trauma* 2006;20(8, Suppl):S1-S146.

This supplement, presented in table format, outlines the commonly used outcome instruments from previous OTA and AAOS trauma session meetings and provides a reference for clinicians to help determine the most appropriate instrument to use.

14. Jurkovich G, Mock C, MacKenzie E, et al: The Sickness Impact Profile as a tool to evaluate functional outcome in trauma patients. *J Trauma* 1995;39(4):625-631.

15. Bergner M, Bobbitt RA, Kressel S, Pollard WE, Gilson BS, Morris JR: The Sickness Impact Profile: Conceptual formulation and methodology for the development of a health status measure. *Int J Health Serv* 1976;6(3):393-415.

16. Bergner M, Bobbitt RA, Carter WB, Gilson BS: The Sickness Impact Profile: Development and final revision of a health status measure. *Med Care* 1981;19(8):787-805.

17. Martin DP, Engelberg R, Agel J, Snapp D, Swiontkowski MF: Development of a musculoskeletal extremity health status instrument: The Musculoskeletal Function Assessment instrument. *J Orthop Res* 1996;14(2):173-181.

18. Engelberg R, Martin DP, Agel J, Obremskey W, Coronado G, Swiontkowski MF: Musculoskeletal Function Assessment instrument: Criterion and construct validity. *J Orthop Res* 1996;14(2):182-192.

19. Engelberg R, Martin DP, Agel J, Swiontkowski MF: Musculoskeletal Function Assessment: Reference values for patient and non-patient samples. *J Orthop Res* 1999;17(1):101-109.

20. Martin DP, Engelberg R, Agel J, Swiontkowski MF: Comparison of the Musculoskeletal Function Assessment questionnaire with the Short Form-36, the Western Ontario and McMaster Universities Osteoarthritis Index, and the Sickness Impact Profile Health status measures. *J Bone Joint Surg Am* 1997;79(9):1323-1335.

21. Swiontkowski MF, Engelberg R, Martin DP, Agel J: Short Musculoskeletal Function Assessment question-naire: Validity, reliability, and responsiveness. *J Bone Joint Surg Am* 1999;81(9):1245-1260.

22. Marsh JL, Slongo TF, Agel J, et al: Fracture and Dislocation Classification Compendium 2007: Orthopaedic Trauma Association Classification, Database and Outcomes Committee. *J Orthop Trauma* 2007;21:S1-S133.

Modification and republication of the OTA fracture classification has reconciled differences with the AO classification and expanded classification of short bones and dislocations. Although not every problem with fracture classification has been solved, this is now a standard reference for fracture classification.

23. Audigé L, Bhandari M, Kellam J: How reliable are reliability studies of fracture classifications? A systematic review of their methodologies. *Acta Orthop Scand* 2004;75(2):184-194.

This article reviews the methodology of reliability studies with emphasis on nonparametric statistics. Level of evidence: III.

24. Anderson DD, Mosqueda T, Thomas T, Hermanson EL, Brown TD, Marsh JL: Quantifying tibial plafond fracture severity: Absorbed energy and fragment displacement agree with clinical rank ordering. *J Orthop Res* 2008;26(8):1046-1052.

The authors demonstrate that they can objectively and quantifiably measure the amount of energy that caused fractures of the distal tibia from CT scans. Furthermore, the severity they measured correlated with clinical rank order of the severity of the injury. Those injuries with higher energy were consistently ranked as more severe by treating surgeons. Level of evidence: II.

25. Slongo TF, Audige L: AO Pediatric Classification Group: Fracture and Dislocation Classification Compendium for Children: The AO Pediatric Comprehensive Classification of Long Bone Fractures. *J Orthop Trauma* 2007;21:S135-S163.

This is a new fracture classification for pediatric bones that was developed by AO using scientific methodology to try to ensure validity and reproducibility.

Delivery of Orthopaedic Trauma Care

Bruce H. Ziran, MD   Timothy Bray, MD   Steven M. Kane, MD   Timothy O'Mara, MD   Peter Althausen, MD

Introduction

Unintentional injury is the leading cause of death in the first four decades of life.[1] In 2000, the costs of health care, coupled with estimated costs of lost lifetime productivity, were estimated to exceed $500 billion.[2] In addition, unintentional injury was responsible for 39.3 million emergency department visits (33% of total visits) in the United States. Overall, emergency department visits increased from 90.3 million to 119.2 million from 1996 to 2006, while the number of emergency departments in the United States dropped from 4,019 to 3,833.[3] The Institute of Medicine, in a 2006 report on the future of emergency care in the United States health system, concluded that "a national crisis in emergency care has been brewing, and is now beginning to come into full view," resulting in issues of overcrowding in hospital emergency departments, fragmentation among the different agencies in the emergency health field, shortage of on-call specialists, and overall lack of emergency preparedness.[4] This, in turn, leads to delays in delivery of emergency care and overcrowding of level I trauma centers as a result of ambulance diversion and transfers of patients with injuries that could be appropriately managed at the local level. With the current political and financial climate in the United States, these issues have become more important, and the care of acute musculoskeletal injuries should be of special interest to all orthopaedic surgeons.

Dr. Bray or an immediate family member is a member of a speakers' bureau or has made paid presentations on behalf of AO and Synthes; and has received research or institutional support from AO and Synthes. Dr. Ziran or an immediate family member is a member of a speakers' bureau or has made paid presentations on behalf of Stryker and Synthes; and serves as a paid consultant to or is an employee of Stryker, Synthes, and Force Medical. Dr. Kane or an immediate family member serves as a paid consultant to or is an employee of SBM; has received research or institutional support from Acumed, Synthes, SBM, and Diatherix; and has stock or stock options held in Johnson & Johnson. Dr. O'Mara or an immediate family member has received research or institutional support from Synthes and Smith and Nephew. Dr. Althausen or an immediate family member has received research or institutional support from Synthes and Smith and Nephew.

Orthopaedic Emergency Care in the United States

One component of the emergency care crisis identified by the Institute of Medicine is the shortage of capable specialists willing to take emergency and trauma calls. This naturally applies to orthopaedic care and represents a multifactorial phenomenon. Reasons for lack of orthopaedic coverage include increasing patient population and increased volume of indigent patients; geographic shortage of orthopaedic surgeons and an overall orthopaedic manpower shortage; inadequate funding for hospitals, emergency departments, and surgeons; increased orthopaedic subspecialization; problems with practice disruption and productivity; and changes in the medicolegal environment. In a survey conducted by the American College of Emergency Physicians, three fourths of emergency department medical directors reported that their hospitals have inadequate on-call specialty coverage; these findings were widespread and affected all geographic areas. Providing emergency orthopaedic care in the community setting has become unattractive for a variety of personal and professional reasons. Both the American Academy of Orthopaedic Surgeons (AAOS) and the American Orthopaedic Association (AOA) have recognized the issue and released position statements on this subject.[5,6]

The AOA established a working committee to review the crisis of access to emergency orthopaedic care. This independent task force, under the direction of the Orthopaedic Institute of Medicine, was assigned the duty of reviewing solutions that could be adopted by the community orthopaedic surgeon. This working committee surveyed the membership of the AAOS and the Orthopaedic Trauma Association (OTA), consulted government experts in health care administration and clinical orthopaedic practices to characterize barriers to emergency department coverage, and eventually published a "call to action" to the orthopaedic community.[6,7]

Based on these survey results, several barriers to emergency care were identified and are outlined in **Table 1**. There have been discussions at the AAOS level regarding emergency care responsibilities; however, the language was never agreed upon by all stakeholders in the solution. The universal theme of the discussion was the encouragement of community orthopaedic surgeons to engage their colleagues and local hospital administrators to establish dialogue in search of a system that would provide emergency care to injured patients within their own community.[5] This practice philosophy does not require that all community surgeons take call. It does, however, encourage all physicians to participate in the decision-making process, and to help design a call coverage program for their specific community. Although the OTA has proposed a system of mandatory call for all AAOS members,[7] the current recommendations of both the AAOS and AOA are that each orthopaedic surgeon participate in developing and implementing community-specific solutions.[7] The two bottom-line recommendations from the task force to address this problem were that orthopaedic surgeons

are the most qualified and capable providers of orthopaedic emergency care, and each community will have unique needs and requirements that must be overcome to create a solution to the problem (**Table 2**).

Alternative Proposals

Although debate on this topic will remain vigorous and divided, a nationally mandated solution may not be possible because practice patterns vary widely in each geographic region. Other possible scenarios may transpire as a result of the call-access problem. The American Association for the Surgery of Trauma has proposed the development of an acute care surgery program in which fellows who are graduates of general surgery residency programs receive training in other subspecialty areas, including orthopaedic surgery emergencies; for example, the acute management of open fractures and compartment syndromes. This movement began as a response to the frustrations expressed by general surgeons who were finding it difficult to locate orthopaedic surgeons willing to provide acute orthopaedic care at their trauma facility. The acute care surgeon would be able to débride and temporarily stabilize open fractures, perform fasciotomies, and reduce simple fractures. Although the OTA initially opposed this track, stating that the orthopaedic surgeon is the most qualified, capable, and cost-effective provider for musculoskeletal care, some individuals in both groups now recognize that there might be a legitimate role for the

Table 1

Barriers to Emergency Care

Lifestyle/time away from family

Poor reimbursement

Perceived increased liability

Disruption of elective surgery practices

Lack of comfort with newer orthopaedic trauma techniques

Inadequate resource commitment from hospital administrations

Table 2

Recommendations of the AOA

- Communities should ensure access to orthopaedic consultation.
- Community-wide teams should evaluate care, assess needs, and recommend solutions.
- All orthopaedic surgeons should recognize a professional obligation to ensure an effective community system for delivery of emergency care.
- Define basic competencies for the care of urgent/emergent orthopaedic conditions.
- Identify specific conditions amenable to definitive management in the community setting.
- Propose methods for maintaining basic trauma competencies.
- Define minimum criteria for emergency orthopaedic care.
- Address care of transfer patients.
- Discussion with orthopaedic training programs regarding core competencies and methods of ensuring appropriate training in orthopaedic trauma care.
- Hospital provision of dedicated daily operating room time and resources for management of orthopaedic trauma cases.
- Collaborate with local orthopaedic surgeons to develop effective emergency department call system and a case transfer system.
- Work with other medical organizations to promote community-based solutions to the crisis.
- Hospitals and orthopaedic professional organizations jointly advocate appropriate reimbursement for emergency musculoskeletal care provided by surgeons and hospitals.
- Local hospitals assess need for emergency coverage by specialty area.
- Negotiate cooperative solutions with third-party payers.
- Involve local physicians to provide unbiased opinions and support for new reimbursement strategies.

acute care surgeon when faced with the crisis in deficient orthopaedic emergency call coverage. Within this debate, nontrauma orthopaedic surgeons have pointed out that hospital administrators often decide to pursue trauma center designation without considering the impact of this pursuit on the orthopaedists' practice. Hospitals counter this notion by declaring that the provision of trauma care is an obligation to the community.

Others remark that this problem is a good reason to support regionalization of trauma care, as found in states such as Maryland, or a single payer system such as the Canadian health care system, as viable alternatives. As the US government debate on health care provisions moves forward, policy makers must assure the US population that government involvement will support access for all patients as well as provide appropriate tools and reimbursement for orthopaedic trauma surgeons expected to provide care.

In regionalized systems, trauma centers usually have sufficient volume and governmental support to ensure that sufficient resources and human capital are available to provide continuous high-quality care. As advocates of such care, trauma surgeons should point out to lawmakers that trauma is best viewed as a public service, much like firefighting and law enforcement, wherein society expects such basic governmental services. Viewed in this light, funding for trauma care does not become encumbered by the arguments that revolve around the health care debate. There are some strong arguments to support regionalized trauma care. Call coverage would not be an issue because there would be a concentrated and adequate number of specialists who are dedicated to trauma and would provide coverage as part of their responsibilities. Additionally, institutional memory and peer-reviewed quality controls would be in place to ensure the highest quality of care. A disadvantage to such a system would be the distances patients would be transported from home and family, appropriate posthospital follow-up care, follow-up for quality control and research, and patient convenience. The vastness of the United States and the reluctance of US citizens to endure such inconveniences may prevent regionalization. However, a solution to this particular disadvantage would be the advent of smaller satellite centers that could support a "community trauma specialist," described elsewhere in this chapter. These centers and individuals would be designated to provide follow-up trauma care as well as help with triage of patients to larger, more resourced centers. Still, there remains a vocal debate among orthopaedic trauma surgeons regarding what each thinks is the best system. The solution is not easy, but governmental mandates may be forthcoming in this regard, and many trauma care providers fear that this development will only worsen and complicate an already difficult situation. It is therefore in the best interest of the orthopaedic community, and moreover, the orthopaedic trauma community, to participate in the debate to find a solution.

Legislative Issues

The federal Emergency Medical Treatment and Active Labor Act (EMTALA) was enacted in 1986 to prevent patient dumping for reasons of inability to pay. Its purpose was to prevent hospitals from turning away people with emergency conditions or transferring people with unstable conditions. The primary impact of EMTALA on orthopaedic surgeons pertains to their on-call responsibilities. It does not require physicians to take call. This service can be mandated only by medical staff bylaws or by contract. Physicians who take call have certain rights. They can provide coverage at several hospitals simultaneously. They can schedule elective surgery while on call. Physicians are subject to direct sanctions for failing to respond or come to the hospital when required. Physicians are subject to monetary penalties for EMTALA violations, up to $50,000 per violation. They can also be excluded from Medicare for flagrant violations. No clear responsibility has been established for follow-up care for patients treated in the emergency department. The EMTALA on-call burden is passed on to the surgeons through medical staff bylaws and regulations.[8]

The Health Insurance Portability and Accountability Act (HIPAA) was finalized in 2002 to create a national standard in protecting patient's medical records and other personal health information. The privacy rules give patients more control over their medical records and limit the way physicians may use and release information. The fines for noncompliance are substantial and the Department of Justice can even impose criminal penalties. This law has had far-reaching implications. Orthopaedic practices and hospitals alike have spent massive amounts of time and money to achieve compliance. More time must now be spent educating patients on their rights so they can make informed decisions regarding their privacy. This is very important with regard to conducting medical research. Prior to initiating any Institutional Review Board–approved studies, most hospital systems mandate completion of HIPAA training or educational courses. Furthermore, with the governmental push toward electronic medical records, there has also been a mandate to ensure security against loss or theft of sensitive medical information. Because trauma patients require involvement of many providers, and often travel long distances for follow-up care, there are potential security risks, and many practices do not yet have adequate information system resources in place to accommodate government regulations.

As health care reform in the United States takes shape, the future of adequate funding for trauma care may be affected in both positive and negative ways. There may be increased funding for institutions and health care systems that provide trauma care, which will help support system infrastructure and hospital-based models. There may also be reductions in reimbursement that may adversely affect the willingness of physicians to provide trauma care.

Trauma System Models

The AAOS, OTA, and AOA have all published multiple position statements regarding the optimal resources for providing orthopaedic trauma care at the community level.[5-7] Hospitals that support the trauma mission typically voluntarily participate in the American College of Surgeons Committee on Trauma (ACSCOT) recommendations for trauma center verification. Although not required, the ACSCOT guideline is the accepted and minimum standard for resources and services of trauma centers at each specific level. Participation is a voluntary effort and has resulted in some state-by-state variances, including some states having their own state verification that closely parallels the ACSCOT recommendations, whereas others do not have any verification process at all. One study of trauma centers around the country found that there is little homogeneity among various level I centers, with wide variations in basic resources recommended for trauma centers.[9]

Community Systems

A community trauma system remains one of the most common methods of trauma care delivery in the United States. There are several different types of hospital-supported orthopaedic community trauma models. One well-described system is a community-based "orthopaedic trauma panel," whereby multiple community orthopedists participate in the care of the trauma patient. This system is coordinated by a fellowship-trained orthopaedic trauma surgeon wherein the panel members care for the most severely injured patients on a rotating basis in conjunction with general surgeons certified by the American College of Surgeons (ACS) program. The hospital financially supports all aspects of the trauma commitment including surgeon stipends, guaranteed payment for the underinsured, institutional support for hospital-based physician assistants (PAs), quality assurance indemnification, call rooms, available and sufficiently sized operating rooms, and yearly continuing medical education. Community orthopaedic surgeons can in turn help to offset some of the hospital costs by participating in cost containment programs, providing teaching opportunities, and coordinating effective, early care to facilitate discharge and decrease hospital stays. Given the appropriate payer mix and commitment to these community orthopaedic trauma programs, both the hospital and physician can create financial rewards to keep these programs solvent while providing excellence in orthopaedic trauma care. Institutions that have implemented such a model have demonstrated revenue positive performance in trauma care. Imaging, surgery, and laboratory charges are particularly revenue productive in these systems.[10-12]

Other similar models are based on hospital "ownership" of the orthopaedic trauma surgeons, either individually or as a group. These are hospital-employed physicians who provide most, if not all, of the care to emergency patients. The advantages of this system for the surgeon are the single location for work, familiarity with the hospital and staff, and financial comfort with monthly base salary and benefits. The disadvantages are the potential conflict with other community orthopaedic providers, cessation of the program on short notice, potential cuts in pay and benefits, and lack of community support for specialty services such as hand and spine. Operationally, however, a panel-type interaction with private surgeons would be similar to the private trauma panel model. Hospital ownership of the orthopaedic trauma practice has been shown also to be very profitable, and certain aspects of practice management costs can be kept to a minimum by using existing hospital resources and staff. Furthermore, downstream revenue from elective cases and outpatient services are kept within the hospital system, whereas with a private model, private surgeons would be free to engage in ventures that compete with the hospital.[10-12]

Another nontraditional model includes utilization of "physician extenders" and functional hospital-to-hospital transfer agreements. In these systems, the extenders are the initial health care providers who stabilize the trauma patient until the trauma physicians arrive. These programs may be more beneficial to the smallest and more remote communities where trauma physicians cover more than one hospital or where there are too few trauma physicians to cover all of the available days. Surprisingly, there remain locations in the United States that do not have 911 service and lack advanced emergency medical services. It is imperative in these systems that the hospital and community physicians work together to create explicit protocols before advertising orthopaedic emergency care. Too frequently, hospitals are quick to market fracture/trauma care and have not taken the time to prearrange the specifics of patient care triage. This is detrimental to the patient, stressful to the emergency physicians, and may create liability for the orthopaedic and trauma surgeons.

If such community programs were to be distributed strategically around tertiary level centers, patients who had been transported long distances to such "regional" centers for acute, life-threatening injuries could then follow up and receive subsequent reconstructive treatment by the community trauma specialist. The community orthopaedic trauma surgeon is a key player in this model because much of the secondary care and treatment required by trauma patients is orthopaedic in scope. Ultimately, each community hospital and its orthopaedic trauma leaders must evaluate together their trauma needs, available physicians, hospital resources, and commitment to the trauma mission to design a trauma system that is effective in caring for these deserving patients. Cost containment, effective patient care, and responsible demands by surgeons can result in quality orthopaedic trauma care.

Academic/University Systems

Universities and other academic medical institutions are usually located in large metropolitan areas and thus benefit from sufficient patient volume to achieve economies of scale. They often have numerous fellowship-trained orthopaedic trauma surgeons on staff, a well-developed general surgical program, and a productive research department. They have experience with trauma care by virtue of their location and mission, as well as institutional memory secondary to having the ability and resources in place to handle problems they have seen multiple times. The model of university care underwent a significant shift in the latter part of the 20th century. In such a system, faculty members were often reimbursed with an academic stipend to compensate them for the inefficiencies of tertiary care, teaching of residents, and poor payer mix. Slowly, these stipends diminished and faculty members were expected to compete with the efficiency of the private sector. More lucrative subspecialties became more valued over trauma, and competition for institutional resources resulted in a less-than-optimal work environment for trauma care. The nontrauma subspecialists often wanted to focus on their specific specialty and not worry about the encumbrances of trauma care. Subsequently, both trauma and nontrauma subspecialists were discouraged from providing trauma care, and the worsening economics and frustrations of providing trauma care were contributory to an anecdotally perceived shift in orthopaedic labor. This created challenges in the structure of many university centers, where most of the faculty had traditionally participated in call coverage.[5-7]

Some systems with 6-year residency programs were able to offer chief residents an opportunity to be hired as instructors during the equivalent of postgraduate year 6. These "superchiefs" gained additional experience under the comfort of their mentor's stewardship, and departments benefited from having the call covered. However, if the instructor/superchief model is used, it is important to also provide the backup and stewardship of fully trained orthopaedic trauma surgeons who can supervise the less experienced surgeons and appropriately take control of the more complex cases. The liability issues of this model of trauma coverage have not yet been well delineated.

Not surprisingly, many orthopaedic trauma surgeons have left academic settings. As a result, community trauma centers benefited from experienced trauma surgeons who helped develop high-quality community programs. The exodus of both trauma and nontrauma talent from the universities and the ability and willingness of trauma surgeons to pursue nontrauma careers resulted in an apparent shortage of orthopaedic trauma surgeons. University and academic centers subsequently implemented changes and new models in an effort to provide a fair and sustainable career path for orthopaedic trauma surgeons. Institutional support to the department and recognition of the value that the orthopaedic trauma surgeons bring to the department and

residency program helped improve retention rates. Additionally, recognition of the unfair payer mix in trauma resulted in the implementation of better reimbursement models. Although numerous compensation formulas exist, many revolve around fair compensation for work done and provide for uncompensated care. This is especially critical in the university setting, because these institutions are considered tertiary centers and as such do not have the liberty of transferring care, a practice more likely at the community centers. EMTALA was an effort to curb the "dumping" process, but the inherent attributes of the trauma population demographic remain an unfair burden to any dedicated trauma practice.

Resource needs at university centers are similar to those at community centers but because of wider variations in volume, they must be able to tolerate idle resources that can be increased to match volume surges. Probably the most important resource requirement is unrestricted access to the operating room. An operating room is considered "at capacity" when utilization is approximately 75% of available room time. In most tertiary level centers, orthopaedic trauma surgeons commonly function at utilization levels of 90% to 120%. Although these percentages may appear to indicate productivity, such overutilization is usually at the expense of the surgeons' time and overtime utilization of hospital staff. Inefficient room turnovers, less optimal equipment availability, less experienced staff during off-hours, and the frequent need for overtime pay can make poor utilization more expensive. Considering the costs of hospitalization, it is easy to estimate that ongoing system inefficiencies could result in hundreds of thousands of dollars of waste that could be recovered through judicious spending on process improvement programs. Theoretical examples of programs that could improve efficiency without compromising safety include available hospitalists who optimize patients for surgery, case management concurrent with clinical treatment, flexible operating room staffing to accommodate surges and ebbs in volume, operating suites that are managed based on clinical needs, and effective modern communication between specialties and dispositions.

Another new resource need within orthopaedic programs with residencies has been midlevel providers, such as PAs. Current resident work-hour restrictions and schedule rotations result in frequent lapses in communication and disruptions in continuity of care. The complexities of the trauma patient require diligent attention to constantly changing patient status, and with published literature demonstrating that the new work-hour restrictions may result in problems with continuity of care, the addition of mid-level providers may be of great benefit. A dedicated orthopaedic trauma PA can greatly improve patient care quality and continuity by serving as a hub of information exchange. Additionally, close working relationships with attending surgeons result in a mirroring and execution of their idiosyncratic techniques and can be a valuable resource for rotating residents and an excellent liaison to other services. The PA may also bill for many provided services, even in the operating room when residents are not available. With proper practice management, the salary of a PA, which commonly exceeds $100,000, may be offset to some extent and, in some cases, completely.[13]

The university programs provide some benefits for trauma surgeons that are not found as frequently in the community setting. There are usually several residents to help with daily patient care as well as colleagues in orthopaedics and other specialties who provide ongoing support for nontrauma issues. The academic setting also provides intellectual stimulation and the challenge to stay current with new surgical techniques and the medical literature. Constant peer review is an excellent method for maintaining one's skills and may help when preparing for the newly implemented Maintenance of Certification programs. There are also the pride and recognition of being affiliated with centers that often have other widely recognized specialists. Such early career benefits make later career aspirations easier due to the accomplishments achieved during one's academic tenure. These accomplishments can be realized only if the department chief provides access to the existing research infrastructure and helps maintain a work environment that allows time for academic endeavors. Also, senior mentoring of junior faculty, when it occurs, is an intangible benefit of the academic environment.

Quality Improvement and Education

System Planning and Improvement

System improvement is usually the responsibility of the general trauma service and includes evaluation of emergency medical services and hospital practices, including rehabilitation. The level of evaluation is usually guided by the ACS accreditation programs or defined by state law. Orthopaedic involvement is critical in all phases of the preliminary protocol development for prehospital care of musculoskeletal injuries, emergency department and transport care, operating room care, orthopaedic trauma floor nursing, and finally, physical therapy and rehabilitation. Monthly quality improvement meetings with representatives of each of these services provide leadership direction and help develop successful best practices for the orthopaedic trauma service.

Quality improvement programs among private practice orthopaedic surgeons within the community setting are extremely difficult to implement, supervise, and enforce sanctions of substandard care. It is especially difficult in community systems where surgeons from different groups may have different training experiences and bring acceptable but alternative methods for review. Hospitals that employ orthopaedic trauma providers have fewer problems with the specifics of a quality assurance process. The experience of senior

community trauma leadership must provide a safe and appropriate educational review program with a primary goal of best serving the trauma patient's improved outcomes. Quarterly meetings to review radiographs, fixation techniques, and complications can be universally educational for all panel members. Morbidity and mortality conference guidelines and documentation have been a part of orthopaedic educational programs for decades and are regarded by ACS review committees as mandatory for maintenance of certification. Although hospitals advise those physicians participating in quality improvement programs that they are legally protected from discovery of the meeting content, those physicians are not protected from character defamation or restraint-of-trade lawsuits. For these reasons, it is imperative that orthopaedic trauma services and their trauma hospitals create indemnity for persons assisting in a professional review action. For the hospital trauma service to ensure quality, the administration must hold harmless all persons assisting in a professional review action conducted by any professional review body of the institution.

Disaster preparedness planning and preparation is of critical importance at the community level. Most states have a department of emergency management, and familiarity with their services for the orthopaedic surgeon is critical in the event of a community catastrophe. Preparedness activities are particularly challenging in practice environments with multiple hospitals and multiple physicians covering emergency services. In the current unstable political environment, orthopaedic trauma surgeons have a community obligation to become involved in the planning process. In most communities, annual meetings to plan disaster management contingencies with the appropriate state agency will help define the orthopaedic surgeon's responsibilities. In general, the guidelines for orthopaedic surgeons are to care for home and family first and then to make one's way to the predesignated hospital. Each community surgeon should have a specified identification card to indicate the hospital to which they are assigned to provide care in the event of an emergency.

Trauma Registry

The creation of a trauma registry is an important aspect of any trauma program. This is a collection of prospectively recorded information about trauma patients. This information is beneficial for physicians, patients, and administrators and serves four major purposes: quality control, timely follow-up, education of residents, and research. It can be used to capture the efficacy of treatments and record adverse events, mortality, and survival rates. Although observational, the trauma registry information can serve to generate a hypothesis or justify future randomized controlled trials. Prior to the implementation of a registry, its purpose should be defined and agreed upon by the users. A full-time, unbiased individual should be hired to collect and oversee the quality of the registry data. All trauma patients must be included, and data should be validated on a regular basis to ensure accuracy and reliability. The OTA also maintains the OTA Trauma Registry Database for Multicenter Studies as a member benefit. The registry is capable of supporting multicenter studies, so any individual or group who desires to use the OTA trauma database for a clinical study is able to do so. Interested individuals can access this information at www.OTA.org.

Trauma Education

Historically, trauma fellowship training has been the responsibility of large, inner-city, university-based hospital systems. University politics, inadequate salaries, research stress, and poor patient teaching populations have created challenges for the university-based programs. The focus of orthopaedic trauma fellowships has always been on surgical technique, research, and supervision of younger resident staff. Many fellows and residents do not end up working in large urban trauma practices. In fact, new graduates are increasingly interested in family and quality of life issues that favor smaller community trauma practices. A new evolution in trauma fellowship education is the possibility of a community trauma fellowship. These fellowships may be tailored for the setting desired by the trainee and thereby provide a bridge between the community generalist and the tertiary specialist. This individual would be trained to repair the common trauma pathologies that a rural community may encounter, and would be able to provide appropriate damage control and transfer for the more complex injuries. In this aspect they may be better suited to serve patients and their communities, and provide a liaison to the tertiary center trauma surgeon, who would then transfer postoperative care back to the community trauma surgeon. This community traumatologist would fill the gaps found in many regions, solve many of the trauma issues raised by orthopaedic surgeons in these private settings, and address some of the geographic challenges of postoperative follow-up for patients transferred long distances for trauma care.

Basic Trauma Competency

All board-certified orthopaedic surgeons should maintain updated certifications to practice musculoskeletal emergency care. During the residency training period, adequate and thorough instruction on care of the emergency orthopaedic patient is one of the requirements for accreditation and for gaining eligibility to sit for the orthopaedic board-certification examination. The basic community practice requirements for orthopaedic trauma care should be an extension of the residency education and are being better defined by ongoing research as well as evaluation by orthopaedic leadership committees. These requirements will certainly include the following: obtain and document a history and physical examination on the injured patient; perform initial care of orthopaedic injuries such as closed reductions, splinting, and basic wound care; obtain and correctly interpret musculoskeletal imaging; provide basic stabilization of fractures when indicated; and provide follow-up and transfer of any postinjury care. In the event that communities or surgeons are unable or unwilling to provide these basic emergency services, transfer agreements should be arranged with nearby referral institutions.[8]

Core Competencies in Orthopaedic Trauma: The Residency Experience Carried Forward

Basic and complex orthopaedic trauma remains the foundation and focus of much of orthopaedic surgery. Trauma education espouses some of the basic aspects of musculoskeletal science and is often the core of many residency programs. Resident performance and learning in orthopaedic trauma care, like all aspects of the residency education process, are evaluated through the Accreditation Council for Graduate Medical Education mandated core competencies. Each residency program defines the goals and objectives essential in orthopaedic trauma care. The ongoing requirement to maintain core competency is reflected in the newly implemented Maintenance of Certification program by the AAOS and American Board of Orthopaedic Surgery. Surgeons are expected to maintain their pursuit of lifelong learning during their orthopaedic career. To this end, the core competencies in trauma care would parallel those of residency to include patient care, medical knowledge, practice-based learning, a systems-based practice, professionalism and ethics, and interpersonal skills and communication.

Patient care remains the mainstay core competency in trauma. Orthopaedic trauma patients are by nature complex and require vigilance, thoroughness, and anticipation. Furthermore, because of the multispecialty aspects of trauma, interactions and collaboration with other medical and surgical specialties are required. Trauma patients are also prone to high levels of fear, pain, and anxiety because of having experienced sudden and unplanned life-threatening or function-altering injuries.

Summary

Delivery of orthopaedic trauma care is a process currently in a period of transition. Undoubtedly, changes in health care administration, funding, and policy will have a dramatic impact on orthopaedic trauma care. The focus of anyone who undertakes trauma orthopaedics as a career path should be to negotiate and procure the resources needed to deliver a successful and sustainable program. The responsibility of surgeons should be not only to provide high-quality surgical care for orthopaedic injuries but also to involve themselves with the challenges and solutions for their community.

1: General Topics and New Technology

Annotated References

1. Centers for Disease Control and Prevention, National Center for Injury Prevention and Control, Web-based Injury Statistics Query and Reporting System (WISQARS): http://www.cdc.gov/injury/wisqars/fatal.html. Published April 2006. Accessed December 2009.

   Statistics that demonstrate the importance of unintentional injury on mortality in the United States are presented.

2. Finkelstein EA, Corso PS, Miller TR: *Incidence and Economic Burden of Injuries in the United States.* New York, NY, Oxford University Press, 2006.

   This article presents an analysis of economic burden of unintentional injuries that evaluates immediate and delayed health care costs, and also estimates effect of long-term morbidity and disability on lost income and productivity.

3. Pitts SR, Niska RW, Xu J, Burt CW: National Hospital Ambulatory Medical Care Survey: 2006 Emergency Department Summary. National health statistics reports, no 7. Hyattsville, MD, National Center for Health Statistics, 2008.

   This statistical report reveals a steady increase in emergency department utilization and corresponding proportional increase in emergency department utilization for ambulatory care.

4. Committee on the Future of Emergency Care in the United States: *Hospital-based emergency care: At the breaking point.* Washington, DC, National Academies Press, 2007.

   Part of a three-volume report by the Institute of Medicine that analyzes the state of emergency care in the United States. This report looks at emergency medical services, emergency care in the hospital, and the delivery of emergency care for children, and tries to identify specific problems and recommend solutions.

5. American Academy of Orthopaedic Surgeons: Position statement: Emergency orthopaedic care. http://www.aaos.org/about/papers/position/1172.asp. Published December 2008. Accessed November 2009.

   The AAOS revised position statement identifies factors contributing to the orthopaedic emergency call crisis and recommends potential actions that may help to alleviate the crisis. This statement deals with coverage for acute trauma care and urgent general orthopaedic care.

6. American Orthopaedic Association, Orthopaedic Institute of Medicine: Report on the crisis in the delivery of orthopaedic emergency care: A call to action. http://www.aoassn.org/filerequestform/index.asp?f=oiomcompletereport.pdf&d=complete%20Report. Published January 2009. Accessed December 2009.

   The position statement of the AOA and Orthopaedic Institute of Medicine makes more descriptive recommendations on potential areas in which change can be effected to alleviate the orthopaedic call crisis.

7. Orthopaedic Trauma Association: On-call position statement. http://www.ota.org/downloads/PositionStatement12-05.pdf. Published December 2005. Accessed November 2009.

   This position statement of the OTA recommends solutions to the orthopaedic emergency call crisis, including potential mandatory call responsibilities for orthopaedic surgeons during their active years at that institution.

8. EMTALA: EMTALA statutes. http://www.emtala.com/law/index.html. Accessed December 2009.

   An explanation of EMTALA regulations is presented.

9. Ziran BH, Barrette-Grischow MK, Hileman B: United States Level I trauma centers are not created equal: A concern for patient safety? *Patient Saf Surg* 2008;2:18.

   Phone surveys of level I trauma centers were performed to identify the types and level of service and resources at each center. There was no homogeneity in the resources at various level I centers, indicating that significant differences exist among various level I centers. University/academic programs seem to be more resourced than community centers.

10. Althausen PL, Coll D, Cvitash M, Herak A, O'Mara TJ, Bray TJ: Economic viability of a community-based level-II orthopaedic trauma system. *J Bone Joint Surg Am* 2009;91(1):227-235.

    The authors outline the economics of a community-based trauma service.

11. Ziran BH, Barrette-Grischow MK, Marucci K: Economic value of orthopaedic trauma: The (second to) bottom line. *J Orthop Trauma* 2008;22(4):227-233.

    The authors demonstrate the financial effects of setting up a hospital-based trauma service, outline the interpretation of service lines, and explain financial concepts used by hospital administrators when evaluating service lines.

12. Bray TJ: Design of the Northern Nevada Orthopaedic Trauma Panel: A model, level-II community-hospital system. *J Bone Joint Surg Am* 2001;83(2):283-289.

    The authors outline the establishment of a community-based trauma service and its pros and cons.

13. Medicare claims processing manual: www.cms.hhs.gov/manuals/Downloads/clm104c12.pdf. Accessed December 2009.

    CMS guidelines for Medicare claims processing are presented.

Chapter 3

Career and Practice Management Issues in Orthopaedic Trauma

Heather A. Vallier, MD   Sam Agnew, MD

Introduction

The Centers for Disease Control and Prevention, the National Center for Statistics and Analysis, and Healthcare Cost and Utilization Project databases indicate that the incidence of fractures (pediatric, adult, and geriatric) increases approximately 11% per year, thus doubling the number of fractures occurring every 5 years for most metropolitan catchment areas. However, 80% of fracture surgery is still performed outside of university-based facilities, and surgeons with increasing lack of interest in being on call or in providing fracture care often work at these centers.[1-3] Trauma in patients with an Injury Severity Score greater than 20 is trending away from seasonal variations in more densely populated areas. Considering all patients with fractures plus trauma admissions, there is little seasonal variation inside a stable population base. Variations, seasonal or otherwise, are a reflection of access, not necessarily diminishing volume of patients. Access to Level I trauma centers curtails the volume of patients as much as any other factor. It is well known that regionalization of trauma care decreases mortality.[1-9] If a hospital system is truly committed to a trauma program, then appropriate resources should be allocated, including infrastructure, capital, and personnel to manage volume. Over time, high-quality programs that are marketed properly can manage the volume and complexity of patients and demonstrate benefits for all: patients receive best-in-class care, while both hospitals and providers maintain a positive revenue stream.

Successful practice improvement requires looking beyond the monetary value of individual compensation to identify key nonsalary components of a meaningful practice, and having an understanding of the methods to achieve and implement them. It is disappointing that many young trauma surgeons are 3 or 4 years into their career and still lack any demonstrable infrastructure to support their work, such as an orthopaedic trauma operating room or team, or even available radiologic equipment and personnel. The methodology of obtaining these components is equally if not more important as what to request during one's negotiation process.

It is important for the physician to focus on the future of his or her practice after partnership with a particular corporation, university, or hospital and to know how the organization is going to help the physician achieve desired goals.

Objectives

Hospitals provide a platform for physicians to practice, and the availability of subspecialty physicians drives patient utilization of services within a facility. For any relationship between physicians and hospital systems to be successful there must be performance metrics and mutual accountability for intended deliverables, both short-term and long-term. With an organized set of deliverables and return on investment, it is completely legal, ethical, and morally sound that when deliverables are achieved the physician should benefit monetarily—provided these benefits are contracted in advance.

Various practice arrangements for orthopaedic trauma surgeons exist. There are intrinsic differences between career performance and business ventures. The advantages and disadvantages of a practice situation for a given provider depend on the provider's goals and priorities. Any arrangement should afford measurement and creation of patient-centric quality improvement, as well as plan for routine review of fiscal performance and professional growth.

In addition, collaborative strategies for operational efficiency and revenue enhancement are developed while optimizing patient care. The interdependence of physicians and facilities needs to be recognized: trauma centers cannot function without orthopaedic trauma surgeons and these individuals require a trauma center to provide the unique services they are capable of. Initiatives to improve business practices will be effective when both parties are engaged from inception through execution and process assessment.

Dr. Vallier or an immediate family member has received research or institutional support from Synthes. Dr. Agnew or an immediate family member serves as a board member, owner, officer, officer, or committee member of Delphi HealthCare Partners and serves as a paid consultant to or is an employee of Delphi HealthCare Partners.

Table 1

Practice Initiation Options

University/academic: Faculty practice plan employee or hospital employee

  Assistant professor template

  Associate professor template

  Full professor template

Private corporation: Private practice; solo or group partnership

  Production (revenue minus expenses) after stipulated time period, with initial base salary guarantee

Hybrid-type: Group practice production model with base compensation and/or call compensation from trauma center

Hospital employee (nonprofit organization): Being a W-2-based employed physician has different if not softer regulations with regard to Stark and antikickback regulations and within the Internal Revenue Service guidelines for nonprofit institutions.

Independent national management corporation: This alternative may assist with long-term survival of a trauma-focused practice.

Selecting a Practice

Initial consideration should be given to the types of patients, injuries, and the volume thereof that a given trauma center has supported or is capable of supporting. Verification by the American College of Surgeons (ACS) for trauma as level I, II, or III will determine to some extent the types of patients and injuries seen, with level I centers providing the most comprehensive trauma care. An understanding of the intensive care unit and operating room capabilities or impediments to access, and the availability of interventional radiology and a range of related surgical specialists such as vascular, plastics, otolaryngology, and maxillofacial will define the scope of musculoskeletal services that can be provided in an institution.[1,10-16]

The geographical location of a trauma center and the catchment area may affect the amount of blunt versus penetrating trauma. Most large urban trauma centers have seen a rise in penetrating trauma over the past 5 years. Patient population characteristics often are linked with payer mix and should be considered when assessing a practice opportunity and the proposed arrangement. The physician should develop an understanding of the needs of the institution and the community, and ensure that both their expectations and the physician's are realistic and in alignment. Practice initiation options are outlined in **Table 1**.

The number of hospital-employed orthopaedic surgeons is now at its highest, and the number is growing steadily. However, one should be aware that in such an arrangement contracts with payers are negotiated by the hospital with little or no input from providers. This inherently leads to contractual rates that favor the facility over the professionals. In the future, development of a national trauma medical group may be more favorable. In an analogous situation the pediatric intensivists (physicians who work in an intensive care unit) have benefited from such an alternative, and the quality of sustained careers has become evident. Using this model, experienced practitioners are responsible for the allocation of manpower, resources, and evidence-based methodology of the practice, and protect the career efforts of the group members.

Another burgeoning practice model is that of a "shift-work" program, which allows the provider to have more control over lifestyle by contracting to cover an emergency department or trauma center for a prescribed amount of time each month (for example, 12 to 15 days), rendering the necessary care and thus reducing or eliminating the on-call burden for the community staff surgeons. This industry is very much in its infancy, but offers vast personal lifestyle freedoms. It is possible that individual surgeons working in such a practice arrangement could more easily participate in humanitarian endeavors (for example, Doctors Without Borders, Orthopaedics Overseas, other missionary work, or the Orthopaedic Trauma Association [OTA]-sponsored Landstuhl Visiting Scholars Program) that otherwise would not be feasible early in their careers.

Professional Service Agreement

The centerpiece of any practice arrangement is the contract, also known as the Professional Service Agreement (PSA). Many if not all of the PSAs currently drafted are based entirely on compliance with Stark II antikickback regulations with little language regarding obligations of the institution or corporation. The contract review arranged by both parties would be based almost entirely on the fair market value nature of the document and on Office of the Inspector General compliance, and typically does not address the forces and factors that guide a successful career. Furthermore, some physicians entering the marketplace are overly concerned with the dollar value of their compensation in the PSA and not the necessary institutional deliverables for a sustainable career. Current physician-centric contracts (limited to term and compensation only) fail to address the core aspects of professional development and career longevity. Physician-centric contracts have a track record of lasting only 2 to 5 years at best, and 36 months on average. Other language standards should include operating room access, orthopaedic trauma room availability, physician extenders, support services, and academic needs. Fiscal validity of such resource allocation may be easily demonstrated with a thorough evaluation and analysis of the halo effect that a viable trauma service creates[13,16-24] (**Table 2**).

Contract terms vary depending on the agreement. In some cases either party may terminate the agreement at

Table 2

Hospital—Physician Contractual Deliverables for the Employed Physician*

Baseline competency of personnel in the operating room and floor for everyday performance of duties. Documented as to present skill set and future expectations

Authority of surgeon over the skill set enhancement of said personnel

Authority over the productivity of the entire service line

Quantifiable and reproducible amount of operating room time each week; does not accept traditional block-time allocation methodology (60 hours of anesthesia time per week as a potential example)

Identifiable plan for practice coverage during continuing medical education, vacation, illness

   Referring hospital notification schema

   Hospital staff notification and policy

   Physical coverage of practice and patients

Annual 3% to 4% cost-of-living increases in base compensation after year 2

Annual reduction in the time per work relative value units generation as attributed to nonsurgical time

   Charting and reporting of said proficiency monthly

   Creation of a baseline minute/work relative value units that must be achieved before any conversion to a production-based model

Evidence-based usage of intraoperative technology drivers:

   Radiologic

   Implants

   Orthobiologic

Continuing medical education for surgeon and entire team each year

Competency of office personnel and skill set assurance each year:

   Master coder in orthopaedics certified annually

   Certified orthopaedic physician's assistant or equivalent

   Certified orthopaedic technician

Annual review of professional fee schedule and authority over its creation or annual modification

Authority over, or significant participation in, vendor contracting for orthopaedic trauma implants, supplies, and capital equipment

Binding terms to contract after 24 months with severance package equivalent to 150% annual salary plus benefits as cash dispersal

If termination without cause: authority over the language of subsequent reference materials

Removal of any noncompete or nonsolicitation language if employed expressly for the purpose of trauma care for the community

*This is an executive position in which a professional is being contracted, not a salesperson who is to work on commission, or simply another employee; therefore, certain baseline deliverables must be in place to ensure stability and a professional career environment

any time with "just cause." Other contracts establish a set term, upon completion of which the contract will expire, unless both parties take action to reach a new agreement. Another type of contract has an "evergreen" clause, automatically renewing for set periods of time unless either party discontinues the agreement.

Restrictive covenants are also becoming more common in contracts. The allowance and enforceability of restrictive covenants varies by state. Noncompete clauses restrict the provider from performing similar services for another employer within the same geographic region for a period of time after the contract has been terminated. There are exceptions to any non-

compete clause being valid or enforceable if one is contracted expressly for the purpose of providing emergency care to patients; the language of the agreement determines the applicability of a noncompete clause. Nonsolicitation clauses are less restrictive, but they prevent a provider from soliciting patients, associates, or referral sources to another practice within the region after the contract has been terminated. Nonsolicitation clauses also prevent a different employer or institution from soliciting the services of the provider.[25]

Contract language should include the definition of trauma, and whether the working definition broadens when most of the fracture work comes under the aus-

Table 3

Program Metrics: Specific Examples of Responsibilities and the Return on Investment

Cost per case reduction for fracture care versus preprogram historical

Cost containment Initiatives created in a manner that can be easily tracked

Personnel attrition within orthopaedics:

Physician

Nurse

Technician

Enhanced ancillary revenue:

Radiology

Physical therapy/occupational therapy

Pharmacy

Home health

Primary care

Medical and surgical specialists

New physicians to medical staff:

Orthopaedic

Radiology

Intensivists

Physician loyalty measurable

Reduction in use of contract nurses, overtime staffing for orthopaedic surgical procedures versus precontract historical

Patient satisfaction grades

Hospital performance-reputation scoring (HealthGrades, US News)

New market acquisition:

Clinical

Geographic

Direct physician revenue over expenses ledger

Facility net contribution margin

Combined value of comprehensive fracture service line: Recovered losses (inpatient + emergency department + outpatient + Emergency Medical Treatment and Active Labor Act) + new revenue (orthopaedic service line)

pices of the "Trauma Service." Such responsibilities for treating trauma patients will be acknowledged by increased support, infrastructure, and reward metrics. Authority issues pertaining to productivity and patient care have to be concrete in the language of the agreement pertaining to call issues (call schedule, call pay if applicable), operating room availability, operating room time and personnel allocation, patient triage, cost containment, procurement of technology, and the creation of designated trauma panels for transparency of care pathways.[18,20] Infrastructure deliverables for both the office and the operating room must be clearly delin-

eated. Cost containment should be considered a means of obtaining resources specifically for the trauma service line: purchasing agreements or "hospital-based cost savings" programs are ethical means of the hospital reinvesting in the trauma service line infrastructure, and hence the career line of the surgeon. Success metrics must be carefully outlined and rewards acknowledged and formally agreed to at the inception of the contract (Table 3). Collections or personal monetary benchmarks alone cannot be the only metric. Several areas should be considered (Table 4).

Contract issues and priorities change over time and are different for physicians at various stages in time and in professional development over the course of their careers. Institutional needs and strategy also evolve over time. Factors that affect the longevity and success of the relationship develop over years and must be addressed in sequential agreements.

Compensation Formulae-Databases

The American Medical Group Association, Medical Group Management Association (MGMA), and the Sullivan-Cotter consulting firm are examples of existing resources that can help determine appropriate compensation levels.[26-28] Trauma patients in most communities have a payer mix with greater numbers of uninsured and Medicaid patients than elective practices.[23,29-32] However, the federal and state subsidy dollars an institution receives (disproportionate share for hospitals and hospital care assistance programs) will be proportional to the volume of indigent patients, and help to offset hospital losses. Although these funds are generally not directly shared with providers, knowledge of the actual amount of funding and the percentage relative to the provision of trauma care can provide leverage for the provider in discussions about compensation. The presence of commitments of individual states to financing of trauma care may also be helpful in job selection. Maryland uses automobile license renewal fees to support trauma care, and New York and New Jersey have insurance requirements for no-fault medical expense coverage after automobile accidents.

Compensation based on the amount, quality, and type of work done (instead of revenue collected) is a fair and appropriate way to measure the effort and value of a trauma surgeon. From the perspective of the contractor, value is (and always will be) simply cost and price, and less about the quality (or perceived quality) of patient care and surgeon expertise. Available objective methods for measuring time and effort for orthopaedic traumatology have shortcomings. Relative value units (RVUs) or work RVUs (wRVUs) for fracture care are an imperfect model when it comes to compensation, as time required to treat a fracture is often two to four times longer than elective orthopaedic procedures for a given number of wRVUs. The RVUs also do not take into account the unique skill of the trauma surgeon, and the element of urgent or emergent availability to provide care. Furthermore, most payers discount the number of wRVUs for multiple procedures done in the same surgical setting—although in many cases it is more efficient, cost-effective, and in the patients' best interest to do so. Negotiation to eliminate multiple procedure discounts or to implement a percentage increase for urgent and emergent care may mitigate this financial impact. The compensation formula between the surgeon and the contracting facility is separate and distinct from what is negotiated by the facility with government or third-party payers. This is perfectly appropriate because provider compensation reflects the provider's expertise and the institutional halo effect, in addition to professional fees and subsequent collections.

Compensation Models

Academic models include fixed salary or salary plus overage opportunities based on collections or RVUs. They also may include opportunities or expectations for compensation based on academic and administrative contributions. Employed physician models include base salary plus overage opportunity based on wRVUs, with a nondiscounted number of RVUs for multiple procedures. Production-physician models include a fee schedule where dollars per wRVU must be on par with nontrauma partners. Hybrid models include base pay plus a bonus or an RVU production model from the physician group, plus institutional support for call coverage. Some examples of hybrid models are base pay (70th percentile MGMA) plus bonus based on wRVU, base pay (median MGMA) plus bonus based on wRVU, or production (wRVU) plus support from the trauma center.

Call Coverage: Options, Solutions, and Authority

All trauma systems must have a clearly defined authority and chain of command with regard to call issues. Because of the ever-increasing challenges associated with being on call as well as taking care of fractures and other injuries, trauma surgeons must prepare for a growing number of patients in need of urgent and emergent care. This mismatch has led to the emergence of two significant factors that affect the career horizon:

1. The expansion in the number of trauma fellowships offered through the OTA match program (82 positions filled for 2010) with large variability in surgical experience (case volume, case mix) and research training among these fellowships. This development may create wide variations in the clinical acumen of the recent graduates. The market will soon be relatively flooded with orthopaedic trauma surgeons compared to years past. However, the presence of a trauma surgeon within an institution may not guarantee that all complex injuries can be successfully managed. Collaborative strategies must be created whereby injured patients can be directed to the specific personnel who are appropriately trained to care for such injuries. For Level II and Level III programs (approximately 1,500

Table 4

Additional Considerations in Formulating a Professional Services Agreement

- Employee retention
- Patient throughput efficiencies
- Length-of-stay metrics for both the emergency department and the inpatient
- Development of service line as Center of Excellence
- Acquisition of new physicians (orthopaedic as well as other interrelated fields) to staff and community
- Technologic advancements that are created as result of trauma care
- Pay-for-performance successes
- Patient satisfaction surveys: internal validated instruments
- Outside evaluations: HealthGrades rating system

---

in the United States) a bona fide triage and transfer program to the region's Level I facility is paramount—protecting both the patient's best interest as well as the interest of the trauma facilities. Algorithms will ensure consistency of expeditious patient care at the appropriate level.

2. The emergence of an entire industry dedicated to on-call solutions (for example, medical staffing: Vista Staffing, Atlanta, GA; Summit Physician Staffing, New York, NY; and orthopaedic emergency department practice management firms: Delphi Healthcare Partners, Morrisville NC). This industry presents an option for the facility facing a diminishing on-call panel of surgeons, and provides the trauma surgeon on site an entire organization dedicated to his or her craft and career, creating various practice and lifestyle improvements not otherwise possible in historical models.[33,34]

A sustainable plan for call coverage must be neither contingent nor reliant on a call stipend to private staff practitioners within the community. Stipends inherently encourage providing a name for the calendar without ensuring any level of surgeon expertise or commitment to actual provision of care. Although a coverage-only model is currently necessary, it is likely not sustainable; the fracture program as a whole must be patient-centric and have a definable end point for each contractual cycle. Patient access and throughput are easily benchmarked. Performance criteria and credentials are requirements of a well-functioning call panel.[35-37] Issues related to call coverage are also discussed in chapter 2.

Benefits

Beyond direct compensation for clinical work, various benefits of employment may be negotiated. Vacation time, sick time, health care benefits, disability insurance, and retirement benefits are often included in hospital employee and academic agreements. Business expenses including travel for academic meetings, licensure and board certification, subscriptions, and memberships in professional societies are negotiable. Cumulatively, these represent a large expense for the average surgeon.

Malpractice coverage consists of occurrence or claims-made policies. When a surgeon leaves the practice, no further action is needed to maintain coverage with an occurrence policy. However, a claims-made policy will require the purchase of tail coverage to protect the provider against any claims made after the surgeon leaves that practice. Malpractice coverage is often a benefit of hospital employee or academic models. Independent trauma contractors or consultants may successfully negotiate for malpractice coverage provided by the hospital system.

Practice Management

The trauma center should consider the providers as stakeholders when addressing operational and financial issues. In well-functioning centers, patients with higher Injury Severity Scores can generate the greatest profit margins, even with more costs of care than those with less severe injuries.[9,18,20,38-40] Specialty trauma services for hand, spine, and pediatrics not only serve an increasing need in most communities, but also may be demonstrably profitable.[29,31,41]

Operational Issues
Operating Room Access
Operating room access is essential for urgent and emergent cases 24 hours per day, 7 days per week, 365 days per year. For other acute and subacute trauma daily access should be possible, but the details for room availability and staffing should incorporate historical volumes and case-mix data. Orthopaedic trauma block time should be exempt from 48- or 72-hour release rules, and should not compete with elective orthopaedic block time. The ACS verification now includes assessment of a protected orthopaedic trauma room. Operating room access and surgeon access and availability must also be consistent, whereby the operating room demand does not compete with the outpatient clinic for a surgeon's time. Operational issues are also discussed in chapter 2.

Resource Allocation
Additionally, the mere presence of a designated operating room is insufficient. There must be adequate personnel in terms of number and expertise, including surgical assistants (physician extenders such as physician assistants, surgical assistants, or nurse clinicians), nursing staff, and radiology technicians. Surgeon input into selection of team members should be welcomed. Experienced and motivated staff are crucial to a well-functioning team. Professional development opportunities for the entire trauma staff should be offered. These

opportunities help increase knowledge and skills and have the added benefits of building team culture while improving morale and job satisfaction. Equipment specific to orthopaedic trauma service should also be readily available, including radiolucent tables and fluoroscopy. Press-Ganey research indicates that the factors listed here account for approximately $18 to $20 million in annual excess costs to any institution with more than 300 beds and with a 22% nurse turnover (national average), and a well-run orthopaedic program can greatly affect that cost.[42] Additional information about resource allocation can be found in chapter 2.

Even with the upfront expenses of investment in an orthopaedic trauma program including physician extenders, other staffing costs, equipment, and call stipend, a positive contribution margin has been demonstrated.[16,23,43,44] Further financial benefit to the hospital exists in the form of downstream revenue from ancillary professional and technical services, offsite facility revenue, and secondary procedural services, as well as the reduction or elimination of private ambulatory surgery center utilization.[14,15] Previous studies have highlighted some of the clinical, operational, and financial benefits of an orthopaedic trauma room. A trauma room with appropriate staffing results in less utilization of expensive off-shift operating room resources and fewer disruptions to elective case scheduling.[18,19,24] Timely access to an operating room for fracture care improves patient throughput, which decreases length of stay and costs, improves patient satisfaction, and likely diminishes the incidence of complications related to recumbency.[11,45-47] Additionally, less operating room time is required to complete trauma procedures when done during the daytime in an orthopaedic trauma room, and fewer complications occur.[24,48] Provider satisfaction is also realized, as trauma providers can work under optimal conditions: daytime hours with an experienced team, and competition with other surgeons and elective procedures (their own or others) is minimized.

Personnel Management
Physician extenders represent a substantial salary commitment, but can generate revenue above their compensation when appropriately managed. Utilization and business plans should be developed accordingly. Skills assessment and documentation of core competencies along with utilization and productivity reviews are necessary elements. Personnel management is discussed in detail in chapter 2.

Patient Relations and Market Development
Patient education brochures may be created for navigating the postoperative period after a trauma situation. Online resources for patient education, scheduling, and logistical information are important features of a successful practice. Such resources are complemented by a patient advocacy program and related personnel and infrastructure, including financial counselors and social workers; these ancillary services improve

patient satisfaction and outcomes. There is significant value to patient-derived evaluation, and a plan for rewarding the service line for such must be crafted, because it is not possible to reward after the fact without a formula in place for doing so. An internal method of measuring patient satisfaction (such as the Health-Grades rating system) should be instituted and reported on a biannual basis. Strategic planning and marketing should incorporate the unique expertise of the traumatology service line and highlight specific providers and services. Various resources exist for market analysis and development.

Information Systems and Technology

Electronic medical records (EMRs) are becoming the expectation of patients and governmental entities. The upfront expense in converting to an EMR and the challenges of implementation and navigating the system are not inconsequential. However, the potential benefits of accessibility and improved communication among providers may be realized. Streamlined EMRs can drastically reduce transcription expenses. A well-functioning EMR is also compatible with billing software, automatically populating electronic claim forms. This expedites billing processes and simplifies the management of denials.

Preferably, a digital imaging system will interface with the EMR.[49] Digital imaging has improved the quality and consistency of radiographic images, which are an integral part of a traumatology practice. Digital images may also be accessed from multiple locations within and outside of a given facility, which is expeditious to patient care. Ideally, a trauma center will have all types of imaging modalities from all locations; for example, emergency department, operating room, inpatient areas, and outpatient clinics, housed within the same computer archiving system.

Compliance and Accreditation

Trauma surgeons should be leaders in the development of trauma policies and processes. Administrative compensation, including participation in hospital quality assurance and ACS accreditation, should be negotiated. ACS verification validates the work and organization that has been put forth and allows an outside agency to authenticate the processes put in place within a trauma center. However, ACS verification is little more than a report card and an internal guideline specific to orthopaedics for such things as an orthopaedic trauma room and acquisition of trauma support personnel and infrastructure, including a data registry and epidemiologist.

Financial Issues

Payer Contracting

Contracting of premier rates with payers for the provision of trauma services represents another substantial financial opportunity for providers and hospital systems. So-called "carve-outs" represent specifically negotiated fees for service that are greater than the stan-

dard fees for that service. If a state-directed or state-supported triage system exists, then trauma carve-outs become much easier to arrange because such services must be provided by statute. In the absence of a state-directed system, carve-outs are possible but require talented negotiators. To maintain budget neutrality, non-trauma providers must be willing to take reduced reimbursement on certain codes. Carve-outs may be most reasonable in a practice arrangement with a heavy emphasis on trauma care, either a private or a hospital-employee model.

Alternatively, in a private or hybrid model, consideration may be given to going out of network with non-governmental payers. This means the payer would be responsible for 100% of charges, as there is no professional contract for the provision of orthopaedic trauma care. Although this method reduces administrative hassles related to contracting and denials, payment is not guaranteed. Furthermore, patients who require staged procedures may not be allowed by their insurer to return to the initial provider for subsequent care.[50]

Coding, Billing, and Charge Capture

Orthopaedic coding has become increasingly complex. A plethora of resources exist specific to this topic, and the AAOS and OTA annual meetings afford opportunities for continuing education on this topic. Ongoing education and familiarity with these constantly changing practices and processes are essential for all providers. Emphasis tends to be placed on coding for surgical procedures, which generate most revenues for a trauma surgeon. Accurate documentation and high-level coding are important in maximizing collections. Notably, although the wRVU and charges for evaluation and management coding and nonsurgical management are smaller, these are generally reimbursed at much higher rates than surgical services.[19,38,44,51,52] Charge capture methodology must be an agreed-upon tactic and one that is measurable in its effectiveness and compliance, as trauma tends to produce a significant number of treated injuries that are not coded for and hence not billed. Every member of the orthopaedic revenue stream (medical doctor, physician assistant, certified orthopaedic physician's assistant, registered nurse, and so on) needs to be involved in charge capture surveillance and monitoring.

Accurate coding and documentation can also reduce the number of insurance denials. ICD-9 codes must match CPT codes. Details of multiple procedures must also be described, including surgical site (same or separate), with appropriate modifiers appended. Expeditious processes to manage denials with appeals should be in place. Most can be successfully undertaken with a letter template. Management of denials can result in substantial revenue recovery, but it requires knowledgeable personnel designated with this responsibility.

Cost Containment

The Advisory Board Company reports that expenses

for medical implants and supplies are now the fastest growing line item. Annual price increases for existing technologies range from 5% to 20%, and new implants or minor implant variations can increase prices by 30% to 70%. Orthopaedic implant choices should be based on quality of patient outcome. However, recent studies have demonstrated shifts in practice to more expensive implants and procedures without proven clinical benefit.[53-57] Physicians should take a lead role in discussions around implant standardization and development of practice guidelines for new technologies. Resultant cost savings should be considered a joint effort of hospital management and physician leaders. Opportunities will arise for gainsharing, which can be ethically and legally acceptable.

Career Development and Practice Growth

The determination of a successful career in orthopaedic trauma surgery has to be distilled to a measurable metric. No other subspecialty of orthopaedic surgery demonstrates such a disparity between career initiation and career completion. Young surgeons in sports medicine, for example, will likely have a similar practice profile at retirement and inception, whereas the trauma surgeon will invariably undergo significant changes in the practice profile over time, and at retirement may have only a small percentage of the practice devoted to fracture or trauma care at all.

Although the cost of an ineffective retention/career development program or process has never been thoroughly tracked for a surgeon practicing trauma exclusively, healthcare experts and MGMA estimates suggest the cost of losing or replacing an orthopaedic trauma surgeon to be approximately $2.5 million (year 1) minus 200% of the value of the compensation package.[27] Beyond the monetary impact, there are employee morale and retention issues, disrupted work flow and patient throughput, damage to the reputation of the facility and its subsequent surgeons on call, and damage to future recruiting efforts (termed in the industry as additive "soft costs"), which are unaccounted for at present. With trauma surgery, the referral base that trauma creates may also be disrupted. This is estimated to be 150 to 200 elective nontrauma-related "word-of-mouth" facility referrals per year from a sustained trauma program. Fewer than 10% of surveyed facilities have identifiable trauma physician retention-career development initiatives. Fewer than 2% had any identifiable exit practices for process improvement and career development, and none used the exit process to effectively change recruiting methods.

Trauma remains a somewhat misunderstood career or service line for such diversified industries within the health care field. Spine, sports medicine, joint arthroplasty, and foot and ankle are service lines within hospitals, practices, and industry; yet trauma invariably has not been considered a career line, and therefore has been underinvested. It stands to reason that similarly trained surgeons performing or asked to perform with similar surgical output with similar patient expectations, outcomes, and efficiencies should have similar work environments and compensation models. Yet traumatology is inherently different from other orthopaedic specialties and should be defined as such. It also stands to reason from a sustainability factor that if a surgeon consistently performs at the 95th percentile for work and patient care parameters, and consistently is compensated at the 50th percentile, this is not fair and is not sustainable. Furthermore, compensation and call pay are selling points and provide great "curb appeal" but there is more than a dollar figure to a successful contract relationship and a subsequent career. Transparency within a practice will foster the development of future leaders. Transparency with regard to financial issues and information is paramount to physician satisfaction, retention, and career development processes. Creation of a career development agreement is critical from the outset—the process of creating value and tracking value must be explicitly spelled out. Clarity of purpose, accountability, communication, and constant mentoring are key factors for success. With the largest number of applicants for trauma fellowships in the history of orthopaedic traumatology, laying the foundation for rewarding long-term careers makes sense for all stakeholders, including patients, surgeons, and hospitals.

Annotated References

1. Mackenzie EJ, Rivara FP, Jurkovich GJ, et al: The National Study on Costs and Outcomes of Trauma. *J Trauma* 2007;63S:54-67.

   This multicenter study examines costs and outcomes of trauma care. Recommendations for practice and future research are given.

2. Newgard CD, McConnell KJ, Hedges JR, Mullins RJ: The benefit of higher level of care transfer of injured patients from nontertiary hospital emergency departments. *J Trauma* 2007;63(5):965-971.

   This retrospective cohort study demonstrates lower mortality with transfer to a trauma center. Level of evidence: III.

3. Sampalis JS, Denis R, Lavoie A, et al: Trauma care regionalization: A process-outcome evaluation. *J Trauma* 1999;46(4):565-579, discussion 579-581.

4. Abernathy JH III, McGwin G Jr, Acker JE III, Rue LW III: Impact of a voluntary trauma system on mortality, length of stay, and cost at a level I trauma center. *Am Surg* 2002;68(2):182-192.

5. Agency for Healthcare Research and Quality: Databases HC: Healthcare Cost and Utilization Project (HCUP). www.hcup-us.ahrq.gov/databases.jsp. (Accessed December 10, 2009.)

The HCUP databases are a free, online query system based on data from the HCUP. It provides access to health statistics and information on hospital inpatient and emergency department utilization.

6. The National Center for Statistics and Analysis: National Highway Traffic Safety Administration. http://www.nhtsa.dot.gov/portal/site/nhtsa/menuitem.a0bd5d5a23d09ec24ec86e10dba046a0. Accessed December 10, 2009.

The National Center for Statistics and Analysis, an office of the National Highway Traffic Safety Administration (NHTSA), is responsible for providing a wide range of analytical and statistical support to NHTSA and the highway safety community at large.

7. Sasser SM, Hunt RC, Sullivent EE, et al; National Expert Panel on Field Triage, Centers for Disease Control and Prevention (CDC): Guidelines for field triage of injured patients: Recommendations of the National Expert Panel on Field Triage. *MMWR Recomm Rep* 2009; 58(RR-1):1-35.

Risk of death for a severely injured patient is 25% lower at a level I center. However, transferring all trauma patients (including the less severely injured) may overburden a trauma center and decrease cost-effectiveness. Level of evidence: II.

8. Taheri PA, Butz DA, Greenfield LJ: Academic health systems management: The rationale behind capitated contracts. *Ann Surg* 2000;231(6):849-859.

9. Utter GH, Maier RV, Rivara FP, Mock CN, Jurkovich GJ, Nathens AB: Inclusive trauma systems: Do they improve triage or outcomes of the severely injured? *J Trauma* 2006;60(3):529-535.

An inclusive model of regionalized trauma care improves outcomes and efficiencies. Clear algorithms, communication, and accountability of providers and facilities underlie the functionality. Level of evidence: II.

10. American College of Surgeons: http://www.facs.org/. Accessed December 10, 2009.

The American College of Surgeons provides survey data and performs accreditation and verification of trauma centers.

11. FitzPatrick MK, Reilly PM, Laborde A, et al: Maintaining patient throughput on an evolving trauma/emergency surgery service. *J Trauma* 2006;60(3):481-486.

Better operational efficiency and shorter length of stay were seen with multidisciplinary trauma service management of all trauma admissions. Level of evidence: II.

12. Hoff WS, Schwab CW: Trauma system development in North America. *Clin Orthop* 2004;422:17-22.

Systems of trauma care should include all phases of care from prehospital through rehabilitation. Shared communication and resource allocation will optimize efficiency and costs. Such a system also meets needs of a mass casualty scenario. Level of evidence: V.

13. Orthopaedic Trauma Association: Available at: www.ota.org. Accessed December 10, 2009.

The Orthopaedic Trauma Association has many resources for orthopaedic trauma surgeons in practice. Minimum requirements for certification as an OTA trauma center (level I) are outlined.

14. Taheri PA, Maggio PM, Dougherty J, et al: Trauma center downstream revenue: The impact of incremental patients within a health system. *J Trauma* 2007;62(3):615-619.

Orthopaedic traumatology provides substantial downstream revenue for the hospital. Downstream facility and professional revenue related to an initial episode of trauma care accounted for 20% and 30%, respectively, of the total receipts related to the trauma episode. Level of evidence: III.

15. Vallier HA, Patterson BM: Economic impact of orthopaedic trauma care on hospitals and hospital systems. *Curr Ortho Prac* 2009;20:475-481.

Trauma care is very sustainable and profitable within regionalized systems that support volume-driven proficiency, productive specialist staffing models, an evidence-based approach to technology, and a high degree of physician-hospital integration. Level of evidence: V.

16. Ziran BH, Barrette-Grischow MK, Marucci K: Economic value of orthopaedic trauma: The (second to) bottom line. *J Orthop Trauma* 2008;22(4):227-233.

Resource allocation to develop an orthopaedic trauma service is described. Impact on the bottom line is realized, providing the reader with knowledge and leverage in negotiation. Level of evidence: III.

17. Accelero Health Partners. http://www.Accelerohealthpartners.com. Accessed December 10, 2009.

Accelero Partners (formerly Human Motion Institute) is a health care management company specializing in orthopaedic and cardiothoracic service line management.

18. Althausen PL, Coll D, Cvitash M, Herak A, O'Mara TJ, Bray TJ: Economic viability of a community-based level-II orthopaedic trauma system. *J Bone Joint Surg Am* 2009;91(1):227-235.

This article is the third in a series of in-depth analyses of the Northern Nevada Trauma System, describing the financial benefits derived from musculoskeletal injuries to the institution supporting a well-run program. Orthopaedic trauma at a busy level II center is profitable to the hospital. Physicians have a hybrid model of compensation: a private group with some hospital support. Practice management details are provided. Level of evidence: IV.

19. Archdeacon MT, Stern PJ: Level-I orthopaedic trauma care: A model for longevity. *J Bone Joint Surg Am* 2006; 88(10):2305-2309.

Elements of a successful working model for academic orthopaedic trauma are described, including recommended resources and commitments from the hospital, orthopaedic department, and providers. Level of evidence: V.

1: General Topics and New Technology

20. Bray TJ, Althausen PL, O'Mara TJ: Growth and development of the Northern Nevada Orthopaedic Trauma System from 1994 to 2008: An update. *J Bone Joint Surg Am* 2008;90(4):909-914.

    A hybrid model for level II trauma care is described, along with physician relationships with the trauma center.

21. Management ECG. http://www.ECG management.com. Accessed December 10, 2009.

    ECG Management has been an expert in physician-hospital alignment strategies.

22. Orthopaedic Trauma Practice Consultants, LLC, Available at http://webotccom/. Accessed December 10, 2009.

    Orthopaedic Trauma Practice Consultants, LLC is an orthopaedic trauma career consulting firm specializing in analysis of career opportunities for dedicated trauma surgeons.

23. Vallier HA, Patterson BM, Meehan CJ, Lombardo T: Orthopaedic traumatology: The hospital side of the ledger, defining the financial relationship between physicians and hospitals. *J Orthop Trauma* 2008;22(4):221-226.

    The experience of orthopaedic traumatologists in a hospital employee model is described. This article characterizes the relationship between physicians and the trauma center and provides leverage in negotiating compensation and resource allocation for trauma care. Level of evidence: III.

24. Wixted JJ, Reed M, Eskander MS, et al: The effect of an orthopedic trauma room on after-hours surgery at a level one trauma center. *J Orthop Trauma* 2008;22(4):234-236.

    An orthopaedic trauma room is cost-effective, improving quality of care and efficiency of care. Trauma care is more often delivered by traumatologists versus other orthopaedic surgeons, and there are fewer disruptions to scheduling. Level of evidence: III.

25. Mishra A, Urquhart AG, Anders GT: Selecting and starting an orthopaedic surgery practice. *Instr Course Lect* 2008;57:729-736.

    This article presents a comprehensive discussion about practice initiation options, including compensation and related legal concerns. Level of evidence: V.

26. American Medical Group Association: http://www.amga.org. Accessed December 10, 2009.

    The American Medical Group Association represents organized medical groups, providing resources for practice management and physician leadership to members and member organizations.

27. Medical Group Management Association: http://www.mgma.com. Accessed December 10, 2009.

    The Medical Group Management Association network is designed to enhance medical group practice performance. Tools for benchmarking, financial planning, practice management, and compensation databases are among available resources.

28. Sullivan, Cotter and Associates, Inc: http://www.sullivancotter. com. Accessed December 10, 2009.

    Sullivan Cotter is a consulting firm that specializes in nonprofit healthcare compensation evaluation and benchmarking.

29. Alderman AK, Storey AF, Chung KC: Financial impact of emergency hand trauma on the health care system. *J Am Coll Surg* 2008;206(2):233-238.

    A hand trauma service is profitable to providers and the facility, although highly sensitive to the amount of indigent care. Level of evidence: III.

30. Bazzoli GJ, Meersman PJ, Chan C: Factors that enhance continued trauma center participation in trauma systems. *J Trauma* 1996;41(5):876-885.

31. Gutweiler JR, Mooney DP: Pediatric trauma care: A profitable enterprise? *J Pediatr Surg* 2007;42(6):1043-1045.

    Pediatric trauma services can be profitable. Inadequate reimbursement from Medicaid and self-pay patients remains a problem, and will result in financial losses if this patient population exceeds 55% of the payer mix. Level of evidence: III.

32. Taheri PA, Butz DA, Greenfield LJ: Paying a premium: How patient complexity affects costs and profit margins. *Ann Surg* 1999;229(6):807-811.

33. Abaris Group: http://www.abarisgroup.com. Accessed December 10, 2009.

    The Abaris Group is a health care consulting firm specializing in emergency department and inpatient program patient flow and capacity building strategies.

34. Delphi HealthCare Partners. http://www.Delphihp.com. Accessed December 10, 2009.

    Delphi HealthCare Partners is a surgeon management firm that specializes in emergency department coverage solutions for facilities.

35. Lachiewicz PF, Dirschl DR, Soileau E: Orthopaedic faculty trauma call policies: A survey of accredited orthopaedic residency programs. *J Orthop Trauma* 2008;22(4):237-240.

    This survey of 106 programs defines trends in physician availability to take calls as well as resource allocation of hospitals for trauma care. Level of evidence: III.

36. McConnell KJ, Johnson LA, Arab N, Richards CF, Newgard CD, Edlund T: The on-call crisis: A statewide assessment of the costs of providing on-call specialist coverage. *Ann Emerg Med* 2007;49(6):727-733.

    Problems with on-call coverage in Oregon are negatively affecting delivery of patient care and hospital costs. Level of evidence: IV.

37. Menchine MD, Baraff LJ: On-call specialists and higher level of care transfers in California emergency departments. *Acad Emerg Med* 2008;15(4):329-336.

Availability of specialists on call has declined rapidly and is delaying patient care. Level of evidence: IV.

38. Fortune JB, Wohltmann C, Margold B, Callahan CD, Sutyak J: Maximizing reimbursement from trauma response fees (UB-92: 68X): Lessons learned from a hospital comparison. *J Trauma* 2005;58(3):482-486.

Effective billing and collection practices for trauma response fees generate substantial additional revenue for the trauma center, without further expense. Level of evidence: III.

39. Hemmila MR, Jakubus JL, Maggio PM, et al: Real money: Complications and hospital costs in trauma patients. *Surgery* 2008;144(2):307-316.

Despite higher costs, patients with complications generated a higher mean contribution margin per day than those patients with an uncomplicated course of care. Level of evidence: III.

40. Taheri PA, Butz DA, Watts CM, Griffes LC, Greenfield LJ: Trauma services: A profit center? *J Am Coll Surg* 1999;188(4):349-354.

41. American Academy of Orthopaedic Surgeons: Practice Management Center Overview. http://www3.aaos.org/member/prac_manag/prac_manage.cfm. Accessed December 10, 2009.

AAOS's practice management center provides a wide scope of pertinent information for various practice settings.

42. Press Ganey: Partners in improvement. http://www.pressganey.com. Accessed December 10, 2009.

Press Ganey is a consulting service on health care performance measurement and management.

43. Breedlove LL, Fallon WF Jr, Cullado M, Dalton A, Donthi R, Donovan DL: Dollars and sense: Attributing value to a level I trauma center in economic terms. *J Trauma* 2005;58(4):668-673, discussion 673-674.

Institutional investment in a level I trauma program contributed favorably to revenue. Details of the model and revenue specific to patients of varying acuity are given. Level of evidence: II.

44. Davis KA, Cabbad NC, Schuster KM, et al: Trauma team oversight improves efficiency of care and augments clinical and economic outcomes. *J Trauma* 2008;65(6):1236-1242.

Trauma team oversight of patient care produces operational efficiency and increased revenue. Shorter hospital stays and lower costs per discharge were seen despite increased patient volumes. The model also describes improvement of documentation and coding practices. Level of evidence: III.

45. Pendleton AM, Cannada LK, Guerrero-Bejarano M: Factors affecting length of stay after isolated femoral shaft fractures. *J Trauma* 2007;62(3):697-700.

Factors the hospital and providers can control to reduce length of stay after femur fracture include time to surgery, time for physical therapy, and radiology delays. Length-of-stay reduction will decrease hospital costs. Level of evidence: IV.

46. Taheri PA, Butz DA, Greenfield LJ: Length of stay has minimal impact on the cost of hospital admission. *J Am Coll Surg* 2000;191(2):123-130.

47. Thomas SN, McGwin G Jr, Rue LW III: The financial impact of delayed discharge at a level I trauma center. *J Trauma* 2005;58(1):121-125.

Increased hospital costs are incurred with delayed discharge. Barriers to discharge occur most often with governmental payers. Level of evidence: III.

48. Bhattacharyya T, Vrahas MS, Morrison SM, et al: The value of the dedicated orthopaedic trauma operating room. *J Trauma* 2006;60(6):1336-1340, discussion 1340-1341.

Surgery done during daytime hours in an orthopaedic trauma room takes fewer minutes and has fewer complications. Level of evidence: III.

49. Kirschenbaum IH, Mabrey JD, Wood GW II, et al: The electronic medical office: Optimizing solutions. *Instr Course Lect* 2008;57:737-745.

This article outlines considerations around implementation of EMR and digital imaging systems. Level of evidence: V.

50. Office of Inspector General: http://www.oig.hhs.gov. Accessed December 10, 2009.

The US office of the Inspector General in May 2009 rendered an advisory opinion on on-call compensation in specific circumstances.

51. American Academy of Orthopaedic Surgeons: http://www.aaos.org. Accessed December 10, 2009.

Educational resources may be purchased. Information on symposia and presentations for practice management, coding/billing, and related issues is available.

52. Barnes SL, Robinson BR, Richards JT, et al: The devil is in the details: Maximizing revenue for daily trauma care. *Surgery* 2008;144(4):670-675.

Standardized documentation for subsequent hospital care has a substantial impact on revenue. Level of evidence: III.

53. The Advisory Board Company: www.advisoryboardcompany.com. Accessed December 10, 2009.

The Advisory Board provides information for practice management and supply chain organization. Physician enfranchisement in supply chain management is encouraged.

54. Anglen JO, Weinstein JN, American Board of Orthopaedic Surgery Research Committee: Nail or plate fixation of intertrochanteric hip fractures: Changing pattern of practice. A review of the American Board of Ortho-

paedic Surgery Database. *J Bone Joint Surg Am* 2008; 90(4):700-707.

Intramedullary hip screw fixation for intertrochanteric femur fractures increased from 3% in 1999 to 67% in 2006 without supporting clinical evidence.

55. Bozic KJ, Jacobs JJ: Technology assessment and adoption in orthopaedics: Lessons learned. *J Bone Joint Surg Am* 2008;90(4):689-690.

Adoption of new technology is a major contributor to healthcare expenses. Better research is needed to help make decisions. Current decision making is influenced by local norms, vendor relationships, direct-to-consumer advertising, and financial incentives. Level of evidence: V.

56. Forte ML, Virnig BA, Kane RL, et al: Geographic variation in device use for intertrochanteric hip fractures. *J Bone Joint Surg Am* 2008;90(4):691-699.

Geographic variation in usage of an intramedullary hip screw compared with a dynamic hip screw is substantial and is unrelated to patient factors. The use of intramedullary hip screws is increasing.

57. Koval KJ, Harrast JJ, Anglen JO, Weinstein JN: Fractures of the distal part of the radius: The evolution of practice over time. Where's the evidence? *J Bone Joint Surg Am* 2008;90(9):1855-1861.

The number of distal radius fractures treated with open reduction and internal fixation versus percutaneous fixation increased from 42% in 1999 to 81% in 2007 despite a lack of improvement in surgeon-perceived functional outcomes. Level of evidence: III.

Chapter 4
Computer-Assisted Surgery

David B. Carmack, MD   David Kahler, MD   Amir Matityahu, MD   Brock T. Wentz, MD

Introduction

Computer-assisted orthopaedic surgery (CAOS) is a developing field using the technologies of fluoroscopy and/or CT, computers, and remote sensing (infrared optical versus electromagnetic signals).[1] It has been in use in orthopaedic surgery since the early 1990s.

Current clinical applications include pelvic and spinal fixation and instrumentation, knee and hip joint arthroplasty, orthopaedic oncologic reconstruction, osteotomy planning/execution, minimally invasive plate placement, insertion of artificial spinal disk replacement, intra-articular knee cruciate ligament bone tunnel placement, knee arthrodesis, minimally invasive hardware removal, diaphyseal fracture treatment, and potentially many other applications.

In general, computer-assisted navigation makes use of stored images, obtained either by preoperative CT or intraoperative C-arm, to assist in the precise insertion of implants, rather than by real-time fluoroscopy. Navigation systems track the positions of surgical tools in relation to the patient's coordinate systems within the field of view of the navigation system. Medical imaging enables less invasive surgery, whereas the position of surgical instruments is monitored on screen. The greatest advance for orthopaedic trauma came in 1999, when fluoroscopic navigation became available; this technology allowed intraoperative storage of C-arm images and real-time navigation, without the use of continuous imaging during implant insertion.[2]

Benefits of CAOS include the ability to decrease radiation exposure to the patient and the surgical team

Dr. Carmack or an immediate family member is a member of a speakers' bureau or has made paid presentations on behalf of AO North America. Dr. Kahler or an immediate family member serves as an unpaid consultant for Brainlab AOTK Computer-assisted Surgery Expert Group. Dr. Matityahu or an immediate family member has received royalties from Synthes; is a member of a speakers' bureau or has made paid presentations on behalf of AO, DePuy, and Synthes; serves as a paid consultant for or is an employee of DePuy; has received research or institutional support from AO, Synthes, Stryker, Zimmer, Medtronic, Smith & Nephew, DePuy, OREF, OTA, and Philips; and owns stock or stock options in Anthem Orthopaedics. Neither Dr. Wentz nor an immediate family has received anything of value from or owns stock in a commercial company or institution related directly or indirectly to the subject of this chapter.

while improving overall surgical accuracy. Specific areas that have benefited from intraoperative use of CAOS are osteotomy planning and execution, comminuted diaphyseal fracture reduction, hardware placement in narrow bony corridors such as the pelvis and spine, and the removal of deep implants (screws) with minimal soft-tissue dissection.

Computer-Assisted Surgery Systems

In the most commonly used systems, an optical tracking system detects static sensors affixed to the patient's skeleton, the reference C-arm, and selected surgical instruments. This infrared sensing system is able to detect the position of trackers with reflectors or light-emitting diodes within the field of view of the tracking camera.

Data can be acquired in three different ways, using fluoroscopic, CT/MRI-guided, or imageless systems. These data points are then used for registration and tracking, as described below. Image-guided systems are somewhat self-explanatory. The imageless systems rely on other information such as centers of rotation of the hip, knee, or ankle, or visual information such as anatomic landmarks.

Registration refers to the necessary process of relating images of anatomic features using radiographs, CT, MRI, or the patient's three-dimensional anatomy to their anatomic position within the surgical field. Early techniques for registration required the placement of pins or "fiducial markers" in the target bone, which necessitated an additional surgical procedure. A surface-matching technique has been used in which the shape of the bone surface is determined using a computer model generated from preoperative images that is matched to surface data points collected during surgery. The most modern techniques using fluoroscopic navigation are self-registering, and require little additional surgical time.

Tracking refers to the sensors and measurement devices that can provide real-time feedback during surgery regarding the orientation and relative position of tools to bone anatomy. For example, optical or electromagnetic trackers can be attached to regular surgical tools, which in turn can provide real-time information of the position and orientation of the tools' alignment with respect to the bony anatomy of interest (**Figure 1**).

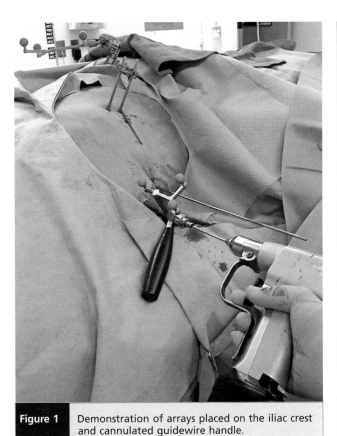

Figure 1 Demonstration of arrays placed on the iliac crest and cannulated guidewire handle.

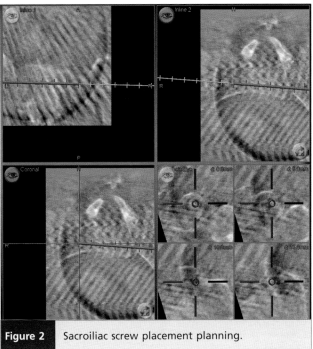

Figure 2 Sacroiliac screw placement planning.

Specific Applications of Image-Guided Orthopaedic Surgery

Iliosacral Screws

The first report of iliosacral screw technique was published in 1978.[2] Other authors performed an open reduction with internal fixation crossing the sacroiliac (SI) joint with a 6% to 25% incidence of wound complications.[3] Several authors demonstrated that placing SI screws into the S1 body is possible with the utilization of fluoroscopic techniques.[4] Several authors have subsequently proposed percutaneous techniques under fluoroscopic[5-7] and CT scan guidance[8,9] and have described the bony corridor that must be traversed to avoid neurologic and vascular complications.

Image-guided navigation systems have been developed in an effort to improve safety, accuracy, and efficiency of many types of surgeries. These systems display patient-specific radiographic data and images while providing real-time feedback regarding the path of surgical instrumentation and implants. The treatment goals for most mechanically unstable injuries of the pelvis include reduction and stable fixation of the pelvic ring. Percutaneous fixation of pelvic fractures with iliosacral screws provides excellent fixation strength in an injured pelvis and reduces the incidence of wound breakdown, infection, and blood loss. However, percutaneous insertion of iliosacral screws using standard multiplanar fluoroscopy can be technically demanding. Safe insertion of screws into the sacrum from the ilium is dependent on adequate fluoroscopic imaging and understanding the anatomic structures that can be seen.

As little as 4° of malposition of SI screws can result in a complication. Screw malposition rates of 13% and neurologic complication rates of 8% have been reported.[10,11] When the sacrum is dysmorphic or has a narrow vestibule for insertion of iliosacral screws, there is an increased risk of malposition and nerve root impingement. Despite an increase in setup time of approximately 10 minutes, computer-aided surgical navigation is a possible solution for SI screw malposition and has been shown to lead to a fourfold decrease in the potential radiation exposure to the patient and surgical team.[12] The diameter, length, and trajectory of iliosacral screws can be planned before insertion. Execution of the preoperative plan is then performed with intraoperative guidance technology. During insertion of SI screws, tools are moved in a preconstructed virtual space without the need for real-time fluoroscopy. Because multiple fluoroscopic views are seen on the computer screen simultaneously, the radiology technician and surgeon do not need to repeatedly adjust the C-arm from one position to another. Consequently, there is an increase in efficiency and decrease in radiation exposure. It has been shown that navigation actually decreases the total surgical time for insertion of iliosacral screws, despite the additional time required for attachment of a tracker at the start of the procedure.[13]

When using fluoroscopic image guidance, the surgeon first reduces the pelvic ring using closed or open

1: General Topics and New Technology

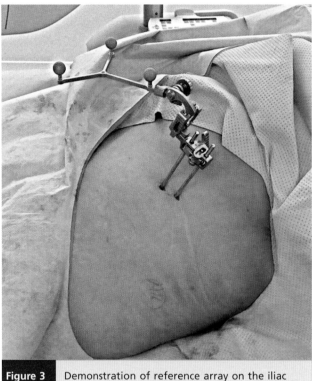

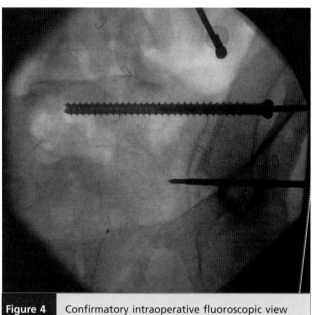

Figure 4 Confirmatory intraoperative fluoroscopic view showing guidewire placement.

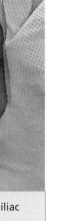

Figure 3 Demonstration of reference array on the iliac crest.

methods, and confirms an adequate reduction with C-arm imagery. Fluoroscopic AP, inlet, outlet, and oblique views can be imaged and stored within the computer workstation (**Figure 2**). The trajectory feature is then used to help identify the optimal starting position on the skin, with the tip of the screw within the center of the S1 or S2 body. The guidewire is inserted to the appropriate depth using the length feature of the software package. Confirmatory images are then obtained to verify that the guidewire has not deflected. The cannulated screw is then placed over the guidewire.

Utilization of intraoperative fluoroscopic-based CT scan (isocentric C-arm) enhances the surgeon's ability to see a virtual slice of the corridor of bone the screws must traverse. This is especially useful in patients who have a dysplastic sacrum. The surgeon first reduces the pelvic ring using closed or open methods, and confirms an adequate reduction with C-arm imaging or intraoperative CT scanning. The CT reconstruction in three different planes is observed, relative to the position of the drill guide. In addition, an extended target view is projected on the screen. The trajectory feature is then used to help identify the optimal starting position on the skin, with the ideal trajectory to the center of the S1 or S2 body. The guidewire is inserted to the appropriate depth using the length feature of the software package. In a study of the placement of 50 consecutive SI screws, no significant deflections of the guidewire were found, and there were no complications or significant screw malpositions using fluoroscopic navigation techniques.[13]

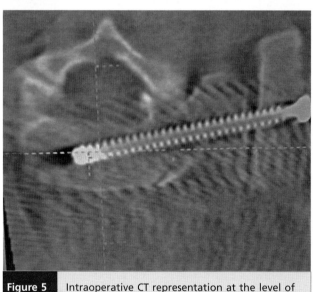

Figure 5 Intraoperative CT representation at the level of the S1 body in the transverse plane.

In a patient with a sacral fracture and dysplasia of the sacrum necessitating placement of S1 and S2 screws, CT-aided pelvis fixation is used to visualize, plan, and direct the screw into small corridors of bone with a trajectory that is from posterior-lateral to anterior-medial. In **Figure 3**, the reflector arrays are placed onto the iliac crest.

Next, CT imaging of the affected area is acquired. The trajectory and screw length are then planned. The guidewires are then placed into the preplanned S1 and S2 bodies (**Figure 4**). Verification images are acquired to assess guidewire deflection and screws are placed (**Figure 4**). In this instance, verification of screw placement was performed intraoperatively using CT scan to

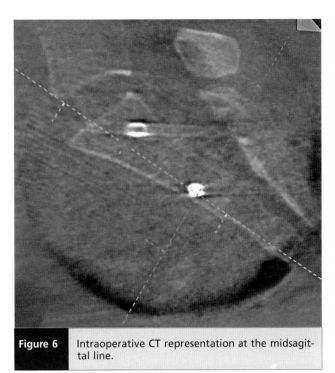

Figure 6 Intraoperative CT representation at the midsagittal line.

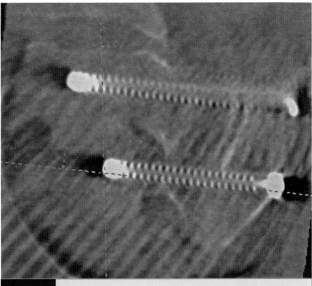

Figure 7 Intraoperative CT representation in the coronal plane.

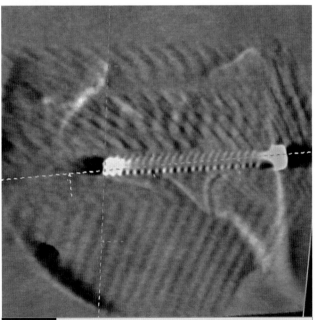

Figure 8 Intraoperative CT representation at the level of the S2 body in the transverse plane.

assess screw position within the S1 and S2 body (Figures 5 through 8).

Pelvic Ring Disruptions

Stabilization of traumatic disruptions of the pelvic ring anterior to the SI joints also can be done using CAOS. Specific applications include the placement of cannulated screws across fractures of the ilium and pubic rami, and the placement of external fixator half pins into the iliac wing and supra-acetabular areas.

It is important to note the strengths and shortfalls of using CAOS to assist in the placement of screws and half-pins during stabilization procedures on pelvic ring disruptions anterior to the SI joints. One strength is the ability to develop the correct trajectory of the guidewire or half-pin in multiple planes simultaneously with first-pass accuracy. An additional strength is the live interactive integrated imaging, surgical instruments, and reference fluoroscopic views that provide the ability to limit dissection required for initiation of bony contact during insertion of the guidewire or half-pin, or during the use of surgical cannulated instruments.

A shortfall is the challenge of visualizing fracture reduction maneuvers of the disrupted pelvic ring in real time on the CAOS-generated images. Integrated software workflows that will allow both fracture reduction and implant placement are in development, and have been successfully used as prototypes (**Figure 9**). Although these techniques are evolving, the use of stored images potentially enables the surgeon to see both fracture reduction and the anatomic pathways that the guidewire or half-pin will be traversing in multiple planes. In essence, CAOS provides an additional benefit

to those surgeons who are already comfortable with percutaneous pelvic fracture management. Any surgeon using these less invasive techniques should be familiar with the corresponding open procedures and approaches, in the event that conversion to a formal open procedure is necessary.

Acetabular Fractures

Open reduction and internal fixation is the standard treatment of unstable fractures of the acetabulum. Recently, percutaneous screw fixation has been de-

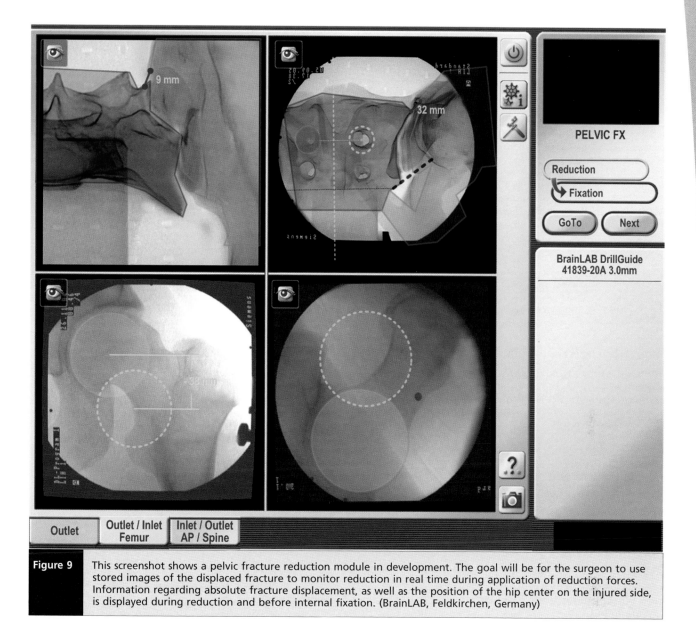

Figure 9 This screenshot shows a pelvic fracture reduction module in development. The goal will be for the surgeon to use stored images of the displaced fracture to monitor reduction in real time during application of reduction forces. Information regarding absolute fracture displacement, as well as the position of the hip center on the injured side, is displayed during reduction and before internal fixation. (BrainLAB, Feldkirchen, Germany)

scribed as an alternative for both acute fractures and nonunions.[14-19] Using this technique, screws are introduced into the anterior and posterior columns of the acetabulum through small incisions, limiting dissection and soft-tissue stripping. Safe corridors for placement of these screws has been studied in the literature.[20] The mean largest diameter corridor of the anterior column screw was 6.4 mm (range, 5 to 7.3 mm), and that of the posterior column was 11.4 mm (range, 9.4 to 13.3 mm). Supra-acetabular screws (**Figure 10, A**) placed from the anterosuperior iliac spine to the posterosuperior iliac spine had a mean largest diameter virtual corridor of 12.1 mm (range, 10.5 to 13.3 mm).[20]

Anterior column screws (**Figure 10, B**) can be placed in either an antegrade (cephalad to caudad) or retrograde (caudad to cephalad) fashion after reduction is achieved. Antegrade insertion is used when the patient is in the supine or lateral position, whereas retrograde insertion requires supine positioning. The fluoroscopic views needed for safe insertion of an anterior column screw include an iliac-inlet oblique view to avoid guidewire penetration of the inner cortex of the superior ramus and an obturator-outlet oblique view to avoid guidewire penetration of the hip joint.[9]

Posterior column screws are placed in either an antegrade or retrograde fashion after reduction is achieved. The fluoroscopic views needed in the supine position for safe posterior column screw insertion include an obturator-outlet oblique view to avoid medial or lateral guidewire penetration and iliac-inlet oblique views to avoid the greater sciatic notch or hip joint breach.

The safe placement of screws without penetration of the hip joint has been well documented both for the complex acetabular fractures and posterior wall frac-

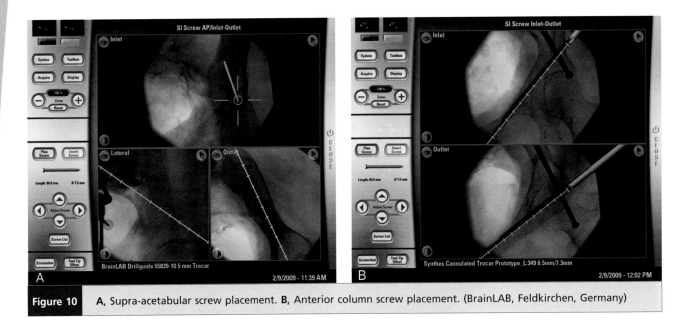

Figure 10 **A,** Supra-acetabular screw placement. **B,** Anterior column screw placement. (BrainLAB, Feldkirchen, Germany)

tures.[21] The insertion of column screws, either percutaneous or open, requires less than 5° of variation to stay within the bony corridors of the pelvis. Unlike SI screws, there are no studies at this time that compare column screws placed via CAOS and two-dimensional fluoroscopy. However, there is a potential for increased precision in column screw placement with fluoroscopic- and CT-guided navigation systems. In a 2004 study, the authors showed that the posterior column screws, retrograde ramus anterior column screws, and supra-acetabular screws inserted via fluoroscopic navigation techniques deviated less than 2 mm and less than 5° from the planned location of these screws.[22] Therefore, navigation may be a viable option for placing acetabular column screws. Experience has shown that navigation has aided in teaching and understanding the correct placement of acetabular column screws. Further, navigation minimizes the need to continually adjust the fluoroscopy machine from one integrated complex view to another. Therefore, in the future, if the current limitations are overcome, the use of navigation systems will increase and allow the surgeon to more precisely and efficiently treat acetabular fractures.

Spine Surgery

The utilization of computer-assisted navigation spine surgery has increased to address the complications associated with pedicle screw placement. Both open and percutaneous placement of pedicle screws can be fraught with complications, such as pedicle wall penetration and neurologic injury. In the thoracic spine, where the pedicles are smaller than in the lumbar spine, pedicle screws are even more likely to be placed in an errant position. Therefore, there is impetus to decrease complications and increase the accuracy of pedicle screw placement. Both CT and fluoroscopy-based navigation systems are available to choose from. Several

studies show that computer-aided navigation increases the accuracy of pedicle screw placement while reducing surgical time and radiation exposure during screw insertion.[23,24] Computer-based navigation has also been shown to decrease fluoroscopy time during screw fixation of an odontoid fracture.[25]

Intramedullary Nailing

Advances in CAOS systems have enabled surgeons to enhance their intramedullary nailing techniques. Navigation can assist the surgeon in choosing the precise starting point for skin incision and nail insertion into the proximal or distal femur, using only a few stored images.

There are three other areas in which CAOS can potentially improve surgical techniques and patient outcomes. The first is the ability to simultaneously visualize both the AP and lateral images of the diaphyseal proximal and distal fracture components during the passing of a guidewire across the fracture. The second is the ability to accurately restore the diaphyseal length and rotation to match the uninjured reference side, if desired. This cannot be easily done during fixation of comminuted fractures using standard techniques; the surgeon who chooses to use navigation can leave the operating room with confidence that the normal anatomy has been restored (**Figures 11 and 12**). The third is the ability to accurately place freehand locking screws either proximally or distally, while visualizing simultaneous AP and lateral images without additional C-arm imaging and radiation exposure.[26]

Fracture Reduction

Computer-assisted orthopaedic surgery can aid the surgeon in reducing two large fracture fragments, such as during diaphyseal fracture nailing. The greatest possible benefit would be the ability to restore the length,

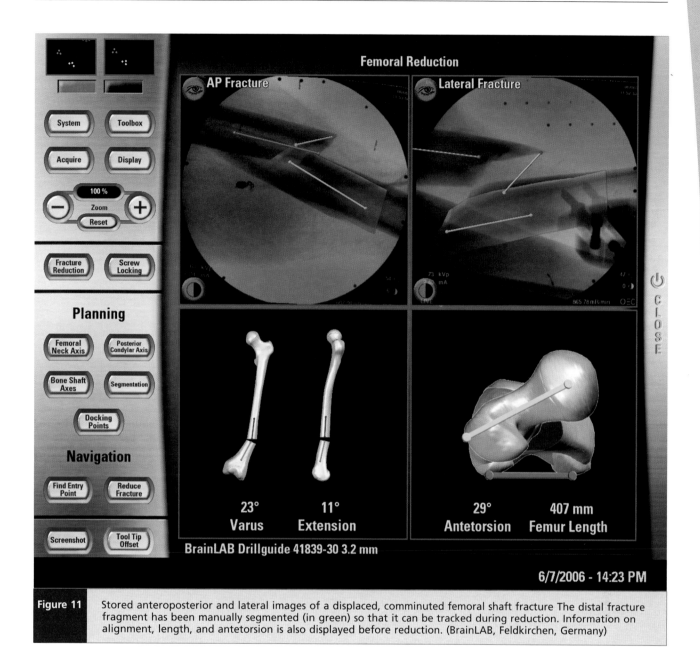

1: General Topics and New Technology

Figure 11 Stored anteroposterior and lateral images of a displaced, comminuted femoral shaft fracture The distal fracture fragment has been manually segmented (in green) so that it can be tracked during reduction. Information on alignment, length, and antetorsion is also displayed before reduction. (BrainLAB, Feldkirchen, Germany)

alignment, and rotation of the fractured diaphysis using the contralateral uninjured limb as a control.

The technology has advanced in the past decade and continues to make progress. Ideally, the work flow of the CAOS program will ultimately increase the speed of the overall procedure, expose the patient and the surgical team to less radiation, and decrease the need for any re-operations resulting from initial fracture malalignment.

Reduction of Radiation Exposure to Patients and Surgeons

Fluoroscopy and radiation exposure are integral aspects of surgical management of fractures. Radiation exposure limits from the International Commission on Radiological Protection are 5 rem/year for a maximal

annual exposure with a 5-year average of 2 rem/year.[26] It has been shown that chronic small increases in altitudinal ionizing radiation dose as seen in airplane pilots has a fivefold increase in hematopoietic malignancies and a threefold increase in skin cancers when compared to the baseline population.[27,28] Further, one study demonstrated that a single CT scan for abdominal trauma and a cervical spine clearance can raise the lifetime cancer risk from 1:8700 to 1:1000.[29] Ionizing radiation exposure is an underappreciated risk for orthopaedic trauma surgeons and trauma patients.

One minute of fluoroscopy exposure is equivalent to 40 mSv (4 rads). Radiation exposure was studied in a population of Italian orthopedists at a small community hospital with poor radiation safety practices. The authors showed that orthopaedic surgeons were five times more likely to develop cancer than other hospital

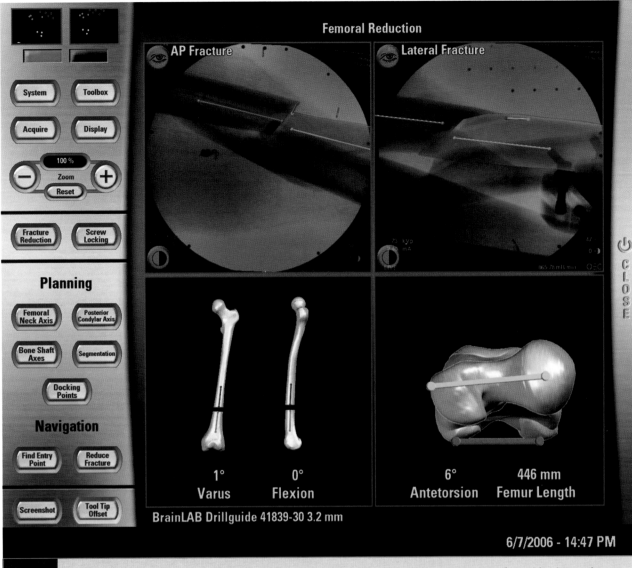

Figure 12 The display shows a virtual image of the reduced fracture following traction, insertion of a guidewire, and correction of rotation. The femoral length and antetorsion now match the contralateral side. (Reproduced with permission from Kahler DM: Navigated long-bone fracture reduction. *J Bone Joint Surg* 2009:91:102-107.) (BrainLAB, Feldkirchen, Germany)

employees who used radiographs.[30] It is obvious that all medical radiation exposure should be kept to a minimum level using the ALARA (as low as reasonably achievable) principle. Therefore, any technology that decreases radiation exposure should be welcomed and encouraged.

In a cadaver study, placement of iliosacral screws with standard fluoroscopic techniques required an average of 26 seconds of fluoroscopy time whereas computer-assisted surgery used 6 seconds of fluoroscopy.[31] This was also shown in other studies where fluoroscopy times were reduced more than fourfold when using computer-assisted surgery compared to standard fluoroscopy for placing pedicle screws and percutaneous acetabular screws.[32] The possible advantage of decreased radiation exposure with the use of computer-assisted navigation techniques may justify the increased

cost and utilization of this technology in the future.

Summary

Computer-assisted musculoskeletal surgical navigational systems allow surgeons to perform complex, traditionally invasive trauma surgeries, such as femoral and pelvic fracture fixation, through small incisions. They help the surgeon to understand the internal anatomy of the pelvis and long bones. Using this navigational technology, surgeons may be able to reduce the amount of time a patient is in surgery, limit radiation exposure, and decrease blood loss and rehabilitation time while increasing surgical accuracy. New work flows that combine both fracture reduction and fixation may soon find favor. Surgical time and radiation exposure when using computer-assisted navigation has shown benefits for specific procedures, but there is little current objective research that corroborates claims of decreased radiation, increased accuracy, increased intraoperative efficiency, and decreased surgical time during routine orthopaedic trauma care. The interface between the user and computer has been continually updated and is becoming more intuitive. However, continued development is needed to increase work flow efficiency and decrease the cost of computer-assisted navigation systems for orthopaedic trauma applications.

Annotated References

1. Ricci WM, Russell TA, Kahler DM, Terrill-Grisoni L, Culley P: A comparison of optical and electromagnetic computer-assisted navigation systems for fluoroscopic targeting. *J Orthop Trauma* 2008;22(3):190-194.

   The authors compared two fluoroscopic navigation tracking technologies, optical and electromagnetic, versus standard freehand fluoroscopic targeting. The optical and electromagnetic systems exhibited improved accuracy and were associated with reduced radiation use.

2. Letournel E: Pelvic fractures. *Injury* 1978;10(2):145-148.

3. Shuler TE, Boone DC, Gruen GS, Peitzman AB: Percutaneous iliosacral screw fixation: Early treatment for unstable posterior pelvic ring disruptions. *J Trauma* 1995;38(3):453-458.

4. Kahler DM: Image guidance: Fluoroscopic navigation. *Clin Orthop Relat Res* 2004;421:70-76.

   This article discusses advantages of fluoroscopic navigation and its use in the treatment of orthopaedic trauma. This technique is often associated with decreased duration of surgery and intraoperative radiation exposure.

5. Matta JM, Tornetta P III: Internal fixation of unstable pelvic ring injuries. *Clin Orthop Relat Res* 1996;329:129-140.

6. Simonian PT, Routt C Jr, Harrington RM, Tencer AF: Internal fixation for the transforaminal sacral fracture. *Clin Orthop Relat Res* 1996;323:202-209.

7. Routt ML Jr, Kregor PJ, Simonian PT, Mayo KA: Early results of percutaneous iliosacral screws placed with the patient in the supine position. *J Orthop Trauma* 1995;9(3):207-214.

8. Remiger A, Engelhardt P: Percutaneous iliosacral screw fixation of vertical unstable pelvic ring fractures. *Swiss Surg* 1996;2(6):259-263.

9. Starr AJ, Reinert CM, Jones AL: Percutaneous fixation of the columns of the acetabulum: A new technique. *J Orthop Trauma* 1998;12(1):51-58.

10. Moed BR, Ahmad BK, Craig JG, Jacobson GP, Anders MJ: Intraoperative monitoring with stimulus-evoked electromyography during placement of iliosacral screws: An initial clinical study. *J Bone Joint Surg Am* 1998; 80(4):537-546.

11. Templeman D, Schmidt A, Freese J, Weisman I: Proximity of iliosacral screws to neurovascular structures after internal fixation. *Clin Orthop Relat Res* 1996;329:194-198.

12. Zwingmann J, Konrad G, Kotter E, Südkamp NP, Oberst M: Computer-navigated iliosacral screw insertion reduces malposition rate and radiation exposure. *Clin Orthop Relat Res* 2009;467:1833-1838.

    The authors studied whether radiation exposure was reduced and screw position improved in patients with percutaneous iliosacral screw insertion using computer navigation compared with those in whom conventional fluoroscopic screw placement was used. Malposition rate and radiation exposure were reduced in patients in whom computer navigation was used. Level of evidence: II.

13. Kahler DM: Computer-assisted fixation of acetabular fractures and pelvic ring disruptions. *Tech Orthop* 2000;10:20-24.

14. Brown GA, Willis MC, Firoozbakhsh K, Barmada A, Tessman CL, Montgomery A: Computed tomography image-guided surgery in complex acetabular fractures. *Clin Orthop Relat Res* 2000;370:219-226.

15. Gay SB, Sistrom C, Wang GJ, et al: Percutaneous screw fixation of acetabular fractures with CT guidance: Preliminary results of a new technique. *AJR Am J Roentgenol* 1992;158(4):819-822.

16. Parker PJ, Copeland C: Percutaneous fluoroscopic screw fixation of acetabular fractures. *Injury* 1997; 28(9-10):597-600.

17. Routt ML Jr, Simonian PT, Grujic L: The retrograde medullary superior pubic ramus screw for the treatment of anterior pelvic ring disruptions: A new technique. *J Orthop Trauma* 1995;9(1):35-44.

18. Routt ML Jr, Nork SE, Mills WJ: Percutaneous fixation of pelvic ring disruptions. *Clin Orthop Relat Res* 2000; 375:15-29.

19. Simonian PT, Routt ML Jr, Harrington RM, Tencer AF: Internal fixation of the unstable anterior pelvic ring: A biomechanical comparison of standard plating techniques and the retrograde medullary superior pubic ramus screw. *J Orthop Trauma* 1994;8(6):476-482.

20. Attias N, Lindsey RW, Starr AJ, Borer D, Bridges K, Hipp JA: The use of a virtual three-dimensional model to evaluate the intraosseous space available for percutaneous screw fixation of acetabular fractures. *J Bone Joint Surg Br* 2005;87(11):1520-1523.

    Virtual three-dimensional models were created using CT

scans from patients with acetabular fractures, and virtual cylindrical implants were placed intraosseously into the acetabulum. Cross-sectional diameters of the anterior and posterior columns were measured and compared with the maximum diameter of the virtual implant. Study results indicate that the size of the screw used for percutaneous fixation of these fractures should not depend on measurement of cross-sectional diameter. Virtual three-dimensional reconstructions may prove helpful in preoperative assessment.

21. Baumgaertner MR: Fractures of the posterior wall of the acetabulum. *J Am Acad Orthop Surg* 1999;7(1): 54-65.

22. Mosheiff R, Khoury A, Weil Y, Liebergall M: First generation computerized fluoroscopic navigation in percutaneous pelvic surgery. *J Orthop Trauma* 2004;18:106-111.

    Computerized fluoroscopic navigation was used in the percutaneous insertion of 45 cannulated screws in 25 patients. This method is believed to save fluoroscopic radiation time and improve the precision of screw placement.

23. Kim CW, Lee YP, Taylor W, Oygar A, Kim WK: Use of navigation-assisted fluoroscopy to decrease radiation exposure during minimally invasive spine surgery. *Spine J* 2008;8(4):584-590.

    The authors assessed the feasibility and safety of navigation-assisted fluoroscopy during minimally invasive spine surgery in a combined cadaver and human study. Results indicated that patient and surgical team exposure to radiation was decreased.

24. Rajasekaran S, Vidyadhara S, Ramesh P, Shetty AP: Randomized clinical study to compare the accuracy of navigated and non-navigated thoracic pedicle screws in deformity correction surgeries. *Spine* 2007;32(2):E56-E64.

    The accuracy of nonnavigation and Iso-C-based navigation was compared in pedicle screw fixation in thoracic spine deformities in a randomized clinical trial. Level of evidence: I.

25. Battaglia TC, Tannoury T, Crowl AC, Chan DP, Anderson DG: A cadaveric study comparing standard fluoroscopy with fluoroscopy-based computer navigation for screw fixation of the odontoid. *J Surg Orthop Adv* 2005;14(4):175-180.

    The authors compared radiation exposure, surgical time, and accuracy of hardware placement using fluoroscopy versus computer-assisted fluoroscopy-based navigation in two cadaver groups in whom odontoid screws were placed. It was concluded that fluoroscopy-based virtual navigation was as safe as standard fluoroscopy and facilitated a reduction in radiation exposure.

26. Kahler DM: Navigated long-bone fracture reduction. *J Bone Joint Surg Am* 2009;91(suppl 1):102-107.

    This article discusses recent developments in computer-assisted surgery, including the ability to precisely match the anatomy of the injured extremity to that of the contralateral limb with respect to rotational alignment and length.

27. Jayasekera N, Roach R: Exposure to direct and scatter radiation with use of mini-C-arm fluoroscopy. *J Bone Joint Surg Am* 2007;89:2552.

    Routine use of mini-C-arm fluoroscopy is associated with minimal radiation exposure, except in the direct path of the radiation beam.

28. Gundestrup M, Storm HH: Radiation-induced acute myeloid leukaemia and other cancers in commercial jet cockpit crew: A population-based cohort study. *Lancet* 1999;354(9195):2029-2031.

29. Richards PJ, Summerfield R, George J, Hamid A, Oakley P: Major trauma and cervical clearance radiation doses and cancer induction. *Injury* 2008;39:347-356.

    The radiation dose of cervical spine clearance and body CT was compared for three different protocols in a cohort of unconscious patients who had experienced major trauma.

30. Mastrangelo G, Fedeli U, Fadda E: Increased cancer risk among surgeons in an orthopaedic hospital. *Occup Med* 2005;55:498-500.

    One hundred fifty-eight hospital workers were studied to determine whether routine radiation dosimetric assessment led to an increased cancer risk. Results indicated that the potential risk of radiation should not be underestimated and safe work practices should be promoted by health care institutions.

31. Collinge C, Coons D, Tornetta P, Aschenbrenner J: Standard multiplanar fluoroscopy versus a fluoroscopically based navigation system for the percutaneous insertion of iliosacral screws: A cadaver model. *J Orthop Trauma* 2005;19(4):254-258.

    The safety and efficiency of standard multiplanar fluoroscopy and virtual fluoroscopy for percutaneous insertion of iliosacral screws were compared. Most screws were safely inserted using both methods.

32. Crowl AC, Kahler DM: Closed reduction and percutaneous fixation of anterior column acetabular fractures. *Comput Aided Surg* 2002;7(3):169-178.

Chapter 5

Minimally Invasive Fracture Care

Clifford B. Jones, MD, FACS   Reto H. Babst, MD   Marc J. Anders, MD

1: General Topics and New Technology

Introduction: Priority-Driven Evolution of Fracture Care

The desire to minimize further injury to the already-traumatized patient has been present throughout the history of orthopaedic trauma care. Minimal access surgery or minimally invasive surgery (MIS) for fracture fixation was first introduced with the external fixator in the 19th century, followed by the development of intramedullary nailing in the 20th century. The cosmetically appealing small incisions were not the sole factor prompting the rapid progression of these minimally invasive techniques, but more important, it was the biologic advantages such as undisturbed fracture healing, less soft-tissue disruption, and fewer infectious complications. This chapter focuses on fracture stabilization techniques using small approaches and more important, minimal interference with the fracture healing process.

The observation of similarities in the pattern of fracture healing between an intramedullary nail and a plate applied by an indirect reduction technique supported the concept of biologic plating. The approach of bridging the fracture zone without disturbing the soft-tissue envelope led to undisturbed bone healing with callus formation, in contrast to the direct bone healing without callus that occurs following traditional rigid fixation using a compression plate technique. The latter includes the inherent risk of fragment devascularization with an increased potential of infection and disturbed bone healing.

The concept of biologic plating, using an indirect approach to the bone, and leaving the soft-tissue envelope

undisturbed, is characterized by indirect reduction using traction and the plate as a reduction aid. The fixation is elastic, demonstrating relative stability. The implant and the bone share the load. This approach forms the basis of the minimally invasive percutaneous plating (minimally invasive plate osteosynthesis [MIPO]) concept, where small soft-tissue windows remote from the fracture site are created to give access to the bone for submuscular plating as is done for intramedullary nailing.

The length of the skin incision cannot define minimal invasiveness; rather, it is defined by the smallest "footprint" the surgeon leaves at the fracture site using mainly indirect reduction techniques and generating minimal additional trauma to the soft tissue adjacent to the fracture when direct reduction is necessary. The soft-tissue windows must be large enough for the bone to be seen and palpated and to insert a tunneling instrument and the plate. At the joint level, the approaches need to be large enough to allow an anatomic, rigid, and direct reduction of the articular surface. Therefore, several new approaches for addressing intra-articular fractures with metaphyseal extensions have evolved. With the distal femur, the parapatellar approach for direct transarticular reduction of the intra-articular fracture is used to insert the plate alongside the femoral shaft without opening the soft-tissue envelope of the femoral shaft.[1] The articular segment is attached to the diaphysis with minimal soft-tissue disruption compared with the traditional lateral approach to the femoral shaft. The same concept applies to the proximal tibia, the distal tibia, and the proximal humerus where the articular fracture is exposed directly with an incision large enough to visualize the fracture and achieve anatomic joint restoration.[2-4] The plate is then slid underneath the muscle alongside the periosteum of the shaft (submuscular technique), before the fracture is reduced by indirect reduction through traction combined with percutaneous direct fracture manipulation and fixation through small stab wounds.

Anatomic precontoured periarticular plates designed specifically for the epiphyseal/metaphyseal regional anatomy, locking screws, and fluoroscopy accelerated the evolution in plate design. Because of the angular stability afforded by multiple locking screws, the plate-screw-bone complex is an extrapolation of an external fixator, which does not depend on friction at the implant-bone interface. If proper fracture alignment is

Dr. Jones or an immediate family member is a board member, owner, officer, or committee member of Grand Valley Surgery Center, Michigan Orthopaedic Society, the Orthopaedic Trauma Association, AOA Committee, and the AAOS Coding Coverage and Reimbursement Committee. Dr. Babst or an immediate family member is a board member, owner, officer, or committee member of the Orthopaedic Trauma Association and serves as an unpaid consultant to AO and Synthes. Dr. Anders or an immediate family member has received royalties from DePuy; is a member of a speakers' bureau or has made paid presentations on behalf of DePuy and Synthes; serves as a paid consultant for or is an employee of DePuy and Synthes; has received research or institutional support from DePuy; and owns stock or stock options in Johnson & Johnson, Pfizer, and Stryker.

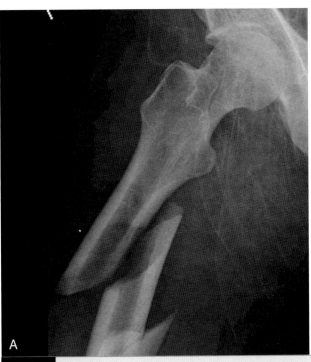
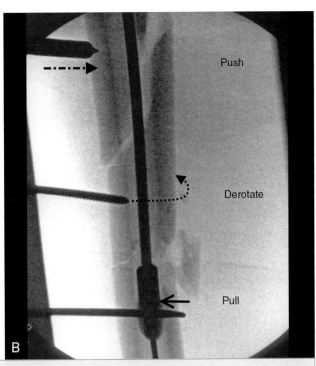

Figure 1 Proximal femoral segmental fracture with varus deformity and displacement (**A**) corrected with percutaneously inserted spike pusher, segmental instability maintained and derotated with a percutaneously inserted unicortical Schanz pin, and translation corrected with a percutaneously inserted shoulder hook while reaming the canal (**B**).

achieved, it will be maintained by the internal fixator. Newer plate designs are multifunctional, allowing for placement of either a standard (nonlocking) or a locked screw through the same hole of the plate. When using a nonlocking screw first, the plate still serves as a reduction tool as in open access surgery. Once reduction is obtained, it can then be definitively fixed using locking head screws without the risk of loss of reduction. This reduction sequence can be remembered with the phrase: "pin-pin, lag-lag, lock-lock." In other words, preliminary fixation on either side of the fracture is temporarily achieved via provisional pins or drill bits, after which the fracture is reduced to the precontoured plate via the lagging of standard screws on each side of the fracture. The final reduction is then locked into position with the locking screws. This is an advantage when treating periarticular fractures with the MIPO technique. With diaphyseal fractures, conventional plating techniques will be sufficient because alignment usually can be achieved without precise plate contouring. The MIPO technique is facilitated not only by new percutaneous reduction instruments, but also by careful preoperative imaging, including CT for articular fractures, as well as a preoperative plan that includes positioning for adequate intraoperative fluoroscopy control, uncovering the contralateral leg as a template to control length, axis, and rotation, and to have an alternative plan if reduction is not achieved through the minimal access surgery.

Problems that have been noted include higher radiation exposure and a long learning curve, malunion, and delayed healing of simple fractures using the bridge plating concept. In the future, computer-assisted navigation, use of biologic stimulation of fracture healing, or new implant designs could help to further improve these new approaches to fracture fixation.

Minimally Invasive Fracture Reduction Techniques

With minimally invasive plate insertion techniques, noninvasive, indirect techniques for fracture reduction are required. Fracture table and boot or skeletal traction are replaced with gentle manual traction or manipulation. Furthermore, shoulder hooks, spike pushers, and Schantz pins inserted percutaneously are used to facilitate fracture reduction, restoration of length, control of rotation, realignment of the limb, and plate or nail insertion[5] (**Figure 1**). Shoulder hooks, which are smaller versions of the bone hook with a longer lever arm, can reapproximate fracture fragments and redirect nail insertion without large incisions or soft-tissue stripping. Furthermore, the hook can expedite plate removal. Spike pushers can be used to realign fracture fragments (**Figure 1**). Schanz pins can be inserted unicortically or bicortically in strategic locations to guide fracture reduction and avoid malrotation, facilitate nail or plate insertion, stabilize segmental fragments while reaming or plating, and can be connected to a temporary external fixator or universal distractor providing temporary fixation.

Fracture Site–Specific Treatment

Techniques of minimally invasive or percutaneous fixation for proximal humeral, pelvic, distal femoral, and distal radial fracture are well established and accepted. Newer and optional techniques for other fractures have recently been described.

Proximal Humeral Fractures

Displaced unstable proximal humeral fractures can be treated in several ways. Osteoporosis, short segment fixation, deforming muscular forces, and overlying musculature interfere with internal fixation. Using MIS techniques, locking plates create immediate stability, and scarring and blood loss are diminished. The plating technique uses a radiolucent table with the fluoroscopic unit on the contralateral side of the table. A small incision with a muscle-splitting approach is created at the junction of the anterior and middle third of the deltoid. With the arm in abduction, the deltoid muscle is gently elevated from the lateral aspect of the proximal humerus. The axillary nerve will be traversing the deltoid distal to the incision. Reduction of the tuberosity and head is achieved via joysticks and temporary fixation. Once the proximal segment is stabilized, it will act as a single fragment. The plate is carefully inserted submuscularly through the incision, beneath the axillary nerve, and finally under the deltoid muscle insertion. If the arm is abducted and a finger is placed under the nerve, plate application is facilitated. A counterincision is created laterally over the distal plate site. Once the appropriate plate position is obtained, the proximal and distal screw insertion is performed through the two small incisions. To avoid injury to the axillary nerve, only the most proximal metaphyseal screws should be used. In a series of 34 consecutive fractures, no loss of fixation or axillary nerve injury was reported.[3]

Humeral Diaphyseal Fractures

The minimally invasive approach to the humeral shaft is well established using antegrade and retrograde nails. Nailing avoids the extensive soft-tissue dissection that is necessary when using standard anterolateral, posterior, or medial approaches to perform open reduction and internal fixation using a plate. In a meta-analysis there was no difference in both treatment modalities regarding infection, secondary radial nerve palsy, or nonunion.[6] However, the risk for a reoperation or for shoulder impingement in these patients was significantly higher using the minimally invasive approach with a nail compared with open reduction and internal fixation (ORIF) using plates.

Anatomic studies[3,4] followed by clinical case series have shown that minimally invasive plating of the humeral shaft is feasible, with a low complication rate.[3-6] The anterior face of the humerus is flat and well suited for a straight plate applied by a minimally invasive submuscular technique. The approach is remote from the fracture site through soft-tissue windows proximally and distally. Using mainly indirect reduction techniques and relatively stable fixation, a bridge plate concept can be applied. Distal fixation has to respect the radial nerve between the brachioradialis and the brachialis muscle either by direct visualization through a mobile soft-tissue window or by protecting it with a pad of the lateral portion of the brachialis muscle.[3,4] Gentle traction is recommended so that the radial and the musculocutaneous nerves are not endangered when working through the distal soft-tissue window.[4]

Minimally invasive plating of humeral shaft fractures is indicated in comminuted or segmental fracture patterns not suited for a nail, in patients with a narrow medullary canal, open physis, or a periprosthetic fracture. In the setting of a primary radial nerve palsy, the radial nerve should be explored to avoid possible entrapment before MIPO is performed.[7] Recently published clinical case series demonstrate that minimally invasive humeral plating is feasible and has a low morbidity. The pooled data in the reported series reveal 8 primary and 3 secondary transient radial nerve palsies in 71 patients. All primary and secondary nerve palsies recovered during the follow-up period.[8] Because bridge plating is nonanatomic by definition, axial malalignment from 13% to 47% has been reporated.[9] The pooled published series demonstrate 2 nonunions and 2 infections in 71 procedures.[9]

Before this approach can be widely recommended, additional comparative studies with a higher level of evidence are needed to appraise the value of this new approach in comparison with the other surgical and nonsurgical treatment modalities.

Femoral Diaphyseal Fractures

Femoral diaphyseal fractures are successfully treated with an antegrade intramedullary nail inserted via piriformis or trochanteric entry or with a retrograde nail inserted through an intercondylar starting site. It is well known that femoral nailing in the supine position in muscular or obese patients is complicated. Starting site accuracy is diminished because the traditional incision over the greater trochanter pushes the trajectory of the initial starting pins and drills from lateral to medial, creating varus alignment. Percutaneous starting sites combined with minimally invasive reduction techniques may enhance alignment, especially avoiding the typical flexion and varus proximal deformities.[5,10] Once the proximal fragment alignment is satisfactory, a percutaneously inserted guide pin is inserted directly into the piriformis fossa or tip of the trochanter. The technique uses a direct alignment without muscle or adipose tissue displacement. In muscular or obese patients, the starting site is usually proximal to the iliac crest because of the intervening soft tissue (**Figure 2**). Newer systems allow for enhanced starting site accuracy with improved modular reamers.[11] Once the starting site is confirmed with fluoroscopy, the remainder of the procedure is performed via a cannulated system or percu-

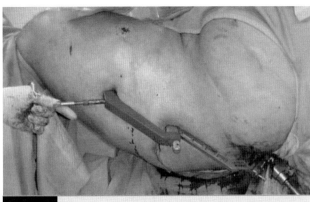

Figure 2 Percutaneous starting site with longer nail guide in an obese patient with segmental femoral diaphyseal fracture.

taneously. Because of the proximal starting site, longer reamers and nail guides facilitate the technique.

Under special circumstances, MIS femoral plating can be used efficiently. Because of blood loss and the potential for overgrowth from open techniques and rotational instability with flexible nailing, submuscular pediatric femoral diaphyseal bridge plating is becoming popular.[12] For the adult population, ipsilateral femoral neck, pertrochanteric, and acetabular fractures, pregnancy, and associated ipsilateral vascular injuries may lessen the indications for femoral nailing. In a retrospective series of 40 fractures in 38 patients, submuscular femoral plating was compared with traditional open plating techniques. Comparable results were noted with either technique; only one nonunion and one infection, both in type III open fractures, were found.[13]

Distal Femoral Fractures

The concept of minimally invasive percutaneous plating was first applied to the distal femur. Plating using MIS techniques can be performed laterally through the iliotibial band or anterolaterally through a lateral parapatellar approach. In a series of 24 fractures in 22 patients with periprosthetic distal femoral fractures around a well-fixed total knee arthroplasty, 86% healed without further intervention and with acceptable alignment maintained and initial stabilization with laterally inserted precontoured locked plates.[14] In a meta-analysis of distal femoral fractures, MIS plating reduced the rates of infection but increased the rates of malalignment and revision surgery compared with traditional open plating.[15]

Proximal Tibial Plateau Fractures

Traditional tibial plateau fracture fixation techniques use large open incisions and are complicated by soft-tissue injury, problems with short segment fixation, and realignment of the limb. Infection rates of greater than 10% are reported with external fixation or dual plating. Newer MIS techniques use small proximal inci-

sions to reduce and stabilize the articular surface, locking plate technology to provide angular stability, and plate jigs that facilitate percutaneous screw insertion. Once the articular surface is reduced and temporarily stabilized, the locking plate is inserted laterally via an iliotibial band-splitting approach and under the anterior tibial musculature. The precontoured plate is then attached to the proximal and diaphyseal tibia with the locking screws. The screws should parallel the joint to avoid the potentially problematic varus reduction. Long plates extending to the distal third or fourth of the tibia should be stabilized only after a counterdistal incision to identify and protect the traversing peroneal nerve and artery.[16]

In early reports of high-energy proximal tibial plateau fractures, high union rates and low infection rates were noted with MIS locked plating.[2,17] Difficulties with alignment were noted in a low number of patients with residual flexion/extension deformities more commonly than varus/valgus malalignment. In a more recent report with longer follow-up, higher rates of malalignment and infection were experienced.[18]

Tibial Diaphyseal Fractures

Tibial diaphyseal fractures are typically and best treated with a tibial nail. Special circumstances such as a total knee arthroplasty or tibial deformity interfere with nail insertion. In an analysis of 20 consecutive patients, minimally invasive plate insertion with a bridge plating technique was studied.[19] Plates were inserted via an approach distant to the fracture site either proximal or distal. The plane of plate insertion was epiperiosteal. Plates are precontoured to allow for appropriate diaphyseal alignment. With plates centered on the fracture site, bridge plating with strategically inserted screws is accomplished. Three screws or six cortices of purchase are desired. The relative stability technique induces callus formation and healing (**Figure 3**). Nineteen of the 20 fractures healed without delay. One nonunion required revision plating to achieve a healed fracture.

Distal Tibial and Tibial Pilon Fractures

Distal tibial fracture fixation has been fraught with problems associated with soft-tissue injuries, infection, and malalignment. Traditional open techniques are now performed in a staged manner, with lower complication rates. Intramedullary nailing reduces complications associated with the soft tissue at the expense of higher malunion rates. MIS plating for the distal tibia can be performed anterolaterally and/or medially depending on the fracture pattern.[4] Most extra-articular fractures can be managed with medial approaches with or without locked plating. With more complex intra-articular patterns, articular surface reduction is essential. The anterolateral approach enhances joint visualization while allowing for submuscular plate application. The approach requires dissection of the superficial peroneal nerve and elevation of the deep peroneal nerve for plate insertion.[20] Standard bridge plating

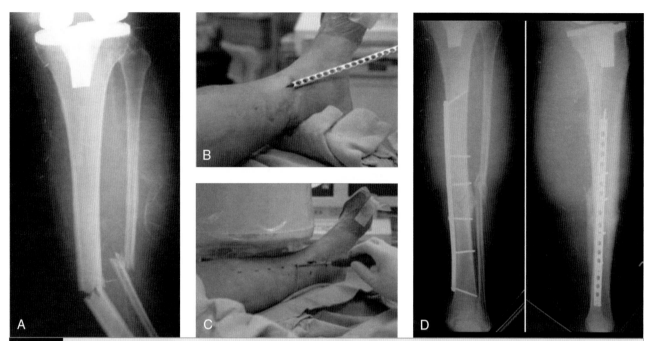

Figure 3 A through D, Percutaneous plate insertion for a displaced tibial diaphyseal fracture distal to a total knee arthroplasty. **A,** Injury radiograph. **B,** Distal incision beginning insertion of the percutaneous retrograde plate. **C,** Plate insertion, percutaneous screw insertion, and plate fixation. **D,** Final AP and lateral radiographs of healed fracture with callus secondary to relative stability fixation.

spanning the area of comminution under the anterior compartment and proximal fixation with an open counterincision away from the zone of injury facilitate the technique. The closure is performed with muscle coverage of the plate both proximally and distally. Advantages of locked submuscular anterolateral bridge plating are the biologic technique, stabilization of short fracture segments, and avoidance of subcutaneous plate position medially, usually under an open wound. In a consecutive series of high-energy tibial plafond injuries with minimal articular involvement, low numbers of infection but higher numbers of secondary surgeries were required to achieve union.[21] Factors affecting healing were comminuted fractures, bone loss, or type III open fractures. Early bone grafting once soft tissues heal would diminish the difficulties with healing.

Problems With MIS

The era of ORIF with anatomic rigid stabilization of fractures has evolved with the advent of minimally invasive relative stability techniques. The MIS technique requires extensive fluoroscopic visualization, which is inherently nonanatomic and imperfect. Even with skilled and experienced surgeons, reduction problems occur. These imperfect reductions alter length, alignment, and rotation, and when used for articular fracture reduction can create articular incongruity. A minimally invasive procedure is not desirable at the cost of a malreduction.

The stability of locked internal fixators inserted submuscularly can be controlled.[22,23] The working length directly influences the axial stiffness and torsional rigidity of the implant. With omission of the screws adjacent to the fracture site (increasing working length), the compression and torsional flexibility are doubled. Therefore, the plastic deformation load of the plate is diminished. The total number of screws directly determines the torsional rigidity. More than three screws on either side of the construct does not affect axial compression rigidity. The placement of the third screw on either side of the construct modulates the axial stiffness in a manner similar to that of the working length. Decreasing distance from the plate to the bone increases construct stiffness. Utilization of a shorter plate with an equal number of screws reduces axial but not torsional stiffness.

Mixing concepts of MIPO can create problems.[24,25] In general, simple fracture patterns require open anatomic reduction and rigid fixation or submuscular relative fixation with screws far apart from the fracture site (increased working length and decreased plastic deformation).[22] For bridging MIPO of the lower extremity, two to three screws on either side of the fracture is sufficient. For upper extremity fractures, the predominantly rotational forces and less axial compression require three to four screws on either side of the fracture. Complex fracture patterns with comminution require indirect reduction, submuscular plating with long plates, and screws adjacent to the fracture site to enhance construct rigidity in the situation of fracture site

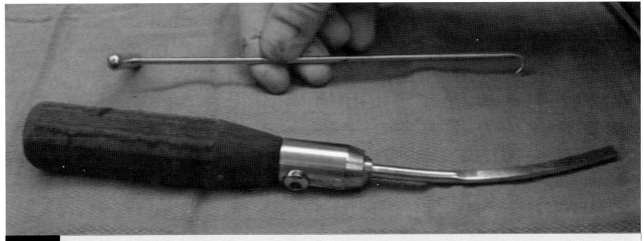

Figure 4   Instruments used for minimally invasive plate removal: shoulder hook (top) and curved bone impacter (bottom).

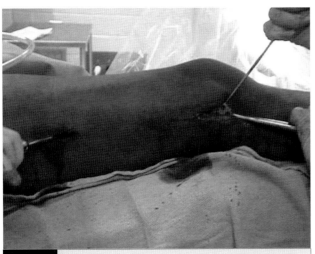

Figure 5   Intraoperative minimally invasive plate removal from the distal femur using push-pull instruments. Note the Cobb elevator under the plate to direct removal and protect the skin.

instability and decreased plate contact secondary to comminution. Relatively short plates or an unstable construct can increase catastrophic implant failure. Osteoporotic fractures require longer plates with bicortical screws to improve the working length, balanced relative stability to match plate-bone compliance, and increased screw number to confirm screw purchase. Newer, stiffer locked plating constructs generate callus, take longer to fail, and with failure may not generate pain until catastrophic failure.[26] If in the setting of osteoporotic bone and locked screw fixation, coronal diaphyseal fractures can be generated from the screws working through the bone similar to a knife through warm butter. Any deviation from these generalities can generate a nonunion with a too-stiff or too-flexible construct.

Precontoured "anatomic" plates are not always individually contoured or anatomic. Furthermore, locked plating requires thicker plates to accommodate the locking mechanism. The combination of imperfect anatomic plate contour and increased plate thickness creates increased plate prominence, especially at the periarticular regions. The plate prominence and surrounding moving structures at the periarticular area can potentially generate plate irritation.

With inserted hardware (intramedullary nail or plate), planned (open physes) or unplanned (nonunion, posttraumatic revision, or prominence) hardware removal can become challenging when attempting to remove the device through the same MIS incisions. Inability to remove all of the soft tissue within the screw head and stripping the fit of the screwdriver within the head can potentially require an open approach to the screw. Gently tapping the screwdriver into the screw head can dislodge the intervening soft tissue and enhance the screwdriver fit into the screw head. Once the screw is removed from the bone and plate, the screw can become dislodged and lost in the soft tissues. Newer screwdriver mechanisms allow for a capturing device in the screw head. Locked screw heads have been noted to become "fused" or "cold worked" into the plate, necessitating drilling the screw head out of the plate and leaving metal debris, or removing the plate by ripping it out of the bone, leaving large screw hole sites. Once the screws have been successfully removed from the plate and soft tissues, plate removal becomes difficult because of soft-tissue ingrowth into more nonused screw hole sites and the submuscular location. Submuscular plate removal can be facilitated with a "push-pull" technique. The plate is pulled out with a bone or shoulder hook and simultaneously is pushed out with a curved bone tamp (**Figures 4 and 5**). Excessive bleeding from the incisions may require opening the area to cauterize bleeding scar tissue or compressive dressings. Hemorrhage control is required to avoid increased compartmental pressures and a potential compartment syndrome.

Summary

Minimally invasive fracture care is based on leaving a small "footprint" in the process of inserting hardware. A small footprint enhances vascular viability of the callus and fracture fragments and potentially lessens scarring and blood loss. Newer plating techniques allow submuscular insertion, thereby reducing the fracture with anatomic precontouring of the plates. Longer plates with strategically inserted screws can optimize a more natural fracture healing deploying relative stability. No matter what technique is used, articular fractures require anatomic rigid fixation, whereas newer, less invasive techniques can improve metaphyseal and diaphyseal fracture or fracture extension healing.

Annotated References

1. Kregor PJ, Stannard JA, Zlowodzki M, Cole PA: Treatment of distal femur fractures using the less invasive stabilization system: Surgical experience and early clinical results in 103 fractures. *J Orthop Trauma* 2004;18(8):509-520.

   Treatment of distal femur fractures with the Less Invasive Stabilization System is associated with high union rates without autogenous bone grafting (93%), a low incidence of infection (3%), and maintenance of distal femoral fixation (100%). Malreductions of the femoral fracture were seen in six fractures (6%). Level of evidence: III.

2. Cole PA, Zlowodzki M, Kregor PJ: Treatment of proximal tibia fractures using the less invasive stabilization system: Surgical experience and early clinical results in 77 fractures. *J Orthop Trauma* 2004;18(8):528-535.

   The Less Invasive Stabilization System provides stable fixation (97%), a high rate of union (97%), and a low (4%) rate of infection for proximal tibial fractures. There were two early losses of proximal fixation, two nonunions, two deep delayed infections, and one deep peroneal nerve palsy. Postoperative malalignment occurred in seven patients with 6° to 10° of angular deformity (one varus/valgus and seven flexion/extension malalignments), and an eighth patient had a flexion deformity of 15°. Level of evidence: III.

3. Laflamme GY, Rouleau DM, Berry GK, Beaumont PH, Reindl R, Harvey EJ: Percutaneous humeral plating of fractures of the proximal humerus: Results of a prospective multicenter clinical trial. *J Orthop Trauma* 2008;22(3):153-158.

   Thirty-four consecutive patients underwent percutaneous plating for treatment of proximal humerus fractures. There were no axillary nerve injuries or loss of reduction. The average Constant score at 1 year was 82 and the Disabilities of the Arm, Shoulder and Hand score was 26. Level of evidence: III.

4. Helfet DL, Suk M: Minimally invasive percutaneous plate osteosynthesis of fractures of the distal tibia. *Instr Course Lect* 2004;53:471-475.

   This technique involves conventional open reduction and internal fixation of the fibula and spanning external fixation of the tibia until the soft-tissue swelling subsides. Subsequently, limited open reduction and internal fixation of displaced articular fragments is performed through small incisions based on CT evaluation followed by minimally invasive percutaneous plate osteosynthesis of the tibia, in which the plafond is attached to the tibial shaft. Level of evidence: V.

5. Rhorer AS: Percutaneous/minimally invasive techniques in treatment of femoral shaft fractures with an intramedullary nail. *J Orthop Trauma* 2009;23(suppl 5) S2-S5.

   Deforming forces of the muscles of the hip, knee, and thigh are neutralized with reduction tools applied percutaneously, blocking screws, and Schanz pins. Mastery of these techniques and appropriate reduction are incumbent on the orthopaedic surgeon treating femoral shaft fractures. Level of evidence: V.

6. Bhandari M, Devereaux PJ, McKee MD, Schemitsch EH: Compression plating versus intramedullary nailing of humeral shaft fractures: A meta-analysis. *Acta Orthop* 2006;77(2):279-284.

   Meta-analysis of three prospective randomized trials from 1969 to 2000, which showed that the risk for a reoperation or a shoulder impingement after nailing is higher, compared with plating. There was no difference between the two treatment modalities regarding nonunion, infection, and radial nerve palsy. Level of evidence: I.

7. Livani B, Belangero W, Andrade K, et al: Is MIPO in humeral shaft fractures really safe? Postoperative ultrasonographic evaluation. *Int Orthop* 2009;33:1719-1723. Epub Aug 13, 2008.

   Nineteen patients underwent postoperative ultrasound examinations after MIPO. Group A comprised midshaft fractures and group B distal third fractures. In group A the distance was between 1.6 and 19.6 mm (mean: 9.3 mm) and in group B between 1.0 and 8.1 mm (mean: 4.0 mm). The ultrasound findings reveal that the radial nerve is quite close to the implant material, especially in the transition between the third and fourth quarters of the humeral shaft. Level of evidence: IV.

8. Livani B, Belangero WD, Castro de Medeiros R: Fractures of the distal third of the humerus with palsy of the radial nerve: Management using minimally invasive percutaneous plate osteosynthesis. *J Bone Joint Surg Br* 2006;88(12):1625-1628.

   Six patients with fractures of the distal third of the humerus complicated by complete lesions of the radial nerve that were entrapped or compressed by bone fragments had complete functional recovery. Healing of the fractures occurred at a mean of 2.7 months (2 to 3 months) and complete neurologic recovery by a mean of 2.3 months. Level of evidence: IV.

9. Zhiquan A, Bingfang Z, Yeming W, Chi Z, Peiyan H: Minimally invasive plating osteosynthesis (MIPO) of middle and distal third humeral shaft fractures. *J Orthop Trauma* 2007;21(9):628-633.

1: General Topics and New Technology

In a prospective, single-center, nonconsecutive clinical series, 13 middle and distal third humeral shaft fractures were reduced by closed means and fixed with long, narrow, 4.5-mm dynamic compression plates introduced through two small incisions away from the fracture sites and placed on the anterior aspect of the humerus. There were no nonunions, radial nerve palsies, or implant failures. According to the UCLA scoring system, results were excellent in 7 cases (53.8%) and good in 6 cases (46.2%). Level of evidence: IV.

10. Bellabarba C, Herscovici D Jr, Ricci WM: Percutaneous treatment of peritrochanteric fractures using the gamma nail. 2000. *J Orthop Trauma* 2003;17(suppl 8)S38-S50.

11. Russell TA, Mir HR, Stoneback J, Cohen J, Downs B: Avoidance of malreduction of proximal femoral shaft fractures with the use of a minimally invasive nail insertion technique (MINIT). *J Orthop Trauma* 2008;22(6): 391-398.

One hundred consecutive proximal femoral shaft fractures (97 patients) were treated with intramedullary nailing with and without the use of a minimally invasive nail insertion technique (MINIT). A total of 72 entry portals were trochanteric, and 28 were piriformis. Seventy-seven percent of the femurs were opened with MINIT, a technique that uses a percutaneous cannulated channel reamer over a guide pin as opposed to the standard method of Kuntscher, in which a femoral awl is used. Malalignment occurred in 26% of fractures treated without the use of the MINIT and in 5.2% when the MINIT was used (*P* < 0.01). There was no statistically significant difference between the different Russell-Taylor fracture types, although there was a trend toward more malalignment in type 2A and 2B fractures (*P* = 0.06). Level of evidence: II.

12. Hedequist DJ, Sink E: Technical aspects of bridge plating for pediatric femur fractures. *J Orthop Trauma* 2005;19(4):276-279.

The submuscular insertion of 4.5-mm, narrow, low-contact dynamic compression plates with minimal exposure for plate entry and percutaneous screw placement has greatly facilitated the treatment of comminuted fractures and allows for stable internal fixation while reducing blood loss and the need for fracture site exposure. The technique creates a stable mode of fixation while maximizing biologic fracture healing potential and also permits early patient mobilization. Level of evidence: IV.

13. Zlowodzki M, Vogt D, Cole PA, Kregor PJ: Plating of femoral shaft fractures: Open reduction and internal fixation versus submuscular fixation. *J Trauma* 2007; 63(5):1061-1065.

Forty acute diaphyseal femoral fractures were studied in 37 patients. Traditional open plating with emphasis on preservation of soft tissue integrity was performed exclusively before February 1999 (n = 19). After that time, of the 21 remaining fractures, submuscular plating techniques were used in all except one. No bone grafting was used for either group. A 2.5% incidence of nonunion and a 5% incidence of infection (2 of 40; both in type III open fractures) were seen in this series of 40 femoral shaft fractures treated with plate application.

Submuscular utilization in the femoral shafts did not have a clear clinical advantage, appears to be more technically challenging, and is associated with a high rate of suboptimal reductions. Level of evidence: III.

14. Ricci WM, Loftus T, Cox C, Borrelli J: Locked plates combined with minimally invasive insertion technique for the treatment of periprosthetic supracondylar femur fractures above a total knee arthroplasty. *J Orthop Trauma* 2006;20(3):190-196.

In a prospective, consecutive case series, 22 consecutive adult patients with 24 (2 bilateral) supracondylar femur fractures (Orthopaedic Trauma Association 33A) above a well-fixed nonstemmed TKA were treated with the Locking Condylar Plate. Nineteen of 22 fractures healed after the index procedure (86%). All three patients with healing complications had insulin-dependent diabetes and were obese (body mass index > 30). Fixation of periprosthetic supracondylar femur fractures with a locking plate provided satisfactory results in nondiabetic patients. Diabetic patients seem to be at high risk for healing complications and infection. Level of evidence: IV.

15. Zlowodzki M, Bhandari M, Marek DJ, Cole PA, Kregor PJ: Operative treatment of acute distal femur fractures: Systematic review of 2 comparative studies and 45 case series (1989 to 2005). *J Orthop Trauma* 2006;20(5): 366-371.

Exploratory subgroup analyses suggest that submuscular locked fixators may reduce infection rates but at an increased risk of fixation failure and revision surgery compared to techniques that require compression of the implant to the femoral shaft (blade plate, dynamic condylar screw, nonlocking condylar buttress plate). Surgeons with increased experience may significantly reduce the risk of revision surgery. Level of evidence: I.

16. Deangelis JP, Deangelis NA, Anderson R: Anatomy of the superficial peroneal nerve in relation to fixation of tibia fractures with the less invasive stabilization system. *J Orthop Trauma* 2004;18(8):536-539.

The superficial peroneal nerve is at significant risk during percutaneous screw placement in holes 11 through 13 of the 13-hole proximal tibia Less Invasive Stabilization System plate. Use of a larger incision and careful dissection down to the plate in this region may minimize the risk of damage to the nerve. Level of evidence: II.

17. Stannard JP, Wilson TC, Volgas DA, Alonso JE: The less invasive stabilization system in the treatment of complex fractures of the tibial plateau: Short-term results. *J Orthop Trauma* 2004;18(8):552-558.

The use of Less Invasive Stabilization System plates appears to stabilize complex fractures of the tibial plateau (n = 34) with a low incidence of complications. The Less Invasive Stabilization System functioned well in maintaining alignment and obtaining union in these high-energy fractures. Level of evidence: IV.

18. Phisitkul P, McKinley TO, Nepola JV, Marsh JL: Complications of locking plate fixation in complex proximal tibia injuries. *J Orthop Trauma* 2007;21(2):83-91.

The complication rate in 37 tibial plateau fractures in a retrospective analysis was 22% deep infection, 22%

malalignment, and 8% loss of alignment. The complication rate, particularly infection, was higher than in previous reports; however, some complications may be inherent in the treatment of high-energy fractures using locking plates. Level of evidence: III.

19. Williams TH, Schenk W: Bridging-minimally invasive locking plate osteosynthesis (Bridging-MILPO): Technique description with prospective series of 20 tibial fractures. *Injury* 2008;39(10):1198-1203.

Excellent final results were obtained in 19 of the 20 cases. Complications included two superficial wound infections, one delayed union, and one fracture requiring revision plating. No loss of reduction was seen in any of the cases. Level of evidence: IV.

20. Wolinsky P, Lee M: The distal approach for anterolateral plate fixation of the tibia: An anatomic study. *J Orthop Trauma* 2008;22(6):404-407.

The distal anterolateral approach can be used to place plates along the anterolateral border of the tibia. The superficial peroneal nerve is always seen in the distal incision and is not at risk. The structures at risk are the deep peroneal nerve and the anterior tibial vessels as they course from a posterior position proximally to a more anterior position distally. Level of evidence: III.

21. Collinge C, Kuper M, Larson K, Protzman R: Minimally invasive plating of high-energy metaphyseal distal tibia fractures. *J Orthop Trauma* 2007;21(6):355-361.

Minimally invasive medial plating will restore limb alignment and yield successful clinical outcomes for high-energy metaphyseal fractures of the distal tibia. Despite the significant reoperation rate and prolonged time to union, most patients can expect a predictable return of function. Strong consideration should be given to adjunctive measures in at-risk patients, including those with highly comminuted fracture patterns, bone loss, or type II or III open fractures. Level of evidence: IV.

22. Stoffel K, Dieter U, Stachowiak G: Biomechanial testing of the LCP: How can stability in locked internal fixators be controlled? *Injury* 2003;34(suppl 2):B11-B19.

23. Stoffel K, Klaue K, Perren SM: Functional load of plates in fracture fixation in vivo and its correlate in bone healing. *Injury* 2000;31(suppl 2S):B37-B50.

24. Strauss EJ, Schwarzkopf R, Kummer F, Egol KA: The current status of locked plating: The good, the bad, and the ugly. *J Orthop Trauma* 2008;22(7):479-486.

The biomechanics of locked plate technology, appropriate indications for its use, laboratory and clinical comparisons to conventional plating techniques, and potential mechanisms of locked plate failure that have been observed are discussed. Level of evidence: IV.

25. Bottlang M, Doornink J, Fitzpatrick DC, Madey SM: Far cortical locking can reduce stiffness of locked plating constructs while retaining construct strength. *J Bone Joint Surg Am* 2009;91:1985-1994.

Far cortical locking significantly reduces the axial stiffness of a locked plating construct. This gain in flexibility causes only a modest reduction in axial strength and increased torsional and bending strength. Level of evidence: II.

26. Kubiak EN, Fulkerson E, Strauss E, Egol KA: The evolution of locked plates. *J Bone Joint Surg Am* 2006;88(suppl 4):189-200.

New plate designs continue to emerge in response to the need to improve current designs and fill niche markets. The development of plates that permit the surgeon to determine screw placement and still maintain the benefits of a fixed-angle device is ongoing, despite the fact that initial variable-angle, fixed-angle devices were plagued with failures of the locking mechanism. Level of evidence: V.

1: General Topics and New Technology

Chapter 6
Soft-Tissue Injury

Jackson Lee, MD   Paul Dougherty, MD   Romney C. Andersen, MD

1: General Topics and New Technology

Introduction

The soft-tissue component of any musculoskeletal injury plays a major role in determining the risk of complications and eventual outcome of the injury, and it is an integral part of the management of orthopaedic trauma. The understanding of the pathophysiology of soft-tissue injury continues to advance and has led to changes in the initial management of these wounds and improvements in skin graft substitutes and biologic dressings. Negative pressure wound therapy (NPWT) is used more often to prepare a wound for definitive management, and there has been greater understanding of the mechanism of action of NPWT at the cellular level. Many previously accepted practices such as techniques of open fracture wound débridement, the 6-hour rule regarding the timing of débridement of open fracture wound, the use of clinical examination to rule in or rule out compartment syndromes, and the type and method of applying an irrigant for open fracture wounds have all been called into question with new investigations. Regarding definitive management, the efficacy of fasciocutaneous flaps as a wound coverage option in comparison with traditional free tissue transfers is a continuing topic of debate.

Pathophysiology

Soft-tissue wounds sustained during a traumatic event result in a cascade of events at the cellular level that promote healing and allow for repair of damaged tissue.

A recent study documented the presence of mesenchymal progenitor cells within traumatized human muscle tissue.[1] The authors were able to isolate dedifferentiated multipotent cells in the débrided tissue. These cells were cultured and were able to produce bone, fat, and cartilage cells within an appropriate inductive medium. Therefore, after injury it may be possible to isolate and expand in culture a population of mesenchymal progenitor cells from the injured tissue and use those cells for host-specific tissue engineering and regeneration applications, facilitating delayed reconstruction of severely traumatized tissue. Another study evaluated the bone produced by induced mesenchymal progenitor cells from the traumatized muscle, comparing that to bone produced from the mesenchymal stem cells present in bone marrow.[2] The authors found the two types of bone had similar genetic expression after induction.

Initial Wound Management

Traumatic open wounds are a window of opportunity for debris and bacteria to both pollute and colonize a wound. Initial treatment of patients with open wounds consists of reducing the bacterial load, as well as removing both debris and dead tissue.

Débridement was originally defined as making an incision extending an open wound along fascial planes to allow for drainage and to allow for the underlying soft tissues to swell. This was in effect a compartment release of a traumatized limb as well as a procedure to allow for unencumbered drainage. Currently, débridement involves wound excision of tissue as well as incisions for exposure and drainage.[3,4]

Compartment syndrome is produced when elevated pressure within a closed myofascial compartment causes microcirculatory failure, rendering the tissues within the compartment ischemic and unable to meet their metabolic needs. Because of the severity of trauma surrounding open fractures, compartment syndrome may occur locally. Extension of the open wound through longitudinal incisions thus helps relieve pressure and allows for inspection of the wound and free drainage if necessary.[3,4]

Surgeons' criteria for excising tissue have been traditionally based on the macroscopic appearance of a wound.[4] For skeletal muscle, the four "C's" (color, consistency, capacity to bleed [or circulation], and contractility) have been used as criteria for excision of tissue. Correlation of the macroscopic and microscopic findings of traumatized skeletal muscle has been done. Scientific analysis of the four criteria has shown corre-

Dr. Andersen or a member of his immediate family has received research or institutional support from the Military Amputee Research Program (MARP), the Orthopaedic Extremity Trauma Research Program (OETRP), and the TRUE Research Foundation. Neither of the following authors or a member of their immediate families has received anything of value from or owns stock in a commercial company or institution related directly or indirectly to the subject of this chapter: Dr. Lee and Dr. Dougherty.

lation between consistency, the ability to bleed, and contractility. The color of tissue was not found to correlate with the microscopic findings of traumatized skeletal muscle. This makes sense, as bruised (discolored) muscle may eventually heal.

Traditionally, the so-called 6-hour rule describes the maximum time allowable for a patient with any open fracture to wait for surgery without increasing the risk of infection.[5] However, studies documenting the necessity for prompt surgical treatment within 6 hours of injury are scarce. Most available studies are retrospective, using infection as an end point to evaluate the timing of initial surgical care from the time of injury. With the available evidence, delays of up to 24 hours may occur without influencing the infection rate.[6,7] Because of small sample size and methodologic limitations, however, the literature does not support elective delay of surgical treatment of open fractures.[8] Likewise, making emergent surgical care of open fractures the priority in the face of physiologic instability is also not justified. Additional large, prospective trials are needed.

Use of sterile irrigation solution has been recommended for the lavage or irrigation of open wounds to reduce the bacterial load in the wound and to help remove dead material or foreign bodies. Mechanical cleansing is also enhanced through the use of irrigation solutions.[5,9-11]

Surgeon preferences for irrigation solutions used for open fracture wounds were recently surveyed.[9] According to members of the Canadian Orthopaedic Association and an AO fracture course, normal saline was preferred by 676 of 984 (70.5%) of the respondents. Bacitracin solution was used by only 161 of 984 (16.8%) of these surgeons, and 695 of 984 (71%) reported using low pressures when delivering the irrigation solution to the wound.

An ideal additive to physiologic irrigation fluid has not been found. Antibiotics that will not degrade in the irrigation solution, most commonly bacitracin, along with neomycin and polymyxin, have been used. Bacitracin interferes with the cell wall synthesis of microbes. Antiseptics, such as those used to prepare skin for surgery and as a hand wash, also have been evaluated. Povidone-iodine and chlorhexidine gluconate are two common additives. At higher concentrations, both cause cell necrosis leading to delayed healing. Sodium hypochlorite and hydrogen peroxide are two other common antiseptics used, which at lower concentrations maintain a bactericidal effect. Sodium hypochlorite (Dakins solution) has been shown to have both bactericidal and cytotoxic effects on fibroblasts. At lower concentration (0.005%), however, the sodium hypochlorite becomes bactericidal only. Hydrogen peroxide has both bactericidal and cytotoxic effects at both regular and decreased concentrations.[12]

Surfactants (soap solutions) have also been recommended for cleansing open wounds. A recent prospective, randomized study compared bacitracin and castile soap in 400 patients with 458 open fractures.[10] The au-thor found that irrigation of open fractures with the antibiotic solution offered no advantage over the use of nonsterile soap solution and may increase the risk of wound healing problems.

The delivery of irrigation solutions has also been studied. Use of high-pressure, pulsed irrigation has been advocated to remove debris and decrease the bacterial load on tissue in open wounds. The optimal pressure for these systems is between 50 and 80 psi. Although more effective in decreasing the bacterial load, the higher pressures decrease fracture and wound healing by damaging bone and soft tissues. A further criticism has been that bacteria may be spread from the wound by jet irrigation. Delivery of fluid by flow or low pressure, such as with a bulb syringe or gravity feed and accompanied by mechanical scrubbing, has been reported to be effective in reducing the bacterial load to tissue.[11,13]

Immediate closure of open wounds is controversial. Recently, success with primary closure has been reported in selected Gustilo-Anderson type IIIA open fractures.[14] Inclusion criteria for immediate wound closure were based on the lack of comorbidities, surgical treatment less than 12 hours after injury, ability to close the wound without tension, and bleeding wound edges.[15]

Intravenous antibiotic use to prevent infection of open wounds is recommended for those associated with open fractures. Traditional recommendations by Gustilo and Anderson, based on the wound severity grade, have also been recently questioned.[16,17] Evidence-based guidelines support the prompt use of first-generation cephalosporins to reduce the infection rate. There is no clear evidence to support the initial use of aminoglycocides or antibiotics specifically for the clostridial species, however. Because of the potential toxicity associated with aminoglycocides, it may be safer to use the first-generation cephalosporin but add an aminoglycocide when cultures or history indicate this addition. Of note, a large prospective trial of antibiotic regimens should be done to help clarify this issue.[18,19]

Flap Coverage

Limb-threatening injuries with significant soft-tissue loss, such as the Gustilo-Anderson type IIIB injuries, continue to be managed successfully using free tissue transfers. The use of vacuum-assisted wound management protocols have helped manage these complex wounds before definitive wound coverage. Although vacuum-assisted wound management is an effective method of early wound management, one study has demonstrated that it does not allow for the delay in timing of definitive flap coverage without an increased infection rate. Early flap coverage, within 7 days of injury, continues to provide lower infection and flap complication rates.[20]

Table 1

Considerations and Contraindications for Using Antibiotic Beads

Considerations

Acute open fractures

Osteomyelitis

Infected nonunions

Management of large soft-tissue dead space

Contraindications

Patient hypersensitivity to the antibiotic

Unsalvageable limb

Small wounds

Osteomyelitis with known slime-forming organisms

The Lower Extremity Assessment Project (LEAP) study group examined the outcomes in patients with limb-threatening type III open tibial diaphyseal fractures. In examining a cohort of patients who underwent either limb salvage or early amputation, the study looked at surgeon-controlled variables that had an effect on outcomes. According to study results, those patients who had simple wound coverage procedures did better than those with flap coverage procedures. Furthermore, patients treated with an external fixator and flap coverage had worse results than those who had early amputations.[21]

Fasciocutaneous flaps continue to gain favor as an alternative to free flap procedures in the lower extremity. Fasciocutaneous flaps are advantageous because they can be mastered by the orthopaedic traumatologist and do not require microsurgical skills. There continues to be debate regarding the superiority of free muscle flaps in the open tibia as compared with fasciocutaneous flaps in regard to fracture healing. Using a mouse model, one group of researchers demonstrated that fasciocutaneous flaps did result in faster fracture healing, more cortical bone content, and a threefold increase in strength of the union at 28 days in comparison with the fasciocutaneous flaps.[22] Additional studies will be needed to define the role of fasciocutaneous flaps for soft-tissue coverage in high-grade open injuries.

Antibiotic Beads

Antibiotic-impregnated polymethylmethacrylate (PMMA) cement beads have been popular for open fracture management in conjunction with surgical treatment and intravenous antibiotic therapy.[23-27] Antibiotic beads have not been approved for manufacture in the United States, and their use in open fractures should be explained to the patient as being off-label. Antibiotic-impregnated cement is most commonly used as a spacer for infected total joint arthroplasty.

Considerations for using antibiotic beads,[23,24] along with contraindications, are outlined in **Table 1**. The use of antibiotic beads is contraindicated in patients with osteomyelitis with known slime-forming organisms, such as *Staphylococcus epidermidis* or *Enterococcus* species. These bacteria may attach to the PMMA, making the bead itself a nidus for infection. The beads can vary in size and shape as well as the type of antibiotic mixed with the PMMA.

The bead pouch technique is often used in the treatment of an open fracture.[23,24] After initial surgical treatment to remove all dead or nonviable tissue, the antibiotic beads are placed within the open wound. The wound is then sealed using a porous barrier, such as Tegaderm (3M, Minneapolis, MN) or Opsite (Smith and Nephew, Memphis, TN). A drain exiting through a separate stab incision is left to dependent or gravity drainage.[28,29] Use of a suction drain elutes the antibiotic quickly from the antibiotic beads and does not produce the same high local concentration. Use of a bead pouch allows for a large increase in the concentration of antibiotics.

Both aminoglycosides (gentamicin or tobramycin) and vancomycin have been used for making antibiotic beads. The aminoglycoside has been used for open fractures. Vancomycin should be used if a resistant staphylococcus organism or methicillin-resistant *Staphylococcus aureus* is present.[24]

Factors that affect local concentration of antibiotics surrounding the antibiotic bead include the size and shape of the bead itself, the concentration of antibiotic within the PMMA, and the amount of flow across the surface of the PMMA.[23,24] By increasing the surface area for elution, a higher local concentration can be generated. Larger spheres elute antibiotics over a greater period of time. Antibiotic beads can vary in size. Bead molds are available from 2 to 8 mm.

A retrospective review of 1,085 patients with open fractures comparing the use of tobramycin-impregnated antibiotic beads and intravenous antibiotics with intravenous antibiotics alone found a decreased infection rate with the more severe open Gustilo-Anderson type IIIB and IIIC fractures when beads were used. Both groups in the series received systemic antibiotic prophylaxis as well using tobramycin, cephalothin, and penicillin.[23] Additional information was presented in a 2008 study.[24]

Because PMMA beads need to be removed, work has been done to allow for placement of antibiotic-impregnated biodegradable osteoconductive substances for long-term implantation. This is especially useful in treating patients with osteomyelitis. Recent work with tobramycin-impregnated calcium sulfate pellets has shown success in treatment of bone infection in both limb and the spine. The use of antibiotic-impregnated osteoinductive or osteoconductive substances shows promise for the future of fracture healing and infection prevention.[25-27]

Negative Pressure Wound Therapy

NPWT continues to expand its roles in the management of acute traumatic wounds. Some of the mechanisms of action of vacuum-assisted wound closure (VAC; KCI, San Antonio, TX) have also been identified. NPWT has several potential benefits that include simplification of wound care for nursing personnel, reduced secondary infection rates, improved wound healing, and decreased wound dehiscence.[30]

Several studies have now demonstrated the effectiveness of NPWT in treating soft-tissue injuries associated with orthopaedic trauma. The VAC has been shown to be beneficial in converting wounds that were initially graded as requiring free tissue transfer or rotational muscle flap coverage to ones that did not need coverage.[31] The VAC was also shown to be beneficial in reducing the cost and need for soft-tissue procedures as well as decreasing morbidity in pediatric patients.[32] VAC dressings have shown promise in decreasing infection rates associated with open fracture care. In a prospective randomized study, the rate of deep infections with the use of a VAC dressing was one fifth that of the control group that received standard wound care.[33]

One aspect of wound management for which the VAC dressing has not been beneficial is in extending the period of time allowable to cover an open fracture. Historically, open fractures covered with either a rotational flap or free flap do better with early coverage. The hope with the VAC dressing was that if the fracture could remain in a sterile environment under negative pressure, flap coverage done later would do as well as early flap coverage. This theory did not prove to be true according to one study; the rate of infection was four times greater in late flap coverage with NPWT than early flap coverage.[20]

VAC dressings have been used extensively by the military and have been safe and effective in routine use and for aeromedical evacuation. In one study assessing transport of patients back from Iraq and Afghanistan to Germany, there was a 19% minor complication rate and a 1% major complication rate with NPWT.[34]

A new technique, instillation therapy, is being used for posttraumatic osteomyelitis with the VAC dressing, whereby the VAC is placed on the wound along with catheters in which polyhexanide antiseptic solution is instilled three times a day. In one study using this technique the recurrence rate of osteomyelitis was one sixth the rate of standard care.[35] The duration of hospital stay was shorter, and there were fewer surgical procedures in the instillation group.

The mechanism of action of the NPWT continues to be studied. Recent work has shown that the combination of the reticulated open cell foam and the negative pressure induces definable changes in the wound healing cascade. In one recent study, VAC therapy was shown to increase levels of interleukin-8 and endothelial growth factor levels in the beds of traumatic wounds.[36] In one small animal study the investigators determined that the vascular response is related to the polyurethane foam, whereas the negative pressure is responsible for the cell proliferation.[37]

Skin Graft Substitutes and Other Biologic Dressings

Split-thickness skin grafting remains the gold standard for covering skin defects.[38] Although significant research is being done to identify an effective inexpensive alternative to split-thickness grafting, these products and techniques have not been used routinely in clinical practice and are usually reserved for massive wounds and large burns.[39] Routine use of keratinocytes embedded in an acellular dermal matrix is still limited by cost and the prolonged time necessary to incubate the cells. The use of temporary cadaver skin grafting to optimize wound beds and prevent infection until permanent coverage is possible is being replaced by the use of skin substitutes.[40] This transition has the advantage of limiting infectious complications of disease transmission from allograft tissue.

The clinical use of skin substitutes has shown promise in areas where standard split-thickness skin grafting has historically been less than optimal. Areas where high skin strain is exhibited, such as on the hands and around joints, also are areas where scar contracture and poor skin quality are well documented. In these high-strain areas, dermal substitutes have shown good functional outcomes.[41] Similarly, the use of skin graft substitutes has also shown promise in areas where traditional skin grafting has been unsuccessful, such as overexposed tendons and bone.[42] In this process, a bilayer dermal substitute consisting of a deep dermal layer composed of a biodegradable matrix of glycosaminoglycan and a superficial layer of semipermeable silicone is placed over the exposed structure and then covered with a negative pressure wound dressing until neodermis formation is present (2 to 4 weeks). Once neodermis formation is evident, the superficial layer of silicone is removed and the wound is then covered with traditional split-thickness skin grafting.

Most of these techniques are expensive and limited to specific indications such as those previously described. For most skin defects, traditional split-thickness skin grafting is an excellent option that has stood the test of time.

Compartment Syndromes

Compartment syndrome continues to be a clinical entity that presents diagnostic challenges to the orthopaedic surgeon. The failure to diagnose and treat compartment syndrome continues to be a common cause of litigation. The diagnosis of compartment syndrome is made based on clinical examination findings in conjunction with an understanding of the nature of the injury. Some surgeons perform a direct measurement of the compartment pressure to help confirm the diagnosis. When the reliability of the clinical examination is in question, compartment pressure monitoring appears to play a major role in diagnosis.

Another study reviewed published series on compartment syndromes to calculate the sensitivity, specificity, positive predictive value, and negative predictive value of clinical findings in the diagnosis. It was determined that sensitivity and positive predictive value in the diagnosis of compartment syndromes of the lower extremity are extremely low, whereas the specificity and negative predictive value are quite high, thus implying that clinical findings are more helpful in excluding compartment syndrome when they are absent than when they are present. It was also observed that when three or more positive signs are present simultaneously, the probability of compartment syndrome is increased substantially.[43]

In an effort to limit the subjectivity of clinical diagnosis, the use of a pulsed-phased, locked-loop ultrasound device shows some potential in the noninvasive detection of elevated compartment pressures and compartment syndrome.[44] In this novel experiment, the authors simulated increased intramuscular pressures created by thigh cuff occlusion in human volunteers and subsequently measured the intramuscular pressures using an invasive slit catheter. These data were compared with readings obtained noninvasively using a phase-locked loop ultrasound device. This comparison also was done with three patients with clinical compartment syndrome. The authors found that the phase-locked loop ultrasound device was able to detect the increased intramuscular pressures, and it was concluded that this device may have a future role in providing objective data for the diagnosis of compartment syndrome.

An issue to consider is the diagnosis of compartment syndrome under general anesthesia. A 2007 study examined the behavior of diastolic blood pressures in patients undergoing tibial nailing under general anesthesia and how it may affect determination of perfusion pressure, which is most often calculated from the difference between the diastolic blood pressure and the compartment pressure. Under general anesthesia, the diastolic blood pressure is often decreased, thereby causing what could be an inaccurate estimation of perfusion pressure when the patient is awake. The diastolic blood pressure was found to return to the preanesthetic level after completion of surgery, and it was suggested that if the length of time the patient is under anesthesia is short, then the decision whether to perform a fasciotomy should be made using the preanesthesia diastolic blood pressure to calculate the perfusion pressure, rather than the intraoperative blood pressures. If the patient is to be under anesthesia for a prolonged period of time, then the perfusion pressure should be calculated based on the intraoperative diastolic blood pressure.[45]

It is clear that when invasive compartment pressure measurement is used to help make or confirm the diagnosis, decisions should not be based on an absolute pressure data point. A classic study has shown that when phosphorus nuclear magnetic resonance spectroscopy is used, muscle begins using anaerobic metabolism when related to inadequate oxygen delivery, not at an absolute pressure but at a pressure difference between the tissue pressure and mean arterial pressure, termed the delta.[46] This information has been well validated in a clinical study of tibial nailing. Using continuous pressure measurements during tibial nailing, patients who had a delta P of 30 mm Hg or greater did not experience compartment syndrome and did not require fasciotomy, whereas those with a delta P less than 30 mm Hg required fasciotomy. The delta P was calculated as a difference between diastolic blood pressure and compartment pressure.[47]

Once the diagnosis of compartment syndrome is made, fasciotomy continues to be the treatment of choice. In a cadaver study, a novel combined approach of transverse fasciotomies combined with a limited longitudinal dermatofasciotomy was shown to be as effective as a standard 16-cm longitudinal release in the anterior compartment.[48]

In a study of induced compartment syndromes in porcine hind limbs, the use of a compartment syndrome ultrafiltration catheter was shown to be able to reduce intramuscular pressures. These ultrafiltration catheters have the potential to be used prophylactically in patients at risk for developing acute compartment syndrome. Furthermore, sampling of the interstitial fluids may allow earlier diagnosis and treatment of acute compartment syndrome, whereas the reduction of interstitial fluids may prevent compartment syndrome from occurring.[49] Although much of this work is in preliminary stages, it shows great potential in allowing practitioners to alter the clinical course of compartment syndrome.

VAC has been shown to decrease the time to definitive wound closure or coverage of both the medial and lateral wounds with compartment release from an average of 6.7 days in the VAC group compared to 16.1 days in the control group. The difference was statistically significant.[50]

Summary

Advances continue in the understanding of the pathophysiology of soft-tissue wounds. These advances have allowed the clinician to alter some of the responses to injury and effect a better outcome for patients. The use of better débridement techniques, more effective irrigation agents and delivery systems, wound management techniques such as VAC therapy, more appropriate use of antibiotic and antibiotic beads, and use of fasciocutaneous flaps have all helped decrease complications and sequelae from severe injuries. Although research is in its early stages, ultrafiltration catheters show great promise in allowing clinicians to alter the course of compartment syndrome.

1: General Topics and New Technology

Annotated References

1. Nesti LJ, Jackson WM, Shanti RM, et al: Differentiation potential of multipotent progenitor cells derived from war-traumatized muscle tissue. *J Bone Joint Surg Am* 2008;90(11):2390-2398.

   The authors isolated mesenchymal progenitor cells from débrided human muscle tissue of war casualties. Reverse transcription chain polymerase reaction demonstrated the ability to differentiate into cell lines of bone and soft tissue.

2. Jackson WM, Aragon AB, Bulken-Hoover JD, Nesti LJ, Tuan RS: Putative heterotopic ossification progenitor cells derived from traumatized muscle. *J Orthop Res* 2009;27(12):1645-1651.

   The authors were able to generate bone tissue from isolated mesenchymal progenitor cells present on débrided muscle tissue from war casualties. These tissue studies provide clues as to how the heterotopic bone forms in war amputees.

3. Fackler ML: Misinterpretations concerning Larrey's methods of wound treatment. *Surg Gynecol Obstet* 1989;168(3):280-282.

4. Scully RE, Artiz CP, Sako Y: An evaluation of the surgeon's criteria for determining the viability of muscle during debridement. *Arch Surg* 1956;72:1031-1035.

5. Werner CM, Pierpont Y, Pollak AN: The urgency of surgical débridement in the management of open fractures. *J Am Acad Orthop Surg* 2008;16(7):369-375.

   The authors discuss the effects of emergent débridement of open fractures.

6. Crowley DJ, Kanakaris NK, Giannoudis PV: Debridement and wound closure of open fractures: The impact of the time factor on infection rates. *Injury* 2007;38:879-889.

   This review article discusses wound incision and excision (débridement) as well as the timing of wound closure. The authors found evidence supporting the "six-hour golden rule" for initial wound surgery to be limited, as well as unclear guidelines for the timing of surgical closure.

7. Reuss BL, Cole JD: Effect of delayed treatment on open tibial shaft fractures. *Am J Orthop* 2007;36:215-220.

   The authors present a retrospective review of 77 patients with 81 open tibia fractures treated with surgical débridement and stabilization at an average time of 13 hours from injury. The authors concluded that time was not a factor for nonunion or infection.

8. Werner CM, Pierpont Y, Pollak AN: The urgency of surgical debridement in the management of open fractures. *J Am Acad Orthop Surg* 2008;16:369-375.

   In this review article, the authors concluded that evidence supporting initial surgical treatment of open fractures within 6 hours from injury in comparison to 6 to 24 hours is limited. Additionally, the effect of delays beyond 24 hours is not clear.

9. Petrisor B, Jeray K, Schemitsch E, et al; FLOW Investigators: Fluid lavage in patients with open fracture wounds (FLOW): An international survey of 984 surgeons. *BMC Musculoskelet Disord* 2008;9:7.

   This study was a survey of AO faculty members and the Canadian Orthopaedic Association as to preferences for fluid use for irrigation of open wounds. Of those surveyed, most (70.4%) preferred normal saline.

10. Anglen JO: Comparison of soap and antibiotic solutions for irrigation of lower-limb open fracture wounds. A prospective, randomized study. *J Bone Joint Surg Am* 2005;87(7):1415-1422.

    The study is a prospective comparison of a bacitracin solution to a castile soap solution for irrigation of 400 patients with 458 open fractures. Wound healing problems occurred more frequently in the bacitracin group than in the castile group ($P = 0.3$). There was no significant difference between the two groups with regard to infection or fracture healing.

11. Svoboda SJ, Bice TG, Gooden HA, Brooks DE, Thomas DB, Wenke JC: Comparison of bulb syringe and pulsed lavage irrigation with use of a bioluminescent musculoskeletal wound model. *J Bone Joint Surg Am* 2006;88(10):2167-2174.

    Bioluminescent *Pseudomonas* species were counted after bulb and pulse lavage irrigation using a goat model. Pulsed lavage reduced the bacteria by 70% and the bulb syringe by 51% at 9 L. Both methods also showed significant reduction of the bacterial count from 6 to 9 L irrigation.

12. Lineaweaver W, McMorris S, Soucy D, Howard R: Cellular and bacterial toxicities of topical antimicrobials. *Plast Reconstr Surg* 1985;75:394-396.

13. Crowley DJ, Kanakaris NK, Giannoudis PV: Irrigation of the wounds in open fractures. *J Bone Joint Surg Br* 2007;89(5):580-585.

    In this review article, the authors concluded that normal saline is an effective irrigant for open fractures with regard to cost and treatment. Use of other irrigants or additives does not appear to enhance the ability to decontaminate a wound.

14. Rajasekaran S, Dheenadhayalan J, Babu JN, Sundararajan SR, Venkatramani H, Sabapathy SR: Immediate primary skin closure in type III A and B open fractures: Results after a minimum of five years. *J Bone Joint Surg Br* 2009;9:217-224.

    The authors selected 153 of 557 Gustilo-Anderson type IIIA or IIIB open tibia fractures for primary closure using strict criteria, which included débridement within 12 hours of injury, no sewage or organic contamination, no primary or secondary skin loss during débridement, a Ganga Hospital open injury skin score of 1 or 2 with a total score of 10 or less, bleeding skin margins, the ability to approximate wound edges without tension, and the absence of peripheral vascular disease.

15. Rajasekaran S, Dheenadhayalan J, Babu JN, Sundararajan SR, Venkatramani H, Sabapathy SR: Immediate primary skin closure in type-III A and B open fractures: Results after a minimum of five years. *J Bone Joint Surg Br* 2009;91(2):217-224.

    The authors prospectively evaluated 185 patients with Gustilo-Anderson type IIIA fractures who had closure of the wounds at the time of initial surgery. There were 33 complications in 23 patients, including deep infection in 5 and superficial infection in 10.

16. Brumback RJ, Jones AL: Interobserver agreement in the classification of open fractures of the tibia: The results of a survey of two hundred forty-five orthopaedic surgeons. *J Bone Joint Surg Am* 1994;76:1162-1166.

17. Bowen TR, Widmaier JC: Host classification predicts infection after open fracture. *Clin Orthop Relat Res* 2005;433:205-211.

    In this retrospective review, there were 174 patients with open fractures classified as having host immune capability. The authors found an increased rate of infection when immune capability was decreased, as well as in the presence of other variables such as tobacco use, severity of fracture, and fracture location. Evidence-based guidelines support the prompt use of first-generation cephalosporins to reduce the infection rate. There is no clear evidence to support the initial use of aminoglycosides or antibiotics specifically for the clostridial species.

18. Hauser CJ, Adams CA Jr, Eachempati SR; Council of the Surgical Infection Society: Surgical Infection Society guideline: prophylactic antibiotic use in open fractures: An evidence-based guideline. *Surg Infect* 2006;7(4):379-405.

    This evidence-based medicine review on the use of antibiotics with open fractures demonstrates there is insufficient evidence to make strong recommendations concerning any extensive treatment regimen. The authors recommend a short course of first-generation cephalosporins given as soon as possible after injury.

19. Holtom PD: Antibiotic prophylaxis: Current recommendations. *J Am Acad Orthop Surg* 2006;14:S98-S100.

    This review article provides a brief overview of both the prophylactic use of antibiotics and the treatment of infections with antibiotics, along with current recommendations for the use of antibiotics in fracture care.

20. Bhattacharyya T, Mehta P, Smith M, Pomahac B: Routine use of wound vacuum-assisted closure does not allow coverage delay for open tibia fractures. *Plast Reconstr Surg* 2008;121(4):1263-1266.

    The authors found a 57% infection rate in open tibia fracture treated in a delayed fashion with NPWT and a flap, compared with 10% in the early flap group.

21. Bosse MJ, MacKenzie EJ, Kellam JF, et al: An analysis of outcomes of reconstruction or amputation after leg-threatening injuries. *N Engl J Med* 2002;347(24):1924-1931.

22. Harry LE, Sandison A, Paleolog EM, Hansen U, Pearse MF, Nanchahal J: Comparison of the healing of open tibial fractures covered with either muscle or fasciocutaneous tissue in a murine model. *J Orthop Res* 2008;26(9):1238-1244.

    Using an animal model, fracture healing using either a muscle flap or fasciocutaneous flap was studied, along with vascular density after application of both types of flaps.

23. Ostermann PA, Seligson D, Henry SL: Local antibiotic therapy for severe open fractures. A review of 1085 consecutive cases. *J Bone Joint Surg Br* 1995;77(1):93-97.

24. Decoster TA, Bozorgnia S: Antibiotic beads. *J Am Acad Orthop Surg* 2008;16(11):674-678.

    Indications and contraindications, specific characteristics, and surgical technique for antibiotic beads are discussed.

25. Wright BA, Roberts CS, Seligson D, Malkani AL, McCabe SJ: Cost of antibiotic beads is justified: A study of open fracture wounds and chronic osteomyelitis. *J Long Term Eff Med Implants* 2007;17(3):181-185.

    The authors present a retrospective review of 125 patients with open fractures and 16 patients with chronic osteomyelitis treated with antibiotic beads followed for an average of 30 weeks (minimum 6 weeks). At last follow-up, the infection rate was 3.2% for the open fracture group and 25% for the osteomyelitis group.

26. Beardmore AA, Brooks DE, Wenke JC, Thomas DB: Effectiveness of local antibiotic delivery with an osteoinductive and osteoconductive bone-graft substitute. *J Bone Joint Surg Am* 2005;87(1):107-112.

    Using a Spanish goat animal model with a colonized tibia defect, the authors found that the use of tobramycin-impregnated calcium sulfate mixed with demineralized bone matrix did not result in positive cultures after 21 days. In comparison, goats with demineralized bone matrix alone did develop infection in seven of eight cases. Level of evidence: I.

27. Wenke JC, Owens BD, Svoboda SJ, Brooks DE: Effectiveness of commercially-available antibiotic-impregnated implants. *J Bone Joint Surg Br* 2006;88(8):1102-1104.

    Using this Spanish goat animal model with an inoculated tibial defect, the authors had four treatment groups: no treatment, handmade tobramycin PMMA beads, commercially available tobramycin-impregnated calcium sulfate pellets, and commercially available tobramycin-PMMA beads. The authors found all antibiotic substances prevented infection at day 21.

28. Henry SL, Ostermann PA, Seligson D: The antibiotic bead pouch technique: The management of severe compound fractures. *Clin Orthop Relat Res* 1993;295:54-64.

29. Henry SL, Ostermann PA, Seligson D: The prophylactic use of antibiotic impregnated beads in open fractures. *J Trauma* 1990;30:1231-1238.

1: General Topics and New Technology

30. Pollak AN: Use of negative pressure wound therapy with reticulated open cell foam for lower extremity trauma. *J Orthop Trauma* 2008;22(10, Suppl):S142-S145.

    The use of NPWT in the treatment of lower extremity trauma is reviewed.

31. Dedmond BT, Kortesis B, Punger K, et al: The use of negative-pressure wound therapy (NPWT) in the temporary treatment of soft-tissue injuries associated with high-energy open tibial shaft fractures. *J Orthop Trauma* 2007;21(1):11-17.

    The authors of this study found that 10 of 24 fractures initially classified as type IIIB eventually did not need a free or rotational flap. Infection and nonunion rates with the use of NPWT were similar to historical controls.

32. Dedmond BT, Kortesis B, Punger K, et al: Subatmospheric pressure dressings in the temporary treatment of soft tissue injuries associated with type III open tibial shaft fractures in children. *J Pediatr Orthop* 2006;26(6):728-732.

    The authors found a 50% decrease in the need for rotational or free flaps from the initial classification of the fracture.

33. Stannard JP, Voglas DA, Stewart R, McGwin G, Alonso JE. Negative pressure wound therapy after severe open fractures: A prospective randomized study. *J Orthop Trauma* 2009;23:552-557.

    The authors found that control patients with standard wound care had a deep infection rate of 28%, whereas patients who received NPWT treatment had a 5.4% infection rate. For open tibia fractures, the same trend continued, with a 36% infection rate for controls and 8% in the NPWT group.

34. Pollak AN, Powell ET, Fang R, Cooper EO, Ficke JR, Flaherty SF: Use of negative pressure wound therapy during aeromedical evacuation of patients with combat related blast injuries. *J Surg Orthop Adv* 2010;19(1):44-48.

    The authors found a very low rate of complications associated with NPWT in use during aeromedical evacuation.

35. Timmers MS, Graafland N, Bernards AT, Nelissen RG, van Dissel JT, Jukema GN: Negative pressure wound treatment with polyvinyl alcohol foam and polyhexanide antiseptic solution instillation in posttraumatic osteomyelitis. *Wound Repair Regen* 2009;17(2):278-286.

    The authors found that with this technique there was a 10% recurrence rate of osteomyelitis and with standard care it was 58.5%. In addition, there was a decrease in the number of surgical interventions needed to eradicate the infection.

36. Labler L, Rancan M, Mica L, Härter L, Mihic-Probst D, Keel M: Vacuum-assisted closure therapy increases local interleukin-8 and vascular endothelial growth factor levels in traumatic wounds. *J Trauma* 2009;66(3):749-757.

    In this prospective randomized study of wounds treated with NPWT, significantly higher levels of IL-8 and VEGF were noted and were thought to induce angiogenesis.

37. Scherer SS, Pietramaggiori G, Mathews JC, Prsa MJ, Huang S, Orgill DP: The mechanism of action of the vacuum-assisted closure device. *Plast Reconstr Surg* 2008;122(3):786-797.

    In this study on mice immunohistiochemical staging systems, bases on blood vessel density (CD31) and cell proliferation (Ki67) were used to determine that the foam was responsible for the endothelial growth while the negative pressure was responsible for the cell proliferation.

38. Föhn M, Bannasch H: Artificial skin. *Methods Mol Med* 2007;140:167-182.

    This article provides an excellent review of the history of skin substitutes.

39. Brusselaers N, Lafaire C, Ortiz S, Jacquemin D, Monstrey S: The consensus of the surgical treatment of burn injuries in Belgium. *Acta Chir Belg* 2008;108(6):645-650.

    This consensus statement of the Belgian Association of Burn Injuries noted the trends in massive skin loss, the new (often expensive) techniques that have been commercialized, and the wide variety of treatment modalities.

40. Schurr MJ, Foster KN, Centanni JM, et al: Phase I/II clinical evaluation of StrataGraft: A consistent, pathogen-free human skin substitute. *J Trauma* 2009;66(3):866-873, discussion 873-874.

    The authors of this phase I/II clinical evaluation showed that a commercial skin graft substitute was comparable to cadaver allograft skin, but without the infection risks.

41. Haslik W, Kamolz LP, Manna F, Hladik M, Rath T, Frey M. Management of full-thickness skin defects in the hand and wrist region: First long-term experiences with the dermal matrix Matriderm. *J Plast Reconstr Aesthet Surg* 2010;63(2)360-364.

    The authors of this study found that the use of Matriderm (a bovine-based collagen I, II, V, and elastin hydrolysate-based dermal substitute) led to no limitations in hand function and produces excellent hand function as measured by DASH-scores.

42. Helgeson MD, Potter BK, Evans KN, Shawen SB: Bioartificial dermal substitute: A preliminary report on its use for the management of complex combat-related soft tissue wounds. *J Orthop Trauma* 2007;21(6):394-399.

    The authors found excellent results with the use of a bioartificial dermal substitute for covering exposed tendon and bone in a military population. Fifteen of 16 wounds were successfully treated with this technique.

43. Ulmer T: The clinical diagnosis of compartment syndrome of the lower leg: Are clinical findings predictive of the disorder? *J Orthop Trauma* 2002;16(8):572-577.

This review of published studies in the English literature on compartment syndrome of the lower leg determined the specificity, sensitivity, and the positive and negative predictive value of clinical indicators of compartment syndrome.

44. Wiemann JM, Ueno T, Leek BT, Yost WT, Schwartz AK, Hargens AR: Noninvasive measurements of intramuscular pressure using pulsed phase-locked loop ultrasound for detecting compartment syndromes: A preliminary report. *J Orthop Trauma* 2006;20(7):458-463.

The authors developed a human model for compartment tamponade and tested the use of an ultrasonic pulsed phase-locked loop fascial displacement waveform analysis for the measurement of intramuscular pressure.

45. Kakar S, Firoozabadi R, McKean J, Tornetta P III: Diastolic blood pressure in patients with tibia fractures under anaesthesia: Implications for the diagnosis of compartment syndrome. *J Orthop Trauma* 2007;21(2): 99-103.

A prospective cohort with a consecutive series of 242 patients with a tibia fracture undergoing intramedullary nailing under general anesthesia were studied with regard to preoperative, intraoperative, and postoperative diastolic blood pressure. They found a predictable response of diastolic blood pressure in these patients and noted that the preoperative diastolic blood pressure is a good indicator of postoperative diastolic blood pressure and that this number should be used to calculate the delta P during routine intramedullary nailing.

46. Heppenstall RB, Sapega AA, Scott R, et al: The compartment syndrome: An experimental and clinical study of muscular energy metabolism using phosphorus nuclear resonance spectroscopy. *Clin Orthop Relat Res* 1988;226:138-155.

47. McQueen MM, Christie J, Court-Brown CM: Compartment pressure monitoring in tibia fractures. *J Bone Joint Surg Br* 1996;78:99-104.

48. Teng AL, Huang JI, Wilber RG, Wilber JH: Treatment of compartment syndrome: Transverse fasciotomy as an adjunct to longitudinal dermatofasciotomy. An in vitro study. *J Orthop Trauma* 2005;19(7):442-447.

The authors performed a cadaver study to determine the efficacy of a transverse fasciotomy incision to decrease compartment pressures in comparison with the standard two-incision fasciotomy.

49. Odland R, Schmidt AH, Hunter B, et al: Use of tissue ultrafiltration for treatment of compartment syndrome: A pilot study using porcine hindlimbs. *J Orthop Trauma* 2005;19(4):267-275.

Using an animal compartment syndrome model, the use of an ultrafiltration catheter was studied for its ability to remove interstitial fluid and effect a reduction in compartment pressure.

50. Yang CC, Chang DS, Webb LX: Vacuum-assisted closure for fasciotomy wounds following compartment syndrome of the leg. *J Surg Orthop Adv* 2006;15(1): 19-23.

The authors evaluated the efficacy of vacuum-assisted management of traumatic fasciotomy wounds in a matched series of 34 patients with or without use of a VAC. Those managed with the VAC yielded a definitive time to closure of 6.7 days, compared to a control group with an average time to closure of 16.1 days.

1: General Topics and New Technology

Chapter 7

The Mangled Lower Extremity

James R. Ficke, MD   Lisa K. Cannada, MD

Introduction

Estimates of the frequency of limb-threatening lower extremity injuries range from 15,000 to 35,000 patients annually.[1] These injuries are among the most severe that orthopaedic surgeons will encounter and certainly can be among the most difficult to treat, requiring clear evaluation of the overall patient and the individual severity of injury and a candid assessment of capabilities of both the surgeon and facility involved in the care of these patients. Although the graphic severity of these injuries can be distracting, the patient with limb-threatening injuries often also has sustained severe systemic trauma that can be life threatening (**Figures 1 and 2**). The principles of advanced trauma life support and overall trauma resuscitation are paramount and must take precedence over attempts at limb salvage or complex surgical procedures. Several studies over the past two decades have attempted to address, in a logical fashion, algorithms directed at guiding treatment.

Patient Characteristics

Patients with devastating lower extremity injuries are by definition high-energy trauma patients. The largest prospective study published to date evaluating high-energy lower extremity trauma, the Lower Extremity Assessment Project (LEAP) study, characterizes the patient population experiencing these injuries.[1] Although there is no single "typical" mangled extremity injury, the injury spectrum involves severe damage to bone and soft tissue, as well as compromise of circulation or extremity perfusion, neurologic injury, and, commonly, severe contamination. The pathway to success in initial management is to recognize the severity of the injury, identify associated injuries requiring priority treatment, and understand patient factors contributing to success along any chosen pathway.

In the LEAP study, the investigators have shown that the most significant prognostic factors for outcomes of limb salvage or amputation were not related to injury severity or type of treatment (limb salvage or amputation). These factors included low educational level (noncompletion of high school), a household income below poverty level, nonwhite racial background, lack of insurance, poor social support network, low self-efficacy, smoking history, or pending injury litigation.[2,3] At 7 years, outcomes of the amputation and limb salvage groups demonstrated very little difference, with both groups reporting more than 40% of patients with severe disability.[4]

Another population with a historically high risk for amputation is patients with popliteal arterial injury. According to a 2006 study, 1,395 patients were identified in the National Trauma Data Bank as having popliteal artery injury.[5] Of these patients, 61% sustained blunt trauma and 39% experienced penetrating trauma. With an overall amputation rate of 14.5%, 18% of patients with blunt injury and 9% of those with penetrating injury had subsequent limb loss. Popliteal arterial injuries were associated with venous injury in 24% of patients, tibia fracture in 46%, femur fracture in 25%, and knee dislocation in 20%. Additionally, 49% of patients underwent fasciotomy for compartment syndrome. Patients with a penetrating injury appeared to have more successful vascular restoration whereas those with blunt injury had less frequently successful reconstructive surgery. Twenty-one percent of patients with associated femur fractures and 20% with associated tibia fractures underwent amputation, but most significant was the finding that blunt injury with fracture and popliteal injury was 2.5 times more likely to result in amputation than a penetrating injury with similar fracture.[5]

Combat-Related Injury

Patients injured during combat sustain multiple injuries nearly 100% of the time, and these injuries are quite often the result of high-energy trauma. A mangled extremity in combat often can be caused by an explosion (**Figure 3**), a gunshot wound or other penetrating injury, and, less commonly, road or traffic accidents,

Dr. Ficke or an immediate family member serves as a board member, owner, officer, or committee member of American Orthopaedic Foot and Ankle Society, Society of Military Orthopaedic Surgeons, and Extremity War Trauma Research Foundation. Dr. Cannada or an immediate family member serves as a board member, owner, officer, or committee member of Orthopaedic Trauma Association; is a member of a speakers' bureau or has made paid presentations on behalf of Smith & Nephew; and has received research or institutional support from Zimmer, Synthes, DePuy, and Smith & Nephew.

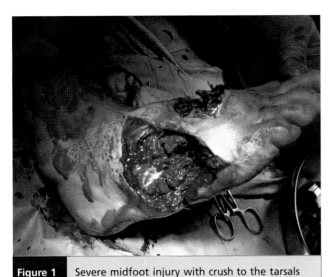

Figure 1 Severe midfoot injury with crush to the tarsals and loss of perfusion to the forefoot.

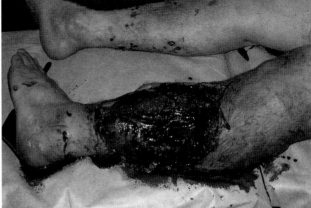

Figure 2 Mid-distal tibia fracture with extensive bone loss and soft-tissue destruction, and gross contamination but isolated injury. Initial débridement, external fixation, and serial assessment are safe alternatives when the patient tolerates them and is able to participate in decision making.

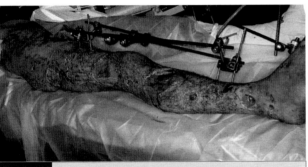

Figure 3 Common appearance of an explosion injury. Multiple soft-tissue injuries with contamination are seen. Each skin violation should be individually assessed but may not require formal excision or débridement. Bridging external fixation stabilizes a periarticular fracture for evacuation and definitive management.

crush injuries, or falls. Patients injured during combat present a challenge to medical care providers because of the high number of patients sustaining these types of severe injuries. As many as 82% of all injured military personnel evacuated from current conflicts have sustained at least one extremity injury.[6] Of these patients, approximately 21% had open fractures, and therefore limb salvage or amputation may be possible. These open injuries are often highly contaminated and associated with neurologic and vascular injuries (Figure 3), requiring massive débridement and damage control techniques for stabilization before the patient is evacuated from the area of combat and transported to the United States for extended care.

Decision Making

In the initial assessment, the physician must quickly evaluate the patient's overall condition, including he-

modynamic status and overall health. As with any polytrauma patient, the fundamentals of acute severe hemorrhage, airway patency, breathing, and circulation are first priority. A secondary survey includes a thorough assessment of the contralateral limb as well as other associated injuries. The graphic severity of the mangled extremity often draws providers' attention, and associated injuries with more ominous prognosis may be missed. Evaluation and primary management of life-threatening injuries should occur before treatment of the severely injured limb. Recent studies documenting early prehospital use of tourniquets in the face of devastating limb injury clearly show higher survival rates.[7,8] At this point, during the secondary survey, an assessment of the injury personality by surgeons experienced with general trauma, orthopaedics, vascular surgery, and plastic surgery should be done. Soft-tissue considerations including coverage requirements, contamination, perfusion, and neurologic status are evaluated and documented. The pattern of bony injury is likewise important, with grade III B and C fracture patterns having higher complication rates and association with amputation. When the patient's overall condition and mental status allow a medical history to be obtained, an assessment of preinjury health status as well as function can be determined.

One of the earliest decisions to be made when evaluating a mangled extremity is the urgency of management. Often, associated injuries, ongoing hemorrhage, or coagulopathy may necessitate emergent amputation as a life-saving procedure. In these circumstances expeditious débridement and damage control techniques are advised. However, in a stable patient with a perfused limb, definitive decisions about limb salvage or amputation can be delayed until the patient and family members are counseled on the relative advantages and possible disadvantages associated with each option. A frank, informative discussion with the patient and family is nearly always beneficial for acceptance of the treatment plan and ultimate outcome of function. A delay in decision making also may enable the patient to be transferred to a center where limb salvage is performed regularly by experienced surgeons. Whenever possible, specialists in vascular and plastic surgery, as well as orthopaedic partners, should be consulted during decision making. Factors to consider before a staged amputation include restoration of alignment, stability, perfusion, and reduction of gross contamination. Only one study has reported criteria for absolute indications for amputation.[9] These criteria included total or near total leg amputation or complete confirmed tibial or sciatic nerve transection. Other reported recommendations have included nonreconstructable vascular injury or ischemia time over 6 hours, devastating unreconstructable soft-tissue loss, or a life-threatening triad of hypothermia, coagulopathy, and hypovolemia in the face of a mangled extremity with exsanguinating hemorrhage. A relatively strong indication for amputation historically has been complete tibial nerve transection observed during surgical exploration. According to a 2005 study, there was no significant difference in outcomes in the LEAP population when plantar sensation was impaired.[10] A subset of the LEAP population (55 patients with insensate lower extremities: 26 underwent amputation and 29 underwent salvage) was compared with a matched cohort of 29 sensate salvage patients, and equivalent outcomes were demonstrated after 24 months. The three groups were compared using social, psychosocial, and occupational measures. Furthermore, the insensate salvage group recovered intact sensation in 67%, and only one patient in the entire group had persistent absent sensation. The study results refuted previous studies recommending absent foot sensation as an absolute indication for amputation.[9]

Presently, sensation of the foot does not appear to affect functional outcome and therefore should not serve as a primary indication for amputation. Several prognostic scoring systems have been described and are detailed in the next section. Ultimately, the decision for limb salvage or amputation is based on assessment of the patient and the injury, along with the surgeon's capabilities and the patient's preinjury function and choice whenever possible.

Limb Salvage Scores

The goal of a fracture classification system is to be able to communicate in a universal language with other surgeons and provide information regarding treatment and prognosis. In a patient with a mangled lower extremity, the ability to guide treatment, whether limb salvage or amputation, and provide a prognosis is ideal. The decision to amputate or to salvage a limb remains challenging. A patient with a mangled lower extremity may have other injuries, severe soft-tissue damage, and medical comorbidities. In addition, the social background and economic status of the patient influence the outcome, and this information is not included in any scoring system.

Although there are several existing scoring systems,[11-15] their validity has not been thoroughly evaluated. Only one has been evaluated prospectively.[12] Ideally, the scoring system for limb salvage would have a high sensitivity; that is, all patients with amputated limbs would have scores at or above the threshold.[16] With high specificity, all patients with salvaged limbs would have scores below the threshold.[16] It is impossible to have 100% sensitivity and specificity. Many factors are not included in the scoring systems regarding other injuries to the patient, such as preexisting medical conditions, quality of surgical débridements and treatment of the fracture, resuscitation requirements, and morbidities of the trauma that may contribute to the outcome. Patients with severe injuries should be transferred to a center capable of handling the treatment and complications that can occur with a mangled extremity. In addition, the availability of plastic surgeons, or others skilled in microvascular tissue transfer, may be crucial to the outcome in providing essential soft-tissue coverage in a timely fashion.

Another factor to consider with the scoring systems is that most indices are based on points assigned to factors beyond the physician's direct control, such as patient age, mechanism of injury, contamination, and specifics of the injury. A surgeon has no control over the energy of injury, the severity of the fracture, and accompanying injury to the muscle, soft tissue, nerve, and blood vessels. However, the surgeon does have some control over the time to reperfusion with a vascular injury, minimizing the warm ischemia time. Surgeons also have some control over shock in that they can regulate fluids and resuscitation, which may also affect the outcome. The scoring systems do not account for the duration of shock, often using a single systolic blood pressure reading.

The most commonly used lower extremities scoring systems include the Mangled Extremity Severity Score (MESS),[11,12] the Predictive Salvage Index (PSI),[13] the Limb Salvage Index (LSI),[14] the Nerve Injury, Ischemia, Soft-Tissue Injury, Skeletal Injury, Shock, and Age of Patient Score (NISSSA),[15] and the Hannover Fracture Scale-97 (HFS-97).[17,18] The scoring systems vary in terms of the scored items, timing of scoring (in the emergency department in comparison with the operating room) and the introduction of bias. The scoring systems were derived from small studies conducted at single institutions, and there is significant difficulty extrapolating the results elsewhere. The MESS is perhaps the most well-known index, assigning points for age, shock, mechanism of injury, and limb ischemia (**Table 1**). A score of 7 or higher is the cutoff point for proceeding with amputation. Only two of the scored variables in the MESS (hypotension, ischemia time) are under the physician's control. Treatment variables are not

Table 1

The Mangled Extremity Severity Score of Points

Age (years)	Points
< 30	0
30-50	1
> 50	2
Shock	**Points**
Systolic blood pressure > 90	0
Transient hypotension	1
Persistent hypotension	2
Extremity Injury	**Points**
Low energy	1
Medium energy	2
High-energy crush	3
High-energy contamination	4
Limb Ischemia	**Points**
Normal perfusion	0
Pulseless, paresthesias	1
Cool, paralyzed	2

accounted for. The benefits of this scoring system are that it is simple and the information needed for scoring is available at the time of the initial evaluation.

The LSI comprised a retrospective study of 70 limbs with an arterial injury and was based on the injury to the skin, muscle, bone, nerve, vein, and artery and on the warm ischemia time. Of the 70 limbs, 51 were salvaged. All limbs that had a score lower than 6 had a 100% salvage rate, and a score greater than or equal to 6 resulted in amputation.[14] However, this scoring system requires extensive evaluation in the operating room, and it can be difficult to apply in the acute evaluation of the injury.

The NISSSA, a modification of the MESS, was a review of 24 patients with grade III injuries. Emphasis was placed on loss of plantar sensation, and greater weight was placed on soft-tissue and skeletal injury. This scoring system is more sensitive and specific than the MESS in predicting amputation.[15]

The PSI was used in patients who had both an orthopaedic and a vascular injury. In this study, 21 limbs were retrospectively studied to determine the factors affecting the salvage risk of amputation. The score was weighted to the level of vascular injury and the degree of bone, muscle, and soft-tissue injury.[13]

The HFS-97 fracture scale was initially developed to identify the risk factors for injury complications in lower extremity high-energy trauma in 1983. It was evaluated retrospectively on 182 open upper and lower extremity fractures, and then prospectively applied. The scoring system encompasses 8 domains, ranging from 0 to 22 points. The cutoff point for amputation

was 11 or higher, and the scoring system was found to have a high positive predictive value (specificity of 0.99).[17,18]

The five scoring systems have been significantly critiqued over the years, specifically regarding subjective assessment of each scoring system and the inability to obtain the same results. The LEAP authors could not validate the clinical utility of any of the five scoring systems they evaluated for a mangled extremity.[16] They also examined whether the five scoring systems would be useful for predicting functional outcome in a subgroup of 407 subjects. None of the scoring systems were useful for predicting outcome as measured at 6 and 24 months in the physical or psychosocial domain of the Sickness Impact Profile (SIP).[19] Overall, authors have concluded that the scoring systems should not be sole criterion on which an amputation decision is based and should not be used to predict outcomes.[16,20]

Functional Outcomes: Limb Salvage Compared With Amputation

In the patient with a mangled extremity, treatment decisions should be made as soon as possible. Because the scoring systems are of limited value, other factors including age, whether the patient smokes, social support, educational level, and preexisting medical conditions have been shown to be important in affecting outcome. Prior to the LEAP study, many articles reporting the results of limb salvage versus amputation were often small cases series. Such studies provide some basis for decision making, but the choice of amputation or reconstruction is a complex decision affected by a multitude of factors.

There have been advances in wound care over the past decade with vacuum-assisted closure (Kinetic Concepts International, San Antonio, TX). In addition, with the multiple disciplines available to both the civilian and military populations and advances in prosthetic design, there may be a push to attempt limb salvage. Just because the means exist does not mean the outcome will be worth the attempt. In evaluating patients with mangled extremities, 92% of patients at initial surgery were in favor of limb salvage over amputation. It has been reported that failure after limb salvage was worse than initial amputation, and that 75% of those patients wished they had elected early amputation.[21,22]

It has been reported that the result of limb salvage in patients with tibia fractures accompanied by vascular injury was nearly always worse than the result of early amputation, leaving the patient with what is now referred to as the 3 Ds: demoralized, divorced, or destitute.[23] The LEAP study prospectively compared the outcomes of patients who underwent amputation versus limb salvage. The hypothesis was that patients with amputation would have a better functional outcome than limb-reconstruction patients. Several evaluations were completed, including the SIP as a primary out-

Table 2

Demographic, Social, and Economic Variables That Affect Lower Extremity Injury Outcomes

Age

15 to 45 years	More likely to screen positive for psychological disorder
Older than 45 years	At 7-year follow-up, 64% patients were older than 45 years; association with poor outcome increases with age

Sex

Female	Other studies support women more likely to have depression, psychological stress, sexual dysfunction

Race

Nonwhite	Poorer outcomes at 2 and 7 years no matter what treatment option chosen (limb salvage versus amputation); more likely to lack health insurance; less likely to have completed high school

Poverty status (per US Census Bureau definition)

Poor households	More likely to have a poorer outcome at 2- and 7-year follow-up; more likely to be associated with having a psychological disorder

Health insurance

Insured	More likely to undergo a delayed amputation

Smokers

Current smokers	Poor outcomes at both 2- and 7-year follow-up (independent of treatment option)
Current and former smokers	Rate of nonunion and infection is increased
Limited social support	More likely to have a psychological disorder Associated with psychological distress Poorer SIP score at 2 years

Education

Lower educational level	Poorer outcome on SIP scores at 2 and 7 years; likely psychological disorder in those at lower educational levels
Personality	Decrease in extroversion was noted at 2-year follow-up through NEO Five-Factor Inventory
Workers' compensation	Poorer result at both 2 and 7 years independent of treatment group
Involvement with legal system	Poorer result at both 2 and 7 years independent of treatment group

1: General Topics and New Technology

come measurement and the NEO Five-Factor Inventory for personality disorders. Overall, patients undergoing amputation rather than reconstruction had a similar SIP outcome.[1] However, several characteristics were identified as predictors of poor SIP scores. Some of these factors may be controlled, whereas others may be able to be addressed with programs/referrals in the hospital. Factors associated with a poor SIP score included rehospitalization for complication, lower educational level, poverty, lack of health insurance, a poor social support network, low self-efficacy, smoking, and involvement in workers' compensation litigation[1,3,24] (Table 2). Interestingly, those with health insurance were more likely to undergo a delayed amputation.[24] However, a delayed amputation can result in more hospitalizations and can contribute to mortality.

The hypothesis that amputation will be a better outcome was not substantiated at 2 or 7 years.[2,4] In those patients with limb salvage, there was an increased num-

ber of hospitalizations and complications. Both the limb salvage and the amputation groups had complications. In the amputation group, the revision amputation rate was 5.4%, and wound infection in the early period (3 months) was the most common complication (34.2%).[25] In the limb salvage group, 3.9% required late amputations. The limb salvage patients had complications of nonunion (31%), wound infection (23.2%), and osteomyelitis (8.6%).[25]

In those patients who undergo amputation, there are additional factors to consider, including timing and level of amputation and the total cost of care in comparison with limb salvage. Patients tend to be less satisfied when the decision to amputate is delayed. Amputation should be considered a reconstructive surgery to improve patient function. The soft-tissue coverage and/or closure options may not always be typical. The LEAP study found that atypical soft-tissue coverage options did not worsen results of below-knee amputation.[26] Thus, because there may be injured soft tissue and lack of soft tissue for a desired approach toward a below-knee amputation, the lowest possible level of amputation should be attempted before proceeding higher because good results can be obtained. The LEAP study found that both patients and physicians were less satisfied with through-knee amputations.[26] Amputation should be performed at the lowest level to preserve function.[27]

The return to work (RTW) rate for patients in both groups in the LEAP study at 2 and 7 years was low, at fewer than 50% of the patients who underwent reconstruction and 53% of the patients who underwent amputation.[4] The authors found higher rates of RTW in patients who were younger, Caucasian, nonsmokers, of average to high self-efficacy, and with preinjury job tenure, higher job involvement, and no pending litigation.[24] Patients with unilateral injuries were found to have a better chance of returning to work than those with bilateral limb-threatening trauma.[28] It is important to understand these factors and try to develop programs to address RTW as that contributes to the overall burden of the trauma to society.[29]

The LEAP authors found projected lifetime health care costs for amputees to be three times higher than for those who underwent limb salvage ($509,275 compared with $163,282).[30] The ability to obtain a prosthesis can be quite difficult for patients with limited resources. In addition, physicians may want to prescribe the most technologically advanced prosthesis to maximize patient function, but this availability may be limited even in patients with insurance.

Both limb salvage patients and amputees require physical therapy to maximize outcome.[31] When analyzing both groups, gait difficulties initially can be expected during recovery. In those patients who undergo limb salvage, reduced walking speed and gait deviation lead to impaired mobility.[32] Decreased ankle range of motion and knee flexion strength and nonreciprocal stair climbing were associated with impaired mobility.[33] This information can be useful when planning rehabilitation protocols.

Functional Outcomes in the Military Population

As of June 2009, there had been more than 875 major limb amputations in a population of more than 15,000 military personnel evacuated from Iraq or Afghanistan.[34] The injuries have been well described, as have the management strategies for this special population.[35] The significance of this review lies in the application of social, psychological, and occupational interventions, and very low inclusion of the negative prognostic factors from the LEAP population. RTW rates have been described for amputees and are related to seniority in military service, military specialty, and amputation level. Overall, RTW rates in the military for a single-limb amputee are approximately 22% for transtibial amputation and 18% for transfemoral amputation.

Clinical Practice Considerations

The LEAP study is a model in multicenter research studies. It is important to realize that personnel familiar with the treatment of these injuries were present at all participating centers. Thus, the best of all possible resources and experience was available to treat these injuries.

Surgeon-controlled variables were evaluated in the treatment of the limb-threatening open tibia fractures (type III). From the LEAP study, a cohort of 156 patients treated with an external fixator (as a definitive treatment) was evaluated regarding the timing to débridement, soft-tissue coverage, and bone graft placement along with the techniques used in the limb salvage procedure.[36] Timing of débridement did not affect the outcome. The timing of the soft-tissue coverage was thought to be predictive of infection but not subsequent complications, and it did not affect the outcome. For patients who required bone graft placement, the timing of this intervention did not affect the outcome. The patients who were treated with an external fixator had more surgical procedures, took a longer time than those treated with an intramedullary nail to achieve full weight bearing, and had more readmissions to the hospital for treatment of infection and nonunion. The authors found that the patients undergoing external fixation who also had a muscle flap for wound coverage had more physical impairment and worse functional outcomes than patients who had an amputation.[36] Definitive treatment with an external fixator instead of an intramedullary nail contributed to a worse outcome in comparison with other treatments.

The outcome of a vascular repair is closely related to total ischemic time. In combat-related extremity vascular injuries, good results have been reported with a temporary vascular shunt (TVS). In a 2008 study, 37 combat patients with 73 major vascular injuries were explored; 26 TVSs were placed in 18 patients; 3 vessels were primarily repaired, and 44 vessels were ligated. Twenty-two shunts were patent upon arrival to a center capable of completing revascularization procedures, and all shunt patients survived their injuries with limb preservation at short-term follow-up.[37] In a case control report of extremity injuries, the amputation-free survival rate at a mean of 22 months was 78% and 77% in the TVS patients and in the control group, respectively.[38] The use of a TVS may be advantageous in damage control orthopaedics in the combat situation, based on these results. TVS use in civilian trauma has application in certain instances, such as a damage control technique and maintaining limb perfusion to allow stabilization of the fracture. A 2008 study reviewed 10-year experience of the use of TVS at a Level 1 trauma center, reporting the results of 67 patients with 101 shunts. The thrombosis rate was 5%, amputation rate 18%, survival rate 88%, and overall limb/patient survival rate 73%[39] (**Figure 4**). Temporary vascular shunting can play an important role in specific instances of limb salvage with good results. In mangled

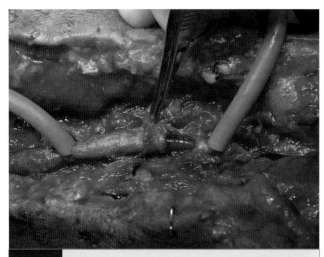

Figure 4 Placement of a TVS permits perfusion while more urgent procedures or resuscitation can be completed.

extremities, wound coverage with a flap is often done when soft-tissue coverage is needed. In the LEAP study, 190 patients with 195 limbs required flap coverage, with 88 limbs treated with rotational flaps and 107 limbs treated with a free flap.[40] There were complications in 53 of the flap procedures (27%), and 46 of the 53 complications required additional surgical treatment. The Injury Severity Score was significantly higher in the patients requiring a free flap than those in the rotational flap group, perhaps indicating that the patients had more substantial overall injury. Of those with the more severe bone injury (Orthopaedic Trauma Association type C), 44% of the limbs treated with a rotational flap had a wound complication, compared with 23% of the limbs treated with a free flap. Those who were treated with a rotational flap for coverage were 4.3 times more likely to have a wound complication requiring surgical intervention.[40] This suggests that perhaps the rotational flaps were harvested from the zone of injury. The use of a free flap to treat open tibia fractures with severe bony injury was less likely to lead to a wound complication. Thus, it is important that the plastic surgeon or wound coverage team understand the concept of the zone of injury to minimize the complication rate and select the correct flap coverage.

Another consideration is posttraumatic stress and its effect on overall patient outcome. The trauma itself is a life-altering experience. The LEAP study evaluated patients for 2 years following the injury. Sixty-eight of the patients in the LEAP study completed four brief symptom inventories over a 2-year period; 48% of the patients screened positive for likely psychological disorder 3 months after the injury, and at 2 years the percentage remained high at 42%.[41] Thus, a severe lower limb injury is associated with severe distress. Only 12% of the patients at 3 months and 22% at 24 months received treatment for psychological distress.[41] Overall, trauma portends high rates of posttraumatic stress. According

to a 2004 study, more than half of orthopaedic trauma patients reported symptoms of posttraumatic stress.[42] Therefore, it is important to understand the nonorthopaedic factors and their impact on overall outcome (Table 2) and perhaps not only develop programs for patients with severe lower extremity trauma but also facilitate the return of trauma patients to premorbid routine.

Summary

Limb-threatening trauma is a dramatic, life-altering event. For those with a mangled lower extremity, the outcomes at 2 and 7 years were similar, and neither limb salvage nor amputation led to a high RTW rate or satisfactory outcome. Several injury-related and surgeon- and patient-derived factors can adversely affect outcomes. The development of programs that provide support to these patients is crucial, and is the next logical step. The ultimate return to function depends on many factors, and begins with frank discussion between the surgeon, patient, family, and specialists in surgical reconstruction. No option is without limitations, complications, and challenges, but a rational, informed approach, involvement of potential surgical specialists, and early intervention with behavioral and pain medicine specialists may be helpful regardless of the particular treatment path chosen.

Annotated References

1. MacKenzie EJ, Bosse MJ, Kellam JF, et al: Characterization of patients with high-energy lower extremity trauma. *J Orthop Trauma* 2000;14(7):455-466.

2. Bosse MJ, MacKenzie EJ, Kellam JF, et al: An analysis of outcomes of reconstruction or amputation after leg-threatening injuries. *N Engl J Med* 2002;347(24):1924-1931.

3. Cannada LK, Jones AL: Demographic, social and economic variables that affect lower extremity injury outcomes. *Injury* 2006;37(12):1109-1116.

   This article summarizes the data from the LEAP study and other investigations regarding the behavioral, demographic, and social factors known to affect outcome following severe lower extremity trauma. Level of evidence: III.

4. MacKenzie EJ, Bosse MJ, Pollak AN, et al: Long-term persistence of disability following severe lower-limb trauma: Results of a seven-year follow-up. *J Bone Joint Surg Am* 2005;87(8):1801-1809.

   This follow-up study confirmed that limb reconstruction and amputation have equivalent outcomes at 7 years after injury. The functional results are poor for both groups. Further studies should concentrate on postinjury social services. Level of evidence: I.

1: General Topics and New Technology

5. Mullenix PS, Steele SR, Andersen CA, Starnes BW, Salim A, Martin MJ: Limb salvage and outcomes among patients with traumatic popliteal vascular injury: An analysis of the National Trauma Data Bank. *J Vasc Surg* 2006;44(1):94-100.

    Popliteal artery injury is a risk factor for limb loss. In this review of the National Trauma Data Bank, 1,395 patients were identified. Amputation rates varied from 12% to 21% depending on associated injuries. Specifically, limb salvage failed in 21% with associated femur fracture and 20% with tibia fractures. Overall, there were significant rates of limb loss, functional disability, and mortality. Level of evidence: III.

6. Owens BD, Kragh JF Jr, Macaitis J, Svoboda SJ, Wenke JC: Characterization of extremity wounds in Operation Iraqi Freedom and Operation Enduring Freedom. *J Orthop Trauma* 2007;21(4):254-257.

    This study described the distribution of extremity fractures during Operation Iraqi Freedom and Operation Enduring Freedom. There were 1,281 soldiers sustaining 3,575 extremity combat wounds. Most were soft-tissue wounds and fractures with results similar to those reported for injuries sustained during previous wars. Level of evidence: IV.

7. Dorlac WC, DeBakey ME, Holcomb JB, et al: Mortality from isolated civilian penetrating extremity injury. *J Trauma* 2005;59(1):217-222.

    This study evaluated the outcomes of civilian patients who experienced exsanguination from penetrating injuries. Proximal injuries of the lower extremities led to immediate death. Eight patients (57%) had bleeding from a site that may have been amenable to tourniquet control. Level of evidence: III.

8. Kragh JF Jr, Walters TJ, Baer DG, et al: Survival with emergency tourniquet use to stop bleeding in major limb trauma. *Ann Surg* 2009;249(1):1-7.

    This study was conducted to determine whether emergency tourniquet use saved lives. The results demonstrated the value of tourniquet use in saving lives, even when shock was absent. There were no limbs lost to tourniquet use. Level of evidence: II.

9. Dagum AB, Best AK, Schemitsch EH, Mahoney JL, Mahomed MN, Blight KR: Salvage after severe lower-extremity trauma: Are the outcomes worth the means? *Plast Reconstr Surg* 1999;103(4):1212-1220.

10. Bosse MJ, McCarthy ML, Jones AL, et al; Lower Extremity Assessment Project (LEAP) Study Group: The insensate foot following severe lower extremity trauma: An indication for amputation? *J Bone Joint Surg Am* 2005;87(12):2601-2608.

    The authors found that the insensate foot should not be a criterion for determining whether limb salvage should be attempted rather than amputation. More than one half of the patients with an insensate foot had regained sensation at 2-year follow-up. Initial plantar sensation is not prognostic of outcome. Level of evidence: I.

11. Johansen K, Daines M, Howey T, Helfet D, Hansen ST

Jr: Objective criteria accurately predict amputation following lower extremity trauma. *J Trauma* 1990; 30(5):568-572, discussion 572-573.

12. Helfet DL, Howey T, Sanders R, Johansen K: Limb salvage versus amputation: Preliminary results of the Mangled Extremity Severity Score. *Clin Orthop* 1990;256: 80-86.

13. Howe HR Jr, Poole GV Jr, Hansen KJ, et al: Salvage of lower extremities following combined orthopedic and vascular trauma: A predictive salvage index. *Am Surg* 1987;53(4):205-208.

14. Russell WL, Sailors DM, Whittle TB, Fisher DF Jr, Burns RP: Limb salvage versus traumatic amputation: A decision based on a seven-part predictive index. *Ann Surg* 1991;213(5):473-480, discussion 480-481.

15. McNamara MG, Heckman JD, Corley FG: Severe open fractures of the lower extremity: A retrospective evaluation of the Mangled Extremity Severity Score (MESS). *J Orthop Trauma* 1994;8(2):81-87.

16. Bosse MJ, MacKenzie EJ, Kellam JF, et al: A prospective evaluation of the clinical utility of the lower-extremity injury-severity scores. *J Bone Joint Surg Am* 2001;83(1):3-14.

17. Suedkamp NP, Barbey N, Veuskens A, et al: The incidence of osteitis in open fractures: An analysis of 948 open fractures (a review of the Hannover experience). *J Orthop Trauma* 1993;7(5):473-482.

18. Krettek C, Seekamp A, Köntopp H, Tscherne H: Hannover Fracture Scale '98: Re-evaluation and new perspectives of an established extremity salvage score. *Injury* 2001;32(4):317-328.

19. Ly TV, Travison TG, Castillo RC, Bosse MJ, MacKenzie EJ, LEAP Study Group: Ability of lower-extremity injury severity scores to predict functional outcome after limb salvage. *J Bone Joint Surg Am* 2008; 90(8):1738-1743.

    The authors present a cohort analysis of 407 patients from the LEAP study. The injury severity of the cohort was assessed with the use of five scoring systems, and the functional outcome was assessed with the physical and psychosocial domain of the SIP. The authors found that none of the five limb-scoring systems were predictive of the SIP outcomes at 6 and 24 months. Thus, it was concluded that injury severity scoring systems are not predictive of functional recovery. Level of evidence: I.

20. Cannada LK, Cooper C: The mangled extremity: Limb salvage versus amputation. *Curr Surg* 2005;62(6): 563-576.

    A close evaluation of the existing multiple scoring systems indicates they should not be the sole determinant for amputation versus limb salvage procedures in the mangled lower extremity. Level of evidence: V.

21. Busse JW, Jacobs CL, Swiontkowski MF, Bosse MJ, Bhandari M, Evidence-Based Orthopaedic Trauma Working Group: Complex limb salvage or early amputation for severe lower-limb injury: A meta-analysis of observational studies. *J Orthop Trauma* 2007;21(1): 70-76.

   Functional outcome is not that different whether a patient undergoes limb salvage or amputation. There should be focus on research to avoid failed limb salvage because these patients would choose amputation if they had to decide all over again. Level of evidence: III.

22. Dahl B, Andersson AP, Andersen M, Andersen GR, Ebskov LB, Reumert T: Functional and social long-term results after free tissue transfer to the lower extremity. *Ann Plast Surg* 1995;34(4):372-375.

23. Hansen ST Jr: The type-IIIC tibial fracture: Salvage or amputation [editorial]. *J Bone Joint Surg Am* 1987; 69(6):799-800.

24. MacKenzie EJ, Bosse MJ, Kellam JF, et al: Early predictors of long-term work disability after major limb trauma. *J Trauma* 2006;61(3):688-694.

   Higher RTW rates were associated with younger age, Caucasian race, higher education, nonsmokers, average to high self-efficacy, preinjury job tenure, higher job involvement, and no pending litigation. In addition, earlier assessment of pain and physical function can be a significant predictor of RTW. Level of evidence: I.

25. Harris AM, Althausen PL, Kellam J, Bosse MJ, Castillo R, Lower Extremity Assessment Project (LEAP) Study Group: Complications following limb-threatening lower extremity trauma. *J Orthop Trauma* 2009;23(1):1-6.

   This is another study from the LEAP group. In patients with amputations, the most frequent complication was wound infection (34.2%). In those patients with limb reconstruction, complications included wound infection (23.2%), nonunion (31%), and osteomyelitis (8.6%). Level of evidence: I.

26. MacKenzie EJ, Bosse MJ, Castillo RC, et al: Functional outcomes following trauma-related lower-extremity amputation. *J Bone Joint Surg Am* 2004;86(8):1636-1645.

   This was an analysis of amputation level on outcome and an evaluation of additional factors (patient, injury, and prosthetics). Physical function was most affected by amputation level. A through-knee amputation had poor outcome secondary to soft-tissue and prosthetic issues. Level of evidence: I.

27. Waters RL, Perry J, Antonelli D, Hislop H: Energy cost of walking of amputees: The influence of level of amputation. *J Bone Joint Surg Am* 1976;58(1):42-46.

28. Smith JJ, Agel J, Swiontkowski MF, Castillo R, et al: Functional outcome of bilateral limb threatening: Lower extremity injuries at two years postinjury. *J Orthop Trauma* 2005;19(4):249-253.

   With severe, bilateral extremity trauma, the function of each limb was found to be similar at 24 months. A patient with a unilateral limb-threatening injury is more likely to return to work. Level of evidence: I.

29. MacKenzie EJ, Bosse MJ: Factors influencing outcome following limb-threatening lower limb trauma: Lessons learned from the Lower Extremity Assessment Project (LEAP). *J Am Acad Orthop Surg* 2006;14(10 Spec No., Suppl)S205-S210.

   This article summarized the LEAP study; specifically, outcomes are more often influenced by socioeconomic factors than treatment. This study can be used to identify opportunities for interventions that may influence outcomes. Level of evidence: II.

30. MacKenzie EJ, Jones AS, Bosse MJ, et al: Health-care costs associated with amputation or reconstruction of a limb-threatening injury. *J Bone Joint Surg Am* 2007; 89(8):1685-1692.

   This study compared 2-year direct and projected lifetime costs of amputation versus reconstruction. The 2-year costs were similar, but when prosthetic costs were added in, the difference was significant. The projected lifetime costs were three times higher for amputees. Level of evidence: I.

31. Castillo RC, MacKenzie EJ, Webb LX, Bosse MJ, Avery J, LEAP Study Group: Use and perceived need of physical therapy following severe lower-extremity trauma. *Arch Phys Med Rehabil* 2005;86(9):1722-1728.

   Physical therapy is thought to be a part of recovery following a mangled extremity. The authors found both amputated and limb salvage groups used similar amounts. The perceived need increased during follow-up: up to 68% at 2 years. Level of evidence: I.

32. Archer KR, Castillo RC, Mackenzie EJ, Bosse MJ; LEAP Study Group: Physical disability after severe lower-extremity injury. *Arch Phys Med Rehabil* 2006; 87(8):1153-1155.

   This subgroup evaluation of the LEAP study concluded decreased walking speed and gait deviation provide a valid measure of physical disability among the patients with limb reconstruction. Level of evidence: II.

33. Archer KR, Castillo RC, Mackenzie EJ, Bosse MJ: Gait symmetry and walking speed analysis following lower-extremity trauma. *Phys Ther* 2006;86(12):1630-1640.

   This study involved 381 patients to identify clinical measures associated with walking speed and contributing factors to gait asymmetry following lower extremity reconstruction. Decreased range of motion arc of the ankle, knee flexion strength, and nonreciprocal stair-climbing pattern were the most significant factors. Level of evidence: II.

34. Department of Defense Casualty Report 2009. http://www.defenselink.mil/news/casualty.pdf. Accessed January 13, 2010.

35. Gajewski D, Granville R: The United States Armed Forces Amputee Patient Care Program. *J Am Acad Orthop Surg* 2006;14(10 Spec No., Suppl):S183-S187.

   There are excellent outcomes in military amputees fol-

1: General Topics and New Technology

lowing the practices of the Armed Forces Amputee Patient Care Program. However, more research is needed to determine optimal treatment. Level of evidence: V.

36. Webb LX, Bosse MJ, Castillo RC, MacKenzie EJ, LEAP Study Group: Analysis of surgeon-controlled variables in the treatment of limb-threatening type-III open tibial diaphyseal fractures. *J Bone Joint Surg Am* 2007; 89(5):923-928.

    This study evaluated surgeon-controlled variables in the outcome of open tibial shaft fractures. Definitive treatment with an external fixator resulted in more complications. Those with an external fixator and muscle flap did worse than patients with an amputation. Level of evidence: II.

37. Taller J, Kamdar JP, Greene JA, et al: Temporary vascular shunts as initial treatment of proximal extremity vascular injuries during combat operations: The new standard of care at Echelon II facilities? *J Trauma* 2008; 65(3):595-603.

    This study reviewed the placement of the TVS in a combat situation prior to transfer to a facility that could complete the revascularization (Echelon II). There were 23 proximal vascular shunts placed in 16 patients with a mean Injury Severity Score of 25 (range, 17 to 43). Twenty-two shunts were patent upon arrival to the Echelon II facility. All shunt patients survived their injuries with a 100% early limb preservation rate. Level of evidence: III.

38. Gifford SM, Aidinian G, Clouse WD, et al: Effect of temporary shunting on extremity vascular injury: An outcome analysis from the Global War on Terror vascular injury initiative. *J Vasc Surg* 2009;50(3):549-555.

    Vascular injury in a case control cohort was studied during the current war on terrorism. There were 64 cases with a TVS compared with 61 control subjects. Mean follow-up was 22 months (range, 1 to 54 months). Overall, there were 26 amputations. The fracture sever-

ity and MESS scores were associated with amputation rate. There was an amputation-free survival rate of 78% in the TVS group and 77% in the control group. The results suggest that TVS can be an adjunct in limb salvage. Level of evidence: IV.

39. Subramanian A, Vercruysse G, Dente C, Wyrzykowski A, King E, Feliciano DV: A decade's experience with temporary intravascular shunts at a civilian level I trauma center. *J Trauma* 2008;65(2):316-324.

    In this review of a 10-year experience with the use of vascular shunts at a Level 1 trauma center, the results of 67 patients with 101 shunts were reported. There were 72 arterial shunts and 29 venous shunts. The thrombosis rate was 5%, amputation rate 18%, survival rate 88%, and overall limb/patient survival rate 73%. Temporary vascular shunting can play an important role in specific instances of limb salvage, with good results. Level of evidence: IV.

40. Pollak AN, McCarthy ML, Burgess AR, The Lower Extremity Assessment Project (LEAP) Study Group: Short-term wound complications after application of flaps for coverage of traumatic soft-tissue defects about the tibia. *J Bone Joint Surg Am* 2000;82(12):1681-1691.

41. McCarthy ML, MacKenzie EJ, Edwin D, et al: Psychological distress associated with severe lower-limb injury. *J Bone Joint Surg Am* 2003;85(9):1689-1697.

42. Starr AJ, Smith WR, Frawley WH, et al: Symptoms of posttraumatic stress disorder after orthopaedic trauma. *J Bone Joint Surg Am* 2004;86(6):1115-1121.

    More than 50% of orthopaedic trauma patients surveyed in the short term after their return to clinic may possibly meet criteria for posttraumatic stress disorder. Level of evidence: IV.

Chapter 8

Amputation of the Extremities

Roman A. Hayda, MD   William J.J. Ertl, MD

1: General Topics and New Technology

Introduction

Amputation of the extremities has been practiced for millennia. Prehistoric cave drawings have depicted amputations; classic Greek and Roman physicians described indications and surgical approaches for amputation; and armed conflicts throughout history have promoted and advanced the care of the amputee. Outside of the military, emphasis on proper surgical care and rehabilitation of the amputee has declined because amputation is often viewed as a procedure of failure. Recent examples of highly functional amputees, both at the recreational and competitive level, have served to destigmatize amputation and make it a more routinely considered clinical option. Amputation should not be viewed merely as an ablative procedure but one that is reconstructive, providing the patient with a stable foundation for prosthetic application and functional restoration. Successful amputation mandates attention to detail during surgery. Advances in techniques and prosthetic options have provided further options in the recovery of the amputee.

General Principles of Amputation

Adhering to the surgical principles of amputation allows for the maximal potential for recovery regardless of the level of amputation in the upper and lower extremity. Preservation of major joints, even with a short residual limb distal to the joint, is preferable to a higher amputation level. Preservation of residual limb length when possible increases the surface area for prosthetic fitting and load distribution. It also provides a better lever arm for prosthetic function and facilitates contracture prevention. In the transfemoral setting, length also improves sitting balance.

The limiting factor for residual limb length is typically not the bone but the presence of a reasonable tissue to provide soft-tissue cover. In the traumatic amputee, a myodesis is critical in achieving muscle balance and providing cushion at the end of the residual limb. Using heavy suture, the muscle is sutured to bone through drill holes or to the periosteum. This process reestablishes resting muscle tension, allows for better limb control, helps avoid contractures, and provides a cushion at the end of the residual limb. Even in the upper extremity, a poorly done myodesis can impair function. In the transhumeral amputee, the myodesis provides important padding to allow more comfort during abduction and flexion. In the transradial amputee, the myodesis can allow for a better myoelectric signal to direct terminal limb function. An alternative method to providing soft-tissue stabilization is myoplasty, which involves suturing and anchoring antagonistic muscles to one another, providing distal coverage and restoring the muscle's length-tension relationship.

Native innervated skin is the preferred tissue to cover an amputated limb because it is the most resistant to shear forces and skin breakdown. Skin grafting, once considered taboo for amputations, is acceptable provided there is a sufficiently healthy soft-tissue bed to accept a skin graft. Silicone gel liners applied directly to the residual limb and used within prosthetic sockets dissipate shear and avoid skin breakdown. Unlike vascular and diabetic amputations, atypical flaps and skin grafts used in the otherwise healthy trauma patient allow for maintenance of limb length and preservation of joints, in turn allowing more vigorous activity levels (**Figure 1**).

Identification of major nerves at the time of amputation is important to prevent the formation of painful neuromas. Both cutaneous sensory nerves and motor nerves are individually identified and sectioned proximally while gentle traction is applied, and then allowed to retract under muscle proximal to the terminal end of the limb. A neuroma inevitably forms as part of the normal nerve healing process, but will be away from the irritation present at the end of the limb. Preemptive efforts to prevent the formation of painful neuromas such as burying the nerve in fat, muscle, or bone have not been consistently successful. Major vessels are ligated at the level of amputation.

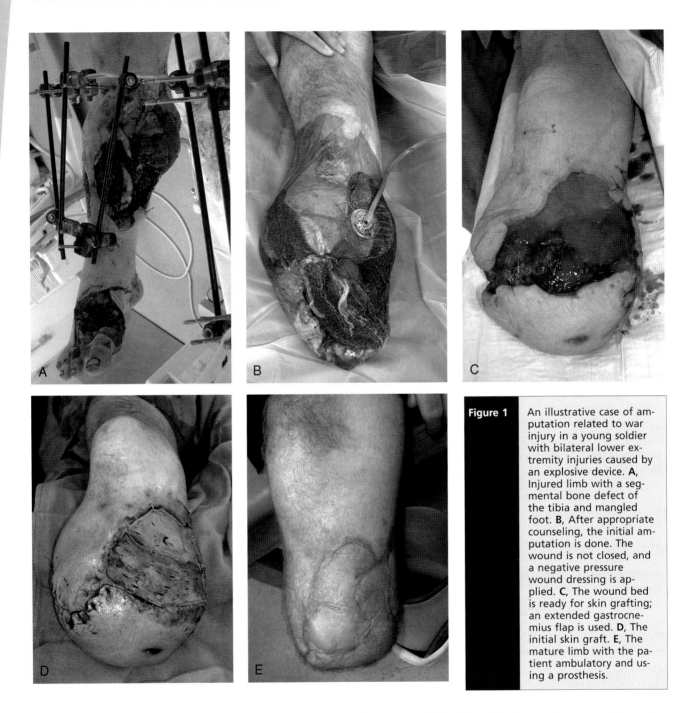

Figure 1 An illustrative case of amputation related to war injury in a young soldier with bilateral lower extremity injuries caused by an explosive device. **A,** Injured limb with a segmental bone defect of the tibia and mangled foot. **B,** After appropriate counseling, the initial amputation is done. The wound is not closed, and a negative pressure wound dressing is applied. **C,** The wound bed is ready for skin grafting; an extended gastrocnemius flap is used. **D,** The initial skin graft. **E,** The mature limb with the patient ambulatory and using a prosthesis.

What's New in Lower Extremity Amputation?

Lower extremity amputations continue to be the most common amputation. Surgeons, prosthetists, and therapists are most familiar with this level, and the prosthetic options are expanding.

Below the ankle, partial foot amputation involving a central ray or lateral rays or forefoot transmetatarsal amputation results in near-normal function. Midfoot amputation at the Lisfranc or Chopart levels is generally not advocated. When such midfoot amputations are performed, an Achilles tenotomy is advised in addition to tenodesis of the tibialis anterior to avoid a painful equinus contracture. Midfoot amputations are more likely to be useful in the multilimb amputee or when access to prosthetics is limited by financial, geographic, or other constraints. The Syme amputation has similar indications because ambulation without a prosthesis, its principal advantage, rarely occurs. Prosthetic options for this level are also very limited due to lack of space between the end of the limb and the floor.

The transtibial amputation is the most commonly performed amputation when the foot, ankle, or distal tibia are not deemed reconstructible. The soft tissues are the most critical element in determining the length of the amputation. Fortunately, the gastrocnemius and soleus muscles are often relatively spared in trauma situations, allowing safe amputation at this level. The extended posterior flap has been suggested to better cover the anterior end of the residual limb[1] (**Figure 1**). The optimal level of bone section is best determined by measurement from the floor rather than from the knee. Bone section 20 to 22 cm from the floor will generally allow for the most current energy-storing terminal components to be used. As long as there is a functioning knee extensor mechanism and adequate soft-tissue cover, no tibial amputation is too short, because the advantages of retaining the patient's native knee generally outweigh potential problems with prosthetic fit and function in comparison with the transfemoral amputee or knee disarticulation. A case series of lengthening of short transtibial and transfemoral amputation was reported in a young patient population (average age, 15 years). Although the procedure was successful in allowing more traditional prosthetic fitting, it was associated with a high complication rate. In patients who had undergone tibial lengthening, half developed knee contracture, with most requiring surgery. However, all patients had improved prosthetic wear and improved energy efficiency in ambulation.[2]

The ongoing debate on the role of the Ertl osteomyoplastic technique or bone bridge procedure is not yet resolved.[3,4] The Ertl procedure for transtibial amputations combines soft-tissue reconstruction with creation of an osseous bridge at the distal end of the limb. A tibiofibular synostosis is created with osteoperiosteal flaps, and soft-tissue stability is maintained by myoplasty. Indications for the Ertl procedure include fibular instability and disruption of the interosseous membrane to avoid a painful, unstable fibula. The technique has been used as both a primary and revision technique. Advocates argue the procedure not only stabilizes the fibula but also creates a larger surface area at the end of the limb. This creates an end-bearing stump, which theoretically translates to greater comfort in socket wear and higher levels of function. Few studies have consistently confirmed these outcomes, whereas other authors have cited increased operation times in performing this procedure.[5]

Discussion also continues on the merits of the through-knee level amputation compared with transfemoral level amputation. The Lower Extremity Assessment Project (LEAP) study found that through-knee amputations had worse outcomes than transfemoral amputations.[6] Unfortunately, the numbers were too small to draw firm conclusions, but it was thought that the poor results could be attributed to compromised soft-tissue coverage in through-knee amputations. If bulkier and asymmetric joint levels are acceptable, through-knee amputations offer an end-bearing stump with good muscle balance, and the retained femoral condyles allow for good suspension of the prosthetic leg socket.

Perhaps the most tantalizing development in lower extremity amputation is the potential for osseointegration of the prosthesis.[7] This novel procedure involves a device akin to a dental post that is implanted in the bone at the distal end of the limb and deliberately protrudes from the skin. The prosthetic limb is then attached to this external post. This experimental procedure is being performed in several centers in Europe but has yet to consistently avoid infectious and mechanical complications. Almost all lower extremity amputees at some point experience problems with socket-limb interface because limb volume and contour change constantly and may result in friction and pressure points during prosthetic wear. This procedure may circumvent these issues related to the socket-limb interface, and this possibility is being actively investigated.

What's New in Upper Extremity Amputation?

Upper extremity amputations most often are the result of limb-threatening trauma. Preservation of a functional elbow joint is an important goal as prosthetic use and satisfaction increase, because the patient can directly position the terminal device in space. The unique application of surgical flaps to provide an adequate and stable soft-tissue envelope may be necessary to ensure preservation of the elbow joint. Soft-tissue stabilization may be accomplished by myodesis, myoplasty, or a combination of these two techniques. If possible, a midlevel transradial amputation would be ideal. However, in trauma, the most proximal level should be about 4 to 5 cm distal to the elbow skin crease. A more proximal amputation compromises prosthetic socket stability and function.

Elbow disarticulations may have the theoretical advantage of more reliable prosthetic suspension. However, the distal limb may be more bulbous or rounded, and the prosthetic elbow joint will be distal to the contralateral elbow. Transhumeral amputations often lead to poor prosthetic use because of the challenges related to prosthetic use. The length of the residual limb is important when considering prosthetic choices. Currently, when a myoelectric prosthesis is desired, a midhumeral amputation may be indicated to allow for adequate space for prosthetic componentry.

Targeted nerve reinnervation is a new technique for transhumeral amputees and shoulder disarticulations that redirects terminal nerves of the brachial plexus into available regional musculature of the shoulder or arm. This allows for natural neural pathways to simultaneously control elbow, wrist, and hand functions by myoelectric signals generated by the terminal nerves. Instead of requiring sequential commands to position the limb and operate the terminal device as is typically required, these operations occur simultaneously and take advantage of the normal function of the sectioned nerves. This technique was first reported in a patient with bilateral shoulder disarticulations.[8] Subsequently, a small case series has been reported with patients of

1: General Topics and New Technology

various upper extremity amputations.[9] Results appear to be promising; however, utilization of this technique has not been widely disseminated.

Lessons Learned From Recent Military Conflicts

Amputation is a signature injury in war as the destructive nature of munitions either amputate limbs or render them unreconstructible, even with current techniques. The current conflict in Iraq and Afghanistan is no exception. At present, approximately 900 amputations have occurred; most have been to the lower extremity but a significant number of upper extremity amputations have also been done.[10] Multiple extremity amputations in various combinations have also been seen. As in previous conflicts, the advantages of specialized centers devoted to amputee care coupled with peer support have assisted in the recovery of these patients. A multidisciplinary approach involving the orthopaedic surgeon, physiatrist, psychiatrist, physical therapist, prosthetist, and case manager has helped these war wounded to adjust to their new lives and maximize their function. An intensive inpatient and outpatient therapeutic regimen whereby wounded warriors in various stages of recovery help each other has resulted in 17% of these individuals choosing to stay on active duty while many others have regained high levels of function; some have even returned to the battlefield. Some patients who initially underwent lower limb salvage with extensive reconstructions are asking for elective amputation when they see their amputated colleagues achieving high levels of function comparatively early following injury. Although some amputees function at a high physical level over a long period, the ability to maintain these high levels of activity for the long term has not been consistently demonstrated in any large cohort of patients. Routine elective amputation to return patients to their desired high levels of activity following severe trauma cannot be recommended at this time in otherwise successful limb reconstructions.

At the inception of the recent military conflict, a panel of military and civilian experts convened to establish policies and priorities governing the care of amputees and defined the 'open length-preserving amputation' technique, in which all nonviable tissues are débrided and the limb stabilized with all wounds left open during the evacuation.[11] No consideration is given to the definitive level of amputation. Definitive closure, often with atypical flaps as shown in Figure 1, was performed at three centers stateside designated to care for amputees. With this method the maximal number of options was left available, particularly in severely mangled limbs, where reconstructive options may be unclear initially. Additionally, tissues from a viable but unreconstructible limb may be used for reconstruction of other injured limbs. Such techniques also may be applicable in the civilian setting.

Advanced methods of pain control, which include peripheral nerve blocks and the use of neural membrane stabilizers such as gabapentin, have facilitated patient transport and allowed for early physical therapy. These pain protocols are initiated very early in the treatment course and appear to assist in the management of complex regional pain syndrome and phantom limb pain.[12]

As a result of attempting to preserve the maximal length of an amputated limb, amputations were often performed within the zone of injury while allowing for the preservation of adjacent joints. Negative pressure dressings were commonly used in soft-tissue management (**Figure 1**, *B*). Advantages of negative pressure dressings include containment of the wound, evacuation of exudates, and the formation of granulation tissue. When combined with vessel loops, negative pressure dressings allow skin traction, minimizing skin retraction and advancing the skin over the muscle as the edema subsides. In select cases, fractures were fixed in the amputated limb to preserve length, provided that there was a possibility fixation could contribute to function with limited surgical risks.[13] Critical in this decision making is the availability of soft-tissue coverage and limited contamination at the open fracture site.

An unintended consequence of amputations within the zone of injury was the development of heterotopic ossification in the amputated limb.[14] Investigators found an 80% prevalence of heterotopic ossification when the amputation was performed in the zone of injury. Fortunately, most cases were managed by prosthetic modification and only 12% required resection. In those requiring resection, it is important to consider dead space management following excision. When the heterotopic bone was underneath skin grafts, infection and wound healing problems were commonly observed. The use of negative pressure dressings, infection, and number of operations were not found to be associated with the development of heterotopic bone. In another study, additional risk factors for heterotopic bone were elucidated to include an Injury Severity Score of 16 or greater, infection, multiple operations, and head injury.[15]

To allow for frequent wound inspection, rigid dressings that have been previously advocated were not routinely used. Typically a soft figure-of-8 wrap was applied, with occasional splint augmentation. Physical therapy was instituted immediately after surgery. This protocol resulted in rare contractures while allowing optimal wound management.

For the transhumeral and shoulder disarticulation war amputee, the new technique of targeted reinnervation was performed at several centers.[8,9] This technique appears promising, but limb function compared to traditional amputation has not yet been reported.

In the military system, the prosthetists were intimately involved in the multidisciplinary team at all stages of recovery. Such conditions may be difficult to replicate in the civilian sector, but they facilitated communication between the patient, therapist, surgeon, and prosthetist. Prosthetic modifications are readily performed before problems develop and allow continuation of rehabilitation. Multiple types of suspensions and terminal devices can be trialed to best fit the needs of the patient. In the upper extremity amputee, both myoelectric and body-powered prostheses were provided to use each limb to its maximal advantage.

Immediate Postoperative Rehabilitation

General Goals
A team consisting of the surgeon, prosthetist, physical therapist, occupational therapist, and a mental health professional assist the patient to establish rehabilitation goals and a timeline of recovery and to adapt to potential setbacks. Additionally, peer support from trained and qualified amputees provides the patient with unique insight and support when coping with an acute amputation. Ideally, rehabilitation goals should be discussed before the completion/formalization of an amputation. However, in the setting of an acute traumatic amputation, the patient may not have participated in treatment decision making and may require the support and services of a mental health professional.[16]

Immediately following surgery, the primary goal is to prevent surgical complications to allow early rehabilitation. Early complications include wound infection, delayed wound healing, swelling, contracture, and deep venous thrombosis (DVT). Meticulous handling of tissue and layered closure of the wounds is mandated at the time of surgery. In traumatic amputations, regardless of the surgical technique applied, closure through the zone of injury has a high incidence of wound failure requiring revision surgery.[5] Edema control begins first with elevation and protection of the limb, regardless of the indication for an amputation. Various techniques for edema control have included elastic bandaging, polymer gel socks, shrinker socks, rigid dressings, and immediate casting. Their application should be individualized to avoid complications of pressure ulcers and wound dehiscence. Rigid dressing may enhance wound healing, prevent flexion contractures of the knee, and provide distal protection to the residual limb in transtibial amputees.[17] The occurrence of DVT in lower extremity amputees has recently been investigated. The incidence of DVT in amputees ranges from 9.4% to 12%.[18,19] Risk factors for DVT in the amputated limb appear to be associated with increased age (older than 70 years), peripheral arterial disease, and transfemoral level of amputation.[20]

Rehabilitation of the amputee requires not only a quality reconstructed residual limb but the expertise and input of physical/occupational therapists, prosthetists, rehabilitation physicians, and potentially, mental health professionals. A generalized conditioning and strengthening program for all amputees should be developed to prevent secondary physical complications related to the amputation.[21] This program needs to be coordinated with a competent and qualified therapist familiar with amputee care. A generalized treatment plan should be developed for upper and lower extremity amputees and tailored to meet the needs of the individual patient.

Upper Extremity
Mobilization of the residual limb should be instituted as early as possible, depending on soft-tissue healing and swelling. Movements should include active, active assisted, and passive range-of-motion modalities of all joints of the residual limb to prevent any contracture that may limit the application of an upper extremity prosthesis. Maintaining elbow motion in the transradial amputee is critical in maximizing function. In transhumeral amputees, prosthetic use typically decreases with fitting delays as most patients adapt to use of a single upper extremity and have increased difficulty in efficiently using a transhumeral prosthesis. Isometric muscle contraction exercises can be instituted once soft-tissue healing is advanced, allowing the limb to maintain volume and muscle function, which will be important qualities if a myoelectric prosthesis is chosen. Computer-assisted training of the myolectric signal may also be useful for regaining volitional control of specific muscle groups. Once the residual limb has stabilized, usually within 4 weeks, application of a prosthesis should be instituted, teaching the patient basic tasks for activities of daily living, advancing tasks as the patient gains confidence with the prosthesis. A phased plan of rehabilitation may enhance patient education and acceptance of an upper extremity prosthesis.[22]

Lower Extremity
As with the upper extremity, the ultimate goal is to provide the patient with a functional residual limb that will accept and support a prosthesis to improve the amputee's ability to function on a daily basis. For lower extremity amputees, the basic goal is ambulation. Early limb protection can be facilitated by rigid dressings to prevent flexion contracture of the knee and early mobilization to maintain joint function. Desensitization modalities such as superficial and deep massage and towel pulls over the end of the residual limb can be instituted at approximately 3 to 4 weeks after surgery. Transfer skills and assisted ambulation should be started as soon as the patient can move the limb. If a rigid dressing is used in the immediate postoperative period, it should be removed by 5 days after surgery to assess the wound and determine the need for additional rigid dressing.[23] To avoid hip flexion contractures associated with prolonged sitting during recovery, patients must be educated in hip stretching. Daily prone stretching while extending the residual limb and/or raising the torso effectively counteracts this problem. Uncomplicated wound healing for transfemoral amputees is usually sufficient by 4 to 5 weeks after surgery to institute a prosthetic fitting and delivery program and ready the

patient's preparatory socket and begin gait training. For transtibial amputees, uncomplicated wound healing may be sufficient by 6 to 8 weeks after surgery to institute fitting and to advance rehabilitation.

Management of Complications

Phantom Pain

Phantom limb sensation and phantom limb pain are common in amputees at later follow-up and can become problematic if not addressed.[24] The patient should be made aware that almost all traumatic amputees initially report phantom limb sensations or pain. Certain patients encounter significant difficulty in the management of phantom pain. Aggressive pain management techniques are helpful and include use of peripheral nerve blocks, sustained-release narcotic medications, and neural membrane stabilizers such as gabapentin, which may curtail the development of established pain pathways.[25] Social reintegration to include vocational training and adaptive sports programs that have become much more common nationwide assist patients to develop methods of adjusting to their new extremities. There have been isolated reports of the use of novel techniques such as mirror therapy,[26] ketamine,[27] and surgical nerve splitting and reanastomosis[28] to break the pathway of phantom limb pain. The role of these techniques in routine recovery of patients is currently unknown.

Nerves and Neuromas

Amputation of any extremity requires the transection of the major peripheral nerves of that limb, resulting in formation of neuromas. However, not all neuromas are painful. Unfortunately, a symptomatic neuroma may cause disabling pain for the amputee, preventing effective use of the prosthesis. Prevention of symptomatic neuromas begins during surgery as described earlier. Cauterization, ligation, or capping appear to have no benefit over simple high transection. When the amputee does develop clinical symptoms of discrete pain, most often the diagnosis of a symptomatic neuroma can be made clinically by the presence of a Tinel sign in the area of question. Often, a palpable nodule or firm structure can be appreciated in the subcutaneous tissue and often elicits the patient's symptoms or can worsen phantom pain when stimulated. Treatment of postsurgical amputation neuromas should begin with an evaluation of the prosthetic socket and liners that interface with the residual limb of the patient. An ill-fitting prosthesis may be causing increased focal pressure, and simple modifications to complete socket revision may change the load experienced by the nerve and reduce or potentially relieve the patient's symptoms. Volume changes that occur during daily use of a prosthesis may also contribute to limb-socket instability, creating focal pressure on peripheral nerves that in turn generate neurogenic pain. Simple patient reeducation on how to

manage sock wear may reduce these neurogenic symptoms. Once it is clinically established that a neuroma is symptomatic despite nonsurgical interventions, the neuroma may be treated via sclerosing injection therapy or by surgical excision. Identification of neuromas can be done via ultrasound or MRI[29-31] while other potential causes are determined.[32] Sclerosing therapy with high-resolution ultrasound-guided injections of phenol have proven to be successful in a case series of patients.[33] This therapy may be an ideal treatment option for patients not desiring to undergo surgical excision or in patients who are physiologically unable to undergo surgical excision. Local injection of the tumor necrosis factor inhibitor etanercept in a small case series has shown promise, but this technique is not widespread.[34] If prosthetic modification or minimally invasive techniques fail to relieve neurogenic pain, the patient may require surgical excision of the peripheral neuroma. Attention should be directed at isolating and freeing the entire neuroma and tracing it proximally to ensure a complete neurolysis and excision of the offending nerve.

Amputation Outcomes

Despite the evolution of amputation techniques and prosthetic hardware, amputation remains associated with significant disability. Some amputees have achieved high levels of function comparable to the function of individuals with normal limbs. However, such results are not consistently achieved. Recent studies have shown significant levels of disability in amputees. The landmark LEAP study provides significant outcomes data for amputees. This multicenter prospective study, using the Sickness Impact Profile outcome score, showed significant disability in physical and psychosocial domains among amputees that worsened 7 years after amputation.[35,36] Only 35% had physical subscores within the population norm. Half had scores indicating severe disability and 25% had scores indicating very severe disability. In this series poorer outcomes were associated with older age, female sex (for physical functioning only), nonwhite race, lower education level, living in a poor household, current or previous smoking, low self-efficacy, poor self-reported health status before the injury, and involvement with the legal system for the purpose of obtaining disability payments. Several smaller studies confirm similar levels of disability.[3,4]

In the lower extremity, prosthetic advances such as energy-storing feet and processor control joints have been assumed to improve patient function. However, supporting biomechanical data are lacking.[37] According to a 2006 study, although patient satisfaction rates with advanced prostheses were high, biomechanical performance was not improved with similar activity levels in transtibial and transfemoral amputees, regardless of the level of sophistication of the prosthetic component.[38] According to results of a 2004 study, no differences in function were found based on the sophistication of the prosthesis.[6] In a recent study of 15 transfemoral amputees, satisfaction rates and daily activity rates were higher with a microprocessor-controlled knee in comparison with a mechanical limb, but no difference in energy efficiency with walking was found.[39]

Functional outcomes following an upper extremity amputation are varied. Patients who undergo upper extremity amputation may require additional psychosocial support and may require insight regarding coping mechanisms to adjust to their amputated limb. Depression and anxiety related to the amputation are prevalent and may lead to avoidance behavior, resulting in poor adaptation.[40] Providing the patient with effective coping modalities and creating a sense of worth may also minimize poor outcomes in upper extremity amputations.[41] Finally, improving prosthetic use may be increased by enhancing the function of the upper extremity prosthesis. Novel materials have reduced the weight and size of the prostheses, and improving suspension may play a role in increased upper extremity amputation prosthetics. Targeted muscle reinnervation that provides an electromyographic signal that can be captured allows for potential complex coordinated prosthetic function.[8,9] Upper extremity prosthetic use is less predictable than that of the lower extremity. Novel prosthetic construction and interfacing may increase functional outcome in the future, but will require larger studies in this patient population.

Summary

Amputation surgery continues to be a necessary option in the armamentarium of the trauma surgeon despite advances in reconstruction surgery. Skillful surgical technique, progressive rehabilitation, and careful application of prosthetic technology will assist in maintaining maximal function among patients.

Annotated References

1. Assal M, Blanck R, Smith DG: Extended posterior flap for transtibial amputation. *Orthopedics* 2005;28(6): 542-546.

   The technique of an extended posterior flap is described with the authors' experience with its use in 17 patients. At a mean follow-up period of 28 months, no healing complications were noted, and subjectively the patients had fewer socket-related complaints. However, it took 4 to 6 months to resolve the bulbous contour of the gastrocnemius. Level of evidence: IV.

2. Bowen RE, Struble SG, Setoguchi Y, Watts HG: Outcomes of lengthening short lower-extremity amputation stumps with planar fixators. *J Pediatr Orthop* 2005; 25(4):543-547.

   The authors performed 14 femoral and 8 tibial lengthening procedures in 20 patients with an average age of 15.1 years with an average follow-up of 4.1 years. Average residual limb length at the time of femoral and tibial surgery was 10.3 cm and 4.8 cm, respectively, and did

not allow the use of a standard prosthesis. Following lengthening, 85% of patients were able to use a standard prosthesis. However, there were an average of 1.4 major complications such as contracture, angulatory deformity, poor soft-tissue coverage, and nonunion per patient. Level of evidence: IV.

3. Pinzur MS, Beck J, Himes R, Callaci J: Distal tibiofibular bone-bridging in transtibial amputation. *J Bone Joint Surg Am* 2008;90(12):2682-2687.

   The authors compared outcomes as rated on the Prosthetic Evaluation Questionnaire, a validated outcomes measure, of 8 trauma patients who were treated with a bone bridge technique and 15 who were not. No outcomes difference was noted between groups. Level of evidence: III.

4. Pinzur MS, Pinto MA, Saltzman M, Batista F, Gottschalk F, Juknelis D: Health-related quality of life in patients with transtibial amputation and reconstruction with bone bridging of the distal tibia and fibula. *Foot Ankle Int* 2006;27(11):907-912.

   The authors evaluated 32 patients treated with a bone bridge technique by a single surgeon. The group included 12 diabetic patients. The authors found a favorable outcome using this technique. Level of evidence: IV.

5. Gwinn DE, Keeling J, Froehner JW, McGuigan FX, Andersen R: Perioperative differences between bone bridging and non-bone bridging transtibial amputations for wartime lower extremity trauma. *Foot Ankle Int* 2008; 29(8):787-793.

   In a group of 42 war-related transtibial amputees in whom bridged versus nonbridged amputation were compared, 66.7% of amputations performed within the zone of injury had wound complications regardless of the type of amputation (bridge or nonbridge). The authors recommend caution when closing wartime amputations. Bone bridge patients had longer surgery times and tourniquet times (179 minutes and 115 minutes, respectively) when compared with nonbridge patients (112 minutes and 78 minutes, respectively). Level of evidence: IV.

6. MacKenzie EJ, Bosse MJ, Castillo RC, et al: Functional outcomes following trauma-related lower-extremity amputation. *J Bone Joint Surg Am* 2004;86(8):1636-1645.

   In an analysis of the 161 individuals in the LEAP cohort who underwent amputation (109 below-knee, 18 through-knee, and 34 above-knee), Sickness Impact Profile scores were equivalent between above-knee and below-knee amputees. However, self-selected walking speeds were faster among below-knee amputees. Through-knee amputees had the worst outcomes in terms of Sickness Impact Profile scores and walking speed. Level of evidence: I.

7. Bryant PR, Huang ME, Roberts TL, Nelson VS, Flood KM: Advances in amputee care. *Arch Phys Med Rehabil* 2006;87(3, Suppl 1):S34-S43.

   The authors discuss current advances in amputee care to include advanced pain management, decision making in amputation levels, new prosthetic design, osseointegration, and experimental interface systems for prosthetic control. Level of evidence: V.

8. Dumanian GA, Lipschutz RD, Miller LA, Stubblefield KA: The use of targeted muscle reinnervation for improved myoelectric prosthesis control in a bilateral shoulder disarticulation amputee. *Prosthet Orthot Int* 2004;28(3):245-253.

    This case study summarizes the results of transferring four nerves of the brachial plexus to various residual musculature in a bilateral shoulder disarticulation patient. Five months after surgery, the patient had three successful functional nerve-muscle units on objective testing. The patient was able to use a myoelectric prosthesis more efficiently when objectively tested.

9. Kuiken TA, Li G, Lock BA, et al: Targeted muscle reinnervation for real-time myoelectric control of multifunction artificial arms. *JAMA* 2009;301(6):619-628.

    Five patients with various proximal upper extremity amputations were tested following targeted muscle reinnervation. All patients showed improvement with use of a myoelectric prosthesis. Three patients were able to demonstrate proficient use of an advanced upper extremity prosthesis. The investigators concluded that targeted muscle reinnervation provided sufficient electromyogram signaling to control advanced upper extremity prosthetics. Level of evidence: IV.

10. Stansbury LG, Lalliss SJ, Branstetter JG, Bagg MR, Holcomb JB: Amputations in U.S. military personnel in the current conflicts in Afghanistan and Iraq. *J Orthop Trauma* 2008;22(1):43-46.

    The authors reviewed records of all injured casualties from 2001 to June 2006. Of these, 5.2% required amputation, similar to rates seen in Vietnam and other recent conflicts. Explosive devices were the most common cause of injury. Of the 423 patients with amputations, 328 had lower extremity amputation and 105 had upper extremity amputation; 18% had more than one extremity amputation and 2.4% had upper and lower amputation. Only 3% of upper extremity injuries resulted in amputation, whereas 8% of lower extremities resulted in amputation despite similarities between upper and lower extremity injury rates. These results reflect the ability to reconstruct limbs and the ability to replicate function with prostheses. Level of evidence: IV.

11. Hayda R, Mazurek M, Powell E, et al: From Iraq back to Iraq: Modern combat orthopaedic care. *Instr Course Lect* 2008;57:87-99.

    The authors describe the methods and early results of caring for war casualties. In addition to the method, early results, and challenges of amputee treatment, the evacuation process, reconstruction, and ongoing research are described. Level of evidence: V.

12. Malchow RJ, Black IH: The evolution of pain management in the critically ill trauma patient: Emerging concepts from the global war on terrorism. *Crit Care Med* 2008;36(Suppl 7)S346-S357.

    The authors describe the use of advanced pain management techniques in the critically injured from the global war on terrorism. The use of multimodal techniques combining regional anesthesia with pharmacologic agents of various classes (nonsteroidal anti-inflammatory drugs, acetaminophen, anticonvulsants, ketamine, anxiolytics, and antidepressants) manages pain effectively while reducing complications. Level of evidence: V.

13. Pickard-Gabriel CJ, Ledford CL, Gajewski DA, Granville RR, Andersen RC: Traumatic transfemoral amputation with concomitant ipsilateral proximal femoral fracture. A report of two cases. *J Bone Joint Surg Am* 2007;89(12):2764-2768.

    Two cases of femur fracture fixation in transfemoral amputees are described; length for prosthetic function is preserved.

14. Potter BK: Heterotopic ossification following traumatic and combat-related amputations: Prevalence, risk factors, and preliminary results of excision. *J Bone Joint Surg Am* 2007;89:476-486.

    The authors analyzed 183 patients with 218 amputated limbs. Overall 63% developed heterotopic ossification. When the amputation was performed within the zone of injury, 80% developed heterotopic injury, which was severe in 45% of blast victims; 12% required excision. Level of evidence: IV.

15. Forsberg JA, Pepek JM, Wagner S, et al: Heterotopic ossification in high-energy wartime extremity injuries: Prevalence and risk factors. *J Bone Joint Surg Am* 2009; 91(5):1084-1091.

    War-injured patients requiring surgery were evaluated for factors related to the development of heterotopic ossification. Of the 243 patients who met inclusion criteria, 157 developed heterotopic ossification. Risk factors identified were age younger than 30 years, amputation, multiple extremity injuries, and Injury Severity Score of 16 or greater. Level of evidence: IV.

16. Cavanagh SR, Shin LM, Karamouz N, Rauch SL: Psychiatric and emotional sequelae of surgical amputation. *Psychosomatics* 2006;47(6):459-464.

    Patients who undergo an acute, unplanned amputation have a higher incidence of posttraumatic stress disorder and may require additional emotional support due to the emotional stress caused by the trauma.

17. van Velzen AD, Nederhand MJ, Emmelot CH, Ijzerman MJ: Early treatment of trans-tibial amputees: Retrospective analysis of early fitting and elastic bandaging. *Prosthet Orthot Int* 2005;29(1):3-12.

    The use of a rigid dressing provided enhanced wound healing, prevented contractures, and allowed for earlier application of the first prosthesis in dysvascular patients. Level of evidence: III.

18. Vieira Bandeira FC, Brandão Pitta GB, Araújo Castro A, Miranda F Jr: Postoperative incidence of deep vein thrombosis after major lower extremity amputation. *Int Angiol* 2008;27:489-493.

    In a series of 128 dysvascular amputees (age 44 to 97 years), 9.4% developed DVT diagnosed with duplex ultrasound despite thromboprophylaxis with heparin immediately following amputation.

19. Huang ME, Johns JS, White J, Sanford K: Venous

thromboembolism in a rehabilitation setting after major lower extremity amputation. *Arch Phys Med Rehabil* 2005;86:73-78.

Fifty consecutive patients who were lower extremity amputees admitted to an acute inpatient rehabilitation facility were evaluated for DVT with duplex ultrasound. Twelve percent were found to have DVT. The average patient age was 63 years. Most patients had amputations performed for vascular disease; 17% were related to tumor. There were no traumatic amputees in this cohort. DVT was associated with poor function.

20. Matielo MF, Presti C, Casella IB, Netto BM, Puech-Leão P: Incidence of ipsilateral postoperative deep venous thrombosis in the amputated lower extremity of patients with peripheral obstructive arterial disease. *J Vasc Surg* 2008;48(6):1514-1519.

In a group of 56 patients with peripheral arterial disease who had undergone an amputation, risk of a DVT in the residual limb appears to be related to advanced age (older than 70 years), the diagnosis of peripheral arterial disease, and a transfemoral level of amputation. Ipsilateral DVT occurred early and was diagnosed within 35 days of surgery. The occurrence of an ipsilateral DVT in this group did not appear to affect mortality. The authors suggest routine screening in this group of patients. Level of evidence: IV.

21. Gailey R, Allen K, Castles J, Kucharik J, Roeder M: Review of secondary physical conditions associated with lower-limb amputation and long-term prosthesis use. *J Rehabil Res Dev* 2008;45(1):15-29.

The authors reviewed factors related to secondary complications of amputees such as osteopenia, gait disturbances, low back pain, postural changes, and deconditioning. Level of evidence: V.

22. Smurr LM, Gulick K, Yancosek K, Ganz O: Managing the upper extremity amputee: A protocol for success. *J Hand Ther* 2008;21(2):160-175.

A five-phase program of rehabilitation is outlined for the upper extremity amputee based on the large experience of military-related upper extremity limb loss. Level of evidence: V.

23. Smith DG, McFarland LV, Sangeorzan BJ, et al: Postoperative dressing and management strategies for transtibial amputations: A critical review. *J Rehabil Res Dev* 2003;40:213-224.

24. Ketz AK: The experience of phantom limb pain in patients with combat-related traumatic amputations. *Arch Phys Med Rehabil* 2008;89(6):1127-1132.

The prevalence and characteristics of phantom limb pain are described, along with the use and perceived effectiveness of standard medical and self-treatment methods for patients with combat-related traumatic amputations.

25. Bone M, Critchley P, Buggy DJ: Gabapentin in postamputation phantom limb pain: A randomized, double-blind, placebo-controlled, cross-over study. *Reg Anesth Pain Med* 2002;27(5):481-486.

26. Chan BL, Witt R, Charrow AP, et al: Mirror therapy for phantom limb pain. *N Engl J Med* 2007;357(21): 2206-2207.

The investigators divided 22 patients into a mirror trial group and two control groups. All treated patients reported pain relief whereas control groups did not. Level of evidence: II.

27. Eichenberger U, Neff F, Sveticic G, et al: Chronic phantom limb pain: The effects of calcitonin, ketamine, and their combination on pain and sensory thresholds. *Anesth Analg* 2008;106(4):1265-1273.

The authors describe 20 patients obtaining acute relief of phantom limb pain with the use of ketamine infusion up to 48 hours following treatment. Level of evidence: II.

28. Prantl L, Schreml S, Heine N, Eisenmann-Klein M, Angele P: Surgical treatment of chronic phantom limb sensation and limb pain after lower limb amputation. *Plast Reconstr Surg* 2006;118(7):1562-1572.

The authors describe a method of dividing the sciatic nerve above the popliteal fossa and anastomosing the split ends. Favorable results were seen in 15 patients. Level of evidence: IV.

29. Ernberg LA, Adler RS, Lane J: Ultrasound in the detection and treatment of a painful stump neuroma. *Skeletal Radiol* 2003;32:306-309.

30. Singson RD, Feldman F, Staron R, Fechtner D, Gonzalez E, Stein J: MRI of postamputation neuromas. *Skeletal Radiol* 1990;19:259-262.

31. Henrot P, Stines J, Walter F, Martinet N, Paysant J, Blum A: Imaging of the painful lower limb stump. *Radiographics* 2000;20:S219-S235.

32. Foisneau-Lottin A, Martinet N, Henrot P, Paysant J, Blum A, André JM: Bursitis, adventitious bursa, localized soft-tissue inflammation, and bone marrow edema in tibial stumps: The contribution of magnetic resonance imaging to the diagnosis and management of mechanical stress complications. *Arch Phys Med Rehabil* 2003;84(5):770-777.

33. Gruber H, Glodny B, Bodner G, et al: Practical experience with sonographically guided phenol instillation of stump neuroma: Predictors of effects, success, and outcome. *AJR Am J Roentgenol* 2008;190(5):1263-1269.

The authors describe their clinical results in a case series of 82 patients who had an acceptable reduction of their neurogenic pain following ultrasound-guided injection of painful neuromas. Level of evidence: IV.

34. Dahl E, Cohen SP: Perineural injection of etanercept as a treatment for postamputation pain. *Clin J Pain* 2008; 24(2):172-175.

Five of six military-related painful limbs were successfully treated with local injection of etanercept.

35. Bosse MJ, Mackenzie EJ, Kellam JF, et al: An analysis of outcomes of reconstruction or amputation of leg-

1: General Topics and New Technology

threatening injuries. *N Engl J Med* 2002;347:1924-1931.

36. Mackenzie EJ, Bosse MJ, Pollak AN, et al: Long-term persistence of disability following severe lower limb trauma: Results of a seven-year follow-up. *J Bone Joint Surg Am* 2005;87:1801-1809.

    In a follow-up study to that listed in reference 35, the authors demonstrated that the LEAP cohort did not improve on long-term follow-up. At 7 years, the 397 patients generally deteriorated in function. Over half of the patients who had reconstruction and amputation also had Sickness Impact Profile scores greater than 10, indicating severe disability. Through-knee amputees were 11 times more likely than all other groups to have a physical subscore greater than 5. Factors associated with worse outcomes were older age, female gender, lower education level, and low self-efficacy. Level of evidence: I.

37. Hofstad C, Linde H, Limbeek J, Postema K: Prescription of prosthetic ankle-foot mechanisms after lower limb amputation. *Cochrane Database Syst Rev* 2004; 1(1):CD003978.

    The authors comprehensively reviewed data regarding terminal devices in transfemoral and transtibial amputees. Twenty-three trials were reviewed involving 217 patients. Energy-storing feet demonstrated increased efficiency only during incline or decline walking and increased walking speed in transtibial amputees.

38. Klute GK, Berge JS, Orendurff MS, Williams RM, Czerniecki JM: Prosthetic intervention effects on activity of lower-extremity amputees. *Arch Phys Med Rehabil* 2006;87(5):717-722.

    The authors investigated activity levels of shock-absorbing versus nonshock-absorbing pilons in 12 transtibial amputees and microprocessor controlled and mechanical knees in 5 transfemoral amputees. When measured by an automated step counter, no differences were found in the number of steps per week or sustained activity level regardless of the level of sophistication of the prosthetic limb. Level of evidence: III.

39. Kaufman KR, Levine JA, Brey RH, McCrady SK, Padgett DJ, Joyner MJ: Energy expenditure and activity of transfemoral amputees using mechanical and microprocessor-controlled prosthetic knees. *Arch Phys Med Rehabil* 2008;89(7):1380-1385.

    Fifteen patients, average age 42 years, who were long-term transfemoral amputees, were evaluated for energy efficiency and level of activity with mechanical and microprocessor-controlled knees while controlling the other prosthetic components. Although energy efficiency of walking was not improved, level of activity and patient satisfaction were improved with microprocessor-controlled knees. Level of evidence: III.

40. Desmond DM: Coping, affective distress, and psychosocial adjustment among people with traumatic upper limb amputations. *J Psychosom Res* 2007;62(1):15-21.

    The authors reviewed the responses of 138 patients to a self-questionnaire; 28.3% of the patients had significant depressive symptoms and 35.5% had high anxiety levels. Avoidance behavior was strongly predictive of psychological distress and poor adjustment. The findings suggest the potential benefits of interventions to reduce reliance on avoidant coping and stimulate more problem-focused approaches to coping with difficulties and challenges in order to facilitate adaptation and prevent problems in psychosocial functioning postamputation.

41. Saradjian A, Thompson AR, Datta D: The experience of men using an upper limb prosthesis following amputation: Positive coping and minimizing feeling different. *Disabil Rehabil* 2008;30(11):871-883.

    Eleven male patients with an upper extremity amputation identified a theme of ongoing awareness of difference in appearance and ability. Consequently, participants described themes of psychosocial and functional adjustment to minimize this sense of difference. This was facilitated by the participants' prostheses and their positive coping style. Participants also identified the personal meanings of their prosthesis and highlighted the terms of its use. The minimization of their sense of difference resulted in a renewed sense of worth. Level of evidence: IV.

Chapter 9
New Technologies

Meir Marmor, MD   Eric G. Meinberg, MD   Theodore Miclau, MD

Introduction

Over the past few years, a wide variety of technologic advancements have been introduced to the field of orthopaedics. Some are evolutionary changes that have significantly improved the effectiveness and efficacy of current treatments, whereas others are more revolutionary advances that may fundamentally change the approach to challenging problems. Although the new technologies are too numerous to describe in a single chapter, some of the most clinically applicable advances for care of the orthopaedic trauma patient are reviewed.

Locked Plating

The clinical need for locked plates arose from the need to meet the demands of minimally invasive surgery and indirect bridging fixation, and to provide stable fixation for osteopenic or pathologic bone and periarticular fractures. Locking plates have been likened to external

Dr. Marmor or an immediate family member has received research or institutional support from Association International pour l'Osteosynthese Dynamique, Aleeva Medical, AO, Arthritis Foundation, Arthrocare, Biomet, DePuy, EBI, ISTO Technologies, Kyphon, Medtronic, Novo Nordisk, Smith & Nephew, Spinal Kinetics, Spinal Motion, Stryker, Synthes, TissueLink, TranS1, and Zimmer. Dr. Meinberg or an immediate family member has received research or institutional support from the Association International pour l'Osteosynthese Dynamique, Aleeva Medical, AO, Arthritis Foundation, Arhtrocare, Biomet, DePuy, EBI, ISTO Technologies, Kyphon, Medtronic, Novo Nordisk, Smith & Nephew, Spinal Kinetics, SpinalMotion, Stryker, Synthes, TissueLink, TranS1, and Zimmer. Dr. Miclau or an immediate family member serves as a board member, owner, officer, or committee member of American Orthopaedic Association, Orthopaedic Research Society, Orthopaedic Trauma Association, San Francisco General Hospital Foundation, and Foundation for Orthopaedic Trauma; serves as a paid consultant to or is an employee of AO, National Institutes of Health (NIAMS and NICHD), Orthopaedic Trauma Care Foundation; serves as an unpaid consultant to Amgen; has received research or institutional support from DePuy, Musculoskeletal Transplant Foundation, National Institutes of Health (NIAMS and NICHD), Philips, Stryker, Synthes, Zimmer, Orthopaedic Trauma Care Foundation, Orthopaedic Trauma Association; has stock or stock options held in Johnson & Johnson, Merck, and Pfizer.

fixators placed internally (hence their occasional description as "internal fixators"). By firmly fixing the screw to the plate through a threaded interface between the screw heads and the plate body, the plate-screw construct acts as a fixed-angle device, with the screws functioning as threaded locked bolts. With this inherent device stability, the need for compressing the plate directly to a bony surface is obviated (similar to the bars of an external fixator) thus preserving blood supply, reducing the need for plate contouring, and providing elastic fixation. This facilitates fracture union through secondary bone healing with callus formation and allows indirect reduction using minimally invasive percutaneous plating techniques.[1]

Biomechanical Concepts

Fracture fixation with traditional nonlocked plating techniques relies on the frictional force created between the plate and bone to counteract the external forces experienced at the fracture site. Stability with these traditional plate-and-screw constructs is primarily achieved via high screw torque. Variables such as bone quality and fracture comminution affect the quality of screw thread purchase in the bone, and therefore the resultant fixation stability that can be achieved with nonlocked plating. In contrast, screws in a locked plating system securely engage the plate, eliminating screw toggle and creating a fixed-angle, single-beam construct. Single-beam constructs are four times stronger than load-sharing beam constructs, where motion occurs between the individual components of the beam construct. Because all the screws in a single screw fragment are locked to the plate at fixed angles, they must fail (pull out) as a unit rather than individually and sequentially, as is the case in regular plating (**Figure 1**). The fixed-angle nature of the plate and locking screw construct resists cantilever bending stresses and reduces the risk of angular deformity in metaphyseal fractures that are comminuted, have missing bone, or are otherwise mechanically unstable.[2] When using locked plates in a bridging manner, the edges of the fracture are not compressed together. Acting as an "internal external fixator" to bridge the fracture, the locked plate provides relative stability, allowing enough strain at the fracture site to promote secondary healing with callus formation. Additionally, it has been proposed that the reduced plate to bone compression afforded by locking plates serves to protect the viability of the bone by

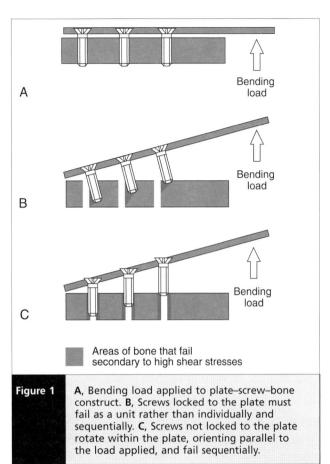

Figure 1 **A,** Bending load applied to plate–screw–bone construct. **B,** Screws locked to the plate must fail as a unit rather than individually and sequentially. **C,** Screws not locked to the plate rotate within the plate, orienting parallel to the load applied, and fail sequentially.

■ Areas of bone that fail secondary to high shear stresses

maintaining microvascular circulation within the cortex and its investing tissues.[3]

Biomechanically, a nonlocked plate system relies on shear forces at the plate-screw junction during loading, whereas a locked plate relies on compressive forces at the screw-bone interface. This force conversion is beneficial in fracture fixation because cortical bone resists compressive loads better than shear loads. Additionally, the inherent angular stability of locked screws allows the applied load to be more evenly distributed among the component screws, avoiding the significant load concentration at a single screw-bone interface that is typical in conventional plating. Thus, the overall fixation strength of the locked plate system equals the sum of fixation strengths of all screw-bone interfaces instead of that of a single component screw, as occurs during conventional plating.[4]

The overall stability provided by the locked plate system across the fracture site becomes dependent on the amount of load applied and the mechanical properties of the plate itself. Acting as an internal external fixator, the fixation rigidity of the locked plate system benefits from the proximity of the plate to the bone and fracture site, with locked screw lengths being significantly shorter than conventional external fixator pins. The extent of the elastic motion that occurs is dictated by the length, the cross-sectional area, and the material properties of the plate, as well as proximity, density, di-

ameter, and cortical configuration (unicortical compared with bicortical) of the inserted screws.[5]

The choice of locked plate length is a key element in the fracture fixation stability provided by the construct and varies according to fracture pattern. Empirically derived recommendations regarding the length of the locked plate typically include using an implant that is 8 to 10 times the length of the fracture in simple patterns and 3 times the length in comminuted fracture patterns. At least two screws per main fragment should be inserted, with three cortices of purchase for simple fractures and at least two screws and four cortices for comminuted fractures. Additionally, a screw-to-hole ratio less than 0.5 limits the bending moments experienced at the most proximal and distal screws. A span of two to three open screw holes over the fracture site may help limit the concentration of stress at the adjacent screw-bone interfaces and provide adequate construct elasticity to allow secondary bone healing.[6]

As with splints, casts, and external fixators, locked plates provide relative stability to the fracture site. When fracture gap strain is kept between 2% and 10%, relative stability leads to secondary bone healing (enchondral ossification) that is characterized by callus formation.[1] Relative stability of the fracture is achieved when the plate is properly sized according to the loading situation and the correct screw density.[6] Newer locked plate designs allow the use of so-called hybrid constructs, in which surgeons use both locked and nonlocking screws together, thus incorporating aspects of locked plating and compression plating into one implant. However, when combining the two fixation methods, the surgeon potentially negates the theoretical advantages of each, creating excessive gap strains at the fracture site potentially leading to nonunion. Often, nonlocking screws can be used to compress fractures and "pull" the plate down to bone, facilitating reduction. The increased stiffness of the locked implant may result in increased rates of periprosthetic fracture in osteoporotic bone. A locked construct, where the outermost screw is a conventional screw, reduces the stress concentration at the plate end and significantly increases the bending strength of the plating construct compared with an all-locked construct.[7]

Indications for Locked Plating
Indications for locked plates include complex periarticular fractures, comminuted metaphyseal or diaphyseal fractures, periprosthetic fractures, and fractures occurring in poor quality bone. Locked plates may also be used as an alternative to dual conventional plating techniques for intercondylar and supracondylar distal femur, bicondylar tibial plateau, and pilon fractures. Additional indications for locked plate systems include metaphyseal fractures of long bones in which intramedullary nail fixation may have a high likelihood of malalignment and poor fixation and fixation after corrective osteotomy procedures.[4]

Designs and Costs

Many locked plating designs are now available. In general, the designs fit into two broad categories—those with fixed-trajectory locking screws and those that allow variable-axis screw locking. Most locking plate systems provide instrumentation to facilitate percutaneous insertion, allow traditional open techniques, provide the option of inserting either unlocked or locked screws through the same plate hole, and allow unicortical or bicortical screw placement. First-generation locked plates relied on unicortical screw fixation. However, monocortical screws require secure purchase in the near cortex and have had insufficient purchase to provide stable fixation in metaphyseal or osteopenic bone with a thin cortex. Additionally, unicortical screw constructs exhibit weakness in torsion, especially in patients with very thin cortices.[4]

The expense of a locked plating construct is substantially higher than that of an equivalent unlocked construct. Much of the cost of such constructs is associated with the locking screws themselves, not the plates. Most systems now offer the surgeon the choice of inserting a locked or unlocked screw through the same hole; thus, the cost of various screw choices should be considered.

Treating Specific Fractures With Locked Plating

Clavicle

Locked dynamic compression plates on the superior surface of the clavicle showed improved bending failure stiffness when compared with nonlocked superior dynamic compression plates in a biomechanical study.[8] There are no clinical reports comparing locked to nonlocked plating in the clavicle.

Proximal Humerus

Biomechanical studies suggest that locked plate fixation of proximal humerus fractures is advantageous in patients who are elderly and have osteoporosis, potentially allowing for earlier postoperative mobilization. Compared to blade plates, locked plates have shown significantly greater stability to torsional loads, a trend toward greater stability in response to bending loads, and significantly less loosening.[9] Compared to unlocked plate fixation, locked plates were shown to be significantly stiffer and provided increased ultimate and cyclic failure strength.[10] Compared to intramedullary nails, locked plates showed significantly less fracture fragment displacement in response to varus cantilever bending, significantly better resistance to torsional loads, and an overall stiffer construct.[11] Clinical studies showed a high rate of fracture union and a low rate of failure.[12] Mechanical support of the medial cortex (recreating a medial buttress) by anatomic reduction or carefully placed inferomedial screws was found to be of critical importance for maintenance of reduction when proximal humerus fractures are treated with locking plates.[13]

Distal Radius

Locked plating of the distal radius appears to offer stable fixation, even for comminuted fractures, allowing early range of motion. In a biomechanical model of dorsally comminuted distal radius fractures, the comparison of dorsally placed, nonlocked T plating compared with volar fixed-angle plating of distal radius fractures showed that the volar locked plate was stiffer than the dorsal plate with respect to both volar and ulnar loading and in all modes of axial loading, with the exception of dorsal loading.[14] In clinical studies, treatment with locking plates is associated with high union rates, low complication rates, and satisfactory clinical outcomes.[15,16]

Distal Femur

In cadaver model biomechanical studies, a locked Less Invasive Stabilization System (LISS; Synthes, USA, Paoli, PA) construct demonstrated greater fixation strength in response to axial loading in comparison with the angle blade plate and the intramedullary nail.[17] Compared to fixation with an angled blade plate, locked plate fixation resulted in significantly less fracture fragment subsidence with cyclic loading and significantly greater ultimate load to failure.[18] Clinical studies have shown high union rates and low failure rates with the use of the locked plating system in distal femoral fractures.[19] Locked plating traditionally is less demanding than blade plating, although careful reduction, surgical technique, and hardware positioning are still necessary.

Proximal Tibia

Laterally-based locked plates provide increased stability in the presence of metaphyseal or metadiaphyseal comminution. This increased stability allows use of a minimally invasive technique, potentially avoiding wound dehiscence and infection associated with extended approaches.[20] When comparing dual plating versus unilateral locked plating for bicondylar tibial plateau fractures, there was similar fracture fragment subsidence with both fixation constructs. However, higher elastic deformation was noted in the unilateral locked plating group.[21] Other studies have found dual plating to have higher strength in controlling the medial fragments.[22,23] In the clinical setting, a high union rate and low failure rate were reported for the treatment of complex tibial plateau fractures with locked plating.[24] Because interfragmentary compression cannot be achieved by locked plates, the supplementary use of interfragmentary screws may be required to prevent loss of reduction and to ensure adequate compression of the fragments.

Calcaneus

In biomechanical studies, locked plate constructs for the treatment of calcaneal fractures demonstrated significantly less plastic deformation with cyclic loading, higher ultimate failure strength,[25] and less fracture fragment displacement in comparison with their nonlocking counterparts.[26] However, clinical studies have not shown that locked plates are superior over conventional plates in treating calcaneal fractures.

Periprosthetic Fractures

Locked plating systems have also been used in the management of periprosthetic fractures around total knee and total hip replacements, with favorable results. In a prospective evaluation of 22 periprosthetic supracondylar femur fractures treated with a locked plate, 86% of fractures went on to uneventful fracture union. Ninety-one percent of fractures had postoperative alignment within 5° of normal, with 88% of patients returning to their baseline ambulatory status. The three fractures that did not heal occurred in patients with comorbid obesity and diabetes.[27] In a series of 11 periprosthetic fractures occurring near total knee replacements, at a mean of 21 weeks, 10 of 11 fractures healed, with 82% of cases healing in anatomic alignment.[28] The use of locked plates often obviates the need for direct exposure of the joint prosthesis, damage to the bearing surface, and complex revision arthroplasty procedures.

Limitations of Locked Plates

Regardless of its success in many fields, locked plating is not a panacea for problems that plague internal fixation of fractures. The reported failure modes of locked plates include plate bending, plate pull-off, plate breakage, and screw breakage at the screw-plate interface.[4] In a retrospective study of 51 patients treated with locked plating of proximal humerus fractures, 8 shoulders in 8 patients (16%) had screws that penetrated the humeral head, suggesting failure of the locked construct to hold the humeral head in the reduced position.[29] A recent prospective multicenter study using locked plates for proximal humerus fractures showed a 35% complication rate (particularly primary and secondary screw perforations into the glenohumeral joint).[30] The use of the LISS system for distal femoral fractures is associated with valgus malalignment. This complication was attributed to loss of reduction, design of the implants, and reduction instruments in first-generation locked plates.[15] In a study of 69 high-energy fractures of the tibial plateau treated by unilateral locked plating, loss of reduction was seen in 13% of the fractures.[31] A subsequent biomechanical study showed that, in the setting of a vertically oriented fracture in a medial tibial plateau without comminution, the medial buttress plate provides significantly greater stability than lateral locked plating in static loading and a trend toward improved stability with cyclic loading.[22] In all but the most osteopenic patients, locked plating likely offers little or no advantage when treating lower energy unicondylar fractures (for example, Shatzker type I, II, III, many type IV). In a biomechanical study of periprosthetic fractures around a stable femoral component of a total hip replacement, a combination of a nonlocked plate with an allograft strut showed superior stiffness when compared with locked plating.[32] Similar results were seen in 14 consecutive patients with Vancouver type B1 periprosthetic fractures of the femur. Of 14 fractures, only 8 (57%) healed uneventfully at a mean of 5.4 months. Six of the locked plate constructs failed: three secondary to plate fracture and three secondary to plate pullout. The authors concluded on the basis of their data that locked plating systems did not offer an advantage over other fixation strategies in the management of fractures distal to the tip of a stable femoral prosthesis.[33] The benefit of locked plates over conventional plates has not been proven by prospective comparative studies in proximal humerus, distal radius, or calcaneus fractures.[15] In a recent study of distal radius fracture, use of a locked volar plate led to better patient-reported outcomes (Disabilities of the Arm, Shoulder and Hand scores) in the first 3 months after fixation. However, at 6 months and 1 year, the outcomes were equivalent to external fixation or a radial column plate.[34] Finally, in a recent meta-analysis of studies comparing locked plates to nonlocked plates in the treatment of distal radius, proximal humerus, or tibial plateau fractures, there were no statistically significant differences in patient-oriented outcomes, adverse events, or complications.[2] Thus, it is prudent to reserve locked plating for problematic fractures for which unlocked plates have demonstrated an increased rate of mechanical failure.

Nanotechnology

Nanotechnology can be defined as the science and engineering involved in the design, synthesis, characterization, and application of materials and devices at the atomic, molecular, and supramolecular levels (at least one dimension on the nanoscale). In the orthopaedic arena, nanotechnology is presently being applied in implants, surgical tools, grafts, cartilage replacement, patient therapy, and patient recovery.[35]

Nanostructured materials are aimed at creating an environment more conducive for osteoblast function and bone ingrowth. Using the process of anodization, a vertically aligned nanotube array of titanium oxide on the surface of titanium substrate can be produced. These tubes produce nanofibers of bioactive sodium titanate structure that induce growth of nanodimensioned hydroxyapatite after immersion in a simulated body fluid.[36] As much as three times more calcium deposition has been displayed by osteoblasts cultured on nanostructured titanium compared with conventional titanium.[37] Helical rosette nanotubes are a new class of self-assembled organic tubes featuring the complementary hydrogen-bonding arrays of guanine and cytosine. These tubular assemblies can allow the attachment of growth factors or specific bone recognition peptide sequences that promote bone cell adhesion.[38] Another approach involves fabrication of a thin nano-dimensioned hydroxyapatite (n-HA) coating on titanium using the soluble gelatin technique and dip-coating method.[39]

Nanostructured ceramics, such as nanostructured diamond, n-HA, and metalloceramic coatings, can improve the friction and wear properties associated with joint arthroplasty components. These are tougher and stronger than coarser-grained ceramics, and they lack common drawbacks attributed to ceramic devices, such as brittleness and geometric limitations. Finally, implants with a surface roughness measured on the nanometer scale are more likely to be colonized with host cells and are less conducive to bacterial adherence than surfaces with micrometer-scale roughness.

Nanotechnology can be applied to improve surgical instruments. The cutting quality of a blade can be improved by the sharpness of the cutting edge and the nanoscale surface roughness of the blade using fabrication techniques such as the plasma sharpening process, which produces diamond-coated carbide blades that have low surface roughness values (20 to 40 nm) and minimize frictional effects.[40] These material properties at the nanoscale allow for lower penetration force, finer dissections, and cleaner cuts leading to more rapid healing. Nanoamorphous coatings have been reported to provide enhanced corrosion and wear properties for medical instruments, using a detonation gun thermal spray process to deposit the nanoamorphous coatings of two compositions: iron-chromium-phosphorus-calcium and tungsten-carbon-cobalt.

Nanostructured biomaterials have the potential to provide unique bone substitute grafts. The nanocomposition of these materials emulates the natural bone's hierarchical organization, to initiate the growth of an apatite (calcium phosphate) layer and to allow for the cellular and tissue responses of bone remodeling. The materials also have the potential to provide analogous mechanical properties to bone, which can then be adapted for different applications. The Young's modulus of a nanocomposite of n-HA with polyamide (polyhexamethylene adipamide), producing n-HA crystals 5 to 26.7 nm in diameter and 30 to 84 nm long, matches well with natural bone. This material can help eliminate stress shielding associated with the mismatch of mechanical properties between graft and bone. In addition to bioactive materials, biodegradable properties in bone grafts also are desirable. When implanted in a marrow cavity, biodegradable n-HA/collagen composites undergo solution-mediated dissolution and giant-cell-mediated resorption at the bone-substitute interface, and promote new bone formation. This process of degradation and consequent bone formation is reminiscent of the known natural process of bone remodeling. Nanofibrous scaffolds fabricated by electrospinning biodegradable polylactic acid (PLA) mixed with single-wall carbon nanotubes showed favorable and promising biologic responses compared to traditional PLA materials.[41,42]

Nanotechnology has also been applied to drug delivery. A water-soluble corticosteroid (betamethasone sodium phosphate) encapsulated into nanospheres with a biodegradable polymer DL-lactide/glycolide copolymer has seemingly prolonged anti-inflammatory action in the joints of arthritic rabbits.[43] Postoperative patient recovery may be improved by applying nanotechnology to wound dressings. A nanofibrous polyurethane membrane prepared by electrospinning has characteristics desirable for an effective wound dressing such as controlled evaporative water loss and excellent oxygen permeability. The dressings also promote fluid drainage, thereby decreasing buildup under the covering to prevent wound desiccation. It has been proposed that the dressings can inhibit exogenous microorganism invasion because of its ultrafine nanoporous structure.[44]

Nanotechnology will be used increasingly in orthopaedics and likely will play a valuable role in future developments. However, at the present time, there is an incomplete understanding of how the costs, risks, and benefits of this technology may affect clinical practice.

Reamer-Irrigator-Aspirator

The reaming process of long bones for intramedullary nail insertion has been associated with pulmonary complications resulting from embolization of medullary elements, such as fat and reaming debris, into the venous system. This embolization is due to highly elevated intramedullary pressures generated by conventional reaming methods.[45]

The Reamer-Irrigator-Aspirator (RIA; Synthes, USA, Paoli, PA) has been developed to reduce medullary embolization. The RIA maintains reduced intramedullary pressure by irrigating the canal and aspirating debris created during the reaming process (**Figure 2**). Animal studies have shown a reduction in the incidence of systemic embolism with the use of RIA.[46] A recent clinical study reported successful use of the RIA for canal débridement to treat osteomyelitis of the tibia and femur.[47] Particles aspirated by the RIA are trapped by a coarse filter, from which they can be recovered and used as an intraoperative source of autologous, osteogenic material. Recent studies confirm the ability of these osseous particles to promote bone healing. The RIA debris filtrate has been shown to contain growth factors important for tissue repair (FGF-2, BMP-2, IGF-I, TGFb1, PDGF), as well as osteoprogenitor cells that respond to these factors.[48] Further evaluation is underway to determine the broader clinical utility of this system.

Negative Pressure Wound Therapy

Negative pressure wound therapy (NPWT) with reticulated open cell foam is a method of temporary protection of soft-tissue defects by polyurethane foam that is sealed with a transparent adhesive drape (**Figure 3**). A negative topical pressure within the wound is generated using a vacuum pump. NPWT has been beneficial for wound healing in a variety of traumatic and nontraumatic soft-tissue defects. It has been shown that NPWT

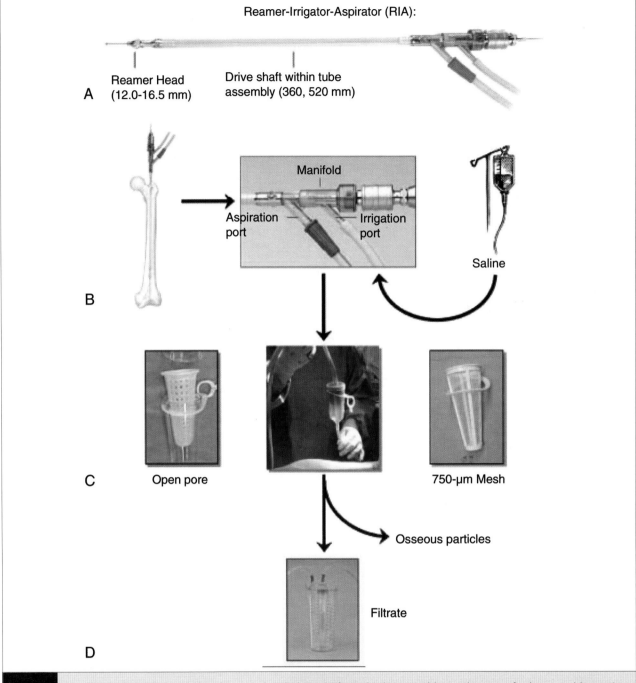

Reamer-Irrigator-Aspirator (RIA):

A, Reamer Head (12.0-16.5 mm) | Drive shaft within tube assembly (360, 520 mm)

B, Manifold | Aspiration port | Irrigation port | Saline

C, Open pore | 750-µm Mesh

Osseous particles

D, Filtrate

Figure 2 RIA system. **A,** System consists of reamer head, drive shaft, and tube assembly. **B,** Close-up of tube assembly manifold, with irrigation and aspiration ports. **C,** Aspirate is typically passed through a filter of optional mesh to collect osseous particles. Examples shown here are as follows: left, open pore; right, 750-mm mesh. Filtrate is collected in a sterile vessel (**D**). Reproduced with permission of Synthes, Inc. Inc. or its affiliates.

optimizes microperfusion and blood flow, increases the partial oxygen pressure within the tissue, and reduces bacterial colonization. The cyclical application of sub-atmospheric pressure alters the cytoskeleton of the cells in the wound bed, triggering a cascade of intracellular signals that increases the rate of cell division and subsequent formation of granulation tissue.[49] NPWT of traumatic wounds leads to increased concentrations of local interleukin-8 (IL-8) and vascular endothelial growth factor, which may trigger accumulation of neutrophils and angiogenesis and, thus, accelerate neovascularization.[50] Other potential mechanisms of action include the removal of excess edematous fluid and alleviation of capillary afterload at the level of the microcirculation, limitation of destructive proteases within the wound, facilitation of bacterial clearance,

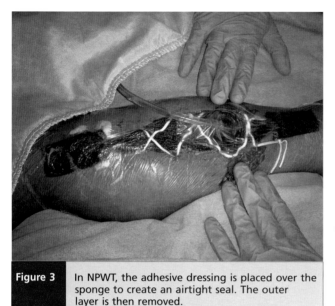

Figure 3   In NPWT, the adhesive dressing is placed over the sponge to create an airtight seal. The outer layer is then removed.

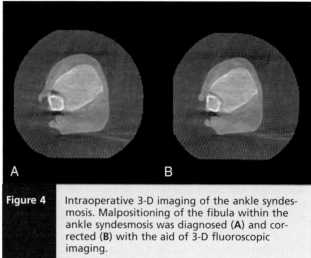

Figure 4   Intraoperative 3-D imaging of the ankle syndesmosis. Malpositioning of the fibula within the ankle syndesmosis was diagnosed (**A**) and corrected (**B**) with the aid of 3-D fluoroscopic imaging.

and limitation of cross-contamination in the hospital environment.[51] The combined effect of these mechanisms may decrease the necessity for further débridement in the "second look" procedure done 48 to 72 hours after the initial procedure.[52]

Wounds for which the use of NPWT may be beneficial include fasciotomy wounds, traumatic wounds associated with initial contamination, open fractures, and surgical incisions made for open reduction and internal fixation of at-risk injuries such as calcaneus, pilon, and tibial plateau fractures. When used in fasciotomy wounds the NPWT has several distinct advantages over conventional dressings. These advantages include the conversion of a wound from an open environment to a closed environment, thus theoretically protecting it from nosocomial infection; the simplification of nursing care by reducing the number of dressing changes needed; the promotion of granulation tissue formation through a microstrain effect that augments muscle healing and allows soft tissue coverage; and the production of a macrostrain on the surrounding tissues that results in collagen relaxation and increased likelihood of primary closure of the wound. NPWT should be applied to a wound after the soft tissue has been thoroughly débrided, explored, and cleaned and after bleeding has been well controlled. Typically NPWT is applied for 48 to 72 hours after which a "second look" procedure is performed.[53]

In a series of 88 high-energy soft-tissue wounds identified in 77 patients treated with NPWT in US facilities in Iraq, both the wound infection rate and the overall wound complication rate were 0%.[54] In a prospective randomized study, NPWT was associated with earlier sealing of seromas or hematomas draining more than 5 days and reduced wound breakdown in high-risk surgical incisions (for calcaneus, pilon, and tibial plateau fractures).[55] The rate of soft-tissue coverage of open

fractures using free flaps has dropped from 42% between 1992 and 1995 to 5% between 2000 and 2003. This change was attributed particularly to the introduction of NPWT to wound care.[56] Further investigations are necessary to fully elucidate the exact mechanisms and kinetics of the wound-healing process as well as the clinical results of NPWT.

Imaging

MRI T1-rho or Cartilage Imaging

Early recognition of traumatic joint injuries and degenerative changes permits interventions that are aimed at delaying the progression of degenerative joint disease. The use of MRI technology to image cartilage has been shown to be very efficacious.

Using arthroscopy as a standard, an MRI fat-suppressed fast spin-echo sequence achieved a sensitivity of 87%, a specificity of 97%, and an accuracy of 92% with minimal interobserver variability (kappa value = 0.93). Newer turbo or fast spin-echo techniques have allowed construction of three-dimensional (3-D) models of cartilage thickness.[57]

Newer quantitative techniques (such as T2 mapping and T1-rho imaging) that measure relaxation times in native cartilage or repair tissue are generally directed toward an assessment of a specific component of articular cartilage biochemistry and ultrastructure. The clinical use of quantitative MRI techniques includes the ability to detect early degenerative changes in cartilage biochemistry that may precede discernible thinning of the cartilage on traditional cartilage-sensitive pulse sequences.

T2 Mapping

Standard T2-weighted MRI highlights the presence of joint fluid and disruption of cartilage structures but may also underestimate the presence of surface defects and surface fibrillation. Direct calculation and mapping of

T2, the transverse relaxation time constant, provides quantitative information on the structure and composition of articular cartilage and local mobile water. Previous investigators have found correlations between T2 and local water content, collagen fiber orientation, and loss of type II collagen. Proteoglycan depletion of articular cartilage using enzymatic degradation of the tissue as a model of osteoarthritis has been shown to have little effect on the T2 value, suggesting some degree of specificity for targeting the collagen component of the matrix.[58] Although water is present in the superficial zone of articular cartilage, the collagen fibers are highly ordered, and this arrangement produces rapid dephasing of the MRI signal, resulting in short T2 values. These reduced T2 values may not be clearly evident on a normal clinical scanner because the superficial zone comprises approximately 10% of the overall tissue depth. Previous investigators have performed scan-rescan protocols on a set of subjects and found a high level of repeatability (precision error of 3%–7%) of calculated T2 values between the scan sessions. In addition, it has been determined that separate examiners can evaluate the same T2 map with a high level of agreement (mean difference of 1 ± 1.4 ms).[58]

T1-rho (T1ρ) Imaging

T1ρ imaging is capable of evaluating "slow-motion" interactions between water and the local macromolecular components within articular cartilage, such as proteoglycans. T1ρ image acquisition produces images with higher signal-to-noise ratio than T2-weighted images. Recent T1ρ imaging research has focused on the evaluation of the quantitative analysis of articular cartilage degeneration. The source of the degeneration has been the application of enzymatic compounds, or in vivo degeneration caused by osteoarthritis. Using enzymatic degradation of proteoglycans by trypsin, a positive linear correlation has been found between the proteoglycan content and the average T1ρ value of cartilage tissue in vitro.[59] In vivo, subjects with clinical osteoarthritis symptoms have been found to have significantly longer T1ρ values than the asymptomatic subjects.[60] In similar subject groups T2 mapping did not show significant differences, suggesting that T1ρ imaging may be more sensitive to cartilage degeneration than T2 mapping alone.[61]

Three-Dimensional Fluoroscopy

Accurate anatomic reconstruction of intra-articular fractures is essential for optimal results in trauma surgery. CT is the standard imaging modality for intra-articular fracture analysis and classification, dedicated treatment planning, and analysis of the results of articular surface reconstruction. Specifically, CT permits the assessment of articular gaps or step-offs, as well as accurate positioning of the implants. However, for intraoperative decision making, the surgeon commonly has to rely on visualization of the approach and two-dimensional imaging provided by conventional C-arm technology. Intraoperative CT is very costly to use, requires designated radiographic technicians, and may be impractical to install in the operating room because of the weight and structure of the technology.

Intraoperative 3-D C-arms were introduced clinically in 2001 (SIREMOBIL Iso-C3D; Siemens Medical Solutions, Erlangen, Germany). The 3-D C-arms consist of a standard mobile C-arm system, a motorized orbital motor, and hardware and software components for 3-D imaging. The 3-D C-arm rotates around the surgical field and, to ensure sterility, an additional draping is usually required. The 3-D C-arm must be positioned so that the region of interest is isocentric on both the AP and lateral projections. Axial scans are first generated, followed by reconstruction into coronal and sagittal slice orientations.[62] When compared with spiral CT images of tibial plateau fractures, 3-D C-arm images were lower in quality and had more prominent metal artifacts, but had a similar clinical value.[63] Iso-C-3D can be useful in planning surgical reconstructions and can verify the reconstruction of articular surfaces, the position of implants, and the accuracy of reduction with diagnostic image quality (**Figure 4**).

The benefits of intraoperative reduction assessment and control of implant positioning have been proven by numerous studies for various indications. In a prospective study of 248 consecutive patients with intra-articular fractures, intraoperative image analysis of 19% resulted in immediate adjustment of the reduction or hardware exchange. These revisions were based on 3-D C-arm views of the articular surface that were not visible using fluoroscopy.[64] 3-D C-arms have also been shown to be superior to conventional fluoroscopy in identifying misplaced acetabular screws.[65]

During arthroscopic reduction and fixation of tibial plateau fractures, 3-D C-arms can provide precise information about the result.[66] In a series of 32 surgically treated calcaneal fractures, 3-D C-arm imaging required an average total time of 610 seconds. The information obtained from the scan led the surgeon to alter the reduction or screw placement in 41% of the patients.[67] Prospective studies are still needed to assess the clinical benefit of this instrument.

Electronic Templating

Traditional pen-on-paper preoperative templating has been likened to a blueprint for major construction and recommended as an important part of preoperative preparation for complex fractures, osteotomies, nonunions, and other complex procedures.[68] Recently, software packages have been developed that use digitized radiographs or CT scans of the affected limb, powerful image manipulation to cut and paste bone segments, and a computerized catalog of implant templates that are scaled to the image (**Figure 5**). These can be used to provide virtual reduction and stabilization, and production of a virtual operative plan.[69] Superior reliability

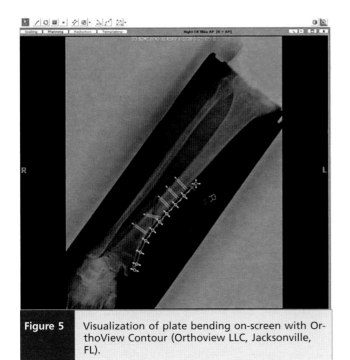

| Figure 5 | Visualization of plate bending on-screen with OrthoView Contour (Orthoview LLC, Jacksonville, FL). |

and accuracy compared to traditional templating has been demonstrated in hip and knee arthroplasty,[70,71] but to date there have been no similar studies in the trauma literature. Electronic templating is useful as an education tool and planning exercise, streamlines implant and equipment needs in the operating room, and ensures a more efficient procedure with reliable outcomes. Given the rapid pace of computer software and hardware development, substantially more improvements will be made in this technology.

Summary

New technologies in orthopaedics are being introduced at a rapid pace. These advancements have the potential to markedly improve the care of patients with musculoskeletal injuries and are highly accessible to the average orthopaedic surgeon (for example, locked plates, NPWT, RIA) or have the potential to change current practice (for example, nanotechnology and imaging breakthroughs). Although it is natural to embrace new technologies to improve patient care, acceptance of these new technologies is often associated with increased costs, and the orthopaedic surgeon is responsible for assessing the merits of each relative to existing standards, based on available evidence.

Annotated References

1. Egol KA, Kubiak EN, Fulkerson E, Kummer FJ, Koval KJ: Biomechanics of locked plates and screws. *J Orthop Trauma* 2004;18(8):488-493.

   The authors review biomechanical principles that guide fracture fixation with plates and screws, comparing and contrasting the function of conventional unlocked plates with that of locked plates in fracture fixation. It is concluded that locked plates and conventional plates provide different biologic environments for healing. Level of evidence: V.

2. Anglen J, Kyle RF, Marsh JL, et al: Locking plates for extremity fractures. *J Am Acad Orthop Surg* 2009; 17(7):465-472.

   The authors reviewed 33 peer-reviewed studies and examined indications for the use of locked plates, their effectiveness in comparison with traditional nonlocked plates, and their cost-effectiveness. Level of evidence: V.

3. Kubiak EN, Fulkerson E, Strauss E, Egol KA: The evolution of locked plates. *J Bone Joint Surg Am* 2006; 88(Suppl 4):189-200.

   This article discusses the history of locked plates, including the impetus for the locked (fixed-angle) plate design, current indications and design trends, the latest clinical and biomechanical data, shortcomings of locked plates, and future applications and directions for locked plates. Level of evidence: V.

4. Strauss EJ, Schwarzkopf R, Kummer F, Egol KA: The current status of locked plating: The good, the bad, and the ugly. *J Orthop Trauma* 2008;22(7):479-486.

   This review focuses on the biomechanics of locked plate technology, appropriate indications for its use, laboratory and clinical comparisons to conventional plating techniques, and potential mechanisms of locked plate failure that have been observed. Level of evidence: V.

5. Gautier E, Perren SM, Cordey J: Effect of plate position relative to bending direction on the rigidity of a plate osteosynthesis: A theoretical analysis. *Injury* 2000; 31(Suppl 3):C14-C20.

6. Gautier E, Sommer C: Guidelines for the clinical application of the LCP. *Injury* 2003;34(Suppl 2):B63-B76.

7. Bottlang M, Doornink J, Byrd GD, Fitzpatrick DC, Madey SM: A nonlocking end screw can decrease fracture risk caused by locked plating in the osteoporotic diaphysis. *J Bone Joint Surg Am* 2009;91(3):620-627.

   The authors studied whether locked plating in osteoporotic diaphyseal bone causes a greater periprosthetic fracture risk than conventional plating because of stress concentrations at the plate end.

8. Celestre P, Roberston C, Mahar A, Oka R, Meunier M, Schwartz A: Biomechanical evaluation of clavicle fracture plating techniques: Does a locking plate provide improved stability? *J Orthop Trauma* 2008;22(4):241-247.

   The authors studied 24 preosteomized synthetic clavicles that were repaired with either contourable dual compression plate (CDCP) or locked CDCP technology (3.5-mm plates) in either the superior or anterior-inferior position to form 4 groups of 6 clavicles. Biomechanically, repairing a midshaft clavicle fracture with a superior plate was more favorable in comparison with anterior-inferior plating in terms of load to failure and bending failure stiffness. Superior locked CDCP plates had improved bending failure stiffness over CDCP plates.

9. Siffri PC, Peindl RD, Coley ER, Norton J, Connor PM, Kellam JF: Biomechanical analysis of blade plate versus locking plate fixation for a proximal humerus fracture: Comparison using cadaveric and synthetic humeri. *J Orthop Trauma* 2006;20(8):547-554.

This study compares the mechanical stability of a fixed-angle blade plate with that of a locked plate in a cadaver proximal humerus fracture fixation model subjected to cyclic loading. Locked plate constructs demonstrated significantly greater torsional stability and similar bending stability than blade plates. In contrast, these same constructs performed similarly with torsional loading when using synthetic humerus specimens.

10. Seide K, Triebe J, Faschingbauer M, et al: Locked vs. unlocked plate osteosynthesis of the proximal humerus: A biomechanical study. *Clin Biomech* 2007;22(2):176-182.

Seven paired humeri were mounted with either a locked or nonlocked proximal humeral plate, followed by a transverse subcapital osteotomy. Because of the optimal load transfer between implant and cancellous bone, a locked screw plate interface was found to reduce fixation failure in proximal humerus fractures.

11. Edwards SL, Wilson NA, Zhang LQ, Flores S, Merk BR: Two-part surgical neck fractures of the proximal part of the humerus: A biomechanical evaluation of two fixation techniques. *J Bone Joint Surg Am* 2006;88(10):2258-2264.

The biomechanical stability of a proximal humeral intermedullary nail was compared with that of a locked plate for the treatment of a comminuted two-part fracture of the surgical neck in a human cadaver model. The locked proximal humeral plate demonstrated superior biomechanical characteristics in comparison with the proximal humeral nail when tested cyclically in both cantilevered varus bending and torsion. The rate of early failure of the proximal humeral nail could reflect the high moment transmitted to the locking proximal screw-bone interface in this implant.

12. Moonot P, Ashwood N, Hamlet M: Early results for treatment of three- and four-part fractures of the proximal humerus using the PHILOS plate system. *J Bone Joint Surg Br* 2007;89(9):1206-1209.

The authors studied 32 patients with acutely displaced three- or four-part proximal fractures of the humerus treated with open reduction and internal fixation using a proximal humeral locked plate. The plate provided stable fixation in young patients with good quality bone sufficient to permit early mobilization. Level of evidence: IV.

13. Gardner MJ, Weil Y, Barker JU, Kelly BT, Helfet DL, Lorich DG: The importance of medial support in locked plating of proximal humerus fractures. *J Orthop Trauma* 2007;21(3):185-191.

Of 35 patients who underwent locked plating for a proximal humerus fracture and who were followed up until healing, 18 with medial support (an appropriately placed inferomedial oblique screw or anatomic humeral head) had a 1.2-mm average loss of humeral head height. In 17 patients without medial support, loss of humeral height averaged 5.8 mm ($P < 0.001$). All fractures in both groups healed without delay, and none required revision to arthroplasty. Achieving mechanical support of the inferomedial region of the proximal humerus was important for maintaining fracture reduction. Level of evidence: IV.

14. Liporace FA, Gupta S, Jeong GK, et al: A biomechanical comparison of a dorsal 3.5-mm T-plate and a volar fixed-angle plate in a model of dorsally unstable distal radius fractures. *J Orthop Trauma* 2005;19(3):187-191.

The authors compared dorsally unstable distal radius fracture fixation with either a standard dorsal non-locked T plate or a volar locked fixed-angle plate in a biomechanical study. The volar locked fixed-angle plate maintained a greater percentage of its initial stiffness after cyclic loading than the dorsal nonlocked plate.

15. Haidukewych GJ, Ricci W: Locked plating in orthopaedic trauma: A clinical update. *J Am Acad Orthop Surg* 2008;16(6):347-355.

The authors reviewed locked plating, with a focus on the limited data available on the efficacy of these new implants, and advised that locked constructs should be reserved for problematic fractures that have demonstrated poor outcomes with unlocked constructs. Level of evidence: IV.

16. Arora R, Lutz M, Hennerbichler A, Krappinger D, Espen D, Gabl M: Complications following internal fixation of unstable distal radius fracture with a palmar locking-plate. *J Orthop Trauma* 2007;21(5):316-322.

The clinical and radiologic outcomes of 114 patients with displaced, unstable distal radius fractures treated with a palmar fixed-angle plate were retrospectively reviewed. Complications arose as a result of very distal palmar plate position, screws that penetrated the extensor compartments, and distal screws in comminuted fracture patterns that cut through the subchondral bone and penetrated the radiocarpal joint. Level of evidence: IV.

17. Zlowodzki M, Williamson S, Zardiackas LD, Kregor PJ: Biomechanical evaluation of the less invasive stabilization system and the 95-degree angled blade plate for the internal fixation of distal femur fractures in human cadaveric bones with high bone mineral density. *J Trauma* 2006;60(4):836-840.

Locked unicortal screw fixation was compared with standard blade plate for fixation of supracondylar femoral fractures using a 4-cm gap fracture model in a biomechanical study. There appeared to be no biomechanical advantage of using the locked plate over the blade plate in bones with high bone mineral density.

18. Higgins TF, Pittman G, Hines J, Bachus KN: Biomechanical analysis of distal femur fracture fixation: Fixed-angle screw-plate construct versus condylar blade plate. *J Orthop Trauma* 2007;21(1):43-46.

Locked unicortical screw fixation was compared to standard blade plate fixation for supracondylar femoral fractures using a fracture gap model. The locking screw-plate construct proved stronger than the blade plate in both cyclic loading and ultimate strength.

19. Kregor PJ, Stannard JA, Zlowodzki M, Cole PA: Treatment of distal femur fractures using the less invasive stabilization system: Surgical experience and early clinical results in 103 fractures. *J Orthop Trauma* 2004;18(8): 509-520.

The treatment of distal femur fractures with LISS was associated with high union rates without autogenous bone grafting (93%), a low incidence of infection (3%), and maintenance of distal femoral fixation (100%). No loss of fixation in the distal femoral condyles was observed despite the treatment of 30 patients older than 65 years. Level of evidence: IV.

20. Musahl V, Tarkin I, Kobbe P, Tzioupis C, Siska PA, Pape HC: New trends and techniques in open reduction and internal fixation of fractures of the tibial plateau. *J Bone Joint Surg Br* 2009;91(4):426-433.

Current surgical approaches and techniques, improved devices for internal fixation, and the clinical outcome after utilization of new methods for locked plating of tibial plateau fractures were reviewed. Level of evidence: V.

21. Gösling T, Schandelmaier P, Marti A, Hufner T, Partenheimer A, Krettek C: Less invasive stabilization of complex tibial plateau fractures: A biomechanical evaluation of a unilateral locked screw plate and double plating. *J Orthop Trauma* 2004;18(8):546-551.

This cadaver study compared the vertical subsidence in a bicondylar tibial plateau fracture model stabilized by either a unilateral locked plate or double nonlocked plating. Both methods of fixation had high resistance to vertical subsidence, and there was no statistically significant difference between either method.

22. Ratcliff JR, Werner FW, Green JK, Harley BJ: Medial buttress versus lateral locked plating in a cadaver medial tibial plateau fracture model. *J Orthop Trauma* 2007;21(7):444-448.

In this cadaver study, the mechanical stability of a medial tibial plateau fracture model secured with a lateral locking periarticular plate was compared with that of a medial buttress plate in cyclic testing and load to failure.

23. Higgins TF, Klatt J, Bachus KN: Biomechanical analysis of bicondylar tibial plateau fixation: How does lateral locking plate fixation compare to dual plate fixation? *J Orthop Trauma* 2007;21(5):301-306.

In this cadaver study, lateral-only locked plating was compared with medial and lateral nonlocked plating in a model of a bicondylar proximal tibial plateau fracture.

24. Stannard JP, Wilson TC, Volgas DA, Alonso JE: The less invasive stabilization system in the treatment of complex fractures of the tibial plateau: Short-term results. *J Orthop Trauma* 2004;18(8):552-558.

Thirty-nine fractures of the tibial plateau that were treated with locked plates and mini-invasive surgical technique were studied in a prospective series. Level of evidence: IV.

25. Stoffel K, Booth G, Rohrl SM, Kuster M: A comparison of conventional versus locking plates in intraarticular calcaneus fractures: A biomechanical study in human cadavers. *Clin Biomech* 2007;22(1): 100-105.

The authors of this cadaver study compared fixation strength obtained using calcaneal plates with and without locking screws in the fixation of osteoporotic fractures. The locking plate showed significantly less irreversible deformation during cyclic loading and a significantly higher load to failure.

26. Richter M, Gosling T, Zech S, et al: A comparison of plates with and without locking screws in a calcaneal fracture model. *Foot Ankle Int* 2005;26(4):309-319.

This biomechanical study compared different plates in an experimental calcaneal fracture model under biocompatible loading. Plates with locked screws provided greater stability during cyclic loading than the plates without locked screws.

27. Ricci WM, Loftus T, Cox C, Borrelli J: Locked plates combined with minimally invasive insertion technique for the treatment of periprosthetic supracondylar femur fractures above a total knee arthroplasty. *J Orthop Trauma* 2006;20(3):190-196.

In this clinical case series, 24 supracondylar femur fractures above a well-fixed nonstemmed total knee arthroplasty were treated with a locking condylar plate; results were satisfactory in nondiabetic patients. Patients with diabetes were at high risk for healing complications and infection. Level of evidence: IV.

28. Raab GE, Davis CM III: Early healing with locked condylar plating of periprosthetic fractures around the knee. *J Arthroplasty* 2005;20(8):984-989.

In a clinical case series of 11 patients with periprosthetic fractures around the knee that were treated with open reduction and internal fixation using a locked condylar plate, there was reliable fracture healing and early motion was permitted in complex fractures. Level of evidence: IV.

29. Egol KA, Ong CC, Walsh M, Jazrawi LM, Tejwani NC, Zuckerman JD: Early complications in proximal humerus fractures (OTA Types 11) treated with locked plates. *J Orthop Trauma* 2008;22(3):159-164.

In a retrospective review, the results of 51 proximal humerus fractures treated with a proximal humeral internal locking system were reported. Screw penetration was the major complication noted. Level of evidence: IV.

30. Brunner F, Sommer C, Bahrs C, et al: Open reduction and internal fixation of proximal humerus fractures using a proximal humeral locked plate: A prospective multicenter analysis. *J Orthop Trauma* 2009;23(3): 163-172.

The authors prospectively evaluated the incidence of complications and functional outcome in 158 proximal humerus fractures treated with a proximal humeral locked plate. The authors recommend accurate length measurement, shorter screw selection, and awareness of anatomic reduction of the fracture. Level of evidence: IV.

31. Gosling T, Schandelmaier P, Muller M, Hankemeier S, Wagner M, Krettek C: Single lateral locked screw plating of bicondylar tibial plateau fractures. *Clin Orthop* 2005;439:207-214.

Of 68 patients in a clinical case series with proximal tibia fractures treated with LISS, 16 had significant malreduction. There were four superficial infections and one deep infection; one fracture did not heal, and nine patients had substantial loss of reduction. Level of evidence: IV.

32. Zdero R, Walker R, Waddell JP, Schemitsch EH: Biomechanical evaluation of periprosthetic femoral fracture fixation. *J Bone Joint Surg Am* 2008;90(5):1068-1077.

Four different constructs for the fixation of periprosthetic femoral shaft fractures after total hip arthroplasty were evaluated. The nonlocked plate with an allograft strut resulted in the highest stiffness of the constructs.

33. Buttaro MA, Farfalli G, Paredes Núñez M, Comba F, Piccaluga F: Locking compression plate fixation of Vancouver type-B1 periprosthetic femoral fractures. *J Bone Joint Surg Am* 2007;89(9):1964-1969.

Fourteen consecutive patients with a Vancouver type B1 periprosthetic femoral fracture were treated with a locking compression plate. Three treatment constructs failed within 12 months after surgery; another three failed because of plate pullout. Level of evidence: IV.

34. Wei DH, Raizman NM, Bottino CJ, Jobin CM, Strauch RJ, Rosenwasser MP: Unstable distal radial fractures treated with external fixation, a radial column plate, or a volar plate: A prospective randomized trial. *J Bone Joint Surg Am* 2009;91(7):1568-1577.

The functional outcomes of treatment of unstable distal radial fractures with external fixation, a volar plate, or a radial column plate were compared. At 6 months and 1 year, the outcomes of all three techniques were excellent, with minimal differences among them in terms of strength, motion, and radiographic alignment. Level of evidence: I.

35. Tasker LH, Sparey-Taylor GJ, Nokes LD: Applications of nanotechnology in orthopaedics. *Clin Orthop Relat Res* 2007;456:243-249.

Current and potential applications of nanotechnology in orthopaedics are reviewed. Level of evidence: V.

36. Oh SH, Finōnes RR, Daraio C, Chen LH, Jin S: Growth of nano-scale hydroxyapatite using chemically treated titanium oxide nanotubes. *Biomaterials* 2005;26(24): 4938-4943.

Titanium oxide nanotube arrays and associated nanostructures can be useful as a well-adhered bioactive surface layer on titanium implant metals for orthopaedic implants.

37. Palin E, Liu H, Webster TJ: Mimicking the nanofeatures of bone increases bone-forming cell adhesion and proliferation. *Nanotechnology* 2005;16:1828-1835.

The role of nanostructured surface roughness of titanium on increasing osteoblastic activity was determined in an in vitro study.

38. Chun AL, Moralez JG, Fenniri H, Webster TJ: Helical rosette nano-tubes: A more effective orthopaedic implant material. *Nanotechnology* 2004;15:S234-S239.

This in vitro study determined the efficacy of helical rosette nanotubes as a bone prosthetic material.

39. Guo L, Hui L: Fabrication and characterization of thin nano-hydroxyapatite coatings on titanium. *Surf Coat Tech* 2004;185:268-274.

The authors examined the effect of firing temperatures on aggregating size of particles of different hydroxyapatite coatings on titanium implants.

40. GFD Gesellschaft für Diamantprodukte mbH Diamaze PSD: Plasma sharpened diamond blades. http://www.gfd-diamond.com/produkte/index_en.htm. Accessed September 3, 2009.

This website provides information on diamond-coated, hard metal blades with plasma-sharpened cutting edges and plasma-sharpened turning tools and drills. The blades combine the hardness of diamonds, exceptional chemical resistance, and extreme sharpness.

41. Venugopal J, Ramakrishna S: Applications of polymer nanofibers in biomedicine and biotechnology. *Appl Biochem Biotechnol* 2005;125(3):147-158.

Recent advancements in electrospinning methods enabling the production of ultrafine fibers with diameters ranging from a few nanometers to a few hundred nanometers with controlled surface and internal molecular structures were reviewed.

42. Zhang Y, Lim CT, Ramakrishna S, Huang ZM: Recent development of polymer nanofibers for biomedical and biotechnological applications. *J Mater Sci Mater Med* 2005;16(10):933-946.

A review of the use of polymer nanofibers for applications such as tissue engineering, controlled drug release, wound dressings, medical implants, nanocomposites for dental restoration, molecular separation, biosensors, and preservation of bioactive agents is presented.

43. Horisawa E, Hirota T, Kawazoe S, et al: Prolonged anti-inflammatory action of DL-lactide/glycolide copolymer nanospheres containing betamethasone sodium phosphate for an intra-articular delivery system in antigen-induced arthritic rabbit. *Pharm Res* 2002;19(4): 403-410.

44. Khil MS, Cha DI, Kim HY, Kim IS, Bhattarai N: Electrospun nanofibrous polyurethane membrane as wound dressing. *J Biomed Mater Res B Appl Biomater* 2003; 67(2):675-679.

45. Müller CA, Green J, Südkamp NP: Physical and techni-

cal aspects of intramedullary reaming. *Injury* 2006; 37(Suppl 4):S39-S49.

The physiologic effects during reaming are reviewed. The authors suggest that intramedullary pressure caused by modern reaming systems can be reduced and perhaps avoided by using a reaming-irrigation-aspiration system. Level of evidence: V.

46. Pape HC, Zelle BA, Hildebrand F, Giannoudis PV, Krettek C, van Griensven M: Reamed femoral nailing in sheep: Does irrigation and aspiration of intramedullary contents alter the systemic response? *J Bone Joint Surg Am* 2005;87(11):2515-2522.

The femurs of 18 sheep were reamed after a unilateral lung contusion was created. The authors found that the presence of a unilateral pulmonary injury and the systemic effects of intramedullary reaming of an intact femur were minimized with use of a reaming-irrigation-aspiration system.

47. Zalavras CG, Singh A, Patzakis MJ: Novel technique for medullary canal débridement in tibia and femur osteomyelitis. *Clin Orthop Relat Res* 2007;461:31-34.

In this retrospective review of 11 patients with intramedullary infections of the tibia or femur treated with débridement, implant removal, and reaming of the medullary canal with a reaming-irrigation-aspiration system, no patients had a recurrence of infection at a minimum 6-month follow-up. Level of evidence: V.

48. Porter RM, Liu F, Pilapil C, et al: Osteogenic potential of reamer irrigator aspirator (RIA) aspirate collected from patients undergoing hip arthroplasty. *J Orthop Res* 2009;27(1):42-49.

The authors assessed whether discarded reaming-irrigation-aspiration system filtrate has osteogenic properties that could be used to enhance the total repair potential of aspirate.

49. Venturi ML, Attinger CE, Mesbahi AN, Hess CL, Graw KS: Mechanisms and clinical applications of the vacuum-assisted closure (VAC) device: A review. *Am J Clin Dermatol* 2005;6(3):185-194.

This article reviews the potential mechanisms of action and applications of subatmospheric pressure dressings. Level of evidence: V.

50. Labler L, Rancan M, Mica L, Härter L, Mihic-Probst D, Keel M: Vacuum-assisted closure therapy increases local interleukin-8 and vascular endothelial growth factor levels in traumatic wounds. *J Trauma* 2009;66(3):749-757.

The impact of VAC therapy and Epigard application on local inflammation and neovascularization in traumatic soft tissue wounds was compared in 32 patients with traumatic wounds. Level of evidence: III.

51. Morykwas MJ, Argenta LC, Shelton-Brown EI, McGuirt W: Vacuum-assisted closure: A new method for wound control and treatment: Animal studies and basic foundation. *Ann Plast Surg* 1997;38(6):553-562.

52. Webb LX, Pape HC: Current thought regarding the mechanism of action of negative pressure wound therapy with reticulated open cell foam. *J Orthop Trauma* 2008;22(Suppl 10):S135-S137.

This review article discusses the main theories regarding the mechanism of action of NPWT with reticulated open cell foam. Level of evidence: V.

53. Pollak AN: Use of negative pressure wound therapy with reticulated open cell foam for lower extremity trauma. *J Orthop Trauma* 2008;22(Suppl 10):S142-S145.

The use of NPWT with reticulated open cell foam in the treatment of complex lower extremity injuries is discussed. Level of evidence: V.

54. Leininger BE, Rasmussen TE, Smith DL, Jenkins DH, Coppola C: Experience with wound VAC and delayed primary closure of contaminated soft tissue injuries in Iraq. *J Trauma* 2006;61(5):1207-1211.

Eighty-eight missile injuries were treated by a novel wound management protocol that included serial aggressive débridement and pulsatile lavage, and were covered with negative pressure (vacuum-assisted closure) dressings. The authors reported wound infection and wound complication rates of 0%. Level of evidence: IV.

55. Stannard JP, Robinson JT, Anderson ER, McGwin G Jr, Volgas DA, Alonso JE: Negative pressure wound therapy to treat hematomas and surgical incisions following high-energy trauma. *J Trauma* 2006;60(6):1301-1306.

Forty-four patients with draining hematomas and 44 patients with open fractures were randomized to either a pressure dressing or NPWT. Significantly less drainage duration was seen in both patient groups with NPWT. Level of evidence: II.

56. Parrett BM, Matros E, Pribaz JJ, Orgill DP: Lower extremity trauma: Trends in the management of soft-tissue reconstruction of open tibia-fibula fractures. *Plast Reconstr Surg* 2006;117(4):1315-1322.

Two hundred ninety patients with open tibial fractures were treated over different 4-year treatment periods using different treatment protocols, demonstrating change in practice, resulting in fewer free flaps and more delayed primary closures and skin grafts with frequent use of the vacuum-assisted closure sponge. Level of evidence: III.

57. Potter HG, Linklater JM, Allen AA, Hannafin JA, Haas SB: Magnetic resonance imaging of articular cartilage in the knee: An evaluation with use of fast spin-echo imaging. *J Bone Joint Surg* 1998;80:1276-1284.

58. Koff MF, Potter HG: Noncontrast MR techniques and imaging of cartilage. *Radiol Clin North Am* 2009;47(3):495-504.

This review article covers recent advances in noncontrast MRI techniques producing images with higher quality for standardized diagnostic interpretation that in many instances obviates the need for intra-articular contrast agents. Level of evidence: V.

59. Akella SV, Regatte RR, Gougoutas AJ, et al: Proteoglycan-induced changes in T1rho-relaxation of

1: General Topics and New Technology

articular cartilage at 4T. *Magn Reson Med* 2001;46(3):419-423.

60. Li X, Benjamin Ma C, Link TM, et al: In vivo T(1rho) and T(2) mapping of articular cartilage in osteoarthritis of the knee using 3 T MRI. *Osteoarthritis Cartilage* 2007;15(7):789-797.

    The results of this study suggest that both in vivo T1-rho and T2 relaxation times increase with the degree of cartilage degeneration. T1-rho relaxation time may be a more sensitive indicator for early cartilage degeneration than T2.

61. Li X, Han ET, Ma CB, Link TM, Newitt DC, Majumdar S: In vivo 3T spiral imaging based multi-slice T(1rho) mapping of knee cartilage in osteoarthritis. *Magn Reson Med* 2005;54(4):929-936.

    Results of this study suggest that T1-rho relaxation times may be a promising clinical tool for osteoarthritis detection and treatment monitoring. Level of evidence: IV.

62. Hüfner T, Stübig T, Citak M, Gösling T, Krettek C, Kendoff D: Utility of intraoperative three-dimensional imaging at the hip and knee joints with and without navigation. *J Bone Joint Surg Am* 2009;91(Suppl 1):33-42.

    Current uses of intraoperative three-dimensional imaging in orthopaedic trauma care are discussed. Level of evidence: V.

63. Kotsianos D, Wirth S, Fischer T, et al: 3D imaging with an isocentric mobile C-arm comparison of image quality with spiral CT. *Eur Radiol* 2004;14(9):1590-1595.

    The image quality of a three-dimensional imaging system (Iso-C-3D) for osteosynthesis of tibial condylar fractures in comparison with spiral computed tomography is evaluated. The image quality of Iso-C-3D was found to be inferior to computed tomography, and metal artifacts were more prominent, but clinical value was the same.

64. Kendoff D, Citak M, Gardner MJ, Stübig T, Krettek C, Hüfner T: Intraoperative 3D imaging: Value and consequences in 248 cases. *J Trauma* 2009;66(1):232-238.

    The utility of three-dimensional imaging in articular fracture reconstruction was evaluated in 248 consecutive patients with intra-articular fractures. Level of evidence: IV.

65. Kendoff D, Gardner MJ, Citak M, et al: Value of 3D fluoroscopic imaging of acetabular fractures comparison to 2D fluoroscopy and CT imaging. *Arch Orthop Trauma Surg* 2008;128(6):599-605.

    The accuracy of three-dimensional fluoroscopic imaging in evaluating acetabular fracture displacement and implant placement with fluoroscopy and computed tomography was assessed in 24 cadaver acetabuli with a transverse acetabular fracture. Three-dimensional fluoroscopic imaging appeared to be more accurate than two-dimensional fluoroscopy in evaluating acetabular fracture constructs.

66. Kendoff D, Pearle A, Hüfner T, Citak M, Gösling T, Krettek C: First clinical results and consequences of intraoperative three-dimensional imaging at tibial plateau fractures. *J Trauma* 2007;63(1):239-244.

    Intraoperative imaging of 19 tibial plateau fractures demonstrated improved ability to identify articular malreduction and implant malposition. Level of evidence: IV.

67. Geerling J, Kendoff D, Citak M, et al: Intraoperative 3D imaging in calcaneal fracture care—clinical implications and decision making. *J Trauma* 2009;66(3):768-773.

    The feasibility and utility of C-arm three-dimensional imaging for calcaneal trauma care in 32 patients over a 2-year period was analyzed in this study. Level of evidence: IV.

68. Mast J, Jakob R, Ganz R: *Planning and Reduction Technique in Fracture Surgery*. Berlin, Germany Springer-Verlag, 1989, pp 1-11.

69. Pilson HT, Reddix RN, Mutty CE, Webb LX: The long lost art of preoperative planning—resurrected? *Orthopedics* 2008;31:1238.

    The advantages of digital surgical planning software enabling the surgeon to formulate a preoperative plan for fracture reduction and fixation are presented.

70. Trickett RW, Hodgson P, Forster MC, Robertson A: The reliability and accuracy of digital templating in total knee replacement. *J Bone Joint Surg Br* 2009;91(7):903-906.

    This study determined the reliability, accuracy, and clinical role of digital templating in the preoperative workup for total knee replacement. Good interobserver and intraobserver agreement was demonstrated for both femoral and tibial templating. The correct size of the implant was predicted in only 48% and 55%, respectively, of the femoral and tibial components.

71. Gamble P, de Beer J, Petruccelli D, Winemaker M: The accuracy of digital templating in uncemented total hip arthroplasty. *J Arthroplasty* 2010;25(4):529-532.

    The reproducibility and reliability of computer templating in primary uncemented total hip arthroplasties compared with standard onlay templating techniques with hard copy radiographs from a digital source was analyzed.

Chapter 10

Disaster and Mass Casualty Preparedness

Christopher T. Born, MD, FACS   Keith O. Monchik, MD

1: General Topics and New Technology

Introduction

Disaster response and management has become an increasingly important aspect of medical care at the local, regional, national, and international levels. Disasters are difficult to predict, but the loss of life, property, and infrastructure can be mitigated by risk analysis, planning, training, and a system of coordinated incident management that has the ability to expand or contract to meet the response needs of any given event. The threat of major mass casualty events is growing, in part because of increased population densities, environmental degradation, proliferation of hazardous materials and technology, and emerging strains of infectious diseases. The global threat of terrorism has added another dimension, and a basic understanding of how to manage injury from weapons of mass destruction has become increasingly important for surgeons.

Government Disaster Response Structure and Relationships

In February 2003, in response to the 2001 terrorist attacks at New York's World Trade Center, President George W. Bush issued Homeland Security Presidential Directive 5. This directive called for the development of a National Incident Management System (NIMS). Its purpose is to improve the coordination of incident response between all levels of governmental (local, state, tribal, territorial, and federal), the private sector (responsible for most of the nation's infrastructure), and

nongovernmental organizations, which are pivotal in providing additional critical humanitarian aid. NIMS is only one part of the larger National Response Framework (NRF). Adherence to NIMS guidelines is a prerequisite for certain organizations to receive federal funds for emergency preparedness. NIMS defines how the nation responds in a unified and coordinated manner through an all-hazards planning approach; from the smallest incidents (for example, an overturned tanker truck carrying a hazardous material on a busy interstate highway) to the largest catastrophes (for example, an earthquake in a major urban area).

The NRF has several components. There is a core document that describes the overall national response doctrine including roles and responsibilities, response actions and organizations, and planning requirements that will lead to an effective national response. Addendum documents, which provide practitioners with detailed information on implementation, include the emergency support function annexes, which address the 15 federal resources most commonly enlisted in response to an incident (for example, transportation, communications, and emergency management) (Table 1). The emergency support function annexes describe the scope, policies, and concept of operations of each emergency support function and identify the coordinators, the primary federal agencies that can provide resources, and ancillary support agencies that have more specific capabilities. Any or all of the emergency support functions can be mobilized in response to a given incident, depending on the nature and breadth of the event. Support annexes define several supporting aspects commonly needed to successfully manage most incidents (for example, financial management, and volunteer and private sector/nongovernmental organization coordination). Incident annexes address the response to several specific, broad incident categories (for example, nuclear/radiologic, biologic, cyber, or mass evacuation).

There are several key concepts embodied by the NRF. Along with NIMS, it is always in effect. Response elements can be implemented at any level and at any time. It seeks to improve coordination among all response partners, and helps to ensure that they use standard command and management structures that allow for flexible, scalable, and adaptable operational capa-

Table 1

Emergency Support Function Annexes

ESF 1 - Transportation

ESF 2 – Communications

ESF 3 – Public Works and Engineering

ESF 4 – Firefighting

ESF 5 – Emergency Management

ESF 6 – Mass Care, Emergency Assistance, Housing, and Human Services

ESF 7 – Logistics Management and Resource Support

ESF 8 – Public Health and Medical Services

ESF 9 – Search and Rescue

ESF 10 – Oil and Hazardous Materials Response

ESF 11 – Agriculture and Natural Resources

ESF 12 – Energy

ESF 13 – Public Safety and Security

ESF 14 – Long-Term Community Recovery

ESF 15 – External Affairs

bilities. Incident response is tiered and is managed at the lowest jurisdictional level (for example, town, county, or state), but is supported by additional capabilities as needed. Partnerships between responder organizations ensure that leaders have shared goals and capabilities that are aligned so that no one is overwhelmed in a crisis. A unified command structure allows for a cooperative effort through the establishment of common sets of objectives and strategies between responding agencies and the development of a single action plan for the incident.

The NRF defines the key response partners and their interrelationships. At the local level, community public safety is in the hands of police, fire, emergency medical services, medical providers, emergency management officials, and numerous others who manage the day-to-day incidents that commonly occur. Key players include the chief elected/appointed official and a local emergency manager, who work with department and agency heads. Nongovernmental organizations assist in providing shelter, clothing, food supplies, counseling, and other services. The private sector is a key partner in that it oversees much of the nation's infrastructure and can provide critical services during and after an event as a part of the recovery process. Incident responses are tiered and scalable depending on the nature and scope of the event, and states may be asked to play a supplementary role to local efforts as they have significant resources of their own. Coordination may need to take place between states through mutual aid and assistance agreements such as the Emergency Management Assistance Compact, by which a state can request and receive assistance from other member states.

At the federal level, when local, state, or tribal resources are exhausted, assistance may be provided for major incidents through the congressionally legislated Stafford Act. In these situations the state's emergency plan must have been activated and the governor of a particular state must make the request through one of the Federal Emergency Management Agency's 10 regional administrators. There was a significant delay in this request after Hurricane Katrina hit New Orleans in 2005. The President ultimately commands the federal response effort, which is coordinated by the secretary of the US Department of Homeland Security with the assistance of a Federal Emergency Management Agency regional administrator.

The organizational components of the NRF have been developed and tested over time. Most incidents begin and end at the local level. The Incident Command System is a key feature of NIMS and is the standard for emergency management across the country. Adaptation of this system is a prerequisite to receiving federal emergency preparedness funding. The need for additional resources will be determined by the incident commander and requests made via the local Emergency Operations Center (EOC). The EOC coordinates information and resources and provides support for the Incident Commander at the scene of the event. If the situation requires resources that are beyond the scope of those that are locally available, state EOCs may be activated and additional assistance requested from neighboring states through the Emergency Management Assistance Compact. In all instances, the concept of a unified command structure is in place by which various agencies or jurisdictions involved in the response are also integrated into the management structure. There are five major management functions of the Incident Command System (**Figure 1**). The size of each component can expand or contract depending on the scope and requirements of the incident. The incident commander has overall responsibility for the management of the incident and is supported by a command staff consisting of the public information officer, a safety officer, and a liaison officer. The other management functions are those of the general staff and comprise four sections: operations, planning, logistics, and finance/administration. It is the operations section that carries out all of the tactical efforts needed to manage medical care, search and rescue, hazardous waste removal, power restoration, and so on. The planning, logistics, and finance/administration sections provide the support functions necessary for the operations section to carry out the physical aspects of the response, all under the direction of the incident commander.

Disaster Definitions and Classifications

The mechanism or etiology of the disaster can be categorized as natural or man-made, with the former term including weather and geophysical calamities, and the

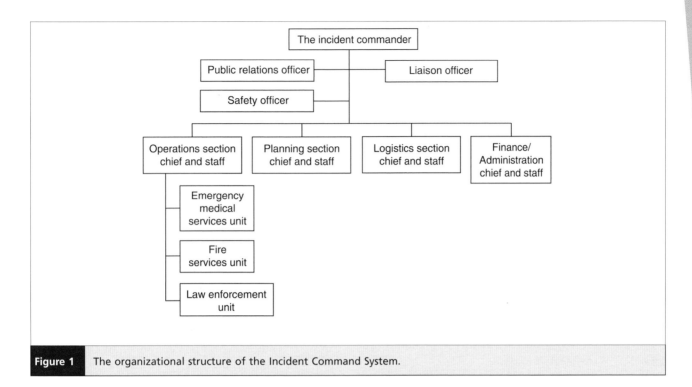

Figure 1 The organizational structure of the Incident Command System.

latter term including unintentional events related to industry and technology and intentional events most frequently related to acts of terrorism.

Disasters can also be classified by their extent and duration. Disasters can exist within a defined, closed area or expand across regional geography. They can be time limited or ongoing. The number of casualties generated and the types of injuries involved are important considerations with respect to the anticipated requirement of response assets. Resource utilization and deployment is a basic factor that distinguishes disaster care from routine medical care. A Level I response requires the use of local resources only. A Level II response necessitates the addition of regional resources. A Level III response includes national/international aid in addition to the regional and local resources.

Recent examples of disaster situations underscore the breadth and variety of event types that must be considered by disaster response planners. For example, the 2003 wildfires in California destroyed more than 400,000 acres and 1,100 homes. Although only 13 people died, the infrastructure of this highly populated area was seriously disrupted. The 2004 tsunami resulted in at least 230,000 deaths around the perimeter of the Indian Ocean. The debacle in New Orleans that followed Hurricane Katrina in 2005, during which 1,800 people died, underscores the problems of political complacency as well as failures in preventive engineering, disaster planning, and response.[1]

Acts of terrorism also call for a well-planned response. In 2005, there were 758 terrorist events in 45 countries, more than half of which were bombings. These events resulted in more than 3,000 deaths and 8,000 injured persons, including 400 first responders. In the United States, the FBI has reported 324 confirmed terrorist bombings between 1980 and 2001. Threats from the classic weapons of mass destruction (chemical, biologic, and radiologic/nuclear weapons) are cause for concern, but these threats tend to be overstated relative to the actual probability of their implementation. Bombs are by far the most common weapon because they are inexpensive, are easy to make and transport, and readily achieve the terrorist's aim of maximum casualty generation with maximum lethality.[2]

What distinguishes mass casualty events from routine patient care is the relationship between total casualty needs and available local resources. True mass casualty events are quite different from routine care of patients, even in the emergency setting. A multiple casualty event is characterized by strained resources over a limited time. A mass casualty event is one in which the needs for casualty care far exceed the available resources.

Planning

Although disasters can be random and unpredictable, there is a widespread misperception that planning and preparation cannot take into account all the possible events. Most disaster types have predictable common patterns and elements that allow them to be analyzed and compared, and from which "lessons learned" can prove helpful in dealing with future events, thereby allowing preparation and planning and enabling successful disaster management and response.

Many stakeholders must be integrated into the overall planning process for responding to a disaster or mass casualty incident, including hospitals, local and regional/state agencies, nongovernmental organizations and volunteer organizations, and the federal government.

Nationally and regionally, the planning process is performed by what is referred to as an all-hazards approach, whereby all potential threats are considered and a single, overall response structure is developed. This means that there is one plan, but the plan is modular, flexible, and scalable and can be appropriately modified to manage a specific event by drawing on various response assets as needed. This plan is more effective and efficient than having several plans for different situations. It is important that any response plan incorporate lessons learned from past experience, define the roles and responsibilities of the participants, be continuously updated, and avoid complacency.[3] Training and rehearsal are critical. Failure to practice and exercise the response components can be a key barrier to successful response outcome. Financial and time investments necessary for adequate disaster preparation and rehearsal are often disincentives to the planning process.

Medical planning has three fundamental components critical for effective health care preparation and response to disasters: competency, capability, and capacity. The keys to implementation are the coordinated efforts among the public health sector, emergency management agencies, and the health care delivery system. The health care delivery system is most commonly associated with the medical response, yet this response will be incomplete without public health and emergency management integration. Such interfaces promote a competent, capable response with the capacity for care appropriate to the event.

Response starts not with the detection of an event, but rather with advance risk identification, planning, and mitigation of possible threats (for example, intensified airport passenger and baggage screening). Mitigation reduces the possibility that these preidentifiable hazards will occur, and preparation lessens the impact of such events when they do occur. A response must be in place for disasters that involve all types of mechanisms and hazards, recognizing elements common to all disasters types (for example, the basic needs of large numbers of victims) and unique facets of particular hazards. A building collapse will generate fundamentally different response needs than an influenza pandemic. Flexibility and adaptability are required to successfully meet these unique demands. All-hazards planning can address these issues by determining the credible threats to the community. A careful look at potential threats from private industry to public venues should be undertaken. For example, farming communities traversed by a major rail line may have different planning issues than a waterfront city with a liquid nitrogen gas terminal. A hazard vulnerability analysis identifies these potential risks and assigns an estimate of the likelihood of occurrence to each risk. These pri-

oritized risks are then matched to an assessment of preparedness, and targets for improvement are identified. Disaster plans then develop around the hazard vulnerability analysis.

Prehospital and Hospital Response

Disaster and mass casualty events require a medical care paradigm change that shifts the use of unlimited resources for each individual to the greatest good for the greatest number of casualties. In the face of limited resources, their use must be conserved for the management of the greatest number injured, rather than using them all on each individual casualty. This approach leads to the best outcome across the affected population. It means that some casualties who would normally be treated may go untreated for the sake of salvaging many more injured patients with lower resource requirements, in the setting of limited resources. In a hospital flooded with casualties, the "acceptable" level of care may have to be lowered to manage the incapacitating surge of patients. This change of focus may challenge ethical views, yet is necessary to help as many of the injured population as possible.

Patient care will frequently begin far from the confines of the hospital. Prehospital response to disasters generally can be categorized into four fairly distinct, yet overlapping, phases: notification, response, recovery, and restoration.

Notification
The notification phase begins with the recognition that an incident has occurred and continues until the first emergency vehicle arrives and site management begins. This phase frequently begins with a period of confusion or chaos. The notification may be made by anyone, including untrained individuals who happen to be on the scene and notice the development of a mass casualty situation.

Response
Casualties who are alive are quickly identified, moved to a casualty collection point, and eventually evacuated during the site-clearing or response phase. Casualties should receive only minimal interventions at the scene—stopping obvious bleeding, for example. Once rescued and determined to be alive, they are transported to casualty collection points away from the scene for triage and further brief life-saving care before being sent to hospitals.

Triage begins early in the response phase and is the process of assigning priorities for treatment of the injured when resources are limited.[3] The goal of triage is to identify the critically injured, based on two factors—the severity of the injury and the urgency of the treatment needs. Triage effectiveness improves when the nature of triage errors is understood. Undertriage is the assignment of a critical casualty to a noncritical category, which could result in unnecessary death. Overtriage is the assignment of a noncritical casualty to the critical category. Overtriage is routinely seen in everyday trauma system management, where expansive resources are generally made available to all of the injured. However, in a true disaster, overtriage is as dangerous to the casualty population as undertriage, because it masks and delays identification of critical casualties and leads to the use of scarce resources for non–critically injured casualties.

Most disaster casualties have minor, noncritical injuries and may be capable of evacuating themselves. Critically injured casualties correlate with an anatomic Injury Severity Score greater than 15. The critically injured statistically constitute approximately 20% of the casualty population. The best measure of mass casualty response medical outcome is the mortality rate only among those who are critically injured and truly at risk of death (critical mortality rate). The overall casualty mortality rate only dilutes the critically injured outcome—most casualties will survive without treatment.[4]

Triage of casualties should begin when the event is recognized. Care focuses on minimal interventions that produce acceptable outcomes for the time being. Triage decisions generate casualty movement, and can lead to triage errors under these chaotic circumstances. The effect of triage errors can be minimized because the triage process is repeated across all levels of care and thus becomes a built-in safety net to minimize the consequences of any errors that do occur.

Good clinical documentation enhances continuity of care and reduces redundant care when resources are scarce. Key elements of the documentation include the triage level, primary survey findings and interventions, and identified injuries.

Many personnel will be involved in the entire triage process, but overall responsibility and decision making should rest with the designated triage officer. Usually this position is filled by the most experienced medical provider available who is familiar with well-established triage systems.[5] The triage officer does not need to be a physician; therefore, this position may be filled by a critical care nurse, paramedic, or, in the event of an unconventional disaster such as a radiation exposure, a radiation physicist. It is important that the triage officer be experienced in treating the types of injury the disaster has caused. However, recent literature suggests that primary triage, even when performed by experienced trauma physicians, can be unreliable in a mass casualty incident.[6] Thus, such a system must be error tolerant.

Casualty prioritization results from placing casualty factors, such as urgency, injury severity, and salvageability, into the context of resources (including capacity and capability) and the disaster situation (marked by geography, time, and evacuation possibilities).

It must be emphasized that safety at the disaster scene for responders, the uninjured, and the injured is paramount. Site safety improves conditions for successful triage: triage that begins before safety at the site is secured will simply generate more casualties.

The presence of hazardous materials always needs to be considered, whether in building materials or biohazardous terrorist weapons. Setting up a decontamination station is an exercise of triage decision making. Further, second hits (for example, an explosion followed by a late building collapse) can occur either as a consequence of the initial mechanism of the disaster or as part of a terrorist plan involving sequential explosions that also target the first responders.

Triage includes the distribution of casualties from the scene to receiving facilities. All disasters are associated with a geographic effect in which the hospital in closest proximity to the incident is inevitably swamped with a disproportionate number of casualties. This overload leads to a rapid drain of resources and personnel. Therefore, it is essential in the earliest phases of prehospital triage to distribute the casualty load to as many hospitals as possible in accordance with the resources available at each hospital and any specialty care offered (for example, burn centers, pediatric hospitals, Level I trauma centers). This process of casualty distribution beyond the closest hospital is known as leapfrogging.

In the event of a suspected terrorist or nuclear/biologic/chemical event, strict care must be taken to protect the hospital from an intentional or accidental second hit whereby a destructive or biohazardous agent is somehow physically introduced into the facility. Initial triage and decontamination areas should be external to the building, personal protective equipment (PPE) should be distributed, and casualty flow should be unidirectional with patients systematically identified, registered, evaluated, and placed into management pathways. These pathways will be initially determined by the triage officer. The triage officer will need to be continuously updated on the expected volume of patients, injury types and severity levels, the hospital's capacity to manage various injuries and availability of operating rooms, intensive care units, respirators, and so on. Minimally acceptable care becomes the standard of care when confronted by large volumes of patients. Laboratory and imaging studies are minimized because these will create bottlenecks that will negatively affect victims who are farther down the chain. Temporizing stabilization and damage control–type management techniques are implemented. Systems for the tracking of patients and record keeping allowing for continuity of care need to be worked out and trialed in advance.

The challenges presented by the response phase include ensuring the safety of emergency responders (making sure the responders do not enter the area without proper protection), gathering information about the incident (number of victims, types of injuries, involvement of chemical or biologic materials), and establishing security around the site, where access is controlled into and out of the general area around the incident. In the situations involving chemical or biologic weapons, challenges include approaching the site from an upwind and upgrade direction, identifying signs and symptoms of the agents, and establishing decontamination areas.

Decontamination and PPE are essential to all responders who come in contact with, or have the potential to come in contact with, casualties contaminated or exposed to chemical, ordnance, biologic, radiologic (COBRA) or other hazardous materials. PPE use is specified in Occupational Safety and Health Administration regulations and reinforced in US Environmental Protection Agency regulations. The National Institute for Occupational Safety and Health (NIOSH) testing certifies PPE appropriate for responding to COBRA incidents. Not all PPE available in the marketplace is NIOSH approved, will not have a NIOSH certification label, and therefore has not been approved by the Occupational Safety and Health Administration for protecting against COBRA hazards.[7] PPE has four levels of protection. Level A requires full encapsulation and bottled air. Level B requires full coverage, head to foot and either a self-contained breathing apparatus or supplied air respirator. Level C requires full coverage including a purifying air respirator or powered air-purifying respirator. Level D consists of a duty uniform/scrubs (street clothes) with routine protective gear such as gown, gloves, and face shield. Training in the use of PPE is essential and will ensure the required familiarity with the equipment, and that it is being used within the limits of manufacturers' approved specifications for protection. Wearing PPE puts responders at considerable risk of developing heat stress. Therefore, regular medical surveillance of providers and short shifts are recommended.[8]

The safety of victims and rescuers in a hostile environment, regardless of the source of danger, is roughly defined by zones. The hot zone is immediately dangerous, such as being in the line of hostile fire, adjacent to damaged and unstable structures, or close to the site of a toxic release. Medical intervention is not generally performed, and efforts are confined to the rapid evacuation of casualties. The highest levels of PPE are indicated, as determined by the identified threat (for example, projectiles, toxins, biologic agents, radioactivity), and the length of time any individual rescuer spends in the hot zone is minimized. The warm zone is potentially dangerous, but sufficiently safe to permit performance of life-saving procedures. PPE is also required in this zone, but usually at a decreased level in comparison to the hot zone. The cold zone is defined as being without a direct environmental threat, and medical care can be rendered with a minimal level of PPE, typically no more than would be required for a hospital bedside procedure.

There are two levels of decontamination—emergency and technical. These combine to cover the rapid decontamination of victims and the more deliberate decontamination of the responders. Emergency decon-

tamination is used to save lives of potential casualties by neutralizing agents on the skin and physically removing the agent hazard. Technical decontamination is performed to remove contamination from the PPE or responders as well as facilities in a deliberate fashion. Decontamination occurs in the warm zone—located at least 300 yards (preferably uphill and upwind) from the hot zone. Clothing and all personal effects are removed and left within the hot zone. Victims then move through the decontamination process in one direction, referred to as the decontamination corridor, to the cold zone where treatment and transport functions take place. A large area is required and it should be upwind, uphill, and upstream of the hot zone, to provide protection for and to handle decontamination of large numbers of people while controlling water runoff. Approximately 80% of the contamination will be removed with the clothing. Bagged clothing should be placed in sealed containers. Casualties should be wet down before removing individual clothing if the hazard is biologic or radiologic to assist in preventing re-erosolizing the agent. Modesty and the public eye (media) should be taken into account. Male and female decontamination corridors can be quickly established and sealed off to ensure privacy.

Search and rescue involves identifying and moving casualties who are alive from the scene. Search and rescue is a specific skill set developed by teams trained in extrication. Casualties trapped beneath collapsed structures pose several risks. First, survival of the casualties themselves is related to the time to extrication. Survival is extremely unlikely if a person is trapped beyond 24 hours. Second, search and rescue is hazardous for rescuers: 70% of fatalities in confined space rescue are the rescuers themselves. Technical specialists may assist the search and rescue teams by providing expertise in hazardous materials, structural engineering, and heavy equipment operation. Field medical care for trapped casualties includes management of hypothermia, dehydration, and crush syndrome. Expertise may be needed for the rare field amputation to allow casualty extrication.

Recovery

Once the living have been rescued and moved away from the scene, efforts at the scene move into the late phase and include recovery of bodies. The shift from rescue to recovery can take an emotional toll on the responders and the community. Safety remains an issue, together with recognition that human remains constitute potential forensic evidence and require identification and tracking.

The recovery phase begins when the disaster situation has been stabilized and the last of the living victims has been delivered to a medical facility to receive definitive medical treatment. During this time, the focus is on reestablishing essential services that may have been interrupted by the disaster, all the while recognizing that evidence collection may be required if the event happens to be of a terrorist nature. It is during the re-

Table 2

Hospital Stakeholders

Emergency department	Communications
Physician staff	Engineering
Nursing staff	Housekeeping
Intensive care units	Nutritional services
Operating rooms	Morgue
Laboratories and blood bank	Volunteer and social services
Radiology	Security
Respiratory therapy	Administration

covery phase that state and federal responders may arrive to provide assistance, including the response of a National Disaster Medical System Disaster Medical Assistance Team. Immediate needs include food, water, shelter, utilities, communication, and sanitation. A food source will be needed for both recovery teams and survivors as well as potable water to maintain proper hydration levels. Prevention of secondary disease transmission is essential, through the use of handwashing stations and portable toilets. Temporarily, a generator with a fuel source may be required to provide power for basic utilities such as heat, lighting, and water/sewage. Basic immediate and urgent medical care and supplies will be required because local hospitals, dispensaries, and pharmacies may have been destroyed. Providers can expect to address issues such as gastrointestinal disorders, sunburns, and heat- or cold-related illness in addition to the premorbid medical conditions of the victims who may no longer have their cardiac or asthma medicines, insulin, and so on. Basic immunizations and boosters such as tetanus and hepatitis should be provided to survivors as well as the distribution of home medication. There may be an additional need for specialized care such as pediatrics, women's health, and psychiatry. Response team members must be up to date with their immunizations and may need specialty coverage in areas of disease prevalence such as typhoid, malaria, and yellow fever.

Restoration

As the recovery phase progresses to restoration, delayed and sustainable needs, such as screening for post-traumatic stress disorder, chronic disease care, critical incident stress debriefing, and after-action reporting, will have to be addressed. Pitfalls in recovery include the absence of postevent analysis and critique. Valuable insights are lost, not only for the particular community affected by the disaster, but for the preparedness of all communities. The postevent analysis should include determination of triage accuracy and casualty outcome.

Hospital Preparedness

For hospitals, planning is critical. The hospital nearest to an event will not only see the first (frequently unannounced) victims, but eventually will be flooded by most of the injured.

In the context of a disaster response where the closest hospital may become overwhelmed with injured victims, the ability of those responsible for managing patient flow to either transfer patient volume out of the prime facility or to have it bypassed completely (leapfrog) is important. From an operational standpoint, a hospital must be able to manage its surge capacity (defined as the ability to maintain an acceptable level of care in the face of an increasing casualty load)[9] and its surge capability (defined as the ability to provide specialty care; for example, pediatrics, neurosurgery, ventilator availability). Surge capacity can be increased by canceling clinics and elective procedures, discharging patients, clearing intensive care units, and opening pre-planned expansion/breakout areas such as cafeterias and auditoriums. An awareness of the capacities and capabilities of neighboring institutions is helpful for managing local and regional patient flow and for decompressing an overwhelmed healthcare system.

Questions essential to any hospital planning include how a hospital is to be alerted to a disaster situation, who is responsible for initiating this alert, and who is in charge once activation occurs. Recognition that an event is occurring or has taken place may be the result of fire/emergency medical services notification, the unexpected arrival of casualties, or a television news story seen in the waiting room. On recognition of the possibility of an event that may generate multiple casualties, a facility needs to have in place a system by which someone will monitor these events and make a decision to call either a disaster "standby" or "activation" code for activation of the emergency operations plan.

The most common problem remains communications related either to the structural issues of response (such as power grid outage, destroyed cell towers, or overwhelming system volume), or to technical problems. An unfueled backup generator, lack of system interoperability, and lack of redundancy all can shut down the needed communications network.

The Joint Commission requires that hospitals adhere to Emergency Management Standards[10] when developing an emergency operations plan or disaster plan. A hazard vulnerability analysis for the hospital must be developed and the hospital's incident structure must be integrated into the community's command structure. The plan must describe how the organization will coordinate clinical and support activities; define the communication structure; manage resources, staff, patients, utilities; credential volunteer professionals; carry out rehearsal exercises (disaster drills); and review and update the plan.

To have an effective plan, all of the hospital's stakeholders must be involved in the process (Table 2). The

1: General Topics and New Technology

Table 3

Community Stakeholders

Police

Fire/emergency medical services/hazardous materials

Government

Public health

Media

Medical examiner

Transportation

emergency operations plan must also be integrated with the various community response stakeholders (Table 3). Participant roles and responsibilities must be defined and include an incident command structure.

When a disaster occurs, the hospital's predesignated emergency operations center needs to be opened and the hospital's incident command system should become operational. The hospital's incident command system framework mirrors the structure of the nationally recognized Incident Command System structure (**Figure 2**) and, as such, is also modular, flexible, and scalable. A medical/technical specialist may be added to the command staff (such as an infectious disease physician or radiation safety officer). Positions within the hospital's incident command system structure are filled with those personnel who have been predesignated and trained to take on the responsibilities. Job action sheets that define each position's purpose, reporting links, and other critical parameters may be distributed to the appropriate personnel. Medical care will fall under the operations section as in the Incident Command System. Security should be notified and the hospital placed into a "lockdown" mode with access limited and tightly controlled. Personnel and vehicle identification are mandatory. Advance disaster planning should include designated areas for families and other concerned parties, the ambulatory minimally injured, the media, and any unattached volunteers.

Several potential barriers to reasonable hospital response planning and enactment need to be recognized and overcome. Included among these is a requirement for inclusivity in the planning process. There is really no part of a hospital that should not be involved because an effective response will require a systemwide cooperative effort. In addition, rehearsal or drills are invaluable. Without them, it is difficult to anticipate and resolve problems in advance. Drills highlight flaws in equipment, space considerations, communications issues, storage and resupply problems, and a host of other considerations that cannot be managed effectively (or at all) in the heat of a response. Planning is not an administrative exercise. Staff education and training is paramount, but hospitals may be understandably reluctant to take on the added expenses of overtime, consulting fees, and storage inventory costs if there is a

sense of "it will never happen here." True disaster response planning must transcend the idea that "this is just another Saturday night, but busier."

Complacency can be mitigated through regular training and education to all potential responders/receivers in conjunction with regular drills. Disaster plan formulation remains a dynamic process, and revision is based on after-action review of drills/recent activations or changes in the hazard vulnerability analysis. The impact of Hurricane Hugo, a category 5 storm that struck the Carolinas in September 1989, was studied.[11] The authors noted a loss of essential utilities, coupled with the location of contingency generators in exposed outdoor locations, which precluded access during the storm. This hurricane occurred 16 years before Hurricane Katrina, and yet some fundamental lessons were missed by the New Orleans hospital disaster planners.

Reviews of previous disasters have consistently demonstrated three problem areas that are recurrent themes for many disaster responses: communications, resupply, and lack of awareness of other hospitals' capability. Communication between the command section and the various branches of the response sections becomes critical. Without valid and shared information, the response components are virtually acting independently of one another. This includes not only internal communications, but also those between the hospital and external response components such as police, fire/emergency medical services, and governmental agencies. Rumors can have a particularly negative effect and need to be addressed expeditiously.

Supply needs are consistently underanticipated—particularly with regard to personnel sustainment (water, food) and wound dressings. Computer simulation has shown that existing disaster plans consistently underestimate the number of needed resuscitation beds in the emergency department and the use of radiology, while consistently overestimating the number of critically injured, level of triage expertise, and the need for medical personnel and operating rooms.[5] Many hospitals in an area may contract with the same vendors. In the event of an emergency, they may all press for supplies from the same source, which will result in an inability to meet the spike in demand. Other problems arise when equipment that is stored or brought in on an emergency basis is found to be incompatible with the hospital's existing system. In any given region, hospitals may either be independent or belong to different health systems. These institutions may have little understanding of the capacities and capabilities of neighboring facilities.

Specialty Education/Pathophysiology

Weapons of Mass Destruction

The increased global incidence of terrorism has necessitated specific provisions for dealing with weapons of mass destruction as a part of disaster management response and education. Terrorism uses physical or psy-

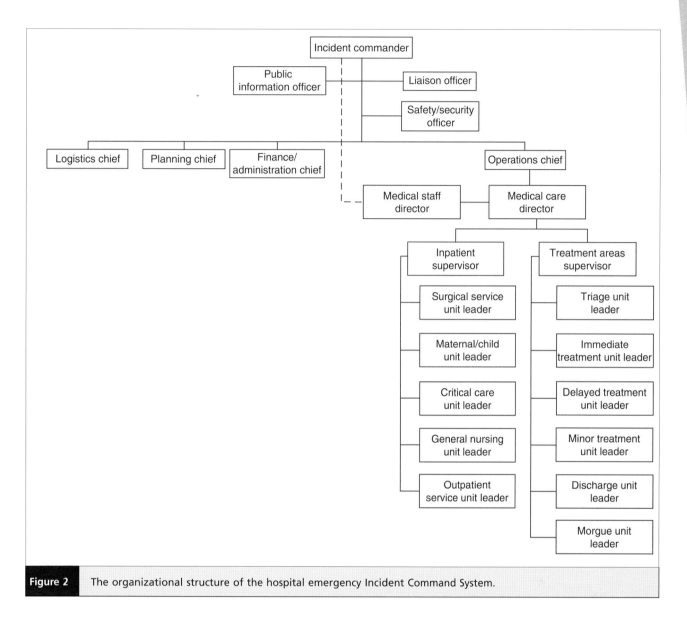

Figure 2 The organizational structure of the hospital emergency Incident Command System.

chological trauma against the civilian population as a means to achieving political goals. Weapons of mass destruction are very effective to this end because they are generally inexpensive, easily transportable, and instill fear and panic in the populace. Chemical, biologic, radiologic, and nuclear attacks remain the most feared, but these agents take significant sophistication to develop into weapons and to deliver. Bombs are the weapon most frequently used around the world as a means to effect political change. It is important to remember also that catastrophic events involving chemical, biologic, radiologic, and nuclear components can take place outside of the context of terrorism. Such industrial accidents have killed or injured thousands of people at one time. Preparation and response must include these nonmilitary explosions as a consideration.

Blast injuries are frequently categorized as primary, secondary, tertiary, and quaternary. Blast physics is described by the rapid transformation of a liquid or solid into a gas that takes place over milliseconds, causing a rapid spike in the local air pressure. This wave moves outward from the explosion source at supersonic speeds as a pressure front (blast overpressure). This pressure front is the source of primary blast injury. It moves through the victim's body in the form of shock, stress, and shear waves that cause implosion, shearing, and acceleration/deceleration injury to tissue and organs. This severe internal damage can sometimes cause death without obvious external damage. Extremity amputation can occur to those in proximity to the blast source and can be used as a marker for triage management following a bombing. The destructive magnitude of the blast has several determinants including the amount and the nature of explosive material used. Explosives can be either low or high energy depending on the rapidity and completeness of the reaction. Chemical components C-4 and nitroglycerine are considerably more powerful than gunpowder or a gasoline-fueled

Table 4

Agents of Chemical Terrorism

Nerve Agents

GA (tabun)

GB (sarin)

GD (soman)

GF (cyclosarin)

VX

Blood Agents

Hydrogen cyanide

Cyanogen chloride

Pulmonary Agents

Chlorine

Phosgene

Blistering Agents (Vesicants)

Mustard agents

Lewisite

Riot Control Agents

Table 5

Category A Biologic Terrorism Pathogens

Anthrax: *Bacillus anthracis*

Botulism: *Clostridium botulinum*

Plague: *Yersinia pestis*

Smallpox: *Variola virus*

Tularemia: *Francisella tularensis*

Viral hemorrhagic fevers: RNA viruses

Molotov cocktail. Ammonium nitrate is a high-energy explosive that is commonly used by terrorists because it is inexpensive and the components are readily available. As the blast wave moves away from the source, its strength deteriorates approximately as the inverse cube of the distance. Blast waves can be reflected off solid objects, thereby increasing their magnitude. Blasts in confined spaces such as a bus or a building are thus predictably more lethal. Positive pressure can also be propagated farther and faster under water.

Primary blast injury to tissue and organ structures can be particularly significant at air fluid interfaces (such as the tympanic membrane or bowel) as well as at the alveolar-capillary interface. Disruption and hemorrhage can cause bowel infarction and blast lung, which can present with symptoms similar to acute respiratory distress syndrome. Those exposed to blast overpressure should be monitored for at least 24 hours because abdominal and lung injury may not be immediately identifiable.

Secondary blast injury is caused by missiles made up of either bomb fragments or imbedded projectiles that are designed to increase wounding (primary fragmentation). Local debris loosened by the blast (glass, pieces of building materials) can also become airborne as secondary fragmentation. Small puncture wounds caused by these forms of shrapnel can be misleading as to the size, amount, and position of imbedded fragments, and liberal use of radiographs is recommended as a part of the evaluation process.

Tertiary injury stems from the victim being thrown by the blast, resulting in potentially significant blunt head and musculoskeletal injury.

Quaternary injury arises from building collapse, which can cause crush, traumatic amputations, and compartment syndromes. Flash burns and other thermal injuries from slow ignition materials and fires as well as smoke or dust inhalation are also considered as quaternary injury.

Chemical weapons are generally considered in five different physiologic agent categories: nerve, blood, pulmonary, blistering (vesicants) and riot control chemicals (Table 4). The 1995 attack on the Tokyo subway system demonstrated the potential problem with chemical agents as victims were allowed unrestricted entry into hospitals. Facilities and personnel became secondarily contaminated with the sarin compound before decontamination procedures could be instituted.

Biologic agents may be difficult to detect and once an outbreak has been realized, it may take even more time to positively identify the infecting agent. Surveillance is critical to the identification of an outbreak.[12] This monitoring is performed by the Centers for Disease Control and Prevention as well as state and local public health offices and emergency departments. School absenteeism, spikes in emergency department admissions for fevers of unknown origin, and sales in over-the-counter pharmaceutical agents are only a few of the epidemiologic parameters that are tracked on a daily basis by monitoring agencies. The Centers for Disease Control and Prevention has identified three different categories of biologic threats based on such factors as ease of dissemination, potential for high mortality, and impact on the public.[13] Category A includes pathogens thought to have the highest potential for use as a weapon (Table 5), whereas category B are only moderately easy to disseminate. Category C threats are those that require bioengineering techniques to develop or are emerging viruses (such as H1N1). The Public Health Security and Bioterrorism Preparedness Act of 2002 established a Select Agents/Toxin List of biologic agents with the potential to pose a severe threat to public health and safety.[14]

Nuclear agents and radiation exposure pose unique threats to the civilian population, whether by nuclear detonation, industrial facility intentional or accidental destruction, dispersal as a "dirty bomb," or dispersal without a bomb component. It must be kept in mind that victims themselves are not radioactive unless they have a contaminating film or dust on their skin. This film or dust can usually be washed off (after clothing removal) with soap and lukewarm water. Medical and surgical care need not necessarily be delayed. Ionizing radiation exposure and lethality is determined by the source type (x-ray versus gamma rays versus α particles, for example) the distance from the source, and the amount of shielding available as protection. The absorbed dose is calculated. 1 Gy is the equivalent of 100 rads. The absorbed dose taken in context with the radiation type will determine the amount of biologic damage as measured in rems. These calculations can be made by a radiation physicist and can aid in the treatment and prognosis of the exposed patient. The prodromal symptoms of significant radiation exposure include nausea, vomiting, diarrhea, central nervous system signs, and skin tingling. The time to symptom onset is the most important factor in determining whether the amount of radiation exposure has been serious. If there are no symptoms within 24 hours and the patient's blood count remains stable, then exposure can be considered minimal and probably not life threatening. In the face of significant exposure, required emergency surgery should be performed in the first 48 hours before the onset of marrow suppression.

Summary

In response to the September 11, 2001, terrorist attacks, the NIMS as part of the NRF was developed to improve the coordination of disaster incident response between all levels of government. Management under a unified command structure allows for a flexible, scalable, tiered incident response with a single action plan. The NRF defines the key response partners and their interrelationships, whereas NIMS defines the organizational components of the ICS that are the standard for emergency management across the country.

Despite the random and unpredictable nature of disasters, most types have predictable, common elements, and planning can be carried out with an "all hazards" approach. Potential risks must be identified in advance before disaster plans and mitigation can be developed. Requisite to disaster response is the integration of public health, medical care, and emergency management. The medical care paradigm shifts to the greatest good to the greatest number of casualties in the face of limited resources. After the safety of victims and rescuers is secured, triage of casualties begins under the responsibility of a designated triage officer who need not be a physician. Decontamination of casualties exposed to chemical, ordnance, biologic, radiologic, or hazardous materials and personal protective equipment for responders are essential. The shift from search and rescue to recovery begins when the disaster situation has been stabilized and patients delivered to medical facilities. If hospitals have been destroyed, recovery will require medical response teams and supplies for immediate and urgent medical care. Hospital preparedness requires an emergency operations plan with hospital and community stakeholders' involvement and a deployable hospital incident command system framework. With global terrorism on the increase, the most feared weapons of mass destruction (chemical, biologic, radiologic, nuclear components) and the most frequently used weapons (bombs) necessitate education and managed disaster response. Catastrophic events and industrial incidents outside the context of terrorism have also killed or injured thousands. Knowledge of blast physics and patterns of injury allows for improvement of diagnostic and treatment strategies, and a basic understanding of chemical, biologic, and nuclear agents, their clinical symptoms, and recommended treatment strategies have become increasingly important for surgeons.

Annotated References

1. Arnold JL: Disaster medicine in the 21st century: Future hazards, vulnerabilities and risk. *Prehosp Disast Med* 2002;17:3-11.

2. Halpern P, Tsai MC, Arnold JL, Stok E, Ersoy G: Mass casualty terrorist bombings: Implications for emergency department and hospital emergency response (Part II). *Prehosp Disast Med* 2003;18:235-241.

3. Auf der Heide E: *Disaster Response: Principles of Preparation and Coordination.* St. Louis, MO, CV Mosby, 1989.

4. Born CT, Briggs SM, Ciraulo DL, et al: Disasters and mass casualties: I. General principles of response and management. *J Am Acad Orthop Surg* 2007;15:388-396.

   This article is the first in a two-part series that covers general principles of disasters and mass casualty incidents including triage and injury severity in disasters. Level of evidence: III.

5. Hirshberg A, Holcomb JB, Mattox KL: Hospital trauma care in multiple-casualty incidents: A critical view. *Ann Emerg Med* 2001;37(6):647-652.

6. Ashkenazi I, Kessel B, Khashan T, et al: Precision of in-hospital triage in mass-casualty incidents after terror attacks. *Prehosp Disaster Med* 2006;21(1):20-23.

   This retrospective study was based on a cohort of patient records that included details of injuries. Level of evidence: II.

7. Centers for Disease Control and Prevention. http://www.cdc.gov/NIOSH. Accessed January 26, 2010.

   This guidance document provides local, state, and federal emergency response entities with comparison information on OSHA/EPA Protection Levels A, B, and C;

and Department of Human Services-adopted PPE performance-based standards.

8. Plante DM, Walker JS: EMS response at a hazardous material incident: Some basic guidelines. *J Emerg Med* 1989;7:55-64.

9. Hirshberg A, Scott BG, Granchi T, Wall MJ Jr , Mattox KL, Stein M: How does casualty load affect trauma care in urban bombing incidents? A quantitative analysis. *J Trauma* 2005;58(4):686-693, discussion 694-695.

10. Understanding Emergency Management Standards Compliance Requirements. Available at http://www.jcrinc.com/common/PDFs/fpdfs/pubs/pdfs/JCReqs/JCP-06-08-S1.pdf. Accessed February 17, 2010.

   Standards for managing resources and assets during emergencies are discussed.

11. Norcross ED, Elliott BM, Adams DB, Crawford FA: Impact of a major hurricane on surgical services in a university hospital. *Am Surg* 1993;59(1):28-33.

12. Grey MR, Spaeth KR: *The Bioterrorism Sourcebook.* New York, NY, McGraw-Hill, 2006.

   This book is a guideline for prevention, identification, and treatment of bioterrorism threats, primarily from the health care worker's perspective.

13. Bioterrorism CDC Agents/Diseases. Available at http://emergency.cdc.gov/agent/agentlist.asp.

   The Centers for Disease Control and Prevention defines and lists biologic agents and diseases as Categories A, B, or C.

14. National Select Agent Registry. http://www.selectagents.gov/Select%20Agents%20and%20Toxins%20List.html. Accessed February 17, 2010.

   The National Select Agent Registry of the Centers for Disease Control and Prevention combines the Select Agents and Toxins lists from the US Department of Health and Human Services and Department of Agriculture, last updated August 31, 2009.

The Polytrauma Patient and Fracture Healing

SECTION EDITOR:

ADAM J. STARR, MD

Chapter 11

Evaluation of the Polytrauma Patient

Kelly Lefaivre, MD, MSc, FRCSC   Craig S. Roberts, MD, MBA   Pierre Guy, MD

Advanced Trauma Life Support

Trauma patients present with a range of potentially life-threatening injuries that vary in severity. An organized approach to trauma patients in which life-threatening injuries are promptly recognized and treated or triaged is the cornerstone of contemporary trauma care. This organized approach has evolved from the Vietnam War experience to the present eighth edition of Advanced Trauma Life Support (ATLS). ATLS is a globally accepted, standardized framework to teach and provide safe initial trauma care by prioritizing the diagnosis and treatment of life-threatening injuries. Taught in 50 countries, the ATLS course has become the most successful training program for the early care of severely injured patients. The interactive teaching format of ATLS has shown sustained levels of performance even 2 years after training. Additional courses have developed from ATLS: Combat Trauma Life Support, adapted to combat situations, and Definitive Surgical Trauma Care (www. iatsic.com), which provides advanced surgical skills for procedures that naturally follow the ATLS protocol.

The ATLS protocol has moved from its initial expert-based consensus approach to an increasingly evidence-based approach. The changes specific to orthopaedics in its eighth edition include the management of exsanguinating pelvic fracture injuries.[1] In the ATLS seventh edition, angioembolization was described for hemodynamically unstable pelvic fractures with negative diagnostic peritoneal lavage, whereas the ATLS eighth edition provides surgical options (external fixa-

tion, pelvic packing) along with angioembolization. The ATLS eighth edition notes that failure to respond to crystalloid and blood administration in the emergency department dictates the need for immediate definitive intervention to control exsanguinating hemorrhage (for example, operation or angioembolization). The ATLS seventh edition also described management based on diagnostic peritoneal lavage (DPL), and recommended that patients with a positive DPL undergo celiotomy, whereas those with a negative DPL instead are managed with angiographic embolization. The ATLS eighth edition states that in the setting of a positive DPL, the pelvis should be temporarily stabilized or "closed" using an available commercial compression device or sheet to decrease bleeding, along with addressing intra-abdominal hemorrhage as required.

Markers for Mortality

Clinicians and researchers have long aimed to identify the individuals at risk of developing severe systemic complications (acute respiratory distress syndrome [ARDS], multiple organ failure and sepsis) or death. Patient factors (demographics), and injury factors (mechanism and severity) are used to guide preventive and/or therapeutic strategies. Means to quantify the risk of morbidity and mortality after trauma include quantifying the number of injured anatomic regions (Injury Severity Score [ISS]), assessing the physiologic response to injury using vital signs and measures of cognitive function available for on-field triage systems (Revised Trauma Score [RTS]), and measurement of biologic markers related to injury and tissue perfusion (hemoglobin level, base deficit, serum lactate, and inflammatory markers).

The factors that predominantly have been associated with mortality are increased patient age, head injury (elevated Glasgow Coma Score [GCS] [Table 1]), an elevated on-field RTS (which combines GCS, respiratory rate, and systolic blood pressure), the presence of multiple system involvement (high ISS), the presence of hemodynamic instability, and base deficit on presentation and throughout resuscitation. A base deficit (negative base excess) is a critical marker of inadequate tissue

Dr. Lefaivre or an immediate family member has received research or institutional support from Stryker, Synthes, and Zimmer. Dr. Roberts or an immediate family member has received research or institutional support from Synthes; has received royalties from Skeletal Trauma; and is a board member, owner, officer, or committee member of the American Academy of Orthopaedic Surgeons, Mid-America Orthopaedic Association, Orthopaedic Trauma Association, and Kentucky Orthopaedic Society. Dr. Guy or an immediate family member serves as a paid consultant for or is an employee of Stryker and has received research or institutional support from Synthes, Stryker, and DePuy.

2: The Polytrauma Patient and Fracture Healing

Table 1

Glasgow Coma Score

	1	2	3	4	5	6
Best Eye Response	Does not open eyes	Opens eyes to pain	Opens eyes to voice	Opens eyes spontaneously	—	—
Best Verbal Response	Makes no sounds	Incomprehensible sounds	Utters inappropriate words	Speaks, but confused/ disoriented	Oriented, converses normally	—
Best Motor Response	Makes no movement	Extension to painful stimuli (decerebrate)	Flexion to painful stimuli (decorticate)	Withdrawal to pain	Localizes to pain	Obeys commands

Table 2

Abbreviated Injury Severity Score

Score	Description
0	None
1	Minor
2	Moderate
3	Serious
4	Severe
5	Critical
6	Maximal, possibly fatal

perfusion which, in the setting of trauma, is most commonly but not always caused by hemorrhage. Because the ISS information is usually collected during the course of hospitalization and at discharge, its use in the acute setting has been limited. Studies have linked mortality to acute clinical information; namely, a trauma patient who is normotensive has a mortality rate of 3% to 6%. With hypotension at admission this rate would rise to 21% to 42%; an associated head injury requiring treatment or a required laparotomy would increase the risk to approximately 50%. A combination of hypotension, pelvic ring injury, head injury, and the need for laparotomy would increase the rate of mortality to more than 90%.

Research has additionally focused on measuring the inflammatory response to trauma and surgery in an attempt to identify at-risk patients in this population.[2,3] The markers measured have included the proinflammatory marker interleukin (IL)-6, IL-8, neutrophil elastase, C-reactive protein, and surface markers for CD 11, along with platelet count and other coagulation measures. Despite large randomized clinical trials, measured levels of inflammatory markers have not yet been associated with mortality. These markers (IL-6) have been able to predict the development of acute lung injury or dysfunction in borderline patients undergoing early femoral fixation. Acute lung injury or dysfunction is a condition differentiated from ARDS by its lesser degree of hypoxemia. The association showed a large odds ratio (6.69), but its wide confidence interval (1.02 to 44.08) with a small event rate advises cautious interpretation. No increased risk of pneumonia, ARDS, systemic inflammatory response, sepsis, multiple organ failure, or mortality have been noted with measured changes in inflammatory markers in trauma.[4]

Scoring Systems

Many scoring systems were initially designed for the purposes of appropriate triage and classification of patients but are now used for quality assurance, evaluation of trauma care systems, research, and reimbursement purposes. These scoring systems have been separated into physiologic, anatomic, and combined scoring systems.[5]

Glasgow Coma Score

Described in 1974 to differentiate injury severity in closed head injury patients, GCS has been expanded to all acute medical and trauma patients, as well as intensive care unit scoring systems. It is used both as an initial assessment tool and to follow changes in neurologic function. The score is a combination of three areas (**Table 1**): best motor response (1-6), best verbal response (1-5), and best eye response (1-4). GCS is observer dependent, and can be greatly affected by other factors including centrally active pharmacologic agents and level of resuscitation. Field GCS is less predictive of mortality than admission GCS, probably because of the effects of early resuscitation.

Abbreviated Injury Severity Score

The Abbreviated Injury Severity (AIS) Score was also developed in 1971 to describe blunt injuries by anatomic body regions. There are nine anatomic areas included: head, face, neck, thorax, abdomen, spine, upper extremity, lower extremity, and external. Each body system is scored from 0 to 6 (**Table 2**). The relative values are consensus driven, and were most recently revised in 1990. This version included scores for 1,300 individual injuries.

Table 3

Revised Trauma Score (A + B + C)

Calculation of Points	Glasgow Coma Score (A)	Systolic Blood Pressure (B)	Respiratory Rate (C)
4	13-15	≥ 90	10-29
3	9-12	76-89	≥ 30
2	6-8	50-75	6-9
1	4-5	1-49	1-5
0	3	0	0

Injury Severity Score

First described in 1974, ISS is calculated using AIS scores. ISS correlates with mortality, morbidity, and length of hospital stay after trauma, is a useful research tool for the comparison of trauma severity between patients and among centers, and is not meant to be used in the field or as a triage tool. It is the score used to define polytrauma, which is defined by an ISS > 17.[6]

For the purposes of calculating ISS, the anatomic regions described previously for the AIS scores are collapsed into six anatomic systems: head and/or neck, face, chest, abdomen, and extremities (including the pelvis). The three highest individual scores are each squared, and the total is added together. The highest possible score is 75 (which correlates with a score of 5 in three body regions). A single score of 6 on any AIS anatomic region results in an automatic score of 75.

Because the calculation of ISS requires the diagnosis of all injuries as well as a quantification of their severity, the ISS is not a useful score at the time of admission to the hospital. However, it is routinely used to prospectively delineate injury severity in trauma registries. One drawback of the ISS is that it only "counts" one injury in any one body area. In a patient with three major abdominal injuries, only the injury with the highest AIS score will be counted. The New Injury Severity Score addresses this issue in that it counts the three highest scoring injuries regardless of anatomic AIS region (a patient could have three abdominal-related scores).

The New Injury Severity Score may be more predictive of complications and mortality than ISS in all patients, and has been convincingly shown to be predictive of extended hospitalization and intensive care unit admission in patients with multiple orthopaedic injuries.[7]

Revised Trauma Score

The original Trauma Score was published in 1981 and was based on the concept that early death in trauma results from compromise of the cardiovascular, respiratory, and nervous systems. The first iteration of this score included five different areas: GCS, respiratory rate, respiratory expansion, systolic blood pressure, and capillary refill. The same lead authors published a revised version of the score in 1989, as capillary refill and respiratory expansion were found to be difficult to evaluate consistently in practice.

RTS included three of the original five physiologic parameters (**Table 3**): GCS, systolic blood pressure, and respiratory rate. Each area is given a score from 0-4, with lower scores being more predictive of mortality. The total score is a sum of the three areas for a total possible score of 12. An RTS of 11 or less identifies 97% of severely injured patients. The RTS is most widely used for triage to determine which patients need to be transported to a trauma center. However, the RTS can underestimate injury severity in patients injured in one body system.

Trauma Injury Severity Score

The Trauma Injury Severity Score (TRISS) combines anatomic (ISS) and physiologic (Trauma Score) information with age, and has been used to develop prediction models for mortality in trauma. Newer versions of the TRISS have since been described using the RTS. These versions recognized the difference between blunt and penetrating injury, and separate models were developed for each mechanism. These amount to simple logistic regression equations to predict the probability of survival.

Although the prediction model based on TRISS can be used to calculate the probability of survival for individual patients, its design is particularly useful for local quality control and the identification of cases that are 'outliers' (unexpected survivors and unexpected deaths). This combined system can also be used to evaluate the performance of trauma populations between centers as well as new protocols.

Orthopaedic Considerations in the Evaluation of Polytrauma Patients

More than half of patients admitted to most trauma centers have musculoskeletal injuries; in general, any musculoskeletal trauma has a strong impact on patient outcome. However, there are certain circumstances in which orthopaedic fractures or conditions can have a dramatic impact on a patient's course after injury. All orthopaedic injuries demand attention and skillful

2: The Polytrauma Patient and Fracture Healing

management to be brought to a successful outcome. Yet, there are some orthopaedic injuries or scenarios that seem to be particularly problematic, especially in the early phases of management. Examples include pelvic ring injuries, single or bilateral femur fractures, traumatic partial or complete amputations, major joint dislocations, or any fracture with neurologic and/or vascular compromise. Only through prompt recognition and expectant management of such conditions will an optimal outcome be ensured.

Evaluation of Patients With Pelvic Fractures

Fractures of the pelvis are life-threatening injuries. Their early recognition and management is an essential part of the management of the multiply injured trauma patient. Initially, assessment for other life-threatening injuries involving the head and chest, major abdominal injuries, and retroperitoneal vascular injuries is critical.

Physical examination findings indicative of major pelvic trauma include abnormal positioning of the lower extremities (shortening, rotation), mechanical instability of the hemipelvis (testing to be performed by one person only, as repeated examinations may dislodge pelvic clots, resulting in hemorrhage), tenderness or palpable gaps of the sacrum or symphysis, flank ecchymosis or hematoma, and perineal trauma (scrotal/labial hematoma or swelling, blood at urethral meatus, rectal laceration or gross blood, abnormal prostate examination, and vaginal laceration or gross blood).

According to ATLS protocols, initial assessment includes an AP pelvis radiograph. This film, as well as the injury mechanism, gives an indication of the stability of the fracture. Those with anterior-posterior compression (APC) II, APC III, lateral compression III, vertical shear, and combined mechanism patterns are more likely to be hemodynamically unstable and require transfusion.[8]

Stable fracture patterns include minimally displaced pubic rami fracture(s), nondisplaced or minimally displaced sacral ala fracture(s), isolated iliac wing fractures not disrupting pelvic ring integrity, and avulsion fractures at muscle insertions. Unstable fracture patterns have more than 2.5 cm of symphysis diastasis, displaced pubic rami fractures, more than 1 cm of sacroiliac joint widening, more than 1 cm of displacement at a sacral fracture, fracture-dislocation of the sacroiliac joint complex, and cephalad hemipelvis migration.

Specific details about the evaluation and acute management of pelvic fractures are provided in chapter 22.

Evaluation of Patients With Femur Fractures

Femur fractures represent a significant injury with the potential for large-volume blood loss, hemodynamic instability, and death. These patients need to be treated according to accepted ATLS and American College of Surgeons trauma protocols.

Two central issues dominate the discussion of the emergent treatment of femur fracture patients: timing of surgery and damage control orthopaedics (external fixation) versus early total care (primary intramedul-

lary nailing). Femur fractures represent a unique injury because of the systemic effects of this injury and its treatment, and the association with ARDS and death.

The mechanism of injury is important in femur fracture patients, specifically to evaluate the likelihood of associated injuries. A complete ATLS-focused physical examination is important, because as many as half of patients with a femur fracture will have an ISS of at least 19.[9] Regardless of whether one is a proponent of early total care or damage control orthopaedics in multiply injured trauma patients, there is consensus that patient resuscitation is pivotal in the minimization of ARDS and death, and this should be the focus of early evaluation and treatment.[9,10]

In the leg specifically, the degree of soft-tissue injury should be assessed, as well as inspection for any open wounds. The thigh carries a large volume of muscle tissue, and crush injuries can be associated with a life-threatening degree of myonecrosis. The size of the thigh hematoma, as well as the neurovascular status, should be followed over time, as the physical findings in the setting of vascular compromise can change over time.[11] Further information regarding the management of femoral fractures is provided in chapters 16 and 33.

Geriatric Trauma

Geriatric patients without hip fracture admitted to a level I trauma center represent approximately 15% to 30% of all admissions, a number that varies based on heterogeneity of age definition (older than 50 or 65 years) and ISS threshold definitions (greater than 10, 12, or 15). Some reports have focused on the cohort older than 80 years because this age group appears to be different from the 65- to 80-year-old group in terms of complication types, mortality, and discharge disposition. This difference in mortality and morbidity in geriatric trauma patients has influenced the care provided to this population.

Increased Mortality of Geriatric Patients

There is a strong relationship between age (older than 65 years) and trauma mortality, with older patients having mortality rates two to three times higher than younger patients in all phases of care[12] (immediate, early: [24 to 48 hours after injury], and delayed [more than 48 to 72 hours after injury]). Common trauma scores (Trauma Score, RTS) correlate well with mortality (**Table 4**). ISS also correlates with mortality in geriatric patients across all ISS groups. The rates differ from matching ISS in younger groups, with the greatest difference noted in the moderate ISS (12 to 15) where mortality of 30% is five times that of the younger patient.

GCS (less than 8) is also uniformly associated with a poor outcome and may guide decision making.[13] Head-injured geriatric patients have higher mortality and poorer outcome than younger patients,[14] and older spinal cord–injured patients have a greater mortality rate than younger patients (27% versus 3.2%), which is ad-

Table 4

Relationship Between Trauma Score and Mortality in Geriatric Patients

Trauma Score	Mortality
15-16	5%
12-14	25%
< 12	65%
< 7-9	Universal

(Adapted with permission from Knudson MM, Lieberman J, Morris JA Jr, Cushing BM, Stubbs HA: Mortality factors in geriatric blunt trauma patients. *Arch Surg* 1994;129:448-453; and Horst HM, Obeid FN, Sorensen VJ, Bivins BA: Factors influencing survival of elderly trauma patients. *Crit Care Med* 1986;14:681-684.)

Table 5

Predictors of Morbidity and Mortality

Factor	Mortality (Odds Ratio)	Morbidity (Complication Predicted)
Transfusion	(1.1)	Sepsis
ISS	(1.04)	ARDS Pneumonia Sepsis Gastrointestinal
GCS	(0.87)	
Fluid requirements	(1.06)	Myocardial infarction

(Adapted with permission from Tornetta P, III, Mostafavi H, Riina J, Turen C, et al: Morbidity and mortality in elderly trauma patients. *J Trauma* 1999;46:702-706.)

ditionally related to American Spinal Injury Association grade (grade A: 66%; D: 23%)[15] The Geriatric Trauma Survival Score calculated an 80% mortality in patients with ISS of 25 or greater and older than 80 years, and identified these two factors and the presence of a cardiac and septic complication as being able to reliably predict mortality (92%).

Increased Morbidity of Geriatric Patients
In-hospital complication rates of 33% (to include pneumonia, myocardial infarction, ARDS, and multiple organ failure) are reported in geriatric trauma patients, compared to 19% in the younger cohort. It has been reported that transfusion, ISS, and fluid requirements were associated with increased risk of morbidity (Table 5).

In-Hospital Management of Geriatric Patients
Early invasive monitoring and liberal use of diagnostic imaging[16] in the diagnosis of potentially life-threatening conditions have improved outcomes among older trauma patients.

Improved outcomes for elderly trauma patients are thought to result from an approach that actively involves an intensive care setting: avoid end organ hypoperfusion/occult hypoperfusion, maximize oxygenation, control blood pressure, correct acidosis (base deficit), stabilize and mobilize patients, and maximize nutrition and rehabilitation. The overall survival rate of geriatric trauma patients is 70% to 90%, whereas the survival rate after intensive care unit admission is 68%.[17]

Additional information about geriatric fractures is provided in chapters 40, 41 and 42.

Transfer to a Higher Level of Care

The process and economics of the transfer of orthopaedic trauma patients between North American hospitals have become more complicated. Several points are noted in the position statement of the Orthopaedic Trauma Association Health Policy Committee (www.ota.org). Transfer of patients with musculoskeletal injuries is often necessary to ensure treatment at an appropriate level of expertise and resource availability. Transfers should not be based on the payer status of the patient. Regional transfer agreements should be established to avoid delays associated with long-distance transfers.

Recent studies of factors that influence the transfer of trauma patients have focused on economics and undertriage. The influence of insurance status on the transfer of femoral fracture patients to a level I trauma center was studied. The authors noted that 58% of patients who were transferred were uninsured, whereas all of the patients who were not transferred were insured.[18] These authors stated that their findings suggested "overtriage," and further noted that insurance status as well as injury severity and orthopaedic surgeon availability influence the decision to transfer femoral fracture patients to a level I trauma center.

Socioeconomic factors, medicolegal issues, and trauma patient transfer trends were examined in a 2006 study, and the authors concluded that there was "a multifactorial reluctance or inability of initial hospitals to care for patients they are theoretically capable of treating, placing undue burden on level I centers."[19]

The characteristics of twice-transferred, rural trauma patients were studied to assess the variables of the phenomenon of undertriage (patients requiring a second transfer to a higher-level trauma center). It was concluded that reducing the number of twice-transferred trauma patients would involve refining protocols concerning the need for specialty care.[20]

A 2008 retrospective study of 10 years of data from the Maryland Ambulance Information System determined whether age bias is a factor in triage errors.[21] It was concluded that even when trauma was recognized by emergency medical services, providers were less likely to consider transporting geriatric patients to

2: The Polytrauma Patient and Fracture Healing

trauma centers. These authors hypothesized that under-triage in this population was the result of unconscious age bias.

Two recent prospective studies provide additional data about the phenomenon of inappropriate transfers to level I trauma centers. In a 2010 study, the authors prospectively assessed the appropriateness, indications, risk factors, and epidemiology of patients with orthopaedic injuries transferred to a level I trauma center, and reported that 16.5% of transfers were deemed completely inappropriate by the accepting orthopaedic traumatologist.[22]

The authors of the second 2010 study prospectively evaluated the appropriateness of transfer of patients with orthopaedic injuries to a level I trauma center from surrounding level II to IV centers.[23] They considered 52% of the transfers to be inappropriate. Sixty-eight percent of the transfers occurred between 6 pm and 5:59 am, and 60% of transfers were on weekends. In addition, 69% of inappropriately transferred patients were discharged directly from the emergency room.

These studies highlight some of the complex issues (for example, Emergency Medical Treatment and Active Labor Act, financial impact of transfers, emergency room orthopaedic coverage, the American College of Surgeons Trauma System, communication) involved in transfer to a higher level of care, and provide data to begin to positively affect the future.

Summary

Refinements in ATLS, identification of markers for mortality, and improvements in scoring systems have the potential to improve the capability of assessing and treating the polytrauma patient. Improved evaluation of the polytrauma patient will undoubtedly improve the ability to stratify patients and link these factors to outcomes. Outcomes assessment in polytrauma continues to move beyond just survival. Orthopaedic entities that affect the outcome of polytrauma patients include pelvic fractures, femur fractures, mangled extremities, and geriatric trauma. Approaches to these entities continue to evolve as a result of linking treatment to outcomes. Transfer of polytrauma patients in North America has become more complicated.

Annotated References

1. Kortbeek JB, Al Turki SA, Ali J, et al: Advanced trauma life support, 8th edition. The evidence for change. *J Trauma* 2008;64(6):1638-1650.

   This paper highlights the evidence-based medicine process by which protocol additions and changes were adopted in the (new) eighth version of the American College of Surgeons' ATLS protocol, and lists the changes in table form.

2. DeLong WG Jr, Born CT: Cytokines in patients with polytrauma. *Clin Orthop Relat Res* 2004;422:57-65.

   This paper reviews the mechanisms that trigger a cytokine response and summarizes the relationship to a traumatic stimulus. It concludes that a cytokine reaction has been recognized after trauma and secondary surgery, but further research is required to determine clinical significance.

3. Roberts CS, Pape HC, Jones AL, Malkani AL, Rodriguez JL, Giannoudis PV: Damage control orthopaedics: Evolving concepts in the treatment of patients who have sustained orthopaedic trauma. *Instr Course Lect* 2005;54:447-462.

   This paper offers a comprehensive review of the clinical and animal scientific work that surrounds the concept of damage control orthopaedics.

4. Pape HC, Rixen D, Morley J, et al; EPOFF Study Group: Impact of the method of initial stabilization for femoral shaft fractures in patients with multiple injuries at risk for complications (borderline patients). *Ann Surg* 2007;246(3):491-499.

   This is a multicenter, randomized, controlled trial comparing intramedullary nailing to external fixation followed by intramedullary nailing in stable and borderline patients. Clinical and laboratory outcomes were measured. Stable patients showed a shorter ventilation time with intramedullary nailing, supporting the emergency trauma care approach to fixing stable patients within 24 hours. 2) Borderline patients showed an increased incidence of acute lung injury, which is a condition that differs from ARDS by its lesser degree of hypoxemia. No difference in the following complications was seen between the groups: pneumonia, ARDS, systemic inflammatory response, sepsis, multiple organ failure, or mortality.

5. Guzzo JL, Bochicchio GV, Napolitano LM, Malone DL, Meyer W, Scalea TM: Prediction of outcomes in trauma: Anatomic or physiologic parameters? *J Am Coll Surg* 2005;201(6):891-897.

   This is a comparison of a new combination system with traditional physiologic and anatomic scoring systems.

6. Keel M, Trentz O: Pathophysiology of polytrauma. *Injury* 2005;36(6):691-709.

   This paper is a recent review of underlying causes of early and late mortality in trauma.

7. Balogh ZJ, Varga E, Tomka J, Süveges G, Tóth L, Simonka JA: The new injury severity score is a better predictor of extended hospitalization and intensive care unit admission than the injury severity score in patients with multiple orthopaedic injuries. *J Orthop Trauma* 2003;17(7):508-512.

8. Magnussen RA, Tressler MA, Obremskey WT, Kregor PJ: Predicting blood loss in isolated pelvic and acetabular high-energy trauma. *J Orthop Trauma* 2007;21(9):603-607.

   An analysis of fracture types and transfusion requirements, which showed that Young and Burgess lateral compression III, APC II, APC III, vertical shear, and combined mechanisms are at high risk of needing transfusion.

9. O'Toole RV, O'Brien M, Scalea TM, Habashi N, Pollak AN, Turen CH: Resuscitation before stabilization of femoral fractures limits acute respiratory distress syndrome in patients with multiple traumatic injuries despite low use of damage control orthopaedics. *J Trauma* 2009;67:1013-1021.

This is a prospective study of all femoral fractures treated at a level I trauma center during a 3-year period. For the most severely injured patients who underwent nailing (ISS > 28, thoracic, Abbreviated Injury Score > 2; *N* = 28), the ARDS rate was only 3.3%. Frequent use of early reamed femoral nailing and infrequent use of damage control orthopaedics showed fairly low ARDS rates.

10. Weninger P, Figl M, Spitaler R, Mauritz W, Hertz H: Early unreamed intramedullary nailing of femoral fractures is safe in patients with severe thoracic trauma. *J Trauma* 2007;62:692-696.

The effect of early definitive fixation of femoral fractures on outcomes in multiply injured patients with severe thoracic trauma was investigated. The authors found that the procedure was safe and appropriate for early definitive care.

11. Kluger Y, Gonze MD, Paul DB, et al: Blunt vascular injury associated with closed mid shaft femur fracture: A cause for concern. *Injury* 1994;36:222-225.

12. Finelli FC, Jonsson J, Champion HR, Morelli S, Fouty WJ: A case control study for major trauma in geriatric patients. *J Trauma* 1989;29(5):541-548.

13. Morris JA Jr, MacKenzie EJ, Edelstein SL: The effect of preexisting conditions on mortality in trauma patients. *JAMA* 1990;263(14):1942-1946.

14. Thompson HJ, McCormick WC, Kagan SH: Traumatic brain injury in older adults: Epidemiology, outcomes, and future implications. *J Am Geriatr Soc* 2006;54(10):1590-1595.

Adults age 75 years and older had the highest rates of traumatic brain injury–related hospitalization and death. Falls were reported as the leading cause of traumatic brain injury (51%) for this population, followed by motor vehicle accidents (5%), with older age negatively affecting outcome. The authors concluded that providing care and predicting outcome was problematic for this population and called for refocusing of research efforts.

15. Fassett DR, Harrop JS, Maltenfort M, et al: Mortality rates in geriatric patients with spinal cord injuries. *J Neurosurg Spine* 2007;7(3):277-281.

The incidence of spinal cord injury was evaluated in patients age 70 years or older. It was concluded that these injuries are more prevalent in this and mortality rate is greater than in younger patients.

16. Loberant N, Rose C: Imaging considerations in the geriatric emergency department patient. *Emerg Med Clin North Am* 1990;8(2):361-397.

17. Battistella FD, Din AM, Perez L: Trauma patients 75 years and older: Long-term follow-up results justify aggressive management. *J Trauma* 1998;44(4):618-623.

18. Archdeacon MT, Simon PM, Wyrick JD: The influence of insurance status on the transfer of femoral fracture patients to a level-I trauma center. *J Bone Joint Surg Am* 2007;89(12):2625-2631.

This was a retrospective cohort study performed within a six-hospital health care system. There was a significant difference in insurance status between patients who had been transferred to the level I trauma center and those who had not, and those who had been definitively managed at the level I center and those who had been managed in community hospitals. The authors concluded that it can be assumed that insurance status as well as injury severity and orthopaedic surgeon availability influence the decision to transfer femoral fracture patients to a level I center.

19. Esposito TJ, Crandall M, Reed RL, Gamelli RL, Luchette FA: Socioeconomic factors, medicolegal issues, and trauma patient transfer trends: Is there a connection? *J Trauma* 2006;61(6):1380-1386.

This retrospective review of a state trauma registry over a 4-year period found that variables most significant for predicting transfer to a level I trauma center included arrival at the initial emergency department between 3 pm and 7 am, and orthopaedic injury or head injury. The authors suggested that their study suggests "a multifactorial reluctance or inability of initial hospitals to care for patients they are theoretically capable of treating ..."

20. Sihler KC, Hansen AR, Torner JC, Kealey GP, Morgan LJ, Zwerling C: Characteristics of twice-transferred, rural trauma patients. *Prehosp Emerg Care* 2002;6(3):330-335.

21. Chang DC, Bass RR, Cornwell EE, Mackenzie EJ: Undertriage of elderly trauma patients to state-designated trauma centers. *Arch Surg* 2008;143(8):776-791.

This retrospective study of 10 years of data from the Maryland Ambulance Information Systems found that even when trauma was recognized by emergency medical services, providers were consistently less likely to consider transporting elderly patients to a trauma center.

22. Crichlow RJ, Zeni A, Reveal G, et al: Appropriateness of patient transfer with associated orthopaedic injuries to a level I trauma center. *J Orthop Trauma* 2010;24:(6)331-335.

The authors present a prospective study of the appropriateness, indications, risk factors, and epidemiology of patients with orthopaedic injuries transferred to a level I trauma center. Of the 546 transfers, 16.5% were deemed completely inappropriate. Whether appropriate or not, most transfers were attributed to either a complete lack of orthopaedic coverage or a lack of expertise at the referring hospital.

2: The Polytrauma Patient and Fracture Healing

23. Thakur NA, Plante MJ, Kayiaros SK, Reinert SE, Ehrlich MG: Inappropriate transfer of patients with orthopaedic injuries to a level I trauma center: A prospective study. *J Orthop Trauma* 2010;24:336-339.

This article describes a prospective study conducted over a 5-month period of the appropriateness of transfer of patients with orthopaedic injuries to a level I trauma center from surrounding level II to IV centers. Of 216 patients transferred, the authors found 52% of the transfers to be inappropriate.

Chapter 12
Pathophysiology of the Polytrauma Patient

David J. Hak, MD, MBA   Philip F. Stahel, MD   Peter Giannoudis, MD, FRCS

Introduction

Trauma remains a leading cause of death and accounts for more than 100,000 deaths in the United States each year. Despite advances in prehospital and hospital care, patients who survive the initial traumatic event are still at risk of death from complications such as acute respiratory distress syndrome (ARDS) and multiple organ failure (MOF).

The orthopaedic surgeon's understanding of the various physiologic responses following multiple trauma has advanced significantly during the past decade, leading to observable changes in clinical practice. In the orthopaedic arena, the management of severely injured patients has evolved from early total care to damage control orthopaedics. Many questions remain, including which patients require staged surgical treatment, how to best limit secondary brain and pulmonary insults, and which parameters most accurately assess resuscitation status.

Physiology of Injury

Severe trauma induces multiple pathophysiologic reactions that are mediated by local tissue injury and by systemic reactions to hypovolemic shock, coagulopathy, ischemia/reperfusion syndrome, and induction of the hepatic acute-phase response.[1,2] In addition, major trauma triggers a profound immunologic dysfunction that is characterized by early activation of the innate immune response (hyperinflammation), followed by delayed attenuation of adaptive immunity with decreased

Dr. Hak or a member of his immediate family is a member of a speakers' bureau or has made paid presentations on behalf of Medtronic and Eisai; serves as a paid consultant to or is an employee of Medtronic; and has received research or institutional support from Synthes and Stryker. Dr. Giannoudis or a member of his immediate family has received research or institutional support from AO, GlaxoSmithKline, Smith & Nephew, Stryker, Synthes, Kuros, and DePuy. Neither Dr. Stahel nor a member of his immediate family has received anything of value from or owns stock in a commercial company or institution related directly or indirectly to the subject of this article.

T cell function (immunosuppression) with enhanced susceptibility to infection.[3-5] These two distinct phases have been defined as the systemic inflammatory response syndrome (SIRS) and the compensatory anti-inflammatory response syndrome, respectively (**Figure 1**). Understanding these pathophysiologic phases is of crucial importance for the orthopaedic trauma surgeon when caring for polytrauma patients, because the inappropriate timing or modality of fracture fixation may induce a "second hit" insult and exacerbate the pathophysiologic cascade leading to sepsis, MOF, and death.[1,6,7]

Immune Response

The innate immune response represents the first line of defense against nonself antigens, including viruses, bacteria, and parasites. Severe trauma has been shown to activate the innate immune response even in the absence of foreign antigens. The endogenous triggers of inflammation induced by major trauma include complement anaphylatoxins and host-generated danger signals, such as pathogen-associated molecular patterns (PAMPs) and the so-called alarmins. Although PAMPs represent microbial molecules recognized by the innate immune system, the alarmins represent nonpathogen-derived danger signals that originate from tissue injury.[2] These include heat-shock proteins, annexins, defensins, S100 protein, and the high mobility group box 1 (HMGB1) nuclear protein.[5,8] Taken together, PAMPs and alarmins constitute the superfamily of damage-associated molecular patterns (DAMPs). Cells of the immune system recognize DAMPs through multiligand receptors, such as Toll-like receptors, expressed on their surfaces. After trauma, DAMPs are potent activators of the innate immune system resulting from major injury alone (alarmins) or after trauma-related infectious complications (PAMPs), including sepsis.[1,7]

Proinflammatory cytokines, such as tumor necrosis factor (TNF) and the interleukins (IL)-1β, -6, -8, -12, -15, and -18 are potent inflammatory mediators released after traumatic tissue injury that bridge the innate and adaptive immune responses.[9] Among multiple immunologic functions, cytokines are potent activators of neutrophils (polymorphonuclear leukocytes [PMNLs]), which are considered the key cellular mediators of the

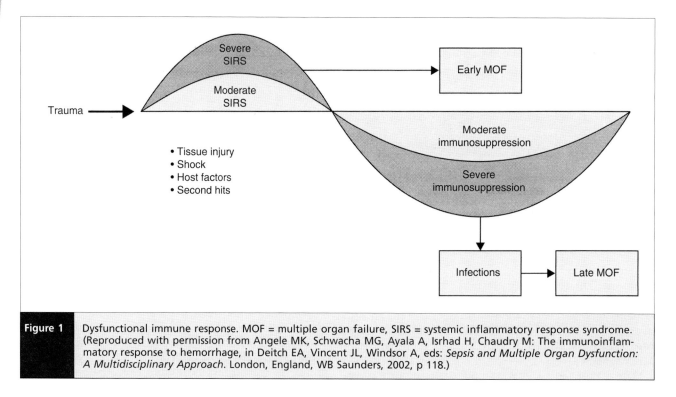

Figure 1 Dysfunctional immune response. MOF = multiple organ failure, SIRS = systemic inflammatory response syndrome. (Reproduced with permission from Angele MK, Schwacha MG, Ayala A, Isrhad H, Chaudry M: The immunoinflammatory response to hemorrhage, in Deitch EA, Vincent JL, Windsor A, eds: *Sepsis and Multiple Organ Dysfunction: A Multidisciplinary Approach.* London, England, WB Saunders, 2002, p 118.)

hyperinflammatory response after major trauma. Neutrophils are recruited from the systemic circulation to the site of tissue injury by chemotactic molecules, such as chemokines (for example, IL-8) and complement anaphylatoxins (C3a, C5a). Priming of neutrophils is the first step of cellular immune activation after trauma, which is mediated by priming molecules including TNF, platelet-activating factor, and complement anaphylatoxin C5a. Primed neutrophils exhibit adhesion, rolling, diapedesis, and the oxidative burst, which leads to the local release of oxygen-derived free radicals and toxic enzymes, leading to "innocent bystander" injury of host tissue. Immune-mediated injury of uninjured tissues by toxic metabolites and enzymes contributes to the development of remote organ failure, including ARDS, MOF, and secondary brain injury related to blood-brain barrier dysfunction and cerebral edema.[1,6,10-13]

In addition to the early activation of innate immune responses, the adaptive immune system recently has been shown to contribute to the immunologic pathophysiology of major trauma. Although PMNLs are the main cellular players of innate immunity, the immunologic memory and specificity of adaptive immune responses are mediated by B- and T-lymphocytes. Natural antibodies are potent initiators of adaptive immune responses after trauma because these immunoglobulins are generated without exposure to external antigens.[14] In contrast to classic antibodies, which are generated in response to specific antigens, natural antibodies are polyreactive and thus bind to multiple antigens exposed after tissue injury, including proteins, polysaccharides, and phospholipids. This self-reactivity may lead to ho-

mologous tissue destruction and autoimmunity. In musculoskeletal trauma and ischemia/reperfusion injury, the alteration of surface epitopes and generation of neoepitopes leads to binding of natural antibodies to host tissue and subsequent activation of the complement cascade. Epitopes are those regions of an antigen capable of eliciting an immune response; neoepitopes are new epitopes present on newly acquired antigens. Activation of complement by natural antibodies represents a bridge to the innate immune response and sets the basis for innate autoimmunity after traumatic injuries to the musculoskeletal system. In addition, T cell activation has been shown to occur in patients with femur fractures. The hyperinflammatory response mediated by natural antibodies and activated T cells early after trauma is usually followed by a phase of severe immunosuppression. Polytrauma patients are highly susceptible to infections and septic complications during this delayed phase of immune compromise, which is characterized by attenuation of T cell–mediated immunity, decreased human leukocyte antigen-DR expression on monocytes, and suppressed natural killer cell activity.[1,4]

Severe trauma induces a deranged immunologic response that renders patients prone to second hit injuries. These additional insults may be induced by inadequate timing and modality of fracture fixation, which may turn the physiologic host defense response into a detrimental host failure disease with secondary tissue insults, infections, and remote organ failure of primarily uninjured tissues (such as the lung, liver, or brain). The ideal time for fracture fixation must therefore take into account the phases of increased vulnerability to

Table 1

Timing of Surgery

Physiologic Status	Surgical Intervention	Timing
Stable (responder)	Early definitive care	Day 1
Unstable (nonresponder)	Damage control	
Hyperinflammation	Second-look surgery	Day 2–4
	Change of tamponades	
Physiologically stable	Scheduled definitive surgery	Day 5–10
Immunosuppression	No surgery!	Week 2–3
Recovery	Secondary reconstructive surgery	> Week 3

second hit insults during the phases of posttraumatic immunologic dysfunction[15] (**Table 1**).

Metabolic Changes

Metabolic changes occurring after major trauma are defined in two phases. The ebb phase has an acute onset after trauma and may persist for several hours. This physiologic reaction is associated with a decline in body temperature, aimed at reducing posttraumatic energy depletion and oxygen consumption. The flow phase occurs after compensation of the state of shock. This phase is characterized by a catabolic state caused by massively increased energy and oxygen consumption associated with an increased metabolic turnover and proteolysis, activation of the innate immune system, and induction of the hepatic acute-phase response. The hypercatabolic phase after major trauma is associated with severe complications related to hyperglycemia (diabetes of trauma), hypoproteinemia, lactate acidosis, and immunosuppression. It is therefore imperative to recognize the presence and significance of these metabolic alterations and to apply early therapeutic strategies for metabolic control, including early enteral nutrition, in addition to the continuing measures of resuscitation with hemorrhage control and securing adequate oxygenation.[16,17]

Acute-Phase Response

Major trauma triggers the hepatic acute-phase response, which contributes to posttraumatic derangement of the immune and coagulation systems. Classic mediators of the acute-phase response released by hepatocytes and Kupffer cells in the liver include proinflammatory cytokines (TNF, IL-1β, IL-6), C-reactive protein, complement component 4 binding protein, procalcitonin, as well as multiple proteases and components of the coagulation cascade, including α1-antitrypsin, prothrombin, and fibrinogen. Thus, the pleiotropic mediators released during the acute-phase response contribute to posttraumatic inflammation,

disseminated intravascular coagulation and coagulopathy, and remote organ failure and septic complications.[1]

Ischemia/Reperfusion Syndrome

Systemic hypotension, hypoxemia, and hypothermia after major trauma, in conjunction with local tissue injury related to contusion, vascular obstruction or injury, and/or compartment syndrome contribute to cellular deficits of oxygen and energy reserve adenosine triphosphate. Fluid resuscitation, warming, limb realignment, and surgical release of increased compartment pressures (for example, by fasciotomies of the extremities or a decompressive craniectomy for severe head injury), will lead to reperfusion of ischemic tissue and initiate a pathophysiologic cascade leading to secondary tissue destruction. The inflammatory reactions induced by ischemia/reperfusion syndrome include activation of the complement cascade and release of reactive oxygen intermediates by activation of xanthine oxidase. Free radicals derived from oxygen and nitrogen, such as hydroxyl ions, hydrogen peroxide, superoxide anion, and peroxynitrite, induce lipid peroxidation that causes cell membrane disintegration and delayed cell death. In addition, activation of the complement cascade by ischemia/reperfusion-related mechanisms results in formation of anaphylatoxins and membrane attack complex, thus exacerbating the pathophysiologic sequelae of host-mediated cell death[3,18] (**Figure 2**).

Traumatic-Hemorrhagic Shock

Hypovolemic (hemorrhagic) shock must be considered to be present, until proven otherwise, in any patient with major trauma, particularly in penetrating and high-energy mechanisms of injury. Shock is a clinical diagnosis, supported by selected laboratory parameters (lactate and base deficit). The American College of Surgeons Committee on Trauma defines four classes of shock depending on the amount of blood loss, physiologic responses, and clinical signs of bleeding (**Table 2**).

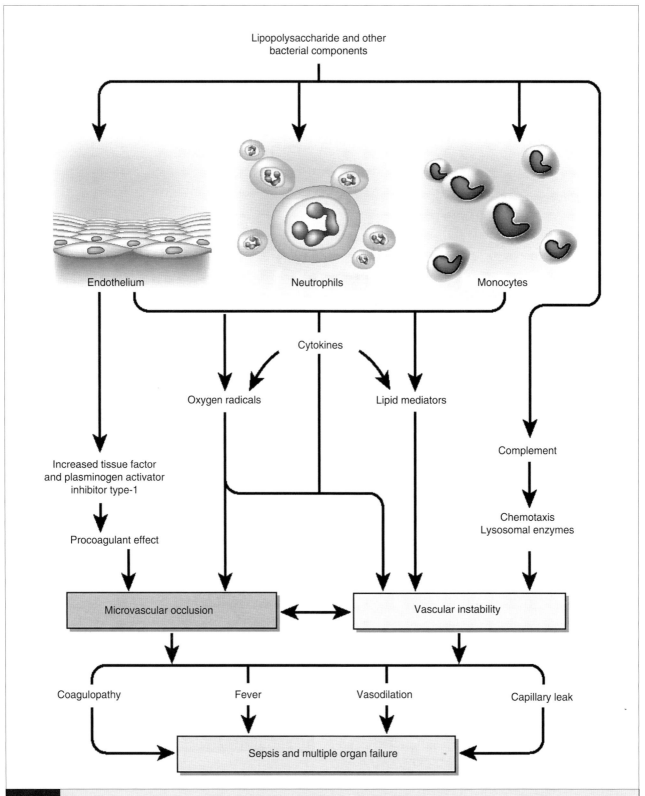

Figure 2 Pathogenetic networks in shock. Lipopolysaccharide and other microbial components simultaneously activate multiple parallel cascades that contribute to the pathophysiology of ARDS and shock. The combination of poor myocardial contractility, impaired peripheral vascular tone, and microvascular occlusion leads to tissue hypoperfusion and inadequate oxygenation, and ultimately to organ failure. (Adapted with permission from Cohen J: The immunopathogenesis of sepsis. *Nature* 2002;420:885–891. http://www.nature.com.)

Table 2

Estimated Fluid and Blood Losses*

	Class I	Class II	Class III	Class IV
Blood loss (mL)	Up to 750	750 to 1,500	1,500 to 2,000	> 2,000
Blood loss (% blood volume)	Up to 15%	15% to 30%	30% to 40%	> 40%
Pulse rate (beats per minute)	< 100	> 100-120	> 120-140	> 140
Blood pressure	Normal	Normal	Decreased	Decreased
Pulse pressure (mm Hg)	Normal or increased	Decreased	Decreased	Decreased
Respiratory rate (breaths per minute)	14 to 20	20 to 30	30 to 40	> 35
Urine output (mL/hr)	> 30	20 to 30	5 to 15	Negligible
Central nervous system/mental status	Slightly anxious	Mildly anxious	Anxious, confused	Confused, lethargic
Fluid replacement (3:1 rule)	Crystalloid	Crystalloid	Crystalloid and blood	Crystalloid and blood

*Based on initial presentation for a 70-kg man.
The guidelines in Table 2 are based on the 3:1 rule. This rule derives from the empiric observation that most patients in hemorrhagic shock require as much as 300 mL of electrolyte solution for each 100 mL of blood loss. Applied blindly, these guidelines can result in excessive or inadequate fluid administration. For example, patients with a crush injury to the extremity may have hypotension out of proportion to their blood loss and require fluids in excess of the 3:1 guidelines. In contrast, patients whose ongoing blood loss is being replaced by blood transfusion require less than 3:1. The use of bolus therapy with careful monitoring of the patient's response can moderate these extremes. (Reproduced with permission from American College of Surgeons' Committee on Trauma: Hemorrhagic Shock in injured patients, in *Advanced Trauma Life Support for Doctors: Student Course Manual*, ed 8. Chicago, IL, American College of Surgeons, 2008, p 61.)

A grading system of severity of shock is useful in the initial assessment of bleeding, particularly because patients with grades I and II hemorrhage do not present with hypotension, and their occult state of shock may be missed.[6] The classic clinical signs of shock are represented by the so-called three windows to microcirculation, which reflect inadequate organ perfusion of the periphery (cold and clammy skin, delayed capillary refill), the kidneys (oliguria or anuria), and the brain (altered mental status or level of consciousness). Despite significant blood loss, young adults, children, and athletes may remain hemodynamically compensated for a prolonged period because of their increased cardiovascular reserves. These patients can initially be frequently misidentified as stable until acute deterioration ensues. Lactate and base deficit have been defined as two highly sensitive laboratory parameters that reflect the true state of hidden shock and correlate with mortality after trauma. The amount of lactate produced by anaerobic glycolysis is an indirect marker of oxygen debt, tissue hypoperfusion, and the severity of hemorrhagic shock. Prospective observational studies have revealed that elevated lactate levels (> 2.5 mmol/L) and decreased base deficit (< -2 mEq/L, eg -3 or -4 mEg/L) independently correlate with mortality after major trauma, particularly at higher thresholds (lactate > 4 mmol/L, base deficit < -6 mEq/L).[19]

Equilibrium Between Inflammatory and Anti-inflammatory Mediators

Systemic Inflammatory Response

Following major trauma, stimuli that initiate the primary reaction (first hit phenomena) include shock, blood loss, hypoxia, acidosis, hypothermia, and acute stress response. In the presence of traumatic-hemorrhagic shock, such changes are induced as peripheral, pulmonary, and splanchnic vasoconstriction, redistribution of blood volume, tachycardia, and widened pulse pressure. The coagulation cascade and the innate immune system are activated early after trauma. Several mediators and cellular elements have been reported to participate in these processes.[20]

The capacity to both characterize and quantify the molecular mediators regulating the priming and responses of target cells and organs has allowed researchers and clinicians to acquire a wealth of knowledge. Multiple alterations in inflammatory and immunologic functions have been demonstrated in clinical and experimental situations following trauma and hemorrhagic shock, supporting the view that a cascade of abnormalities is initiated in the immediate postinjury period that may ultimately lead to ARDS and MOF. There is a vigorous proinflammatory cytokine response following severe injury that involves increased serum levels of IL-1,

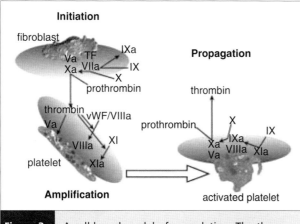

Initiation

Propagation

Amplification

activated platelet

Figure 3	A cell-based model of coagulation. The three phases of coagulation occur on different cell surfaces. Initiation occurs on the tissue factor–bearing cell; amplification, on the platelet as it becomes activated; and propagation; on the activated platelet surface. (Reproduced from Hoffman M, Monroe DM III: A cell-based model of hemostasis. *Throm Haemost* 2001;85:958-965.)

IL-2, TNF-α, IL-6, IL-8, IL-12, and interferon-gamma.[21] These molecules function as acute phase hormones that stimulate a response following stress and are produced by a variety of cells including monocyte/macrophages and T helper-1 lymphocytes. As noted previously, several other host- and microbial-derived molecules are also capable of activating innate immune responses after trauma. The number of molecules categorized in this superfamily is expanding, but their pathophysiologic contribution to the trauma-related systemic inflammatory response is currently under investigation.

In general terms, the liberation of inflammatory mediators after trauma is dependent initially on the severity of trauma (first hit phenomenon) and subsequently on the activation of the various immunologic cascades during therapeutic or diagnostic interventions, surgical procedures, and posttraumatic/postoperative complications (second or third hits).[22] Inflammatory mediators that participate in posttraumatic events are released from local cellular populations and also mediate systemic inflammation. The priming, rolling, activation, and sequestration of PMNLs, monocytes, and lymphocytes trigger multifocal pathophysiologic molecular processes. Chemokines and anaphylatoxins derived from complement activation induce chemotaxis and activation of PMNLs, which are consequently recruited to the site of injury.[23] These inflammatory cells interact and adhere to the endothelium via adhesion molecules, such as L-selectin and ICAM-1.[23] Mediators of PMNL priming include complement anaphylatoxin C5a, TNF, IL-8, granulocyte-macrophage colony-stimulating factor, lipopolysaccharide, and others.

A genetic component has furthermore been implicated in the vulnerability to the immune response and

to second hits after major trauma. It is possible that certain patients will react differently to major injury depending on their underlying genotype.[24] DNA chip technology is already being explored in an effort to clarify the different responses to traumatic first, second, or third hits, and the reasons some patients develop unexpected complications and undesirable clinical outcomes.

Coagulopathy

Postinjury coagulopathy is associated with an increased incidence of MOF and death. About one third of all polytrauma patients are coagulopathic on admission, as determined by an increased international normalized ratio.[25] The pathophysiology of coagulopathy in trauma is complex and not fully understood. The simple explanation of a mechanism related to depletion/dilution of coagulation factors after fluid resuscitation, the so-termed dilutional coagulopathy, has been challenged. Recent data emphasize the role of tissue injury, in conjunction with hemorrhagic shock, as crucial initiators of postinjury coagulopathy after trauma. The complex cascade of events leading to coagulopathy after major trauma furthermore involves immunoactivation and posttraumatic inflammation, related to endothelial cell activation and activation of the complement cascade. The classic views of the intrinsic and extrinsic coagulation cascades were challenged by a cell-based model of coagulation, which emphasizes the unique role of tissue factor and factor VIIa for achieving hemostasis in a bleeding patient[26] (**Figure 3**). The theory behind this model questions the conventional understanding of "test tube" coagulation as outdated and not accurately reflecting in vivo coagulation under pathophysiologic conditions involving both cellular and plasma components of coagulation. Current understanding of the pathophysiology of postinjury coagulopathy includes tissue injury with resulting hemorrhage, tissue hypoperfusion, clotting factor dilution, hypothermia, acidosis, and inflammation (**Figure 4**). Detailed knowledge on how these factors play a part in the development and perpetuation of coagulopathy is a prerequisite for designing optimized treatment strategies for resuscitation and blood component therapy in high-risk trauma patients.[27]

Thromboelastography offers a new method that may provide a more accurate assessment of coagulopathy in the multiply injured trauma patient, and will likely be more commonly used in the future.[28] Unlike international normalized ratio, prothrombin time, or partial thromboplastin time, thromboelastography provides a real-time graphic representation of all aspects of clot formation and lysis.

MOF and Sepsis

An uncontrolled systemic hyperinflammatory response may lead to MOF. Therapeutic strategies to minimize organ dysfunction and organ failure target this systemic hyperinflammatory response and include damage con-

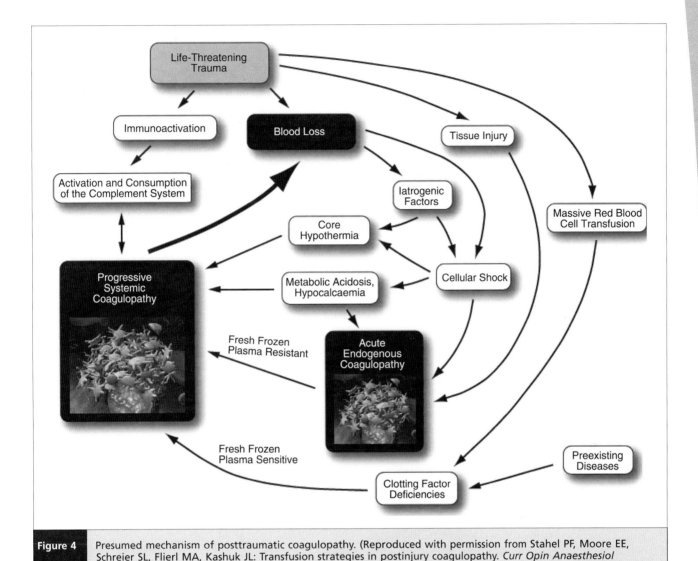

Figure 4 Presumed mechanism of posttraumatic coagulopathy. (Reproduced with permission from Stahel PF, Moore EE, Schreier SL, Flierl MA, Kashuk JL: Transfusion strategies in postinjury coagulopathy. *Curr Opin Anaesthesiol* 2009;22:289-298.)

trol surgery, treatment of abdominal compartment syndrome, protective ventilation techniques, and strict glycemic control. The Denver MOF scoring system was developed in 1987 as a descriptive end point for clinical studies.[13] It evaluates four organ systems (pulmonary, hepatic, renal, cardiac) daily while the patient is in the intensive care unit. The degree of organ dysfunction is graded from 0 (best) to 3 (worst). Using this scoring system, investigators have shown that the incidence, severity, and associated mortality of postinjury MOF has decreased over a 12-year period from 1992 to 2003.[10] These improvements have been attributed to advances in trauma and critical care, including a decreased use of blood transfusion during resuscitation.

Sepsis results from an exaggerated host response to infection. The usually beneficial host response becomes amplified and dysregulated, leading to an overwhelming inflammatory response that can progress to shock and death. In general, coagulation is activated and fibrinolysis is impaired, resulting in microvascular thrombosis that exacerbates tissue hypoxia and may ultimately result in organ failure. Multiple studies have shown that the first 6 hours of early sepsis management are especially important from a diagnostic, pathogenic, and therapeutic perspective, and that steps taken during this period can have a significant impact on outcome.[29]

Compensatory Anti-inflammatory Response Syndrome

While a systemic inflammatory response is evolving at the same time, an anti-inflammatory response is exerted as part of the homeostatic mechanisms.[30] This shift from a T helper-1 proinflammatory response to a Th-2 anti-inflammatory response represents a compensatory process (counter anti-inflammatory response syndrome. This phenomenon represents a host response aimed at maintaining homeostasis and controlling the extent of SIRS. Several mediators have been shown to regulate this compensatory effort, including anti-

Table 3

Parameters for Monitoring the Resuscitation Process

- Stable hemodynamics without the need for vasoactive or inotropic stimulation
- No hypoxemia or hypercapnia
- Serum lactate < 2.5 mmol/L
- Normal coagulation (international normalized ratio, thromboelastography)
- Normothermia
- Normal urinary output (> 1 mL/kg/h)

inflammatory cytokines such as TGF-β, IL-4, IL-10, and IL-13.[31]

The Two Hit Model

The early posttraumatic phase of hyperinflammation between the second and fourth days after trauma (Table 1) is a period of enhanced susceptibility to a second-hit insult.[1,3] Thus, major surgical interventions should be avoided during this vulnerable period. Exceptions are made for second-look surgeries for further débridement of necrotic tissue and reduction of bacterial contamination, sterile dressing changes, and removal of wound packing. The physiologic window of opportunity for orthopaedic procedures lies somewhere between days 5 to 10 after trauma, corresponding to the interval between the hyperinflammatory phase and the delayed period of immunosuppression.[4] Scheduled surgical procedures in fully resuscitated patients include secondary wound closures, the conversion from external to internal fixation for long bone and pelvic fractures, the definitive osteosynthesis of periarticular fractures, and the 360-degree completion fusion for unstable vertebral fractures. Later on, multiply injured patients will again become susceptible to second hits during the phase of immunosuppression. No major surgical procedures should be performed during this vulnerable period because of the high risk of iatrogenic complications that may lead to sepsis and multiple organ failure. Controversy exists concerning when the window of opportunity closes and the risk for secondary hits begins to rise. At present, there are no specific criteria that define the start and end of this "no touch" period. Definitive reconstructive procedures will be performed after a full recovery in the intensive care unit, once the pathology of the immune system has completely resolved.[1,6,7]

Monitoring Resuscitation

The process of resuscitation requires a coordinated effort to restore intravascular volume and provide necessary oxygen for the consumption demands of the tissues. The point at which these demands are met is called the critical oxygen delivery. Under favorable circumstances oxygen delivery can be measured with a pulmonary artery catheter, but resuscitation frequently must be performed without definitive monitoring. Therefore, metabolic surrogates of oxygen delivery are commonly used end points of resuscitation. Hemoglobin level should not be used as a guide to resuscitation, because it is inaccurate while active hemorrhage is still occurring.[19,32,33] Heart rate and blood pressure are not sensitive parameters for determining the severity of shock.[19,32,33] Other clinical signs of organ hypoperfusion include urinary output and altered mental status. Currently, tissue perfusion-related markers are in common usage, including arterial base deficit, serum lactate, arteriovenous oxygen content difference, and mixed venous pH.[19,32,33] Polytrauma patients are considered to be stable when several end points of resuscitation are met,[6] as outlined in **Table 3**.

Optimal resuscitation in the laboratory environment is considered to occur at a mean arterial pressure of 50 to 60 mm/Hg, the point at which the benefit of reducing ischemia by supporting perfusion balances the risk of increased hemorrhage resulting from higher blood pressure.[34] In general terms, the objective is to maintain a lower blood pressure early in the patient's clinical course while maintaining metabolic indicators at reasonable values and thus ensuring that ischemia is not advancing too far.

The Eastern Association of the Surgery of Trauma (EAST) recommends using several different laboratory measures to detect a compensated shock state after hemodynamic parameters are normalized and bleeding is controlled. Laboratory evidence of ongoing metabolic acidosis can help quantify the management of shock. Sampling of arterial blood for base deficit should be done once bleeding has been controlled and hemodynamics are normalized. Analysis of venous blood for lactate should also be performed. A persistent base deficit or elevated lactate suggests ongoing hypoperfusion. It has been reported that base deficit values are reliable predictors of additional fluid and blood requirements in these patients.[35] It is important for the clinician to assess the physiologic state of the patient early after admission so that appropriate treatment strategies can be implemented. Patients can be classified into one of four categories: stable, borderline (patient at risk), unstable, and "in extremis."[36]

Stable patients respond to initial therapy and are hemodynamically stable throughout their initial clinical pathway. These patients are characterized by a low Injury Severity Score.

Borderline patients usually present with combinations of injuries (for example, bilateral femoral shaft fractures) at risk of rapid deterioration. They may respond to initial resuscitation efforts but their condition may change rapidly. Criteria for identifying these patients include the presence of any of the conditions outlined in **Table 4**.

Table 4

Criteria for Identifying Borderline Patients*

- Injury Severity Score ≥ 40 in the absence of any thoracic injury
- Hypothermia below 35°C
- Initial mean pulmonary arterial pressure > 24 mm Hg or a > 6 mm-Hg rise in pulmonary artery pressure during intramedullary nailing or other operative intervention
- Multiple injuries (Injury Severity Score > 20) in association with thoracic trauma (AIS > 2)
- Multiple injuries in association with severe abdominal or pelvic injury and hemorrhagic shock at presentation (systolic blood pressure < 90 mm Hg)
- Radiographic evidence of pulmonary contusion
- Patients with bilateral femoral fracture
- Patients with moderate or severe head injuries (Abbreviated Injury Score 3 or greater)

*The presence of one or more of these criteria may be used to identify the borderline patient.

Table 5

Definition Criteria for Acute Lung Injury and ARDS

Acute onset

Bilateral infiltrates on an AP chest radiograph

Pulmonary capillary occlusion pressure < 18 mm Hg or absence of clinical signs of left atrial hypertension

Arterial hypoxemia (regardless of positive end-expiratory pressure)
P_{AO_2}/F_{IO_2} < 300 mg Hg = Acute lung injury
P_{AO_2}/F_{IO_2} < 200 mg Hg = ARDS

(Adapted with permission from Bernard GR, Artigas A, Brigham KL, et al: The American European Consensus on ARDS: Definitions, mechanisms, relevant outcomes, and clincial trial coordination. *Am J Respir Crit Care Med* 1994;149:818-824.)

Unstable patients remain hemodynamically unstable despite initial resuscitation efforts. Surgical procedures should be limited to lifesaving maneuvers to address hemorrhage, followed by timely transfer to the intensive care unit for ongoing resuscitation and appropriate monitoring.

Patients considered to be in extremis usually present with uncontrollable bleeding. Despite ongoing resuscitation efforts they remain physiologically unstable and are very close to death. Only absolutely life-saving procedures are performed and they are transferred directly to the intensive care unit for invasive monitoring and advanced support of all the vital organ systems. Several different hemodynamic perfusion variables have been established as good indicators in both human and animal studies to help the clinician make appropriate decisions regarding the management of multiply injured patients that present in a physiologic crisis secondary to hypovolemic shock. Parameters that can be used to monitor the resuscitation process[6,36,37] are described in **Table 3**.

Monitoring Pulmonary Function

Blunt thoracic trauma is frequently present in patients with multiple injuries. The extent of underlying damage to the lung parenchyma is often not evident on plain chest radiographs, but can be quantified by chest CT scan.[6,7] Progressive deterioration of lung function is a common finding among trauma patients in the surgical intensive care unit, with a variable degree of respiratory insufficiency leading to ARDS and MOF (**Table 5**). Ventilatory support should be considered if respiration rate is less than 12 or greater than 24 breaths per minute, tidal volume is decreased, and respiratory effort is increased. Other indications for ventilatory support include apnea, hypoventilation, flail chest, spinal cord injury, diaphragmatic injury, head injury with a Glasgow Coma Scale (GCS) score ≤ 8, hypoxia, hypercapnia and hypothermia. Medical treatment is focused on minimizing the risk of atelectasis and/or parenchymal damage. Mechanical ventilation assists alveolar recruitment and improves intrapulmonary gas distribution. It is widely accepted that early ventilation improves pulmonary function and reduces the incidence of ARDS.[12,38] Respiratory monitoring plays a crucial role during the resuscitation process. Simultaneous displays of airway pressure and flow are currently continuously available. Devices such as pulse oximetry to monitor hemoglobin oxygen saturation noninvasively have improved the ability to detect and address any deterioration in oxygenation in a more timely fashion. Better pain management—including the use of regional anesthesia—together with more appropriate sedation regimens have shortened the duration of mechanical ventilation. Some studies have suggested that mortality from ARDS may have decreased,[39] and several factors may be involved, including ventilation using lower tidal volumes, which reduces the inflammatory response and decreases mortality. Experimental studies demonstrate that high transpulmonary pressures may injure even previously normal lungs, especially without sufficient positive end expiratory pressure (PEEP).[38] Given the potential for injury related to aggressive ventilation, hypercapnia has been accepted as a legitimate and usually well-tolerated consequence of lung-protective ventilation. A pressure-controlled ventilation mode, using low tidal volume, is desirable. Modern ventilation strategies with low tidal volume (4 to 8 mL/kg), best PEEP,[38] low airway pressures (< 35 cm H_2O), and an inspiratory oxygen concentration of 55% to 60% often are ideal. Recently, the open lung concept was proposed for the prevention of pulmonary failure. This strategy focuses on the recruitment of alveoli by a temporary increase in PEEP.[40] The evidence with regard to the efficacy of this concept is yet to be determined.

2: The Polytrauma Patient and Fracture Healing

Table 6

Glasgow Coma Scale

Clinical Parameter	Points
Eye Opening (E)	
Spontaneous	4
To speech	3
To pain	2
None	1
BEST Motor Response (M)	
Obeys commands	6
Localizes pain	5
Normal flexion (withdrawal)	4
Abnormal flexion (decorticate)	3
Extension (decerebrate)	2
None (flaccid)	1
Verbal Response (V)	
Fully oriented	5
Disoriented/confused conversation	4
Inappropriate words	3
Incomprehensible words	2
None	1

GCS Score: Σ (E + M + V) = Severity of head injury
14-15 points = Mild
9-13 points = Moderate
3-8 points = Severe

Monitoring of Head Injury

Traumatic brain injury (TBI) remains the leading cause of death in patients younger than 45 years.[41] Patients who survive initial injury are susceptible to secondary cerebral insults initiated by the release of neurotoxic and inflammatory endogenous mediators.[42] Hypoxia and hypotension during the early time period after trauma represent the main contributing factors causing secondary brain injury and adverse outcome.[43] The endogenous neuroinflammatory response in the injured brain contributes to cerebral edema, increased intracranial pressure, and decreased cerebral perfusion pressure. Therefore, the monitoring of intrcranial pressure and cerebral perfusion pressure have been recommended in patients with severe closed head injury.[41] The classification of head injury based on the level of consciousness is assessed by the GCS (Table 6). Postresuscitation GCS has been shown to correlate with the patients' outcome and is thus considered a clinically relevant scoring system.[44] Patients with mild head injury (GCS 14 or 15) represent about 80% of all head-injured patients presenting in the emergency department. These patients usually suffer from a mild cerebral concussion, which corresponds to diffuse brain injury with preserved consciousness but a certain degree of temporary neurologic dysfunction. In contrast, the classic cerebral concussion results in a reversible loss of consciousness, which is always accompanied by posttraumatic amnesia. Approximately 3% of all patients with mild head injury deteriorate later due to a potentially fatal intracranial hemorrhage (patients who "talk and die"). Thus, institutional algorithms must define adequate monitoring strategies for patients with mild head injury, consisting of a generous indication for an early head CT scan and the potential need for clinical observation in patients at risk for secondary deterioration. Patients at risk for secondary deterioration include those with clinical signs of a classic concussion, and those who are taking anticoagulation medication. Moderate head injury corresponds to a GCS score between 9 and 13 and is associated with an increased risk for a delayed intracranial hemorrhage, compared with patients with mild head injury. Therefore, a head CT scan is recommended in all patients with moderate head injury, in conjunction with clinical observation for 24 hours. Severe head injury is defined as a GCS score of 3 to 8, which corresponds to comatose patients by definition. These patients require early endotracheal intubation for mechanical ventilation and monitoring in the intensive care unit.

The ideal timing of fracture fixation in head-injured patients remains a topic of debate, particularly related to the fixation of femur shaft fractures. Although some groups advocate immediate definitive fracture fixation (early total care), others support the concept of damage control orthopaedics with temporary fracture fixation by external fixation, followed by a staged conversion to internal fixation.[45] The latter approach attempts to limit secondary damage to the injured brain due to second hit insults caused by hypoxemia, hypotension, stress, and pain. Currently, there is a lack of high-quality evidence to determine the ideal timing and modality of fracture fixation in patients with severe head injuries. Large, randomized multicenter trials are needed to evaluate the validity of the damage control orthopaedics concept in head-injured patients with associated orthopaedic injuries. Until higher level evidence data are available, the management strategy presented in **Table 7** may represent a safe decision-making strategy for head-injured patients with associated orthopaedic injuries.[46] Additional principles of damage control orthopaedics can be found in chapter 16.

Deep Venous Thrombosis and Pulmonary Embolism

Although abnormalities in the clotting system leading to prolonged hemorrhage occur early following trauma, venous thromboembolism, including deep venous thrombosis (DVT) and pulmonary embolism, are significant problems that develop later. Trauma leads to a significantly increased and persistent generation of thrombin along with disruption of its regulation. Pelvic

Table 7

Decision-Making Strategy for Head-Injured Patients With Orthopaedic Injuries

1. Early total care in patients with *mild* head injury (GCS 14/15), and normal craniocerebral CT scan (if available).

2. Damage control approach with external femur fixation of long bone fractures in patients with *severe* head injury (GCS ≤ 8 points and/or presence of significant intracranial pathology on CT scan, cerebral edema, intracranial hemorrhage).

3. Consider damage control procedure with external femur fixation in all patients with *moderate* TBI, either with a GCS of 9 to 13 points, or in presence of "minor" intracranial pathology on CT scan (eg, traumatic subarachnoid bleeding) in patients with GCS of 14 or 15.

4. Consider conversion from external to internal fixation in awake and alert head-injured patients (GCS > 12) after recovery from a comatose state, or in comatose patients with a stable ICP (< 20 mm Hg) and Cerebral perfusion pressure (> 80 mm Hg) for more than 48 hours.

fractures, lower extremity fractures, spinal fractures, spinal cord injury, head injury, and age have traditionally been noted as key risk factors for DVT development following trauma.

A meta-analysis performed by EAST identified patients with spinal cord injury and spine fractures to be at highest risk, but failed to support inclusion of other traditional risk factors as independent risk factors for thromboembolism. Older age was found to be a risk factor, but investigators were unable to define an exact age at which the risk substantially increases.[47] Age has been repeatedly shown to be an important factor in the risk of DVT following trauma.[48] In a recent study, TBI was found to represent an independent risk factor for the development of DVT regardless of prophylaxis. TBI was defined as any intraparenchymal hemorrhage or extra-axial intracranial bleeding identified on radiographic imaging. Investigators found a threefold to fourfold increased risk of DVT formation in patients with TBI even with chemical prophylaxis.[49]

Controversy exists over the best method of prophylaxis following trauma, and there is limited level I evidence to provide management guidance. Although a few studies have investigated DVT prophylaxis in trauma patients, the recommendations for prophylaxis are largely based on data extrapolated from research in nontrauma patients. The most recent American College of Chest Physicians guidelines recommended routine prophylaxis for all major trauma patients, if possible (grade 1A recommendation).[50] In the absence of contraindication, low molecular weight heparin (LMWH) should be used and started as soon as it is considered safe to do so (grade 1A recommendation). For patients in whom LMWH is contraindicated the guidelines recommend the use of intermittent pneumatic compression

devices or possibly graduated compression stockings alone (grade 1B). The use of inferior vena cava filters is not recommended (grade 1C). The guidelines also recommend against routine duplex ultrasound screening for asymptomatic individuals (grade 1B); however, duplex ultrasound is suggested for high-risk individuals who have received suboptimal or no thromboprophylaxis (grade 1C). Continuation of thromboprophylaxis is recommended until hospital discharge (grade 1C). For patients with impaired mobility requiring prolonged inpatient rehabilitation, continuation of LMWH or conversion to warfarin is recommended (grade 2C).

The use of chemical prophylaxis may be contraindicated in the presence of a closed head injury or ongoing risk of bleeding. Although the use of vena cava filters has been advocated for the severely injured patient at high risk in whom chemical prophylaxis is contra-indicated, their use is not currently recommended.[50] In one recent clinical series, despite a dramatic increase in the use of vena cava filters, the investigators were unable to show a reduction in the rate of pulmonary embolism.[51]

Currently, prolonged prophylaxis requires either daily LMWH injection or conversion to warfarin. Disadvantages of warfarin include its slow onset of action, genetic variation in metabolism, multiple food and drug interactions, and a relatively narrow therapeutic range that requires frequent monitoring and dosage adjustment.

Several new anticoagulants have been developed that target a single coagulation factor and have a predictable dose-response relationship. These include direct thrombin inhibitors and factor Xa inhibitors. While initial investigations focused on parental drugs, several oral direct thrombin inhibitors and factor Xa inhibitors are in clinical development. These oral agents provide the potential for ease of administration and a predictable anticoagulant response that does not require monitoring. Ximelagatran, the first oral direct thrombin inhibitor, was shown to be an effective antithrombotic agent but was associated with potential liver toxicity and an increased risk of cardiac events after prolonged administration, and it did not receive FDA approval in the United States.[52] Fondaparinux is a synthetic pentasaccharide that binds to antithrombin and selectively inhibits factor Xa indirectly. It is injected subcutaneously on a daily basis. Randomized clinical studies comparing fondaparinux to LMWH showed comparable efficacy, and this agent has been approved by the FDA for the prevention and treatment of venous thromboembolism after major orthopaedic surgery.[53,54]

Summary

The understanding of complex physiologic responses following trauma continues to evolve. Clinical and basic science studies have identified the timing during which severely injured patients are at risk for iatrogenic second hits that can be induced by prolonged surgical interventions. Improperly timed surgery during this sus-

2: The Polytrauma Patient and Fracture Healing

ceptible period places patients at increased risk for sepsis and multiple organ failure. Knowledge of these pathophysiologic responses and adherence to staged treatment algorithms will help improve survival and overall outcomes in severely injured patients.

Annotated References

1. Keel M, Trentz O: Pathophysiology of polytrauma. *Injury* 2005;36(6):691-709.

   This is an outstanding review of the pathophysiologic changes occurring in multiply injured patients.

2. Stahel PF, Smith WR, Moore EE: Role of biological modifiers regulating the immune response after trauma. *Injury* 2007;38(12):1409-1422.

   The authors reviewed the pertinent literature on the immunologic changes occurring after major trauma and discussed new therapeutic aspects of immunomodulation, including the attenuation of neutrophil priming, immunonutrition, and the impact of damage control surgery.

3. Hietbrink F, Koenderman L, Rijkers G, Leenen L: Trauma: The role of the innate immune system. *World J Emerg Surg* 2006;1:15.

   This is an excellent review on the current understanding of the role of innate immune system activation after major trauma.

4. Tschoeke SK, Ertel W: Immunoparalysis after multiple trauma. *Injury* 2007;38(12):1346-1357.

   The authors described the pathomechanisms leading to posttraumatic immunosuppression and the concomitant risk of infection in multiply injured patients.

5. Zedler S, Faist E: The impact of endogenous triggers on trauma-associated inflammation. *Curr Opin Crit Care* 2006;12(6):595-601.

   This review article elucidates the mechanisms and pathophysiologic impact of the hyperinflammatory response induced by major trauma.

6. Stahel PF, Heyde CE, Ertel W: Current concepts of polytrauma management. *Eur J Trauma* 2005;31:200-211.

   The authors present the "European concept" of polytrauma management in conjunction with a description of standard protocols, including the ATLS algorithm and damage control strategies.

7. Gebhard F, Huber-Lang M: Polytrauma: Pathophysiology and management principles. *Langenbecks Arch Surg* 2008;393(6):825-831.

   This is an up-to-date overview on the current management principles for polytrauma, based on the underlying pathophysiologic changes.

8. Peltz ED, Moore EE, Eckels PC, et al: HMGB1 is markedly elevated within 6 hours of mechanical trauma in humans. *Shock* 2009;32(1):17-22.

   Postinjury plasma samples were assayed for HMGB1 in 23 trauma patients at risk for multiple organ failure. HMGB1 is a late mediator of the systemic inflammation associated with sepsis. In contrast, following traumatic injury HMGB1 is released early and may be integral to the early inflammatory response to trauma and is a potential target for future therapeutics.

9. Giannoudis PV, Harwood PJ, Loughenbury P, Van Griensven M, Krettek C, Pape HC: Correlation between IL-6 levels and the systemic inflammatory response score: Can an IL-6 cutoff predict a SIRS state? *J Trauma* 2008;65(3):646-652.

   The authors report that an IL-6 level > 200 pg/dL diagnosed a SIRS state with 83% sensitivity and 75% specificity. Both a SIRS state and an IL-6 level > 300pg/dL were associated with a significantly increased risk of complication (pneumonia, MOF, and death).

10. Ciesla DJ, Moore EE, Johnson JL, Burch JM, Cothren CC, Sauaia A: A 12-year prospective study of postinjury multiple organ failure: Has anything changed? *Arch Surg* 2005;140(5):432-438, discussion 438-440.

    The authors report a decrease in the incidence, severity, and associated mortality of postinjury MOF, which they attribute to improvements in trauma and critical care.

11. Schmidt OI, Heyde CE, Ertel W, Stahel PF: Closed head injury: an inflammatory disease? *Brain Res Rev* 2005; 48(2):388-399.

    This review summarizes the known mechanisms of neuroinflammation after closed head injury based on data from clinical and experimental studies.

12. Dewar D, Moore FA, Moore EE, Balogh Z: Postinjury multiple organ failure. *Injury* 2009;40(9):912-918.

    This review describes the current understanding of the pathophysiology of MOF, discusses strategies for prevention and treatment, and provides future directions for research.

13. Sauaia A, Moore EE, Johnson JL, Ciesla DJ, Biffl WL, Banerjee A: Validation of postinjury multiple organ failure scores. *Shock* 2009;31(5):438-447.

    This study compared the Denver MOF and Marshall MOF scoring systems. Both scoring systems performed well. The Denver MOF system, which is simpler, showed greater specificity.

14. Kulik L, Fleming SD, Moratz C, et al: Pathogenic natural antibodies recognizing annexin IV are required to develop intestinal ischemia-reperfusion injury. *J Immunol* 2009;182(9):5363-5373.

    The authors propose that annexin IV is a key ischemia-related target antigen that is recognized by natural antibodies in a pathologic process required in vivo to develop intestinal ischemia reperfusion injury.

15. Pape HC: Effects of changing strategies of fracture fixation on immunologic changes and systemic complications after multiple trauma: Damage control orthopedic surgery. *J Orthop Res* 2008;26(11):1478-1484.

16. Hasenboehler E, Williams A, Leinhase I, et al: Metabolic changes after polytrauma: An imperative for early nutritional support. *World J Emerg Surg* 2006;1:29.

    This article reviews the pathophysiologic metabolic changes after major trauma that support the current basis for early "immunonutrition" of polytrauma patients.

17. Moore FA, Moore EE: The evolving rationale for early enteral nutrition based on paradigms of multiple organ failure: A personal journey. *Nutr Clin Pract* 2009;24(3):297-304.

    This article discusses why the gut is now recognized to be a very important immunologic organ. It reviews a new paradigm for the use of early enteral glutamine, beginning during active shock resuscitation, to minimize gut injury and to allow for more effective early enteral nutrition, with the goal of a more balanced SIRS/CARS response and faster recovery.

18. Kaczorowski DJ, Tsung A, Billiar TR: Innate immune mechanisms in ischemia/reperfusion. *Front Biosci (Elite Ed)* 2009;1:91-98.

    This article reviews the evolving body of literature, which has provided insight into the early molecular events that activate the innate system after ischemia and repurfusion.

19. Rossaint R, Cerny V, Coats TJ, et al: Key issues in advanced bleeding care in trauma. *Shock* 2006;26(4):322-331.

    The authors present a thorough review article on the current key aspects related to hemorrhage control after major trauma.

20. Giannoudis PV, Dinopoulos H, Chalidis B, Hall GM: Surgical stress response. *Injury* 2006;37(suppl 5):S3-S9.

    This article reviews the characterization and quantification of inflammatory cascades following surgery and trauma, and various methods that have been developed to modulate the immune-inflammatory system and at the same time to prevent overreaction and unexpected complications.

21. Pape HC, Griensven MV, Hildebrand FF, et al; Epoff Study group: Systemic inflammatory response after extremity or truncal fracture operations. *J Trauma* 2008;65(6):1379-1384.

    This prospective, multicenter, nonrandomized cohort study assessed proinflammatory markers in 86 blunt trauma patients, and evaluated their relationship to blood loss and duration of surgery in different fracture locations. A higher increase in cytokine levels occurred when surgeries were performed early (day 1-2) across all patient groups. The level of the released markers seemed to be related to the magnitude of surgery, rather than to the duration of the procedure.

22. Morley JR, Smith RM, Pape HC, MacDonald DA, Trejdosiewitz LK, Giannoudis PV: Stimulation of the local femoral inflammatory response to fracture and intramedullary reaming: A preliminary study of the source of the second hit phenomenon. *J Bone Joint Surg Br* 2008;90(3):393-399.

    The authors assessed whether the femoral canal could be a potential source of the second hit phenomenon by examining the local femoral intramedullary and peripheral release of IL-6 after fracture and subsequent intramedullary reaming. In all patients, the fracture caused a significant increase in the local femoral concentrations of IL-6, and a significant further increase was seen with intramedullary reaming of the femoral canal, providing evidence that intramedullary reaming can cause a significant local inflammatory reaction.

23. Bhatia R, Dent C, Topley N, Pallister I: Neutrophil priming for elastase release in adult blunt trauma patients. *J Trauma* 2006;60(3):590-596.

    The authors reported a significant increase in the capacity of PMNL to release elastase following major trauma, but not in isolated fracture patients, and found that surgery did not further alter polymorphonuclear elastase release.

24. Giannoudis PV, van Griensven M, Tsiridis E, Pape HC: The genetic predisposition to adverse outcome after trauma. *J Bone Joint Surg Br* 2007;89(10):1273-1279.

    This article reviews the current evidence for the genetic predisposition to adverse outcome after trauma.

25. Moore EE, Moore FA, Fabian TC, et al; PolyHeme Study Group: Human polymerized hemoglobin for the treatment of hemorrhagic shock when blood is unavailable: The USA multicenter trial. *J Am Coll Surg* 2009;208(1):1-13.

    This article presents the results of the prospective randomized Polyheme trial designed to assess the role of artificial polymerized hemoglobin for the early resuscitation of hypotensive trauma patients.

26. Hoffman M, Monroe DM III: A cell-based model of hemostasis. *Thromb Haemost* 2001;85(6):958-965.

27. Stahel PF, Moore EE, Schreier SL, Flierl MA, Kashuk JL: Transfusion strategies in postinjury coagulopathy. *Curr Opin Anaesthesiol* 2009;22(2):289-298.

    This review discusses the current literature on coagulopathy and transfusion strategies in patients with traumatic hemorrhage.

28. Kashuk JL, Moore EE, Le T, et al: Noncitrated whole blood is optimal for evaluation of postinjury coagulopathy with point-of-care rapid thromboelastography. *J Surg Res* 2009;156(1):133-138.

    The authors addressed the diagnostic aspects of rTEG as a fast and sensitive tool for the assessment and management of postinjury coagulopathy at the bedside.

29. Rivers EP, Coba V, Visbal A, Whitmill M, Amponsah D: Management of sepsis: Early resuscitation. *Clin Chest Med* 2008;29(4):689-704, ix-x.

    This article reviews the importance of early identification and comprehensive resuscitation of septic patients to improve survival.

30. Miyaoka K, Iwase M, Suzuki R, et al: Clinical evalua-

2: The Polytrauma Patient and Fracture Healing

tion of circulating interleukin-6 and interleukin-10 levels after surgery-induced inflammation. *J Surg Res* 2005;125(2):144-150.

The risk of SIRS and multiple organ dysfunction after orthognathic surgery was studied. Circulating levels of IL-6 and IL-10 were assessed, along with neutrophil function as a marker for organ failure. It was concluded that the ratio of IL-6 to IL-10 may be predictive for SIRS.

31. Flohé S, Flohé SB, Schade FU, Waydhas C: Immune response of severely injured patients: Influence of surgical intervention and therapeutic impact. *Langenbecks Arch Surg* 2007;392(5):639-648.

This article reviews immunomodulating approaches in the treatment of trauma patients and therapeutic strategies avoiding additional immune deterioration.

32. Spahn DR, Cerny V, Coats TJ, et al: Management of bleeding following major trauma: A European guideline. *Crit Care* 2007;11:R17. Erratum in *Crit Care* 2007;11:414.

Guidelines for the management of bleeding after major trauma were created based on a systematic review of published literature. It was concluded that a multidisciplinary approach to management of bleeding after major trauma is needed for optimal care.

33. Stahel PF, Smith WR, Moore EE: Current trends in resuscitation strategy for the multiply injured patient. *Injury* 2009;40(suppl 4):S27-S35.

The authors present an overview of resuscitation protocols for multiply injured patients.

34. Burris D, Rhee P, Kaufmann C, et al: Controlled resuscitation for uncontrolled hemorrhagic shock. *J Trauma* 1999;46(2):216-223.

35. Davis JW, Shackford SR, Mackercie RD, Hoyt DB: Base deficit as required to volume resuscitation. *J Trauma* 1998;28(10):1464-1467.

36. Giannoudis PV: Surgical priorities in damage control in polytrauma. *J Bone Joint Surg Br* 2003;85(4):478-484.

37. McCunn M, Dutton R: End-points of resuscitation: How much is enough? *Curr Opin Anaesthesiol* 2000; 13(2):147-153.

38. Gattinoni L, Caironi P, Cressoni M, et al: Lung recruitment in patients with the acute respiratory distress syndrome. *N Engl J Med* 2006;354:1775-1786.

The authors studied the relationship between the percentage of lung recruitment and clinical and physiologic effects of PEEP. Results indicated that the percentage of potentially recruitable lung is variable, associated with the response to PEEP.

39. Ciesla DJ, Moore EE, Johnson JL, et al: Decreased progression of postinjury lung dysfunction to the acute respiratory distress syndrome and multiple organ failure. *Surgery* 2006;140:640-647.

The authors did a prospective study of data on trauma patients at risk for postinjury MOF.

40. Agrò F, Barzoi G, Doyle DJ, Manieri A: Reduction in pulmonary shunt using the open lung concept. *Anaesthesia* 2004;59(6):625-626.

The authors describe the use of a ventilator software function (Open Lung Tool) to apply optimal ventilation pressures to open the lung and keep it open.

41. Stahel PF, Smith WR: Closed head injury, in Bland KI Csendes A, Garden OJ, Sarr MG, Wong J, eds: *General Surgery: Principles and International Practice*. London, England, Springer, 2009. pp 131-142.

This is an up-to-date review on the current diagnostic and therapeutic modalities for patients with closed head injuries.

42. Elf K, Nilsson P, Enblad P: Prevention of secondary insults in neurointensive care of traumatic brain injury. *Eur J Trauma* 2003;29:74-80.

43. Stahel PF, Smith WR, Moore EE: Hypoxia and hypotension, the "lethal duo" in traumatic brain injury: Implications for prehospital care. *Intensive Care Med* 2008;34(3):402-404.

This editorial discusses the crucial role of hypoxia and hypotension in contributing to secondary brain injury, and cautions from the generous application of permissive hypotension in the management of bleeding trauma patients with head injuries.

44. Healey C, Osler TM, Rogers FB, et al: Improving the Glasgow Coma Scale score: Motor score alone is a better predictor. *J Trauma* 2003;54:671-678.

45. Roberts CS, Pape HC, Jones AL, Malkani AL, Rodriguez JL, Giannoudis PV: Damage control orthopaedics: Evolving concepts in the treatment of patients who have sustained orthopaedic trauma. *Instr Course Lect* 2005; 54:447-462.

This article reviews the concepts of damage control orthopaedics, which emphasizes the stabilization and control of the injury rather than repair in a subgroup of severely injured patients, particularly those with chest injuries, head injuries, or mangled extremities.

46. Flierl MA, Stoneback JW, Beauchamp KM, et al: Femur shaft fracture fixation in head-injured patients: When is the right time? *J Orthop Trauma* 2010;24:107-114.

This review article outlines the rationale of damage control orthopaedics and staged conversion to definitive fracture fixation in patients with severe head injuries and associated femur shaft fractures.

47. Rogers FB, Cipolle MD, Velmahos G, Rozycki G, Luchette FA: Practice management guidelines for the prevention of venous thromboembolism in trauma patients: The EAST practice management guidelines work group. *J Trauma* 2002;53(1):142-164.

48. Selby R, Geerts W, Ofosu FA, et al: Hypercoagulability after trauma: Hemostatic changes and relationship to

venous thromboembolism. *Thromb Res* 2009;124(3): 281-287.

The authors prospectively examined several markers of in vivo coagulation and fibrinolysis for 2 weeks after multisystem trauma in a prospective cohort of patients who received no anticoagulant prophylaxis. They concluded that major trauma leads to significantly increased and persistent thrombin generation with disruption of its regulation, that coagulation markers do not appear to add independent predictive value in detecting venous thromboembolism, and that increasing age was the most important clinical predictor of venous thromboembolism after trauma.

49. Reiff DA, Haricharan RN, Bullington NM, Griffin RL, McGwin G Jr, Rue LW III: Traumatic brain injury is associated with the development of deep vein thrombosis independent of pharmacological prophylaxis. *J Trauma* 2009;66(5):1436-1440.

The authors report that the incidence of DVT among injured patients with TBI is significantly higher than those patients without head injury independent of anticoagulation therapy.

50. Geerts WH, Bergqvist D, Pineo GF, et al; American College of Chest Physicians: Prevention of venous thromboembolism: American College of Chest Physicians Evidence-Based Clinical Practice Guidelines (8th Edition). *Chest* 2008;133(suppl 6):S381-S453.

Evidence-based guidelines for the prevention of venous thromboembolism were approved by the American College of Chest Physicians.

51. Cherry RA, Nichols PA, Snavely TM, David MT, Lynch FC: Prophylactic inferior vena cava filters: Do they make a difference in trauma patients? *J Trauma* 2008; 65(3):544-548.

The authors report on their prospective review of 244 trauma patients receiving a prophylactic inferior vena cava filter over a 3-year period. While the incidence of filter use increased in each year there was no significant impact on the overall pulmonary embolism rate, with a 1.6% pulmonary embolism rate among the filtered patients.

52. Agnelli G, Eriksson BI, Cohen AT, et al; EXTEND Study Group: Safety assessment of new antithrombotic agents: Lessons from the EXTEND study on ximelagatran. *Thromb Res* 2009;123(3):488-497.

The EXTEND study assessed the safety and efficacy of extended administration (35 days) of ximelagatran or enoxaparin for the prevention of venous thromboembolism after elective hip replacement and hip fracture surgery. Prolonged administration of ximelagatran was associated with an increased risk of liver toxicity.

53. Eikelboom JW, Quinlan DJ, O'Donnell M: Major bleeding, mortality, and efficacy of fondaparinux in venous thromboembolism prevention trials. *Circulation* 2009;120:2006-2011.

The authors used Cox proportional hazards to study the association between major bleeding and death using patient data from eight large randomized trials.

54. Turpie AG, Bauer KA, Eriksson BI, Lassen MR: Fondaparinux vs enoxaparin for the prevention of venous thromboembolism in major orthopedic surgery: A meta-analysis of 4 randomized double-blind studies. *Arch Intern Med* 2002;162(16):1833-1840.

2: The Polytrauma Patient and Fracture Healing

Chapter 13

Advances in the Enhancement of Bone Healing and Bone Graft Substitutes

Aaron Nauth, MD, FRCSC   Paul R. Kuzyk, MD, MSc, FRCSC   Thomas A. Einhorn, MD
Emil H. Schemitsch, MD, FRCSC

Introduction

An understanding of fracture healing biology is fundamental to the practice of orthopaedic trauma. Advances in plating techniques and bone graft substitutes, along with newly available systemic agents and biophysical methods for stimulating bone healing, provide the trauma surgeon with an array of options for treating acute fractures, nonunions or delayed unions, and bone defects.

Critical Components of Fracture Healing

Five critical components are necessary for fracture healing to occur (**Figure 1**): osteoconduction, osteogenesis, osteoinduction, mechanical stability, and vascularity.

Dr. Nauth or an immediate family member has received research or institutional support from Stryker, Synthes, and Zimmer. Dr. Einhorn or an immediate family member has received royalties from Osteotech; is a member of a speakers bureau or has made paid presentations on behalf of Stryker; serves as a paid consultant to or is an employee of Amgen, Eli Lilly, National Institutes of Health (NIAMS and NICHD), Novartis, Osteotech, Smith & Nephew, Stryker, Zelos, Biosurface Technologies, Procter and Gamble, and Anika; has received research or institutional support from National Institutes of Health; and owns stock or stock options in Osteogenix, Biomineral Holdings, Healthpoint Capital, and Implant Protection. Dr. Schemitsch or an immediate family member serves as a board member, owner, officer, or committee member of Canadian Orthopaedic Association, Orthopaedic Trauma Association, Osteosynthesis, and Trauma Care Foundation; has received royalties from Stryker; is a member of a speakers bureau or has made paid presentations on behalf of Smith & Nephew and Stryker; serves as a paid consultant to or is an employee of Stryker, Pfizer, Smith & Nephew, Zelos, Biomimetic, Amgen, and Bayer; and has received research or institutional support from Biomimetic, Smith & Nephew, Stryker, Synthes, Zimmer, and Linvatec. Neither Dr. Kuzyk nor an immediate family member has received anything of value from or owns stock in a commercial company or institution related directly or indirectly to the subject of this chapter.

Osteoconduction provides an appropriate scaffold for the migration, adherence, and proliferation of osteoprogenitor cells and blood vessels that is required for fracture healing. Autograft bone, allograft bone, and calcium phosphates represent examples of osteoconductive materials. Osteogenesis represents an appropriate population of cells capable of forming bone. These cells arise from mesenchymal stem cells, which arrive via the bone marrow, periosteum, muscle, and circulation to the fracture site, differentiate into osteoprogenitor cells, and ultimately form bone. Autogenous cancellous bone graft and autogenous bone marrow both contain viable populations of osteogenic cells. Osteoinduction represents appropriate signaling from growth factors and cytokines necessary to initiate the fracture healing process. This process is primarily accomplished by signaling the migration, proliferation, and differentiation of stem cells and progenitor cells from the surrounding soft tissues, bone marrow, and periosteum. Numerous growth factors have been implicated in this process, including bone morphogenetic proteins (BMPs), vascular endothelial growth factor (VEGF), and platelet-derived growth factor. The component of this process that involves the influence of a growth factor on an undifferentiated mesenchymal stem cell, causing it to differentiate along a chondro-osteogenic pathway, is known as osteoinduction. To date, only specific BMPs have been shown to exert this effect on cells. This signaling cascade is depicted in **Figure 1**. Appropriate stability at the fracture site is also necessary for fracture healing to occur. Different graft materials and fixation techniques contribute differing degrees of mechanical stability to a fracture. For instance, cancellous autograft or allograft contributes little mechanical stability, whereas cortical autograft or allograft can significantly enhance the stability of a fracture. Similarly, calcium phosphate cement demonstrates excellent compressive strength in the setting of metaphyseal defects (**Figure 2**). The relative effects of differing degrees of mechanical stability are discussed in the subsequent section. Finally, an adequate blood supply for the delivery of oxygen, nutrients, and pro-

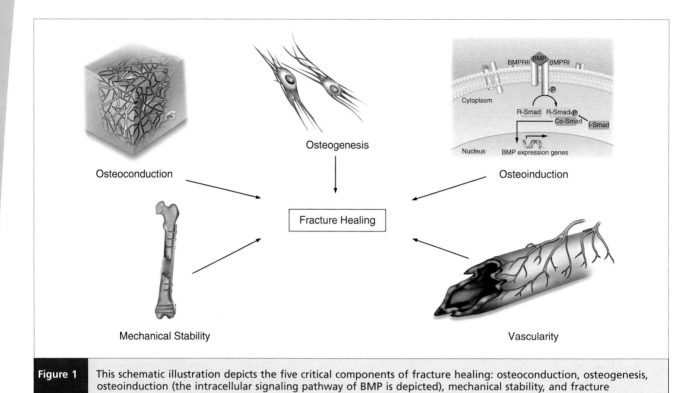

Figure 1 This schematic illustration depicts the five critical components of fracture healing: osteoconduction, osteogenesis, osteoinduction (the intracellular signaling pathway of BMP is depicted), mechanical stability, and fracture vascularity.

genitor cells is critical for fracture healing to occur. The use of intramedullary nails and percutaneous plate fixation represents a clinical method of minimizing disruption to fracture vascularity and enhancing fracture healing. Vascularized bone grafts and tissue transfer can increase vascularity at the site of fracture; however, their use is limited by technical issues and donor site morbidity. Basic science work has demonstrated that the application of angiogenic growth factors (for example, VEGF) or angiogenic cell populations (for example, endothelial progenitor cells) can increase vascularity in animal models of fracture healing; however, clinically available methods of increasing fracture vascularity are currently lacking.[1,2]

An understanding of these five components allows the trauma surgeon to assess the clinically available bone grafts and bone graft substitutes based on their ability to provide one or more of these components. Moreover, it allows the assessment of individual clinical situations and the selection of the appropriate graft material based on its properties and the needs of the specific situation. For instance, in the setting of a metaphyseal defect following a depressed tibial plateau fracture, the use of an osteoconductive substance with compressive strength, such as calcium phosphate cement, is appropriate. In contrast, in the setting of an atrophic nonunion, an osteoinductive or osteogenic material, such as BMP or autogenous cancellous bone graft, is necessary. Finally, when faced with a significant traumatic bone defect, a material with both osteoconductive and osteoinductive properties, such as au-

togenous cancellous bone graft, or BMP combined with cancellous allograft bone, is likely required.

Phases of Fracture Healing

In the presence of the previously mentioned elements, fracture healing follows a reliable cascade of events that restores the bone to its preinjury state. The initial stage involves hematoma formation from disruption of the local endosteal and periosteal blood supply. A subsequent inflammatory stage occurs, characterized by the release of inflammatory mediators from local cells and platelets. This results in a progressive increase in blood flow that peaks approximately 2 weeks after fracture. The subsequent revascularization phase is characterized by the formation of new blood vessels by endothelial progenitor cells, which arrive via the bone marrow and circulation. This phase is followed by the infiltration and proliferation of mesenchymal stem cells, which then differentiate based on the local conditions of the fracture site.

The degree of stability (inversely related to strain), in combination with the oxygen tension and signals from local growth factors, influences the type of fracture healing that occurs, primarily via the effects on the differentiation of local progenitor cells. High strain with low oxygen tension promotes the differentiation of cells that produce fibrous tissue, leading to fibrous nonunion. Low strain and high oxygen tension tend to promote the formation of woven bone directly (hard cal-

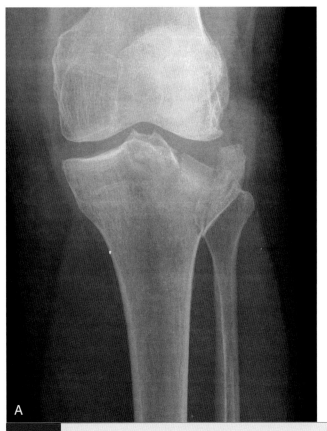

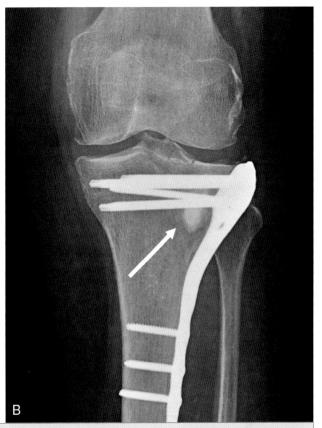

| Figure 2 | Preoperative radiograph (**A**) and 3-month follow-up radiograph (**B**) of a split-depression lateral tibial plateau fracture in a 61-year-old woman. The fracture was treated with open reduction and internal fixation with subsequent grafting of the subarticular metaphyseal defect with calcium phosphate cement (arrow). |

lus), through a process referred to as intramembranous bone formation. Regions of intermediate strain and low oxygen tension promote chondrocyte differentiation and cartilage formation (soft callus). The cartilage callus stabilizes the fracture site, reducing strain and allowing the calcification of the cartilage matrix and bone formation by osteoblasts in a process known as endochondral bone formation. Endochondral and intramembranous bone formation occur in fractures with varying degrees of relative stability. Relative stability occurs clinically in the setting of fractures stabilized with intramedullary nails (load-sharing devices) or bridge plates. A third type of fracture healing occurs in fractures with cortical contact and direct compression (absolute stability), such as might occur in the situation of a humeral shaft fracture that is anatomically reduced and stabilized with a compression plate. In this setting primary healing occurs via direct haversian remodeling, whereby osteoclasts resorb bone and create cutting cone channels across the fracture site, allowing blood vessels and osteoblasts to follow.

Fracture healing finally progresses to the repair phase, usually with a combination of intramembranous and endochondral bone formation. The final phase involves remodeling of the immature woven bone to mature lamellar bone, which occurs over months to years.

Advances in Biologic Fracture Fixation

The concept of biologic fracture fixation has evolved dramatically over the past two decades. There has been a distinct shift away from full fracture exposure and direct anatomic fracture reduction, in favor of limited soft-tissue stripping and indirect fracture reduction. This development can be considered an advance in fracture biology because it is rooted in biologic concepts. Although primary fracture healing can be achieved by the methods of absolute stability discussed above, an adequate blood supply and soft-tissue bed are necessary for primary healing to proceed. Often anatomic reduction and compression of the fracture (absolute stability) occur at the expense of extensive soft-tissue stripping and devascularization of the fracture, especially in situations of fracture comminution. This development has led to a shift toward using methods of relative stability such as intramedullary nails or bridge plating techniques, which incorporate the use of longer plates and fewer screws. These implants can be used in a percutaneous manner, which limits the disruption of fracture vascularity and fracture hematoma. The relative stability of these implants favors fracture healing through callus formation. Clinically, these techniques have resulted in increased callus formation, increased

Table 1

Summary of the Grades of Recommendation for the Different Options for the Enhancement of Fracture Healing

Recommendation	Grade of Recommendation
There is fair evidence to support the use of intramedullary nailing or percutaneous plate fixation for the treatment of long bone fractures.	B
There is fair evidence to support the use of autogenous cancellous bone graft in the treatment of fractures.	B
There is poor-quality evidence to support the use of autogenous bone marrow aspirate in the treatment of fractures.	C
There is poor-quality evidence to support the use of allograft bone in the treatment of fractures.	C
There is good evidence to support the use of calcium phosphate cement in the treatment of subarticular, metaphyseal defects associated with fractures.	A
There is insufficient/inconclusive evidence to support the use of calcium sulfates in the treatment of fractures.	I
There is poor-quality evidence to support the use of demineralized bone matrix (DBM) in the treatment of fractures.	C
There is good evidence to support the use of BMPs as an alternative to autograft in the reconstruction of traumatic bone defects and the treatment of nonunion.	A
There is fair evidence to support the use of BMPs in the acute management of high-grade (IIIA or IIIB) open tibia fractures.	B
There is insufficient/inconclusive evidence to support the use of platelet concentrates in the treatment of fractures.	I
There is insufficient/inconclusive evidence to support the use of parathyroid hormone (PTH) in the treatment of fractures.	I
There is insufficient/inconclusive evidence to support the use of electrical stimulation in the treatment of fractures.	I
There is insufficient/inconclusive evidence to support the use of ultrasound in the treatment of fractures.	I
There is insufficient/inconclusive evidence to support the use of extracorporeal shock wave therapy (ESWT) in the treatment of fractures.	I

A = good evidence from level I studies with consistent findings, B = fair evidence from level II or III studies with consistent findings, C = poor-quality evidence from Level IV or V studies with consistent findings, I = insufficient or conflicting evidence.

union rates, decreased time to union, and fewer infectious and soft-tissue complications. Although randomized studies comparing percutaneous plate fixation to traditional open techniques are lacking, numerous prospective studies have shown favorable results compared with historical controls, and systematic reviews have supported their use (levels II and III evidence).[3-6] In addition, there is basic science evidence to support the contention that they cause less disruption of fracture vascularity.[7,8] Overall, a grade B recommendation can be made for the use of intramedullary nailing and percutaneous plate fixation in the treatment of long bone fractures. A summary of grades of recommendation is presented in **Table 1**.

Advances in Bone Grafting

Autogenous Bone Graft
Autogenous cancellous bone graft possesses the properties of osteogenesis, osteoconduction, and osteinduction, and accordingly is the gold standard against which all grafting materials are compared. Its osteogenic capacity is due to the fact that autogenous cancellous bone graft contains a viable population of osteoblasts as well as osteoprogenitor and mesenchymal stem cells that can differentiate to form bone. Its cancellous nature makes it an ideal osteoconductive scaffold. It also contains osteoinductive proteins, such as BMPs, albeit in limited quantities. Transplanted autogenous bone graft is rapidly infiltrated by blood vessels and osteoprogenitor cells because of its porous structure. Bone resorption by osteoclasts and bone formation by osteoblasts occurs concomitantly in a process known as creeping substitution. Advantages of autogenous cancellous graft include its strong biologic activity, complete histocompatibility, and no risk of disease transmission. However, cancellous autograft provides little mechanical stability and does not contribute to vascularity at the fracture site. Further limitations of autogenous bone graft include donor site morbidity and limit-

ed amounts of graft material available for use. Complications such as chronic donor site pain, hematoma, infection, and fracture have been reported in up to 30% of patients.[9] Cortical autografts are rarely used in orthopaedic trauma surgery. Nonvascularized grafts provide osteoconduction and mechanical strength; however, their mechanical strength is progressively degraded by resorption and revascularization after implantation. Vascularized cortical autografts provide osteoconduction, mechanical strength, and vascularity; however, their use is limited by the requirement of specialized techniques and donor site morbidity.

Overall, there is very little direct clinical evidence to support the use of autogenous bone graft in orthopaedic trauma, although autogenous bone graft has been used in numerous level I studies as the gold standard of treatment and has shown efficacy in those studies. Overall, a grade B recommendation can be made for the use of autogenous cancellous bone graft in the treatment of fractures.

Autogenous Bone Marrow

The use of bone marrow aspirate represents another way to transplant osteoprogenitor and mesenchymal stem cells for the promotion of bone healing. As a graft material, it provides osteogenic properties and possible osteoinduction from growth factor secretion by transplanted cells. It may also secrete factors that stimulate angiogenesis. The ability of bone marrow aspirate to enhance healing recently has been correlated with the concentration of stem cells contained in the aspirate.[10] Advantages of bone marrow aspirate include low donor site morbidity and the potential for percutaneous application. As a graft material it lacks osteoconductivity, mechanical strength, and vascularity. Bone marrow aspirate can be combined with osteoconductive materials such as DBM, allograft bone, or calcium phosphates. Clinical evidence for the use of bone marrow aspirate is limited to a few level IV studies and a single level III study, and its use remains controversial.[11] Overall, a grade C recommendation for the use of bone marrow aspirate in fracture treatment can be made.

Allograft Bone

Allograft bone is bone tissue harvested from deceased tissue donors and represents a versatile and convenient source of bone graft. These grafts are available off the shelf, avoid donor site morbidity, and can be obtained in cortical or cancellous form. Because of the sterilization process, they primarily act through osteoconduction because there are no viable cells contained in the graft and the retained osteoinductive proteins are very limited. Based on these properties, most surgeons limit their use of cancellous allograft to use as a bone graft extender. In the cortical form, they can be used to contribute mechanical stability to constructs, although their long-term stability is limited by poor revascularization relative to cortical autograft. The major concerns with the use of allograft bone are the risks of dis-

ease transmission and immune response. The evidence supporting their use in orthopaedic trauma surgery is confined to level IV studies, and a grade C recommendation can be made for their use.[11]

Advances in Bone Graft Substitutes

Calcium Phosphates

Ceramics are a class of compounds with a highly crystalline structure that is ideally suited to act as osteoconductive scaffolds. The most widely studied of these compounds is calcium phosphate. Calcium phosphate is available in a variety of forms ranging from blocks and pellets to self-setting cements. Calcium phosphate cement acts as a custom bone-void filler that can provide both mechanical compressive strength and osteoconductivity. Advantages of this bone graft substitute include osteoconductivity, mechanical strength in compression, low morbidity, no risk of disease transmission, and the fact that it is readily available as an off-the-shelf product in unlimited amounts. Disadvantages include its lack of osteoinductive and osteogenic properties as well as its poor tensile strength. Because of its lack of tensile strength and osteoinductivity, calcium phosphate is not recommended for diaphyseal defects or nonunions. Calcium phosphate cement has been extensively investigated in the setting of fractures with subarticular metaphyseal defects, including distal radius fractures, tibial plateau fractures, calcaneal fractures, and femoral neck fractures. In a randomized controlled trial, calcium phosphate cement was shown to be superior to autogenous iliac crest bone graft in the management of subarticular metaphyseal defects associated with tibial plateau fractures (level I evidence).[12] In addition, a recent meta-analysis of randomized trials of the use of calcium phosphate cement in fracture treatment concluded that their use in metaphyseal defects was associated with decreased pain, improved maintenance of fracture reduction, and improved functional outcomes (level I evidence).[13] Overall, a grade A recommendation can be made for the use of calcium phosphate cement as a bone graft substitute in the management of subarticular metaphyseal defects.

Calcium Sulfates

Calcium sulfate represents one of the oldest bone graft substitutes in orthopaedics. Because of differences in its composition, calcium sulfate is resorbed much more rapidly than calcium phosphate (4 to 12 weeks for calcium sulfate compared with up to 1 year for calcium phosphate cement). Concerns that it resorbs too rapidly to be replaced by bone have caused some authors to question its osteoconductive capacity. In addition, high rates of sterile wound drainage in studies of calcium sulfates have been attributed to osmotic loads generated by its rapid resorption. Calcium sulfate is available in combination with antibiotics, and most think that its use should be restricted to osteomyelitic defects.[14]

2: The Polytrauma Patient and Fracture Healing

There is currently inconclusive evidence in the literature for the use of calcium sulfates in orthopaedic trauma, and as such, a grade I recommendation can be made for its use.[15]

Demineralized Bone Matrix

DBM is formed by acid extraction of the mineralized extracellular matrix of allograft bone. After the acid extraction process, what remains is collagen and noncollagenous proteins, including osteoinductive proteins such as the BMPs. DBM is available in multiple forms including gels, putties, pastes, and granules. DBM is highly osteoconductive, but its osteoinductivity is relatively limited and highly variable among the different preparations and donors. It does not provide any mechanical stability and has the theoretical potential for disease transmission because it is obtained from allograft bone. The clinical evidence for its use is limited to level IV studies, and most authors recommend that it be used only as a bone graft extender in combination with autogenous bone graft or autogenous bone marrow.[11] Overall, a grade C recommendation can be made for the use of DBM in orthopaedic trauma.

Bone Morphogenetic Proteins

BMPs represent one of the most well-studied bone graft substitutes in orthopaedic trauma. They comprise a large family of structurally related proteins, which belong to the transforming growth factor-β (TGF-β) superfamily. BMPs have been shown to play important roles in embryonic organ development, limb formation, and fracture healing. In the context of fracture healing, BMPs bind to mesenchymal stem cells and promote their proliferation and differentiation into osteoprogenitor cells, making them truly osteoinductive. Recombinant technology has allowed their mass production, and two BMPs are currently commercially available in the recombinant form: rhBMP-2 and rhBMP-7. Both of these recombinant BMPs have been shown to induce bone formation in a dose-dependent fashion. Although BMPs are not osteoconductive, they can be readily combined with an osteoconductive material, such as allograft or ceramics. Further advantages of the BMPs include off-the-shelf availability, low morbidity, and no risk of disease transmission. The safety of their use has been documented in numerous clinical studies. Lack of mechanical strength, high expense, and questionable effects on fracture vascularity represent some of their disadvantages. In orthopaedic trauma, BMPs have been evaluated clinically in randomized studies in the setting of traumatic bone defects, nonunion, and open tibia fractures. In a randomized study of the use of rhBMP-2 combined with allograft for the delayed reconstruction of traumatic tibial bone defects, the BMP/allograft combination was compared with autogenous iliac crest bone graft (AICBG).[16] That study showed equivalence of the two treatments with respect to defect healing and reintervention, with the avoidance of iliac crest harvest morbidity in the BMP/allograft group (level I evidence).

A randomized study of tibial nonunion comparing treatment with rhBMP-7 or AICBG also showed equivalence between the two groups (level I evidence).[17] The BESTT trial evaluated the use of BMP in a randomized trial of 450 patients with open tibia fractures (level I evidence).[18] Patients were randomized to one of three groups: insertion of 6 mg of rhBMP-2 at time of definitive wound closure, insertion of 12 mg of rhBMP-2 at time of definitive wound closure, or standard of care (no bone graft). The patients in the high-dose BMP group demonstrated significantly reduced rates of secondary intervention and significantly faster wound and fracture healing. However, there was a disproportionate number of reamed nails in the BMP group despite randomization. In a subgroup analysis of patients from the BESTT trial combined with patients from a concurrent randomized trial in the United States, the insertion of rhBMP-2 at time of definitive wound closure was compared with standard of care (no bone graft) in the management of high-grade (Gustilo 3A or 3B) open tibia fractures.[19] The BMP group demonstrated significant decreases in reintervention rates and infection rates (level I evidence). Overall, a grade A recommendation can be made for the use of BMPs as an alternative to AICBG in the reconstruction of traumatic bone defects or in the treatment of nonunion. Given that BMP use in high-grade open tibia fractures has been evaluated only in a post-hoc fashion, a grade B recommendation for the use of BMPs in the acute management of such injuries can be made.

Platelet Concentrates

In the native fracture hematoma, platelets aggregate and subsequently degranulate, releasing several growth factors that influence wound and fracture healing, including platelet-derived growth factor, TGF-β, VEGF, and fibroblast growth factor. Collectively, these growth factors have been referred to as "osteopromotive" by many authors, because they do not directly stimulate bone formation and cannot be considered truly osteoinductive.[20] Platelet-rich plasma is easily obtained from whole blood using commercially available devices and can form a platelet gel with the addition of thrombin. Platelet concentrates can be mixed with osteoconductive substances such as DBM or allograft bone for use as a bone graft substitute. Advantages of platelet concentrates include its low cost, ease of use, autologous nature, and potential effects on stimulating vascularity. Disadvantages are that it is not truly osteoinductive, requires combination with an osteoconductive material, and lacks mechanical strength. In addition, there is a paucity of clinical studies evaluating the efficacy of this material in fracture healing. There has been considerable promise shown with the use of platelet concentrates in animal models of diabetic fracture healing; however, clinical studies are lacking.[21] Overall, a grade I recommendation for the use of platelet concentrates in orthopaedic trauma can be made.

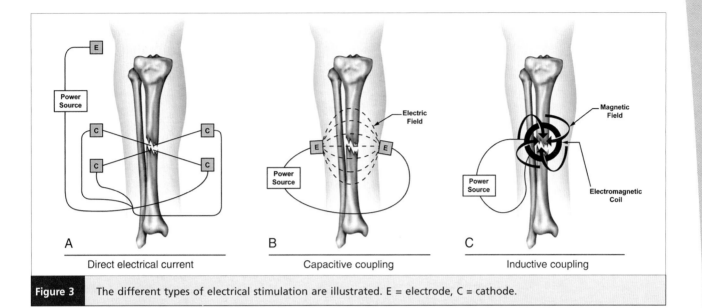

Figure 3 The different types of electrical stimulation are illustrated. E = electrode, C = cathode.

Systemic Agents

It is well understood that systemic factors play an important role in fracture healing. Advancing patient age, diabetes, anemia, malnutrition, smoking, nonsteroidal anti-inflammatory drug use, and long-term steroid use have all been shown to adversely affect fracture healing, and it is important that these factors are optimized as much as possible in the orthopaedic trauma patient.[22] There has been significant interest in developing systemic therapies for fracture healing, whereby fracture healing could be enhanced by the systemic administration of an agent rather than a locally invasive therapy. PTH is one such agent that has generated significant interest recently. PTH is a major systemic regulator of calcium, phosphate, vitamin D, and bone turnover. PTH (1-34), also known as teriparatide, has been shown to be clinically effective in treating osteoporosis and preventing osteoporosis-related fractures. In addition, a growing body of preclinical evidence supports the use of PTH (1-34) as an anabolic agent for the enhancement of fracture healing.[23] In a recent observational cohort study of 145 fracture patients who received a standard dose of PTH (1-34) administered by subcutaneous injection, radiographic and clinical fracture healing was observed in 93% of patients after 12 weeks of treatment (level IV evidence).[24] Of particular note is the fact that 88% of the patients in this cohort had either nonunion, delayed union, or significant medical comorbidities known to be detrimental to fracture healing. In a recent randomized study, 8 weeks of once-daily PTH (1-34), administered subcutaneously at a dose of 20 µg or 40 µg, was compared with placebo injection in postmenopausal patients with a conservatively managed distal radius fracture.[25] The primary outcome measure in that study was time to radiographic union as assessed by CT. The results showed a statistically significant shorter time to healing in the 20-µg group, but not the 40-µg group (level I evidence).

Although preclinical evidence and early clinical evidence are encouraging, there is currently insufficient evidence to recommend the use of PTH in orthopaedic trauma patients, rendering it a grade I recommendation.

Advances in the Physical Enhancement of Bone Healing

The relationship between physical forces and bone biology has been recognized since the development of Wolff's law over a century ago. Mechanical forces (compression, distraction, and shear), electrical forces, and ultrasonic waves have all been found to exert some level of effect on bone growth and fracture healing. Electrical stimulation and ultrasound devices have been developed in an effort to apply these physical forces for the enhancement of fracture healing.

Electrical Stimulation

An applied mechanical stress on a bone results in the generation of electrical potentials. Compression results in the generation of electronegative potentials, whereas tension results in the generation of electropositive potentials. Bone has been shown to form under electronegative potentials and resorb under electropositive potentials. It is thought that this generation of electrical potentials is the pathway through which bone forms in response to an applied load. There is basic science evidence to suggest that electrical stimulation results in the upregulation of growth factors such as TGF-β and the BMPs, suggesting that its effect may be due to enhanced osteoinduction.[26] Three clinical techniques for the application of electrical stimulation to promote fracture healing are commonly used: direct electrical current, capacitive coupling, and inductive coupling (**Figure 3**).

Direct electrical current techniques are somewhat invasive, as they involve the implantation of one or more cathodes into the bone (**Figure 3, A**). An anode is typically placed on the skin and an external power source is used to deliver a 5- to 100-μA current. An electrochemical faradic reaction occurring at the cathode is thought to be primarily responsible for the osteogenic effect of direct electrical stimulation. This reaction at the cathode lowers oxygen concentration, increases pH, and produces hydrogen peroxide. The net result is an increase in osteoblastic activity, a decrease in osteoclastic activity, and the release of growth factors, such as VEGF. Several case series have suggested that high rates of healing (72.5% to 99%) may be achieved for uncomplicated fracture nonunions (level IV evidence).[27]

Capacitive coupling is a noninvasive technique that involves placing two electrodes on the skin overlying the fracture site (**Figure 3, B**). An alternating current is then used to create an electrical field within the fracture site. Potentials of 1 to 10 V at frequencies of 20 to 200 kHz are applied to the electrodes, resulting in the development of electric fields of 1 to 100 mV/cm at the fracture site.[28] Electrical field strength and the duration of bone cell exposure to the electrical field (or "duty cycle") are thought to be the most significant factors in bone cell proliferation. A randomized trial showed that significantly more fracture nonunions healed with capacitive coupling therapy compared with placebo (level II evidence).[29] In addition, case series have suggested rates of healing ranging from 68.8% to 96% for uncomplicated fracture nonunions (level IV evidence).[30]

The third type of electrical stimulation used to enhance fracture healing is inductive coupling. Inductive coupling relies on the use of a pulsed electromagnetic field (PEMF) device that is placed on the skin over the fracture site (**Figure 3, C**). The PEMF consists of a wire coil through which a current is passed. This current generates a magnetic field that in turn induces an electrical field within the fracture site. The size of the electrical field is dependent on the magnitude of the magnetic field and the physical characteristics of the tissues surrounding and within the fracture site. The variability of the current flowing through the PEMF results in an induced magnetic field that is time variable, and thus, an electrical field within the bone whose magnitude varies with time. This variable electrical field is thought to stimulate a physiologic response from bone cells that is similar to that elicited by mechanical stress. A recent meta-analysis concluded that current evidence from randomized clinical trials is insufficient to suggest a clinical benefit for the use of inductive coupling for fresh fractures, osteotomies, delayed unions, and nonunions (level I evidence).[31]

Overall, the clinical evidence for electrical stimulation is conflicting and inconclusive, rendering it a grade I recommendation.

Ultrasound

An ultrasound machine uses a piezoelectric transducer to generate an acoustic pressure wave with a frequency that is greater than human hearing (greater than 20 kHz). Ultrasound machines used to enhance fracture healing typically generate waves with frequencies in the range of 1 to 12 MHz. These waves are transmitted through the body's tissue by the vibration and collision of molecules. The ultrasonic waves used for medical applications may be high-intensity (energies of 1 to 300 W/cm2) or low-intensity (energies of 1 to 50 mW/cm2) waves. High-intensity ultrasound causes considerable heating of the tissue with resulting necrosis. In contrast, low-intensity ultrasound leads to temperature changes of less than 1°C within tissues and has been used to enhance bone healing with fresh fractures, stress fractures, nonunions, and distraction osteogenesis.

Proposed mechanisms for the enhancement of fracture healing by low-intensity ultrasound include enhancements in intracellular calcium levels, cell signal transduction, gene expression, blood flow, and bone remodeling. Although the forces generated by an ultrasound wave are several orders of magnitude less than those generated by weight bearing, the frequencies of the ultrasound wave are several orders of magnitude greater than those experienced with an activity such as walking. Low strain, high frequency forces have been shown to act within the fracture callus to speed healing. Ultrasound also results in a minor increase in tissue temperature (approximately 1°C). Some enzymes that are active within the fracture callus, such as matrix metalloproteinases, display enhanced function with a small increase in temperature.

Despite the success of the low-intensity ultrasound to accelerate fracture healing in basic science studies, clinical studies have yet to show a clear benefit. A meta-analysis on low-intensity ultrasound identified 13 randomized trials that evaluated the use of ultrasound for treatment of operatively and nonsurgically treated fractures.[32] The authors concluded that the evidence for the effect of low-intensity ultrasound on healing of fractures is moderate to very low in quality and provides conflicting results. Although there was some evidence from randomized trials included in that review that ultrasound accelerates fracture healing in the closed management of fractures in the tibia, distal radius, and scaphoid, those trials failed to show a significant benefit in terms of functional outcome. Overall, a grade I recommendation can be made for the use of ultrasound in the treatment of fractures.

Extracorporeal Shock Wave Therapy

Extracorporeal shock wave therapy (ESWT) relies on the generation of a single-impulse acoustic wave with a high amplitude and short wavelength. When the acoustic wave enters the body, it is transformed into a mechanical force at the boundary of tissues with different rigidities (for example, the boundary between muscle and bone). This causes microtrauma within the cortex of the bone on which ESWT has been applied. This microtrauma is thought to stimulate neovascularization and the differentiation of cells into the osteogenic lineage. Clinical studies on ESWT have focused mainly on its use for fracture nonunions. A review of the basic science and clinical literature on the use of ESWT for fracture nonunions suggests that clinical studies are of a poor level and do not provide strong evidence for the use of ESWT to treat fracture nonunion.[33] A randomized clinical trial investigating the use of ESWT for the treatment of fracture nonunion or for the acceleration of fresh fracture healing would be helpful to substantiate the use of this treatment modality. Overall, a grade I recommendation can be made for the use of ESWT in the treatment of fractures.

Summary and Future Directions

Successful fracture management requires an understanding of the biology of fracture healing, a knowledge of available treatments for enhancing fracture healing, and an appreciation of the evidence for their use. By understanding the critical components of fracture healing and how available treatment options address these components, orthopaedic trauma surgeons can make informed and educated decisions about the treatment of their patients.

Treatment methods continue to evolve, and it is possible that future therapies will involve cell-based strategies, sophisticated scaffolds, or the delivery of growth factors by the use of gene therapy. These techniques have been extensively studied in preclinical models of fracture healing and have shown promising results. With continued research, it is possible that such therapies will enter the clinical realm and be a component of future fracture management.

Annotated References

1. Li R, Stewart DJ, von Schroeder HP, Mackinnon ES, Schemitsch EH: Effect of cell-based VEGF gene therapy on healing of a segmental bone defect. *J Orthop Res* 2009;27(1):8-14.

   Using a rabbit model, the authors demonstrated enhanced healing of bone defects in the tibia with the use of fibroblasts transfected to overexpress VEGF, compared with treatment with nongenetically modified fibroblasts. They were also able to show histologic evidence of increased vascularity in the defects treated with the VEGF-transfected cells.

2. Mifune Y, Matsumoto T, Kawamoto A, et al: Local delivery of granulocyte colony stimulating factor-mobilized CD34-positive progenitor cells using bioscaffold for modality of unhealing bone fracture. *Stem Cells* 2008;26(6):1395-1405.

   Using a rat nonunion model, the authors demonstrated that the transplantation of human endothelial progenitor cells resulted in a dose-dependent increase in fracture healing and angiogenesis.

3. Schütz M, Müller M, Krettek C, et al: Minimally invasive fracture stabilization of distal femoral fractures with the LISS: A prospective multicenter study. Results of a clinical study with special emphasis on difficult cases. *Injury* 2001;32(suppl 3):SC48-SC54.

4. Papakostidis C, Grotz MR, Papadokostakis G, Dimitriou R, Giannoudis PV: Femoral biologic plate fixation. *Clin Orthop Relat Res* 2006;450:193-202.

   The authors systematically reviewed the literature on femur fractures treated with percutaneous plate fixation. Compiling the data from 19 studies, they were able to review the results of 697 femoral fractures managed with minimally invasive techniques. Their analysis demonstrated high union rates (98.4%) and low infection rates (2%) with the use of biologic techniques. The authors concluded that biologic plating is a viable alternative to modern nailing techniques. Level of evidence: II.

5. Herrera DA, Kregor PJ, Cole PA, Levy BA, Jönsson A, Zlowodzki M: Treatment of acute distal femur fractures above a total knee arthroplasty: Systematic review of 415 cases (1981-2006). *Acta Orthop* 2008;79(1):22-27.

   The authors systematically reviewed the literature on the surgical treatment of acute distal femur fractures above a total knee arthroplasty. Compiling the data from 29 studies, they were able to review the results of 415 cases that were managed surgically. Their analysis showed improved results with the use of retrograde nailing or locked plating when compared to traditional plating methods. The differences were statistically significant for fractures treated with retrograde nailing, whereas those treated with locked plating only showed a trend toward improved outcomes. The authors concluded that modern-day treatment options are superior to conventional treatment options in the management of distal femur fractures above total knee arthroplasty. Level of evidence: II.

6. Wright JG, Swiontkowski MF, Heckman JD: Introducing levels of evidence to the journal. *J Bone Joint Surg Am* 2003;85(1):1-3.

7. Farouk O, Krettek C, Miclau T, Schandelmaier P, Guy P, Tscherne H: Minimally invasive plate osteosynthesis: Does percutaneous plating disrupt femoral blood supply less than the traditional technique? *J Orthop Trauma* 1999;13(6):401-406.

8. Perren SM: Evolution of the internal fixation of long bone fractures. The scientific basis of biological internal fixation: Choosing a new balance between stability and biology. *J Bone Joint Surg Br* 2002;84(8):1093-1110.

9. Sen MK, Miclau T: Autologous iliac crest bone graft: Should it still be the gold standard for treating nonunions? *Injury* 2007;38(suppl 1):S75-S80.

   This article reviews the scientific basis for the use of AICBG and discusses the risks and benefits of its use. Level of evidence: V.

10. Hernigou P, Poignard A, Beaujean F, Rouard H: Percutaneous autologous bone-marrow grafting for nonunions: Influence of the number and concentration of

progenitor cells. *J Bone Joint Surg Am* 2005;87(7): 1430-1437.

In this study, the authors treated 60 noninfected, atrophic nonunions of the tibia with a percutaneous injection of concentrated bone marrow that was aspirated from the iliac crests of the patients. Fifty-three of the nonunions went on to fracture union. The number of progenitor cells contained in the concentrated aspirate was estimated by counting fibroblast colony-forming units. The authors were able to demonstrate a positive correlation between the number of progenitor cells contained in the concentrated aspirate and the amount of fracture callus. There were significantly lower concentrations of progenitor cells in the seven patients whose nonunions failed to unite. Level of evidence: IV.

11. De Long WG Jr, Einhorn TA, Koval K, et al: Bone grafts and bone graft substitutes in orthopaedic trauma surgery: A critical analysis. *J Bone Joint Surg Am* 2007; 89(3):649-658.

This recent review examines the available evidence for the use of bone grafts and bone graft substitutes in orthopaedic trauma. A critical appraisal of the literature is presented along with grades of recommendation for the use of bone grafts and bone graft substitutes in orthopaedic trauma.

12. Russell TA, Leighton RK; Alpha-BSM Tibial Plateau Fracture Study Group: Comparison of autogenous bone graft and endothermic calcium phosphate cement for defect augmentation in tibial plateau fractures: A multicenter, prospective, randomized study. *J Bone Joint Surg Am* 2008;90(10):2057-2061.

In this randomized trial of 120 fractures, the authors compared the use of calcium phosphate cement versus AICBG in the management of subarticular metaphyseal defects of the proximal tibia associated with tibial plateau fractures. The defects treated with calcium phosphate cement showed significantly less articular subsidence when compared to the AICBG group. Level of evidence: I.

13. Bajammal SS, Zlowodzki M, Lelwica A, et al: The use of calcium phosphate bone cement in fracture treatment: A meta-analysis of randomized trials. *J Bone Joint Surg Am* 2008;90(6):1186-1196.

The authors systematically reviewed available randomized studies on the use of calcium phosphate cement in fracture treatment. Fourteen studies were included in the analysis, including trials on the use of calcium phosphate cement in the management of distal radius fractures, femoral neck fractures, intertrochanteric hip fractures, calcaneus fractures, and tibial plateau fractures. From their pooled analysis, the authors concluded that the use of calcium phosphate cement in the management of fractures is associated with decreased postoperative pain, improved maintenance of fracture reduction, and improved functional outcomes. Level of evidence: I.

14. McKee MD, Wild LM, Schemitsch EH, Waddell JP: The use of an antibiotic-impregnated, osteoconductive, bioabsorbable bone substitute in the treatment of infected long bone defects: Early results of a prospective trial. *J Orthop Trauma* 2002;16(9):622-627.

15. Hak DJ: The use of osteoconductive bone graft substitutes in orthopaedic trauma. *J Am Acad Orthop Surg* 2007;15(9):525-536.

This article reviews the scientific basis for the use of osteoconductive bone graft substitutes in orthopaedic trauma and provides a comprehensive review of the available osteoconductive graft substitutes.

16. Jones AL, Bucholz RW, Bosse MJ, et al; BMP-2 Evaluation in Surgery for Tibial Trauma-Allograft (BESTT-ALL) Study Group: Recombinant human BMP-2 and allograft compared with autogenous bone graft for reconstruction of diaphyseal tibial fractures with cortical defects: A randomized, controlled trial. *J Bone Joint Surg Am* 2006;88(7):1431-1441.

In this randomized trial of 30 fractures, the authors compared the use of rhBMP-2 combined with allograft versus AICBG in the delayed reconstruction of posttraumatic, diaphyseal defects of the tibia. The defects treated with rhBMP-2/allograft showed no significant differences versus the AICBG group with respect to union or complication rates. The authors concluded that rhBMP-2/allograft is a viable alternative to AICBG that avoids the complications associated with graft harvest. Level of evidence: I.

17. Friedlaender GE, Perry CR, Cole JD, et al: Osteogenic protein-1 (bone morphogenetic protein-7) in the treatment of tibial nonunions. *J Bone Joint Surg Am* 2001; 83-A(pt 2, suppl 1):S151-S158.

18. Govender S, Csimma C, Genant HK, et al; BMP-2 Evaluation in Surgery for Tibial Trauma (BESTT) Study Group: Recombinant human bone morphogenetic protein-2 for treatment of open tibial fractures: A prospective, controlled, randomized study of four hundred and fifty patients. *J Bone Joint Surg Am* 2002;84(12): 2123-2134.

19. Swiontkowski MF, Aro HT, Donell S, et al: Recombinant human bone morphogenetic protein-2 in open tibial fractures: A subgroup analysis of data combined from two prospective randomized studies. *J Bone Joint Surg Am* 2006;88(6):1258-1265.

In this subgroup analysis of two randomized trials, a total of 131 high-grade open tibia fractures were identified. These high-grade open fractures were randomized to receive either rhBMP-2 at the time of definitive wound closure or no treatment (standard of care). The results demonstrated a significantly lower rate of invasive secondary interventions (the primary outcome measure of both studies) and a significantly lower rate of infection in the rhBMP-2 group. The authors concluded that the acute use of rhBMP-2 in high-grade open tibia fractures results in improved outcomes and lower infection rates. Level of evidence: I.

20. Watson JT: Overview of biologics. *J Orthop Trauma* 2005;19(10, suppl):S14-S16.

This article reviews several currently available bone graft substitutes and discusses the evidence available for their use.

21. Gandhi A, Doumas C, Dumas C, O'Connor JP, Parsons JR, Lin SS: The effects of local platelet rich plasma delivery on diabetic fracture healing. *Bone* 2006;38(4):540-546.

    Using a diabetic rat fracture model, the authors demonstrated that the percutaneous delivery of platelet-rich plasma resulted in enhanced fracture healing.

22. Gaston MS, Simpson AH: Inhibition of fracture healing. *J Bone Joint Surg Br* 2007;89(12):1553-1560.

    This article reviews the current literature regarding the importance of systemic factors in modulating fracture healing.

23. Barnes GL, Kakar S, Vora S, Morgan EF, Gerstenfeld LC, Einhorn TA: Stimulation of fracture-healing with systemic intermittent parathyroid hormone treatment. *J Bone Joint Surg Am* 2008;90(suppl 1):120-127.

    This article reviews the scientific basis for the modulation of fracture healing by PTH administration and reviews the growing body of preclinical evidence for the use of PTH in animal models of fracture healing.

24. Bukata S, Kaback L, Reynolds D, O'Keefe R, Rosier R: 1-34 PTH at physiologic doses in humans shows promise as a helpful adjuvant in difficult to heal fractures: An observational cohort of 145 patients. *Trans Orthop Res Soc* 2009;34:paper 227.

    This observational cohort study of 145 patients with a variety of fractures demonstrated a 93% rate of clinical and radiographic union with 12 weeks of subcutaneous PTH 1-34 administration. Eighty-eight percent of the patients treated had either a nonunion, delayed union, or significant medical comorbidities known to be detrimental to fracture healing. Level of evidence: IV.

25. Aspenberg P, Genant HK, Johansson T, et al: Teriparatide for acceleration of fracture repair in humans: A prospective, randomized, double-blind study of 102 postmenopausal women with distal radial fractures. *J Bone Miner Res* 2010;25(2):404-414.

    In this randomized trial of 102 patients with a conservatively managed distal radius fracture, the authors compared the once daily subcutaneous administration of two doses of teriparatide (20 μg or 40 μg) to placebo. The primary outcome measure was time to radiographic union as assessed by CT scan. There was a statistically significant decreased time to healing in the 20 μg group compared to placebo. Similar effects were not statistically significant in the 40 μg group. There were no significant differences in final radiographic outcome measures (such as ulnar variance or dorsal angulation) or functional outcome measures between the groups. Level of evidence: I.

26. Aaron RK, Boyan BD, Ciombor DM, Schwartz Z, Simon BJ: Stimulation of growth factor synthesis by electric and electromagnetic fields. *Clin Orthop Relat Res* 2004;419:30-37.

    This article reviews the scientific basis for electrical stimulation and reviews the basic science evidence that demonstrates upregulation of numerous growth factors by the application of electrical stimulation.

27. Brighton CT, Black J, Friedenberg ZB, Esterhai JL, Day LJ, Connolly JF: A multicenter study of the treatment of non-union with constant direct current. *J Bone Joint Surg Am* 1981;63(1):2-13.

28. Aaron RK, Ciombor DM, Simon BJ: Treatment of non-unions with electric and electromagnetic fields. *Clin Orthop Relat Res* 2004;419:21-29.

    This article reviews the clinical literature on the use of electromagnetic fields for treatment of nonunions.

29. Scott G, King JB: A prospective, double-blind trial of electrical capacitive coupling in the treatment of non-union of long bones. *J Bone Joint Surg Am* 1994;76(6):820-826.

30. Abeed RI, Naseer M, Abel EW: Capacitively coupled electrical stimulation treatment: Results from patients with failed long bone fracture unions. *J Orthop Trauma* 1998;12(7):510-513.

31. Mollon B, da Silva V, Busse JW, Einhorn TA, Bhandari M: Electrical stimulation for long-bone fracture-healing: A meta-analysis of randomized controlled trials. *J Bone Joint Surg Am* 2008;90(11):2322-2330.

    This meta-analysis examined four randomized controlled trials that evaluated the clinical use of inductive coupling electrical stimulation to treat delayed union and nonunion of fractures. The authors concluded that the current evidence from randomized clinical trials is insufficient to suggest a clinical benefit for the use of this therapy for fresh fractures, osteotomies, delayed unions, and nonunions. Level of evidence: I.

32. Busse JW, Kaur J, Mollon B, et al: Low intensity pulsed ultrasonography for fractures: Systematic review of randomised controlled trials. *BMJ* 2009;338:b351.

    This meta-analysis on low-intensity ultrasound identified 13 randomized trials that evaluated the use of ultrasound for treatment of operatively and nonsurgically managed fractures. The fractures were from varied anatomic sites, and studies focused on fresh fractures, fracture nonunions, stress fractures, and distraction osteogenesis. Authors of the meta-analysis ranked the quality of these studies to range from moderate to very low. Pooled results from three low quality studies suggest a reduction of 36.9% (95% CI of 25.6% to 46.0% with $I^2 = 41.6\%$) in time to radiographic union with the use of low-intensity ultrasound for nonsurgically treated fresh fractures. The use of ultrasound showed a benefit to functional outcome in only one study. Authors concluded that evidence is moderate to poor in quality and provides conflicting results. Level of evidence: I.

33. Biedermann R, Martin A, Handle G, Auckenthaler T, Bach C, Krismer M: Extracorporeal shock waves in the treatment of nonunions. *J Trauma* 2003;54(5):936-942.

2: The Polytrauma Patient and Fracture Healing

Chapter 14

Nonunions and Malunions

Brett R. Bolhofner, MD   Maureen Finnegan, MD   Douglas W. Lundy, MD, FACS

Introduction

Bone must heal nearly completely with bone for the skeleton to regain its ability to withstand mechanical load and for fracture outcome to be successful from a functional perspective. Few other tissues are capable of such self-regeneration after injury and instead heal with scar. When a fracture fails to heal clinically and radiographically and when the reparative process has ceased on a cellular level, then nonunion can be said to occur. Frequently it is not possible to say, except retrospectively, exactly when a nonunion is established. Somewhat arbitrarily, fractures are frequently considered nonunions when they have not healed by 6 months.

Different healing rates occur according to fracture pattern, mechanism, the particular bone involved, and the bone region (that is, diaphysis or metaphysis). When healing, as judged by clinical and radiographic parameters, is thought to be proceeding at a slower rate than would be expected from similar fracture circumstances but has not altogether halted, then delayed union can be considered to be present.

Fractures that heal in any position less than anatomic could critically be considered malunions. Whether a malunion is clinically significant, acceptable, or requires additional treatment should be individualized to the particular bone and patient.

Etiology

The etiology of nonunion may at times be enigmatic but frequently one or more basic contributing factors can be identified. These factors can most simply be categorized as prefracture host, fracture/injury, treatment, and postfracture host.

Dr. Bolhofner or an immediate family member is a board member, owner, officer, or committee member of the Florida Orthopaedic Society. Dr. Lundy or an immediate family member serves as an unpaid consultant to Synthes, and has stock or stock options in Livengood Engineering. Neither Dr. Finnegan nor an immediate family member has received anything of value from or owns stock in a commercial company or institution related directly or indirectly to the subject of this chapter.

Prefracture Host Factors

By definition, prefracture host factors exist before the time of the injury. In some instances such factors actually predispose the patient to the fracture incurred (for example, poor bone quality, poor balance, or syncope), and they certainly create problems in achieving subsequent fracture union. Smoking (probably the most widely studied host issue), diabetes, endocrinopathy,[1] HIV, medications including steroids and chemotherapeutic agents, and nutritional issues may exist alone or in combination at the time of the fracture, and they create less-than-optimal conditions.

In a recent series, 37 patients with persistent nonunion after fracture treatment were referred for endocrinologic evaluation. Thirty-one of these patients had a previously unrecognized underlying endocrine abnormality including hypogonadism, thyroid and parathyroid disorders, or calcium imbalance. Eight of these patients achieved union by correction of the underlying endocrinopathy without additional surgery.[1]

Bisphosphonates, commonly used for the treatment of osteoporosis, have recently been shown to contribute to an increased incidence of nonunion.[2]

Fracture/Injury Factors

The injury itself may or may not define the prospects for uneventful healing. High-energy injuries, soft-tissue damage, and especially open fractures with bone loss frequently define the healing prospects beginning at the time of injury. These scenarios frequently require a staged approach to achieve healing and avoid nonunion. Any injury, closed or open, that devitalizes bone will have a detrimental effect on healing potential and rate.

Treatment Factors

Nonunion may develop despite completely appropriate treatment but is encouraged by less-than-appropriate treatment. Both surgical and nonsurgical treatment can have a role, and choosing the appropriate treatment must be individualized to the specific fracture and the patient. The stability achieved by the chosen treatment method should be adequate for healing to progress for that particular fracture. The basic principles of treatment selected should be adhered to whether it is something as simple as functional bracing or as complex as major surgical intervention. To the extent possible, surgical treatment should minimize additional bone injury or devitalization of fragments or the introduction of bacteria because both may lead to healing problems. Ideally, the selected treatment should enhance the possibility of fracture union or at least not diminish it.

Postfracture Host Factors

In general, prefracture host issues remain present during the healing period and should be optimized to the extent possible. This would include correction of metabolic and endocrine disorders or nutritional deficiencies and smoking cessation. In addition, host issues that develop during the postfracture period can be problematic and include compliance, psychosocial and economic issues, and infection. All of these host issues may have a direct or indirect influence on fracture healing. It has recently been shown that cell viability, differentiation, and gene expression of osteoblasts may be altered in patients with nonunions. It cannot be stated with certainty at this time whether these alterations are present before or develop after the establishment of nonunion.[3] Angiogenesis, which is critical in bone formation, has been shown to be altered in patients with nonunions. Specific angiogenic factors may be lower in the initial phases of healing in patients who go on to develop nonunions compared to those with normal healing.[4]

Evaluation

Nonunion occurs at the cellular level; unfortunately, it cannot be readily and directly appreciated when evaluating a patient. Clinical skill including examination and history taking along with radiographic and other diagnostic tests can be relied on to infer what is happening at the fracture site biologically.

History

All of the factors that may impair fracture healing must be reviewed in the history of the patient being evaluated for nonunion, delayed union, or malunion. These include the prefracture and postfracture host issues discussed previously and any medical management directed at optimization of these conditions. The injury mechanism and circumstances as well as the rendered treatments must also be known to the greatest degree possible. Ongoing issues related to compliance, habits, social factors, and employment should be defined whenever possible.

Physical Examination

Although the physical examination is focused around the affected limb, the importance of a complete physical examination cannot be overlooked. Pertinent conditions that may not be known to the patient or disclosed in the history, such as nicotine staining, heart failure, peripheral neuropathy, and poor nutrition, may be detected on general physical examination.

The affected extremity should be evaluated for local tenderness, pain with range of motion, and ability to bear weight. These findings may sometimes be the only clue that there is an issue with healing. Soft-tissue and neurocirculatory status, the condition and function of adjacent joints, and the presence of deformity (including shortening and scarring) are important.

Diagnostic Testing

Plain radiography may be diagnostic. In the past, when hardware was broken, bent, or otherwise failed, nonunion could be presumed or at least highly suspected. The current dilemma is that modern implants maintain their integrity for long periods in the face of nonunion without exhibiting a failure. In a recent series, it was reported that failure of a locked plate in the face of full weight bearing and nonunion did not occur for up to 1 year postoperatively.[5]

In these cases, other diagnostic modalities such as CT reconstruction and MRI may be obtained, but they may be nondiagnostic or their image quality impaired by the metal used for internal fixation. There is no substitute for a high level of clinical suspicion and diligent follow-up.

Nuclear medicine studies may be useful in some instances to define physiologic activity or lack thereof at the fracture site. Labeled white blood cell scans can be useful for differentiating subclinical infection in combination with appropriate serologic studies including erythrocyte sedimentation rate and C-reactive protein.

Assessment of Deformity

One of the puzzles of fracture treatment is that some fractures heal in the face of deformity (malunions) but similar fractures do not heal (nonunions). Although correcting the deformity in a malunion restores length and may prevent adjacent joint arthrosis, correction of nonunion is imperative to restore a mechanical environment favorable to fracture healing. The ideal mechanical environment for fracture healing is compression or axial loading with elimination and minimization of bending and shear stresses. Fracture site motion, biomechanically defined as strain, must be within the tolerance of the local cells in order for fracture healing to occur. Motion (strain) that exceeds cell tolerances will delay or even prevent fracture repair. As deforming forces are more pronounced in weight-bearing extremities, deformity correction is more critical in these limbs. Although most patients bear weight on their lower extremities, there are patients with paraplegia or other neuromuscular diseases who bear weight on their upper extremities.

Three major deforming forces (bending, shear, and axial load) produce three major deformities (angulation, rotation, and shortening). Translation is a minor deforming force that can be associated with any or all of the major forces and can either exaggerate or diminish the resultant deformity. Angulation actually occurs only in one plane but is frequently evaluated and described in two planes because standard radiographs are made in the AP and lateral planes. If the extremity could be continuously rotated and repeat radiographs obtained, the deformity would eventually be demonstrated to be in only one plane, usually best seen on an oblique view. Angular deformity during loading creates a bending moment; conversion of this bending moment to compressive loading is needed for union to occur.

Rotational deformities are functionally disabling in both upper and lower extremities. Assessing the individual's physiologic rotation in the uninjured limb during initial treatment helps avoid this type of deformity; the same uninjured limb assessment is needed to evaluate deformity correction. Nonunions with rotational instability have persistent torsional forces at the fracture site that prevent union. Chronic rotational deformities involving interosseous membrane shortening may not be amenable to complete correction. Rotational deformity is difficult to evaluate on plain radiographs; CT scans of both the involved and uninvolved extremity, with cuts at the proximal and distal ends of the affected long bones, are necessary for accurate quantitative assessment of rotational deformities.

Discrepancies in limb length are not only functionally disabling in the lower extremity, but they also tend to increase both mechanical forces and wear on adjacent joints as well as the spine and the opposite extremity. Evaluation of length inequality can be done either clinically or with radiographs. Clinical evaluation is done in the standing patient by placing premeasured blocks under the short limb until the pelvis is level. Radiographic evaluation can be done using either supine scanogram or a CT scanogram. Because most facilities no longer have the equipment for supine scanograms, the CT version is more commonly used. When assessing limb-length discrepancy, the surgeon needs to take into account any angular deformities because correction of these will affect eventual length. Treatment of length discrepancy, similar to correction for angulation or rotation, can be either immediate or achieved over time. Surgical decision making should depend on the number of deformities as well as types and severity.

Classification

Classification of nonunion is an attempt to group and describe nonunions according to what is, or in some cases, is not occurring biologically at the fracture site. The most basic classification is whether the nonunion is infected (septic or aseptic). Commonly used terms including hypertrophic, oligotrophic, atrophic, and pseudarthrosis are simply ways of relating the radiographic appearance to a biologic status at the fracture site. Failure of fracture healing to progress is commonly related either to an unfavorable biologic environment or nonphysiologic mechanical loads across the fracture site. In certain cases, both biology and mechanical load may be causal factors. Understanding the individual pathophysiology, which may be somewhat defined by classification, aids the surgeon in designing successful treatment plans.

The time at which delayed union becomes nonunion is a controversial issue; time is the ultimate test as the fracture either heals or progresses to a well-established nonunion. When fracture healing fails to progress within a time frame defined by clinical experience and established literature according to the type of fracture and the particular bone involved, the potential for the development of nonunion looms.

Once failure of fracture healing has been determined, understanding the specific biology and mechanics of that fracture environment will allow for design of a successful treatment plan. Defining the characteristics of ununited fracture fragments may require using resources such as CT, MRI, and nuclear medicine studies. This determination is particularly important for periarticular and short-segment metaphyseal nonunions as well as infected nonunions. Fluoroscopy, with stress views to outline the site and degree of motion, may also be a useful tool.

When vascularity at the fracture site is near normal but excess motion is present, a hypertrophic nonunion may occur, which may require only mechanical stability to proceed to union (**Figure 1**). Well-vascularized fracture fragments attempt to heal by forming callus to bridge the gap. This increased callus may progress to the development of the classic elephant's foot callus seen on radiographs of a hypertrophic nonunion.

On the other hand, when blood supply is compromised at the nonunion site, atrophic nonunion may develop. Poorly vascularized fractures will produce minimal to no callus, potentially increasing mechanical instability as a secondary effect. This decreased vascularity may be the result of an open injury or any of the other factors already discussed.

In the case of an infected nonunion, it is usually necessary to eradicate the infection to achieve union; this typically requires surgical débridement, intravenous antibiotics, and/or application of local antibiotics.

The mechanical environment needed for fracture healing includes the application of loads to the fracture that are within physiologic limits, which include consideration of both the magnitude of applied forces and any fracture gaps. Hypertrophic, oligotrophic, and atrophic nonunions all have some degree of unacceptable load. In hypertrophic nonunions, when mechanical factors are the primary problem, both fracture gap and loading should be assessed. Periarticular fractures, which are frequently atrophic, do not tolerate gaps. Bone requires tissue strains that fall within physiologic limits to progress toward fracture healing. The concept of tissue strain relates motion to the width of the gap: high strain occurs from large motion over a small gap, while low strains occur when there is little motion over a large gap. This explains why more comminuted fractures with a larger surface area tolerate flexible fixation (relative stability), while simple transverse fractures do not tolerate motion (high strain) and require rigid fixation (absolute stability). Axial load is well tolerated, whereas shear forces tend to disrupt callus. Bending forces are a combination of compression and tension. The compressive side may load the fracture in the axial

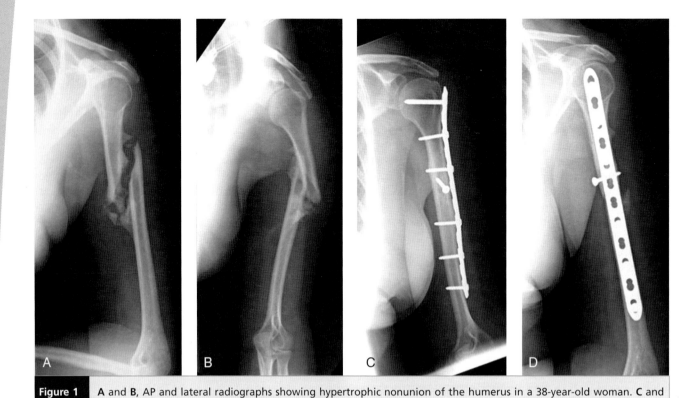

Figure 1   **A** and **B**, AP and lateral radiographs showing hypertrophic nonunion of the humerus in a 38-year-old woman. **C** and **D**, AP and lateral radiographs showing healed nonunion treated with compression without grafting. Because of the hypertrophic nature of the nonunion, only additional stability was required, with no bone grafting.

mode, aiding the healing reaction, while the tension side may disrupt callus formation. Accurate assessment of loads at the nonunion site, as well as fracture gaps, will aid in treatment planning.

Metaphyseal and periarticular fractures present a unique mechanical situation. Contracture of the adjacent joint creates a lever arm at the fracture site, generating abnormal forces on the tissue and impeding healing. Evaluation of potential adjacent joint contractures and subsequent releases combined with rigid fixation to eliminate abnormal forces may be critical for healing. In stark contrast, diaphyseal nonunions can tolerate less rigid fixations such as intramedullary nails, as long as physiologic load is restored in a well-vascularized environment.

Nonunions with adequate vascularity and excessive mechanical forces, when left untreated for a significant length of time, may result in the formation of a false joint or pseudarthrosis. This is a synovial joint that forms between the two fracture ends. Treatment involves resection of the false synovial joint, reestablishment of the medullary canal, and mechanical stabilization.

Treatment

Matching Patient and Surgeon Goals

Patients with nonunions typically present with significant pain and morbidity. They have often been through several operations and have endured significant pain for 6 to 8 months or more. Patients with nonunions are often unable to work and have significant financial burdens. Many times they are looking for a "quick fix" for their problem.

It is imperative that the overall goals of treatment be understood by the patient and the treating surgeon. Clearly, achieving optimal function of the affected limb is the goal. The surgeon must consider the condition of the surrounding soft tissues as well as the functionality of the associated joints. Sometimes, fracture union is not the most appropriate goal of treatment, and arthroplasty or amputation is the best option. It may require an extended period of time and multiple surgical procedures to accomplish fracture union and realignment or arthrodesis of affected joints.

Deformity Correction

There are multiple surgical techniques available for the treatment of malunited fractures. The surgeon may elect to perform an acute correction of the deformity, or a gradual correction of the malunion may be optimal instead. The indications for surgical management of a malunion differ depending on which bone is affected and many patient variables including age, functional status of the surrounding joints, comorbidities, and the overall desires and expectations of the patient.

Acute Correction

Acute correction of a deformity has the distinct advantage of immediately correcting the malalignment and restoring the function of the extremity. The surgical tactic for the osteotomy is planned before the operation to restore the mechanical axis of the entire limb. The patient is able to immediately appreciate the correction and may begin rehabilitation soon after surgery. There are several disadvantages of this technique. Errors in preoperative planning or surgical execution may result in less than ideal correction and incomplete improvement of the deformity. Rapid adjustment may also cause unintentional injury to neural or vascular structures due to stretch or kinking. It is also wise to monitor for compartment syndrome after performing an acute correction.

The indications for an acute correction of deformity vary according to the location of the deformity and many patient-related variables. Certainly, an opportune time to perform an acute correction may be when treating a delayed union in which deformity developed after the internal fixation failed. Commonly accepted indications for surgical management of lower extremity malunions include 10° of varus or 15° of valgus at the knee or ankle, or 20 mm of medial shift of the mechanical axis. Other indications include deformities that result in ligamentous instability on the convex side of the deformity, inability to place the foot in a plantigrade position, and a limb-length discrepancy greater than 20 mm.[6] Although these values are somewhat arbitrary, they are generally accepted by the surgical community as being predictive in preventing posttraumatic arthritis of the surrounding joints.

Osteotomies may produce lengthening or shortening of the limb depending on the location of the osteotomy and the produced angle (varus or valgus). Generally, all osteotomies that correct varus deformity will subsequently result in lengthening of the limb.[7] An osteotomy may also produce translation of the mechanical axis. Osteotomies usually are best performed at the center of rotation of angulation (CORA),[8] which is determined by measuring the overall alignment of the limb on standard 51-inch radiographs. Osteotomies performed at the CORA will produce angular correction without translation of the affected bone.

Closing-wedge osteotomy is the most commonly used technique in performing corrective surgery for malunions. The surgeon must perform thorough preoperative planning to determine the correct location, orientation, and size of the osteotomy to ensure that the desired result will be achieved. Closing-wedge osteotomies are advantageous because there are large viable bone edges along the cuts that are optimal for osseous union. Closing-wedge osteotomies in the lower extremity may produce lengthening of the extremity even though bone was removed to produce the correction. The overall effect of limb lengthening or shortening is complicated and depends on the location, direction, and angle of the osteotomy. Disadvantages of a closing-

wedge osteotomy include the amount of exposure and dissection that is required to access the area for the osteotomy. If a periarticular closing-wedge osteotomy is performed, traversing ligaments and tendons may be functionally lengthened due to the segment of bone that is removed, potentially causing joint laxity and/or altering myotendinous function.

Opening-wedge osteotomies are advantageous in that they may restore limb length and appropriate tension to the surrounding muscles, tendons, and ligaments. The osteotomy may be performed through smaller incisions than a similar closing-wedge osteotomy. Opening-wedge osteotomies may be more difficult to heal than closing-wedge osteotomies because of the need for healing of the associated gap, which requires some sort of bone grafting. The void produced by the opening wedge is usually filled with autologous bone, allogenic bone, or ceramic bone void fillers. Opening-wedge osteotomy has been combined with intra-articular osteotomy for correction of lateral plateau valgus malunions with depression.[9]

A neutral osteotomy combines a closing and an opening wedge, and this type of osteotomy tends to be length neutral in that it does not produce bone shortening or lengthening. It can be relatively complex and technically difficult to perform. The bone removed from the closing wedge is inserted through the osteotomy to the far side to function as the bone graft for the opening wedge. The obvious advantage of this technique is that bone lengths are left unaffected and autologous bone grafts are used.

Oblique osteotomies may be performed to correct complex and multiplanar deformities. These osteotomies can correct angular, rotational, and sometimes even limb-length discrepancies. Preoperative planning for these procedures can be complicated, but the resulting correction is elegant in its execution[10,11] (**Figure 2**).

Dome osteotomies are performed by producing a circular osteotomy, usually based on the CORA. This allows rotation of the distal fragment at the CORA and will not lengthen or shorten the bone. These osteotomies can be difficult to perform.

Once the deformity has been corrected with an osteotomy, the bone requires stabilization to maintain the correction. Casting or external fixation can be used, but most surgeons use either internal or intramedullary fixation. Internal fixation with plates and screws provides compression across the osteotomy, and locking constructs provide improved fixation in the metaphyseal bone in the periarticular areas. Periarticular plates cannot be used without contouring because the osteotomy usually results in significant changes in the morphology of the bone. Disadvantages of internal fixation are the exposure required to insert the plates and the need to protect weight bearing. Intramedullary fixation nicely stabilizes osteotomies and allows early weight bearing. Intramedullary fixation can be technically difficult due to changes in the alignment of the intramedullary canal because of the osteotomy. Intramedullary

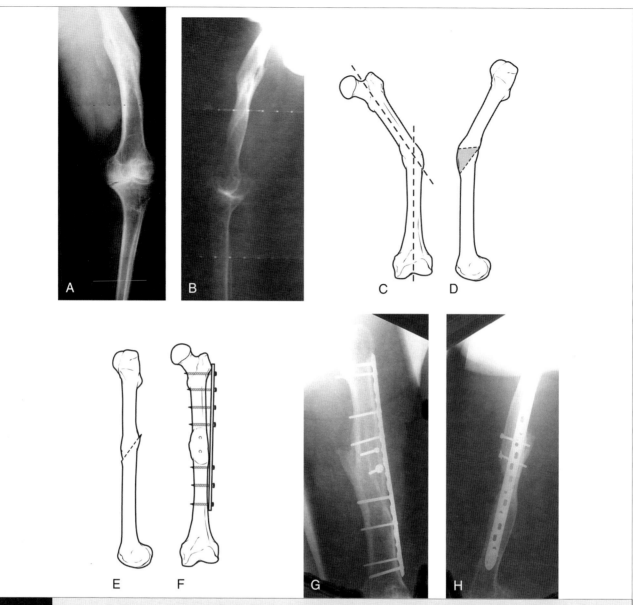

Figure 2 **A** and **B**, AP and lateral radiographs of a malunited femur with angulation and translation. **C** through **F**, Preoperative plans for oblique osteotomy. **C** and **D**, A wedge must be removed to correct the translation in the lateral plane. **E** and **F**, After wedge removal, the oblique surfaces may slide longitudinally to add some length. Fixation is with lag screws and a plate. **G** and **H**, AP and lateral radiographs after oblique osteotomy. Angulation and translation along with length have been restored.

fixation may not adequately stabilize osteotomies through metaphyseal bone without blocking screws or other techniques such as adjunctive plating.

Recently a clamshell osteotomy using an intramedullary nail has been advocated for diaphyseal malunions for deformity correction. As in a Sofield technique, the malunited central segment is osteotomized proximally and distally and again in the central osteotomized segment and longitudinal plane. The proximal and distal segments are then anatomically aligned in all planes and secured with a locked intramedullary nail. The central osteotomized segments or clamshell is bypassed by the nail as if it were an acute fracture fragment.[12]

Gradual Correction

Gradual correction of a malunion can be performed with the Ilizarov fixator. This device uses distraction osteogenesis by slowly stretching the soft callus in the corticotomy site. This method results in new bone that fills the void left after the distraction has corrected the deformity.

The advantage of this technique is that multiple complex corrections can be performed at one time to include angular, translational, and rotational deformities and length discrepancy. These devices can be placed percutaneously, resulting in minimal surgical dissection. The gradual nature of the correction allows the soft tis-

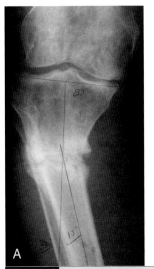
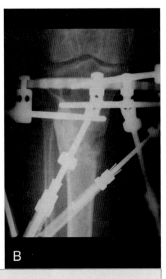

Figure 3 **A,** Radiograph showing angulated nonunion of the proximal tibia in a 46-year-old patient. The CORA is 15° varus. **B,** Same patient with a Taylor spatial frame. Correction was performed without opening the nonunion site.

sues to accommodate to the change in alignment. The correction is assessed in the outpatient setting, allowing fine-tuning of the adjustment.

Disadvantages of this technique include the inconvenience of wearing the external fixator. Some patients are intolerant of the Ilizarov fixator and prefer an acute correction with internal or intramedullary fixation. Patients using an Ilizarov fixator may experience pin tract infections and pin loosening, requiring additional procedures. If the osteotomy does not heal, surgical options are complicated because of the risk of infection when using internal or intramedullary fixation after prolonged external fixation.

The principles applied when using the Ilizarov fixator are similar to those used in acute correction techniques in that preoperative planning is critical for determining the site of the corticotomy. The preoperative plan will determine the angular correction necessary and will also determine if any translational components in the correction. By using 51-inch radiographs of the lower extremities combined with meticulous preoperative planning, the surgeon can restore the mechanical alignment, length, and rotation of the affected extremity.

In 1997, the Taylor spatial frame was introduced, revolutionizing the Ilizarov method. This device uses six struts that attach the Ilizarov rings and allow for correction of multiple deformities. The surgeon uses a computer program to calculate the correction and manage the pace of the correction. The principles of the Ilizarov fixator are still used, but the ease of correction is dramatically improved. There is no difference in lengthening between the Taylor spatial frame and the Ilizarov fixator.[13] **(Figure 3).**

Length

Fractures can be responsible for a loss of limb length because of angular malreduction, segmental bone loss, or comminution. When this occurs, patients may report limb-length discrepancies that they often only notice after fracture union. Patients may easily compensate for a limb-length discrepancy up to 2 cm with a shoe lift. Discrepancies greater than 4 cm tend to be poorly tolerated and require shoe modifications. Surgical options include shortening of the opposite extremity or lengthening of the affected extremity. Lengthening procedures include Ilizarov lengthening, intramedullary lengthening, or sliding osteotomies.

The Ilizarov fixator is nicely suited to limb lengthening through the process of distraction osteogenesis, which may be performed in conjunction with an intramedullary nail. When using this method, the Ilizarov fixator and the intramedullary nail are placed during the initial procedure. When distraction is completed, the nail is locked and the Ilizarov fixator is removed. This technique results in less time in the external fixator, faster consolidation of the regenerate, and quicker return of knee motion.[14] Similar results may be obtained using a unilateral fixator over an intramedullary nail.[15]

The intramedullary skeletal kinetic distractor nail (ISKD, Orthofix, McKinney, TX) is an intramedullary device that can be used to produce limb lengthening through distraction osteogenesis. The advantage of this system is that there are no external components used in the lengthening. Lengthening is achieved through rotation of the extremity that mechanically lengthens the nail. Angular deformities cannot be addressed with this device, but rotational corrections can be done acutely during the initial surgery[16] **(Figure 4).**

Rotation

Rotational malalignment can be corrected acutely through the osteotomy or gradually with the Ilizarov fixator. The extent of the deformity must be determined preoperatively, and the bone needs to be marked before cutting the osteotomy so that the correct amount of rotation can be assessed. Kirschner wires placed in each fragment set to the correction angle desired before cutting the osteotomy can be helpful in determining the appropriate amount of rotation.

Achieving Union

Defining a set period of time before a fracture can be called a nonunion is inappropriate. The time required for a fracture to proceed to solid union is dependent on many variables including location of the fracture, extent of soft-tissue injury, presence of infection, patient age, and comorbidities, as well as many other factors.

Nonsurgical Measures

Optimal therapy for patient factors such as endocrinopathies, metabolic disorders, smoking, and inadequate

2: The Polytrauma Patient and Fracture Healing

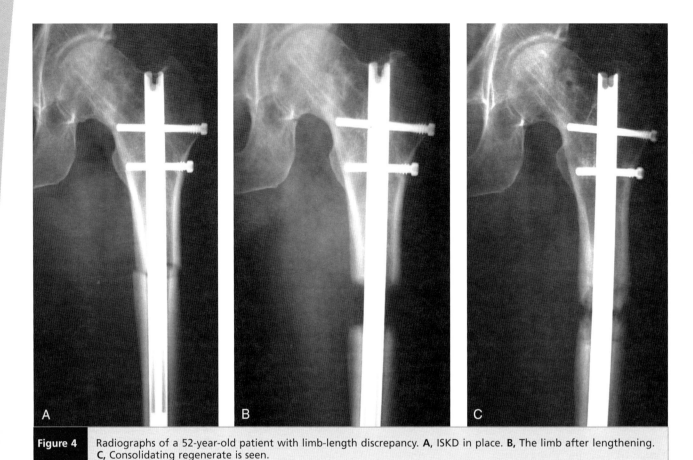

Figure 4 Radiographs of a 52-year-old patient with limb-length discrepancy. **A,** ISKD in place. **B,** The limb after lengthening. **C,** Consolidating regenerate is seen.

nutrition, as well as elimination of possibly offending medications, are paramount nonsurgical measures that should be undertaken whenever possible. Adjuvant therapies such as ultrasound may be effective, but their role in surgically treated fractures with hardware in place requires additional investigation.[17]

Atrophic Nonunion

Atrophic nonunions are characterized by resorption of bone around the fracture site and lack of radiographic signs of callus. These nonunions are believed to occur from a biologic failure in the healing mechanism. Although mechanical stability is important for these nonunions to heal, they mostly need a biologic boost to proceed to union. The local nonunion site must be adequately prepared before application of the bone graft to optimize the biologic stimulus. The fibrous tissue occupying the nonunion site must be excised, and the surrounding bone should be decorticated to encourage the incorporation of bone graft and healing of the nonunion.

Atrophic nonunions are best treated with bone grafts or bone graft substitutes that will stimulate the local environment to improve the healing potential. Autologous bone graft remains the mainstay, and donor sites include the standard locations as well as newer techniques.

Reamer Irrigator Aspirator

The reamer irrigator aspirator (RIA, Synthes, Paoli, PA) is a recent technical development for the harvesting of autogenous bone graft via a less invasive route. The RIA is a one-pass reamer with a self-contained irrigant and suction. The canal reamings are evacuated and trapped or collected.[18] As much as 60 to 80 cm³ of graft material may be obtained.[19,20] The graft material contains both pluripotent cells and significant growth factors.[21] The aspirate also contains growth factors and pluripotential mesencyhmal cells.[22] So far, minimal complications have been reported, and these patients have less pain compared with those who undergo iliac crest bone graft harvesting.[23]

Cancellous allogenic bone graft may be used to extend autologous bone graft to fill large defects. Allogenic bone should not be used alone because it lacks the osteogenic and osteoinductive properties required to stimulate atrophic nonunions. Bone marrow has also been used with success as a graft in the treatment of atrophic nonunions.[24]

Exchange intramedullary nailing is a technique that improves both the mechanical and the biologic environment of the nonunion. The surgeon exchanges the current intramedullary nail for one that is 1 to 4 mm wider than the previous nail, thus improving the mechanical stiffness of the fixation. The reaming of the canal necessary to allow passage of the wider nail is thought to both add bone graft to the canal as well as stimulate the blood supply to the nonunion. Reaming reduces the endosteal blood supply and increases the periosteal blood supply stimulating new periosteal bone formation.[25]

Although expensive, synthetically derived bone morphogenetic proteins (BMPs) are effective in the treatment of atrophic nonunions. The manufacturers of BMP-7 were allowed a human device exemption from the FDA to apply this product in the treatment of tibial nonunions. BMP-7 was as effective as autologous bone graft in the treatment of tibial nonunions, without the associated morbidity of harvesting bone.[26] BMP-7 has also been used to effectively expand the autograft used in a series of 45 atrophic nonunions.[27] Even considering the expense of BMP, cost savings from a decreased number of interventions and fewer hospital days may be realized when BMP is used alone or in combination with bone grafting for nonunions.[28]

Another method of treatment in recalcitrant nonunions is to resect the nonunion area, removing all of the nonviable bone. The surgeon must remove an adequate amount of bone so that there is only viable bone remaining in either fragment. The surgeon then uses bone transport with the Ilizarov fixator to gradually close the defect and restore length through distraction osteogenesis. Vascularized bone grafts may also be used to fill bone voids after resection of the atrophic nonunion.

The role of mesenchymal stem cells in bone repair and the relatively new field of regenerative medicine hold further promise in the treatment of nonunited and metabolically diseased bone.[29]

Hypertrophic Nonunion

Hypertrophic nonunions are characterized by adequate local biology but inadequate mechanical stability at the nonunion site (**Figure 1**). Radiographs demonstrate a widened segment of bone at the nonunion with inability to bridge the bony gap. Revision of the fixation and improvement of mechanical stability at the nonunion site are required for nonunion progress toward healed bone. The mechanical environment of the nonunion can be improved by revision fixation with intramedullary nails, plates and screws, or external fixation. Plate fixation after failed treatment with rods has been shown to be effective in the femur.[30]

Dynamization of nonunions occurs when the surgeon removes interlocking screws from an intramedullary nail or decreases the rigidity of an external fixator. This technique allows more mechanical load across the nonunion. Success rates vary widely depending on the particular bone involved, and the timing of this intervention is not well defined. Dynamizing the fixation improves the bony contact and improves compression at the nonunion site. This technique is minimally invasive and may be the first step in healing a hypertrophic nonunion.

Infection and Nonunion

The presence of infection can inhibit fracture healing. The surgeon must set priorities along the course of treatment toward the ultimate goal of obtaining the maximal function of the patient. This treatment plan may include staged reconstruction with resection of the infected and necrotic bone, application of temporary fixation, and space management with antibiotic beads or spacers followed by definitive fixation and bone grafting as appropriate. Sometimes, the optimal treatment is amputation.

Segmental Bone Loss

Segmental bone loss is a frequently encountered scenario and a problem without a perfect solution. Treatment options currently available include bone transport, primary shortening followed by lengthening, vascularized or nonvascularized free grafts, and most recently, titanium mesh cages and membrane induction.

Limited data consisting of case reports exist for the use of a titanium cage filled with cancellous graft similar to those used in spine surgery for the treatment of segmental defects. Successful consolidation and healing at the host junctions with 1-year follow-up are reported.[31,32]

Membrane induction involves the insertion of polymethylmethacrylate spacers into the bone defect. The bone must previously or concurrently be stabilized by internal fixation and must have a good soft-tissue envelope.[33,34] A membrane then forms around the polymethylmethacrylate spacer and in 4 to 6 weeks is opened but preserved while the cement spacer is removed and replaced with cancellous graft. The mechanism by which the membrane is induced by the spacer is unknown. The membrane serves to both contain the graft and provide growth factors for healing.[35] Treatment of defects up to 25 cm have been successful[33] (**Figure 5**).

Staged Treatment

Treatment plans for any nonunion should consider the need for staging the necessary procedures. A hypertrophic nonunion that only requires mechanical stability is usually treated in a single stage. However, nonunions that are lacking soft-tissue coverage, have length or deformity issues, or are infected frequently require staging of procedures.

With the advent of the vacuum-assisted wound closure system, soft-tissue coverage has become less of a challenge. Wounds covered using vacuum-assisted wound closure usually have clean granulation tissue at the edges and often have granulation tissue on the bone.[36-38] If the vacuum system fails, coverage can be obtained by working in conjunction with a plastic surgeon, using tissue expanders, local flaps, or vascularized flaps. Débridement of the nonunion site at the time of coverage may expedite treatment, but bone grafting should be left until the coverage is mature. The edge of the mature coverage can then be elevated for placement of either bone graft or bone substitutes.

2: The Polytrauma Patient and Fracture Healing

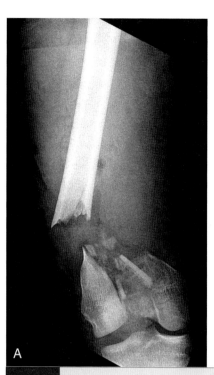
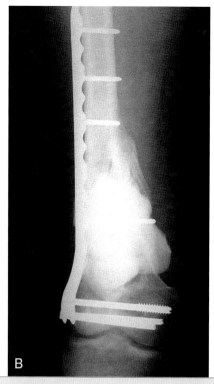
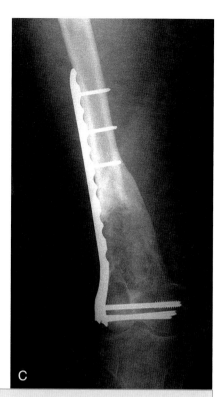

Figure 5 Radiographs showing treatment of segmental bone loss. **A,** Open distal femur fracture with segmental bone loss. **B,** Polymethylmethacrylate spacer and plate. **C,** After membrane induction.

Infected nonunions may be the most difficult nonunions to treat, always require staged treatment, and take the longest time to achieve union. The primary stage must focus on eradicating or at a minimum controlling the infection. Complete excision of infected tissue, placement of local antibiotics (usually via spacers), and coverage of the wound are essential.[39,40] Systemic antibiotics during the initial phase of treatment should be considered. In some instances when the treatment of infection is not progressing, amputation may need to be considered.

Summary

Optimally, nonunion is prevented by obtaining union in every patient. However, with the myriad host, injury, and treatment variables, prevention of nonunion will not realistically occur in the foreseeable future. Nonunion and malunion will invariably occur, and solid treatment plans based on biomechanics and biology will continued to be needed. The basic principles of deformity correction, stable fixation, restoration of a healing environment, and grafting have not significantly changed, but newer and more stable implants, grafting sources, and techniques and improved basic science knowledge are enhancing treatments. Cellular, biochemical, and genetic research is a promising but developing field that is likely to enhance but not replace the current basic principles.

Annotated References

1. Brinker MR, O'Connor DP, Monla YT, Earthman TP: Metabolic and endocrine abnormalities in patients with nonunions. *J Orthop Trauma* 2007;21(8):557-570.
   Previously unknown metabolic or endocrine disorders were diagnosed in 31 of 37 patients with unexplained nonunion. These disorders included vitamin D deficiency, hypogonadism, calcium imbalance, and thyroid and parathyroid conditions. Correction of the underlying disorder can be therapeutic.

2. Solomon DH, Hochberg MC, Mogun H, Schneeweiss S: The relation between bisphosphonate use and nonunion of fractures of the humerus in older adults. *Osteoporos Int* 2009;20(6):895-901.
   A multivariable regression model demonstrates the association of bisphosphonate use and an increased chance of nonunion in an approximately 20,000 patient cohort.

3. Hofmann A, Ritz U, Hessmann MH, et al: Cell viability, osteoblast differentiation, and gene expression are altered in human osteoblasts from hypertrophic fracture non-unions. *Bone* 2008;42(5):894-906.
   The authors analyzed osteoblastic cell activity, formation of alkaline phosphatase, and mineralization-positive units as well as gene expression in osteoblasts with fracture nonunions and compared them to those of control individuals. The authors noted, as the study suggests, that cell viability, differentiation, and gene expressions of osteoblasts are altered in patients who develop recurrent and recalcitrant nonunions.

4. Weiss S, Zimmermann G, Pufe T, Varoga D, Henle P: The systemic angiogenic response during bone healing. *Arch Orthop Trauma Surg* 2009;129(7):989-997.

   The study compares various angiogenic cytokine levels in a healthy control group versus those in a group of patients with nonunions. The serum concentration of these factors was distinctly different between the two groups. The differences were present as early as 2 to 4 weeks after surgery and therefore may eventually provide some prognostic information regarding fracture healing at a relatively time interval.

5. Vallier HA, Hennessey TA, Sontich JK, Patterson BM: Failure of LCP condylar plate fixation in the distal part of the femur: A report of six cases. *J Bone Joint Surg Am* 2006;88(4):846-853.

   Nonunion and implant failure was not noted until 6 months in 2 cases, 7 months in one case, 9 months in 1 case, and a full 14 months in another.

6. Probe RA: Lower extremity angular malunion: Evaluation and surgical correction. *J Am Acad Orthop Surg* 2003;11(5):302-311.

7. Wade RH, New AM, Tselentakis G, Kuiper JH, Roberts A, Richardson JB: Malunion in the lower limb: A nomogram to predict the effects of osteotomy. *J Bone Joint Surg Br* 1999;81(2):312-316.

8. Paley D: Osteotomy concepts and frontal plane alignment, in Paley D (ed): *Principles of Deformity Correction.* Berlin, Germany, Springer-Verlag, 2002, pp 99-154.

9. Marti RK, Kerkhoffs GM, Rademakers MV: Correction of lateral tibial plateau depression and valgus malunion of the proximal tibia. *Oper Orthop Traumatol* 2007;19(1):101-113.

   The technique of opening-wedge osteotomy of the proximal tibia combined with an intra-articular osteotomy for depressed healed tibial plateau fractures is detailed. Fifteen of 23 patients did not have progression of arthritis with average of 14 years of follow-up.

10. Sangeorzan BJ, Sangeorzan BP, Hansen ST Jr, Judd RP: Mathematically directed single-cut osteotomy for correction of tibial malunion. *J Orthop Trauma* 1989;3(4):267-275.

11. Chiodo CP, Jupiter JB, Alvarez G, Chandler HP: Oblique osteotomy for multiplanar correction of malunions of the femoral shaft. *Clin Orthop Relat Res* 2003;406:185-194.

12. Russell GV, Graves ML, Archdeacon MT, Barei DP, Brien GA Jr, Porter SE: The clamshell osteotomy: A new technique to correct complex diaphyseal malunions. *J Bone Joint Surg Am* 2009;91(2):314-324.

    Ten patients with diaphyseal tibial and femoral nonunions were treated successfully using a segmental diaphyseal osteotomy and locked intramedullary nail fixation. Simplicity, multiplanar correction, and early weight bearing are listed as advantages.

13. Kristiansen LP, Steen H, Reikerås O: No difference in tibial lengthening index by use of Taylor spatial frame or Ilizarov external fixator. *Acta Orthop* 2006;77(5):772-777.

    Twenty tibial lengthenings performed with the Taylor spatial frame were compared with 27 tibial lengthenings using the Ilizarov external fixator. There were no differences in lengthening index or complications. The authors noted that the correction of deformity was easier with the Taylor spatial frame.

14. Paley D, Herzenberg JE, Paremain G, Bhave A: Femoral lengthening over an intramedullary nail: A matched-case comparison with Ilizarov femoral lengthening. *J Bone Joint Surg Am* 1997;79(10):1464-1480.

15. Kocaoglu M, Eralp L, Bilen FE, Balci HI: Fixator-assisted acute femoral deformity correction and consecutive lengthening over an intramedullary nail. *J Bone Joint Surg Am* 2009;91(1):152-159.

    These authors describe their experience in 28 femoral deformity corrections and lengthenings with a unilateral fixator over a femoral nail. Average external fixator time was 83 days with an average of 6 cm of lengthening. There were no deep infections. Level of evidence: IV.

16. Cole JD, Justin D, Kasparis T, DeVlught D, Knobloch C: The intramedullary skeletal kinetic distractor (ISKD): First clinical results of a new intramedullary nail for lengthening of the femur and tibia. *Injury* 2001;32(suppl 4):SD129-SD139.

17. Siska PA, Gruen GS, Pape HC: External adjuncts to enhance fracture healing: What is the role of ultrasound? *Injury* 2008;39(10):1095-1105.

    This is a comprehensive review of the theory, mechanics, clinical results, and studies of low-intensity pulsed ultrasound for bone healing.

18. Pape HC, Tarkin IS: Reamer irrigator aspirator: A new technique for bone graft harvesting from the intramedullary canal. *Oper Tech Orthop* 2008;18:108-113.

    A detailed technique for using the RIA is described. Fluoroscopic control of all phases and cessation of suction when not actively reaming is recommended. Reaming should be advanced, paused, withdrawn, and advanced throughout the procedure.

19. Newman JT, Stahel PF, Smith WR, Resende GV, Hak DJ, Morgan SJ: A new minimally invasive technique for large volume bone graft harvest for treatment of fracture nonunions. *Orthopedics* 2008;31(3):257-261.

    The authors discuss the technique for RIA use as a bone graft harvest tool. A low rate of donor site morbidity was documented in a limited number of cases.

20. Stafford PR, Norris B: Reamer irrigator aspirator as a bone graft harvester. *Tech Foot Ankle Surg* 2007;6:100-107.

    The history and technique of RIA graft harvesting are presented. Contraindications are metabolic bone disease, active metastatic disease, previous osteomyelitis, advanced age, osteoporosis, and bleeding disorders.

2: The Polytrauma Patient and Fracture Healing

21. Schmidmaier G, Herrmann S, Green J, et al: Quantitative assessment of growth factors in reaming aspirate, iliac crest, and platelet preparation. *Bone* 2006;39(5): 1156-1163.

    Reamings from RIA are comparable to iliac crest with respect to growth factors. The irrigation fluid itself also contains growth factors.

22. Porter RM, Liu F, Pilapil C, et al: Osteogenic potential of reamer irrigator aspirator (RIA) aspirate collected from patients undergoing hip arthroplasty. *J Orthop Res* 2009;27(1):42-49.

    Aspirate harvested with the RIA from five patients was examined for osteogenic properties. The aspirate demonstrated high levels of fibroblast growth factor-2, insulin-like growth factor-I, and latent transforming growth factor-β1. The harvested cells were sensitive to induction to become osteogenic and chondrogenic cells.

23. Belthur MV, Conway JD, Jindal G, Ranade AR, Herzenberg JE. Bone graft harvest using a new intramedullary system. *Clin Orthop Relat Res* 2008;466(12):2973-2980.

    The average graft volume with RIA was 43.3 mL (25 to 75 mL). Patients who used the RIA, in comparison with those who underwent iliac bone grafting regarding postoperative pain, had less pain intensity and frequency. Level of evidence: III.

24. Hernigou P, Mathieu G, Poignard A, Manicom O, Beaujean F, Rouard H: Percutaneous autologous bone-marrow grafting for nonunions: Surgical technique. *J Bone Joint Surg Am* 2006;88(suppl 1, pt 2):322-327.

    These authors describe their technique of harvesting bone marrow aspirate with a 2.4-mm trocar for use in treating nonunions. They injected an average of 20 mL of aspirate into 60 atrophic tibial nonunions, and 53 went on to union. There was a correlation between the progenitors in the graft and the efficacy.

25. Reichert IL, McCarthy ID, Hughes SP: The acute vascular response to intramedullary reamin: Microsphere estimation of blood flow in the intact ovine tibia. *J Bone Joint Surg Br* 1995;77(3):490-493.

26. Friedlaender GE, Perry CR, Cole JD, et al: Osteogenic protein-1 (bone morphogenetic protein-7) in the treatment of tibial nonunions. *J Bone Joint Surg Am* 2001; 83(suppl 1, pt 2):S151-S158.

27. Giannoudis PV, Kanakaris NK, Dimitriou R, Gill I, Kolimarala V, Montgomery RJ: The synergistic effect of autograft and BMP-7 in the treatment of atrophic nonunions. *Clin Orthop Relat Res* 2009;467(12):3239-3248.

    The authors combined BMP-7 with autograft in the treatment of 45 nonunions. All of the nonunions healed in an average of 5 months. They found BMP-7 to be beneficial as a graft expander. Level of evidence: IV.

28. Dahabreh Z, Dimitriou R, Giannoudis PV: Health economics: A cost analysis of treatment of persistent fracture non-unions using bone morphogenetic protein-7. *Injury* 2007;38(3):371-377.

    Cost savings through a decreased number of procedures and fewer in-patient days when using BMP-7 with or without bone graft were noted. The authors arrived at this conclusion by comparing the cost of previous treatment to the cost of the treatment after the use of BMP-7.

29. Undale AH, Westendorf JJ, Yaszemski MJ, Khosla S: Mesenchymal stem cells for bone repair and metabolic bone diseases. *Mayo Clin Proc* 2009;84(10):893-902.

    The authors review the theory and current state of stem cell therapies in animals and humans as they apply specifically to bone-healing issues. Mesenchymal stem cells from adults and not embryonic marrow are promising.

30. Bellabarba C, Ricci WM, Bolhofner BR: Results of indirect reduction and plating of femoral shaft nonunions after intramedullary nailing. *J Orthop Trauma* 2001; 15(4):254-263.

31. Attias N, Lindsey RW: Case reports: Management of large segmental tibial defects using a cylindrical mesh cage. *Clin Orthop Relat Res* 2006;450:259-266.

    Three patients were treated for segmental tibial defects using a titanium mesh cage packed with cancellous bone graft and demineralized matrix. The constructs were stabilized over a locked intramedullary nail and followed for a minimum of 1 year. The three patients in the series healed and had satisfactory functional outcome.

32. Clements JR, Carpenter BB, Pourciau JK: Treating segmental bone defects: A new technique. *J Foot Ankle Surg* 2008;47(4):350-356.

    Postmortem evaluation of a titanium mesh cage and graft from a patient treated for a distal tibial defect confirmed osseous consolidation of the graft and healing at the host graft interface.

33. Masquelet AC, Fitoussi F, Begue T, Muller GP: Reconstruction des os Longs Par Membrane Induite et Autogreffe Spongieuse. *Arr Chir Plasti Esthet* 2000;45:346-353.

    A series of 35 cases of diaphyseal defects ranging from 4 to 25 cm were treated with a staged induced polymethylmethacrylate membrane technique. Average time to full weight bearing was 8.5 months.

34. Ristiniemi J, Lakovaara M, Flinkkilä T, Jalovaara P: Staged method using antibiotic beads and subsequent autografting for large traumatic tibial bone loss: 22 of 23 fractures healed after 5-20 months. *Acta Orthop* 2007;78(4):520-527.

    The authors treated 23 fractures with average bone loss of 52 mm with a staged polymethylmethacrylate membrane induction technique. Union was achieved in 22 fractures at a mean healing time of 40 weeks.

35. Pelissier P, Masquelet AC, Bareille R, Pelissier SM, Amedee J: Induced membranes secrete growth factors including vascular and osteoinductive factors and could stimulate bone regeneration. *J Orthop Res* 2004;22(1): 73-79.

The authors demonstrated by qualitative and quantitative immunochemistry the production of growth factors and osteoinductive (BMP-2) factors in the polymethylmethacrylate membrane in rabbits. Maximum factors were present at 4 weeks.

36. Wild T, Stremitzer S, Budzanowski A, Hoelzenbein T, Ludwig C, Ohrenberger G: Definition of efficiency in vacuum therapy: A randomised controlled trial comparing with V.A.C. therapy. *Int Wound J* 2008;5(5):641-647.

The study was terminated after the initial 10 patients treated with vaccum-assisted wound closure had significantly better outcomes. The authors found a 54% increase in surface granulation tissue and a 27% reduction in fibrin tissue at the base of the wound.

37. Gabriel A, Shores J, Heinrich C, et al: Negative pressure wound therapy with instillation: A pilot study describing a new method for treating infected wounds. *Int Wound J* 2008;5(3):399-413.

Faster resolution of infection and wound closure with fewer hospital days were the results in patients who had vacuum-assisted wound closure instead of standard moist dressing.

38. Canavese F, Gupta S, Krajbich JI, Emara KM: Vacuum-assisted closure for deep infection after spinal instrumentation for scoliosis. *J Bone Joint Surg Br* 2008;90(3):377-381.

Fourteen pediatric spine infections treated without need for implant removal.

39. Diefenbeck M, Mückley T, Hofmann GO: Prophylaxis and treatment of implant-related infections by local application of antibiotics. *Injury* 2006;37(suppl 2):S95-S104.

A review of the use of antibiotic-ladened spacers in infection is presented.

40. Thonse R, Conway J: Antibiotic cement-coated interlocking nail for the treatment of infected nonunions and segmental bone defects. *J Orthop Trauma* 2007;21(4):258-268.

Twenty patients were studied using antibiotic-coated nails. Infection control was 95% and union rate was 85%.

2: The Polytrauma Patient and Fracture Healing

Chapter 15
Infections

Michael T. Mazurek, MD   Paul J. Girard, MD

The Burden of Infection

Posttraumatic infection remains a challenging problem for the orthopaedist.[1] The incidence of infection after traumatic fracture approaches 16%, depending on the nature of the initial injury and the treatment rendered. Furthermore, posttraumatic infections are being seen more frequently, especially in immunocompromised patients. Although knowledge and the ability to treat musculoskeletal infections continue to increase, treatments are often complex and can be accompanied by problematic late sequelae including nonunion, chronic osteomyelitis, amputation, and death. The extended treatment of posttraumatic musculoskeletal infection (using antibiotics, wound care, multiple surgical procedures, and revision of implants) results in an increased financial burden on an already strained health care system. The personal and emotional impact on the patient and his or her family can lead to chronic intractable pain, depression, discord, and prolonged or permanent disability.

Nosocomial infections are the most common complication affecting hospitalized patients. Nosocomial is defined as denoting a new disorder, not the patient's original condition, associated with being treated in a health care environment. Approximately 5% to 10% of patients (about 2 million patients annually) admitted to acute care hospitals acquire one or more infections. These infections result in as many as 90,000 deaths.[2] Surgical site infections are the second most common cause of nosocomial infection, after urinary tract infections.

Nosocomial infections occur through patient-to-patient transmission via transiently or persistently colonized health care workers. Inadequate hand hygiene and sharing of equipment such as stethoscopes and blood pressure cuffs have been implicated in disease transmission. This problem is magnified when multiple consultants treat seriously injured trauma patients in the surgical intensive care unit setting. Closely related to cross-contamination is the concept of colonization pressure, defined as the proportion of other patients colonized with a problem bacteria in a specific hospital unit.[3]

Pathogenesis

Homeostasis and Symbiosis

When a patient's musculoskeletal tissues are exposed to bacteria, a delicate interplay between the infecting organism and the host eventually dictates the outcome. When patients experience traumatic injury, there is often a disruption of the soft-tissue envelope that contains an intricate network of blood vessels and lymphatics—part of the host's normal defense against infection. This disruption in normal homeostasis provides foreign bacteria an opportunity to begin colonization. Bone fragments stripped of periosteum, foreign bodies, surgical implants, and sutures provide a protected environment, allowing bacteria to avoid normal host defenses. All natural biologic surfaces, with the exception of articular cartilage and teeth, are protected by endothelium, epithelium, or periosteum. These physical barriers decrease the adhesion of bacteria because of the presence of host extracellular polysaccharide molecules and desquamation. If infection progresses, it may further decrease local vascularity through microvascular thrombosis. It is the role of the orthopaedist, based on the condition of the host and the inoculum of microbes, to determine the appropriate intervention in favor of the host.

Host Traits That Potentiate Infection

The immunocompetency of the host is paramount. Certain systemic factors have been associated with an increased risk of infection, including extremes of age, diabetes, renal insufficiency, systemic steroid use, obesity, malnutrition, alcohol and tobacco abuse, immunosuppression for organ transplantation, and the need for disease-modifying antirheumatic drugs such as methotrexate and azathioprine, and new medicines such as infliximab, etanercept, adalimumab, and anakinra.[4]

Local factors that predispose to infection include vascular insufficiency, prior surgical scars, radiation therapy, and the severity of soft-tissue damage. Special

Dr. Mazurek is deceased. At the time this chapter was written Dr. Mazurek or an immediate family member had received research or institutional support from the Orthopaedic Trauma Extremity Research Program. Neither Dr. Girard nor an immediate family member has received anything of value from or owns stock in a commercial company or institution related directly or indirectly to the subject of this article.

consideration of the host's ability to mount a defense must be made before proper treatment can be initiated. Similarly, intraoperative care and surgical technique bring other variables into play, including the use of perioperative antibiotics, effective hemostasis, prevention of hypothermia and hyperglycemia, adequacy of débridement and irrigation with removal of all devitalized tissue, choice of surgical stabilization and local antibiotics, soft-tissue management, optimal placement and use of surgical drains, and postoperative oxygenation. Even the presence of suture increases the susceptibility of host tissue to infection. According to a classic study, 7.5×10^6 staphylococci were required to initiate an intradermal infection in normal tissue, whereas inoculation of only 300 organisms was needed to produce a similar infection in the presence of silk suture.[5] In another study, the attachment of bacteria to 10 different suture materials was examined; it was concluded that the number of adherent bacteria was dependent on the specific bacteria, the duration of contact, and the physical configuration (monofilament versus braided multifilament), surface area, chemical structure, and coating of the suture.[6] These investigators also found that in comparison with *Escherichia coli*, *Staphylococcus aureus* more readily adhered to sutures.

Bacterial Traits That Potentiate Infection

Although *S aureus* is the most consistent cause of musculoskeletal infections, other gram-positive and gram-negative bacilli and anaerobic organisms are commonly isolated. Bacteria have evolved various mechanisms to thwart the host immune system. For example, *S aureus* is a natural colonizer of cartilage and collagen because of its specific surface-associated adhesins for binding sites on collagen.[7]

The ability to create biofilm, a community of bacteria surrounded by an extracellular matrix of glycoproteins, is a notable characteristic of several species.[8] The composition of this extracellular matrix binds secreted antibodies, impairs antibiotic penetration, and inhibits phagocytosis. Organisms within the biofilm upregulate the secretion of factors that impede antibiotic delivery and activity. Bacteria that produce ß-lactamase upregulate this enzyme within the matrix, and catalase-positive organisms express increased concentrations of catalase, preventing effective diffusion of hydrogen peroxide, one of the immune system's primary defense chemicals. The biofilm network also allows for more efficient transmission of virulence factors through bacteriophages and gene transfer.

The complexity of this matrix is mediated by a process known as quorum sensing, a communication mechanism by which bacteria "team up" and develop what has been called a bacterial social network.[9] Bacteria within this network have been shown to modify protein expression to mediate the organization of the biofilm, thus allowing for a unique biofilm phenotype, with a complex structure containing varying microenvironments. This organization facilitates communication among bacteria contained within the biofilm, allowing for signaling to propagate increased resistance and adaptations to the host's defense mechanisms. Although target signals have been developed, the method of communication and defense within the biofilm is redundant, and the likelihood of developing a single on-off gene product to inhibit the formation of biofilm is unlikely. Strategies that are designed to simultaneously target a variety of signaling pathways within this network may provide a more suitable future method for treatment.

Transfer of Resistance Capability and Emergence of Resistant Strains

Multidrug-resistant organisms are defined as microorganisms that are resistant to one or more classes of antimicrobial agents. Although the names of certain multidrug-resistant organisms describe resistance to only one agent (methicillin-resistant *S aureus* [MRSA], vancomycin-resistant enterococci [VRE]), these bacteria are frequently resistant to most available antimicrobial agents. Certain gram-negative bacilli, including *E coli*, *Klebsiella pneumoniae*, and *Acinetobacter baumannii*, produce extended spectrum β-lactamases and are resistant to multiple classes of antibiotics.

S aureus is responsible for 80% of human osteomyelitis. Six months after methicillin was marketed in October 1960, three methicillin-resistant isolates were reported. Methicillin resistance requires an isolate with a minimum inhibitory concentration (MIC) to oxacillin of at least 4 μg/mL. It is encoded on the *mec* gene, producing penicillin-binding protein PBP2a. By the early 1990s, MRSA accounted for 20% to 25% of *S aureus* isolates in hospitalized patients. By 1999, it accounted for more than 50% of *S aureus* isolates in intensive care units, and that percentage increased to 60% by 2003.

Vancomycin, a glycopeptide antibiotic, is the most widely used agent for the treatment of serious gram-positive infections. The first staphylococci with reduced susceptibility to vancomycin were found in Japan in 1997. The MICs of these vancomycin-intermediate *S aureus* (VISA) isolates range from 4 to 8 μg/mL. More common are strains of MRSA that are heteroresistant to vancomycin (hVISA). These strains contain subpopulations that exhibit reduced susceptibility.

Transfer of Van A-mediated vancomycin resistance from VRE to MRSA first occurred in Michigan in 2002. Five isolates have been recovered to date. Enteroccoci possess several systems, including plasmids and transposons, enabling them to transmit genetic material to other bacteria. The prevalence of VRE increased from less than 1% to approximately 15% by 1997, 25% by 1999, and 30% by 2003.

The emergence of new strains of MRSA in the community in patients without known risk factors was first reported in Australia in the early 1990s. Most MRSA strains isolated from patients with community-acquired infections have been distinct from those endemic in health care settings. Differences in strains of MRSA can

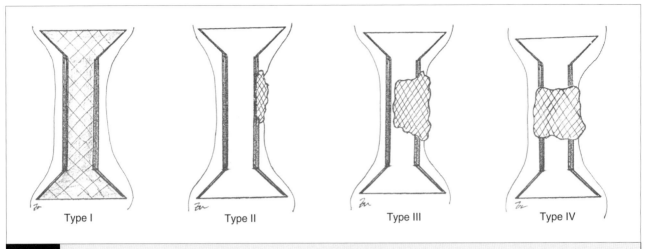

Type I   Type II   Type III   Type IV

Figure 1   Illustration of the Cierny-Mader classification of osteomyelitis. Type I is medullary osteomyelitis (usually hematogenous seeding; intramedullary nail without cortical penetration). Type II is superficial osteomyelitis (external to medullary canal often contiguous with open wound). Type III is invasive/stable osteomyelitis (medullary and external involvement but with axial skeletal stability). Type IV is invasive/unstable osteomyelitis (permeative with unstable segment or segmental loss). (Adapted from Ziran BH, Rao N: Infections, in Baumgaertner MR, Tornetta P III, eds: *Orthopaedic Knowledge Update: Trauma 3*. Rosemont, IL, American Academy of Orthopaedic Surgeons, 2005, p 132.)

be detected on the basis of genotypic analysis with pulsed-field gel electrophoresis, Panton-Valentine leukocidin gene detection, staphylococcal chromosomal cassette (SCC) *mec* typing, multilocus sequence typing, and spa typing. Two pulsed-field types of MRSA, USA 300 and USA 400, account for most community-acquired infections, whereas types USA 100 and USA 200 predominate in health care settings. Community-acquired infections often carry gene complexes for Panton-Valentine leukocidin, a cytotoxin accounting for severe abscesses in otherwise healthy individuals. Another genetic marker found in some strains of MRSA is the SCC *mec* type IVa for methicillin resistance. This genetic cassette is smaller than types I through III, typically found in health care–associated MRSA, and is thought to be more transferable between *S aureus* strains.[10]

Intracellular Persistence of Bacteria

S aureus can remain viable within neutrophils and can invade and survive within osteoblasts.[11] It is likely that these intracellular pathogens are a significant cause of persistent infection and may warrant the use of antibiotics (such as rifampin) that work at the intracellular level.[12]

Classification

A classification system for osteomyelitis was presented in 1970; the information gained with this system is only descriptive and related to pathogenesis.[13] In this classification system, type 1 infections are hematogenous in origin; type 2 are related to a contiguous focus such as an open wound, prior surgical exposure, or fix-

ation; and type 3 are associated with vascular disease and its complications. A more commonly used and helpful classification system is the Cierny-Mader staging system,[14] which integrates the anatomic location and extent of osseous disease as well as the physiologic status of the patient or host, and provides a framework to consider disease beyond osseous pathology. The anatomic portion of the staging system is easiest to apply to the long bones and is divided into four types (**Figure 1**). Type I is limited to medullary involvement; type II is superficial and involves cortical bone; type III is localized and involves both cortical and medullary elements; and type IV is diffuse with extensive involvement. Type IV is further differentiated by inherent skeletal instability following resection.

The staging system is further divided into subtypes that characterize the physiology of the host and its ability to respond in a positive manner physiologically and immunologically to treatment protocols. Type A hosts have normal physiology without significant systemic disease or local tissue factors. Type B hosts can be locally or systemically compromised. Local compromise may involve chronic open wounds or sinus tracts, prior tissue transfers, or compartment syndrome. Systemically compromised hosts have disease that can impair the normal response to infection, such as diabetes, vascular disease, malnutrition, or other causes of immunosuppression. Assessment of patients with local or systemic infection is necessary to make sure that underlying conditions or issues (for example, tobacco use, nutritional deficiencies, blood glucose level, edema) are treated or corrected before resection is undertaken and to improve the host response to treatment. Type C hosts have significant systemic compromise in the face of severe infection. Staged resection and reconstruction

2: The Polytrauma Patient and Fracture Healing

is believed to be too much of a burden for their impaired physiology, making treatment worse than the disease.[15] Appropriate treatment strategies for type C hosts include chronic suppression, ablation via amputation, or coexistence with the pathogen and wound care as needed.[15]

Evaluation of the Patient With Musculoskeletal Infection

Patient History
Assessment of the patient with a musculoskeletal infection should begin with a careful history. Salient points related to determination of the cause and chronicity of the infection should be reviewed, along with a detailed accounting of the patient's history of injury, medical condition, social history, expectations and desires related to treatment outcome. An injury history that includes open fractures, compartment syndrome, staged or definitive treatment in an external fixator, and the presence of transcutaneous pins should arouse suspicion of infection in a patient with a nonunion, chronic unexplained pain, or a new wound or cellulitis in a previously traumatized limb. Patient evaluation may occur within a short time span from injury or surgery to presentation with an osseous or soft-tissue infection, but it is not uncommon for the evaluation to take place many months or years after the inciting event. In addition, prior episodes of cellulitis, wound-healing problems, and prescriptions for antibiotics may be indicative of an underlying infection. Many patients will have undergone multiple bone and soft-tissue procedures. Response to prior treatment should be discussed, and prior records made available for review if possible. In addition, the patient's medical condition should be carefully documented. Comorbidities such as diabetes, malnutrition, vascular disease, malignancy, and other causes of immunosuppression should be sought and documented. A social history to include tobacco and alcohol use, as well as an assessment of the patient's social and financial support network and available resources, is critical in the evaluation and may help guide treatment recommendations. Consultation with an internist, plastic surgeon, infectious disease specialist, and/or a nutritionist may be appropriate following the initial evaluation to coordinate and plan treatment. An appraisal of the patient's desires and expectations begins while taking a history. Work history and goals as well as overall activity level and physical functioning should be discussed. A patient employed as a manual laborer with the goal of returning to this work may be directed to job retraining. A treatment plan will take these factors into consideration, and will involve reinforcing realistic patient goals and expectations or revising those that are unrealistic or not attainable.

Clinical Evaluation
The physical examination of a patient with a suspected musculoskeletal infection may lead immediately to the diagnosis when the patient has an open wound with exposed bone or implants, or the presentation may be more subtle and unimpressive. A careful assessment of the soft tissues is mandatory and includes all native healthy tissues as well as all prior incisions, open wounds, sinus tracts, and graft sites. These areas should be documented or photographed. Local edema, warmth, erythema, and tenderness should be sought. Deformity, gross motion, and pain with stress at a fracture site should be noted and are evidence of a malunited or ununited fracture. Joint range of motion should be assessed. Incisions associated with tissue transfer or vascular repair and reconstruction may be sought when the patient is unsure about what prior procedures were done and there are no records available for review. A careful neurologic and vascular examination should be documented.

Laboratory Evaluation
Initial laboratory studies include an assessment of the systemic inflammatory markers erythrocyte sedimentation rate (ESR) and C-reactive protein (CRP), as well as a complete blood count. Patients who are seen within 3 weeks after trauma or surgery may have an elevated ESR and CRP level.[16] The CRP level is expected to drop to preoperative/preinjury levels 3 weeks after trauma or surgery. The ESR may remain elevated for months and is therefore less reliable as an indicator of infection. The white blood cell count is commonly normal to minimally elevated in patients with chronic indolent infection, but it may be elevated in those with severe infections or an acute presentation. The ESR and CRP level are sensitive but not specific; therefore, they cannot be diagnostic. Elevated ESR and CRP level should heighten suspicion of infection and lead to further testing. Other serum studies that may be useful are a nutritional panel in malnourished patients in whom treatment recommendations can be influenced or those patients who require corrective action before embarking on treatment. Similarly, an elevated level of HbA1C (a serum marker of chronically poor glucose control) in diabetic patients may influence definitive plans or mandate better glycemic control before treatment decisions are made. Blood cultures are unlikely to be helpful unless the presentation includes significant signs or symptoms of systemic illness. In-office culture swabs and/or aspirations of wounds or sinus tracts and needle biopsy specimens have been shown to be unreliable at culturing specific organisms involved in the osseous disease, and isolation of anaerobic organisms, even when present in the bony lesion, is poor.[17-19] Intraoperative cultures have been recommended as the most reliable method of isolating the causative organisms. Multiple bone and soft-tissue specimens should be taken from varying locations in the surgical field and labeled appropriately.

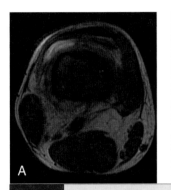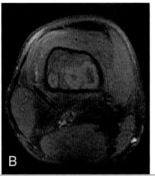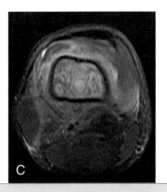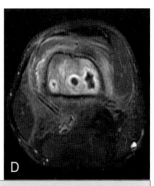

Figure 2 Typical finding on MRI with osteomyelitis. **A,** This T1-weighted fat-sensitive image shows healthy subcutaneous fat. The marrow, which usually has a signal intensity similar to the subcutaneous tissues, has a very low signal intensity. **B,** When the same T1-weighted image has the fat suppressed, the signal intensity of the marrow contents is more similar to that of the surrounding muscle tissue. **C,** This T2 fluid-sensitive image, also with the fat suppressed, demonstrates widespread edema both in and outside of the bone, consistent with a wide inflammatory process. **D,** This last sequence is the same as **B**; however, gadolinium has been added and low signal intensity areas with surrounding enhancement are noted within the marrow. This finding is indicative of the body's attempt to wall off an infection and a pocket of purulent fluid.

Imaging

Conventional radiography is the first-line imaging study when evaluating musculoskeletal infections. Although the imaging workup typically consists of more advanced imaging, plain radiographs offer the ability to follow clinical progress with repeat studies at a lower cost and greater accessibility. Initial radiographs may appear normal, or have subtle changes such as soft-tissue edema, periosteal reaction, and cortical thickening or irregularity. More advanced disease can show sequestrum and involucrum formation, permeative changes, and significant bone resorption and destruction. Evaluation of fracture (if present) healing and alignment along with integrity of associated instrumentation is possible.

MRI can be a very useful adjunct in diagnosing and delineating the extent of osteomyelitis (**Figure 2**). Associated soft-tissue masses and fluid collections as well as sinus tracts can be easily seen, and treatment can be planned based on these findings. One study showed that sensitivities of 98% and specificities of 78% were possible with T1-weighted and short tau inversion recovery sequences, and specificity improved to 82% with the addition of signal change on T2-weighted images as an additional criterion.[20] It can be difficult to obtain quality images after surgery in an orthopaedic patient with metal implants in place. Metal artifact can distort the image, thwarting the ability to assess disease. In addition, healing fractures, bone infarcts, and healed or healing infections can mimic osteomyelitis on MRI. The addition of intravenous gadolinium contrast can improve the ability to differentiate between infection and reparative fibrovascular scar.

CT is useful for assessing detail in bony lesions and in planning surgical resection of diseased bone. Involucrum and sequestrum, as well as cortical erosions and periosteal reaction, can be easily seen, improving the ability to assess the extent of the disease, especially in patients in whom MRI is not possible because of type and location of hardware. Several nuclear medicine studies are available to assist in making the diagnosis. In patients with a known fracture with increased local bone metabolism, little benefit is gained from a technetium Tc 99m (^{99m}Tc) labeled red blood cell study, as it will likely be positive and nondiagnostic. Patients can be assessed after surgery and postinjury with a tagged white blood cell study using either indium 111 or ^{99m}Tc (**Figure 3**). Although indium 111 is regarded as the gold standard, it is more difficult to handle, has poorer image quality, and a higher radiation dose than ^{99m}Tc. Sensitivities of indium 111-tagged white blood cell studies range from 60% to 84%. In addition, immunoscintigraphy is possible with ^{99m}Tc-MAB (monoclonal antigranulocyte antibodies). This tracer has the benefit of wide distribution and high sensitivity and specificity. Limitations include significant difficulty in imaging the spine, pelvis, and proximal femur with this technique because of the abundant and active marrow elements that often create a falsely positive study.[21]

Fluorodeoxyglucose (^{18}F-FDG) positron emission tomography (PET) may help identify orthopaedic infections. PET scanning has the advantage of higher spatial resolution and multiplanar imaging ability, as in other methods of tomography. Background marrow elements have a low glucose metabolism, allowing for better differentiation between normal and disease states. Also, healing fractures see only a small increase in FDG uptake in PET scanning, and this limits significant false-positive results seen in other studies. Drawbacks of PET include a high cost and lack of anatomic landmarks to help assess the precise location and extent of the infection. Improving protocols and access to PET-CT may eliminate the latter concern and make PET-CT the study of choice in the future.[21]

2: The Polytrauma Patient and Fracture Healing

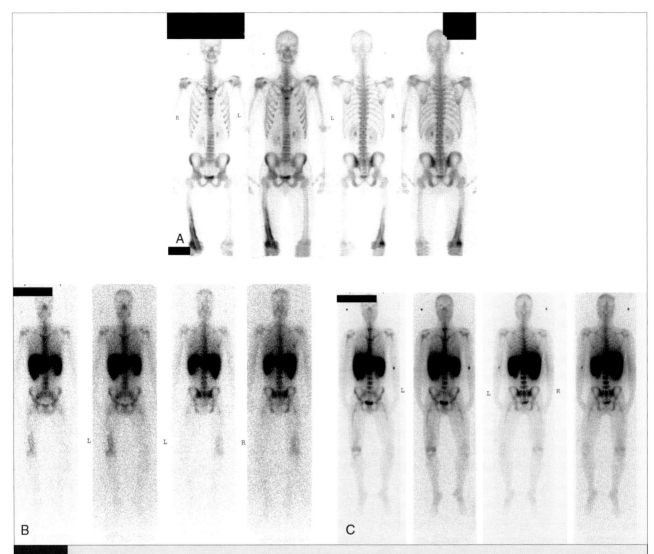

Figure 3 Typical nuclear medicine studies with osteomyelitis. **A**, A bone scan demonstrates areas of high radionucleotide uptake at the distal femur indicative of cellular activity that could be caused by fracture healing, high marrow activity, or infection. **B**, A tagged white blood cell scan also shows high uptake in the distal femur indicative of infection or increased marrow activity. This is not seen with fracture healing or nonunion. Note the uptake in the spleen and liver not seen in the bone scan. **C**, Although there is increased marrow activity in this sulfur colloid study, it does not match that of the white blood cell scan; therefore, all of the uptake cannot be caused by marrow. The diagnosis is osteomyelitis.

Treatment

The treatment of osteomyelitis is complicated and dependent on multiple factors including chronicity of infection, bacterial virulence, host factors, presence of fractures with need for bony stabilization, and integrity of the surrounding soft-tissue envelope. The ultimate goal should be a functional extremity obtained via safe surgical and medical therapy rendered through a multidisciplinary approach.

Principles of Antimicrobial Therapy

Ideally, antibiotic therapy is directed by culture of specific organisms within the infected bone. Unfortunately, osteomyelitis cultures can be negative in as many as 50% of patients, even those with histologically proven osteomyelitis.[22,23] A complete list of antibiotic therapies specific to cultured organisms is provided in **Table 1**. Select oral antimicrobial agents are listed in **Table 2**. Achieving therapeutic levels of antimicrobial agents in bone is difficult. Although cephalosporins and penicillins tend to be the best antibiotics for treating commonly encountered infecting organisms, their concentrations in bone from systemic administration are poor. Quinolones, macrolides, azithromycin, and (most recently) linezolid have been found to have the highest mean bone:serum concentration ratios (commonly between 0.3 and 1.2). By comparison, the ratios are usually between 0.15 and 0.3 for cephalosporins and glycopeptides, and between 0.1 and 0.3 for penicillins.[24-26]

Table 1

Initial Antibiotic Regimens for Patients With Posttraumatic Osteomyelitis

Organism	Antibiotic(s) of First Choice	Alternative Antibiotic(s)
S aureus or coagulase-negative (methicillin-sensitive) staphylococcus	Oxacillin (2 g IV q 6 h) or clindamycin phosphate 900 mg IV q 8 h	First-generation cephalosporin or vancomycin
S aureus or coagulase-negative (methicillin-resistant) staphylococcus	Vancomycin (1 g IV q 12 h) plus rifampin	Linezolid, trimethoprim-sulfamethoxazole, or minocycline plus rifampin
Varied streptococci (groups A and B β-hemolytic organisms or penicillin-sensitive Streptococcus pneumoniae)	Penicillin G (4 million units IV q 6 h)	Clindamycin, erythromycin, vancomycin, or ceftriaxone
Intermediate penicillin-resistant S pneumoniae	Ceftriaxone (2 g IV q 24 h)	Erythromycin, clindamycin, or levofloxacin
Pencillin-resistant S pneumoniae	Vancomycin (1 g IV q 12 h)	Levofloxacin
Enterococcus species	Ampicillin (2 g IV q 6 h) or vancomycin (1 g IV q 12 h)	Ampicillin-sulbactam, linezolid
Enteric gram-negative rods	Fluoroquinolone (such as ciprofloxacin 750 mg orally bid)	Third-generation cephalosporin
Serratia species or Pseudomonas aeruginosa	Levofloxacin (500 mg IV q 24 h), cefepime (2 g IV q 12 h) plus fluoroquinolone	Ertapenem 1 g IV Q 24 h
Anaerobes	Clindamycin (900 mg IV q 8 h)	For gram-negative anaerobes: amoxicillin-clavulanate or metronidazole
Mixed aerobic and anaerobic organisms	Amoxicillin-clavulanate (875 mg and 125 mg, respectively, orally bid)	Ertapenem (1 g IV q 24 h)

IV = intravenously, q = every, bid = twice daily, h = hours.
(Reproduced from Ziran BH, Rao N: Infections, in Baumgaertner MR, Tornetta P III, eds: Orthopaedic Knowledge Update: Trauma 3. Rosemont, IL, American Academy of Orthopaedic Surgeons, 2005, p 137.)

Table 2

Selected Oral Antimicrobial Agents With Excellent Oral Bioavailability Commonly Used to Treat Patients With Musculoskeletal Infection

Fluoroquinolone

Ciprofloxacin

Levofloxacin

Gatifloxacin

Metronidazole

Linezolid

Rifampin

Trimethoprim-sulfamethoxazole

Fluconazole

Itraconazole

(Reproduced from Ziran BH, Rao N: Infections, in Baumgaertner MR, Tornetta P III, eds: Orthopaedic Knowledge Update: Trauma 3. Rosemont, IL, American Academy of Orthopaedic Surgeons, 2005, p 138.)

From a treatment perspective, this makes antimicrobial therapy alone and in short durations impossible for eradication of most bone infections, particularly those that are subacute or chronic. Often, antimicrobial therapy is used as an adjunct to surgical treatment of osteomyelitis, requiring therapy lasting at least 6 weeks or longer, concurrent use of multiple synergistic antibiotics, and prolonged intravenous administration.

Antibiotic suppression is the use of antibiotics to arrest bacterial growth without complete eradication. One common scenario involves suppression in the presence of an infected but incompletely healed fracture following internal fixation. Suppressive therapy is commonly used in such situations to control the infection while awaiting fracture union. Retention of hardware in the face of infection remains a topic of debate among orthopaedists and infectious disease consultants. Although most agree that successful treatment can be attained with retention of implants, recent literature suggests rates of chronic infected nonunion as high as 32% despite antibiotic suppression.[27] Suppressive therapy is also used when eradication of osteomyelitis would require the morbidity of multiple surgeries and is thus

2: The Polytrauma Patient and Fracture Healing

deemed unacceptable in certain patients because of medical comorbidities or advanced age. In these patients, chronic administration of antibiotics is appropriate to suppress the infection and allow for a reasonably functional extremity.

Monitoring of Antimicrobial Therapy

ESR and CRP level are commonly used to assess and follow adequacy of treatment. When these markers fail to demonstrate a predictable decline following medical and surgical treatment, an assessment is made to determine the need for prolonged antibiotics or further surgical débridement. In those patients requiring grafting of bony defects following extensive débridement for osteomyelitis, it is preferable to repeat laboratory analysis 2 to 3 weeks after completion of antibiotics to ensure that a suppressed infection is not present before placing a potential nidus for infection (bone graft) into a previously infected area, though no level I to IV evidence exists to support this practice.

Proper monitoring for toxic effects of antibiotic therapy is essential. Chronic antibiotic therapy often has adverse effects on the kidneys and hematopoietic system. Periodic chemistry panel with measurement of creatinine for renal toxicity and complete blood counts are therefore appropriate throughout the duration of antibiotic treatment.[28-30] In addition, vancomycin and aminoglycosides are associated with ototoxicity.

Antibiotic Depot Devices: Cement and Membrane Formation

Initially popularized in the total joint literature, placement of antibiotic in cement is an excellent mechanism to deliver superconcentrated antibiotics to an area of infected bone. Multiple antibiotic formulations, including the addition of vancomycin, tobramycin, gentamicin, and ciprofloxacin to bone cement, have been studied.[31] Typically, these antibiotics are eluted from the cement for 2 to 6 weeks in concentrations higher than the MIC for bacteria, depending on the antibiotic used. Factors such as bead size (creating an optimal surface area) and brand of cement have been implicated in producing the best environment for bacterial eradication. It has been recognized that the membrane formed around an antibiotic-impregnated spacer may have properties conducive to eventual healing. After artificial diaphyseal defects in rabbits were filled with an antibiotic cement spacer, the spacer was carefully removed, leaving the surrounding membrane intact. Bone graft was placed within this membrane and histologic studies were performed 2, 4, 6, and 8 weeks after implantation. Analysis revealed rich vascularization of the graft adjacent to the membrane. Qualitative and quantitative immunochemistry showed production of growth factors (vascular endothelial growth factor, transforming growth factor-ß1) and osteoinductive factors (bone morphogenetic protein-2), suggesting biologic activity in the membrane formed around antibiotic spacers.[32,33] Antibiotic cement has also been used as a stabiliza-

tion device in long bone diaphyseal infection, using a chest tube or another mold to form an antibiotic-impregnated cement intramedullary nail that can elute antibiotics locally and provide some stability, while obviating concerns of biofilm formation.[34]

Most recently, biodegradable calcium-based antibiotic spacers that elute antibiotics at high concentrations and are later replaced by new bone formation in defects made in animal models have been developed.[35] Application of this technique could decrease the total number of procedures required for reconstruction of bony defects.

Irrigation

After removal of all infected and devitalized tissue, the zone of disease is irrigated to remove bacteria from the remaining tissue. There has been considerable debate over the best irrigation solution and delivery method. A contaminated model was created in a goat with genetically altered luminescent bacteria, and four different irrigation solutions (normal saline, castile soap, bacitracin, and benzalkonium chloride) were tested.[36] All the solutions were delivered with low-pressure pulsed lavage after surgical débridement. Using a photon counting camera, bacterial counts were evaluated. All groups had a significant immediate decrease in bacterial count, with castile soap and normal saline having the best and worst performance, respectively. However, all groups experienced an increase in bacterial counts at 48 hours (rebound effect) that was lowest for the normal saline group. In addition, pulse lavage was compared with bulb irrigation in this same model using only normal saline. Although a similar significant decrease in bacterial counts was noted postoperatively in both groups, the rebound effect at 48 hours was greatest in the pulsed lavage group. These findings suggest that normal saline delivered at the lowest pressure may be superior to all other irrigation fluids and methods of delivery, though a clinical trial would be beneficial to confirm these results.

Hyperbaric Oxygen

Hyperbaric oxygen has been suggested as an adjunct in the treatment of osteomyelitis, especially when compromised oxygenation of tissue exists due to local trauma or vascular disease. Although several case series support the use of this modality to promote wound healing, few have control groups and none delineates which patient factors would predict a favorable response to this treatment, which in some locations may be difficult to access.[37] There is one case series looking specifically at hyperbaric oxygen as an adjunct for treating osteomyelitis, in which this modality was used to treat recalcitrant disease in 13 femurs along with débridement and antibiotics.[38] Success was reported in 12 (92%) of the patients treated. Better clinical trials with control groups are needed to determine the benefit of hyperbaric oxygen in the treatment of osteomyelitis.

Surgical Treatment

Osteomyelitis is a disease of devitalized bone and soft tissue, occasionally existing in the presence of foreign surgical hardware, where bacteria can attach and be protected from the body's natural defense systems. The cornerstone of treatment is débridement of infected bone and surrounding necrotic tissue.[21] Complete treatment of osteomyelitis mandates extensive excision of this tissue to include all devitalized bone and surrounding soft tissue.[1] To date, no better intraoperative assessment of bone and tissue viability exists than the presence of bleeding tissue (the paprika sign).[39] Bony defects are filled with antibiotic spacers, and soft-tissue defects are covered using rotational or free tissue transfer flaps.[40] Most of the adjuncts mentioned in this chapter are applied before bony defects are filled. Although the topic of bone defects is beyond the scope of this discussion, options include grafting (vascularized and nonvascularized), bone graft substitutes, and distraction osteogenesis. Each of these techniques has been reported in the literature with varying degrees of success. The bone must be stabilized throughout treatment and can be accomplished with internal fixation, although biofilm formation and incomplete eradication of bacteria is cause for concern. External fixation has also been advocated, although pins can be a source of new infection and can limit the use of subsequent fixation devices. Intramedullary nails should be used only in a staged fashion if an external fixator has been in place longer than 3 weeks, because of risk of infection. Casting can be used but may limit the clinician's ability to access wounds and is often less stable than other forms of fixation.

Ultimately, the limb may prove to be unsalvageable, making amputation necesssary. The best indications for amputation involve situations where the function of the salvaged limb is inferior to anticipated function following amputation and subsequent prosthetic fitting. When treatment has been so prolonged as to limit the individual from continuing a productive life or the extremity infection results in life-threatening systemic illness, amputation should be considered. Although sepsis is rare in osteomyelitis, amputation must also be considered when limb salvage becomes a threat to patient survival.

Summary

Diagnosis and treatment of osteomyelitis is challenging and requires an individualized and multidisciplinary approach for successful treatment. A thoughtful assessment of the patient and his or her goals will assist in developing an individualized treatment plan. Involving colleagues across disciplines to prepare the patient for and assist with treatment can improve disease eradication and outcomes.

Annotated References

1. Lazzarini L, Mader JT, Calhoun JH: Osteomyelitis in long bones. *J Bone Joint Surg Am* 2004;86(10):2305-2318.

   The features of osteomyelitis are discussed, along with a description of etiology, pathogenesis, experimental data, clinical manifestations, and treatment methodology.

2. Pollack A: Rising threat of infections unfazed by antibiotics. *New York Times*, February 27, 2010.

3. Marc JM, Bonten MJM, Slaughter S, et al: The role of colonization pressure in the spread of vancomycin-resistant enterococci: An important infection control variable. *Arch Intern Med* 1998;158:1127-1132.

4. Cierny G III, Mader JT, Penninck JJ: A clinical staging system for adult osteomyelitis. *Clin Orthop Relat Res* 2003;414:7-24.

5. Elek SD, Conen PE: The virulence of Staphylococcus pyogenes for man: A study of the problems of wound infection. *Br J Exp Pathol* 1957;38(6):573-586.

6. Chu CC, Williams DF: Effects of physical configuration and chemical structure of suture materials on bacterial adhesion: A possible link to wound infection. *Am J Surg* 1984;147(2):197-204.

7. Patti JM, Bremell T, Krajewska-Pietrasik D, et al: The Staphylococcus aureus collagen adhesion is a virulence determinant in experimental septic arthritis. *Infect Immun* 1994;62:152-161.

8. Fux CA, Costerton JW, Stewart PS, Stoodley P: Survival strategies of infectious biofilms. *Trends Microbiol* 2005;13(1):34-40.

   This review article discusses the current concepts of biofilms and the related strategies that bacteria use to evade host defenses. The overall structure and defense mechanisms of organisms using biofilms are described. The concept of quorum sensing, and how it applies to the organization of biofilms at the microcellular level, is explained.

9. Ng WL, Bassler BL: Bacterial quorum-sensing network architectures. *Annu Rev Genet* 2009;43:197-222.

   The authors review the mechanisms concerning quorum sensing and discuss the differences between two quorum-sensing systems, and how they are different from other paradigmatic bacterial signal transduction systems.

10. Healthcare Infection Control Practices Advisory Committee (HICPAC): Management of multidrug-resistant organisms in healthcare settings, 2006. Centers for Disease Control and Prevention. http://www.cdc.gov/hicpac/mdro/mdro_3.html

11. Garzoni C, Kelley WL: Staphylococcus aureus: New evidence for intracellular persistence. *Trends Microbiol* 2009;17(2):59-65.

2: The Polytrauma Patient and Fracture Healing

This article discusses some of the more recent literature providing evidence that *Staphylococcus* species maintain the ability to persist intracellularly in host epithelial cells and even after phagocytosis by neutrophils, contributing to the persistence of orthopaedic infections.

12. Ellington JK, Harris M, Hudson MC, Vishin S, Webb LX, Sherertz R: Intracellular Staphylococcus aureus and antibiotic resistance: Implications for treatment of staphylococcal osteomyelitis. *J Orthop Res* 2006;24(1):87-93.

   This is an experimental study in which mouse osteoblasts were allowed to be invaded by *S aureus*. Rifampin was useful in helping to eradicate infection, and if *S aureus* was allowed to prevail longer than 12 hours intracellularly, the bacteria would develop antibiotic resistance through various mechanisms, including observed structural changes in the form of an intracellular capsule.

13. Waldvogel FA, Medoff G, Swartz MN: Osteomyelitis: A review of clinical features, therapeutic considerations and unusual aspects. *N Engl J Med* 1970;282(4):198-206.

14. Cierny G, Mader JT: Adult chronic osteomyelitis: An overview. *Orthopedics* 1984;7:1557-1564.

15. Cierny G III, Mader JT: Approach to adult osteomyelitis. *Orthop Rev* 1987;16(4):259-270.

16. Neumaier M, Scherer MA: C-reactive protein levels for early detection of postoperative infection after fracture surgery in 787 patients. *Acta Orthop* 2008;79:428.

   The authors present a prospective study of 787 patients undergoing surgical treatment of fractures. Findings included a peak C-reactive protein level on postoperative day 2 in comparison with preoperative levels, then gradually returning to normal. In 17 of the 787 patients, a postoperative infection (culture positive) developed. These patients showed a persistent rise or a second peak developed in the C-reactive protein level beyond postoperative day 4. The authors concluded that the postoperative C-reactive protein levels are a reliable indicator of infection if compared with preoperative levels, and if abnormal levels persist beyond the fourth postoperative day.

17. Perry CR, Pearson RL, Miller GA: Accuracy of cultures of material from swabbing of the superficial aspect of the wound and needle biopsy in the preoperative assessment of osteomyelitis. *J Bone Joint Surg Am* 1991;73(5):745-749.

18. Agarwal S, Zahid M, Sherwani MK, Abbas M, Huda N, Khan AQ: Comparison of the results of sinus track culture and sequestrum culture in chronic osteomyelitis. *Acta Orthop Belg* 2005;71(2):209-212.

   A prospective study compared the bacterial flora obtained from sequestrum culture versus sinus track culture. Sinus track cultures were done and the results were compared with culture of the sequestrum. There was a discrepancy between the bacterial flora grown from sinus track and sequestrum cultures in 33 of 62 patients.

19. Akinyoola AL, Adegbehingbe OO, Aboderin AO: Therapeutic decision in chronic osteomyelitis: Sinus track culture versus intraoperative bone culture. *Arch Orthop Trauma Surg* 2009;129(4):449-453.

   The authors assessed the concordance of sinus track culture with that of intraoperative bone culture to guide antibiotic therapy in patients with chronic osteomyelitis in a prospective comparative study. Intraoperative bone culture appears to predict more reliably the complete etiologic organisms than sinus track culture in chronic osteomyelitis.

20. Erdman WA, Tamburro F, Jayson HT, Weatherall PT, Ferry KB, Peshock RM: Osteomyelitis: Characteristics and pitfalls of diagnosis with MR imaging. *Radiology* 1991;180(2):533-539.

21. Kaim AH, Gross T, von Schulthess GK: Imaging of chronic posttraumatic osteomyelitis. *Eur Radiol* 2002;12(5):1193-1202.

22. Floyed RL, Steele RW: Culture-negative osteomyelitis. *Pediatr Infect Dis J* 2003;22(8):731-736.

23. Wu JS, Gorbachova T, Morrison WB, Haims AH: Imaging-guided bone biopsy for osteomyelitis: Are there factors associated with positive or negative cultures? *AJR Am J Roentgenol* 2007;188(6):1529-1534.

   The authors present a retrospective review of 800 consecutive patients undergoing imaging-guided core bone biopsies. Forty-one patients had histologically proven osteomyelitis; 14 (34%) had positive cultures. It was concluded that the rate of positive culture results in histologically proven osteomyelitis obtained from imaging-guided bone biopsies is low.

24. Landersdorfer CB, Bulitta JB, Kinzig M, Holzgrabe U, Sörgel F: Penetration of antibacterials into bone: Pharmacokinetic, pharmacodynamic and bioanalytical considerations. *Clin Pharmacokinet* 2009;48(2):89-124.

   The authors present an excellent review of multiple classes of antibiotics and their concentration levels attained in various tissue types, including bone (subdivided into cortical and cancellous).

25. Rao N, Ziran BH, Hall RA, Santa ER: Successful treatment of chronic bone and joint infections with oral linezolid. *Clin Orthop Relat Res* 2004;427:67-71.

   The authors present the results of a prospective, observational study of 11 patients with culture-positive osteomyelitis or periprosthetic joint infections treated with linezolid between 1999 and 2001. All patients were not candidates for vancomycin chemotherapy because of prior adverse reaction, allergy, or failure of treatment. After surgical treatment, patients received intravenous linezolid and were transitioned to oral linezolid for a minimum of 6 weeks. All 11 patients had clinical remission after a mean follow-up of 27 months.

26. Razonable RR, Osmon DR, Steckelberg JM: Linezolid therapy for orthopedic infections. *Mayo Clin Proc* 2004;79(9):1137-1144.

The authors present a retrospective review of 20 consecutive patients who took linezolid for the treatment of orthopaedic infections. Fifty-five percent (11 patients) achieved clinical cure, and 7 (35%) had clinical improvement but received long-term antimicrobial suppressive therapy. It was concluded that linezolid may be an effective alternative therapy for orthopaedic infections due to linezolid-susceptible gram-positive bacteria.

27. Rightmire E, Zurakowski D, Vrahas M: Acute infections after fracture repair: Management with hardware in place. *Clin Orthop Relat Res* 2008;466(2):466-472.

The effectiveness of hardware retention, antibiotic suppression, as well as irrigation and débridement in the face of acute osteomyelitis, was evaluated. Of 69 patients, successful results were reported in 68% and unsuccessful results in 32%. Patients who smoked were 3.7 times more likely to have unsuccessful results. The overall success rates of treating infection with hardware retention is questioned.

28. John R, Herzenberg AM: Renal toxicity of therapeutic drugs. *J Clin Pathol* 2009;62(6):505-515.

Several therapeutic agents can adversely affect kidney function, resulting in tubulointerstitial, glomerular, or vascular disease. This review describes the morphologic patterns of drug-induced disease in the kidney.

29. Whitman CB, Joseph JM, Sjoholm LO: Cephalosporin-induced leukopenia following rechallenge with cefoxitin. *Ann Pharmacother* 2008;42(9):1327-1332.

The authors describe a case of cefazolin-induced leukopenia in a critically ill patient who developed this adverse reaction upon rechallenge with cefoxitin.

30. Segarra-Newnham M, Tagoff SS: Probable vancomycin-induced neutropenia. *Ann Pharmacother* 2004;38(11):1855-1859.

A case report of vancomycin-induced neutropenia and a review of the literature are presented.

31. Zalavras CG, Patzakis MJ, Holtom P: Local antibiotic therapy in the treatment of open fractures and osteomyelitis. *Clin Orthop Relat Res* 2004;427:86-93.

A bioabsorbable vehicle is impregnated with antibiotic(s) active against the suspected pathogens, aminoglycoside and/or vancomycin. Local antibiotic therapy is a safe technique resulting in high local concentration of antibiotics with minimal systemic levels. Nonabsorbable vehicles may eliminate the need for reoperation and removal.

32. Pelissier P, Masquelet AC, Bareille R, Pelissier SM, Amedee J: Induced membranes secrete growth factors including vascular and osteoinductive factors and could stimulate bone regeneration. *J Orthop Res* 2004;22(1):73-79.

This study evaluated the histologic and biochemical characteristics of membranes induced by the placement of antibiotic impregnated cement spacers in rabbits. Histologic studies revealed rich vascularization. Immunochemistry showed production of growth factors (vascular endothelial growth factor, transforming growth factor-ß1) and osteoinductive factors (bone morphogenetic protein-2).

33. Viateau V, Guillemin G, Calando Y, et al: Induction of a barrier membrane to facilitate reconstruction of massive segmental diaphyseal bone defects: An ovine model. *Vet Surg* 2006;35(5):445-452.

The authors used an ovine model to evaluate membrane formation in staged treatment of segmental diaphyseal bone defects. Histologic examinations at 6 months demonstrated that the induced membrane had vascularized CBFA1+ cells, and very few macrophages entrapped in a collagenous tissue were positive for type I collagen. It was concluded that polymethylmethacrylate-induced membrane constrained the graft, was well vascularized, and may have osteogenic properties.

34. Thonse R, Conway JD: Antibiotic cement-coated nails for the treatment of infected nonunions and segmental bone defects. *J Bone Joint Surg Am* 2008;90(suppl 4):163-174.

The technique and results for using a local antibiotic delivery system to get high antimicrobial concentrations and stability to long bone osteomyelitis are described.

35. Lazarettos J, Efstathopoulos N, Papagelopoulos PJ, et al: A bioresorbable calcium phosphate delivery system with teicoplanin for treating MRSA osteomyelitis. *Clin Orthop Relat Res* 2004;423:253-258.

The effectiveness of calcium phosphate as a delivery system of teicoplanin for treating MRSA was studied. Bacterial eradication signified a considerable decrease of the total histologic scores of osteomyelitis compared with control subjects, accompanied with newly growing host bone. The calcium phosphate with teicoplanin delivery system seems promising for treatment of bone infection attributable to MRSA.

36. Owens BD, White DW, Wenke JC: Comparison of irrigation solutions and devices in a contaminated musculoskeletal wound survival model. *J Bone Joint Surg Am* 2009;91(1):92-98.

Four different irrigation fluids and two different irrigation techniques (pulsed lavage versus bulb) were compared in a contaminated animal model. The quantity of bacteria immediately after treatment and at 48 hours was compared.

37. Wang C, Schwaitzberg S, Berliner E, Zarin DA, Lau J: Hyperbaric oxygen for treating wounds: A systematic review of the literature. *Arch Surg* 2003;138(3):272-279, discussion 280.

38. Chen CE, Ko JY, Fu TH, Wang CJ: Results of chronic osteomyelitis of the femur treated with hyperbaric oxygen: A preliminary report. *Chang Gung Med J* 2004;27(2):91-97.

Hyperbaric oxygen therapy has been used as an adjunct in the management of chronic osteomyelitis in many hospitals in Taiwan. This retrospective study investigated the clinical results of hyperbaric oxygen therapy for chronic refractory osteomyelitis of the femur. Hyperbaric oxygen therapy is an effective and safe adjunctive therapy for the management of chronic refractory osteomyelitis of the femur.

39. Sachs BL, Shaffer JW: A staged Papineau protocol for chronic osteomyelitis. *Clin Orthop Relat Res* 1984;184: 256-263.

40. Tulner SA, Schaap GR, Strackee SD, Besselaar PP, Luitse JS, Marti RK: Long-term results of multiple-stage treatment for posttraumatic osteomyelitis of the tibia. *J Trauma* 2004;56(3):633-642.

A retrospective analysis of 47 patients treated for post-traumatic osteomyelitis of the tibia is presented. Using the Cierny-Mader classification, most patients had a localized osteomyelitis. A staged approach involved débridement, antibiotics, flap coverage, and late bone grafting. The average follow-up was 94 months, and only 9% of patients had a recurrence of osteomyelitis requiring additional surgical interventions. Staged surgery proved to be an excellent method of treating osteomyelitis.

Chapter 16

Damage Control Orthopaedics: Practical Issues

Philip R. Wolinsky, MD   Michael T. Charlton, MD

Introduction

Damage control orthopaedics (DCO), or the staged stabilization of long bone fractures, is an emerging area with treatment recommendations that are still being developed. The systemic effects of orthopaedic surgery and trauma, the interactions between them, and current treatment recommendations regarding the timing and type of fracture fixation for trauma patients are the focus of this chapter. A more thorough discussion of the pathophysiologic principles that support the treatment concepts herein is presented in chapter 12.

Benefits of Early Fracture Stabilization

Historically, long bone fractures were initially treated with traction. Definitive fixation was performed on a delayed basis, after the peak of fat embolization (FE) and fat embolization syndrome had passed. During the 1970s, due to improvements in intensive care, anesthesia, and surgical techniques, many fracture patients underwent earlier surgery. Studies published during the 1980s and 1990s demonstrated the benefits of early stabilization of long bone fractures, particularly for patients with multiple injuries. The incidence of fat embolization syndrome or adult respiratory distress syndrome (ARDS), the mortality rate, and the length of intensive care unit and hospital stay decreased as a result of early long bone fracture stabilization and had the greatest effect on the most severely injured patients.

These findings led to the era of early total care. In this paradigm, lower extremity long bone fractures, and femur fractures in particular, were stabilized as early as possible regardless of length of surgery or consideration of the status of the patient. However, some patients did not tolerate early total care well, leading to the concept that certain patient groups were "at risk" for complications after immediate definitive fracture management. Although the general consensus remains that long bone fractures should be stabilized acutely, a topic of current debate centers around the optimal method of the initial stabilization that should be used, that is, definitive nailing or staged treatment with a provisional external fixator. The latter approach is referred to as DCO. Extensive research is under way to determine which patients can tolerate early definitive stabilization and which benefit from a staged, DCO approach.[1]

Risks of Early Stabilization and the Immune System Response to Trauma

The initial injury leads to damage that can include soft-tissue injuries, fractures, hypoxia, hypotension, reperfusion injury, and head injuries. This constellation is referred to as the "first hit." Physicians have no control over the extent of the first hit. Later stressors, including episodes of sepsis or interventions such as anesthesia and surgery, are referred to as a "second hit." As discussed in chapter 12, a second hit can further activate the systemic inflammatory response and compound the initial damage. Surgery, while beneficial in the repair of fractures, also stimulates the immune system. Surgical procedures, particularly intramedullary femoral instrumentation, cause the release of inflammatory mediators and prime circulating polymorphonuclear white blood cells as well as depression of monocyte function.[2-4] The effect of the surgical procedure seems to be greater if blood loss is high and the procedure is performed earlier after injury.[5] By making decisions about the timing and method of surgical treatment of fractures, surgeons can limit further physiologic insult to the already-injured patient and influence the patient's hospital course.

The interactions between the initial and secondary injuries are mediated by the immune system and the systemic inflammatory response, which are discussed in chapter 12.

Dr. Wolinsky serves as a paid consultant to Zimmer and Biomet, has received research or institutional support from Zimmer and Synthes, and has received nonincome support (such as equipment or services), commercially derived honoraria, or other non–research-related funding (such as paid travel) from AO North America. Dr. Charlton or an immediate family member has received research or institutional support from Synthes and has received nonincome support (such as equipment or services), commercially derived honoraria, or other non–research-related funding (such as paid travel) from AO North America.

2: The Polytrauma Patient and Fracture Healing

How to Evaluate Patients and Limit Risks

All long bone fractures are not the same and may occur as isolated injuries or in combination with other system derangements, and the patient may be completely or incompletely resuscitated. Research has sought to define the best treatment strategy in the face of commonly encountered injury combinations. Patient groups that have been studied extensively include those with long bone fractures and thoracic injuries or head injuries, underresuscitated/hypoperfused patients, and those with a combination of these factors.

Thoracic Injuries

Patients with thoracic injuries were the initial focus of studies performed in Europe in the early 1990s, which suggested that early reamed nailing of femoral shaft fractures in these patients led to an increase in ARDS. Because it was known that femoral reaming caused embolization of marrow contents to the lungs, this conclusion seemed logical. However, other studies, including some from North America, concluded that it was the severity of the pulmonary injury, and not the treatment method of the femoral fracture, that determined the risk of ARDS. To date, a definitive association between reamed femoral nailing and development of ARDS in the setting of thoracic injury remains unproven and continues to be a topic of extensive debate. Based on current evidence, it is reasonable to individualize the timing and method of long bone stabilization according to the patient's clinical condition. Patients who are incompletely resuscitated undergo damage control procedures in many centers, that is, external fixation, which provides rapid fracture stabilization with little blood loss, in order to minimize the second hit. This approach can be considered in any patient for whom definitive fixation with nailing is not yet appropriate, whether it is due to patient-related factors or surgeon-institutional resources that may dictate that a delay is necessary. Other centers continue to rely primarily on early stabilization with definitive reamed intramedullary nails. Recently, a provocative study reported on a damage control strategy in which rapid retrograde nailing without reaming is carried out simultaneously with other emergency procedures, such as exploratory laparotomy. The surgeons who reported their clinical experience with this approach note that in multiply injured patients undergoing surgery for other injuries, retrograde nailing of the femur with small-diameter nails placed without reaming can be accomplished expeditiously in about the same time as placement of an external fixator, avoiding some of the problems with external fixation of the femur such as pin tract infection and the need for early conversion to a definitive method of fixation.[6] However, although unreamed retrograde nailing may be applied as rapidly as external fixation, it still results in potentially more blood loss and marrow embolization than placement of an external fixator, and these factors, rather than time in the operating room,

correlate with the amount of stimulation to the immune system.[5] It must be emphasized that there is no widespread experience with this technique, and further validation must be obtained before it can be recommended as an acceptable practice.

Head-Injured Patients

Numerous studies support both sides of the controversy regarding early fracture stabilization in patients with head injuries. At issue is the possibility of a secondary injury to the brain caused by intraoperative hypotension or hypoxia. Even one such episode can result in a higher mortality rate and a higher incidence of a vegetative state.[7] Patients with a severe head injury (defined as a Glasgow Coma Score of 8 or lower) experience disruption of the autoregulation of their cerebral blood flow. When this occurs, cerebral perfusion pressure becomes dependent on mean arterial pressure. A decrease in mean arterial pressure leads to reduction in cerebral blood flow; therefore, any hypotensive episodes during early fracture fixation, or any other procedure, can lead to cerebral ischemia, secondary brain injury, and a compromised neurologic outcome. Patients who undergo early stabilization of their fractures have associated blood loss and fluid resuscitation needs that could affect the brain in the setting of associated head injury. Nevertheless, the current literature is inconclusive and controversy remains as to whether early long bone stabilization in patients with mild, moderate, or severe brain injury either enhances or worsens outcome.[8]

Indisputably, in order to safely carry out early fracture surgery in head-injured patients, cerebral perfusion pressure must be maintained and often requires invasive monitoring, may require the use of vasoactive drugs, and often mandates the resuscitation of the patient by the infusion of blood products. If these techniques are not available, definitive early surgery should not be performed, and the patient should be considered for transfer to a tertiary trauma center with neurosurgical support.

Compensated Shock

Some evidence exists that patients in compensated shock (normal vital signs) are at risk for complications after early definitive surgery. In a retrospective review, patients with an Injury Severity Score (ISS) $\geq$ 18 and a femur fracture that was stabilized within 24 hours of admission with a reamed nail, who at the time of surgery did not have any clinical signs of shock (normotensive, not tachycardic, and adequate urine output) were retrospectively divided into two groups based on lactate levels (normal and abnormal).[9] The group with a lactate level greater than 2.5 mmol/L had a higher pulmonary and infectious complication rate. This study highlights the importance of monitoring more sensitive parameters such as lactate to assess response to resuscitation.[9]

Fat Embolism Syndrome

Substantial data in the literature demonstrate that reamed femoral nailing results in systemic FE. Normal femoral canal pressures in humans measure approximately 65 mm Hg. Because the femur has no venous valves, canal contents will drain into the bloodstream when the driving pressure exceeds the normal intramedullary (IM) pressure. Animal and human studies have shown that reamed femoral nailing causes development of pressures that are high enough to generate FE and that pulmonary FE occurs during the procedure. Animal studies have shown that IM canal instrumentation leads to an increased IM pressure, which causes bone marrow contents to enter the blood and then move to the lung. On the way to the lung the thrombi become surrounded by activated platelets. In the lung, bone marrow contents and thrombi stimulate an intense inflammatory response. Fat has been shown to activate inflammatory cells in laboratory studies. Pulmonary FE also causes a transient increase in pulmonary artery pressure that is likely mediated via vasoconstrictive agents liberated in the lung. The pulmonary effects of FE may be potentiated by other systemic injuries, such as systemic hypotension and/or a lung injury.[10]

Studies have also shown that reamed femoral nailing stimulates the immune system. Patients with femur fractures have elevated cytokine levels at admission, and cytokine levels rise even further after reamed femoral nailing. A prospective, randomized study of "stable" patients who were randomized to early intramedullary nailing versus external fixation followed by later IM nailing found that an early IM femoral nail was associated with increased systemic inflammation, while an initial external fixator was not.[3]

There is recent evidence that blood loss, length of the procedure, and earlier postinjury procedures may be important in stimulation of the immune system in multiply injured patients. The longer the operation, the more blood that is lost; the sooner after injury the procedure is done, the greater the stimulation of the immune system.[11,12]

Timing of Fracture Repair

Recent studies have examined the effect of immediate definitive long bone stabilization (early total care) on the systemic inflammatory response, compared with damage control procedures. One of the first randomized prospective trials addressing this issue, as mentioned previously, demonstrated that the proinflammatory markers interleukin (IL)-6 and IL-8 were both significantly elevated in multiply injured patients undergoing immediate femoral IM nailing as opposed to external fixation, with peak IL-6 values occurring at 24 hours following early total care. No effect on clinical outcome was noted.[13] Levels of these markers were not shown to increase following conversion of external fixation to IM nailing, even though conversion took place

at an average of 2.9 days after injury. Other studies have shown the peak inflammatory response occurs within 2 to 4 days after injury. Sample size and selection criteria (patients with severe chest trauma were excluded) are possible reasons for these discrepancies.[14]

A more recent study retrospectively evaluated the effect of early total care versus DCO on the systemic inflammatory response syndrome (SIRS) scores and the incidence of multiorgan system failure.[3] The SIRS score is a validated scoring system that is composed of four variables scored at 0 or 1, for a final maximum score of 4 points. These variables include leukocyte count above 12 or below 4, pulse greater than 90 beats per minute, respiratory rate above 20 breaths per minute (or $Pco_2 <$ 33 mm Hg), and core body temperature above 38° or below 34°C. A score above 1, in the absence of sepsis, constitutes a systemic inflammatory response. Despite higher initial New Injury Severity Scores in the DCO group, patients undergoing DCO procedures had a smaller and shorter postoperative systemic inflammatory response than those undergoing immediate IM nailing. Patients undergoing conversion from external fixation to IM nailing at the height of their systemic inflammatory response showed the most pronounced subsequent inflammatory response, which was correlated with organ failure. This finding suggests that the risk of organ failure and the detrimental effects of the so-called second hit phenomenon are not mitigated by damage control procedures alone. Rather, the timing of conversion may play a pivotal role in reducing morbidity and mortality in these critically injured patients, and likely is related to the period and intensity of the individual patient's systemic inflammatory response. Many factors likely contribute to SIRS in individual patients, including injury severity, the number of organ systems initially involved, preexisting medical comorbidities, age and overall health of the patient, and the quality and immediacy of the resuscitative measures. Additionally, although the direct effect of IM reaming on pulmonary status remains controversial, it is possible that the burden of prolonged surgical care associated with early definitive fixation and the attendant risks of hypothermia, acidosis, blood and fluid loss, and coagulopathy serve to exacerbate the cascade of systemic inflammation that is associated with multisystem organ failure.[15]

Although most of the recent literature advocating damage control procedures has done so in the context of severely injured polytrauma patients, DCO strategies are being increasingly used in the management of simple isolated injuries in which immediate definitive management poses little additional risk. This misapplication adds to the burden of financially strapped trauma centers and, more importantly, potentially places patients at undue risk associated with multiple procedures, in addition to the obvious associated risks of delaying definitive care. The use of DCO should be reserved for critically injured polytrauma patients for whom the immediate burden of early total care is likely to have deleterious effects. After

2: The Polytrauma Patient and Fracture Healing

appropriate stabilization, as measured by markers of the systemic inflammatory response (not readily available in most centers), ISS (mostly used for research), or continued metabolic derangement (base deficit, plasma lactate, persistent coagulopathy), expedient conversion to definitive forms of fixation is desirable.

Management strategies, therefore, should be individually focused and predicated on identifying those factors that may place the polytrauma patient at an unacceptably high risk for early definitive care. Even so, the decision to use damage control measures universally in critically ill patients has not been shown to improve outcomes with regard to mortality. A meta-analysis of 63 controlled trials assessing the timing for surgical treatment of femoral shaft fractures in multiply injured patients revealed that no consistent definition existed for "early" versus "late" treatment arms.[16] Furthermore, widespread recommendations across the treatment spectrum, mostly unsupported by biochemical data, were noted. A subanalysis of 27 studies providing data on mortality in patients definitively treated in less than versus greater than 24 hours revealed an odds ratio of 0.89 (95% confidence interval, 0.51-1.53), suggesting no clear benefit to either treatment strategy. Of note, however, is that an additional analysis of four studies comparing surgical treatment within 24 hours versus nonsurgical management revealed a combined odds ratio of 0.07 (95% confidence interval: 0.03-0.14), highly favoring the surgical treatment group ($P<$ 0.00001). These data clearly support some form of early fracture stabilization, either with a damage control procedure or through definitive early total care. The same article also reviewed the management strategies used through a retrospective review of cases collected through the German Trauma Society Registry. A forward stepwise logistic regression analysis revealed that Glasgow Coma Scores, Abbreviated Injury Severity Scores for the Thorax, and prothrombin time were the three best predictors of femoral shaft treatment initially by external fixation. The German Trauma Society Registry study revealed that most surgeons applied what the authors described as "risk adaptive DCO," with wide variation in the criteria used in the decision making process and perhaps treatment decisions influenced by the level of support at the various hospital trauma centers.[17]

Timing of Conversion: External Fixation to Reamed IM Nailing of the Femur

The timing of conversion from DCO external fixation to definitive fixation has been investigated by multiple authors. A recent study prospectively evaluated potential advantages and complication rates associated with the staged management of fractures in critically injured patients (75 patients with ISS = 37.3). The fractures underwent conversion at an average of 13.7 days (range, 3 to 46 days). The authors concluded that external fix-

ation was faster than early total care procedures and resulted in significantly less blood loss. The risks of complications including pin tract infections, deep infections, and nonunions were no higher for the patients who underwent staged fixation. There were no adverse effects on reduction quality and time to mobilization, rehabilitation, or functional treatment in patients treated in a staged fashion. DCO strategies were thought to be effective, time saving, and safe.[18]

Unresolved Controversies

The following questions remain unanswered: 1. Do readily available, objective criteria exist at the time of injury that can be used to assess which patients are at unacceptably high risk for early total care? 2. What are the optimal specific biochemical markers that can characterize the individual patient's response to resuscitative measures? 3. Are these tests available and practical in the clinical setting? 4. Do treatment strategies based on these criteria affect mortality, risk of further complications, or long-term functional results in multiply injured patients?

Experience Gained From the Wars in Iraq and Afghanistan

Similar to previous wars, the current conflicts in Southwest Asia have yielded valuable information regarding the management of trauma victims. Unlike in past wars, the use of highly effective body armor has reduced the number of fatal wounds caused by penetrating trauma to the chest and abdomen. This increased survivability, in addition to higher proportions of wounds due to blast injury and burns from improvised explosive devices, has necessitated the treatment of severe orthopaedic injuries in casualties who may not have survived in previous conflicts.

Hemorrhage Control

Local Agents

Exsanguination is the leading preventable cause of combat-related death in 50% of those killed in action (those dying before reaching a medical facility).[19] As a result, the military medical community has undertaken an extensive effort to prevent exsanguination. At the field level, personnel carry first aid kits containing combat application tourniquets, clot-promoting bandages, fibrin sealant dressings, and powder-formulated hemostatic agents for direct wound application.[20,21] All combat troops receive "self aid and buddy care" training in the use of these devices before deployment. Upon reaching medical personnel, casualties receive whole blood or the 1:1 use of packed red cells in conjunction with plasma.

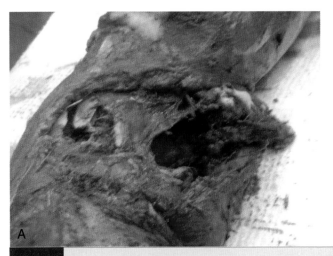
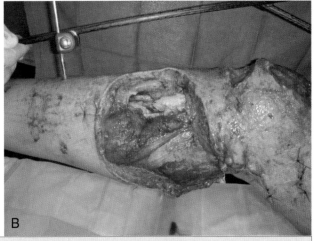

Figure 1 The quality of the initial débridement is paramount. **A,** Photograph of a blast wound prior to initial débridement. **B,** The same wound after serial débridements 4 days later, showing a mostly viable muscle bed with skip areas of muscle and bone necrosis.

Recombinant Activated Factor VIIa

Recombinant activated factor VIIa (rFVIIa) has been increasingly used to treat and potentially mitigate bleeding at the site of injury. The drug's mechanism of action theoretically makes it an ideal candidate for use in trauma because its effects are believed to be limited to the site of injury with no effect on the overall systemic coagulation cascade. In a series of seven critically injured patients with massive transfusion requirements (25 to 49 units of packed red blood cells), cessation of diffuse bleeding and a decrease in transfusion requirements following rFVIIa administration were reported, and it was concluded that rFVIIa may play a role as an adjunctive hemostatic measure.[22] Subsequently, a recent review of six large animal studies and one prospective randomized study in elective surgery revealed reduced blood loss and a decreased need for transfusion.[23] Further research to better determine systemic and localized effects, optimum dosing regimens, safety profiles, and efficacy in preventing life-threatening hemorrhage is needed.

Hypotensive Fluid Resuscitation

The revived strategy of controlled resuscitation has gained favor among military medical outfits in the forward deployed setting. Because bleeding is the most recognized preventable cause of mortality, emphasis is placed on first controlling hemorrhage directly followed by the execution of controlled fluid resuscitation designed to restore a functional yet hypotensive circulating volume that will not disrupt previously formed clots. This strategy is born out of the vastly different prehospital setting found in combat as opposed to urban civilian trauma and is based on the premise that hemorrhage control is paramount and logistic constraints abound.[24] Battlefield casualties are given intravenous fluids such as high molecular weight hetastarch

(500 mL) in the prehospital setting based solely on the presence of obvious massive blood loss with the absence of a radial pulse and incoherent mental status. Because 500 mL of high molecular weight hetastarch is equivalent to 3,000 mL of lactated Ringer solution, no more than 1,000 mL of hetastarch is administered to a single patient. Although intravenous access is emphasized (single 18 gauge), it is primarily used for the administration of pain medication and antibiotics and used only for fluid resuscitation when all of the above criteria are met. Patients are categorized as responders, transient responders, and nonresponders and are triaged and evacuated accordingly based on the tactical scenario. Hypotensive resuscitation is not applicable to patients with obvious head injuries. Applicability of this strategy to civilian settings is not currently known.

Application of Damage Control Orthopaedics

Wound Management

War injuries in general are notable for marked contamination and soft-tissue cavitary effects resulting from penetrating projectiles and blast injury. Consequently, these wounds are almost never closed primarily. The quality of the initial débridement, expedient fracture stabilization, and the rapid restoration of blood flow to the extremity are critical to limb salvage in theater (**Figure 1**).

Accordingly, damage control procedures are commonplace in the management of these critically injured patients while they remain in the combat theater. Additionally, mass casualty events; constraints on time, manpower, and resources; and the battle scenario itself often dictate that external fixation be used to stabilize fractures in casualties who may have been eligible for early total care based on patient factors alone. Injuries

2: The Polytrauma Patient and Fracture Healing

of this nature are rare, however, and levels of contamination and the extremely high-energy nature of these extremity wounds almost always mandates the execution of damage control strategies acutely in combat. As a result, external fixators or simple splinting are used almost universally while casualties remain within the combat theater.

Fasciotomies

Prophylactic fasciotomies are performed liberally in theater to prevent compartment syndrome because of the high-energy nature of these injuries, concerns for reperfusion injury secondary to restoration of blood flow through temporary vascular shunts or as a result of tourniquets, and long transit times at altitudes that are required to evacuate casualties out of the combat zone. It is difficult to predict if these strategies have contributed to limb salvage rates, increased morbidity, or functional outcomes because the development of randomized controlled trials and even retrospective reviews are problematic in this environment.

Vacuum-Assisted Wound Closure

Vacuum-assisted wound therapy is routinely applied in civilian centers for managing soft-tissue wounds, and its use and efficacy are well described.[25] Early problems using the device in combat and aeromedical evacuation have largely been resolved, and its use has become the standard of care in the acute management of these soft-tissue wounds as vacuum pump units approved for flight have been developed and battery life has been extended.

Soft-Tissue Coverage Procedures

The care of host nation civilian casualties, necessary in the prolonged stabilization phases of these conflicts, has necessitated that some soft-tissue coverage procedures be performed in theater by American military surgeons. Skin grafting and rotational and free flap coverage are performed as early as possible and often in conjunction with antibiotic bead pouches, but only after thorough serial débridements have reduced the risk of wound sepsis to acceptable levels. Unfortunately, free flap failure rates in theater have been high. Further investigation into the causes of these unacceptably high failure rates, namely the extensive zone of injury associated with blast trauma and venous outflow problems leading to flap congestion, is an ongoing area of intensive research.

Military conflicts often yield innovation out of necessity. The current wars in Iraq and Afghanistan have been no different in that regard. Recent methodologies used in the combat setting and their applicability to the modern-day practice of civilian trauma management, from the prehospital setting to the definitive resuscitative phases, should be the subject of intense future study.

Summary

DCO has gained widespread acceptance as a greater understanding of the deleterious proinflamatory effects associated with extensive trauma have become better understood. Attempts to limit the second hit phenomena have become the focus of current treatment strategies, with special attention given to specific injury patterns and the attendant risks uniquely associated with each of them. Damage control procedures and treatment strategies should be reserved for critically ill patients in whom prolonged surgical intervention places them at undue risk. In the absence of severe trauma—that is, low-energy, isolated mechanisms of injury—early definitive management is appropriate and often preferred. Further investigation into future strategies that could enable surgeons to provide earlier definitive management in the critically ill is warranted. The experiences gained from the current wars in Iraq and Afghanistan have led to a greater understanding of the profound physiologic derangements associated with severe trauma.

Annotated References

1. Scalea TM: Optimal timing of fracture fixation: Have we learned anything in the past 20 years? *J Trauma* 2008;65(2):253-260.

   The evolution of thinking about long bone fracture fixation and timing of fixation is summarized.

2. Bhatia R, Dent C, Topley N, Pallister I: Neutrophil priming for elastase release in adult blunt trauma patients. *J Trauma* 2006;60(3):590-596.

   Evidence of polymorphonucleocyte "priming" in patients after major trauma is discussed.

3. Harwood PJ, Giannoudis PV, van Griensven M, Krettek C, Pape HC: Alterations in the systemic inflammatory response after early total care and damage control procedures for femoral shaft fracture in severely injured patients. *J Trauma* 2005;58(3):446-452.

   Despite a higher ISS, patients with femur fractures treated with damage control procedures had a smaller and shorter postoperative systemic inflammatory response compared with those treated with early total care.

4. Morshed S, Miclau T, Bembom O, Cohen M, Knudson MM, Colford JM Jr: Delayed internal fixation of femoral shaft fracture reduces mortality among patients with multisystem trauma. *J Bone Joint Surg Am* 2009;91: 3-13.

   The authors performed a restrospective cohort study to assess the effect of timing of internal fixation on the mortality of patients who have had multisystem trauma. Results indicated that those with serious abdominal injury benefit most from delayed treatment.

5. Pape HC, Griensven MV, Hildebrand FF, et al; Epoff Study Group: Systemic inflammatory response after extremity or truncal fracture operations. *J Trauma* 2008; 65(6):1379-1384.

    Cytokine releases were higher after operation with higher blood loss that were performed on the first or second day after injury.

6. Higgins TF, Horwitz DS: Damage control nailing. *J Orthop Trauma* 2007;21(7):477-481.

    The authors discuss strategies for minimizing the risk of acute intramedullary nailing in trauma patients.

7. Flierl MA, Stoneback JW, Beauchamp KM, et al: Femur shaft fracture fixation in head-injured patients: When is the right time? *J Orthop Trauma* 2010;24:107-114.

    The authors outlined the underlying immunopathophysiology of traumatic brain injury and presented clinical recommendations on timing of fixation.

8. Dunham CM, Bosse MJ, Clancy TV, et al: Practice management guidelines for the optimal timing of long-bone fracture stabilization in polytrauma patients: The EAST practice management guidelines work group. *J Trauma* 2001;50:958-967.

9. Pape HC, Giannoudis PV, Krettek C, Trentz O: Timing of fixation of major fractures in blunt polytrauma: Role of conventional indicators in clinical decision making. *J Orthop Trauma* 2005;19(8):551-562.

    The authors summarize the clinical parameters that can be used to assess the treatment of trauma patients.

10. Pape HC, Rixen D, Morely J, et al: Impact of the method of initial stabilization for femoral shaft fractures in patients with multiple injuries at risk for complications (borderline patients). *Ann Surg* 2007;246(3): 491-501.

    Early (less than 24 hours after injury) stabilization of femoral shaft fractures in "borderline" patients led to a higher incidence of acute lung injury.

11. Probst C, Probst T, Gaensslen A, Krettek C, Pape HC; Polytrauma Study Group of the German Trauma Society: Timing and duration of the initial pelvic stabilization after multiple trauma in patients from the German trauma registry: Is there an influence on outcome? *J Trauma* 2007;62(2):370-377.

    Keeping the initial surgery short and delaying surgery are associated with a lower rate of organ failure and mortality in patients with an ISS of 16 or greater.

12. Tschoeke SK, Hellmuth M, Hostmann A, Ertel W, Oberholzer A: The early second hit in trauma management augments the proinflammatory immune response to multiple injuries. *J Trauma* 2007;62(6):1396-1403.

    Proinflammatory cytokines were increased in multiple trauma patients after early surgical procedures (second hit).

13. Pape HC, Grimme K, Van Griensven M, et al; EPOFF Study Group: Impact of intramedullary instrumentation versus damage control for femoral fractures on immu-noinflammatory parameters: Prospective randomized analysis by the EPOFF Study Group. *J Trauma* 2003; 55(1):7-13.

14. Waydhas C, Nast-Kolb D, Trupka A, et al: Posttraumatic inflammatory response, secondary operations, and late multiple organ failure. *J Trauma* 1996;40(4): 624-630.

15. Pape HC, Giannoudis PV, Krettek C: The timing of fracture treatment in polytrauma patients: Relevance of damage control orthopedic surgery. *Am J Surg* 2002; 183(6):622-629.

16. Pape HC, Tscherne H: Early definitive fracture fixation, pulmonary function and systemic effects, in Baue AE, Faist E, Fry M, eds: *Multiple Organ Failure*. New York, NY, Springer Verlag, 2000, pp 279-290.

17. Rixen D, Grass G, Sauerland S, et al; Polytrauma Study Group of the German Trauma Society: Evaluation of criteria for temporary external fixation in risk-adapted damage control orthopedic surgery of femur shaft fractures in multiple trauma patients: "Evidence-based medicine" versus "reality" in the trauma registry of the German Trauma Society. *J Trauma* 2005;59(6):1375-1394.

    This meta-analysis concluded that management strategies for multiply injured patients with femoral shaft fractures were largely based on unvalidated criteria, although external fixation was more likely to be initially used in patients with increasing severity of ISS, Glasgow Coma Score, thorax trauma, base excess, coagulation abnormalities, and initial probability of death.

18. Taeger G, Ruchholtz S, Waydhas C, et al: Damage control orthopedics in patients with multiple injuries is effective, time saving, and safe. *J Trauma* 2005;59:409-416.

    The authors performed a prospective analysis of 1,070 patients over a 3.5-year period and compared complication rates from initial damage control procedures with subsequent conversion procedures, concluding the staged management is a safe treatment strategy.

19. Alam HB, Burris D, DaCorta JA, Rhee P: Hemorrhage control in the battlefield: Role of new hemostatic agents. *Mil Med* 2005;170(1):63-69.

    This article is a summary of newly introduced clotting agents used in the combat setting.

20. Holcomb JB: The 2004 Fitts Lecture: Current perspective on combat casualty care. *J Trauma* 2005;59(4):990-1002.

    This article highlights recent advances in combat casualty care delivered in Iraq and Afghanistan.

21. Acheson EM, Kheirabadi BS, Deguzman R, Dick EJ Jr, Holcomb JB: Comparison of hemorrhage control agents applied to lethal extremity arterial hemorrhages in swine. *J Trauma* 2005;59(4):865-874.

    This study compared three hemorrhage control agents and concluded that fibrin sealant dressings were superior in controlling lethal arterial hemorrhage.

2: The Polytrauma Patient and Fracture Healing

22. Martinowitz U, Kenet G, Segal E, et al: Recombinant activated factor VII for adjunctive hemorrhage control in trauma. *J Trauma* 2001;51(3):431-438.

23. Holcomb JB: Use of recombinant activated factor VII to treat the acquired coagulopathy of trauma. *J Trauma* 2005;58(6):1298-1303.

    This article reviews recombinant factor VII effectiveness in six large animal studies and one prospective randomized study in elective surgery.

24. Holcomb JB: Fluid resuscitation in modern combat casualty care: Lessons learned from Somalia. *J Trauma* 2003;54(suppl 5):S46-S51.

25. Herscovici D Jr, Sanders RW, Scaduto JM, Infante A, DiPasquale T: Vacuum-assisted wound closure (VAC therapy) for the management of patients with high-energy soft tissue injuries. *J Orthop Trauma* 2003; 17(10):683-688.

Section 3

Upper Extremity

SECTION EDITOR:

JOHN T. CAPO, MD

Chapter 17

Shoulder Trauma

James C. Krieg, MD   Andrew Green, MD   Peter A. Cole, MD

Scapula Fractures

Scapula fractures have traditionally been thought of as rare injuries that can be treated by benign neglect without functional compromise. Part of the rationale for this approach is that the shoulder has universal motion and can compensate for deformity and loss of glenohumeral rotation. By definition, however, some sort of functional compensation must occur after malunion, possibly resulting in loss of motion, strength, and/or endurance. Internal fixation of scapula fractures was first discussed in 1910, and surgical approaches to the lateral border of the scapula in 1932. The most commonly used approach for surgical repair of scapula fractures is the extensile posterior approach, first described in 1964.

Although it should be acknowledged that no prospective comparative outcome studies on the treatment of scapula fractures exist, there has been significant interest in documenting the outcomes of scapula fractures and in developing techniques of internal fixation of displaced scapular fractures, giving orthopaedic surgeons much-needed information regarding epidemiology, diagnosis, functional consequence of deformity, and surgical approaches.

Epidemiology, Associated Morbidity, and Mortality

Partly because of the oblique orientation of the scapula on the thorax, its surrounding muscular envelope, and the presence of adjacent bones such as the clavicle and ribs that dissipate energy by fracturing more easily, the scapula typically breaks only in the setting of high-energy collisions. Thus, it is not surprising that only approximately 20% of these fractures occur in females and the average age for patients with scapula fractures is in the mid 40s; mean ages for patients with surgically treated scapula fractures range from 35 to 38 years in two recent systematic reviews.[1,2]

Scapula fractures are associated with injuries to other organ systems in approximately 90% of cases, as well as ipsilateral extremity lesions in approximately 50% (**Figure 1**). Spine injuries occur in approximately 15%, with slightly higher rates of significant traumatic brain injury. After controlling for injury severity, the following injuries occurred with greater frequency in combination with scapula fractures: rib fractures, pneumothorax, lung injury, ipsilateral extremity injury, and spine injury.[3]

Imaging and Classification

All patients with scapula fractures should have true AP, Y scapular view, and axillary lateral radiographs. In addition, fractures suspected of being intra-articular, those that are significantly displaced, and those whose patterns are indeterminate should have CT scans. Three-dimensional reconstructions are particularly helpful in interpreting CT data. Multiple measures of displacement exist. Glenopolar angle is determined by the angle between a line from cranial to caudal limits of

Dr. Krieg or an immediate family member has received royalties from Synthes Craniomaxillofacial and SAM Medical Products; serves as a paid consultant for or is an employee of Synthes; has received research or institutional support from AO Spine North America, AO-Stiftung-ASIF Foundation, Bank of America Foundation, The Center, Orthopaedics and Neurological Surgeons, Fidelity Investments, Helena Orthopaedics Clinic, Illinois Orthopaedics & Hand Center, Inland Orthopaedics of Spokane, JMS Hand Associates, Northwest Biomet, Pacific Rim Orthopaedics, Proliance Surgeons, Proliance Orthopaedics & Sports Medicine, The Seattle Foundation, Seattle Christian Foundation, Silicon Valley Community Foundation, Simonian Sports Medicine Clinic, SKS Plastic Surgery, Spectrum Research, Synthes, Synthes Spine, Washington Research Foundation, Washington State Orthopaedics Association, Webber Lawn & Yard Care, National Institutes of Health, National Science Foundation, Veterans Affairs Rehabilitation Research and Development Service, Orthopaedic Research and Education Foundation, AO North America Amgen, Bayer AG, BioAxone Therapeutique, CeraPedics, Christopher Reeve Paralysis Foundation, DePuy, Foundation for Orthopedic Trauma, Integra, Lifesciences Corporation, National Science Foundation, Ostex International, Orthopaedic Trauma Association, Paradigm Spine, Smith & Nephew, Synthes Spine, the Boeing Company, US Army Research Office, and the US Department of Education; and owns stock or stock options in Johnson & Johnson. Dr. Green or an immediate family member serves as a board member, owner, officer, or committee member of the American Academy of Orthopaedic Surgeons; has received royalties from Tornier; serves as a paid consultant to or is an employee of Tornier and Illuminoss; has received research or institutional support from Arthrex, Smith & Nephew, and Tornier; owns stock or stock options in Illuminoss; and has received nonincome support (such as equipment or services), commercially derived honoraria, or other non–research-related funding (such as paid travel) from Elsevier. Dr. Cole or an immediate family member serves as a paid consultant for or is an employee of Synthes and has received research or institutional support from Synthes and DePuy.

the glenoid fossa and a line from the superior aspect of the glenoid fossa to the most caudal point of the scapular body. Normal values are 30° to 45°. It is a measure of malrotation of the glenoid neck around the axis from front to back. Glenoid version is best measured with CT and compared with that of the opposite shoulder. Other measures of displacement include intra-articular step-off or gap displacement (seen on CT scan). Often there is lateral displacement of the lateral border of the scapula relative to the glenoid fossa and scapular neck, making the glenoid appear to be medialized. However, the incidence or degree of true glenoid medialization relative to the midline has not been clearly defined. Lateral border displacement does affect the morphology of the scapula, potentially affecting muscle length-tension relationships, and can be measured off of an anteroposterior radiograph of the shoulder, although it is of uncertain clinical significance. True medial-lateral displacement of the glenoid relative to the midline can be measured on an AP chest radiograph or CT scan in a symmetrically positioned patient. Angulation of the scapular body is seen on a Y-scapular view.

Although several classifications of scapula fractures have been proposed, no comprehensive classification system correlates very well with typical fracture patterns. Given the complex three-dimensional anatomy of the scapula and overlying structures of the thorax that are radiographically superimposed on the scapula, it is difficult to understand how the scapula is fractured and displaced (**Figure 2**).

A recent study detailed topographic information on fracture patterns and frequency detected on three-dimensional CT reconstructions of the scapula in 90 patients.[4] This scapula fracture map suggests that fractures of the scapular neck and body are highly re-

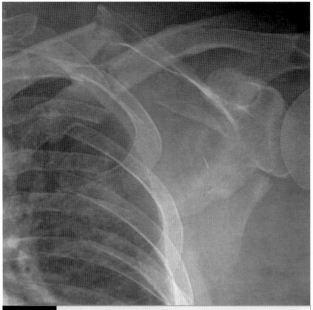

Figure 1 This AP radiograph of the shoulder demonstrates common findings associated with scapula fractures, including a markedly decreased glenopolar angle, multiple displaced fractured ribs, and an ipsilateral clavicle fracture.

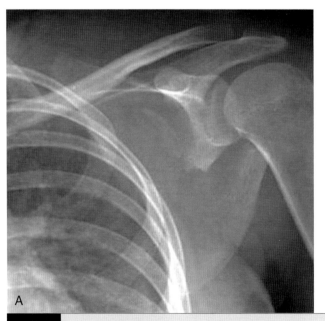
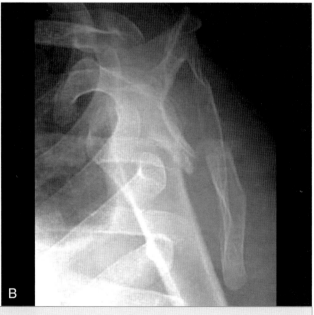

Figure 2 **A,** An AP shoulder view indicating severe displacement at the lateral border, such that the glenoid is significantly medial and likely rotated relative to the scapular body. The degree of lateral border offset, often called medialization, can be measured between a vertical line at the lateralmost edge of the proximal to the lateralmost edge of the distal scapula body. **B,** A Y scapular view showing a high degree of translation of the two main fragments as well as what is commonly referred to as angulation.

producible, whereas fractures involving the articular surface are associated with a much more random pattern of fractures of the scapular neck and body. The fracture pattern that occurred most commonly (in more than two thirds of cases) extended from the lateral border just below the glenoid and exited the vertebral border just caudal to the spine of the scapula (**Figure 3**). Additionally, 22% of fractures involved the spinoglenoid notch, and 17% involved the articular surface.[4]

Because of the complex anatomy and difficulty in imaging the scapula, the interrater agreement of measurements of the morphology of scapula fractures and fracture classification is low. In a recent study, two examiners assessed 44 three-dimensional CT scans. Whereas standard radiographs of the shoulder were adequate for assessing scapular body and acromion fractures, they demonstrated little accuracy for glenoid, coracoid, or scapular neck fractures. In such cases, three-dimensional CT scans detected all such fractures and thus had a higher sensitivity.[5]

To date, there are no adequately defined methods for measuring displacement of the glenoid or angular deformity in different planes. For example, in many scapula fractures the glenoid appears to be translated medially, but differentiating true glenoid medialization (which may be an indication for surgery) from lateral displacement of the lateral border of the scapula (creating a false impression of glenoid medialization) can be very difficult. Thus, communication on indications for surgery, and the rendering of meaningful clinical outcomes based on such indications, will remain nebulous at best, until validated methods of assessment are defined.

Outcomes

Two recent systematic reviews summarized the published literature on scapula fractures.[1,2] The first study analyzed 520 surgically treated and nonsurgically treated patients collected from 22 level IV retrospective case series. The authors reported that 80% of isolated glenoid fractures were being treated surgically, and good to excellent results were achieved in 82% of patients, based on an assessment of clinical outcome. Although 99% of isolated scapular body fractures were being treated conservatively, 14% of this group went on to have a fair or poor result. Additionally, 83% of fractures described as scapular neck were treated nonsurgically, but 23% of these resulted in a fair or poor clinical outcome.[1] These results clearly demonstrate that there are subgroups of extra-articular scapular fractures that do poorly when treated nonsurgically, although the reasons for this are not understood. This systematic review however, could not perform valid comparisons between surgically treated and nonsurgically treated scapulas because of the variability between studies, outcome measures, definitions, and associated injuries. The second systematic review included an analysis of 243 surgical cases from 17 studies. Seventy-eight percent of patients were treated with a posterior

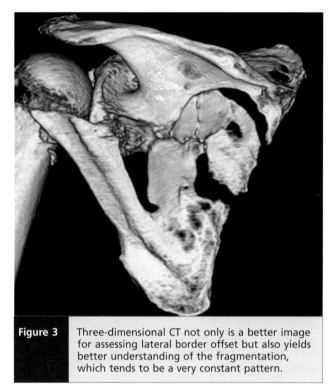

Figure 3 Three-dimensional CT not only is a better image for assessing lateral border offset but also yields better understanding of the fragmentation, which tends to be a very constant pattern.

approach, 18% with an anterior approach, and 4% with a combined approach. Internal fixation of an associated ipsilateral clavicle fracture was performed in only 27% of the cases involving fractures of both the scapula and clavicle. Complications in these surgical series included infection in 4.2% of patients, though only one patient had a deep infection. Suprascapular nerve injury was reported in 2.6% of patients, although it was unclear whether nerve insult occurred at injury or at surgery. The most commonly reported complication was hardware removal in 7.1% (15 patients), although in 3 patients the symptomatic hardware was clavicular plates. Overall, 83.4% of patients reported good to excellent results after surgical treatment.[2]

Scapular Neck and Body Fractures

Two recent studies reported an association of poor clinical outcomes with a decreased glenopolar angle after conservative treatment.[6,7] In both studies, there was a statistically significant positive correlation between Constant scores and the glenopolar angle.[6] In addition, there was a significant difference in outcome between patients with glenopolar angles more than or less than 30°.[7] In a German study of 51 patients who were treated conservatively and followed for more than 5 years, motion (forward flexion, abduction, and external rotation) was significantly decreased in the injured shoulder, but did not necessarily correlate with lower functional outcomes. However, the authors did find a statistically significant correlation between restricted range of motion and diminution of muscular strength.[8] A biomechanical model for assessing the effect of dif-

3: Upper Extremity

ferent degrees of scapular neck malunion on the biomechanics of the glenohumeral joint was developed. Additional muscle efforts due to changes in moment arms were recorded in the pectoralis major and biceps muscles, along with shortening of the rotator cuff musculature. The authors effectively showed the increase in work required of these muscles to execute the function of glenohumeral constraint in the setting of scapular malunion.[9]

One recent surgical series composed of 22 patients who had sustained a displaced fracture of the scapular neck (associated with displaced articular fragments in 11) and were surgically treated 3 weeks to 3 months after injury demonstrated good functional outcomes approaching normative values, even after delayed treatment.[10] In a recent review of nonsurgical treatment of extra-articular scapular body fractures, injuries healed and shoulder function returned to normal or nearly normal. However, polytraumatized patients scored worse on general health measures, likely because of their concomitant injuries.[11]

Intra-articular Glenoid Fractures

Surgical reduction and stabilization of displaced intra-articular glenoid fossa fractures is a well-established procedure.[30] A recent study reported the clinical outcome of 14 patients with low-energy shoulder dislocations associated with a glenoid rim fracture (mean age, 53 years) with radiographically documented concentric reductions of the glenohumeral joint.[12] All patients had anterior avulsion fractures, maintained shoulder stability through the course of follow-up (mean, 5.6 years), and had good outcomes according to Constant score (98%) and no pain, despite two manifesting radiographic signs of osteoarthritis. This study generally supports current recommendations for nonsurgical treatment in older patients with glenoid fractures small enough that humeral subluxation does not occur, although this scenario requires relative immobilization for a period of 6 weeks.[12] Recently, arthroscopic methods for treatment of isolated glenoid rim and/or glenoid fossa fractures have been described, though these reports lack sufficient data for critical analysis.[13]

Coracoid and Acromion Fractures

In a series documenting the surgical treatment of scapular process fractures, the results of 27 consecutive fractures (13 acromion and 14 coracoid), including the functional outcome in a subset of 13 at a mean 11-month follow-up period were studied.[14] All patients had fracture healing and painless range of motion, although three required hardware removal because of irritation. Indications for surgery included painful nonunions, fractures displaced more than 1 cm, and associated multiple disruptions of the superior shoulder suspensory complex. The mean final Disabilities of the Arm, Shoulder and Hand (DASH) score was 7, and all eight parameters of the Short Form-36 (SF-36) were comparable to normative scores.[14]

Surgical Indications

The orthopaedic literature regarding scapular fractures has significant limitations, and methodologically rigorous studies are lacking to allow for the determination of definitive treatment recommendations. There are five main categories of fractures for surgical consideration, sometimes occurring in combination: articular glenoid fractures, extra-articular fractures of the scapular neck, scapular body fractures, a scapula fracture associated with an ipsilateral injury to the superior shoulder suspensory complex (generally an acromioclavicular dislocation or clavicle fracture), and displaced process fractures (acromion and coracoid). The term scapular neck is not clearly defined or agreed upon.

Although different authors have used different criteria for surgical management, it seems reasonable to consider displaced scapular process fractures (1 cm), displaced articular fractures (> 5 mm), and articular glenoid fractures associated with humeral subluxation as injuries best treated with open reduction and internal fixation (ORIF) (Figure 4). More controversial is the threshold for ORIF of extra-articular fractures involving the displaced lateral border of the scapula or scapular neck. With these injuries, typical indications for surgeons who advocate surgery are 2 cm of lateral border–glenoid offset (medialization), 40° of scapular body angulation (measured on a Y scapular radiographic view), or a glenopolar angle (in the plane of the scapula) less than 20°. Although clinical data are lacking, in the case of ipsilateral injuries to the scapula and clavicle–acromioclavicular joint complex (known as floating shoulder), fixation of one or all components of the injury should be considered.

Surgical Techniques
Approaches

Because surgical intervention for scapula fractures is occurring more frequently, there has been recent interest in surgical approaches to the scapula. A modification of the traditional Judet approach has been described (Figure 5). This approach uses the same skin incision as reported by Judet, but intermuscular intervals are used to access the scapular borders for reduction and fixation instead of elevating the muscles off of the scapula en masse. The infraspinatus fascia is mobilized along with the deltoid muscle, as the latter is detached from the spine of the scapula. This should decrease the risk of neurovascular compromise, especially as it relates to the suprascapular nerve. It also minimizes muscle stripping and potential devitalization of the scapula.[15] The largest surgical series to date describes 37 intra-articular and extra-articular scapula fractures treated through a modified Judet approach, using 2.7- and 2-mm implants for the lateral scapular border.[16] Critical structures, including the medial circumflex artery and suprascapular neurovascular bundle must be protected during these posterior approaches.

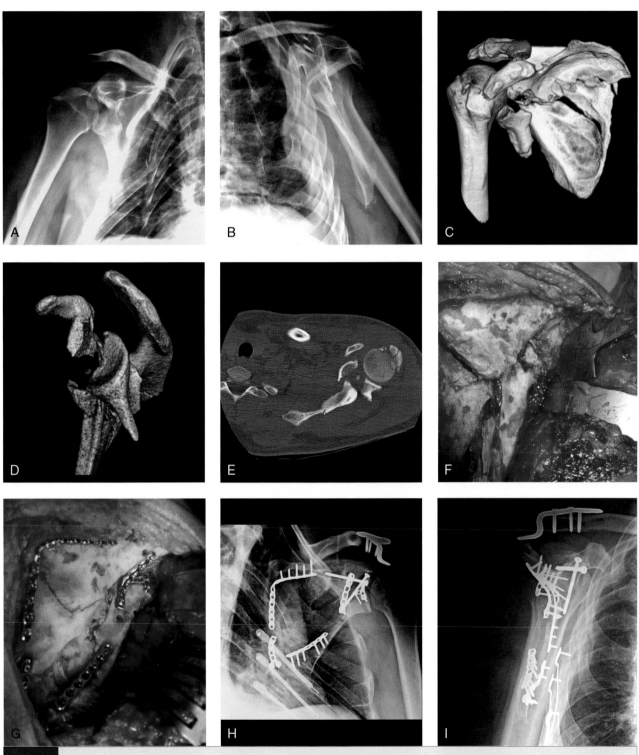

Figure 4 **A,** AP radiograph revealing a displaced intra-articular fracture of the glenoid fossa and a dislocated acromioclavicular joint. **B,** A Y scapular radiograph depicting the injury in **A** with minimal angular deformity of the body, but displacement of the coracoid. **C,** Three-dimensional CT allowing discernment of a large posterior glenoid as well as extension into the body of the scapula. **D,** Three-dimensional CT of the patient in **C** rotated to a Y scapular position to appreciate the morphology of the glenoid fossa fragments. **E,** Two-dimensional CT demonstrating axial alignment of the fragments and their displacement. **F,** At 1 month after the injury, it was decided to use a posterior Judet approach in which the rotator cuff is elevated to access the body, neck, and posterior glenoid. The suprascapular neurovascular bundle is being protected by a large retractor oriented so its edge does not impale the suprascapular nerve and vessels. **G,** The scapula in **F** after fixation with 2.7- and 2-mm implants. **H,** Postoperative AP radiograph after fixation of the scapula, the acromioclavicular joint, and three ribs. **I,** Postoperative Y scapular radiograph showing the fixation in **H.**

3: Upper Extremity

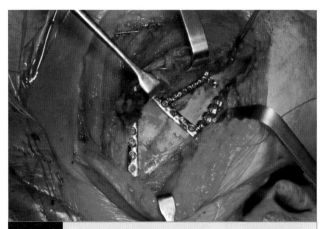

Figure 5 Intraoperative photograph demonstrating access to the posterior lateral border of the scapula using the intramuscular approach between the teres minor and infraspinatus, which is less invasive than a standard Judet approach.

Scapulothoracic Dissociation

Scapulothoracic dissociation is a devastating condition caused by a traction force applied to the upper extremity, resulting in neurovascular compromise. Because patients are often obtunded or intubated during initial evaluation, this limb-threatening condition can remain undetected. It is critical to maintain clinical suspicion for this injury during the secondary survey of trauma patients. Inspection and palpation of the shoulder can reveal that the entire shoulder from the neck distally, including the axilla, is swollen and boggy from hematoma. Uneven pulses in the upper extremities should prompt an arterial pressure index measurement, as well as palpation and auscultation in the supraclavicular region and axilla, where a bruit can be detected after an injured subclavian or axillary artery. The chest may show lateral displacement of the scapula. Side-to-side differences in the position of the scapula should be measured to the midline spinous process and are quantified by the scapula index, which is the ratio of the injured side to the uninjured side.

When scapulothoracic dissociation is considered, work-up includes establishing arterial and neurologic integrity. If the arterial pressure index is abnormal (< 0.9), an arteriogram should evaluate for intimal tears or frank avulsions. If significant suspicion exists for a neurologic injury, MRI with contrast is warranted to evaluate the cervical spine and brachial plexus. CT myelograms are useful for assessing whether nerve root avulsions have been sustained.

The outcome of scapulothoracic dissociation is uniformly poor. One series reported functional outcomes in 25 patients at a mean of 12.3 years after injury.[17] There were 9 complete and 10 incomplete neurologic lesions, and 6 patients died. Six patients eventually underwent below-elbow amputation. There were signifi-

cantly worse SF-36 and Subjective Shoulder Rating Scores in patients with complete compared to incomplete brachial plexus injuries. The authors found no correlation between functional outcome scores and the scapula index or the presence or absence of a vascular injury.[17] The authors of another recent study established a correlation between the level of vascular injury and partial versus complete neurologic lesions. Axillary arterial injuries were more frequently associated with incomplete brachial plexus lesions, whereas subclavian arterial injuries were more frequently associated with complete plexus lesions.[18] Another study documented functional outcomes in 29 patients with brachial plexus lesions, and divided these into a group with scapulothoracic dissociation (11 patients) and those without (18 patients). There were striking and significant differences, with much worse outcomes in patients with associated scapulothoracic dislocation.[19]

Clavicle Fractures

Clavicle fractures represent one of the more common injuries encountered in orthopaedic practice.[20] Although there is little debate that nonsurgical treatment yields generally excellent results in minimally displaced fractures, recent trends indicate that certain subpopulations of injured patients may be better treated surgically. As surgical indications continue to evolve, newer techniques are being explored to better treat these common injuries.

Nonsurgical Treatment

Use of a sling for protection and comfort remains the mainstay of closed treatment. A recent review of the literature reveals no compelling evidence that any other treatment is more effective than a sling.[21] The same review also concludes that there is inadequate evidence to support the routine use of low-intensity pulsed ultrasound to speed healing or reduce risk of nonunion.

Despite the historical success of nonsurgical management, several concerns remain. Nonunion occurs more frequently than had previously been considered. In a prospective review of 868 consecutive patients, nonunion occurred in 6.2% of clavicular fractures treated nonsurgically.[22] Risk factors for nonunion include displacement greater than 100%, female sex, advanced age, and comminution. A 2005 study reported 7% nonunion in a series of 222 patients followed prospectively.[23] Perhaps more impressively, 42% of patients had fracture sequelae, including pain and functional impairment. Risk factors for adverse sequelae included complete displacement, advanced age, and comminution. In this study, shortening of the clavicle was not related to outcome.

Malunion of the clavicle can be associated with symptoms of pain and muscle weakness. A 2004 study showed that corrective osteotomy for symptomatic malunions was associated with significant improvement of symptoms after minimum follow-up of 12 months.[24]

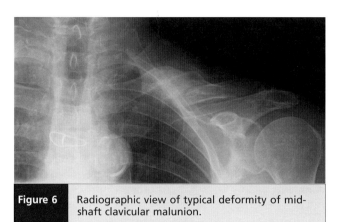

Figure 6 Radiographic view of typical deformity of mid-shaft clavicular malunion.

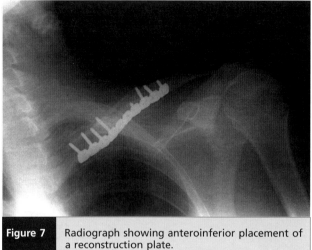

Figure 7 Radiograph showing anteroinferior placement of a reconstruction plate.

The typical deformity includes shortening and inferior displacement (**Figure 6**).

In a study of lateral clavicle fractures, 21% had a nonunion after nonsurgical treatment.[25] Despite the fact that 14% of all patients had symptoms severe enough to seek delayed surgical treatment, there was no difference in function between those with nonunion and those whose fractures had healed. Nor was there any functional difference between those treated nonsurgically and those who had delayed surgical intervention, after their treatment was completed.

Open Reduction and Internal Fixation

ORIF has historically been the mainstay of surgical treatment of displaced clavicle fractures. Traditionally, compression plates are applied to the superior aspect of the clavicle.[26] More recent series have documented the efficacy of anteroinferior plate placement, using either a 3.5-mm limited contact dynamic compression plate or a 3.5-mm reconstruction plate[27] (**Figure 7**). Advantages are purported to be safer screw placement, less irritability due to implant prominence, and less need for reoperation for plate removal.

Typically, reconstruction plates are favored because they are easy to contour to fit the complex anatomy of the clavicle. However, these plates are less stiff and weaker than compression plates. Generally, 3.5-mm screw-plate systems are recommended because of their strength relative to size. However, 2.7-mm screw-plate systems have also been used with success.[28] Although weaker in bending strength, advantages of the latter are lower profile plates and more screws per fragment for similar length plates.

Current advances in plate design include precontoured plates with a stiffness and strength similar to most 3.5-mm compression plates. The advantages of bone-specific plates include a better fit of the plate on the clavicle.[29] In addition, many plates have incorporated designs that use a cluster of holes to accommodate smaller screws in the distal end of the plate. This increases the number of points of fixation in the lateral clavicle, helping to minimize the risk of screw failure (**Figure 8**). Indications for locking plate technology are

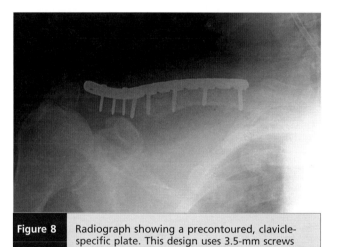

Figure 8 Radiograph showing a precontoured, clavicle-specific plate. This design uses 3.5-mm screws medially and 2.7-mm screws laterally to optimize screw strength and number.

incompletely understood in the clavicle. Although some simulated biomechanical data show improved fixation when tested in torsion and compression, there are few clinical data to guide its use, and other modes of failure have not been fully investigated.[30,31]

Plating of lateral third clavicle fractures has traditionally been a challenge, in large part because of the inability to gain adequate fixation in the lateral fragment. In the past, strategies have included spanning the acromioclavicular joint to gain the added advantage of fixation in the acromion, or supplemental coracoclavicular fixation with screws and/or sutures. Another strategy that has evolved is the use of a clavicular hook-plate.[32] The plate hooks under the acromion, posterior to the acromioclavicular joint, to improve lateral fixation (**Figure 9**). It is recommended that this plate be removed to prevent impingement symptoms and osteolysis of the acromion. Clinically, this plate has been reported to have results that compare favorably to other modes of fixation.[33]

3: Upper Extremity

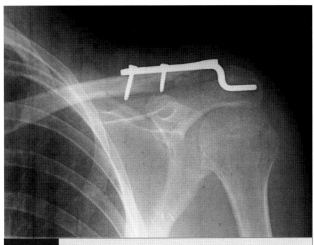

Figure 9 Radiograph showing a lateral hook-plate for a Neer type II lateral clavicle fracture.

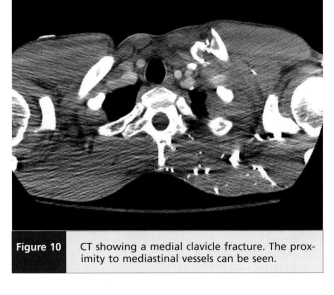

Figure 10 CT showing a medial clavicle fracture. The proximity to mediastinal vessels can be seen.

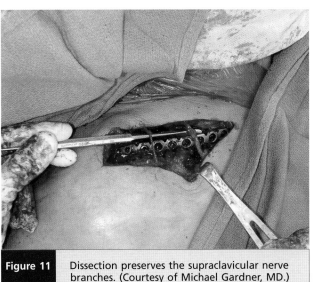

Figure 11 Dissection preserves the supraclavicular nerve branches. (Courtesy of Michael Gardner, MD.)

Although rare, medial clavicle fractures are often associated with significant chest trauma. Their proximity to mediastinal structures increases the risk associated with displacement and may create additional risk of iatrogenic vessel injury with surgical fixation (**Figure 10**).

ORIF of clavicle fractures often requires an incision that passes through the course of the supraclavicular nerves. Dissection should be performed carefully in the subcutaneous layer to identify and preserve these nerves, in order to minimize the risk of iatrogenic cutaneous nerve injury (**Figure 11**). In addition, studies have shown the importance of periosteal blood supply in the middle third of the clavicle. Periosteal stripping must be avoided to allow for uneventful bone healing. The challenges of infection in the clavicle are significant.

Intramedullary Fixation

The tight intramedullary canal of the clavicle together with its complex shape present unique challenges to medullary fixation. Techniques have been introduced that use flexible intramedullary implants.[34] Titanium nails have been used from a medial starting point. The technique is dependent on adequate fluoroscopic imaging (**Figure 12**). Safe passage of the nail across the fracture site is dependent on fracture reduction and appropriate imaging. A significant number of fractures may need to be opened to reduce the fracture and safely pass the nail into the lateral fragment (**Figure 13**). Results with this technique have been comparable to other surgical treatment methods. Indications continue to be defined.

Comparative Studies

In 2007 the Canadian Orthopaedic Trauma Society published the results of a prospective, randomized study of treatment of displaced, midshaft clavicle fractures in adults.[35] This collaborative effort evaluated outcomes of 132 patients randomized to receive closed treatment versus open plating of this subgroup of patients with clavicle fractures. In comparison with patients who did not undergo surgery, patients who had undergone ORIF had lower nonunion rates (2 of 67 versus 7 of 65 patients), shorter time to union (16.4 weeks versus 28.4 weeks), and no symptomatic malunions (9 in the nonsurgical group). These level I data provide support for surgical treatment of a select group of patients with clavicle fractures. Although the complication rate was low in this study (one mechanical failure, three wound infections, five reports of local irritation due to hardware), the overall risk of surgical treatment and the ideal indications remain incompletely understood. Furthermore, ideal indications for the various modes of surgical care remain the subject of investigation.

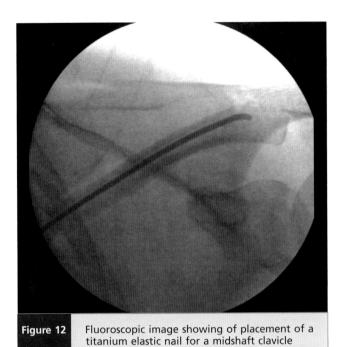

Figure 12 Fluoroscopic image showing of placement of a titanium elastic nail for a midshaft clavicle fracture. The fracture pattern is simple and reduces well during nailing. (Courtesy of Michael Gardner, MD.)

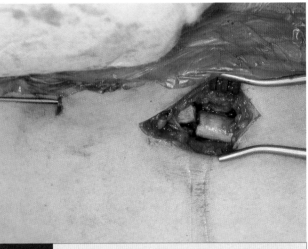

Figure 13 Clinical photograph showing open reduction required for safe passage of the intramedullary nail. (Courtesy of Michael Gardner, MD.)

Acromioclavicular Joint Injuries

The acromioclavicular joint complex is the only point of ligamentous attachment of the upper extremity to the clavicle and consequently the thorax. The scapula is fixed to the distal clavicle by both the acromioclavicular and coracoclavicular ligaments. The acromioclavicular joint is a diarthrodial joint and has an inclination that varies from vertical to oblique and overriding the medial acromial articular surface. The lateral clavicular epiphysis forms at about age 5 years and fuses to the distal clavicle as late as the early 20s.

Acromioclavicular joint stability is primarily provided by the acromioclavicular and coracoclavicular ligaments. The acromioclavicular ligaments provide anterior posterior stability, while the coracoclavicular ligaments are the primary restraints to superior displacement (conoid) and acromioclavicular joint compression (trapezoid). In addition, the deltoid and trapezius muscles provide some dynamic stability that becomes important in the setting of an unstable acromioclavicular joint.

Most acromioclavicular joint injuries occur in males and are the result of a traumatic force to the lateral or superior aspect of the shoulder that drives the acromion and scapula inferiorly.

Classification

Acromioclavicular joint injuries are classified into six types. The clinical evaluation is usually straightforward, especially if there is prominence of the distal clavicle. Type III and V injuries involve superior dis-

placement of the clavicle relative to the acromion. In type IV injuries the distal clavicle is displaced posteriorly into the trapezius muscle. Nondisplaced acromioclavicular joint sprains and impactions usually present with some local swelling and tenderness specifically over the joint. In more severe high-energy trauma, acromioclavicular joint injuries can be associated with other shoulder girdle injuries such as clavicle fractures, scapulothoracic dissociations, and intra-articular glenohumeral joint injuries.[36] Dedicated plain radiographic views of the acromioclavicular joint provide sufficient imaging in most cases. Advanced imaging can be considered based on the clinical setting.

Treatment Strategies

Type I and II injuries are treated nonsurgically with relatively rapid functional recovery and little expectation of long-term sequelae. Nevertheless, late complications, such as posttraumatic arthritis, can occur and may require treatment.[37] Early surgical treatment is usually considered for type IV and V injuries. Type VI injuries are very rare and also require surgical treatment. The treatment of type III injuries is somewhat controversial. There are many publications that support nonsurgical treatment because of relatively rapid functional recovery, minimal significant long-term functional sequelae, and avoidance of surgical risk.[38] Nevertheless, there are proponents of acute surgical treatment of type III acromioclavicular joint dislocations. Despite all of the literature there is little evidence-based research that definitively clarifies this issue. Consequently, it is likely that individual consideration will remain an important factor in the management of these injuries. Nonsurgical treatment has been associated with more rapid recovery and fewer unsatisfactory results. However, in patients with acromioclavicular displacement of 2 cm or more, early surgery produced better results.

Several studies have evaluated the biomechanics of a variety of techniques for repair and reconstruction of the acromioclavicular joint. Most studies find that coracoclavicular fixation provides superior strength compared to coracoacromial ligament transfer (Weaver-Dunn reconstruction) although normal joint anatomy and stability usually are not completely restored.[39,40] One study demonstrated that a modified Weaver-Dunn reconstruction augmented with coracoclavicular fixation provides better initial stability and also restores acromioclavicular kinematics.[41]

Surgical treatment of acute acromioclavicular dislocation can be performed with and without distal clavicle resection. Coracoclavicular fixation with any number of techniques, including coracoclavicular screw or coracoclavicular suture with and without suture anchors, appears to provide satisfactory stability to allow ligament healing.[42] Refinement of technique can improve the congruity of the acromioclavicular joint.[43] In addition, acromioclavicular fixation with pins, as well as clavicle hook-plates, is reported to give good results.[44] Arthroscopically assisted techniques or both acute and chronic acromioclavicular joint dislocations have been developed.[45]

According to some reports, complications of surgical treatment are emphasized as a rationale for advocating nonsurgical treatment.[46] Wound infections can occur and care must be taken to avoid neurologic injury. Loss of reduction can occur and may be more common than actually reported.

Reconstruction

Reconstruction for chronic acromioclavicular joint dislocation requires ligament reconstruction. The most recent focus has been on the use of tendon autograft or allograft reconstruction of the coracoclavicular ligaments. The in vitro biomechanics of tendon graft reconstruction are superior to coracoclavicular ligament transfer, and early reports are encouraging.[40,47,48]

Sternoclavicular Joint Injuries

Sternoclavicular joint dislocation is a rare injury. Classification has primarily been descriptive. Injuries are acute or chronic, partial (subluxation) or complete (dislocation), and anterior or posterior. Clinical examination is often adequate for diagnosis of an anterior dislocation, yet posterior dislocation may be clinically subtle and may require CT or MRI for accurate assessment. Posterior dislocation carries with it the risk of thoracic vessel injury. Angiography may be prudent for identification of these injuries.

Anterior Dislocation

Few series exist with sufficient numbers to provide firm treatment guidelines on sternoclavicular dislocations. Anterior dislocations seem to result in few long-term problems, regardless of the ultimate stability or reduction of the joint. Although most of these injuries result in an unstable sternoclavicular joint, an attempt at closed reduction is recommended. Reduction is performed with a bump of towels under the medial scapula while pressure is directed posteriorly over the medial aspect of the clavicle and traction is applied to the abducted arm.

Posterior Dislocation

Posterior dislocation is less frequent than anterior dislocation. However, the consequences are more significant, due to the proximity of the great vessels. Closed reduction of posterior sternoclavicular dislocation is also done with a bump between the scapula, and may require anesthesia so that the medial clavicle may be gripped with a towel clip in order to pull it forward. If closed reduction fails, an open reduction should be done without delay. A chest surgeon should be available during open reduction. After exposure of the sternoclavicular joint, the medial clavicle can be directly reduced and should be stabilized. Typically, stabilization has involved reconstruction of the capsule and supporting ligaments. One method uses the semitendinosus tendon as material for reconstruction.[49]

Glenohumeral Dislocation

The glenohumeral joint is the most commonly dislocated large joint. Because of the limited contribution of the bony anatomy, glenohumeral stability is highly dependent on the integrity and functioning of the soft-tissue restraints provided by the labrum, capsule, and rotator cuff. Anterior dislocations account for approximately 98% of glenohumeral dislocations, whereas posterior dislocations are much less common, which is why many posterior fracture-dislocations are missed and become chronic injuries. Although glenohumeral dislocations are commonly considered to afflict younger patients, they occur throughout adolescence and adulthood and present a variety of treatment challenges.

Evaluation

Most glenohumeral dislocations are the result of a traumatic event, and most patients present to an emergency department setting for evaluation. Less commonly, patients sustain a traumatic shoulder injury with a glenohumeral dislocation or subluxation that spontaneously reduces. These patients often forego formal evaluation and treatment until they have a recurrent episode.

The initial evaluation includes obtaining a history and performing a careful physical examination. Although the history is usually straightforward, it can sometimes be unclear. For example, it is not uncommon for elderly patients to present for an "emergent" evaluation of what is really a chronic glenohumeral dislocation that was previously unrecognized. Knowledge of the mechanism of injury can be helpful. Posterior dislocations usually result from an adduction and axial load force to the shoulder or a direct blow to the anterior aspect of the shoulder. Seizures are implicated in up to 50% of reported cases of posterior dislocation.

The physical examination must be thorough, including both musculoskeletal and neurovascular evaluation, to avoid errors in diagnosis. Patients with an anterior dislocation usually have anterior prominence of the humeral head and a sulcus under the posterior acromion. In contrast, patients with posterior dislocations have flattening of the anterior shoulder and classically are unable to internally rotate the shoulder.

Plain radiographs should be obtained before reduction to confirm the diagnosis and identify associated injuries. The standard series of radiographs includes a true AP, axillary lateral, and Y-scapular views. Radiographic examination is especially important in older patients, who are much more likely to have an associated fracture. Inadequate imaging is the major reason that posterior dislocations are missed. The typical AP view of the shoulder normally projects the humeral head over the glenoid and cannot be used to rule out a posterior dislocation. If plain radiographs cannot be obtained, CT is especially valuable to determine the extent of anterior humeral impression fracture in cases of posterior dislocation.

Associated Injuries

Glenohumeral dislocations can be complicated by several associated injuries. Tearing of the anteroinferior glenoid labrum occurs in more than 90% of younger patients who sustain a traumatic anterior glenohumeral dislocation. With increasing age, especially beyond 40 years, rotator cuff tears are more common. In patients older than 40 years, early imaging with MRI should be considered. Weakness of internal rotation, as indicated by positive lumbar lift-off and belly press tests, suggests subscapularis tearing; external rotation weakness suggests a large posterosuperior rotator cuff tear.

Displaced glenoid rim and greater tuberosity fractures are usually the result of an anterior glenohumeral dislocation. ORIF should be considered for large displaced glenoid rim fractures. CT should be used to assess displacement, the size of the bone fragment, and glenohumeral congruity. Surgical treatment with open or arthroscopic reduction and internal fixation is reported with generally satisfactory outcomes.[50] Greater tuberosity fractures occur in up to one third of anterior glenohumeral dislocations, are more common in older patients, and frequently reduce anatomically with closed reduction of the dislocation. More extensive proximal humerus fractures with associated glenohumeral dislocations typically occur in geriatric patients but can also occur as a result of high-energy trauma. Posterior dislocation can occur with surgical neck fracture. These fractures should be identified with appropriate imaging and treatment adjusted to avoid further iatrogenic trauma.

Nerve injuries are more common in older patients and when there is an associated fracture. The anatomy of the axillary nerve places it at risk of injury. It is tethered anterior and posterior to the glenohumeral joint and has limited excursion. In a younger patient an axillary nerve injury may not be initially evident because with an intact rotator cuff, weakness of shoulder elevation can be difficult to appreciate in the early evaluation. Subsequent careful examination of the shoulder will generally demonstrate deltoid weakness. Brachial plexus injuries are less common.

Patients involved in high-energy trauma often have more extensive associated injuries, and careful evaluation is required to avoid errors in diagnosis.[51] In the setting of polytrauma, glenohumeral dislocations can be missed as a result of more focused attention on other life-threatening injuries.

Anterior Dislocation
Nonsurgical Treatment
Many dislocations can be reduced with minimal anesthetic requirement.[52] Several methods including the Kocher, traction-counter traction, Stimson, Milch, and scapular manipulation can be used, with gentle techniques preferred. Several studies report that most anterior glenohumeral dislocations can be reduced with intra-articular lidocaine. As a result, the complications of intravenous medication (oversedation, nausea, and vomiting) are avoided and the duration of time spent in the emergency department is significantly reduced. Occasionally, greater relaxation is required, and it should be considered in patients with nondisplaced proximal humeral fractures to avoid iatrogenic displacement.

After closed reduction the shoulder is typically immobilized for 2 to 4 weeks. Most studies demonstrate that immobilization in internal rotation does not affect the recurrence rate. A Cochrane database study concluded that there was essentially no evidence to determine the best method of conservative management following closed reduction of traumatic anterior dislocation of the shoulder.[53]

Recently there has been increasing interest in external rotation immobilization after primary anterior glenohumeral dislocation. An in vitro study with a simulated Bankart lesion found that external rotation of the shoulder increased the contact force between the glenoid labrum.[54] Another study used MRI to evaluate coaptation of a Bankart lesion in 19 shoulders with anterior glenohumeral instability.[55] The authors found that separation and displacement were significantly less when the shoulder was in an external rotation position compared to the typical immobilization position of internal rotation. However, despite these findings, recent comparative series have been contradictory regarding benefits to immobilization in external rotation. Early arthroscopic evaluation after traumatic anterior dislocation concluded that internal rotation immobilization of the shoulder malreduces the Bankart lesion and contributes to the incidence of recurrent instability.[56] Conversely, immobilization in external rotation seems to improve redislocation rates.[57]

Recurrent dislocation is the most common complication or sequela of anterior glenohumeral dislocation. Early recurrence within the first week after injury is indicative of more extensive injury, possibly including a large rotator cuff tear or disruption of the normal osseous restraints to dislocation due to either an isolated fracture of the glenoid rim or fractures of both the glenoid rim and the greater tuberosity. Early surgical stabilization for these patients is indicated.[58]

Surgical Treatment

Advances in the understanding of the natural history of primary anterior glenohumeral dislocation have led to increased consideration of primary surgical stabilization. The negative correlation between patient age at the time of initial dislocation and the rate of recurrence has long been recognized. Nevertheless, the traditional indication for surgical treatment was recurrent dislocation or instability. Initial favorable reports of primary surgical stabilization in young, high-risk populations stimulated further investigation of both the natural history of anterior shoulder instability and the effect of primary surgical treatment.

A prospective nonrandomized study of mostly rugby players found that 95% of the patients treated nonsurgically had a recurrent dislocation within 18 months.[59] In contrast, only 5% of the patients treated with an arthroscopic repair had a recurrent dislocation. A small randomized prospective study of a young military population also compared nonsurgical and acute arthroscopic repair.[60] The authors found that at an average follow-up of 36 months, 75% of the nonsurgical patient group had recurrent instability, whereas only 12 percent of the patients who underwent repair had recurrent instability.

A Cochrane database systematic review reported in 2004 found that surgical treatment resulted in statistically significant lower recurrent instability rates.[61] However, it was concluded that there was insufficient evidence available to determine whether nonsurgical treatment should not remain the prime treatment option. A more recent prospective, randomized, double-blinded study of 88 patients younger than 35 years compared the outcome of arthroscopic lavage with arthroscopic Bankart repair and found that surgical repair reduced the risk of redislocation by 76% and the risk of recurrent instability by 82%.[62] They also found that the functional scores of the surgical repair group were better with lower treatment costs and greater satisfaction. Nevertheless, the treatment of primary anterior glenohumeral dislocation remains controversial.

Understanding the natural history of primary anterior glenohumeral dislocation is of paramount importance. The 25-year follow-up of a prospective multicenter study of 257 Swedish patients was recently reported.[63] The rate of surgical treatment of recurrent dislocation was correlated with patient age at the time of initial dislocation. Seventy percent to 75% of patients younger than 20 years had at least one recur-

rence. Of those patients who had a recurrence, approximately 45% underwent surgical stabilization. Overall, 22% of the patients had recurrent dislocations and were not surgically stabilized. Of these, 65% did not have a recurrent event within 10 years and were considered to be stable. Another prospective observational study of 252 patients between age 15 and 35 years used survivorship analysis to determine that the rate of recurrence was 55.7% at 2 years and 66.8% at 5 years.[64]

Posterior Dislocation

Closed Reduction

The management of posterior dislocations depends on timely diagnosis and the extent of the anterior impression fracture. Closed reduction is more likely to be successful when the humeral head defect involves less than 20% of the articular surface. When there is greater involvement of the humeral head, the reduction is more likely to be unstable, and surgical treatment may be required. Closed reduction can be performed under local anesthesia, intravenous sedation, or general anesthesia. The goal is to minimize resistance from the patient to easily obtain the reduction and avoid iatrogenic fracture. The arm is flexed forward, internally rotated, and adducted to disengage the head from the posterior glenoid rim. With longitudinal traction and anterior pressure on the humeral head from behind, reduction is achieved. The arm is externally rotated, lowered to the side, and then immobilized in 15° of extension and 15° of external rotation for 4 to 6 weeks in a light fiberglass cast or prefabricated brace. Contraindications to closed reduction are a fixed dislocation that is not easily reducible or a fracture at the surgical neck or greater tuberosity.

If the glenohumeral joint is unstable after closed reduction, temporary percutaneous fixation can be considered. This procedure is more reliable when the articular segment injury involves 20% or less of the articular surface but can also be considered when 20% to 40% of the articular segment is involved and there are contraindications to more extensive surgical treatment. Fixation from the acromion into the humeral head is preferable to transarticular glenohumeral fixation. The pins should be buried to avoid pin tract infection and removed 4 to 6 weeks later.

Surgical Treatment

Open reduction is indicated when the humeral head defect is larger. Open reduction is usually performed through an anterior deltopectoral approach, which permits evaluation of the anterior impression fracture. The humeral head is carefully disengaged from the posterior aspect of the glenoid with a wide flat elevator. A superior deltoid-splitting approach can also be used for open reduction. There are several alternatives to reconstruct the anterior humeral head impression defect to restore glenohumeral stability and shoulder function. In rare cases the impacted articular surface of the humeral head can be disimpacted. Bone graft is packed underneath the reduced articular surface to support it and prevent collapse.[65] Transfer of the subscapularis tendon into the impression defect, as described by McLaughlin, or Neer's modification in which the lesser tuberosity is transferred, is effective in preventing recurrent posterior dislocation. The results of tuberosity transfer have been superior to those of subscapularis transfer.[66]

Femoral head and humeral head allograft can be used to reconstruct large humeral head defects. Femoral head allograft has the advantage of better bone quality.[67] When the humeral head defect is large or greater than 40% or when significant degeneration of the articular surface has occurred, humeral head replacement is also an option that avoids the longer term risk of allograft collapse.[68]

Brachial Plexus Injuries

Although neurologic injury is relatively uncommon, when associated with musculoskeletal trauma it can have a substantial effect on the outcome. The general proximity of these structures to the skeletal elements of the shoulder girdle, as well as specific anatomic relationships, place the brachial plexus and proximal peripheral nerves at risk of injury. Nerve injury can occur as a result of blunt injury, stretch injury, and direct contact with fracture fragments. Studies with electrodiagnostic testing demonstrate that the prevalence of nerve injuries associated with glenohumeral dislocations and humeral neck fractures ranges from 20% to 30%. In patients older than 50 years, it is as high as 50%. Vascular injury should always be considered when there is a neurologic injury.

The brachial plexus is particularly vulnerable in high-energy trauma. Brachial plexus injuries are reported to occur in up to 5% of motorcycle and snowmobile accidents and are more common among males.[69] Closed head injuries, rib fractures, and intrathoracic injury are commonly associated with brachial plexus injuries. Musculoskeletal shoulder girdle injuries including scapulothoracic dissociation, comminuted proximal humerus fractures, and clavicle fractures are associated with brachial plexus injuries but are not necessarily always present. Brachial plexus injuries are classified as either supraclavicular or infraclavicular. The cervical roots and upper trunk of the brachial plexus are fixed at the neck and by attachment to the proximal peripheral nerves of the upper extremity and are typically injured by traction mechanisms. Most brachial plexus injuries are supraclavicular and are often mixed injuries with a variety of root, cord, and peripheral nerve involvement due to the extensive length of injury.[70] Supraclavicular injuries often involve nerve root avulsion and have a poor prognosis for recovery.

The proximal peripheral nerves including the spinal accessory nerve, long thoracic nerve, suprascapular nerve, axillary nerve, and musculoskeletal nerve can be injured with shoulder girdle trauma. The axillary nerve is the most commonly injured peripheral nerve. It is fixed by connection to the posterior cord and the deltoid, and passes through the quadrilateral space inferior to the glenohumeral joint. Although anatomic variants of the proximal peripheral nerves are uncommon, there is considerable variability in the precise anatomic locations and positions. The location of the axillary nerve is on average 5 cm (range, 4 to 7 cm) lateral to the acromion, and the distance from the coracoid to the musculocutaneous nerve is on average 5 cm (range, 2 to 8 cm).

Axillary nerve injury is the most common nerve injury associated with glenohumeral dislocation and occurs in as many as 5% to 10% of cases. Most axillary nerve injuries associated with dislocation are neurapraxias and recover within 4 to 6 months. The suprascapular nerve is at risk of injury from scapula fracture. The suprascapular nerve passes through the suprascapular and spinoglenoid notches and can be injured in association with scapular neck fractures. The motor branches to the supraspinatus muscle are about 3 cm medial to the supraglenoid tubercle, whereas the motor branches to the infraspinatus are about 2 cm from the posterior glenoid. Isolated musculocutaneous nerve injuries are rare but are reported in association with anterior glenohumeral dislocation. The presence of a peripheral nerve injury should lead one to perform a more detailed evaluation of the brachial plexus and other peripheral nerves.

A detailed physical examination is the preliminary means of evaluating the neurologic status of the upper extremity. Even in the initial evaluation setting a reasonably good determination of the neurovascular status is possible. If the patient is cooperative, palpation of voluntary muscle contraction is usually possible. In the acute setting all peripheral nerves from the axillary to more distal nerves can usually be assessed for both motor and sensory function. The examination is organized so that identification of a distal deficit prompts investigation for more proximal injury at the cord, trunk, or root level. Management of life-threatening injuries takes precedence over the treatment of brachial plexus injuries. Associated shoulder girdle injuries are initially treated with the expectation that the neurologic injury will recover. Further investigation with advanced imaging and electrodiagnostic studies is pursued if there are no signs of recovery. Electrodiagnostic studies are used to document the extent of an injury as well as to monitor recovery. They can be obtained after 3 weeks when wallerian degeneration has occurred and denervation patterns can be detected.

Most brachial plexus and proximal peripheral nerve injuries are neurapraxic and undergo substantial spontaneous recovery within a few months. Axonotmetic injuries in which the epineurium and perineurium remain intact recover through nerve regeneration at the rate of 1 to 4 mm per day.[70] Neurotmetic lesions with complete axonal disruption have no capacity to recover spontaneously. Surgical exploration is indicated when there is failure of spontaneous recovery of a peripheral nerve injury after 3 months. Most recent literature suggests consideration of early surgical treatment of severe brachial plexus injuries.[71] Surgical treatment of patients with brachial plexus injuries consists of several nerve procedures, muscle transfers and transplantation, osteotomies, and joint arthrodesis. Nerve repair and reconstructive procedures include neurolysis, intraplexus ipsilateral and contralateral neurotization, extraplexus neurotization, and nerve transfers, all with or without nerve grafting. Restoration of elbow flexion is a priority, followed by shoulder stability and more distal function.

Summary

Shoulder trauma management continues to evolve. As with other articular injuries, glenoid fractures often warrant open reduction and internal fixation. As the understanding of shoulder trauma improves, the importance of restoration of anatomic relationships becomes clearer. At the same time, surgical interventions become more refined. The goal of anatomic restoration and improved methods of surgical care may increase surgical indications. As outcomes studies become available, they help refine decision making.

Annotated References

1. Zlowodzki M, Bhandari M, Zelle BA, Kregor PJ, Cole PA: Treatment of scapula fractures: Systematic review of 520 fractures in 22 case series. *J Orthop Trauma* 2006;20(3):230-233.

   The authors reviewed 22 series of scapula fracture treatment. Data were compiled on 520 fractures from these series to identify relative occurrence of fracture types, treatments selected, reported results of treatment, and complications including infection and secondary surgical care.

2. Lantry JM, Roberts CS, Giannoudis PV: Operative treatment of scapular fractures: A systematic review. *Injury* 2008;39(3):271-283.

   The authors retrospectively reviewed 17 series of surgically treated scapula fractures, totaling 243 cases. Most commonly treated were glenoid fossa and glenoid neck fractures. Most had undergone posterior surgical approaches and were fixed with plates and screws. Approximately 25% had ipsilateral clavicle fracture. Most patients had excellent outcomes, and complications were infrequent.

3. Baldwin KD, Ohman-Strickland P, Mehta S, Hume E: Scapula fractures: A marker for concomitant injury? A retrospective review of data in the National Trauma Database. *J Trauma* 2008;65(2):430-435.

   This review of the National Trauma Database, undertaken from 1992 to 2002, sought to correlate injury patterns with scapula injury. The authors controlled for overall injury severity in order to identify those concomitant injuries that seemed more commonly associated with scapula fractures and were not merely reflective of overall injury severity. After adjusting for severity, injuries associated with scapula fractures were upper extremity, thoracic, and pelvic injury.

4. Armitage BM, Wijdicks CA, Tarkin IS, et al: Mapping of scapular fractures with three-dimensional computed tomography. *J Bone Joint Surg Am* 2009;91(9):2222-2228.

   The authors sought reproducible patterns of fracture in a series of patients, all of whom had surgical treatment for fractures of the scapula. Although fractures varied, the most common pattern is the lateral border fracture immediately inferior to the glenoid and extending to the superior aspect of the medial scapula. Less common are intra-articular fractures.

5. Tadros AM, Lunsjo K, Czechowski J, Corr P, Abu-Zidan FM: Usefulness of different imaging modalities in the assessment of scapular fractures caused by blunt trauma. *Acta Radiol* 2007;48(1):71-75.

   The authors of this study found CT to be more useful than plain radiographs in identifying discrete aspects of scapula fracture. Three-dimensional CT was found to be most useful.

6. Bozkurt M, Can F, Kirdemir V, Erden Z, Demirkale I, Başbozkurt M: Conservative treatment of scapular neck fracture: The effect of stability and glenopolar angle on clinical outcome. *Injury* 2005;36(10):1176-1181.

   This series of 18 patients with extra-articular scapula fractures treated nonsurgically found that older patients had more displacement as seen on glenopolar angle, that Constant score was positively associated with glenopolar angle, and that outcome was significantly affected by associated injuries.

7. Kim KC, Rhee KJ, Shin HD, Yang JY: Can the glenopolar angle be used to predict outcome and treatment of the floating shoulder? *J Trauma* 2008;64(1):174-178.

   This series of seven patients, all of whom had ipsilateral clavicle and scapula fractures (floating shoulder) examined displacement as measured by glenopolar angle and outcome as measured by Constant score. There was a statistically significant decrease in Constant score with decreasing glenopolar angle.

8. Schofer MD, Sehrt AC, Timmesfeld N, Stormer S, Kortmann HR: Fractures of the scapula: Long-term results after conservative treatment. *Arch Orthop Trauma Surg* 2009;129(11):1511-1519.

   This long-term outcome study evaluated 50 patients with 51 scapula fractures for an average of 65 months after closed treatment. There were some limitations in motion and strength, but overall functional results were quite good.

9. Chadwick EK, van Noort A, van der Helm FC: Biomechanical analysis of scapular neck malunion: A simulation study. *Clin Biomech* 2004;19(9):906-912.

   The authors sought an explanation for loss of shoulder function after scapular neck malunion according to biomechanical changes around the glenohumeral joint. A loss of force in the rotator cuff muscles and changes in muscle activation can lead to loss of arm function in patients with scapular neck malunion.

10. Herrera DA, Anavian J, Tarkin IS, Armitage BA, Schroder LK, Cole PA: Delayed operative management of fractures of the scapula. *J Bone Joint Surg Br* 2009; 91(5):619-626.

    Twenty-two patients with fractures of the scapula were treated surgically more than 3 weeks after injury. Sixteen of 22 had radiologic and functional follow-up, a mean time of 12 months postoperatively. Thirteen of 16 returned to previous employment and recreational activities without limitation. No wound complications or nonunions occurred.

11. Gosens T, Speigner B, Minedus J: Fracture of the scapular body: Functional outcome after conservative treatment. *J Shoulder Elbow Surg* 2009;18:443-448.

    The authors present a strong argument that the poor results of some patients with scapula fractures are caused by associated injuries. Truly isolated scapula fractures had good outcomes according to DASH, (Simple Shoulder Test), and SF-36 scores.

12. Maquieira GJ, Espinosa N, Gerber C, Eid K: Nonoperative treatment of large anterior glenoid rim fractures after traumatic anterior dislocation of the shoulder. *J Bone Joint Surg Br* 2007;89(10):1347-1351.

    This study followed 14 consecutive patients with large (greater than 5 mm), displaced (greater than 2 mm) anteroinferior glenoid rim fractures associated with dislocation. All had conservative care. There were no redislocations or subluxations, and no arthritis seen after a mean follow-up of 5 to 6 years. The authors concluded that anteroinferior glenoid fractures can be treated nonsurgically if concentric shoulder reduction can be achieved on the AP radiograph.

13. Bauer T, Abadie O, Hardy P: Arthroscopic treatment of glenoid fractures. *Arthroscopy* 2006;22(5):569, e1-e6.

    Arthroscopic reduction and suture fixation techniques for the treatment of displaced glenoid fractures are described.

14. Anavian J, Wijdicks CA, Vang S, Schroder LK, Cole PA: Surgery for scapula process fractures: Good outcome in 26 patients. *Acta Orthop* 2009;80(3):344-350.

    The authors describe a case series of 26 patients with 27 fractures of the coracoid or acromial process of the scapula. After mean follow-up of 11 months the only complications observed were painful hardware, leading to its removal in three patients. All fractures united and all shoulders regained full motion.

15. Nork SE, Barei DP, Gardner MJ, Schildhauer TA, Mayo KA, Benirschke SK: Surgical exposure and fixation of displaced type IV, V, and VI glenoid fractures. *J Orthop Trauma* 2008;22(7):487-493.

    The authors describe a modification of the extensile surgical approach of Judet that allows for exposure of the intra-articular glenoid as well as the medial scapular body. Also described is a reduction and fixation strategy used in commonly encountered fracture patterns.

16. Jones CB, Cornelius JP, Sietsema DL, Ringler JR, Endres TJ: Modified Judet approach and minifragment fixation of scapular body and glenoid neck fractures. *J Orthop Trauma* 2009;23(8):558-564.

    The authors describe their modification of the Judet extensile approach to intra-articular glenoid fractures. Fracture fixation was provided by 27-mm minifragment plates.

17. Zelle BA, Pape HC, Gerich TG, Garapati R, Ceylan B, Krettek C: Functional outcome following scapulothoracic dissociation. *J Bone Joint Surg Am* 2004;86(1): 2-8.

    The authors report on the functional outcome of 24 patients with scapulothoracic dissocation, an average of 12.6 years after injury. Patients who sustained concomitant complete brachial plexus palsy had significantly worse outcomes on the SF-36 and Subjective Shoulder Rating System scales.

18. Sen RK, Prasad G, Aggarwal S: Scapulothoracic dissociation: Level of vascular insult, an indirect prognostic indicator for the final outcome? *Acta Orthop Belg* 2009; 75(1):14-18.

    The authors retrospectively reviewed scapulothoracic dissocation in 8 patients and combined data with 37 patients previously reported in the literature. They correlated proximal arterial injury (subclavian artery) with risk of complete brachial plexus palsy versus more distal arterial injury (axillary artery) with risk of partial plexus palsy.

19. Riess KP, Cogbill TH, Patel NY, Lambert PJ, Mathiason MA: Brachial plexus injury: Long-term functional outcome is determined by associated scapulothoracic dissociation. *J Trauma* 2007;63(5):1021-1025.

    This retrospective review of 29 patients treated for brachial plexus injury caused by blunt force were divided into those with and without associated scapulothoracic dissociation. Those with scapulothoracic dissociation had significantly worse functional outcomes as they related to muscle function and disability.

20. Postacchini F, Gumina S, De Santis P, Albo F: Epidemiology of clavicle fractures. *J Shoulder Elbow Surg* 2002; 11(5):452-456.

21. Lenza M, Belloti JC, Andriolo RB, Gomes Dos Santos JB, Faloppa F: Conservative interventions for treating middle third clavicle fractures in adolescents and adults. *Cochrane Database Syst Rev* 2009;2:CD007121.

    This Cochrane database study compiled data for three randomized and quasirandomized studies of nonsurgical treatment protocols for clavicle fracture. Outcomes included pain, shoulder function, and health-related quality of life, as well as return-to-activity information. The authors found no significant benefit to ultrasound treatment, nor any benefit to either figure-of-8 bandage or simple sling in comparison with each other.

3: Upper Extremity

22. Robinson CM, Court-Brown CM, McQueen MM, Wakefield AE: Estimating the risk of nonunion following nonoperative treatment of a clavicular fracture. *J Bone Joint Surg Am* 2004;86(7):1359-1365.

This was a prospective observational study of clavicle fractures treated closed. Over 51 months there were 868 patients, 8 of whom were treated with immediate surgery. At 24 weeks there were 6.2% nonunions. Risk factors for nonunion included advancing age, female gender, displacement of fracture (lack of cortical apposition), and presence of comminution.

23. Nowak J, Holgersson M, Larsson S: Sequelae from clavicular fractures are common: A prospective study of 222 patients. *Acta Orthop* 2005;76(4):496-502.

24. McKee MD, Wild LM, Schemitsch EH: Midshaft malunions of the clavicle: Surgical technique. *J Bone Joint Surg Am* 2004;86(suppl 1):37-43.

Fifteen patients underwent corrective osteotomy for malunion of the clavicle following closed treatment. The technique included osteotomy through the fracture site, and internal fixation with plate and screws. Patients reported improvements in DASH scores from an average of 32 points to 12 points. Complications included one nonunion and two patients requiring plate removal. All patients, except the one with nonunion, reported a high degree of satisfaction.

25. Robinson CM, Cairns DA: Primary nonoperative treatment of displaced lateral fractures of the clavicle. *J Bone Joint Surg Am* 2004;86(4):778-782.

One hundred twenty of 127 patients with displaced fractures of the lateral clavicle were treated nonsurgically. Eighty-six patients were seen an average 6.2 years after injury. Fifteen more were interviewed by phone. Fourteen percent had symptoms severe enough to warrant surgical intervention. Of the remaining 87 patients, 21 had a nonunion. The average Constant score on the nonsurgically treated group was 93 points. There were no significant differences in Constant score between those with early surgery, late surgery, or no surgery. None of the groups differed from age-matched control subjects on the SF-36.

26. McKee MD, Seiler JG, Jupiter JB: The application of the limited contact dynamic compression plate in the upper extremity: An analysis of 114 consecutive cases. *Injury* 1995;26(10):661-666.

27. Collinge C, Devinney S, Herscovici D, DiPasquale T, Sanders R: Anterior-inferior plate fixation of middle-third fractures and nonunions of the clavicle. *J Orthop Trauma* 2006;20(10):680-686.

Eighty consecutive patients with a middle third fracture or painful nonunion of the clavicle underwent open reduction and internal fixation using an anteroinferior plating technique with a precontoured 3.5-mm plate and lag screw(s). Clinical and radiographic union was present at a mean of 9.5 weeks for patients treated for acute fracture and 10.5 weeks for those treated for nonunion. Complications included one failure of fixation, one nonunion, and three infections. Two patients underwent implant removal for bothersome hardware. Func-

tional results (American Shoulder and Elbow Surgeons and SF-36) were good or excellent for the vast majority of patients, except those with neurologic injury.

28. Schwarz N, Höcker K: Osteosynthesis of irreducible fractures of the clavicle with 2.7-mm ASIF plates. *J Trauma* 1992;33(2):179-183.

29. Huang JI, Toogood P, Chen MR, Wilber JH, Cooperman DR: Clavicular anatomy and the applicability of precontoured plates. *J Bone Joint Surg Am* 2007; 89(10):2260-2265.

Clavicular anatomy was examined in 100 pairs of bones using mapping software. Axial radiographs were taken, and a template for a commercially available precontoured clavicular plate was examined. The plate, designed to fit the superior surface of the clavicle, fit poorly in 38% of specimens. The best fit for this plate was found to be along the medial aspect of the superior surface.

30. Celestre P, Roberston C, Mahar A, Oka R, Meunier M, Schwartz A: Biomechanical evaluation of clavicle fracture plating techniques: Does a locking plate provide improved stability? *J Orthop Trauma* 2008;22(4):241-247.

Biomechanical testing was performed on synthetic clavicle models with simulated fractures, comparing superior and inferior placement as well as locking and nonlocking screw constructs. In bending failure, superior plate placement was superior to inferior placement. Superior locked plate-screw constructs had improved bending stiffness compared with nonlocked constructs.

31. Robertson C, Celestre P, Mahar A, Schwartz A: Reconstruction plates for stabilization of mid-shaft clavicle fractures: Differences between nonlocked and locked plates in two different positions. *J Shoulder Elbow Surg* 2009;18(2):204-209.

This study evaluated the biomechanical stability of locking and nonlocking clavicle reconstruction plates for treating midshaft, transverse fractures, comparing anteroinferior to superior plate position. Repaired constructs were tested in axial compression, axial torsion, and cantilever bending failure. In compression, anteroinferior plates were significantly stiffer than superior plates and locked plates stiffer than nonlocked. In torsion, anteroinferior plates were stiffer, with a significant interaction term that favored anteroinferior locked and superior nonlocked plates. In cantilever bending, superior plates had a significantly higher bending failure load and stiffness. Anteroinferior plates failed at a significantly lower load (approximately 40 N or approximately 4 kg), which could potentially occur in the postoperative period.

32. Renger RJ, Roukema GR, Reurings JC, Raams PM, Font J, Verleisdonk EJ: The clavicle hook plate for Neer type II lateral clavicle fractures. *J Orthop Trauma* 2009; 23(8):570-574.

Forty-four patients, average age 38.4 years (18 to 66 years), with a Neer type II lateral clavicle fracture were treated with the clavicle hook plate. All 44 implants were removed after consolidation, at a mean of 8.4 months (2 to 33 months) postoperatively. At an average follow-up of 27.4 months (13 to 48 months), the average Constant score was 92.4 (74 to 100). Complications included one dislocation of an implant (2.2%), two cases of pseudarthrosis (4.5%), two superficial wound infections (4.5%), two patients with hypertrophic scar tissue (4.5%), and three instances of acromial osteolysis (6.8%). Thirty patients (68%) reported discomfort caused by the implant. These implant-related complaints and the acromial osteolysis disappeared after removal of the hook plate. Removal of all implants was recommended.

33. Flinkkilä T, Ristiniemi J, Lakovaara M, Hyvönen P, Leppilahti J: Hook-plate fixation of unstable lateral clavicle fractures: A report on 63 patients. *Acta Orthop* 2006;77(4):644-649.

Sixty-three patients with unstable lateral clavicle fixation were treated with open reduction and internal fixation with a plate that attached to the clavicle with screws and had a hook designed to be placed under the acromion. There were three nonunions and one delayed union, only one of which required surgery. Fifty-nine fractures healed uneventfully.

34. Jubel A, Andermahr J, Schiffer G, Tsironis K, Rehm KE: Elastic stable intramedullary nailing of midclavicular fractures with a titanium nail. *Clin Orthop Relat Res* 2003;408:279-285.

35. Canadian Orthopaedic Trauma Society: Nonoperative treatment compared with plate fixation of displaced midshaft clavicular fractures: A multicenter, randomized clinical trial. *J Bone Joint Surg Am* 2007;89(1):1-10.

This randomized clinical trail compared plate fixation to nonsurgical treatment in 132 displaced midshaft clavicle fractures, emphasizing patient-oriented outcomes and complications. DASH and Constant scores were dramatically better in the surgery group at all time points, while the mean time to union was 28.4 weeks in the nonsurgical group compared to 16.4 weeks in the surgery group. Most complications in the surgery group were hardware-related.

36. Tischer T, Salzmann GM, El-Azab H, Vogt S, Imhoff AB: Incidence of associated injuries with acute acromioclavicular joint dislocations types III through V. *Am J Sports Med* 2009;37(1):136-139.

The authors performed diagnostic arthroscopy on 77 patients who were undergoing surgical treatment of an acute type III, IV, or V acromioclavicular dislocation. Fourteen percent of the patients had an associated superior labral anterior-posterior (SLAP) tear. There was one full-thickness rotator cuff tear. The mean age of the patients with SLAP tears was 42.1 versus 35.5 years (*P* = 0.058) for patients without SLAP tears. Although the authors treated the SLAP tears arthroscopically in all cases they did not determine whether the SLAP tears were preexisting or whether the treatment of the SLAP tear affected the outcome.

37. Mouhsine E, Garofalo R, Crevoisier X, Farron A: Grade I and II acromioclavicular dislocations: Results of conservative treatment. *J Shoulder Elbow Surg* 2003;12(6):599-602.

38. Bannister GC, Wallace WA, Stableforth PG, Hutson MA: The management of acute acromioclavicular dislocation: A randomised prospective controlled trial. *J Bone Joint Surg Br* 1989;71(5):848-850.

39. Deshmukh AV, Wilson DR, Zilberfarb JL, Perlmutter GS: Stability of acromioclavicular joint reconstruction: Biomechanical testing of various surgical techniques in a cadaveric model. *Am J Sports Med* 2004;32(6):1492-1498.

Concerns exist about the strength of traditional Weaver-Dunn reconstructions. The mean anterior-posterior and superior laxity of an unaugmented Weaver-Dunn reconstruction was four to five times greater than in its native state. Although the laxity of coracoclavicular fixation with coracoclavicular suture fixation was significantly less than the laxity of unaugmented Weaver-Dunn, the laxity of coracoclavicular fixation was also significantly greater than in its native state. The authors did not evaluate the laxity of coracoacromial ligament transfer with coracoclavicular augmentation.

40. Mazzocca AD, Santangelo SA, Johnson ST, Rios CG, Dumonski ML, Arciero RA: A biomechanical evaluation of an anatomical coracoclavicular ligament reconstruction. *Am J Sports Med* 2006;34(2):236-246.

In this study, the authors compared the strength of three surgical repairs for acromioclavicular dislocation. The anatomic coracoclavicular ligament repair with tendon graft had significantly less laxity than a modified Weaver-Dunn reconstruction.

41. LaPrade RF, Wickum DJ, Griffith CJ, Ludewig PM: Kinematic evaluation of the modified Weaver-Dunn acromioclavicular joint reconstruction. *Am J Sports Med* 2008;36(11):2216-2221.

The authors used a cadaver model with intact, cut state, and reconstruction with coracoacromial ligament transfer and coracoclavicular suture fixation to evaluate translational motion of the acromioclavicular during passive shoulder elevation. The modified Weaver-Dunn reconstruction restored acromioclavicular translation to near-intact values. However, the reconstruction fixed the clavicle in a more anterior and inferior position. Because the distal clavicle is resected in this reconstruction, the slight malposition of the clavicle is probably not clinically significant.

42. Dimakopoulos P, Panagopoulos A, Syggelos SA, Panagiotopoulos E, Lambiris E: Double-loop suture repair for acute acromioclavicular joint disruption. *Am J Sports Med* 2006;34(7):1112-1119.

The authors report the results of the surgical treatment of 34 patients (24 type III, 10 type V). They used coracoclavicular suture fixation. At a mean follow-up period of 33.2 months, the mean Constant-Murley score was 93.5 points. There were no patients with posttraumatic acromioclavicular joint degeneration. There was slight loss of reduction in only two patients.

43. Baker JE, Nicandri GT, Young DC, Owen JR, Wayne JS: A cadaveric study examining acromioclavic-

3: Upper Extremity

ular joint congruity after different methods of coraco-clavicular loop repair. *J Shoulder Elbow Surg* 2003; 12(6):595-598.

The authors compared the congruity of the acromio-clavicular after coracoclavicular fixation with subcoracoid sutures through drill holes. Drill holes placed more anteriorly improved the acromioclavicular congruity, although none fully restored normal joint congruity. The findings are most relevant to acromioclavicular joint repairs and reconstructions that do not resect the distal clavicle. The importance on precise acromioclavicular joint alignment has not been determined.

44. Gstettner C, Tauber M, Hitzl W, Resch H: Rockwood type III acromioclavicular dislocation: Surgical versus conservative treatment. *J Shoulder Elbow Surg* 2008; 17(2):220-225.

The authors compared the results of two treatment cohorts; 17 patients treated nonsurgically and 24 patients treated surgically with a clavicle hook plate. The patients were provided with information regarding the treatment of type III acromioclavicular dislocations and elected their treatment. At mean follow-up of 37 months the mean Constant score for the nonsurgical group was 80.7 compared to 90.4 ($P < 0.05$) for the surgical group. Ten of 17 nonsurgically treated patients (58.8%) achieved excellent or good results while 21 of 24 surgically treated patients (87.5%) achieved excellent or good results. In this study, patients who selected surgical treatment of acute type III acromioclavicular dislocations with a clavicle hook plate appeared to have superior outcomes when compared to patients who elected nonsurgical treatment.

45. Chernchujit B, Tischer T, Imhoff AB: Arthroscopic reconstruction of the acromioclavicular joint disruption: Surgical technique and preliminary results. *Arch Orthop Trauma Surg* 2006;126(9):575-581.

The authors report the results of arthroscopic-assisted repair of acute type IV and V acromioclavicular dislocations. The mean Constant score was 95, and 12 of the 13 patients considered the result to be good or excellent.

46. Calvo E, López-Franco M, Arribas IM: Clinical and radiologic outcomes of surgical and conservative treatment of type III acromioclavicular joint injury. *J Shoulder Elbow Surg* 2006;15(3):300-305.

In a retrospective chart review, the authors compared the minimum 12-month outcomes of 32 patients treated with open reduction and acromioclavicular transarticular pin fixation to those of 11 patients who had nonsurgical treatment of type III acromioclavicular dislocations. There was no statistically significant difference in the clinical outcomes. The acromioclavicular joint remained anatomically reduced in only half of the surgically treated patients, and surgically treated patients had a greater incidence of acromioclavicular arthritis. Consequently, the authors recommended nonsurgical treatment of type III acromioclavicular dislocations.

47. Lee SJ, Keefer EP, McHugh MP, et al: Cyclical loading of coracoclavicular ligament reconstructions: A comparative biomechanical study. *Am J Sports Med* 2008; 36(10):1990-1997.

Recent developments in reconstruction of acromioclavicular dislocations have focused on coracoclavicular ligament reconstruction with tendon grafts. In this study, the authors compared reconstruction of acromioclavicular dislocations with coracoacromial transfer without and with augmentation with either no. 5 coracoclavicular suture fixation or semitendinosus graft. All of the isolated coracoclavicular ligament transfers failed under low load cycling. At the higher loads all of the suture-augmented repairs failed while the semitendinosus graft augmented specimens did not.

48. Nicholas SJ, Lee SJ, Mullaney MJ, Tyler TF, McHugh MP: Clinical outcomes of coracoclavicular ligament reconstructions using tendon grafts. *Am J Sports Med* 2007;35(11):1912-1917.

The authors report the results of nine cases of type V acromioclavicular dislocation that were treated with coracoclavicular ligament reconstruction using a semitendinosus allograft passed under the coracoid and through a drill hole in the clavicle. The distal 1 cm of the clavicle was resected and the repair was augmented with a suture tape that was passed with the tendon allograft. Follow-up radiographs demonstrated maintenance of the distal clavicle reduction, and the patients regained near normal shoulder motion and strength.

49. Tauber M, Gordon K, Koller H, Fox M, Resch H: Semitendinosus tendon graft versus a modified Weaver-Dunn procedure for acromioclavicular joint reconstruction in chronic cases: A prospective comparative study. *Am J Sports Med* 2009;37(1):181-190.

Two consecutive cohorts (nonrandomized) of 12 patients had treatment of a chronic type III, IV, or V acromioclavicular dislocation with a modified Weaver-Dunn procedure or a semitendinosus graft reconstruction of the coracoclavicular ligaments. Supplemental coracoclavicular fixation was provided with a cerclage wire in both procedures. The outcomes as determined with the American Shoulder and Elbow Surgeons and Constant scores were significantly better with the tendon graft reconstruction. In addition there was mean loss of reduction in the Weaver-Dunn group of about 2.5 mm.

50. Osti M, Gohm A, Benedetto KP: Results of open reconstruction of anterior glenoid rim fractures following shoulder dislocation. *Arch Orthop Trauma Surg* 2009; 129(9):1245-1249.

The authors reported the outcome of open reduction and internal fixation of anterior inferior glenoid fractures. The mean age of the patients was 49.4 years, somewhat older than the usual patients who have surgical treatment of anterior glenohumeral dislocations. The repairs were performed with an anterior arthrotomy and cannulated screw fixation of the fracture fragment.

51. Singh S, Tan CK, Sinopidis C, et al: Missed posterior dislocations of the shoulder after intramedullary fixation of humeral fractures: A report of three cases. *J Shoulder Elbow Surg* 2009;18:33-37.

The authors discuss three cases in which posterior dislocations were missed after fracture fixation.

52. Eachempati KK, Dua A, Malhotra R, Bhan S, Bera JR: The external rotation method for reduction of acute an-

terior dislocations and fracture-dislocations of the shoulder. *J Bone Joint Surg Am* 2004;86(11):2431-2434.

The authors reported successful closed reduction in 29 of 40 patients in an emergency department setting with minimal premedication using the external rotation method. This experience contrasts recent trends that favor the use of monitored conscious sedation. This approach provides faster reduction in many cases and avoids potential complications and resource requirements of conscious sedation.

53. Handoll HH, Hanchard NC, Goodchild L, Feary J: Conservative management following closed reduction of traumatic anterior dislocation of the shoulder. *Cochrane Database Syst Rev* 2006;1:CD004962.

In this meta-analysis, the authors identified only one report of a quasirandomized controlled trial that studied nonsurgical management after traumatic anterior dislocation of the shoulder. They reviewed the study by Itoi et al[57] that compared external and internal rotation immobilization. In contrast to the conclusions of Itoi et al, these authors concluded that there was no statistically significant difference in the rates of recurrent instability between the two groups. They also found no difference in the failure to return to preinjury sports by previously active athletes. Lastly, they noted that Itoi et al have presented additional results from continued studies that have yet to be published.

54. Miller BS, Sonnabend DH, Hatrick C, et al: Should acute anterior dislocations of the shoulder be immobilized in external rotation? A cadaveric study. *J Shoulder Elbow Surg* 2004;13(6):589-592.

The authors used a cadaver shoulder model of a Bankart lesion to assess the effect of humeral rotational position on the contact force between the anterior inferior labrum and the glenoid. When the arm was in neutral rotation there was no detectable contact force. The contact force increased as the arm passed through neutral rotation and reached a maximum at 45° of external rotation. The contact force returned to zero when the arm was returned to neutral rotation. Based on the findings, the authors concluded that the external rotation position might improve the healing rate of a Bankart lesion after closed reduction of an anterior glenohumeral dislocation.

55. Itoi E, Sashi R, Minagawa H, Shimizu T, Wakabayashi I, Sato K: Position of immobilization after dislocation of the glenohumeral joint: A study with use of magnetic resonance imaging. *J Bone Joint Surg Am* 2001;83(5):661-667.

56. Hart WJ, Kelly CP: Arthroscopic observation of capsulolabral reduction after shoulder dislocation. *J Shoulder Elbow Surg* 2005;14(2):134-137.

Twenty-five patients with an acute traumatic anterior shoulder dislocation underwent arthroscopic evaluation at a mean of 10 days after injury. The authors evaluated the effect of shoulder position on the reduction of the anteroinferior capsulolabral complex. The reduction of the labrum onto the glenoid was improved in 22 patients (92%). The reduction of the inferior labrum was

further improved with abduction of the arm. Overall, the best reduction was consistently found when the arm was put into a position of 30° of abduction and external rotation of approximately 60°. The authors concluded that immobilization of the shoulder with the arm in internal rotation probably contributes to healing of the Bankart lesion in a malreduced position; this may contribute to the incidence of recurrent instability.

57. Itoi E, Hatakeyama Y, Sato T, et al: Immobilization in external rotation after shoulder dislocation reduces the risk of recurrence: A randomized controlled trial. *J Bone Joint Surg Am* 2007;89(10):2124-2131.

In a randomized controlled trial, the authors studied the benefit of immobilization in external rotation. The risk of recurrence of shoulder dislocation was reduced in comparison with that associated with the conventional method of immobilization in internal rotation.

58. Robinson CM, Kelly M, Wakefield AE: Redislocation of the shoulder during the first six weeks after a primary anterior dislocation: Risk factors and results of treatment. *J Bone Joint Surg Am* 2002;84(9):1552-1559.

59. Larrain MV, Botto GJ, Montenegro HJ, Mauas DM: Arthroscopic repair of acute traumatic anterior shoulder dislocation in young athletes. *Arthroscopy* 2001;17(4): 373-377.

60. Bottoni CR, Wilckens JH, DeBerardino TM, et al: A prospective, randomized evaluation of arthroscopic stabilization versus nonoperative treatment in patients with acute, traumatic, first-time shoulder dislocations. *Am J Sports Med* 2002;30(4):576-580.

61. Handoll HH, Almaiyah MA, Rangan A: Surgical versus non-surgical treatment for acute anterior shoulder dislocation. *Cochrane Database Syst Rev* 2004;1: CD004325.

This meta analysis of studies comparing surgical and nonsurgical treatment of acute anterior shoulder dislocation identified five studies that reported the results of treatment of 239 patients. The authors' analysis found that surgical treatment resulted in statistically significant lower rates of recurrent instability, dislocation, or subluxation. Nevertheless, they also concluded that there was insufficient evidence available to determine whether nonsurgical treatment should remain the prime treatment option for other categories of patients. They emphasized that this is especially true of patient categories at lower risk of activity-limiting recurrence.

62. Robinson CM, Jenkins PJ, White TO, Ker A, Will E: Primary arthroscopic stabilization for a first-time anterior dislocation of the shoulder: A randomized, double-blind trial. *J Bone Joint Surg Am* 2008;90(4):708-721.

The authors compared the 2-year outcome of arthroscopic lavage to arthroscopic repair in a randomized, double-blinded study of 88 patients younger than 35 years who had sustained a primary anterior glenohumeral dislocation. Surgical repair reduced the risk of recurrent dislocation by 76% and recurrent instability by 82%. They also reported that the functional scores were better, the treatment costs lower, and the level of satisfaction greater in the surgical repair group.

63. Hovelius L, Olofsson A, Sandström B, et al: Nonoperative treatment of primary anterior shoulder dislocation in patients forty years of age and younger: A prospective twenty-five-year follow-up. *J Bone Joint Surg Am* 2008;90(5):945-952.

This is the most recent reporting of the findings of the authors' long-term prospective study of the outcome of primary anterior shoulder dislocations in younger patients who were initially treated with immobilization. The rate of surgical treatment of recurrent dislocation correlated with the patient's age at the time of initial dislocation. In patients younger than 20 years, 70% to 75% had at least one recurrence. Of those patients who had a recurrence, approximately 45% underwent surgical stabilization; 30% to 35% of patients from age 20 to 25 years had surgical stabilization. Approximately 15% of patients age 30 to 40 years had surgical stabilization. Overall, 22% of the patients had recurrent dislocations and were not surgically stabilized. Of these, 65% did not have a recurrent event within the past 10 years and were considered to be stable. The long-term outcomes that the authors report should be considered when determining treatment, and they suggest that the current emphasis on early surgical treatment of primary anterior dislocation in younger patients may be overly aggressive.

64. Robinson CM, Howes J, Murdoch H, Will E, Graham C: Functional outcome and risk of recurrent instability after primary traumatic anterior shoulder dislocation in young patients. *J Bone Joint Surg Am* 2006; 88(11):2326-2336.

The authors designed a prospective observational outcome study of 252 patients between age 15 and 35 years. One hundred thirty-four patients had a repeat dislocation and 16 had recurrent subluxation. Recurrent instability occurred at a mean of 13.3 months after the initial injury. Based on survivorship analysis, the rate of recurrence was 55.7% at 2 years and 66.8% at 5 years. One hundred ten of the 134 patients (82%) who had a redislocation were treated with surgical stabilization after the first redislocation. The authors note that this study does not clarify the natural history of primary shoulder dislocation. They support the use of surgical repair to treat after a single recurrent episode.

65. Assom M, Castoldi F, Rossi R, Blonna D, Rossi P: Humeral head impression fracture in acute posterior shoulder dislocation: New surgical technique. *Knee Surg Sports Traumatol Arthrosc* 2006;14(7):668-672.

The authors describe a new surgical technique to treat posterior shoulder dislocation with humeral head impression fracture that is only slightly invasive, where the depressed chondral surface is raised to regain a normal articular contour. The chondral surface is supported by an interference biabsorbable screw, and the insertion of the subscapularis tendon is left intact. Two male patients with an acute shoulder posterior dislocation associated with anteromedial impression fracture of about 40% and 50%, respectively, of the articular humeral shape were treated. The average follow-up was 26 months where plain radiograph and CT scan showed an anatomic humeral surface free from signs of arthritis or necrosis. Functional results were excellent in both cases. This new technique is easy, less invasive than others, and ensures a stable cartilage and subchondral support without the use of grafts.

66. Finkelstein JA, Waddell JP, O'Driscoll SW, Vincent G: Acute posterior fracture dislocations of the shoulder treated with the Neer modification of the McLaughlin procedure. *J Orthop Trauma* 1995;9(3):190-193.

67. Gerber C, Lambert SM: Allograft reconstruction of segmental defects of the humeral head for the treatment of chronic locked posterior dislocation of the shoulder. *J Bone Joint Surg Am* 1996;78(3):376-382.

68. Sperling JW, Pring M, Antuna SA, Cofield RH: Shoulder arthroplasty for locked posterior dislocation of the shoulder. *J Shoulder Elbow Surg* 2004;13(5):522-527.

The authors reviewed 12 patients who underwent arthroplasty for locked posterior dislocation of the shoulder. Follow-up occurred at a minimum of 5 years. Pain relief and restoration of motion were predictable. Three patients underwent revision for instability, all of whom had recurrent dislocations in the early postoperative period. One other patient underwent revision for component loosening.

69. Midha R: Epidemiology of brachial plexus injuries in a multitrauma population. *Neurosurgery* 1997;40(6): 1182-1188.

70. Narakas A: Brachial plexus surgery. *Orthop Clin North Am* 1981;12(2):303-323.

71. Bentolila V, Nizard R, Bizot P, Sedel L: Complete traumatic brachial plexus palsy: Treatment and outcome after repair. *J Bone Joint Surg Am* 1999;81(1):20-28.

Chapter 18

Fractures of the Humerus

Matt Graves, MD   Sean E. Nork, MD

Proximal Humerus Fractures

Introduction and Epidemiology

Proximal humerus fractures are relatively common injuries, and are typically defined as either minimally displaced or displaced. Minimally displaced fractures have been defined as those in which no segment is displaced more than 1 cm or angulated more than 45°; they are more common than displaced fractures. Nonsurgical treatment of these fractures is globally accepted, with good to excellent outcomes noted in most cases.[1] Displaced fractures, which are challenging to treat, occur in two specific subsets of the population. High-energy displaced fractures are seen most often in young adults age 18 to 40 years after accidents involving a motor vehicle or a fall from a significant height. Lower energy displaced fractures are seen most often in patients older than 65 years with osteoporosis, after a fall from a standing position.

Although many articles on displaced proximal humerus fractures have been published, treatment is controversial. In young patients, this controversy involves the surgical approach to the fracture and the most appropriate implant for fixation. In older patients, management controversies revolve around not just surgical approach and implant choice, but also the role of hemiarthroplasty, and even whether surgical treatment is justified.

The treatment of displaced proximal humerus fractures is gaining considerable attention because of the sheer volume of fractures anticipated over the upcoming decades. A recent update on the epidemiology of proximal humerus fractures suggests that the number of proximal humerus fractures in older patients will triple over the next three decades.[2] The relevance of defining best practice protocols is obvious. To ideally accomplish this, long-term outcome data from well-designed trials will be necessary. In the meantime, knowledge of currently available information drives decision making.

Anatomy

Knowledge of the four basic osseous segments of the proximal humerus and their soft-tissue attachments assists with understanding the deforming forces that cause displacement of each fragment, devising means to counteract those forces to restore normal anatomic relationships, and creating a construct to maintain those relationships until healing occurs (**Figure 1**). Considerable attention has been given to defining the normal relationships among segments of the proximal humerus.[3,4] In the coronal plane, the humeral head is inclined with respect to the shaft by a neck-shaft angle that varies from 130° to 150°. The center of the humeral head is offset medially from the center of the canal by 4 to 14 mm, and -2 to 10 mm posteriorly. The most cephalad point on the humeral head articular surface is approximately 8 mm proximal to the tip of the greater tuberosity. In the sagittal plane, the humeral head is retroverted approximately 0° to 55° with respect to the shaft, depending on the methodology used for measurement.

The anterolateral ascending branch of the anterior humeral circumflex artery perfuses the humeral head. This vessel runs parallel and lateral to the tendon of the long head of the biceps and terminates as the arcuate artery, entering the humeral head anteriorly at the proximal end of the intertubercular groove.[5] This finding led many to question how the humeral head remains viable after fracture of the proximal humerus, because this location is commonly involved in proximal humerus fracture lines. A four-part fracture model was created in an anatomic cadaver study to assess the effect of common fracture lines on the arterial supply to the humeral head.[6] It was noted that the humeral head could remain perfused after ligation of the anterolateral ascending branch at its entry point into the humeral head. Although there were no extraosseous anastomoses with the arcuate artery, the humeral head remained

Dr. Graves or an immediate family member is a member of a speakers' bureau or has made paid presentations on behalf of Synthes; serves as paid consultant for or is an employee of Synthes; has received research or institutional support from Synthes and Stryker; and is a board member, owner, officer, or committee member of Orthopaedic Trauma Association. Dr. Nork or an immediate family member is a member of a speakers' bureau or has made paid presentations on behalf of Synthes, AO North America, and Orthopaedic Trauma Association; serves as a paid consultant for or is an employee of Synthes, AO North America, and Orthopaedic Trauma Association; has received research or institutional support from Synthes, AO North America, and Orthopaedic Trauma Association; and is a board member, owner, officer, or committee member of Orthopaedic Trauma Association and the American Academy of Orthopaedic Surgeons.

3: Upper Extremity

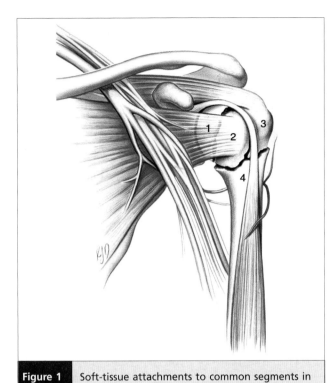

Figure 1 Soft-tissue attachments to common segments in proximal humerus fractures predict typical displacements. 1 = humeral head; 2 = lesser tuberosity; 3 = greater tuberosity; 4 = shaft. (Reproduced with permission from Neer CS II: Four-segment classification of proximal humeral fractures: Purpose and reliable use. *J Shoulder Elbow Surg* 2002;11:389-400.) http://www.sciencedirect.com/science/journal/10582746.)

perfused via the abundant intraosseous anastomoses from the metaphyseal and posteromedial vessels. This finding has subsequently been supported by a prospective surgical evaluation that noted the importance of medial and posteromedial metaphyseal extension of the humeral head in fracture patterns.[7] In this study, good predictors of humeral head ischemia were metaphyseal head extension length less than 8 mm, disruption of the integrity of the medial hinge between the humeral head and shaft, and an anatomic neck component.

Evaluation

Clinical Examination

The extremity examination begins with inspection of the soft-tissue envelope of the shoulder and arm. Swelling and ecchymosis are common with proximal humerus fractures, often extending down fascial planes into the mid or even lower portions of the arm. If the fracture meets surgical indications, further attention should be focused on the soft tissue overlying the proposed surgical incision. Palpation of osseous landmarks assists with defining local associated injuries, such as scapula, clavicle, and humeral shaft fractures.

The neurologic examination is focused on the brachial plexus and the peripheral nerves that extend from this region. A high incidence of associated nerve injury

has been reported. The axillary, suprascapular, radial, and musculocutaneous nerves are most commonly injured in the setting of a proximal humerus fracture. Nerve injuries are more common in older patients and those with hematoma formation (possibly reflecting greater displacement of the fracture). Most nerve injuries demonstrate partial or complete recovery within 4 months. Axillary nerve sensation is tested on the lateral aspect of the upper arm. The sensory portion of the axillary nerve arises from the posterior branch of the axillary nerve, along with one or two motor branches supplying the posterior head of the deltoid muscle. Most of the motor supply of the axillary nerve arises from the anterior branch, which wraps around the neck of the humerus in close proximity to many of the common proximal humerus fracture patterns. Motor function of the axillary nerve is very challenging to test during the acute postinjury period.

Although associated vascular injuries are less common after proximal humerus fractures, they create a dire situation, historically resulting in an upper extremity amputation rate of 30%. The axillary artery passes medial to the humeral head and surgical neck area of the proximal humerus, and can be injured in either high- or low-energy trauma. Potential causes of injury include direct intrusion from a bony spike secondary to fracture displacement or a traction injury to the upper extremity. Clinical presentation ranges from obvious acute arm ischemia to more subtle findings including persistent or worsening pain, delayed onset of nerve palsy or worsening of nerve palsy present at the initial evaluation, and localized axillary swelling and bruising.[8] Complete injury to the vessel negates blood flow to the upper extremity and must be handled as a surgical emergency in concert with a vascular surgeon.

Radiographic Evaluation

Good-quality imaging is essential for understanding and defining the pathoanatomy of proximal humerus fractures. The radiographic series consists of three images: the AP view, the lateral or Y scapular view, and the axillary view (**Figure 2**). The AP view reveals the relationship of the humeral head with respect to the glenoid, the humeral neck-shaft angle, the offset of the center of rotation of the head with respect to the shaft, and the relationship of the greater tuberosity to the humeral head. The ability to see the relationship of the greater tuberosity to the humeral head is often improved with external rotation of the arm.[9] Fracture lines between the head and shaft, head and greater tuberosity, and greater tuberosity and shaft are typically visible if present. The Y scapular view provides additional information about the relationship between the humeral head and glenoid, visualization of sagittal plane translation of the humeral head with respect to the shaft, and additional information regarding greater tuberosity displacement. The superimposed scapula often obscures specific details of fracture pathoanatomy. The axillary view is the most difficult to

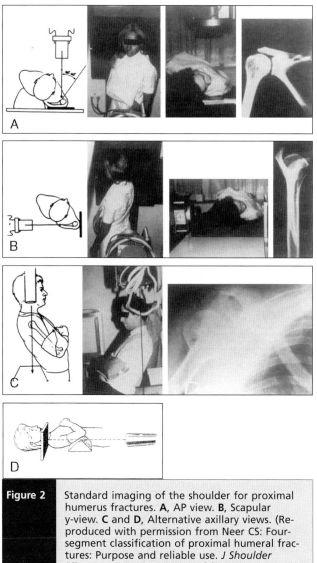

Figure 2 Standard imaging of the shoulder for proximal humerus fractures. **A**, AP view. **B**, Scapular y-view. **C** and **D**, Alternative axillary views. (Reproduced with permission from Neer CS: Four-segment classification of proximal humeral fractures: Purpose and reliable use. *J Shoulder Elbow Surg* 2002;11:389-400.) http://www.sciencedirect.com/science/journal/10582746.)

Minimal displacement	Displaced Fractures		
	2 part	3 part	4 part
Anatomic neck			
Surgical neck			
Greater tuberosity			
Lesser tuberosity			Articular surface
Fracture-dislocation Anterior			
Posterior			

Figure 3 The Neer classification system for proximal humerus fractures. (Reproduced with permission from Neer CS II: Four-segment classification of proximal humeral fractures: Purpose and reliable use. *J Shoulder Elbow Surg* 2002;11:389-400.) http://www.sciencedirect.com/science/journal/10582746.)

obtain in the trauma setting, secondary to the need for arm abduction. Alternative axillary views that require less abduction of the arm are possible. The axillary view does provide information about the relationship of the humeral head and glenoid, making dislocations more easily recognizable; visualization of associated glenoid rim pathology; and evaluation of tuberosity displacement.

Although not routinely indicated, CT scans can provide additional information about the pathoanatomy of some proximal humerus fractures.[10] They assist in delineating the fracture fragments and the major fragment relationships, and axial CT cuts can substitute for an inadequate axillary radiograph. CT is most useful when the plain radiographs are inconclusive or when humeral head involvement is notable, such as in impaction fractures and head-splitting fractures. Although not a standard part of proximal humerus fracture imaging, both two-dimensional and three-dimensional reformatting assists with preoperative planning and occasionally alters the surgical plan.

Classification

The well-known Neer classification system was developed to allow for consistency in diagnosing the pathoanatomy of proximal humerus fractures. It is based on displacement of segments rather than fracture lines and was proposed to describe the soft-tissue pathoanatomy as well as that of the bone. It was originally designed to be based on clinical, surgical, and radiographic findings, but has been commonly used to classify fractures based on radiographic interpretation alone.[11] Making the classification in the evaluation stage allows for treatment to be defined a priori. Unfortunately, this transition has led to multiple studies questioning the interobserver reliability of the classification system.

The Neer system consists of four major types, defined by the number of parts noted in the fracture (**Figure 3**). To allow for categories to be developed, a part was defined by an arbitrarily set displacement of 1 cm or 45° of angulation. A one-part (minimally displaced)

Humerus proximal segment, extra-articular unifocal

1. Avulsion of tuberosity
2. Impacted metaphysis
3. Non-impacted metaphysis fracture

Humerus, proximal segment, extra-articular bifocal

1. With metaphyseal impaction
2. Without metaphyseal impaction
3. With glenohumeral dislocation

Humerus, proximal segment, articular fractures

1. Articular fracture with slight displacement impacted valgus fracture
2. Articular fracture impacted with marked displacement
3. Articular fracture with glenohumeral dislocation

Figure 4 AO-OTA classification of proximal humerus fractures. (Reproduced with permission from Marsh JL, Slongo TF, Agel J, et al: Fracture and Dislocation Classification Compendium 2007: Orthopaedic Trauma Association Classification, Database and Outcomes Committee. *J Orthop Trauma* 2007;21(suppl 10):1-163.).

fracture can consist of multiple fracture lines—regardless of the level or number—with none of the parts meeting the displacement criteria. In two-part fractures, the named segment is the one that is displaced. In three-part fractures, one tuberosity is displaced, whereas the other tuberosity remains attached to the head. In the updated Neer system, four-part fractures are subdivided into four-part valgus-impacted fractures and four-part nonvalgus-impacted fractures (lateral fracture-dislocations). True fracture-dislocations are placed into a separate category and named according to the number of parts (two, three, or four) and the direction of dislocation of the head fragment (anterior, posterior, inferior, and so on).

The AO-Orthopaedic Trauma Association (OTA) system is an alphanumeric system divided into three basic groups, each containing many subgroups (**Figure 4**), which was updated in 2007. The AO-OTA classification system was designed to provide a more expanded classification of proximal humerus fractures—based on Neer's scheme—but allowing for more detailed subgrouping. There were four main concerns with the initial Neer system that led to this more expanded system: lack of separation of valgus-impacted four-part fractures from other four-part fractures in the original Neer system (this has been corrected in the updated system as noted previously); a perceived underemphasis on the severity of the displaced anatomic neck fracture; a perceived inadequacy of subgrouping for detailed analysis; and concern that the arbitrarily set displacement criteria of the Neer system might not denote the amount of displacement that led to functional compromise or vascular discontinuity between segments. The detail of this classification system has led to its use mainly as a research tool.

A proximal humerus fracture classification system based on three-dimensional CT has been published recently.[12] This system was developed in response to the advances in imaging techniques and to the lack of interobserver agreement in other systems. More research is required to determine the validity of this CT-based classification system.

Treatment

Minimally Displaced Fractures

The treatment of minimally displaced fractures has been nonsurgical, with variation in the length and type of physiotherapy. Evaluation criteria for the results of nonsurgical treatment have also varied. Whatever the outcome criteria used, most patients experience functional recovery, with most obtaining good or excellent results.

One study evaluated the epidemiology and outcome of 507 consecutive minimally displaced proximal humerus fractures using a standard physiotherapy regimen.[1] Five main findings were noted: there is variation in the incidence of minimally displaced fractures in the different AO-OTA subgroups, with most falling into type A; age is the main determinant of outcome according to the Neer outcome score; older patients subjectively think that the results of treatment are better than the objective functional measurements would indicate; comorbidities seem to affect the overall outcome; and there is a positive correlation between length of physiotherapy and outcome.

Displaced Fractures in Physiologically Young and Active Patients

Evidence-based treatment decisions are limited in the care of proximal humerus fractures. Methodologic study flaws were consistently noted in a recent systematic review of treatment modalities, leading to an inability to produce treatment-guiding conclusions.[13] In spite of this limitation, surgical treatment of displaced fractures is accepted in the physiologically young, active patient population. The goal is to restore function by restoring and maintaining preinjury anatomy until union, while allowing for early physiotherapy during the healing process. Maintenance of the humeral head is thought to be a requisite for lasting functional recovery in this population. Many different surgical options have been proposed; the three most common are closed reduction and percutaneous pinning, intramedullary rodding, and plate osteosynthesis.

Closed Reduction and Percutaneous Pinning

Closed reduction and percutaneous pinning is a minimally invasive surgical procedure that minimizes the risk of additional vascular insult that might affect fracture healing and humeral head viability. Disparate results have been published, highlighting the technical variability and difficulty of the procedure. A recent anatomic study improved the understanding of safe pin placement.[14] This study provided three important findings: the starting point of the lateral pins should be at least twice the distance from the superior to inferior margin of the humeral head cartilage; the greater tuberosity pins should engage the medial cortex at least 2 cm from the inferior margin of the humeral head cartilage; and the shoulder should be held in external rotation when placing the greater tuberosity pins (**Figure 5**).

Limitations of the procedure include the inability to allow for early unrestricted passive motion secondary to pins traversing gliding anatomic planes. Complications specific to this technique include pin loosening, pin migration, and pin site infection. The stability afforded by this technique is somewhat limited and the complication of pin migration can be very severe. Logical indications would include reliable patients with fracture patterns that had some inherent stability after reduction and were amenable to closed reduction techniques. These include two-part fractures with minimal neck comminution and valgus-impacted three-part and four-part fractures with minimal tuberosity comminution.

Intramedullary Rodding

Intramedullary rodding is also a minimally invasive technique, maintaining maximal vascularity to the fracture fragments and humeral head. In addition, the intramedullary position of the implant potentially provides some mechanical advantage to maintaining stability between the head and shaft fragments by limiting the moment arm for bending. A recent article revealed that rodding could provide effective stability to union for the appropriately selected fracture pattern.[15] Failure was recognized specifically for fractures involving an unstable or comminuted lateral metaphysis with extension into the entry site of the implant. Complications specific to this technique include impingement secondary to proximal implant prominence, loosening of proximal interlocking screws, and difficulty maintaining tuberosity position without additional implant support. Implant placement also involves supraspinatus violation in line with its fibers. The stability afforded by this implant is excellent for maintaining the restored relationship between the humeral head and shaft, especially in the absence of tuberosity involvement. It addi-

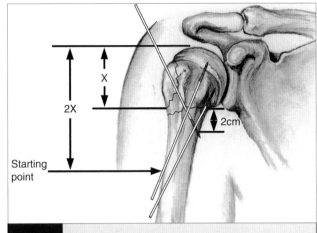

| Figure 5 | Guide for percutaneous pin placement in proximal humeral fracture treatment. Arrows represent the distance from one horizontal line to the next. (Reproduced with permission from Rowles DJ, McGrory JE: Percutaneous pinning of the proximal part of the humerus: An anatomic study. *J Bone Joint Surg Am* 2001;83:1695-1699.) |

tionally provides the advantage of supporting humeral shaft fracture extension without additional dissection or deltoid release. Logical indications include two-part shaft (surgical neck) fractures, especially when humeral shaft fracture extension is noted. Technique diligence is required as the position for manipulative closed reduction of the proximal humerus fracture (abduction) is at odds with the arm position required for implant insertion (adduction).

Plating

With the advent of precontoured, locking proximal humeral implants, plating has gained popularity (**Figure 6**). Open plating is typically performed through either a deltopectoral or deltoid-splitting approach. Advantages of open plating include its wide applicability, allowing for the treatment of nearly any fracture pattern. In addition, it is versatile, providing for direct or indirect reduction techniques and traditional or locking implant placement. Disadvantages include the potential vascular embarrassment created by soft-tissue dissection and the potential for scar tissue formation created by disturbing gliding tissue planes. Recent advances in plating have been made in the areas of construct stability and the application of minimally invasive osteosynthesis.

Construct stability is a combination of many factors including bone quality, fracture pattern, fracture reduction, implant type, and implant placement. For proximal humerus fractures treated with locking plates, common failure modes include varus failure (**Figure 7**) and intra-articular screw penetration (**Figure 8**). Progress in preventing varus failure has centered around an improved understanding of the importance of the stability provided by restoration of the medial neck of the humerus.[16] Laterally based implants are stressed by off-

3: Upper Extremity

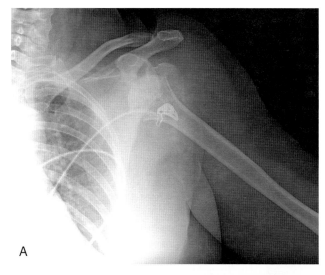

A

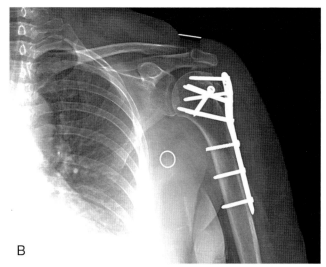

B

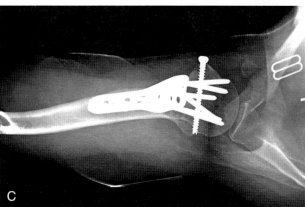

C

Figure 6 Radiographic studies of the shoulder of a 55-year-old woman with a valgus-impacted four-part fracture-dislocation. **A,** The injury. **B,** 1-year follow-up AP view. **C,** 1- year follow-up axillary lateral view.

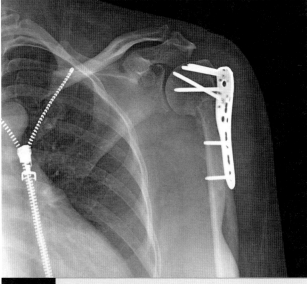

Figure 7 Radiograph showing varus failure of proximal humerus fracture fixation.

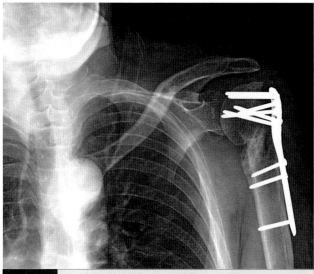

Figure 8 Radiograph showing intra-articular screw penetration associated with proximal humerus fracture fixation.

axis, cyclical bending loads. This stress is limited by restoration of the far cortex. With proximal humerus fractures, the far cortex is the medial neck. Restoration of the medial neck can be accomplished by achieving an anatomic or slightly impacted reduction that possesses some inherent stability. If medial neck comminution makes this impossible, the placement of fixed-angle screws along the inferomedial portion of the neck provides artificial support to resist varus failure. Another recognized form of limiting this failure mode has been to incorporate the rotator cuff into predrilled holes in the laterally based implant. In addition to limiting varus failure, this technique limits tuberosity escape.

Intra-articular locking screw penetration has been noted in multiple series of locked plate fixation, with an incidence of approximately 20%.[17,18] Intra-articular screw penetration takes four main forms: intraoperative lack of recognition of excessively long screws; postoperative varus failure leading to superior screw "cutout;" postoperative humeral head collapse into a pattern of inherent stability along the fixed-angle relationship of the rigid implant; and postoperative humeral head osteonecrosis. The clinical significance of intra-articular screw penetration varies and is affected by its location and preinjury functional demands of the patient. Further work is necessary to discover preventive solutions, especially for the latter two failure modes.

Along with the recent focus on construct stability, there has been a recent interest in advancing minimally invasive insertion techniques. The goal has been to combine the mechanical advantages of locked plating with the biologic advantages of limited incision surgery. The extended anterolateral acromial approach has provided a safe passage for lateral plate insertion, with a clearly defined localization of the anterior motor branch of the axillary nerve, approximately 35 mm distal to the proximal prominence of the greater tuberosity.[19,20] Although useful for two-part shaft (surgical neck) fractures, two-part greater tuberosity fractures, and three-part greater tuberosity fractures, some limitations arise from the minimal access offered through this approach. First, access to the lesser tuberosity segment or a dislocated head segment is restricted. Second, care must be taken not to use locking guides that were created for the deltopectoral approach, because these can place excessive pressure on the anterior motor branch of the axillary nerve. Third, placement of screws in the plate holes near the anterior motor branch is challenging and potentially dangerous. Unfortunately, the anterior motor branch passes next to the screw holes typically required to support the inferomedial neck.[21] Despite these limitations, early prospective results of the technique are promising.

Displaced Fractures in Older Patients
Nonsurgical management of displaced proximal humerus fractures is globally accepted for patients who have limited need of shoulder function and for those who are unable to undergo surgery. In addition, nonsurgical management has been shown to produce mostly good outcomes for certain fracture patterns. Specifically, the results of nonsurgical management of the impacted varus fracture (AO-OTA A2.2), the impacted valgus fracture (AO-OTA B1.1), and the translated two-part fracture (AO-OTA A3.2) have been evaluated.[22] Certain commonalities were noted for all of these fracture patterns: age was found to be a determinant of outcome, with increasing age typically resulting in decreased shoulder function; the subjective impression of the patient was consistently better than the objective evaluation of glenohumeral movement and strength would suggest; outcome scores tend to steadily improve throughout the first year; and nonunion was a rare finding, whereas what could be considered malunion was very common. Some differences were also noted. For the impacted valgus fracture and the translated two-part fracture, the degree of displacement was noted to be a determinant of outcome, with more displacement leading to poorer results. This finding was not noted for the impacted varus fracture. Although the impacted varus fracture continues to displace during the initial treatment phase, there was surprisingly no correlation between increasing varus angulation and decreased shoulder function.

Surgical treatment of displaced fractures in older patients is controversial, but has been shown to produce good to excellent results in multiple series.[17,18] Surgical treatment consists of fracture fixation and hemiarthroplasty. Although the goal of restoring pain-free function is the same in the active older patient as in younger patients, the surgical prerequisite is different. Maintaining the humeral head is no longer a primary concern. In addition, osteoporotic bone challenges construct stability. Because of these premises, hemiarthroplasty is a favorable option when osteonecrosis is likely or there is a high likelihood of being unable to obtain and maintain an acceptable reduction until union. These scenarios include: two-part articular segment (anatomic neck) fractures, complex three-part fractures, true four-part fractures (nonvalgus-impacted), three-part and four-part fracture-dislocations, head-splitting fractures, and severely osteoporotic fractures in which construct stability is questionable.

A recent comprehensive systematic review of proximal humerus fracture hemiarthroplasty revealed that pain relief was nearly universal but marked limitation of function was common.[23] Rehabilitation protocols typically allowed for immediate passive motion and active motion after tuberosity union. Mean active forward flexion and abduction were 106° and 92°, respectively. Superficial and deep infections were rare, with incidences of 1.5% and 0.6%. The most common complications noted were tuberosity malposition, displacement, or nonunion. The incidence of tuberosity complications was 11%. Heterotopic ossification and proximal migration of the humeral head were noted in

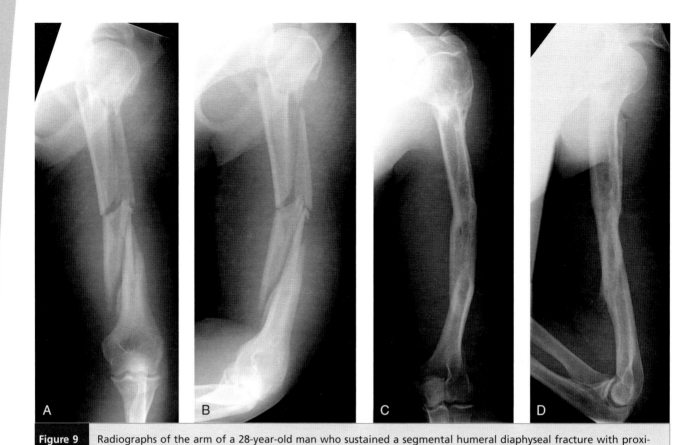

Figure 9 Radiographs of the arm of a 28-year-old man who sustained a segmental humeral diaphyseal fracture with proximal extension (**A** and **B**). The extent of fracture is noted in each view. Despite the extensive involvement, the patient was treated with a coaptation splint followed by functional bracing for 3 months. Healing progressed uneventfully with acceptable alignment at 6 months (**C** and **D**).

8.8% and 6.8%, respectively. The mean Constant score was 56. Although hemiarthroplasty prevents the complications associated with fracture fixation, it is clearly not without its own set of complications. Patients should be counseled before surgery as to the proposed goals and expected outcomes based on currently available data and individual surgeon-specific results. Surgeons should be intimately aware of the common failure modes and complications and proactively work to prevent those from occurring. Prospective, randomized trials comparing nonsurgical treatment, fracture fixation, and hemiarthroplasty are needed to define the best approach to these complex injuries in the older population.

Humeral Shaft Fractures

Introduction and Epidemiology
Humeral shaft fractures are among the most common fractures treated, representing up to 5% of all fractures seen by orthopaedic surgeons. In young patients, these injuries are frequently the result of high-energy trauma such as a motor vehicle crash, fall from height, motorcycle crash, gunshot wound, or skiing accident. Low-energy falls predominate in the older population, espe-

cially in women. Most humeral shaft fractures can be managed without surgery; however, certain patient, injury, and fracture characteristics suggest the need for surgical treatment.

Radiographic Evaluation
The radiographic evaluation begins with orthogonal images of the entire humerus, including images of the shoulder and elbow joints. CT is not indicated for fractures confined to the humeral diaphysis. Traction films may be useful for fractures with extension proximally or distally but are typically not indicated for routine humeral shaft fractures. Repeat radiographs of the humerus following a manipulative reduction are necessary and may add information regarding the fracture pattern.

Treatment
Nonsurgical Treatment
Most humeral shaft fractures can be successfully treated without surgery. Nonsurgical treatment is an extremely active process for both the surgeon and the patient. Initially, a simple reduction maneuver and placement of a coaptation splint will generally allow for improved patient comfort and an improved position of the extremity (**Figure 9**). The coaptation splint is ideally molded to

counteract the observed deformities, with varus and extension being most common. A careful neurologic examination is performed after any fracture manipulations and splint applications. Although rare, if a change in neurologic status occurs with fracture manipulation and repositioning, the splint should be removed and the arm reevaluated. It remains controversial whether a radial nerve palsy following closed manipulative reduction requires surgical exploration, because the nerve recovery rate is similar to that seen with primary traumatic radial nerve palsies in closed humeral fractures. Nevertheless, the presence of a radial nerve palsy is often used as an indication for surgical stabilization and nerve exploration. Because the coaptation splint is primarily for comfort and to prevent any further soft-tissue injury, a perfect reduction is unnecessary. Minimizing the deformity may reduce muscle spasm and discomfort and certainly minimizes the pressure on the soft tissues and skin from the underlying fracture ends.

Ideally, the arm is placed into a functional brace within 1 to 2 weeks after injury. The brace consists of an adjustable plastic shell with multiple Velcro straps that can be tightened to maximize the hydrostatic pressure within the arm to help realign the humerus and allow for functional movement of the upper extremity during healing. The patient is instructed to perform co-contraction exercises of the biceps and triceps. Range-of-motion exercises at the shoulder, elbow, wrist, and fingers are encouraged to help with swelling and to maintain mobility. The patient should be taught to adjust the brace daily as swelling subsides, and radiographs should be obtained at frequent intervals to ensure adequate alignment and healing. Occasionally, an abduction pillow or a brace extension (proximally or distally) may be required to improve the alignment, especially in the coronal plane. Given the range of motion at the shoulder joint, some angular deformity is generally well tolerated at the humeral diaphysis. Historically, the following parameters are used for acceptable alignment: less than 30° of varus or valgus angulation, less than 20° of anterior or posterior angulation, and less than 2 cm of shortening. These values are based on marginal science, and the patient's body habitus and arm size may contribute to the definition of acceptability. The fracture should demonstrate consolidation, decreased motion, and decreased pain by 4 to 8 weeks. Once there is clinical (decreased or no pain at the fracture site) and radiographic evidence of healing, the patient can begin to decrease brace usage. Brace use is typically continued for an average of 11.5 weeks.

Historically, reported union rates with nonsurgical treatment of humeral shaft fractures have been as high as 98%. Subsequent studies indicate that the union rate with nonsurgical treatment may not be that predictable, with nonunions reported in the range of 10% to 20%. In two recent studies reviewing functional bracing for humeral diaphyseal fractures, the nonunion rate was 10%.[24,25] This is valuable information in setting patient expectations regarding nonsurgical treatment,

Table 1

Relative Indications for Surgical Treatment of Humeral Shaft Fractures

Multiple injuries
- Bilateral humeral fractures
- Lower extremity fractures that limit weight bearing
- Floating elbow
- Concomitant head injury
- Other injuries where nursing care is facilitated by internal stabilization

Open fractures

Burns or soft tissue injury that precludes humeral bracing

Vascular injury

Brachial plexus injury

Displaced pathologic fracture

Radial nerve dysfunction following manipulative closed reduction

Specific fracture characteristics and patterns
- Significant distraction at the fracture site
- Long proximal spiral fractures
- Joint extension distally

Inability to maintain an adequate reduction with bracing

Body habitus that precludes bracing

Note: Pathologic fracture, open fracture, an associated vascular injury, and failure to maintain an acceptable reduction with bracing are strong indicators for surgical treatment.

the expected success, and the need to proceed to surgical treatment in carefully selected individuals. Although the definition of success following nonsurgical treatment is frequently limited to fracture union and acceptable alignment, recent studies have sought to evaluate functional outcomes following functional bracing.[24]

Surgical Treatment

Indications for surgical treatment are summarized in **Table 1.** It should be emphasized that there are very few absolute indications for the surgical stabilization of humeral diaphyseal fractures. Severe associated soft-tissue trauma is a strong indication for surgical stabilization. Displaced pathologic fractures should be treated surgically, ideally with an intramedullary nail, because it allows stabilization and support for the entire humerus. Most of the remaining indications for surgery are relative and should be combined with other aspects of the injury and the patient. Most open fractures are treated with surgical stabilization at the time of surgical débridement. However, open humeral fractures have been successfully treated with an appropriate irrigation and débridement followed by functional bracing. Patients with multiple injuries or where nursing care can be facilitated with humeral stabilization may be opti-

3: Upper Extremity

mally treated with early surgical treatment. Similarly, patients with associated upper extremity vascular or brachial plexus injuries may be optimally treated with early surgery to minimize additional neurovascular injury and to allow osseous apposition if muscle function will not allow dynamic compression with nonsurgical management. On occasion, the fracture pattern itself, even in isolated humeral fractures, may influence treatment.[26] For instance, extensive segmental fractures may be difficult to treat with functional bracing. According to a recent study, it was observed that simple fracture patterns had a higher rate of nonunion compared to the remaining cohort of patients treated nonsurgically.[24] Approximately 20% of simple (type A) fracture patterns did not unite. Poorer outcome scores were observed following surgical repair of the nonunions that occurred following failed nonsurgical treatment. In another study of humeral fractures treated with functional bracing, a higher average risk of nonunion in patients with proximal-third long oblique fractures was observed.[25] Although not statistically significant given the small study size, nonunions were reported in 29% of proximal third fractures, suggesting that these patterns may deserve special attention and consideration. These studies indicate that early identification of fracture patterns that are likely to fail nonsurgical treatment can be helpful in the decision-making process. This finding does not suggest, however, that all simple (type A) fracture patterns or proximal fractures require surgical treatment, but should be used as additional information that helps the surgeon and the patient decide on the optimal treatment method.

Surgical treatment of humeral fractures can be accomplished with plate fixation, intramedullary nailing, or external fixation. External fixation has limited indications and is most suitable as a temporary measure for high-energy open fractures with significant soft-tissue injury that requires repeated débridements. The decision to proceed with plating and nailing remains controversial (and often contentious); there are proponents for each. The results of comparison studies of these two methods will be discussed further after the description of each method.

Plate Osteosynthesis

Open reduction and internal fixation (ORIF) with application of a plate is a predictable procedure that yields high union rates and acceptable complications. Union rates of 90% to 95% have been routinely reported, and alignment can be obtained and maintained. The main disadvantages of plate fixation are the need for a large surgical approach with the negative cosmetic consequences, iatrogenic radial nerve injury, the possibility of deep infection, and failure of fixation, especially in osteoporotic bone. With knowledge of the local anatomy, the incidence of iatrogenic nerve injury should be minimized. The path of the radial nerve relative to the various surgical approaches has been investigated in detail and should minimize iatrogenic injury during treatment.

Multiple surgical approaches to the humeral shaft including anterior, anterolateral, lateral, posterior, and medial are well known and described in most standard texts. The choice of approach is determined by the fracture location, the fracture configuration, and the comfort of the surgeon with the anatomy. For fractures proximal to the deltoid tuberosity, a deltopectoral combined with an anterior or anterolateral approach is often used. For fractures in the middle third of the humerus, the anterolateral, the direct lateral, and the modified posterior triceps-sparing approach are most often used. For distal fractures, the modified posterior approach and the triceps-splitting approach are most often used.

Recently, as in other anatomic sites, there has been interest in minimally invasive surgical approaches to the humerus. Such approaches demand knowledge of the position of the radial nerve, and the relationship of the radial nerve to the humerus was simplified based on the length of the humerus.[27] This situation allows for correction based on the relative size of the patient, and is easy to recall based on a one third–two thirds relationship. The results of 20 cadaver dissections yielded the finding that the nerve almost universally pierced the lateral intermuscular septum within 5 mm of the junction of the middle and distal thirds of a line extending from the lateral epicondyle to the lateral acromion process.[27]

The typical recommendation for the size of the plate necessary to stabilize a humeral shaft fracture originally was a 4.5-mm broad implant, which was modified to a 4.5-mm narrow implant, and is now generally assumed to be the plate that is sized appropriately for the patient's humerus. In most instances, a 4.5-mm narrow plate of appropriate length is recommended (**Figure 10**). In particularly small patients, a 3.5-mm plate may be appropriate, and a biomechanical study does suggest that these implants are of sufficient size to support axial loads during weight bearing.[28] However, clinical studies are necessary before 3.5-mm implants can be routinely recommended for the treatment of humeral diaphyseal fractures. In terms of plate length and screw density, extrapolation from other biomechanical studies yields the general recommendation that increasing plate length (a minimum of four screw holes of plate length, preferably five, completely on either side of the fracture) combined with at least three bicortical screws with maximal spread per side allows for a construct of adequate strength and stiffness.

Fixation strength remains a concern in some humerus fractures, and this is amplified in osteoporotic bone. Although locking plates have been introduced and used in humeral diaphyseal fractures, biomechanical studies do not universally support the use of locking implants. In a study evaluating torsional stiffness after locked or hybrid plating of humeral shaft fractures in synthetic bone, the authors found that both the locking screw construct and the hybrid construct (a combination of locking and conventional screws) offered a sig-

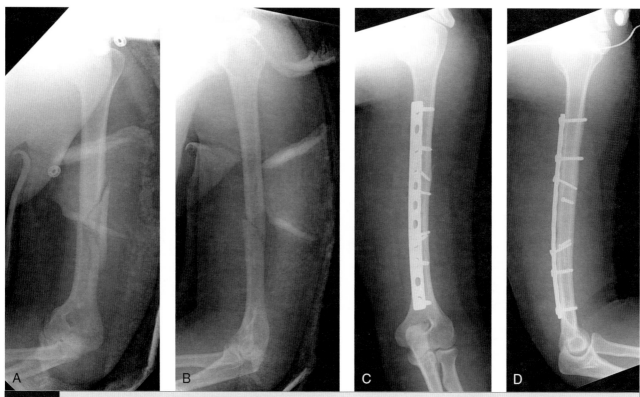

Figure 10 Radiographs of a 23-year-old man who sustained a closed humerus fracture in addition to bilateral lower extremity injuries after a motorcycle crash. **A** and **B**, AP and lateral views. **C** and **D**, Postoperative radiographs showing the spiral fracture with an associated butterfly fragment. A modified posterior triceps-sparing exposure was used, allowing protection and mobilization of the radial nerve. A 4.5-mm narrow plate was contoured and applied to the posterior surface of the humerus. Alignment and stability were restored.

nificant biomechanical advantage over conventional screws in their bone model of osteoporosis.[29] However, in a study evaluating a gap defect in both cadaver and synthetic bone, no particular advantage was demonstrated with locking screws compared to conventional screws in axial loading.[28] Axial loading was chosen as the loading method to demonstrate that early weight bearing is possible in a humeral shaft fracture stabilized with a plate of adequate length. Although locking implants have been shown to offer improved fixation in osteoporotic bone models, further clinical studies are necessary as this applies to humeral shaft fixation.

Largely driven by the cosmetic appearance of the large surgical approaches necessary for plate fixations, minimally invasive approaches for humeral shaft plating (minimally invasive plate osteosynthesis have been introduced. Anterior and lateral approaches have been described, studied, advocated, and used for minimally invasive plating of humeral fractures. The anterior approach was first identified as feasible and safe,[30] and then reported in a series of 13 patients with middle or distal humeral diaphyseal fractures.[31] This initial report demonstrated rapid healing, no nonunions, and no iatrogenic nerve injuries. These findings have been confirmed in subsequent studies that compared open and minimally invasive methods. Faster healing was observed in patients treated with minimally invasive plate

osteosynthesis and there were no iatrogenic radial nerve palsies (RNP). Surprisingly, the authors reported an incidence of iatrogenic RNP in more than 30% of patients treated with standard open plating techniques.[32] The high incidence of iatrogenic RNP in open plating cannot be adequately explained (or understood), but these reports do suggest that minimally invasive techniques are possible and safe. Further study is necessary before this method can be recommended routinely.

Intramedullary Nailing
Intramedullary nailing has been used with success for the treatment of humeral shaft fractures (**Figure 11**). However, the same principles that apply to intramedullary nailing of lower extremity fractures do not necessarily translate to the upper extremity. Although intramedullary nails are certainly strong enough to allow weight bearing, upper extremity usage following fixation typically does not involve weight bearing. The main advantages with intramedullary nailing are that it can be accomplished through a smaller incision, does not disrupt the fracture hematoma, and requires less soft-tissue dissection of the humerus. Antegrade and retrograde techniques have been described. Reported union rates are high, although inferior to plating. However, there are several complications that are unique to

3: Upper Extremity

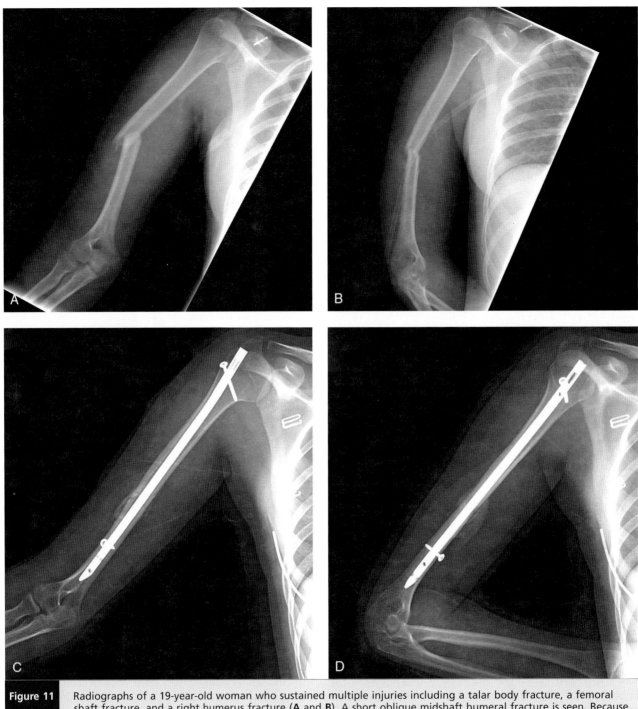

Figure 11 Radiographs of a 19-year-old woman who sustained multiple injuries including a talar body fracture, a femoral shaft fracture, and a right humerus fracture (**A** and **B**). A short oblique midshaft humeral fracture is seen. Because of the need for early mobilization and weight bearing, combined with optimizing the cosmetic appearance, an antegrade, reamed, statically locked humeral nail was placed, with predictable healing at 2 months. **C** and **D**, AP and lateral radiographs reveal healing in acceptable alignment.

humeral nailing and this should be used in the decision-making process regarding treatment options.

Shoulder pain, injury to the rotator cuff, and shoulder stiffness all are associated with antegrade nailing. These factors may be related to the surgical approach (anterior versus direct lateral), disruption or injury to the rotator cuff tendons, or variability in the proximal humeral geometry. The anterior (or anterolateral acromial) approach for antegrade humeral nailing uses an incision extending from the tip of the acromion, and the deep dissection is ideally placed between the anterior and middle portions of the deltoid muscle. This approach is actually more colinear with the proper nail starting point in both planes and may give better access to the rotator cuff tendon for protection during the procedure. Additionally, this approach allows for identification and protection of the anterior motor branch of the axillary nerve before placement of proximal interlocking bolts. Regardless of the skin incision and the deep dissection chosen, the rotator cuff tendons should be protected and repaired following nail placement. Retrograde nailing minimizes the risk of shoulder-related complications; however, elbow pain and supracondylar fracture at the nail entry site are of concern. Iatrogenic radial nerve injury is certainly a concern with humeral nailing, and has been reported in numerous series. In a patient whose nerve status is unknown, or in a patient with a neurologic deficit following intramedullary nailing, the exact pathology would remain a mystery to the surgeon if a closed nailing was performed. Therefore, in patients with unknown neurologic examination findings or in patients with a known deficit, nerve exploration or nerve monitoring is warranted. For closed nailing procedures in patients with an intact radial nerve, maintaining an accurate reduction of the fracture and avoiding reaming across the fracture have been suggested as methods of minimizing iatrogenic injury.

Comparison Studies of Plating and Nailing

A recent meta-analysis compared compression plating and intramedullary nailing of humeral shaft fractures.[33] In a pooled analysis of three studies and 155 patients, the authors concluded that plate fixation was associated with a 74% risk reduction for reoperation and a 90% risk reduction for shoulder impingement. Although this meta-analysis appears to support plate fixation for humeral shaft fractures, a much larger study population would be necessary to make strong recommendations, and the results should be interpreted with caution.

Radial Nerve Injury

Radial nerve injury following humeral shaft fracture is commonly observed and deserves special attention. In closed fractures, the incidence of associated traumatic RNP is typically estimated at 8 to 15%. In a systematic review of 21 studies and 4,517 humeral fractures, the overall prevalence of RNP was 11.8%.[34] Fractures located in the middle and middistal portions of the humerus had a higher incidence of nerve palsy, as did transverse and spiral patterns (compared to oblique and comminuted patterns).

Spontaneous recovery of a traumatic RNP in a closed fracture treated without surgery is typically estimated at 85% to 90%. Therefore, early exploration for closed humeral shaft fractures with an associated RNP will not change the neurologic outcome in most patients (that is, the nerve will typically recover with surgical or nonsurgical treatment). However, advantages of early exploration and nerve repair are that it allows for identification of any nerve injury before the nerve becomes encased in scar tissue, allows for shortening of the humerus if necessary, and minimizes the chance of

nerve entrapment in fracture callus.[34] These advantages contribute to the controversy regarding the management of closed humeral fractures with an associated RNP that occurs at the time of the traumatic accident. In a systematic review, an overall recovery rate of 88.1% was observed (consistent with other studies); however, spontaneous recovery was reported in only 70.7% of patients treated conservatively.[34] Given the similar rate of recovery in the patients treated conservatively and those who underwent exploration, it is likely that many of the early nerve explorations were unnecessary and did not affect the nerve recovery rate. Based on their data, the authors found that a limited waiting period for nerve recovery had no effect on the final recovery. This again confirms the generally held belief that in most closed humeral fractures with an associated RNP, spontaneous recovery is likely and observation is indicated, assuming that no other factors drive the decision for surgical treatment.

The time interval for nerve recovery is an important consideration for both the patient and the surgeon. Obviously, from the patient's perspective, maximizing timely recovery of nerve function is desired. In two publications, the average time to spontaneous recovery was 7 weeks.[34,35] This finding suggests that some period beyond 7 weeks is necessary to allow a reasonable percentage of patients to declare nerve recovery, and to avoid unnecessary nerve exploration in patients in whom spontaneous recovery will occur. However, the optimal waiting period remains a subject of intense debate, with some authors recommending a waiting period based on nerve regeneration rates of 6 months.[34]

In open fractures, the incidence of RNP is higher and the predicted rate of spontaneous recovery is much lower. Early exploration may be indicated in this patient population. In a study of 24 high-energy humeral diaphyseal fractures with associated complete sensory and motor radial nerve deficits, open injuries were observed in 11.[35] Radial nerve exploration was performed in all of the open fractures and in 3 of the 13 patients with closed fractures. Six patients in this group (25%) were found to have a radial nerve transection, all were in patients with open injuries, and none of the five who underwent primary repair of the nerve recovered. All of eight intact and explored nerves, as well as 90% of the unexplored nerves (in closed fractures) recovered. The authors, based on their experience with these high-energy injuries, reported that primary nerve repairs in these patients do poorly; intact nerves and nerve palsies in closed fractures recover in most patients; there is not a clear indication for nerve exploration, even in high-energy injuries; and complete recovery can be delayed, with a range of 1 to 21 months. Because the average time to full recovery was 6 months, patience in observation, before undertaking tendon transfers or other procedures, is prudent.[35]

The Holstein-Lewis (H-L) fracture pattern remains an area of concern given its reported increased incidence of an associated RNP. The H-L pattern is charac-

3: Upper Extremity

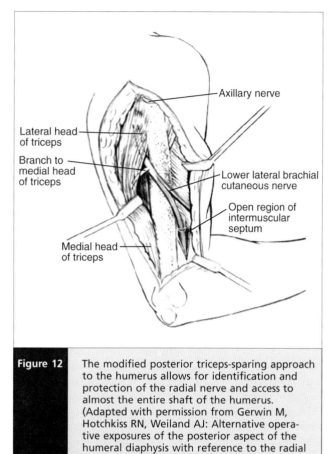

Figure 12 The modified posterior triceps-sparing approach to the humerus allows for identification and protection of the radial nerve and access to almost the entire shaft of the humerus. (Adapted with permission from Gerwin M, Hotchkiss RN, Weiland AJ: Alternative operative exposures of the posterior aspect of the humeral diaphysis with reference to the radial nerve. *J Bone Joint Surg Am* 1996;78: 1690-1695.)

terized by a spiral or oblique fracture in the distal third of the humerus with varus angulation around a relatively intact lateral intermuscular septum (**Figure 12**). Although previous small series suggested a high association, a large systematic review perhaps softened the association between this fracture pattern and the incidence of an RNP.[34] To better understand the incidence of the H-L fracture pattern, the incidence of an associated RNP, and the outcomes after treatment, 361 humeral shaft fractures were reviewed.[36] The H-L pattern was noted in 7.5% of patients, along with a significantly higher incidence of acute RNP (22% versus 8%). Although these values represent only six radial nerve palsies, all recovered whether the fracture was treated surgically (n = 4) or nonsurgically (n = 2). Good results were obtained with regard to healing, function, and radial nerve recovery independent of the treatment method. The authors conclude that primary surgical intervention is relative in this pattern, even with an associated RNP.[36]

The management of an RNP associated with a humerus fracture remains complicated and must be based on multiple factors including the fracture pattern, the fracture location, the associated soft-tissue injury, and whether the nerve injury was due to the trauma or a manipulation of the arm (**Figures 13** and **14**). A careful

discussion with the patient regarding the potential risks and benefits of surgical versus nonsurgical treatment as they relate to the radial nerve is typically required. In an interesting expected-value decision analysis, in which potential outcomes were gleaned from the published literature and presented to patients for their input, a decision tree was constructed. These authors ultimately concluded that initial observation was the preferred strategy in cases where the expected rate of recovery was high.[37] With regard to treatment of radial nerve injuries associated with humeral shaft fractures in specific circumstances, some general recommendations can be made. A secondary RNP that occurs during closed fracture treatment or manipulation warrants consideration and discussion with the patient regarding immediate exploration. The concern is that the nerve is either stretched around a fracture end or incarcerated within the fracture itself. However, in published series, the rate of spontaneous nerve recovery in secondary nerve palsies is virtually identical to that in primary traumatic radial nerve palsies. In open fractures, because the incidence of nerve laceration is sufficiently high and the need for an open débridement already exists, nerve exploration is warranted at the time of fracture cleaning and stabilization. For fracture patterns or situations that already require surgical intervention in a patient with an associated RNP, then surgical treatment and radial nerve exploration (preferably with plating) is a logical treatment strategy. In the common scenario where there is an RNP in a closed fracture that is amenable to nonsurgical treatment, the rate of recovery is sufficiently high that following these patients for at least 3 to 12 weeks (or based on electrophysiologic studies) is reasonable.[34,38]

Extra-articular Distal Third Fractures

The treatment of extra-articular distal third fractures of the humerus deserves special mention because good results have been obtained with both surgical and nonsurgical treatment methods. In the previously mentioned study of the H-L fracture pattern, surgical and nonsurgical treatment yielded similar functional results according to measured range of motion, strength, and the Short Musculoskeletal Function Assessment.[36] However, in a larger retrospective review of 40 patients with distal third humeral diaphyseal fractures treated with either functional bracing or plate fixation, the authors found measurable and quantifiable differences between the two groups.[39] Surgical treatment was associated with more predictable alignment and a more rapid return to function, but there were three patients with an iatrogenic nerve injury in the surgically treated group. In patients treated nonsurgically, skin breakdown occurred in two patients and alignment was less optimal than in the surgically treated patients. However, no functional deficits related to angular deformities were found. This study suggests that both surgical and nonsurgical treatment methods can be used in dis-

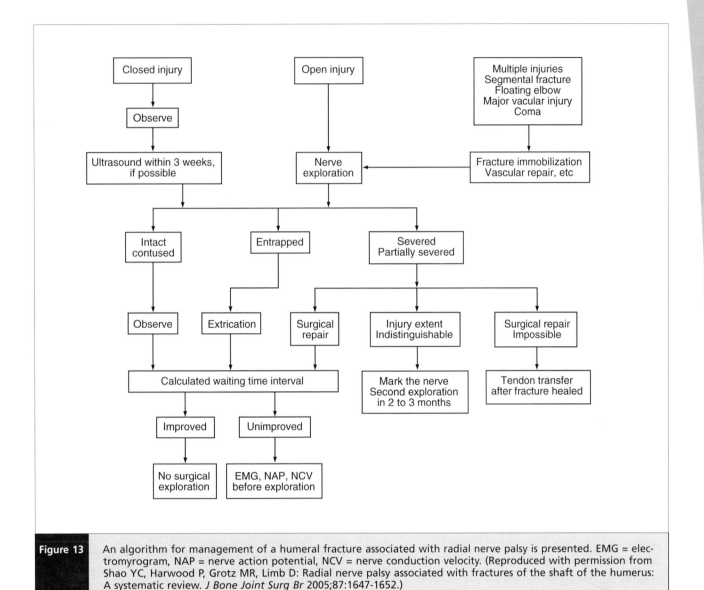

Figure 13   An algorithm for management of a humeral fracture associated with radial nerve palsy is presented. EMG = electromyrogram, NAP = nerve action potential, NCV = nerve conduction velocity. (Reproduced with permission from Shao YC, Harwood P, Grotz MR, Limb D: Radial nerve palsy associated with fractures of the shaft of the humerus: A systematic review. *J Bone Joint Surg Br* 2005;87:1647-1652.)

tal third fractures, and a careful discussion with the patient regarding the potential risks is required.[39]

Distal Humerus Fractures

Introduction
Fracture of the distal humerus remains one of the most challenging articular injuries to treat because of a combination of factors, including the multiple complex articulations that exist at the elbow joint, the desire for early joint motion, and the limited access to the articular surface. Surgical treatment is typically required for intra-articular fractures. Despite a careful surgical procedure, an accurate reduction, and improved implant designs, complications are commonly encountered. An understanding of the injury, the anatomy, and the optimal treatment options can help to minimize these potential complications.

Anatomy
The distal humerus is roughly triangular in shape with medial and lateral columns of bone that connect the articular segment to the diaphysis. The articular component of the distal humerus is composed of the trochlea and the capitellum. The articular surface of the distal humerus articulates with the ulna at the ulnohumeral joint and with the radius at the radiocapitellar joint. Just proximal to the trochlea are the olecranon and coronoid fossae; this is a region of thin unicortical bone that accommodates the tip of the olecranon posteriorly (with elbow extension) and the coronoid process anteriorly (with elbow flexion). The medial epicondyle is the origin for the flexor-pronator muscles as well as the medial collateral ligament. The lateral epicondyle is the origin for the extensor-supinator muscles as well as the lateral collateral ligament complex. The ulnar nerve is located posterior to the medial epicondyle and passes through the cubital tunnel at the elbow before giving

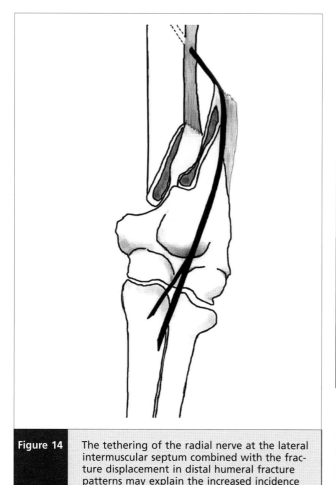

Figure 14 The tethering of the radial nerve at the lateral intermuscular septum combined with the fracture displacement in distal humeral fracture patterns may explain the increased incidence of an associated radial nerve palsy in some reviews.

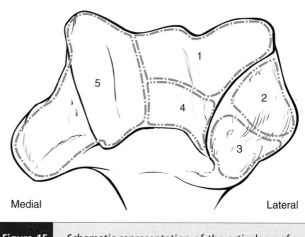

Medial   Lateral

Figure 15 Schematic representation of the articular surface of the distal humerus showing the constituent parts of the articular fracture. 1 = capitellum and lateral portion of the trochlea; 2 = lateral epicondyle; 3 = lateral epicondyle (posterior metaphyseal portion); 4 = posterior aspect of the trochlea; 5 = medial aspect of the trochlea and medial epicondyle. (Reproduced with permission from Ring D, Jupiter JB, Gulotta L: Articular fractures of the distal part of the humerus. *J Bone Joint Surg Am* 2003;85:232-238.)

off sensory and motor branches to the elbow joint and the forearm musculature.

Evaluation and Classification

Physical examination should include evaluation of the entire upper extremity. The focused portion of the clinical evaluation in a patient with a distal humerus fracture should include a comprehensive assessment of the neurovascular status of the arm with special attention placed on the function of the ulnar, radial, and median nerves. The arm should be circumferentially inspected for any skin disruptions, especially posteriorly where open fractures typically occur.

Orthogonal radiographs in the AP and lateral planes are required. Traction films in both planes can be extremely helpful in revealing the extent of the fracture(s), the articular displacement, and any metaphyseal involvement. CT is not routinely required but may be helpful in capitellar fractures and anterior coronal shear fractures and in fracture patterns that are poorly understood based on plain radiographic imaging. Contralateral elbow radiographs may be useful for comparison and preoperative planning.

Distal humerus fracture classification schemes are typically descriptive and based on fracture morphology and location. Anatomic pattern descriptions are useful and include transcondylar, supracondylar, intercondylar, and capitellar fractures. The AO-OTA classification is divided into extra-articular (type A), partial articular (type B), and complete articular (type C) injuries. Complete articular fractures are further divided based on the amount of comminution in the supracondylar and articular regions. Some fractures are totally confined to the articular segment at or distal to the olecranon fossa. These fractures have been subdivided based on their involvement of the five main articular fragments (**Figure 15**). Unfortunately, no classification scheme has been shown to reliably predict treatment or outcomes. Communication regarding the injury pattern is optimized by a careful anatomic description of all of the fracture components, with particular attention to displacement and comminution of the articular segments, the medial epicondyle, and the supracondylar region.

Treatment

Nonsurgical Treatment

With the advances in surgical technique and implant design, surgical treatment is the current standard for displaced, unstable supracondylar fractures. However, nonsurgical treatment has historically yielded reasonable results in very limited circumstances.[40] Nonsurgical treatment is currently reserved for nondisplaced, stable fractures and patients who are unable or unwilling to undergo surgical treatment.

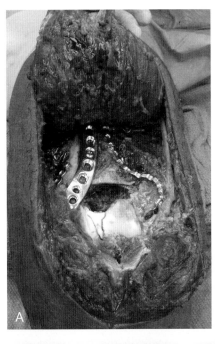
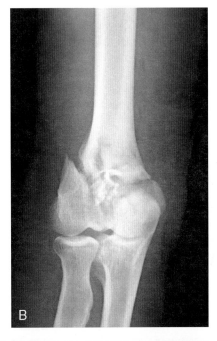
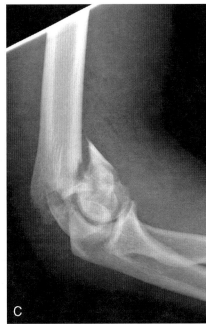
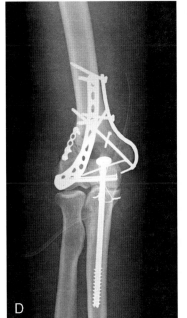
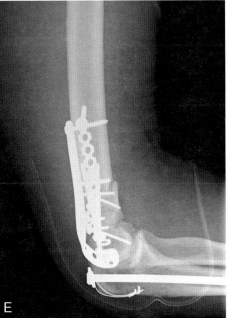

Figure 16	A 43-year-old man sustained an intra-articular distal humerus fracture (type C3) after a fall from a height. **A**, Intraoperative photograph of the olecranon osteotomy. **B** and **C**, AP and lateral injury radiographs. **D** and **E**, AP and lateral postoperative radiographs. Medial and lateral column plates were used, and the osteotomy was fixed with an intramedullary screw combined with a tensioned wire.

Surgical Treatment

The goals of surgical treatment are the same as for other periarticular fractures: anatomic articular reduction of joint fragments; stable internal fixation to meet local biomechanical demands; preservation of blood supply through atraumatic soft-tissue technique; and early functional motion for rehabilitation.

To achieve these goals, attention has been focused on the surgical approach, reduction techniques, fixation constructs, and rehabilitation protocols. Over the past 5 years, understanding of the implications of the surgical approach, the biomechanics of fracture fixation constructs, the expected outcomes of surgical treatment, and the decision to use ORIF or total elbow arthroplasty (TEA) has improved.

Surgical approaches can be divided into soft-tissue mobilization procedures and the olecranon osteotomy approach. The choice of surgical approach has significant consequences that revolve around the ability to visualize the articular surface to obtain an anatomic reduction and the potential complications associated with creating another fracture (the olecranon osteotomy). In general, soft-tissue mobilization procedures do not allow for the same visualization of the articular surface as the olecranon osteotomy because it is the olecranon that covers the distal humeral articular surface.[41] While allowing for premium visualization of the articular surface, the olecranon osteotomy has the incipient risk of nonunion, which has historically been reported at approximately 10%. The choice of surgical approach should be made by weighing the risks of osteotomy complications against the benefit of enhanced articular visualization. With simple articular fracture patterns, the goal of an anatomic joint reduction can be reached with more limited visualization. However, if expanded exposure is needed for accurate reduction of a complex intra-articular fracture, then an olecranon osteotomy should be performed (**Figure 16**).

Soft-Tissue Mobilization Procedures

Many soft-tissue mobilization procedures that avoid olecranon osteotomy have been reported in the literature; each varies in the way it addresses the triceps. Three common approaches are the triceps sparing (paratricipital), triceps splitting, and triceps reflecting.

The triceps-sparing approach is especially useful for the treatment of extra-articular and simple articular fracture patterns, regardless of the metaphyseal fracture configuration.[42] A posterior midline skin incision allows for mobilization of the triceps and anconeus off the posterior humerus, capsule, and intermuscular septae. Working windows can be developed on the lateral and medial sides of the triceps tendon. Visualization is typically adequate to reduce the metaphyseal segment to the shaft and to reduce simple articular fractures. Column-specific plating is easily undertaken.

The triceps-splitting approach has been popularized for use in distal humeral shaft fractures, but it can be extended distally with midline splitting and medial/lateral elevation of the tendinous attachment to the olecranon. Visualization of the articular surface is aided via longitudinal distraction of the ulna along the axis of the humerus and flexion of the elbow. Column-specific plating is possible through the split in the triceps muscle. A specific advantage for this approach is its utility with an open fracture combined with a significant injury to the triceps aponeurosis. This approach has the disadvantages of splitting the triceps muscle and still having limited articular visualization because of the location of the olecranon process.

Triceps-reflecting approaches have been popularized for both ORIF and TEA. These approaches reportedly preserve triceps function, leading to minimal postoperative weakness. Like the other soft-tissue mobilization procedures, they maintain the continuity of the olecranon, making them advantageous when TEA is a possibility.

Olecranon Osteotomy

Original enthusiasm for transolecranon exposures has been tempered by the complications of nonunion and implant prominence. However, more recent reviews of outcomes after an olecranon osteotomy approach for the distal humerus have found much lower rates of nonunion and complications associated with the osteotomy itself.[43-45] Still a popular approach because of improved articular visualization, the technique has been recently evaluated in the literature.[41] Advances in both the shape of the osteotomy and stabilization techniques have been suggested. Currently an intra-articular chevron-shaped osteotomy pointing distally is preferred.[43-45] Stabilization with low-profile plating, modified tension-band wiring, intramedullary screw fixation, and the combination of intramedullary screw fixation with dorsal ulnar wiring all have been successful. Regardless of which type of fixation is chosen, ensuring secure stabilization is of utmost importance. The incidence of nonunion has decreased substantially in all recent studies. At this point, implant prominence seems to be the main concern.

The effect of the approach on the functional outcome of surgical fixation of supracondylar-intercondylar humerus fractures has been evaluated,[46,47] although not with a well-controlled, prospective study trying to isolate this treatment variable. Currently, there does not seem to be an overwhelming advantage to either the soft-tissue mobilization procedures or the olecranon osteotomy. The decision is still reasonably made at the discretion of the surgeon. Important patient and fracture variables that may influence the decision include osteoporosis, the severity of the articular injury, the presence of a triceps aponeurosis injury, and the presence of associated fractures about the elbow.

The Biomechanics of Fracture Fixation Constructs

The distal humerus is subject to axial, bending, and torsional loads. Fracture fixation constructs are designed to resist these loads, while allowing early functional motion. The constructs are numerous and include multiple permutations of locking, nonlocking, precontoured, surgeon-contoured, titanium, stainless, parallel, and perpendicular plating.[48,49] Although there is no single standard plating construct, some accepted principles are listed in **Table 2**.

Recent biomechanical literature has addressed stability in comminuted fracture models. In a fracture gap model, the position of implant placement (perpendicular versus dorsal plating) was found to be more important than the type of implant (locking compression versus conventional reconstruction plating) when cyclically loaded in compression, bending, and torsion.[48] While the indications for locking constructs are still in evolution, the use of locking implants has increased. A recent biomechanical study compared the stability of parallel versus perpendicular double-locking plating systems in an osteoporotic fracture model. Both

Table 2

Accepted Principles for Fracture Fixation Constructs

Independent screw or wire constructs are inadequate in adult fractures.

Dual plating is preferred to single plate constructs.

Column plating is preferred, whether perpendicular or parallel.

One third tubular plates are inadequate.

Screw placement into articular surface fragments through plates is desirable (rather than independent screw placement outside of plates).

systems seemed to provide adequate stability for early mobilization of the elbow in patients with osteoporotic bone, with higher stability in compression and torsion noted in the parallel system.[49]

Expected Outcomes of Surgical Treatment

Outcomes following ORIF of distal humerus fractures have evolved with time and improved surgical approaches and reductions[45,50-52] and can be measured in many ways. Although long-term functional outcomes are similar to those reported in the short term, residual deficiencies are the norm rather than the exception.[51] The average flexion-extension arc is typically around 100° to 110°, with an average pronation-supination arc of 160° to 170°. Regaining terminal extension is difficult, with an approximate mean flexion contracture of 25°. Muscle weakness is also common, with strength typically reaching approximately 75% of the contralateral, normal side. Although current ORIF techniques provide reliable results, both limb-specific questionnaires (such as Disabilities of the Arm, Shoulder and Hand) and general health-status questionnaires (such as Short Form-36) reveal postoperative limitations.[47]

Older Patients, Osteoporosis, and the Decision Between ORIF and TEA

The principle of stable fixation for the allowance of early functional motion is severely tested in the subpopulation of older patients with osteoporotic, comminuted fractures. As a result, abandoning ORIF in favor of TEA is a common scenario.[53-55] Two studies have compared the results of these two treatment options. In a retrospective review, the Mayo Elbow Performance Score and the need for revision surgery were used as primary outcome measurements.[53] TEA was found to be a viable alternative to ORIF, with better outcome scores and fewer revision surgeries noted in this patient group. A more recent multicenter, prospective, randomized, controlled trial echoed these findings.[55] TEA was found to be the preferred alternative in complex distal humerus fractures not amenable to stable fixation. Ar-

throplasty resulted in more predictable and improved 2-year functional outcomes compared with ORIF.

Rehabilitation and Postoperative Care

Optimally there should be sufficient stability to allow early elbow range of motion following ORIF of a distal humerus fracture. Extended immobilization is associated with unacceptable elbow stiffness and should be avoided. Initially the arm is placed in a well-padded posterior splint to protect the surgical wound and to minimize discomfort for the initial 24 to 48 hours. Longer immobilization may be required in patients with posterior open fractures, extensive soft-tissue injuries, or wounds that were difficult to close after a lengthy procedure. Proponents exist for initial splinting in extension or at 90° of flexion. Early active and active-assisted range-of-motion exercises are initiated. Exercises that allow active extension against resistance are typically avoided during the first 6 weeks after surgery if an osteotomy approach was used or in cases with a triceps repair or disruption. Overly aggressive passive range-of-motion exercises are generally avoided because of the possibility of creating more inflammation and stiffness by pushing through a painful arc, and the potential for creating elbow instability by the loss of the stabilizing function of active muscle contraction. Weight bearing for articular injuries is delayed for 12 weeks. Prophylaxis for heterotopic ossification is not routinely used. However, there is some evidence that a significant (more than 48-hour) delay to surgery, an associated head injury, and a prolonged period of mechanical ventilation may be associated with increased ectopic bone formation postoperatively.

Complications

Complications following ORIF of distal humerus fractures include stiffness, heterotopic ossification, nonunion, failure of fixation, malunion, ulnar neuritis, and infection. Elbow stiffness is the most common of these complications, and most patients lose some component of elbow extension. Early surgical intervention, stable fixation allowing early and consistent range-of-motion exercises, and avoiding prolonged postoperative immobilization can help to minimize elbow stiffness. Heterotopic ossification, although uncommon, may limit elbow motion. Surgical contracture release and/or heterotopic bone resection may be necessary in patients who do not obtain a functional arc of elbow motion.

Early failure of fixation is frequently the result of inadequate surgical fracture stabilization, although patient factors such as noncompliance and osteopenia may also contribute. Nonunion, especially in the supracondylar region, may occur and is more common after an open fracture. Management of a nonunion in the supracondylar region typically involves an open repair with revision fixation and bone grafting. Intra-articular nonunions can be difficult to manage and usually require a complete revision of the surgical procedure with adequate joint visualization to restore the articular surface.

3: Upper Extremity

Ulnar neuritis can occur as a result of the distal humerus fracture, because of the surgical procedure or postoperative hardware irritation. Atraumatic identification and protection of the ulnar nerve throughout the surgical procedure should be performed, with avoidance of excessive traction. The necessity for transposition of the ulnar nerve following fixation remains controversial, and superior results have not been demonstrated with either approach.

Fortunately, infection after ORIF of the distal humerus is rare, despite lengthy surgical procedures and a significant amount of soft-tissue dissection necessary in a relatively subcutaneous anatomic location. Open fractures are at higher risk for infection and should be managed using the usual principles of treating open injuries.

Annotated References

1. Gaebler C, McQueen MM, Court-Brown CM: Minimally displaced proximal humeral fractures: Epidemiology and outcome in 507 cases. *Acta Orthop Scand* 2003;74(5):580-585.

2. Palvanen M, Kannus P, Niemi S, Parkkari J: Update in the epidemiology of proximal humeral fractures. *Clin Orthop Relat Res* 2006;442:87-92.

   This study examines the current trends in the number of proximal humerus fractures from low-energy accidents in elderly Finns over the last three decades. Level of evidence: IV.

3. Iannotti JP, Gabriel JP, Schneck SL, Evans BG, Misra S: The normal glenohumeral relationships: An anatomical study of one hundred and forty shoulders. *J Bone Joint Surg Am* 1992;74(4):491-500.

4. Pearl ML: Proximal humeral anatomy in shoulder arthroplasty: Implications for prosthetic design and surgical technique. *J Shoulder Elbow Surg* 2005;14(1, suppl S)99S-104S.

   This is a review paper highlighting different studies in shoulder anatomy relevant to prosthetic geometry.

5. Gardner MJ, Voos JE, Wanich T, et al: Vascular implications of minimally invasive plating of proximal humerus fractures. *J Orthop Trauma* 2006;20(90):602-607.

   The authors studied the relationship of a direct surgical approach to the lateral plating zone of the proximal humerus and to the penetrating vascular supply of the humeral head. A direct approach may minimize iatrogenic vascular injury during treatment of fractures of the proximal humerus.

6. Brooks CH, Revell WJ, Heatley FW: Vascularity of the humeral head after proximal humeral fractures: An anatomical cadaver study. *J Bone Joint Surg Br* 1993; 75(1):132-136.

7. Hertel R, Hempfing A, Stiehler M, Leunig M: Predictors of humeral head ischemia after intracapsular fracture of the proximal humerus. *J Shoulder Elbow Surg* 2004; 13(4):427-433.

   Predictors of fracture-induced humeral head ischemia were evaluated. The most relevant predictors were length of the dorsomedial metaphyseal extension, integrity of the medial hinge, and basic fracture type.

8. Stenning M, Drew S, Birch R: Low-energy arterial injury at the shoulder with progressive or delayed nerve palsy. *J Bone Joint Surg Br* 2005;87(8):1102-1106.

   A retrospective case series of 20 patients with delayed nerve palsy or deepening of initial palsy secondary to an arterial injury from low-energy shoulder trauma is discussed.

9. Parsons BO, Klepps SJ, Miller S, Bird J, Gladstone J, Flatow E: Reliability and reproducibility of radiographs of greater tuberosity displacement: A cadaveric study. *J Bone Joint Surg Am* 2005;87(1):58-65.

   A cadaver study using fluoroscopic images of prepositioned osteotomized greater tuberosity fragments was done to determine the best view for recognition of greater tuberosity displacement.

10. Bahrs C, Rolauffs B, Sudkamp NP, et al: Indications for computed tomography (CT) diagnostics in proximal humeral fractures: A comparative study of plain radiography and computed tomography. *BMC Musculoskel Dis* 2009;10:33.

    In comparison with conventional radiographs with an AP view and high-quality axial views, CT with thin-slice technology and three-dimensional imaging always provides a clear presentation of the fractured region.

11. Neer CS II: Four-segment classification of proximal humeral fractures: Purpose and reliable use. *J Shoulder Elbow Surg* 2002;11(4):389-400.

    A review of the thought process behind the original Neer classification system is presented, along with updates on the criteria for the categories and outlines requirements for reliable use.

12. Edelson G, Kelly I, Vigder F, Reis ND: A three-dimensional classification for fractures of the proximal humerus. *J Bone Joint Surg Br* 2004;86(3):413-425.

13. Lanting B, MacDermid J, Drosdowech D, Faber KJ: Proximal humeral fractures: A systematic review of treatment modalities. *J Shoulder Elbow Surg* 2008; 17(1):42-54.

    A systematic review of 66 studies including 2,155 patients with proximal humerus fractures provides very few conclusions secondary to inadequacies of studies.

14. Kamineni S, Ankem H, Sanghavi S: Anatomic considerations for percutaneous proximal humeral fracture fixation. *Injury* 2004;35:1133-1136.

15. Agel J, Jones CB, Sanzone AG, Camuso M, Henley MB: Treatment of proximal humeral fractures with Polarus

nail fixation. *J Shoulder Elbow Surg* 2004;13(2):191-195.

16. Gardner MJ, Weil Y, Barker JU, Kelly BT, Helfet DL, Lorich DG: The importance of medial support in locked plating of proximal humerus fractures. *J Orthop Trauma* 2007;21(3):185-191.

    A retrospective review of 35 patients with proximal humerus fractures treated with locked plating with the goal of determining which factors influenced maintenance of fracture reduction after locked plating is presented.

17. Owsley KC, Gorczyca JT: Fracture displacement and screw cutout after open reduction and locked plate fixation of proximal humeral fractures. *J Bone Joint Surg Am* 2008;90(2):233-240.

    The authors present a radiographic and clinical review of 53 patients treated with a proximal humeral locking plate with an informative discussion on common failure modes. Level of evidence: IV.

18. Südkamp N, Bayer J, Hepp P, et al: Open reduction and internal fixation of proximal humeral fractures with use of the locking proximal humerus plate: Results of a prospective, multicenter, observational study. *J Bone Joint Surg Am* 2009;91(6):1320-1328.

    The authors present a prospective, multicenter, observational study of 187 patients treated with a proximal humeral locking plate. Level of evidence: IV.

19. Gardner MJ, Griffith MH, Dines JS, Briggs SM, Weiland AJ, Lorich DG: The extended anterolateral acromial approach allows minimally invasive access to the proximal humerus. *Clin Orthop Relat Res* 2005;434:123-129.

    The authors present a cadaver dissection and case study describing the extended anterolateral acromial approach for use in the treatment of proximal humerus fractures. Level of evidence: IV.

20. Robinson CM, Khan L, Akhtar A, Whittaker R: The extended deltoid-splitting approach to the proximal humerus. *J Orthop Trauma* 2007;21:657-662.

    The authors concluded that the extended deltoid-splitting approach provides enhanced surgical exposure and is an alternative to the deltopectoral approach, which has limited surgical access.

21. Laflamme GY, Rouleau DM, Berry GK, Beaumont PH, Reindl R, Harvey EJ: Percutaneous humeral plating of fractures of the proximal humerus: Results of a prospective multicenter clinical trial. *J Orthop Trauma* 2008;22(3):153-158.

    The safety and functional outcome of percutaneous plating of two-part surgical neck and three-part impacted proximal humerus fractures is evaluated in a prospective clinical trial.

22. Court-Brown CM, McQueen MM: The impacted varus (A2.2) proximal humeral fracture: Prediction of outcome and results of nonoperative treatment in 99 patients. *Acta Orthop Scand* 2004;75(6):736-740.

    The authors performed a prospective analysis on 99 impacted varus proximal humerus fractures. Nonsurgical treatment sometimes caused an increase in varus angulation, but overall outcomes were good 1 year after fracture.

23. Kontakis G, Koutras C, Tosounidis T, Giannoudis P: Early management of proximal humeral fractures with hemiarthroplasty: A systematic review. *J Bone Joint Surg Br* 2008;90(11):1407-1413.

    A systematic review of hemiarthroplasty for treatment of proximal humerus fractures provides insight into expected results and potential complications.

24. Ekholm R, Tidermark J, Törnkvist H, Adami J, Ponzer S: Outcome after closed functional treatment of humeral shaft fractures. *J Orthop Trauma* 2006;20(9):591-596.

    The authors observed healing in 90% of closed fractures treated with a functional brace. Nonunions were more frequent (trend only) in simple fracture patterns and the functional outcome of nonunion treatment, despite healing, was worse. Selected closed fractures may be appropriately treated with plate fixation initially.

25. Rutgers M, Ring D: Treatment of diaphyseal fractures of the humerus using a functional brace. *J Orthop Trauma* 2006;20(9):597-601.

    Isolated humeral diaphyseal fractures treated with functional bracing had union in 90%, with excellent functional results in these patients. However, nonunion was observed in 29% of proximal-third long oblique fractures.

26. Castella FB, Garcia FB, Berry EM, Perello EB, Sanchez-Alepuz E, Gabarda R: Nonunion of the humeral shaft. Long lateral butterfly fracture: A nonunion predictive pattern? *Clin Orthop Relat Res* 2004;424:227-230.

    Thirty patients with nonunion of the humeral shaft were reviewed retrospectively; nine had an initial fracture pattern that had not been previously described. Eight of the fractures went on to nonunion after initial nonsurgical treatment.

27. Fleming P, Lenehan B, Sankar R, Folan-Curran J, Curtin W: One-third, two-thirds: Relationship of the radial nerve to the lateral intermuscular septum in the arm. *Clin Anat* 2004;17(1):26-29.

    In a cadaver dissection study, the radial nerve was found to enter the anterior compartment consistently (within 5 mm) at the junction of the middle and distal thirds of the humerus (defined by a line from the lateral epicondyle to lateral acromion).

28. O'Toole RV, Andersen RC, Vesnovsky O, et al: Are locking screws advantageous with plate fixation of humeral shaft fractures? A biomechanical analysis of synthetic and cadaveric bone. *J Orthop Trauma* 2008;22(10):709-715.

    This biomechanical study evaluated a comminuted midshaft humeral fracture in synthetic bone models and cadaver humeri stabilized with a 3.5-mm locking plate using either locked or unlocked screws. No biomechanical

3: Upper Extremity

advantage could be demonstrated with the use of locking screws in torsion, bending, and axial stiffness and load to failure.

29. Gardner MJ, Griffith MH, Demetrakopoulos D, et al: Hybrid locked plating of osteoporotic fractures of the humerus. *J Bone Joint Surg Am* 2006;88(9):1962-1967.

Locked plates were found to be significantly more stable than unlocked constructs when tested with torsional cyclic loading. Hybrid constructs did not compromise the mechanical characteristics of the construct and may be advantageous.

30. Apivatthakakul T, Arpornchayanon O, Bavornratanavech S: Minimally invasive plate osteosynthesis (MIPO) of the humeral shaft fracture. Is it possible? A cadaveric study and preliminary report. *Injury* 2005; 36(4):530-538.

In an anatomic study in cadavers, the authors investigated the relationship between the radial nerve and a plate placed using a minimally invasive anterior technique. No nerve entrapment was found, although the average distance to the nerve was small. Forearm supination was useful for maximizing safety.

31. Zhiquan A, Bingfang Z, Yeming W, Chi Z, Peiyan H: Minimally invasive plating osteosynthesis (MIPO) of middle and distal third humeral shaft fractures. *J Orthop Trauma* 2007;21(9):628-633.

Thirteen patients (nonconsecutive) with a middle third or distal third humerus fracture were treated with a minimally invasive plating technique. The fractures united rapidly and there were no iatrogenic radial nerve palsies in this small series.

32. An Z, Zeng B, He X, Chen Q, Hu S: Plating osteosynthesis of mid-distal humeral shaft fractures: Minimally invasive versus conventional open reduction technique. *Int Orthop* 2010;34:131-135.

33. Bhandari M, Devereaux PJ, McKee MD, Schemitsch EH: Compression plating versus intramedullary nailing of humeral shaft fractures: A meta-analysis. *Acta Orthop* 2006;77(2):279-284.

In a review of the three prospective and randomized studies comparing plates and nails for humeral shaft fractures, the authors concluded that plate fixation may reduce the risk of reoperation and shoulder impingement compared to intramedullary nails.

34. Shao YC, Harwood P, Grotz MR, Limb D, Giannoudis PV: Radial nerve palsy associated with fractures of the shaft of the humerus: A systematic review. *J Bone Joint Surg Br* 2005;87(12):1647-1652.

In a systematic review of 35 manuscripts, the prevalence of radial nerve palsy after humeral shaft fracture was 11.8%, and it was associated with fractures of the middle and distal thirds and with transverse and spiral patterns. The overall nerve recovery rate was 88.1%, and early exploration was not associated with improved recovery.

35. Ring D, Chin K, Jupiter JB: Radial nerve palsy associated with high-energy humeral shaft fractures. *J Hand Surg Am* 2004;29(1):144-147.

In 24 patients with high energy diaphyseal humeral fractures with complete neurologic deficits, the authors confirmed the high incidence of nerve transection in open humeral fractures and the poor result with primary repair in these patients. Intact nerves and closed fractures were associated with a high recovery rate, although it was often quite delayed.

36. Ekholm R, Ponzer S, Törnkvist H, Adami J, Tidermark J: The Holstein-Lewis humeral shaft fracture: Aspects of radial nerve injury, primary treatment, and outcome. *J Orthop Trauma* 2008;22(10):693-697.

An increased incidence of radial nerve palsy (22% versus 8%) was demonstrated with the Holstein-Lewis fracture pattern. Return of radial nerve function, healing, and overall outcome were predictably good whether surgical or nonsurgical treatment was performed.

37. Bishop J, Ring D. Management of radial nerve palsy associated with humeral shaft fracture: A decision analysis model. *J Hand Surg Am* 2009;34:991-996.

A systematic review was undertaken to determine outcomes and treatment for a radial nerve palsy associated with a humeral shaft fracture. The authors concluded that initial observation was the preferred strategy in most clinical situations. However, if spontaneous nerve recovery is thought to be extremely low, early surgery may optimize outcome.

38. Lambert S: Further opinion: Radial nerve palsy associated with fractures of the shaft of the humerus. A systematic review. *J Bone Joint Surg Br* 2005;87(12):1-3.

39. Jawa A, McCarty P, Doornberg J, Harris M, Ring D: Extra-articular distal-third diaphyseal fractures of the humerus: A comparison of functional bracing and plate fixation. *J Bone Joint Surg Am* 2006;88(11):2343-2347.

Extra-articular distal third humeral diaphyseal fractures treated with either plate fixation or functional bracing were retrospectively compared. The authors concluded that surgical treatment achieved better alignment and return of function but had an increased risk of nerve injury or infection. Closed treatment, although associated with deformity, yielded excellent functional results.

40. Srinivasan K, Giannoudis P, Agarwal M, Patil V, Matthews SJE: Fractures of the distal humerus in the elderly (aged 75-100): Analysis of results after operative and nonoperative treatment. *J Bone Joint Surg Br* 2008; 90B(suppl 1):8.

The authors analyzed functional outcome after surgical and nonsurgical treatment of fractures of the distal humerus in patients older than 75 years. Results were better after surgical treatment.

41. Wilkinson JM, Stanley D: Posterior surgical approaches to the elbow: A comparative anatomic study. *J Shoulder Elbow Surg* 2001;10-4:380-382.

42. Schildhauer TA, Nork SE, Mills WJ, Henley MB: Extensor mechanism-sparing paratricipital posterior ap-

proach to the distal humerus. *J Orthop Trauma* 2003; 17(5):374-378.

43. Ring D, Gulotta L, Chin K, Jupiter JB: Olecranon osteotomy for exposure of fractures and nonunions of the distal humerus. *J Orthop Trauma* 2004;18(7):446-449.

    Fixation of an apex distal chevron osteotomy with a modified tension band technique yielded predictable results in 45 patients. The authors reported a single nonunion and low hardware removal rate for symptoms (13%).

44. Coles CP, Barei DP, Nork SE, Taitsman LA, Hanel DP, Bradford Henley M: The olecranon osteotomy: A six-year experience in the treatment of intraarticular fractures of the distal humerus. *J Orthop Trauma* 2006; 20-3:164-171.

    The authors reviewed their experience with the use of a chevron osteotomy of the olecranon in complex distal humerus fractures, most of which were open injuries. All 67 osteotomies healed. Osteotomy fixation hardware removal was performed in 30% overall, but in only 8% for symptoms. The authors concluded that an osteotomy can be useful and has an acceptable rate of complications.

45. Hewins EA, Gofton WT, Dubberly J, MacDermid JC, Faber KJ, King GJ: Plate fixation of olecranon osteotomies. *J Orthop Trauma* 2007;21(1):58-62.

    The use of a 3.5-mm reconstruction plate to stabilize an apex distal chevron osteotomy resulted in predictable union, low complications, and the infrequent need for hardware removal in a series of 17 consecutive patients with fractures of the distal humerus.

46. Ek ET, Goldwasser M, Bonomo AL: Functional outcome of complex intercondylar fractures of the distal humerus treated through a triceps-sparing approach. *J Shoulder Elbow Surg* 2008;17:441-446.

    The authors studied functional outcome of complex intercondylar fractures of the distal humerus treated with ORIF via a triceps-sparing approach. The triceps-sparing approach provided adequate exposure of the fracture site and facilitated early rehabilitation, leading to a satisfactory functional outcome.

47. McKee MD, Wilson TL, Winston L, Schemitsch EH, Richards RR: Functional outcome following surgical treatment of intra-articular distal humeral fractures through a posterior approach. *J Bone Joint Surg Am* 2000;82(12):1701-1707.

48. Korner J, Diederichs G, Arzdorf M, et al: A biomechanical evaluation of methods of distal humerus fracture fixation using locking compression plates versus conventional reconstruction plates. *J Orthop Trauma* 2004; 18(5):286-293.

    In a biomechanical study, the authors compared different plate configurations and the use of locking implants. Perpendicular plate applications were found to be superior to two dorsally applied implants.

49. Stoffel K, Cunneen S, Morgan R, Nicholls R, Sta-

chowiak G: Comparative stability of perpendicular versus parallel double-locking plating systems in osteoporotic comminuted distal humerus fractures. *J Orthop Res* 2008;26(6):778-784.

    Two locking plate systems with two different plating configurations were compared in paired cadaver bones. Both configurations were found to produce adequate stability, although the parallel configuration showed improved stability compared to the perpendicular system.

50. Russell GV Jr, Jarrett CA, Jones CB, Cole PA, Gates J: Management of distal humerus fractures with minifragment fixation. *J Orthop Trauma* 2005;19(7):474-479.

    This is an excellent technical report on the treatment of complex intra-articular distal humerus fractures using a combination of small screw fixations and standard plating techniques.

51. Doornberg JN, van Duijn PJ, Linzel D, et al: Surgical treatment of intra-articular fractures of the distal part of the humerus: Functional outcome after twelve to thirty years. *J Bone Joint Surg Am* 2007;89(7):1524-1532.

    Thirty patients were followed for an average of 19 years after fixation for a distal humerus fracture. The good short-term results were durable in the long term using multiple measures of functional outcomes. Radiographic signs of arthrosis did not predict outcomes or disability.

52. Reising K, Hauschild O, Strohm PC, Suedkamp NP: Stabilisation of articular fractures of the distal humerus: Early experience with a novel perpendicular plate system. *Injury* 2009;40(6):611-617.

    In this retrospective review of 40 patients, treatment consisted of a fixed angle plating system with two perpendicular anatomically contoured implants. Good functional results were observed. Implant failure and nonunion were rare.

53. Frankle MA, Herscovici D Jr, DiPasquale TG, Vasey MB, Sanders RW: A comparison of open reduction and internal fixation and primary total elbow arthroplasty in the treatment of intraarticular distal humerus fractures in women older than age 65. *J Orthop Trauma* 2003;17(7):473-480.

54. Kamineni S, Morrey BF: Distal humeral fractures treated with noncustom total elbow replacement: Surgical technique. *J Bone Joint Surg Am* 2005;87(Pt 1, suppl 1):41-50.

    The surgical technique and results followed a total elbow replacement were described in detail in a group of 48 patients with an average age of 67 years with distal humerus fractures. Range of motion, elbow scoring, complications, and durability were predictable and good in these properly selected patients.

55. McKee MD, Veillette CJ, Hall JA, et al: A multicenter, prospective, randomized, controlled trial of open reduction: Internal fixation versus total elbow arthroplasty for displaced intra-articular distal humeral fractures in elderly patients. *J Shoulder Elbow Surg* 2009;18(1):3-12.

    In a comparison study of 42 patients older than 65 years

randomized to treatment with either a semiconstrained total elbow or ORIF of a distal humerus fracture, the arthroplasty patients were found to have more predictable and improved 2-year outcomes. Range of motion was similar between the groups, and reoperations were required in 12% of the arthroplasty group and 27% of the ORIF group.

Chapter 19

Fractures and Dislocations of the Elbow

Gregory J. Della Rocca, MD, PhD, FACS   Murray J. Beuerlein, MD, MSc, FRCS(C)

Olecranon Fractures

Fractures of the olecranon often result in complete loss of active elbow extension, as the main olecranon fracture fragment contains the insertion of the triceps brachii. They almost invariably involve the ulnohumeral articulation. Anatomic restoration of the greater sigmoid notch of the ulna is vital, both for normal elbow function and to diminish the risk of future arthrosis. Multiple methods of fixation have been described, all of which are variably successful for the treatment of olecranon fractures. Although good results can be expected after proper diagnosis, treatment, and rehabilitation of olecranon fractures, complications can occur, and often are related either to implant prominence (caused by the subcutaneous nature of the olecranon) or inadequate fixation technique.

Classification

No single classification system of olecranon fractures has gained wide acceptance. Instead, it is useful to classify these injuries simply as either nondisplaced or displaced, and simple transverse versus comminuted fracture patterns.

Nonsurgical Treatment

Nonsurgical treatment of olecranon fractures is reserved primarily for nondisplaced or minimally displaced fractures (those with less than 2 mm of displacement). The patient normally is able to actively extend the elbow in this situation. No consensus exists for type of immobilization (with the elbow flexed to 90° or with the elbow fully extended), length of immobilization (days to weeks), early exercise regimen (active, active-

assisted, or passive range of motion), and time to initiate resisted elbow extension (6 to 12 weeks) in the setting of an acute, nondisplaced olecranon fracture. Good results can be expected, but patients should be warned that a slight loss of motion might occur even after full healing.

Surgical Treatment

Multiple methods of fixation for olecranon fractures exist, including tension band wiring, intramedullary screw fixation, and plate-and-screw fixation. Olecranon fracture fragment excision is also an option. Prior to embarking on an strategy for surgical treatment of olecranon fractures, the surgeon must have a complete understanding of the injury pattern. Poor surgical tactics with inappropriate fixation strategies can result in poor outcomes. For example, failure to recognize and treat associated coronoid fractures, radial head fractures, or elbow instability associated with olecranon fractures can lead to dismal outcomes, such as chronic elbow dislocation, despite perfect anatomic reduction of the olecranon component of the fracture.

Surgical Approach

A standard posterior approach is generally used for exposure, reduction, and fixation of olecranon fractures. The patient may be positioned lateral or prone, with the arm suspended by an arm board or bolster beneath the ventral brachium, or supine, with the arm draped across the chest. There is adequate space for application of a tourniquet about the superior brachium, if desired. The incision parallels the dorsal border of the ulna and begins a few centimeters proximal to the olecranon tip. The incision can be performed in a straight fashion across the olecranon process itself, curve medially around the olecranon process to allow for visualization of the ulnar nerve if desired, or curve laterally around the olecranon process to minimize the likelihood of a tender scar in a medial location (where patients may rest the elbow on a table or armrest). Fascia between the extensor carpi ulnaris and the flexor carpi ulnaris is incised directly off the subcutaneous border of the ulna, and the muscles medial and lateral to the border are elevated as necessary for exposure. The frac-

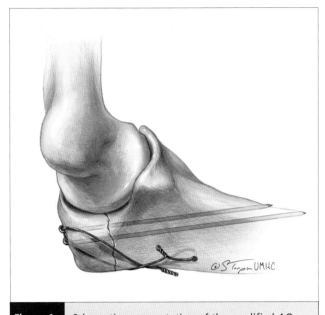

Figure 1 Schematic representation of the modified AO technique of tension band wiring of a simple transverse olecranon fracture. Note that the wire tips emanate from the ventral cortex of the proximal ulna, distal to the base of the coronoid process. (Copyright Curators of the University of Missouri, Columbia, MS, 2009.)

ture site is viewed and cleaned of interposed periosteum and organizing hematoma. Often, the chondral surface of the distal humeral trochlea is readily visible and can be inspected for chondral injury. Reduction of the fracture is accomplished with a variety of aids, such as sharp hooks, Kirschner wires, and reduction forceps. Elbow extension can often facilitate this reduction.

Tension Band Wiring

Tension band wire constructs are generally reserved for noncomminuted transverse olecranon fractures. The function of the tension band, theoretically, is to convert eccentric distraction forces across the fracture site, in this case generated by the pull of the triceps, to compressive forces at the articular surface (opposite the tension band). This theory has been challenged, however, by a biomechanical study that failed to demonstrate the conversion of tensile forces from the pull of the triceps to compressive forces at the articular surface in the presence of a tension band.[1]

Careful preoperative planning is necessary before utilization of a tension band wire construct for fixation of an olecranon fracture. A tension band wire construct alone is insufficient fixation for complex fracture-dislocations of the elbow; injury radiographs should be carefully scrutinized for elbow subluxation, coronoid fractures, and radial head fractures.[2] Comminution of the olecranon is also a contraindication to treatment with a tension band wire construct. Impaction or bone loss at the articular surface can result in narrowing of the greater sigmoid notch with use of a tension band

construct, resulting in incongruity between the ulnar notch and the trochlea of the distal humerus. Conversely, bone loss or comminution at the dorsal cortex can result in angulation at the fracture site with concomitant gapping of the articular surface. A fracture that extends more distally in an oblique fashion also may not be ideal for stabilization with a tension band construct and be more amenable to lag screw and plate fixation.

The classic method of tension band wire application included two parallel medullary Kirschner wires and a cerclage or figure-of-8 wire passed through a dorsal bone tunnel. A modified AO technique has been developed in which the Kirschner wires are passed bicortically beneath the ulnohumeral articulation, emanating from the ventral cortex of the proximal ulna just distal to the base of the coronoid process (**Figure 1**). The bicortical method of tension band wiring appears to have improved biomechanical strength over the medullary method and reduces the risk of implant prominence because of wire migration.[3] An alternative technique involving a single medullary screw with a supplemental dorsal figure-of-8 wire has also been advocated for fixation of olecranon fractures or osteotomies.[4] Figure-of-8 constructs using suture to minimize implant-related irritation instead of stainless steel wire or cable have been examined. Braided polyester suture has been demonstrated to lack stiffness and results in increased displacement of the fracture under physiologic loads.[5] More recently, the use of a suture of braided polyester with a polyethylene core (#2 FiberWire, Arthrex, Naples, FL) for the figure-of-8 portion of the tension band construct was demonstrated to be biomechanically equivalent to 18-gauge stainless steel wire in a cadaver transverse olecranon fracture model.[6]

Plate-and-Screw Fixation

Fixation of comminuted olecranon fractures is often accomplished with plate-and-screw constructs (**Figure 2**). Open reduction and internal fixation with plates and screws is also used for simple fractures of the olecranon that occur distal to the midportion of the greater sigmoid notch. Plating techniques have been shown to be successful in the setting of comminuted olecranon fractures and for fixation of olecranon osteotomies.[4,7,8] Plates are often applied in neutralization mode for comminuted olecranon fractures; compression techniques risk narrowing the greater sigmoid notch. Interfragmentary screws, placed either in positioning mode or compression mode outside of the plate, are often used to supplement the plate fixation. Allograft, autograft, or osteobiologic void fillers can be used in the setting of depressed olecranon fracture fragments to provide support of the articular surface. Plate choice is according to surgeon preference; reconstruction-style plates[8] or precontoured plates[7] are commonly used. One-third tubular plates may prove insufficiently strong, and dynamic compression plates are difficult to contour, but both have also been used successfully. Medial and lateral plating of olecranon fractures has been

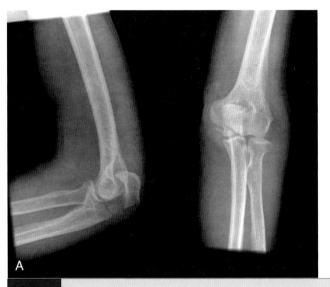
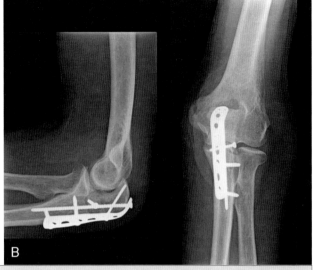

Figure 2 **A,** Injury radiographs of an isolated, widely displaced, comminuted olecranon fracture. **B,** Postoperative radiographs of the same elbow after application of a plate-and-screw construct with an independent positioning screw used for the comminuted fragment.

advocated; however, a dorsal plate (with or without a supplemental medullary screw, which may add more stability) has been demonstrated to be more biomechanically sound.[9]

Medullary Screw Fixation

Use of a single medullary screw for fixation of olecranon fractures requires extreme care to ensure a good outcome. Small-diameter screws may fail to gain purchase opposite the fracture site in the medullary canal. Larger-diameter screws may gain excellent purchase with apparent high torque required for further advancement as the screw threads engage the endosteum of the medullary canal; this high torque generation may not be related to seating of the screw head or washer on the fracture fragment. In other words, high torque can be developed as the screw threads engage the endosteum, despite minimal or no fracture compression. Careful visual scrutiny of the fracture site coupled with adequate radiographic analysis is necessary to guarantee full lag screw seating. Also, eccentric placement of the screw may be required so that full seating of the (straight) screw in the (curved) proximal ulna does not create a coronal plane deformity with distraction at the fracture site (**Figure 3**). Nevertheless, a single, partially threaded, 7.3-mm cancellous medullary screw with or without a supplemental figure-of-8 tension band wire was biomechanically advantageous over a standard tension band wiring technique for fixation of olecranon fractures in a cadaver model.[1]

Excision

Excision of the tip of the olecranon in combination with triceps advancement is primarily of historical interest, although it can be used for patients with limited functional demands. Abnormally elevated joint stresses

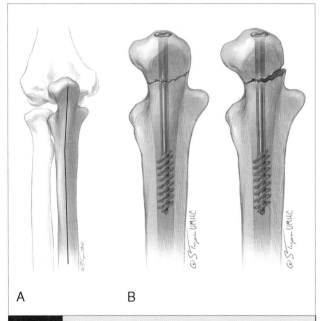

Figure 3 **A,** The intact proximal ulna has a slight varus curve. **B,** Seating of a straight medullary screw can result in gapping of the fracture site, as the screw aligns with the medullary canal, on the medial or lateral side if the screw is not placed eccentrically and carefully. (Copyright Curators of the University of Missouri, Columbia, MS, 2009.)

have been noted with olecranon fracture fragment excision and triceps advancement.[10] No more than 50% of the olecranon should be excised so that stability of the elbow is maintained. Generally, the triceps tendon is advanced and attached anteriorly to provide a smooth gliding surface for the distal humeral trochlea during

3: Upper Extremity

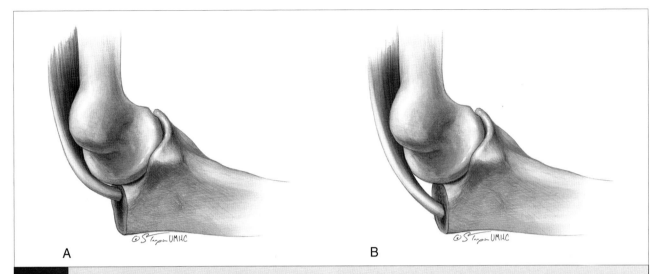

Figure 4 Schematic representation of anteriorly placed (**A**) and posteriorly placed (**B**) triceps tendon advancement. Anterior advancement results in a smoother transition between the tendon and the remaining articular surface of the greater sigmoid notch. Posterior advancement may result in a stronger extensor mechanism, but a residual step-off is left between the tendon and the edge of the articular surface. (Copyright Curators of the University of Missouri, Columbia, MS, 2009.)

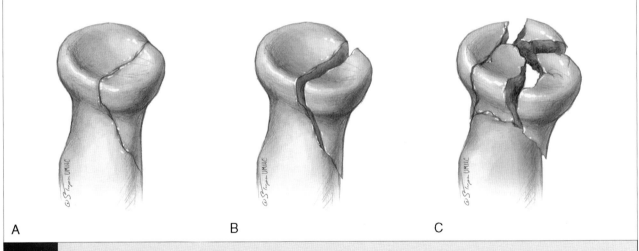

Figure 5 The Mason classification of radial head fractures. **A**, type I, nondisplaced. **B**, Type II, displaced, partial articular. **C**, Type III, displaced, complete articular, minimum of two articular fragments. (Copyright Curators of the University of Missouri, Columbia, MS, 2009.)

elbow motion (**Figure 4**). Posterior advancement, however, may be associated with increased elbow extension strength.[11]

Radial Head Fractures

Management of radial head fractures is dictated by the presence or absence of concomitant elbow instability, the degree of comminution of the radial head fragment(s), and the demands of the patient. The goal of treatment is to restore (or maintain) the flexion-extension arc of the elbow as well as the pronation-supination arc of the forearm. The radial head is an important contributor to elbow stability, especially in the setting of other injuries to the elbow (ligament disruptions, olecranon fractures, coronoid fractures, or dislocation); excision of a comminuted radial head without replacement should be considered cautiously.[12]

Classification

The Mason classification system is commonly used for radial head fractures (**Figure 5**). Type I fractures are nondisplaced; type II fractures are partial articular, displaced fractures; and type III fractures are comminuted, complete articular fractures. Simple fracture of the radial neck, with separation of the (intact) radial head from the radial shaft, is not addressed in the Mason classification. A fracture of the radial head with an associated dislocation of the elbow is often referred to as a Mason type IV injury; this was not originally included in Mason's classification scheme and is of limited value because of the vast diversity of elbow fracture-dislocations that involve fracture of the radial head.

Nonsurgical Treatment

Nonsurgical management is generally reserved for nondisplaced (Mason type I) and some partial articular (minimally displaced Mason type II) fractures of the radial head. Radiographic guidelines that dictate nonsurgical management of minimally displaced Mason type II fractures do not exist, and a biomechanical study exists that questions the reliability of correlating radial head fracture fragment size with radiocapitellar stability.[13] Radial head fractures can result in significant elbow stiffness and can block pronation and/or supination of the forearm. In the acute setting, an examination of forearm rotation is essential. Often, this is not tolerated during the acute phase following injury; a week of rest followed by repeat examination, or aspiration of the elbow hemarthrosis followed by infiltration of the joint with anesthetic, can allow for a more reliable examination. Mechanical blocks to passive forearm pronation and supination are considered indications for surgical intervention. However, a recent study has questioned the frequency of true mechanical blocks in displaced Mason type II radial head fractures, and showed that patients who underwent open reduction and internal fixation did not have improved long-term (22 years) outcomes over published outcomes data on those with similar injuries treated nonsurgically.[14]

Nonsurgical management of Mason type III radial head fractures should be undertaken with great caution; these fractures are often part of a fracture-dislocation complex of the elbow or part of the so-called Essex-Lopresti lesion (disruption of the interosseous ligament of the forearm, resulting in longitudinal forearm instability if not recognized and addressed appropriately), and outcomes are likely to be poor with nonsurgical management of these injury complexes.[15] Delayed excision of the radial head for patients with poor outcomes from nonsurgical management of acute radial head fractures may be unreliable at improving those outcomes.[16]

Properly executed open reduction and internal fixation[17] or radial head replacement[18] in the appropriate patient is associated with better results. However, a recent study of Mason type II radial head fractures with between 2 to 5 mm of displacement revealed pain-free elbows in nearly 80% and motion similar to the contralateral, uninjured side. Six patients with poor early outcomes benefited from delayed excision of the radial head.[19] Also, a long-term uncontrolled study of 100 "uncomplicated" Mason type II and type III radial head fractures, treated by various nonsurgical means, with 19 years of follow-up revealed overall good results

in most patients, with 9 patients undergoing late radial head excision resulting in improvement of symptoms.[20]

Surgical Treatment
Surgical Approach
Exposure of the radial head can be accomplished either through the Kocher interval between the anconeus and the extensor carpi ulnaris or through a more anterior split approximately between the extensor digitorum communis and the extensor carpi radialis brevis (Kaplan approach).[21,22] An oblique incision in the skin between the lateral humeral epicondyle and the dorsal border of the ulna, parallel to the Kocher interval, is used for the Kocher approach. Alternatively, a direct posterior exposure can be used, with elevation of full-thickness cutaneous flaps to reach the Kocher interval, if there is an associated fracture of the proximal ulna that requires exposure and fixation. Exposure through the Kocher interval should avoid dissection posterior to the anterior border of the anconeus to avoid injury to the lateral collateral ligament complex. If the Kaplan interval is used, the skin incision is from the lateral epicondyle to the radial neck, taking care to keep the dissection anterior to the equator of the radial head. With all exposures, if the radial neck must be exposed for plate fixation, pronation of the forearm should be accomplished to protect the posterior interosseous nerve.

Open Reduction and Internal Fixation
Open reduction and internal fixation of radial head fractures is often performed for Mason type II fractures with an associated block of forearm rotation. Small fragments occasionally will require excision, especially if little or no subchondral bone is present on the fracture fragment(s). Small lag screws and/or buttress plates have been used successfully. A 110° "safe zone" for implant application, such that implants will not block forearm rotation, has been described[23] (**Figure 6**). Often, impaction of the articular surface will be present; elevation of this impaction with placement of supportive bone graft or osteobiologic material is sometimes necessary. Multiple studies have demonstrated good results with open reduction and internal fixation. Some authors advocate fixation with crossed interfragmentary screws only, even for complete (Mason type III) radial head fractures, finding that outcomes are improved over similar fractures treated with plate-and-screw constructs.[24]

Mason type III fractures historically have been treated by radial head excision or arthroplasty, as open reduction and internal fixation has resulted in high failure rates and poor outcomes. However, newer implant availability (miniature blade plates, locking plates) has prompted further study of surgical fixation of these difficult injuries. One study of 28 Mason type III fractures demonstrated that improved strength and function and similar joint motion were noted in those patients undergoing open reduction and internal fixation in comparison with radial head excision.[25] Multiple other studies

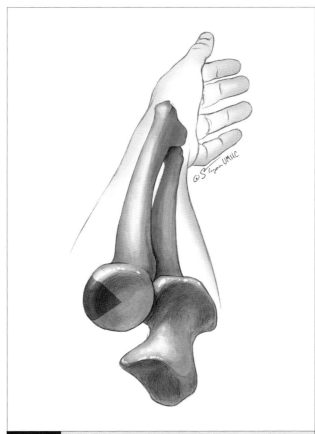

have evaluated the biomechanics of different fixation constructs for repair of radial head and neck fractures.[26,27]

Excision

Partial radial head excision is often performed when fracture fragments are too small to be adequately secured after reduction but the remainder of the radial head is intact. Excision of radial head fracture fragments can affect elbow stability, and this should be carefully assessed when contemplating this treatment regimen.[13] Excision of the entire radial head in the setting of highly comminuted complete fractures should be undertaken cautiously and perhaps should be restricted to low-demand patients. Even in stable elbows, resection of the radial head can lead to altered kinematics, and it has been shown to increase varus-valgus laxity in a cadaver model.[28] Long-term studies of radial head resection in the setting of isolated radial head fractures revealed good functional outcomes at the elbow with regard to motion, but a high number of patients were noted to have residual elbow and/or wrist

pain or to have radiographic evidence of elbow arthrosis.[29] Symptomatic late posterolateral rotatory instability can also result from radial head resection in some patients.[30] Nevertheless, a recent small study points to good long-term results of excision.[31]

Arthroplasty

Radial head arthroplasty for highly comminuted fractures of the radial head and/or neck has become popular. Historically, poor results were noted after radial head arthroplasty, perhaps related to synovitis in the setting of arthroplasty implants made of silicone.[32] However, current methods of radial head replacement, using monoblock or modular metal radial head components, appear to be associated with good short- and medium-term outcomes.[18,33] Long-term outcomes are unknown.

Radial head replacement may prevent long-term adverse sequelae of excision in some patients. Cadaver modeling has demonstrated restoration of normal kinematics and laxity in stable elbows (those without ligament disruption) after replacement of a resected radial head.[28] Late replacement of the radial head may also help ameliorate symptoms associated with posttraumatic elbow arthrosis after radial head fracture or excision.[34] Attritional radial shortening, which has been associated with negative consequences at the wrist and distal radioulnar joint,[35] may perhaps be prevented by radial head arthroplasty in lieu of excision for radial head fractures that cannot be reconstructed.

Radial head arthroplasty can be technically challenging. Multiple implants are available, including monoblock and modular types, the latter of which can be assembled before implantation or implanted part-by-part and assembled in situ. Care must be taken not to overstuff the radiocapitellar joint with a component that is too large because this can lead to cartilage wear, elbow stiffness (typically, a lack of flexion), and pain.[36,37] Widening of the lateral ulnohumeral articulation on direct AP radiography can be indicative of overstuffing with an oversized implant. However, this is not always the case; the ulnohumeral articulation occasionally may have the radiographic appearance of lateral widening at baseline, and contralateral images of the uninjured elbow can be beneficial if doubt exists regarding placement of a component that may result in overstuffing of the radiocapitellar joint.[38] Also, variability of arthroplasty components exists, with loose-fitting, cemented, and porous-ingrowth necks available, along with round versus anatomically contoured head surfaces. As native radial head anatomy is difficult to reproduce accurately during fracture treatment with arthroplasty, loose radial head components may provide more flexibility in treatment. A recent clinical study of loose modular radial head implants revealed good short-term results and no symptoms attributable to radiographic lucency around such a loose implant.[39]

Elbow Dislocations

The elbow is a highly stable joint that is composed of three distinct articulations: the ulnohumeral joint, radiocapitellar joint, and proximal radioulnar joint. Flexion-extension of the elbow occurs via the ulnohumeral articulation, whereas rotation occurs about the radioulnar articulation. Despite inherent stability, isolated, closed elbow dislocations are thought to be the second most common joint dislocation, after the shoulder. Because of the conformity of the ulnohumeral and radiocapitellar joints, there is a high incidence of associated fracture when the elbow dislocates, which must be detected and treated to maximize outcomes. Elbow instability is categorized as simple instability (dislocation in the absence of fracture) and complex instability (dislocation with associated fracture).

Most commonly, elbow dislocation occurs posteriorly. Treatment of simple elbow dislocation normally consists of closed reduction with nonsurgical treatment, followed by early range of motion within a stable arc of motion. Surgical treatment of simple elbow dislocation is reserved for open injuries and for dislocations that fail to remain reduced with nonsurgical treatment. Complex elbow dislocations (those associated with fracture) have much worse outcomes in general and almost always benefit from surgical reconstruction.

The stability of the elbow is conferred by a complex interplay of bony and soft-tissue constraints. The primary stabilizers of the elbow consist of the ulnohumeral articulation including the coronoid process, the anterior band of the medial collateral ligament (MCL), and the lateral collateral ligament complex (LCLC). The secondary stabilizers of the elbow include the radial head, common flexor and extensor origins, and the joint capsule. Injury or deficiency of these primary restraints is necessary but not sufficient to render the elbow unstable. If the corresponding secondary constraints are intact, the elbow will remain stable. For example, the anterior band of the MCL is the primary restraint to valgus loading; however, if the elbow is MCL deficient, an intact radial head will resist valgus forces and confer stability.

The mechanism of injury for elbow dislocation is often a fall onto an outstretched hand that becomes fixed, with a rotation moment about the elbow. This causes a progressive soft-tissue injury that begins on the lateral aspect of the elbow with disruption of the LCLC and progresses both anteriorly and posteriorly to the medial aspect of the elbow. As such, the MCL may remain intact and act as the central fulcrum around which the elbow dislocates. In the final stage of the continuum, the MCL is also injured.[40]

Nonsurgical Treatment

Isolated, closed elbow dislocations are generally treated closed. After conscious sedation of the patient, the elbow is reduced, often involving pressure on the olecranon tip with gentle traction and forearm supination.

Stability is then assessed by taking the elbow gently through a range of motion, first with the forearm in pronation and then in supination. The point of posterior instability with progressive extension should be noted. Further examination of elbow stability (with varus or valgus stress) is of little use, as it is expected that the elbow will redislocate with stress (because of the ligament injuries that are invariably present). Pronation of the forearm may impart greater stability to the elbow, although this has not been proved. Postreduction radiographs should be obtained and a concentric reduction documented. Any associated fracture seen on radiographs may need to be further investigated with a CT scan of the elbow.

Dislocations that remain reduced throughout the postreduction motion examination are occasionally splinted for 7 to 10 days at 90° of flexion to allow pain and swelling to subside. A recent small study, however, demonstrated that early motion and sling use, in lieu of splinting, is associated with earlier return to normal activity without an increased subluxation/dislocation rate.[41] Unrestricted range of motion is then allowed, with restricted weight bearing for 6 to 12 weeks. Immobilization longer than 2 to 3 weeks may result in increased pain and stiffness and more difficulty regaining normal motion.[42] Elbows noted to be unstable in supination and/or in full extension can be placed into a hinged elbow brace with a 30° extension block and with the forearm held in a neutral or pronated position, after a short period of immobilization. This requires careful monitoring, because the elbow that remains somewhat unstable may redislocate during outpatient management. Elbows with gross instability (easy redislocation) despite a successful reduction should prompt a more thorough examination for incarcerated chondral fragments or soft tissues within the ulnohumeral joint or for small associated fractures, sometimes better evaluated with CT or with open exploration.

Routine surgical repair for closed, simple elbow dislocations is not recommended.[40] In one prospective study, no difference was noted in outcome between two groups of elbow dislocation patients who underwent either closed reduction or open reduction with ligament repair.[42] However, for open injuries, as well as for dislocations that cannot be maintained reduced, surgical intervention is necessary.

Surgical Treatment

Open repair of soft-tissue disruptions in the setting of elbow dislocations is often dependent on the type of injury, where open wounds may be present, and on stability that is achieved after repair of only one side (medial or lateral). The presence of an open wound over either the medial or lateral elbow helps guide treatment; that is, if an open wound is present, irrigation and débridement followed by ligament repair and musculotendinous repair is easily accomplished through the wound. Medially, either ligament rupture or ligament avulsion appears to occur at nearly equal rates.[43] Lat-

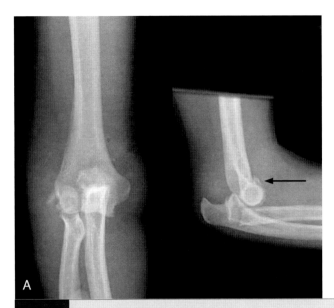
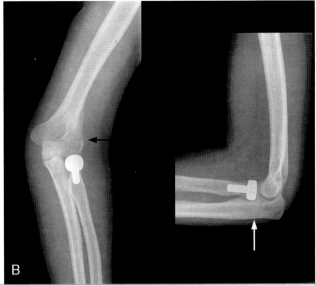

Figure 7 **A,** Injury radiographs of a terrible triad fracture-dislocation of the elbow, demonstrating posterior elbow dislocation with associated coronoid fracture (*black arrow*) and radial head fracture. **B,** Postoperative radiographs of the same elbow after radial head replacement, coronoid and capsular repair with suture placed through proximal ulna drill tunnels (*white arrow*), and lateral collateral ligament repair with bioabsorbable suture anchor (*black arrow*).

eral collateral ligament disruption, however, appears primarily to occur by avulsion from the lateral epicondyle of the humerus.[43,44] Repair of either ligament is tailored to the type of injury (rupture or avulsion), and as near-anatomic a reconstruction as can be achieved is sought. Repair of tears/avulsions of the flexor-pronator mass medially or of the extensor mass laterally are normally accomplished; significant injury to one or both of these masses sometimes is noted in elbow dislocations in which nonsurgical treatment has failed.

In the setting of a closed and highly unstable injury, the lateral side is approached first; often, repair of the lateral collateral ligament and associated musculotendinous injury proves sufficient for stability in the setting of simple elbow dislocation unable to be treated by closed means. Residual instability after ligament and soft-tissue repair occasionally requires treatment with a hinged external fixator[45] or ulnohumeral joint transfixion with crossed pins or screws.

Elbow Fracture-Dislocations

Dislocations of the elbow with associated fractures create so-called complex elbow instability. Fracture-dislocations of the elbow have historically done very poorly with nonsurgical treatment. Surgical treatment also has resulted in historically poor outcomes, perhaps because of a lack of understanding of the injury complex. The four commonly accepted types of elbow fracture-dislocations are the terrible triad, the Monteggia-variant elbow fracture-dislocation, the trans-olecranon fracture-dislocation, and the varus posteromedial elbow fracture-dislocation.

Terrible Triad

The terrible triad of the elbow refers to a posterior dislocation of the elbow with associated radial head and coronoid fractures (**Figure 7**). Abysmal outcomes have been documented for patients with terrible triad injuries when treated nonsurgically; this treatment method should be discouraged. The surgical approach for treatment of this injury complex involves a lateral approach to the elbow through the Kocher or Kaplan interval. Often, a bare lateral humeral epicondyle is encountered, consistent with avulsion of both the LCLC and the extensor origin.[44] The radial head may be variably comminuted and partially versus completely fractured. Coronoid fracture morphology varies from a "fleck" with attached anterior elbow joint capsule to large fragments fractured through the coronoid base with or without the sublime tubercle of the ulna.[46] Chondral or osteochondral fragments may be incarcerated within the ulnohumeral joint.

The mainstay of therapy involves repair of the anterior elbow capsular attachment, repair or replacement of the radial head, and repair of the lateral ligamentous and musculotendinous complex.[46,47] Resection of unreconstructable radial head fractures (with planned prosthetic replacement before closure) can improve exposure of the coronoid fracture bed. Small coronoid fracture fragments will often be attached to the anterior elbow capsule. This injury may be repaired with heavy suture repair of this capsular disruption through bone tunnels drilled into the coronoid fracture bed from the dorsal proximal ulna. Small, transversely oriented coronoid fracture patterns seem to be common in terrible triad injuries.[48] Anatomic reduction of the coronoid fracture fragment may not be necessary, although this

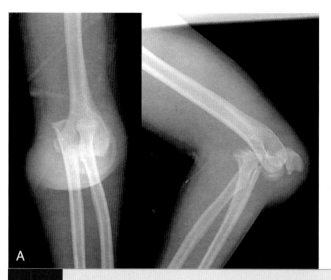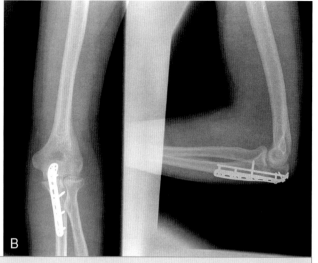

Figure 8	**A**, Injury radiographs of a transolecranon fracture-dislocation of the elbow. Note the maintained relationship between the radius and the ulnar shaft. **B**, Radiographs of the same elbow 6 months after open reduction and internal fixation of the ulna only.

has not been proved. Larger coronoid fracture fragments may be captured with proximal ulnar lag screws or may require medial plating if the sublime tubercle is involved in the fracture. Radial head repair or replacement can then be completed, followed by lateral soft-tissue repairs. Exploration and repair of associated MCL injuries is not routinely necessary.[49] However, for residual significant instability after these repairs have been accomplished, MCL repair and/or hinged external fixator application may be necessary.[50]

Results of surgical treatment of terrible triad injuries are variable, and patients should be counseled regarding the severity of the injury and difficulty in achieving a good outcome, even with skilled surgical management. A recent study demonstrated unsatisfactory patient-reported results at 1 year using multiple validated outcomes instruments, despite restoration of elbow joint stability in all patients.[51] Another recent study described good restoration of elbow motion and forearm rotation, although 8 of 36 patients in the series required a second surgical intervention because of stiffness, instability, or infection.[47] Another recent series comparing acute with subacute treatment of terrible triad injuries found good results with a standard method of surgical treatment but found improved elbow flexion arcs and more straightforward management when the injuries were addressed within 2 weeks.[52]

Transolecranon Fracture-Dislocation

So-called transolecranon fracture-dislocations of the elbow are injuries in which the proximal ulna is fractured and displaced, and the elbow has dislocated anteriorly without disruption of the proximal radioulnar joint (**Figure 8**). This injury is not to be confused with a Monteggia lesion, in which the ulna is fractured, the radiocapitellar joint is dislocated, and the proximal radioulnar joint is also disrupted. In the transolecranon fracture-dislocation, the ligaments are often spared, and anatomic reduction with stable fixation of the olecranon fracture will restore stability to the elbow.[53] The term transolecranon was adopted because of the appearance of the humeral trochlea having been driven through the olecranon process. These fractures have a high incidence of associated open wounds.[53]

Surgical treatment of transolecranon elbow fracture-dislocations requires methodical attention to all components of the injury. Coronoid fractures may be present, and they often are large in size. Stabilization of the coronoid fracture fragment to the ulnar shaft may be accomplished via lag screw fixation or, for small fragments, nonabsorbable heavy sutures passed through bone tunnels. It is often easier to address the coronoid fracture before reducing the olecranon fracture component because the displaced olecranon fracture allows for direct visualization of the coronoid fracture reduction. Plate-and-screw constructs are often used for stabilization of the (often comminuted) olecranon component of the fracture-dislocation. Good restoration of the anatomy of the greater sigmoid notch of the ulna is key to restoration of elbow stability and motion.[53] Radial head fractures, which are present occasionally, can be addressed through the same dorsal surgical incision by elevating a full-thickness subcutaneous flap and accessing the fracture site through the Kocher interval. The radial head fracture should not be repaired through the same deep approach as the proximal ulna because this may lead to a proximal radioulnar synostosis.

Results after proper treatment of this injury pattern are good. Good-to-excellent results have been demonstrated in 15 of 17 patients at an average of 25 months.[53] In another small series, outcomes were eval-

3: Upper Extremity

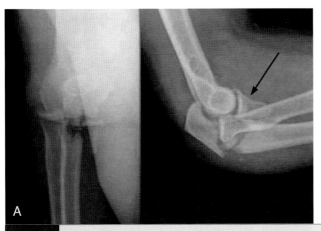
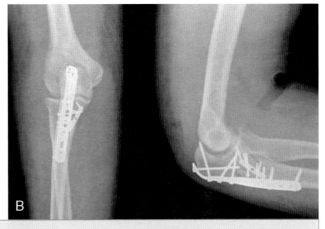

Figure 9 **A,** Injury radiographs of a Monteggia-variant fracture-dislocation of the elbow. Note the large coronoid fracture fragment associated with this particular patient's injury (*black arrow*) and small radial head fracture. **B,** Postoperative radiographs of the same elbow after open reduction and internal fixation of the proximal ulna with excision of radial head fracture fragment. Note that the radiocapitellar joint is reduced in both views.

uated using validated outcomes instruments, and demonstrated overall good results obtained with satisfactory restoration of the greater sigmoid notch of the ulna.[54] Interestingly, the unique patient in this series treated with tension band wiring for the olecranon fracture component required revision surgery because of loosening of fixation and loss of reduction. In a different recent series, 10 of 14 patients had good-to-excellent results after surgical treatment of transolecranon elbow fracture-dislocations. Three patients required reoperation after early implant failure—all had been treated with tension band wiring constructs.[55] Although these study failure numbers are small, surgical treatment of these injuries using tension band wiring constructs should be undertaken with great caution.

Monteggia-Variant Fracture-Dislocation

Posterior olecranon fracture-dislocations are commonly termed Monteggia-variant fracture-dislocations. Key characteristics of this injury include an apex-posterior fracture of the olecranon, which is often comminuted, posterior radiocapitellar dislocation, and (often) radial head fracture[56] (**Figure 9**). Although the proximal radioulnar joint may be relatively spared in this injury complex (unlike in a classic Monteggia complex involving fracture of the ulnar shaft with dislocation of the radiocapitellar and proximal radioulnar joints), proper management of this injury is vital for restoration of normal elbow and forearm function. Improper treatment of this injury can result in elbow instability and/or forearm rotational dysfunction. Complications in treatment of these injuries include malunion of fractures, radioulnar synostosis, and pain and mechanical dysfunction of the forearm because of failure to address associated radial head fractures.[56]

Adequate treatment of this injury parallels that of the classic Monteggia complex: anatomic reduction of

the ulna should result in reduction of the radiocapitellar joint. This is often accomplished through a dorsal approach to the ulna, with a plate-and-screw construct for fixation of the fracture. The ulnar fracture can be highly comminuted, perhaps requiring multiple interfragmentary screws either independent of or through the plate. Coronoid fractures can be present, and these often are more easily addressed before performing the olecranon fragment repair, as the coronoid fracture can be seen through the displaced olecranon fracture. Large coronoid fragments may require buttress plating medially. Radial head fractures can be addressed through the Kocher interval, after elevating a full-thickness subcutaneous flap laterally from the dorsal ulnar incision. At the conclusion of fixation, careful examination of forearm rotation and of elbow motion is necessary. Any residual subluxation of the radiocapitellar joint should lead the surgeon to question the adequacy of reduction of the ulnar component of the fracture.

Few studies have concentrated on outcomes of this particular injury complex. Results of treatment algorithms, as previously discussed, have been published.[56] In addition, a successful technique of salvage of these complex injuries in the setting of malreduction or failure of fixation has been documented, which involves revision of ulnar reduction and fixation and may also involve necessary treatment of radial head or coronoid fractures with or without hinged elbow external fixation.[57] A complex of proximal ulna fracture (not involving the ulnohumeral articulation), radiocapitellar dislocation with or without radial head fracture, and frank posterior dislocation of the ulnohumeral joint has also been described recently. Patients with this posterior ulnohumeral dislocation associated with Monteggia lesions demonstrated increased elbow stiffness and greater disability than did patients with posterior Monteggia lesions not associated with ulnohumeral dislocation, at an average of 29 months.[58]

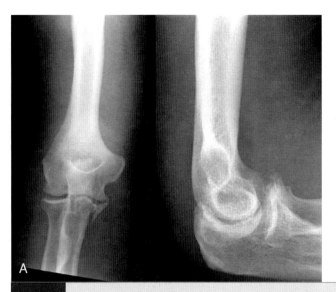
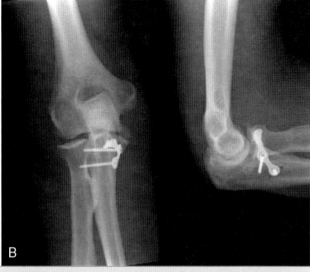

Figure 10 **A**, Injury radiographs of a varus posteromedial fracture-dislocation of the elbow. Stress examination intraoperatively revealed significant varus instability and radiocapitellar joint widening consistent with disruption of the lateral collateral ligament (not shown). **B**, Postoperative radiographs of the same elbow after open reduction and internal fixation of the anteromedial coronoid fracture and suture repair of the lateral collateral ligament, revealing good reduction of the elbow joint.

Posteromedial Varus Fracture-Dislocation

Fracture-dislocations of the elbow, in which the fracture primarily involves the coronoid process, can result in a recently recognized pattern of elbow instability termed posteromedial varus fracture-dislocation (**Figure 10**). In this injury, coronoid fractures associated with elbow dislocations may extend distally along the MCL insertion. The coronoid fracture often occurs at the anteromedial facet, with loss of the buttress effect of this portion of the coronoid to varus stress. When this occurs, rupture of the lateral collateral ligament (most commonly, avulsion from the humeral origin) is no longer countered by an intact anteromedial coronoid facet, and elbow instability ensues. Coronoid fracture type (in this case, anteromedial facet fracture) has been shown to correlate with elbow injury type (in this case, posteromedial varus instability pattern).[48] This relationship has also been verified in an ex vivo cadaver biomechanical study.[59] Proper management of this injury, with repair of the coronoid fracture and of the lateral collateral ligament, results in good outcomes.[60]

Summary

Fractures and dislocations of the adult elbow are difficult injuries to treat. Because the adult elbow is relatively intolerant of injury and immobilization, only diligent care will provide patients with the best outcomes. The surgeon must have a complete understanding of the injury complex and of the bony and soft-tissue anatomy around the elbow. Judicious soft-tissue handling and anatomic reduction, with stable fixation, are important to allow for early, unrestricted elbow motion. Aggressive and early rehabilitation of the injured elbow is vital in order to maximize patient outcomes. Careful attention to detail in the management of complex elbow injuries will lead to rewarding outcomes for both the patient and surgeon.

Annotated References

1. Hutchinson DT, Horwitz DS, Ha G, Thomas CW, Bachus KN: Cyclic loading of olecranon fracture fixation constructs. *J Bone Joint Surg Am* 2003;85(5):831-837.

2. Villanueva P, Osorio F, Commessatti M, Sanchez-Sotelo J: Tension-band wiring for olecranon fractures: Analysis of risk factors for failure. *J Shoulder Elbow Surg* 2006;15(3):351-356.

   The authors present a retrospective review of 37 olecranon fractures treated with tension band wiring with a 4-year average follow-up. Mild disability was common. Arthritis was more common in the setting of instability. Satisfactory outcomes were seen in the majority of patients. Level of evidence: IV.

3. Mullett JH, Shannon F, Noel J, Lawlor G, Lee TC, O'Rourke SK: K-wire position in tension band wiring of the olecranon: A comparison of two techniques. *Injury* 2000;31(6):427-431.

4. Coles CP, Barei DP, Nork SE, Taitsman LA, Hanel DP, Bradford Henley M: The olecranon osteotomy: A six-year experience in the treatment of intraarticular fractures of the distal humerus. *J Orthop Trauma* 2006; 20(3):164-171.

3: Upper Extremity

The authors reviewed 70 distal humerus fracture patients treated with olecranon osteotomy. Sixty-seven patients with adequate follow-up healed, with only one delayed union. Eighteen of 61 patients with sufficient follow-up required implant removal. Level of evidence: IV.

5. Harrell RM, Tong J, Weinhold PS, Dahners LE: Comparison of the mechanical properties of different tension band materials and suture techniques. *J Orthop Trauma* 2003;17(2):119-122.

6. Carofino BC, Santangelo SA, Kabadi M, Mazzocca AD, Browner BD: Olecranon fractures repaired with Fiber-Wire or metal wire tension banding: A biomechanical comparison. *Arthroscopy* 2007;23(9):964-970.

A biomechanical cadaver study of four different transverse olecranon osteotomy fixation techniques comparing FiberWire suture (Arthrex, Naples, FL) with 18-gauge metal tension band is presented. No significant strength difference was noted.

7. Anderson ML, Larson AN, Merten SM, Steinmann SP: Congruent elbow plate fixation of olecranon fractures. *J Orthop Trauma* 2007;21(6):386-393.

A retrospective review of 32 olecranon fractures treated with the Mayo Congruent Elbow Plate system is discussed. Outcomes measures were good to excellent in 92% of those with available data. Few implant removals were required. Level of evidence: IV.

8. Hewins EA, Gofton WT, Dubberly J, MacDermid JC, Faber KJ, King GJ: Plate fixation of olecranon osteotomies. *J Orthop Trauma* 2007;21(1):58-62.

The authors present a retrospective review of 17 olecranon osteotomies repaired with 3.5-mm reconstruction plates at a 32-month average follow-up. One implant complication occurred (screw penetration of proximal radioulnar joint) and one implant removal was required. Healing occurred in 100%. Level of evidence: IV.

9. Gordon MJ, Budoff JE, Yeh ML, Luo ZP, Noble PC: Comminuted olecranon fractures: A comparison of plating methods. *J Shoulder Elbow Surg* 2006;15(1):94-99.

A cadaver biomechanical study compared medial and lateral plating of simulated comminuted olecranon fractures with single dorsal plate with or without a medullary screw. A single dorsal plate with medullary screw had significantly more strength than dual plates.

10. Moed BR, Ede DE, Brown TD: Fractures of the olecranon: An in vitro study of elbow joint stresses after tension-band wire fixation versus proximal fracture fragment excision. *J Trauma* 2002;53(6):1088-1093.

11. Didonna ML, Fernandez JJ, Lim TH, Hastings H II, Cohen MS: Partial olecranon excision: The relationship between triceps insertion site and extension strength of the elbow. *J Hand Surg Am* 2003;28(1):117-122.

12. O'Driscoll SW, Jupiter JB, Cohen MS, Ring D, McKee MD: Difficult elbow fractures: Pearls and pitfalls. *Instr Course Lect* 2003;52:113-134.

13. Beingessner DM, Dunning CE, Beingessner CJ, Johnson JA, King GJ: The effect of radial head fracture size on radiocapitellar joint stability. *Clin Biomech* 2003;18(7):677-681.

14. Lindenhovius AL, Felsch Q, Ring D, Kloen P: The long-term outcome of open reduction and internal fixation of stable displaced isolated partial articular fractures of the radial head. *J Trauma* 2009;67(1):143-146.

Sixteen patients with Mason type II radial head fractures without associated elbow dislocation were evaluated 22 years after open reduction and internal fixation. Five complications of surgery occurred, and 14 patients underwent implant removal. Compared to results published in other reports of nonsurgical treatment of these injuries, surgery appears to offer no benefit. Level of evidence: IV.

15. Davidson PA Jr, Moseley JB Jr, Tullos HS: Radial head fracture: A potentially complex injury. *Clin Orthop Relat Res* 1993;297:224-230.

16. Broberg MA, Morrey BF: Results of delayed excision of the radial head after fracture. *J Bone Joint Surg Am* 1986;68(5):669-674.

17. Ring D, Quintero J, Jupiter JB: Open reduction and internal fixation of fractures of the radial head. *J Bone Joint Surg Am* 2002;84(10):1811-1815.

18. Moro JK, Werier J, MacDermid JC, Patterson SD, King GJ: Arthroplasty with a metal radial head for unreconstructible fractures of the radial head. *J Bone Joint Surg Am* 2001;83(8):1201-1211.

19. Akesson T, Herbertsson P, Josefsson PO, Hasserius R, Besjakov J, Karlsson MK: Primary nonoperative treatment of moderately displaced two-part fractures of the radial head. *J Bone Joint Surg Am* 2006;88(9):1909-1914.

In a retrospective review, 49 patients were treated nonsurgically for a 2- to 5-mm displaced Mason type II radial head fracture involving ≥ 30% of the joint surface. Average follow-up was 19 years. Six patients underwent delayed radial head excision. Predominantly favorable outcomes were noted. Level of evidence: IV.

20. Herbertsson P, Josefsson PO, Hasserius R, et al; Long-Term Follow-Up Study: Uncomplicated Mason type-II and III fractures of the radial head and neck in adults: A long-term follow-up study. *J Bone Joint Surg Am* 2004;86(3):569-574.

The authors report 19-year follow-up of 100 patients with Mason type II or III radial head fractures managed nonsurgically. Predominantly favorable outcomes were noted, with delayed radial head excision being effective in those with poor early outcomes. Level of evidence: IV.

21. Kaplan EB: Surgical approach to the proximal end of the radius and its use in fractures of the head and neck of the radius. *J Bone Joint Surg Am* 1941;23:86-92.

22. Hotchkiss RN: Displaced fractures of the radial head: Internal fixation or excision. *J Am Acad Orthop Surg* 1997;5(1):1-10.

23. Smith GR, Hotchkiss RN: Radial head and neck fractures: Anatomic guidelines for proper placement of internal fixation. *J Shoulder Elbow Surg* 1996;5(2, pt 1): 113-117.

24. Smith AM, Morrey BF, Steinmann SP: Low profile fixation of radial head and neck fractures: Surgical technique and clinical experience. *J Orthop Trauma* 2007; 21(10):718-724.

    A surgical technique of crossed-screw fixation of radial head and neck fractures is described.

25. Ikeda M, Sugiyama K, Kang C, Takagaki T, Oka Y: Comminuted fractures of the radial head: Comparison of resection and internal fixation. *J Bone Joint Surg Am* 2005;87(1):76-84.

    The authors retrospectively compared radial head resection versus fixation for Mason type III fractures at 10 years (resection) or 3 years (fixation). Improved results were noted with fixation over resection, and fixation was recommended as the technique of choice. Level of evidence: III.

26. Capo JT, Svach D, Ahsgar J, Orillaza NS, Sabatino CT: Biomechanical stability of different fixation constructs for ORIF of radial neck fractures. *Orthopedics* 2008; 31(10):pii.

    The authors performed a cadaver biomechanical study of five different fixation techniques for radial neck fractures. Plates and screws versus screws alone offer differing strength advantages, and addition of lag screws improves strength in torsion and bending.

27. Burkhart KJ, Mueller LP, Krezdorn D, et al: Stability of radial head and neck fractures: A biomechanical study of six fixation constructs with consideration of three locking plates. *J Hand Surg Am* 2007;32(10):1569-1575.

    The authors performed a cadaver biomechanical study of six different fixation techniques for simulated radial neck fracture gap fixation. Plate-and-screw constructs with angular stability (locking plates or blade plates) were comparable or stronger than nonlocked implants or crossed screws alone.

28. Beingessner DM, Dunning CE, Gordon KD, Johnson JA, King GJ: The effect of radial head excision and arthroplasty on elbow kinematics and stability. *J Bone Joint Surg Am* 2004;86(8):1730-1739.

    The authors performed a cadaver biomechanical study of elbows, with and without collateral ligaments attached, with increasing wedges removed from radial head. Subtle deterioration of elbow stability was seen after removal of wedges of all sizes, even with intact ligaments.

29. Herbertsson P, Josefsson PO, Hasserius R, Besjakov J, Nyqvist F, Karlsson MK: Fractures of the radial head and neck treated with radial head excision. *J Bone Joint Surg Am* 2004;86(9):1925-1930.

    The authors studied 61 patients with Mason types II, III, or IV fractures who were treated either with acute or delayed radial head excision. Inferior outcomes were seen with those undergoing excision after Mason type IV fracture (elbow fracture-dislocation). Timing of radial head excision had no effect on any fracture subgroup. Level of evidence: III.

30. Hall JA, McKee MD: Posterolateral rotatory instability of the elbow following radial head resection. *J Bone Joint Surg Am* 2005;87(7):1571-1579.

    Forty-two patients with elbow-related complaints after radial head resection were evaluated; 7 patients (17%) were noted to have posterolateral rotatory instability. This diagnosis should be considered in patients with elbow complaints after radial head resection. Level of evidence: IV.

31. Karlsson MK, Herbertsson P, Nordqvist A, Hasserius R, Besjakov J, Josefsson PO: Long-term outcome of displaced radial neck fractures in adulthood: 16- to 21-year follow-up of 5 patients treated with radial head excision. *Acta Orthop* 2009;80(3):368-370.

    Five patients with Mason type III radial head fractures were treated with radial head excision and evaluated at an average of 18 years. Two patients reported occasional weakness, but none had major complaints. All had radiographic changes consistent with arthrosis. Level of evidence: IV.

32. Vanderwilde RS, Morrey BF, Melberg MW, Vinh TN: Inflammatory arthritis after failure of silicone rubber replacement of the radial head. *J Bone Joint Surg Br* 1994;76(1):78-81.

33. Grewal R, MacDermid JC, Faber KJ, Drosdowech DS, King GJ: Comminuted radial head fractures treated with a modular metallic radial head arthroplasty: Study of outcomes. *J Bone Joint Surg Am* 2006;88(10):2192-2200.

    A prospective case series of 26 patients with radial head arthroplasties evaluated at 2 years is presented. The bulk of recovery appears to occur within 6 months. Mild weakness and loss of motion remain in most patients at 2 years. All elbows were stable, and five elbows had evidence of arthrosis. Level of evidence: IV.

34. Shore BJ, Mozzon JB, MacDermid JC, Faber KJ, King GJ: Chronic posttraumatic elbow disorders treated with metallic radial head arthroplasty. *J Bone Joint Surg Am* 2008;90(2):271-280.

    A retrospective review of radial head arthroplasty for 32 patients with failed prior silicone arthroplasty, radial head excision, or nonunion/malunion of radial head fractures, at a mean follow-up of 8 years is presented. Good results were seen. Level of evidence: IV.

35. Ikeda M, Oka Y: Function after early radial head resection for fracture: A retrospective evaluation of 15 patients followed for 3-18 years. *Acta Orthop Scand* 2000;71(2):191-194.

3: Upper Extremity

36. Birkedal JP, Deal DN, Ruch DS: Loss of flexion after radial head replacement. *J Shoulder Elbow Surg* 2004; 13(2):208-213.

Six patients with loss of flexion after radial head arthroplasty were retrospectively reviewed; four who underwent removal of the prosthesis recovered some flexion. A cadaver biomechanical study demonstrated narrowing of the radiocapitellar joint with increasing flexion. Overstuffing the radiocapitellar joint with a radial head prosthesis may therefore inhibit elbow flexion. Level of evidence: IV.

37. Doornberg JN, Linzel DS, Zurakowski D, Ring D: Reference points for radial head prosthesis size. *J Hand Surg Am* 2006;31(1):53-57.

A CT-based, anatomic evaluation of 17 elbows revealed significant variability in the position of the radial head articular surface relative to the coronoid process. The authors suggest that contralateral elbow radiographs may be helpful for preoperative planning of radial head arthroplasty.

38. Rowland AS, Athwal GS, MacDermid JC, King GJ: Lateral ulnohumeral joint space widening is not diagnostic of radial head arthroplasty overstuffing. *J Hand Surg Am* 2007;32(5):637-641.

Plain AP radiographs of 50 normal elbows were reviewed to evaluate medial and lateral ulnohumeral joint spaces. The lateral joint space was noted not to be parallel, and therefore widening of this space may not be diagnostic of overstuffing of the radiocapitellar joint with a radial head prosthesis.

39. Doornberg JN, Parisien R, van Duijn PJ, Ring D: Radial head arthroplasty with a modular metal spacer to treat acute traumatic elbow instability. *J Bone Joint Surg Am* 2007;89(5):1075-1080.

Twenty-seven patients with a loose (noncemented and noningrowth) radial head arthroplasty demonstrated good elbow stability, range of motion, and good-to-excellent results in most patients at 40 months. Lucencies noted about the stem of the component did not correlate with increased short-term complaints. Level of evidence: IV.

40. O'Driscoll SW, Morrey BF, Korinek S, An KN: Elbow subluxation and dislocation: A spectrum of instability. *Clin Orthop Relat Res* 1992;280:186-197.

41. Maripuri SN, Debnath UK, Rao P, Mohanty K: Simple elbow dislocation among adults: A comparative study of two different methods of treatment. *Injury* 2007; 38(11):1254-1258.

A retrospective review of 42 closed elbow dislocations treated either with splinting and delayed motion or with sling and immediate motion demonstrated slightly better functional outcomes in the sling with the early motion group. Level of evidence: III.

42. Josefsson PO, Gentz CF, Johnell O, Wendeberg B: Surgical versus non-surgical treatment of ligamentous injuries following dislocation of the elbow joint: A prospec-

tive randomized study. *J Bone Joint Surg Am* 1987; 69(4):605-608.

43. Micic I, Kim S-Y, Park I-H, Kim P-T, Jeon I-H: Surgical management of unstable elbow dislocation without intra-articular fracture. *Int Orthop* 2009;33(4):1141-1147.

Twenty-four patients with unstable elbow dislocations were reviewed; the medial collateral ligament was found avulsed from the humerus 55% of the time, and the lateral collateral ligament was found avulsed from the humerus 80% of the time. This may have implications for surgical methods of repair/reconstruction. Level of evidence: IV.

44. McKee MD, Schemitsch EH, Sala MJ, O'Driscoll SW: The pathoanatomy of lateral ligamentous disruption in complex elbow instability. *J Shoulder Elbow Surg* 2003; 12(4):391-396.

45. McKee MD, Bowden SH, King GJ, et al: Management of recurrent, complex instability of the elbow with a hinged external fixator. *J Bone Joint Surg Br* 1998; 80(6):1031-1036.

46. Ring D, Jupiter JB, Zilberfarb J: Posterior dislocation of the elbow with fractures of the radial head and coronoid. *J Bone Joint Surg Am* 2002;84(4):547-551.

47. Pugh DM, Wild LM, Schemitsch EH, King GJ, McKee MD: Standard surgical protocol to treat elbow dislocations with radial head and coronoid fractures. *J Bone Joint Surg Am* 2004;86(6):1122-1130.

Thirty-six patients with terrible triad injuries of the elbow were retrospectively reviewed. A consistent method of surgical treatment is proposed consisting of repair/replacement of the radial head, repair of anterior capsular structures with or without coronoid, and lateral ligament repair. Overall good results were noted, with stable elbows noted in 34 patients at 34 months. Level of evidence: IV.

48. Doornberg JN, Ring D: Coronoid fracture patterns. *J Hand Surg Am* 2006;31(1):45-52.

Sixty-seven coronoid fracture patterns were analyzed after fracture-dislocation of the elbow. A high correlation of coronoid fracture pattern was seen with this type of elbow fracture-dislocation. This may have implications for surgical planning and treatment. Level of evidence: IV.

49. Forthman C, Henket M, Ring DC: Elbow dislocation with intra-articular fracture: The results of operative treatment without repair of the medial collateral ligament. *J Hand Surg Am* 2007;32(8):1200-1209.

Thirty-four fracture-dislocations of the elbow were treated surgically without repair of the medial collateral ligament. Two noncompliant patients had continued instability, but the others all had stable elbows with good range of motion and reasonable results at an average of 32 months following injury. Repair of the MCL does not appear to be necessary if fractures and lateral ligaments are repaired. Level of evidence: IV.

50. Ring D, Hannouche D, Jupiter JB: Surgical treatment of persistent dislocation or subluxation of the ulnohumeral joint after fracture-dislocation of the elbow. *J Hand Surg Am* 2004;29(3):470-480.

Thirteen patients with persistent instability of the elbow after repair of fracture-dislocation were successfully treated with ligament and fracture repair/reconstruction and hinged external fixation. Level of evidence: IV.

51. Egol KA, Immerman I, Paksima N, Tejwani N, Koval KJ: Fracture-dislocation of the elbow: Functional outcome following treatment with a standardized protocol. *Bull NYU Hosp Jt Dis* 2007;65(4):263-270.

Twenty-nine patients with terrible triad fracture-dislocations of the elbow were reviewed at least 1 year after surgical repair. All had motion and strength deficits and poor outcomes scores relative to normal individuals. Elbow stability, however, was restored in all patients. Level of evidence: IV.

52. Lindenhovius AL, Jupiter JB, Ring D: Comparison of acute versus subacute treatment of terrible triad injuries of the elbow. *J Hand Surg Am* 2008;33(6):920-926.

A comparison between terrible triad injuries treated within 2 weeks and those treated at ≥ 3 weeks was conducted. Both groups recovered flexion arc and strength, but improved results were noted in those patients treated within 2 weeks of injury. Level of evidence: III.

53. Ring D, Jupiter JB, Sanders RW, Mast J, Simpson NS: Transolecranon fracture-dislocation of the elbow. *J Orthop Trauma* 1997;11(8):545-550.

54. Mortazavi SM, Asadollahi S, Tahririan MA: Functional outcome following treatment of transolecranon fracture-dislocation of the elbow. *Injury* 2006;37(3):284-288.

Eight patients with transolecranon elbow fracture-dislocation were retrospectively reviewed. Only one was treated with tension band wiring, which failed. The other seven were treated with plate and screws. Reasonable outcomes were noted at an average of 37 months. Level of evidence: IV.

55. Mouhsine E, Akiki A, Castagna A, et al: Transolecranon anterior fracture dislocation. *J Shoulder Elbow Surg* 2007;16(3):352-357.

Fourteen transolecranon fracture-dislocations were retrospectively identified from a total of 93 olecranon fractures. Treatment failures were noted in patients with inadequate fixation, including several tension band wiring constructs. Stable fixation of this underdiagnosed injury pattern is imperative for good outcomes. Level of evidence: IV.

56. Ring D, Jupiter JB, Simpson NS: Monteggia fractures in adults. *J Bone Joint Surg Am* 1998;80(12):1733-1744.

57. Ring D, Tavakolian J, Kloen P, Helfet D, Jupiter JB: Loss of alignment after surgical treatment of posterior Monteggia fractures: Salvage with dorsal contoured plating. *J Hand Surg Am* 2004;29(4):694-702.

A review of 17 patients with failed fixation for posterior Monteggia-variant elbow fracture-dislocations was accomplished at an average of 5 years after revision of fixation. All patients healed and had concentric elbow reductions. Range of motion was good, and good-to-excellent outcomes were noted in most of these patients. Level of evidence: IV.

58. Strauss EJ, Tejwani NC, Preston CF, Egol KA: The posterior Monteggia lesion with associated ulnohumeral instability. *J Bone Joint Surg Br* 2006;88(1):84-89.

Twenty-three patients with posterior Monteggia-variant elbow fracture-dislocations were examined. Inferior results were seen in the six patients with associated complete posterior elbow dislocations with the Monteggia complex. Level of evidence: III.

59. Pollock JW, Brownhill J, Ferreira L, McDonald CP, Johnson J, King G: The effect of anteromedial facet fractures of the coronoid and lateral collateral ligament injury on elbow stability and kinematics. *J Bone Joint Surg Am* 2009;91(6):1448-1458.

A cadaver biomechanical study was performed on intact elbows followed by progressively increasing simulated coronoid fractures, with and without lateral collateral ligament disruption and repair. The size of the anteromedial coronoid fracture may be a determinant of elbow stability in the traumatic situation.

60. Doornberg JN, Ring DC: Fracture of the anteromedial facet of the coronoid process. *J Bone Joint Surg Am* 2006;88(10):2216-2224.

Eighteen patients with anteromedial facet coronoid fractures were reviewed at an average of 26 months after injury. All six patients treated nonsurgically or with failed fixation developed arthrosis and varus elbow subluxation, with fair-to-poor results. The other 12 patients had good-to-excellent results. Level of evidence: IV.

Chapter 20

Fractures of the Forearm and Distal Radius

Alexandra Schwartz, MD   Melvin Rosenwasser, MD   Neil White, MD   Eric Swart, MD

Forearm Fractures

The forearm should be considered as a functional unit where the radius rotates about the fixed ulna. The forearm is a dynamic and dependent "functional joint"[1] whose purpose is to position the hand in space. The radius and ulna are connected by the proximal and distal radioulnar joints, and a longitudinal structure between the bones, the interosseous membrane. The interosseous membrane is a fibrous sheath that divides the forearm into anterior and posterior compartments and also serves as a restraint to migration of the radius relative to the ulna. Proximally, the radial head articulates with the ulna and is stabilized by the annular ligament and elbow capsule. Distally, the ulna articulates with the sigmoid notch of the radius. The distal radioulnar joint (DRUJ) is stabilized by the triangular fibrocartilage complex (TFCC). All these structures together form a ring. This ring structure allows for the two bones to function as a unit. To restore proper function to the forearm, almost all adult both-bone forearm fractures and forearm fracture/dislocations must be treated surgically.

Patients with a forearm fracture typically present after a traumatic event with pain, deformity, and swelling. Careful examination of the radial, ulnar, median, pos-

Dr. Schwartz or an immediate family member is a member of a speakers' bureau or has made paid presentations on behalf of Synthes; is a paid consultant to or an employee of Zimmer; has received research or institutional support from Synthes; and has stock or stock options held in Zimmer. Dr. Rosenwasser or an immediate family member has received royalties from Biomet; is a member of a speakers' bureau or has made paid presentations on behalf of Biomet and Stryker; is a paid consultant to or is an employee of Biomet and Stryker; and has received research or institutional support from Kinamed. Dr. White or an immediate family member is a member of a speakers' bureau or has made paid presentations on behalf of Synthes; is a paid consultant to or an employee of Zimmer; has received research or institutional support from Synthes; and has stock or stock options held in Zimmer. Neither Dr. Swart nor an immediate family member has received anything of value from or owns stock in a commercial company or institution related directly or indirectly to the subject of this chapter.

terior interosseous, and anterior interosseous nerves is critical. Pulse examination of the radial and ulnar arteries is also important. High suspicion for compartment syndrome must be maintained both preoperatively and postoperatively. The skin and soft tissues must be closely assessed for open wounds. Palpation for tenderness at the DRUJ and proximal radioulnar joint (PRUJ) is important to rule out associated injuries.

Radius Fractures

Isolated radius fractures are uncommon in adults. These fractures have previously been thought to represent a Galeazzi-type fracture with subtle injury to the DRUJ. Fractures within the 7.5 cm closest to the distal radius are at higher risk of being a Galeazzi injury. Isolated radial shaft fractures should be treated surgically with open reduction and internal fixation to allow for early range of motion as well as to restore the anatomy required for proper function.

Ulna Fractures

Isolated ulna fractures, also known as "nightstick fractures," frequently result from a direct blow to the ulna. Soft tissues must be closely examined with this injury mechanism to rule out an open fracture. If the fracture is less than 10° angulated and less than 50% translated, it may be treated nonsurgically.[2] Immobilization options include short arm cast, long arm cast, and/or fracture bracing. Surgical treatment is indicated for fractures with greater than 10° of angulation, greater than 50% translation, PRUJ or DRUJ instability, or proximal ulna fractures. Fracture fixation is achieved with internal fixation.

Galeazzi Fractures

The Galeazzi fracture is a fracture of the radius (usually middle or distal third) with an associated disruption of the DRUJ. The mechanism by which these injuries occur is still unclear. This type of fracture is difficult to reproduce in laboratory settings. Common theories include a fall onto an outstretched and pronated hand, axial load with extreme wrist extension and pronation, and/or a direct blow to the dorsoradial forearm.

3: Upper Extremity

On physical examination, the patient will present with pain, swelling, and deformity of the forearm and likely the wrist. The DRUJ is tender with palpation, and the ulnar head may be prominent. There is a broad spectrum to the severity of the injury, and a DRUJ injury must be suspected at the time of examination of any patient with an isolated radial shaft fracture, because this aspect of the injury may not be apparent on plain radiographs.

Radiographic evaluation of Galeazzi fractures should include AP and lateral views of the forearm and dedicated wrist views. A true lateral view of the wrist is required to properly assess the DRUJ. Contralateral radiographs may be obtained if the diagnosis is not clear. CT may also be used for complex injury patterns. Radiographic findings that suggest rupture of the DRUJ include (1) fracture at the base of the ulnar styloid; (2) widening of the DRUJ on the AP view of the wrist; (3) dislocation of the ulna relative to the radius on a true lateral view of the wrist; and (4) more than 5 mm of shortening of the radius relative to the ulna (ulna positive) when compared to the contralateral wrist.[3]

Treatment: Nonsurgical treatment in adults results in poor outcome in most patients and therefore should be reserved for very rare situations in which the patient is unable to tolerate any surgery or has a very limited life expectancy.

Surgical treatment is indicated for all Galeazzi fracture/dislocations because nonsurgical treatment has yielded unsatisfactory results. Therefore, the Galeazzi fracture is also known as "the fracture of necessity," meaning it necessitates surgical treatment.

The goal of surgical treatment is to achieve an anatomic reduction of the radius and to restore a stable, functional DRUJ. The standard treatment of the radius fracture is open reduction using the volar approach of Henry and plate fixation with a 3.5-mm compression plate. Another method of fixation is intramedullary fixation. In adults this requires an interlocking nail to avoid malunion in a malrotated and shortened position. Otherwise prolonged external immobilization is required until union is achieved. In addition, an intramedullary nail for a metaphyseal radius fracture does not allow for fill of the medullary canal at the level of the fracture, allowing translation and shortening of the fracture. For this reason, intramedullary nailing is not recommended for metaphyseal or metadiaphyseal radius fractures. Once the radius is reduced and stabilized in an anatomic position, the DRUJ must be critically assessed. Because of variance of laxity between patients, the contralateral DRUJ should be examined to determine the baseline stability. If it is stable after fixation of the radius, the extremity is immobilized with a long arm splint or cast in the position of greatest stability (most often supination) for 6 weeks. If the ulna can be dislocated from the sigmoid notch with the forearm in supination, the DRUJ is unstable. If the DRUJ is unstable or irreducible, it requires fixation with two Kirschner wires (K-wires) that transfix the ra-

dius and ulna, repair of the ulnar styloid if the fragment is large enough, or soft-tissue repair. If K-wires are used, two wires are placed to lessen the risk of K-wire breakage. Four cortices are crossed in case the wires break, to help facilitate removal of the broken portion of K-wire. If the ulna is not able to be reduced closed, interposed extensor carpi ulnaris, extensor digitorum communis, or extensor minimi may result. Other structures impeding closed reduction can include a metaphyseal fragment buttonholed through the capsule, periosteum, or an avulsion fracture from the fovea. Postoperative management of a Galeazzi fracture usually involves immobilization with a long arm cast/splint for 4 to 6 weeks. Postoperative radiographs in plaster should be obtained to ensure the DRUJ is reduced.

Complications after treatment of Galeazzi fractures include nonunion, malunion with resultant restricted pronation and supination, damage to nerves or vessels, infection, complex regional pain syndrome, and subluxation of the DRUJ with subsequent degenerative changes.

Monteggia Fracture-Dislocation

This injury pattern was first described in 1814 as a fracture of the proximal third of the ulna and an anterior dislocation of the proximal radius. This eponymic term currently is commonly applied to any ulna fracture, usually proximal, that is associated with a subluxation or dislocation of the radial head and disruption of the proximal radioulnar joint. The Monteggia fracture-dislocation must be distinguished from a transolecranon fracture-dislocation. This latter injury is best described as an olecranon fracture associated with an intact proximal radioulnar joint, so that the radial head, which is still attached to the proximal ulna, dislocates as a unit (**Figure 1**).

Monteggia fractures are classified into four types according to the direction of displacement of the radial head as described by Bado: type 1, ulna fracture with anterior radial head subluxation-dislocation; type 2, ulna fracture with posterior radial head subluxation/dislocation; type 3, ulna fracture with lateral radial head subluxation/dislocation; and type 4, ulna fracture with associated radial head fracture-dislocation.

One should be aware that type 2 posterior fracture-dislocations typically are accompanied by unstable ulna fractures and may be associated with an anterior triangular or quadrangular fracture of the ulna at or just distal to the coronoid process. These posterior dislocations are most often seen in middle-aged and elderly adults.

The history and physical examination is important for patients with Monteggia fracture-dislocations. As with all upper extremity fractures, age, hand dominance, functional demands, and occupation are all vital parts of the history. Careful attention must be paid to the neurologic examination, especially the radial nerve/posterior interosseous nerve.

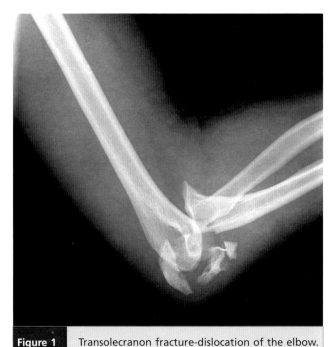

Figure 1   Transolecranon fracture-dislocation of the elbow.

Radiographic workup of a patient with a suspected Monteggia fracture includes AP and lateral views of the forearm and dedicated AP and lateral views of the elbow. These views are required for diagnosis and classification, as well as formulation of a treatment plan. If there is an associated fracture of the radial head, or in case of a complex fracture-dislocation, CT may be indicated to further delineate the fracture pattern. Contralateral elbow views are also helpful for complex injury patterns.

Treatment: As with Galeazzi fracture-dislocations, Monteggia fracture-dislocations require surgical fixation to restore anatomic alignment of the forearm and thereby the proximal radioulnar joint. The ulna must be reduced anatomically to allow for a stable radiocapitellar and radioulnar joint. The patient may be positioned supine, lateral, or prone. The lateral and prone positions eliminate the need for an assistant holding the arm. The ulna fracture is exposed through the interval between the extensor carpi ulnaris and flexor carpi ulnaris. Metadiaphyseal and diaphyseal ulna fractures are stabilized with a 3.5-mm compression plate placed on the dorsal surface. For more proximal ulna fractures, a periarticular olecranon plate may be used or a compression plate can be contoured to fit around the tip of the olecranon. Especially for apex-posterior injury patterns, plates should be placed on the dorsal surface, not the radial or ulnar side of the ulna. Intramedullary devices should not be used for fixation of adult Monteggia fractures. Anatomic restoration of the ulna generally allows for concentric reduction of the radial head. If the radial head does not reduce, the ulnar reduction must be critically reassessed. If anatomic restoration is still possible, there may be soft tissue interposed at the

proximal radioulnar joint. Anatomic structures that may block reduction of the proximal radioulnar joint include the capsule, the annular ligament, radial nerve, or biceps tendon.[4] Intraoperative radiographs must be evaluated so that a line down the center of the radial shaft and head intersects the capitellum in all positions of flexion and extension on any view.

The prognosis for patients with a Monteggia fracture-dislocation is worse with the posterior type 2 fracture-dislocations, concomitant fractures of the radial head and coronoid, fractures of the ulna at the level of the coronoid, or fractures that are associated with comminution in the region of the coronoid, or both.[5]

Complications of Monteggia fractures include elbow stiffness, subluxation-dislocation of the radial head, malunion, nonunion, synostosis, infection, and damage to nerves.

Fixation of Forearm Fractures

Standard fixation for adult forearm fractures are nonlocking 3.5-mm limited contact dynamic compression plates. For very distal or proximal fractures, 2.7-mm compression plates, locking plates, or specialty plates may be used. Traditionally, six cortices of fixation are achieved on both sides of the fracture. A recent study assessed 53 patients with forearm fractures that were treated with a plate that was three holes longer than the fracture both proximally and distally.[6] Two screws were placed in each fragment, with one screw in the holes just proximal and just distal to the fracture and the other screw in the most proximal and distal holes. With this technique, the union rate was 97% with no refractures and no change in alignment. There were two delayed unions and one nonunion. Another study using minimal screw plate fixation found a nonunion rate of 9%, all atrophic and in open fractures.[7] They concluded that technical emphasis should be placed on plate length, not number of cortices of fixation. Segmental fractures may require two plates (**Figure 2**). These should be placed so that there is overlap between the plates to prevent a stress riser.

Locking plates have become more frequently used in many different fractures over the last several years. A biomechanical study evaluated comminuted ulna fractures in synthetic, osteoporotic model bones.[8] The authors assessed various constructs and tested cyclic axial loading and three-point bending. Bicortical locked screws withstood significantly more cycles to failure compared to bicortical nonlocked screws, as well as unicortical locked screws. Less distance between plate and bone also increased stability. However, these biomechanical advantages have to be considered in light of the increased expense of locking technology and the decades of clinical success that have been achieved with nonlocked screws and plates in adult forearm fractures.

Intramedullary fixation can be used for selected adult forearm fractures; common indications include pathologic fractures/impending pathologic fractures,[9]

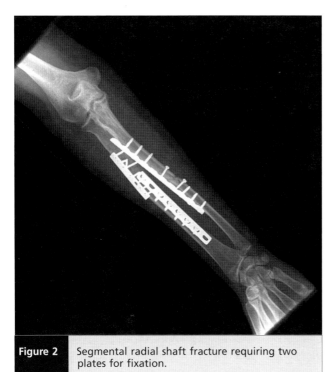

Figure 2 Segmental radial shaft fracture requiring two plates for fixation.

segmental fractures, fractures secondary to gunshot wounds, and certain refractures after plate removal. Theoretic advantages of intramedullary nailing include decreased periosteal stripping (often done to apply a plate), decreased rate of refracture, and less prominent hardware. A recent retrospective study evaluated 38 intramedullary nails placed into 27 forearm fractures.[10] Monteggia fractures, Galeazzi fractures, osteoporotic fractures, and segmental comminuted fractures were excluded. The authors found that fluoroscopy time was increased early in their experience. They reported an average healing time of 14 weeks (9 to 32 weeks range) and one nonunion. Mean pronation and supination was 85° and 87°, respectively. Ninety-two percent had excellent or good results. Postoperative immobilization was continued until bridging callus was seen.[10]

External fixation may be used temporarily for grossly contaminated fractures or those with severe soft-tissue injury. It is rarely used for definitive treatment of adult both-bone forearm fractures or fracture-dislocations.

Nonunions

With current fixation techniques, nonunion of diaphyseal forearm fractures is rare, with rates quoted as less than 5%. Nonunion is usually associated with a complex injury pattern, infection, bone defect, or inadequate fixation.[11] Hypertrophic nonunions are uncommon, representing only 9% of nonunions. Atrophic nonunions are much more common and associated with open fractures, inadequate fixation, infection, and fracture-dislocation. Infected nonunions require a staged protocol to eradicate the infection. The hard-

ware and any infected necrotic bone is removed, a temporary antibiotic spacer and/or temporary spanning external fixator can be used to maintain length, and then bone grafting and internal fixation is performed, all in conjunction with appropriate antibiotics.

Risk factors for ulnar nonunions include fracture displacement, polytrauma, and comminution. In addition, most ulnar nonunions are seen at the junction of the middle and distal third where the blood supply is poorest. In addition, the ulna may be predisposed to nonunion because it is subject to torsional forces as the radius rotates around it during pronation and supination.

Malunion

Malunion can be caused by failure to restore length, rotation, and axial alignment. Careful assessment of intraoperative imaging can decrease the risk of malreduction of the radius. The bicipital tuberosity should be 180° from the radial styloid. In addition, intraoperative rotation of the forearm should be carefully assessed and, if needed, compared to the other arm. Failure to restore the radial bow is associated with loss of forearm rotation as well as decreased grip strength. Change in the location of the maximal radial bow is of greater functional significance than the change in its magnitude; if the location of the maximum radial bow is restored compared to that of the normal arm, near-normal rotation and grip strength can be expected. Up to 10° of angulation in any plane can be tolerated without much clinical significance. However, 20° or more angulation in either the radius or ulna results in significant loss of pronation/supination.

Refracture

The rate of refracture after plate removal from the forearm has been reported to be between 16% and 26%. Protective splinting and protected activity should be routine after hardware removal, and the plates should not be removed for at least 1 year after the initial injury.

Bone Defects

Although initial reports supported the use of autogenous bone grafting in forearm fractures with greater than 33% of shaft diameter comminution, studies have demonstrated no difference in union rates between comminuted fractures treated with and without bone grafting.[12,13]

Outcomes

Diaphyseal forearm fractures in patients older than 18 years treated surgically with plate fixation were studied retrospectively.[14] Thirty patients with both-bone forearm fractures at a mean follow-up of 5.4 years were included. Mean Disabilities of the Arm, Shoulder and Hand (DASH) score for these patients was significantly increased compared to normal values. Disability was

Table 1

Normal and Acceptable Postreduction Radiographic Values

Measurement	Normal	Acceptable Postreduction§	
		Literature	Author's Opinion⁺
Volar tilt	11°	0 to 15° dorsal	10° dorsal tilt
Ulnar variance*	Equal to other side or ± 2 mm	2 to 4 mm shortening	3 mm shortening
Radial inclination	22°	10° to 17°	15°
Articular displacement	Congruous	1 to 2 mm step or gap	2 mm step 1 mm gap⁺⁺

* Lunate facet to ulnar head, as compared to contralateral side
⁺ Predicting fracture stability is more important than minding any specific parameters. If the fracture is unstable, no cast will maintain reduction.
⁺⁺ While preventing point contact is important, containing the lunate is paramount for achieving a good outcome. As such, only 1 mm of gap is acceptable.
§ Note that the goal of surgical intervention is anatomic restoration of the distal end of the radius. The acceptable postreduction values vary widely by report and opinion and are also related to the functional demands of the individual patient. This is most noted by recent literature that shows increased tolerance to malunions in the elderly. The senior author's preferences are outlined in bold.

determined largely due to pain, not objective findings. Strength was on average 30% less than the contralateral arm even years after the injury.

Distal Radius Fractures

The diagnosis and management of distal radius fractures has been varied and controversial since Colles' first description in 1814. Recent innovations in internal fixation approaches and implants have fueled a wave of enthusiasm for volar locked plating, which to date has not been supported by rigorous multicenter clinical trials. Disagreement still exists with respect to classification, indications, surgical approaches, and treatment despite the publication of more than 1,000 peer-reviewed articles on the subject within the past 5 years.

Distal radius fractures account for 20% of all fractures seen in the emergency department. Fractures occur in a bimodal distribution with high-energy mechanisms for young adult males and low-energy falls from standing height for osteopenic postmenopausal females. Osteoporosis is a strong independent predictor of susceptibility to distal radius fracture and has also been shown to correlate with loss of radial length and poor clinical outcome.

Restoration of the distal radius anatomy is the rationale for surgical treatment and has been correlated with improved functional outcome, although the elderly low-demand patient may tolerate malunion and deformity.[15-17] Bone quality is directly related to the capacity to reduce and maintain reduction and thus is one of the most significant factors in indicating and guiding treatment plans. Fracture classification systems are based on describing fracture patterns and parts and are often linked to treatment algorithms, but are not sufficiently predictive of outcome. Bone quality and carpal alignment may be more useful in sorting through the

treatment options and informing patients about their injury and prognosis.[18]

Evaluation

After a distal radius fracture is identified, the patient and affected limb must be carefully evaluated. This evaluation should include the skin, adjacent joints, and the neurovascular system. Documentation of the mechanism of injury and energy absorbed is important, as is the assessment of the patient's general health, functional requirements, living accommodations, and expectations.

Upon recognition of injury, gross deformity should be corrected with gentle traction and the fracture should always be splinted. When symptoms of acute carpal tunnel syndrome are present, fracture reduction may be sufficient to decompress the median nerve and should be done urgently. Following this, high-quality radiographs in the AP, lateral, and oblique planes should be obtained. Although rarely indicated in the acute setting, contralateral films may be helpful in judging radial length. Special views have become widely used, especially the tilted lateral view, which eliminates the overlap of the radial styloid and enhances the view of the articular facets. Radiologic indices to be measured include radial height and inclination, volar tilt, and articular displacement (Table 1). The radiographs should be carefully assessed for associated injuries such as intercarpal injury with scapholunate or lunotriquetral instability patterns, dorsal intercalated segment instability (DISI), volar intercalated segment instability (VISI), and carpal diastasis or incongruence. Another feature to note is the presence of carpal translation, which is characterized by the lunate facet fragment and lunate translating off axis with the radial shaft (for example, volar or dorsal Barton fractures). This denotes fracture instability and is correlated with poor outcomes if not corrected.

CT may be useful in pattern recognition of complex

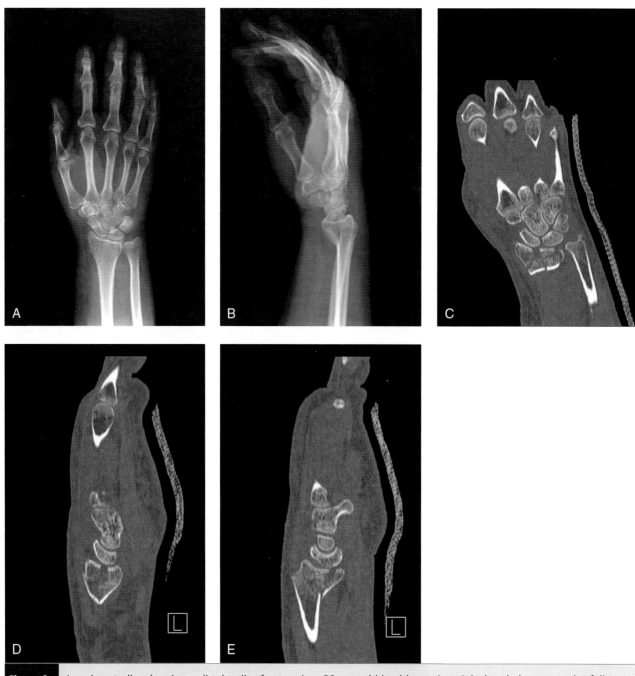

Figure 3 Imaging studies showing a distal radius fracture in a 56-year-old healthy, active, right-handed woman who fell onto an outstretched hand. **A** and **B**, Radiographs reveal minimal displacement and well-maintained radiographic parameters. However, closer inspection of the lateral view reveals a large intra-articular gap and suspicion of volar shear component, suggesting instability. CT confirms significant articular incongruity (**C** and **D**), and unstable volar component (**E**). In this case, CT unveiled clear surgical indications.

intra-articular distal radius fractures, as well as in the assessment of displacement. This is especially true with regard to fragment rotation at the sigmoid notch and distal radioulnar joint. CT is more helpful after a closed reduction is obtained, as even a partial realignment of the fragments will aid in the interpretation of the CT images. Three-dimensional CT reconstructions have increased sensitivity and specificity of fracture patterns and injury severity, leading to improved surgical indications and planning. Although CT has been shown to alter treatment plans, it has not been shown to affect outcome. Nevertheless, it should be used whenever there is concern about the adequacy of closed reduction or after limited percutaneous techniques that may not be sufficiently confirmed by standard radiographs. **Figure 3** demonstrates an unstable and displaced volar ulnar lunate facet fracture identified by CT but not obvious on plain radiographs.

Associated Injuries

Clinical and anatomic studies have shown that injuries to adjacent soft-tissue structures occur in approximately half of distal radius fractures,[19] and in almost all intra-articular fractures. The most common and potentially significant causes of persistent symptoms include injuries to the ulnocarpal ligaments or TFCC, and/or ulnar styloid fracture.

Concomitant scapholunate interosseous ligament injury has been identified in many distal radius fractures, as well as injury to the lunotriquetral interosseous ligament. These diagnoses may be made via arthroscopy and include partial tears that do not lead to chronic instability. When significant destabilizing ligament injuries are observed, they require additional reduction and stabilization via suture repair supplemented by K-wire fixation. Clinically significant ligament injuries may be missed unless the treating physician maintains a high index of suspicion and looks for evidence of carpal instability.

The treatment of ulnar styloid fractures has been influenced by recent literature,[20] which has challenged the dogma that basal, or type 3, fractures must be internally fixed and that lesser fractures need not be addressed. Recent treatment algorithms have instead focused on the evaluation of DRUJ stability.

Two recent clinical studies support nonsurgical management of associated ulnar styloid fractures. The first, a retrospective cohort study, compared 76 surgically treated distal radius fractures with 76 control fractures that were not accompanied by ulnar styloid fracture. All ulnar styloid fractures were treated closed. There was no significant difference in outcome between those with and without styloid fractures at 2 years. There was also no statistically significant difference in outcome between patients with styloid fractures with a displacement greater than 2 mm and those with minimally displaced fractures.[20] The second study reviewed 118 consecutive patients treated with volar locked plating. Sixty-eight percent of patients had styloid fractures, and there was no difference at 15 months between those with and without styloid fractures.[19]

This oversimplification has been clarified by the recommendation that all surgically treated distal radius fractures, following stabilization, should have DRUJ stability assessment via a shuck or translation stress test. This test is done by holding the radius and translating the ulna to its dorsal and palmar extremes and assessing both asymmetry and endpoint. The test is done with the extremity in neutral, full pronation, and full supination; a qualitative feel for increased laxity can be appreciated. Assessment of ulnocarpal instability must be performed following distal radius stabilization. There are no firm guidelines, but gross translational instability and asymmetry compared to the contralateral wrist should be addressed. Often this may preclude early mobilization of an internally fixed fracture, because a long arm cast or splint may be necessary in the fully supinated position for at least 3 to 4 weeks. If the supinated position does not confer stability, ulnocarpal instability may be successfully treated by techniques such as tension band wiring of the ulnar styloid, arthroscopic or open TFCC repair, or ulnocarpal pinning.

Classification

There are at least 20 distal radius fracture classification systems, and no consensus exists as to their reliability or value in the planning of treatment. Orthopaedic surgeons prefer eponymous names because fractures tend to overlap and therefore detail is insufficient. Fracture line delineation, or fragment counting, does not denote or connote instability or guide treatment. Several recent studies have shown moderate to poor intraobserver and interobserver reliability of the AO/ASIF, Frykman, Fernandez, Cooney, Melone and other classification systems. In a recent prospective cohort study, 621 radiographs of distal radius fractures were evaluated.[21] The authors found only moderate agreement between surgeons and final evaluators, thus calling into question the validity of the use of these classification systems in therapeutic trials. The same researchers and others have shown moderate agreement with AO/ASIF groupings and only fair agreement within subgroup categories.[21]

Another study evaluated injury characteristics including mechanism, initial displacement, ulnar-sided injury, hand dominance, and other patient characteristics and found that none of these predicted outcome at 1 year.[22]

Commonly used classification systems along with their advantages and disadvantages are summarized in **Table 2**.

Treatment and Related Outcomes

The nine discrete clinical treatments of displaced distal radius fractures have been summarized below. These treatments are closed reduction and casting, closed reduction and percutaneous pinning, bridging and nonbridging external fixation, volar and dorsal plating, fragment-specific fixation, intramedullary nailing, and internal bridge plating. Variations and combinations of techniques are also commonly reported, further muddling any possible assessment of efficacy. For example, external fixation in isolation, with percutaneous pinning, with limited dorsal incisions and percutaneous pins, with volar plate fixation, and with bone graft or bone filler through limited open approaches have all been described. This has yielded a heterogeneous and often conflicting collection of studies, consisting primarily of case series and technique reports. No compelling evidence has elevated any one of these techniques to become the gold standard. Nonetheless, the advances in the use of volar locked plating (VLP) technology and variable axis screws have led to enthusiasm for this technique, despite the paucity of high-level evidence supporting its use.

Table 2

Fracture Classification

Classification	Description	Advantages	Disadvantages
Eponyms	Example: "Colles," "Smith's," "Volar Barton," "Dorsal Barton"	• If used correctly, impart large amount of information with only a few words	• Often used incorrectly (more broadly than intended) and create confusion • Not comprehensive: do not include all fractures
AO/ASIF	Three basic groups with subdivisions based on location and pattern (Table 3)	• Comprehensive • Moderate intra- and inter-observer reliability	• 144 subtypes, making it cumbersome to use • decreased reliability with subtyping
Frykman	Differentiates between intra- and extra-articular fractures of the radiocarpal joint and radioulnar joint, with and without ulnar styloid fractures	• Highlights importance of DRUJ	• No information about metaphyseal comminution or displacement • Low reliability • Does not direct treatment
Melone	Divides fractures into four major parts with increasing grade for increasing comminution and instability	• First classification to highlight importance of the lunate facet and specifically the coronal split within it	• Not comprehensive • Low reliability • Does not direct treatment
Fernandez	Based on mechanism of injury: bending, articular shear, and compression fractures, fracture-dislocations, and combined mechanisms	• Comprehensive • Directs treatment	• Complicated/difficult to understand and use • Poor reliability

Indications

All displaced distal radius fractures should undergo immediate reduction if for no other reason than to relieve any excessive pressure on the soft tissues and alleviate potential stress on adjacent nerves. What has become increasingly clear is that marked initial displacement is predictive of the failure of closed treatment, because widely displaced fractures will frequently collapse and subside even after adequate closed reduction. Similarly, severe osteoporotic fragility fractures that may be easy to reduce closed often cannot be maintained because of poor bone quality.

Assessment of postreduction fracture stability and the risk of redisplacement is difficult to quantify. However, several guidelines have emerged. The Lafontaine criteria for fracture stability state that the amount of dorsal comminution, dorsal displacement, concomitant ulnar fracture, intra-articular extension, and age are all significant risk factors for redisplacement. More recently, a prospective study of 4,000 radiographs found age, metaphyseal comminution, and ulnar variance to be the most significant risk factors for redisplacement.[23] Another study targeted carpal malalignment as a major risk for redisplacement.[24] No instability scoring system has been validated or accepted as the uniform guide for treatment.

Surgical indications include inadequate initial closed reduction or redisplacement after acceptable initial reduction (Table 1). High-energy injuries in younger patients will most often require open treatment to restore correct anatomy and maximize restoration of function.[16] Displacement in osteoporotic fragility fractures may not require the same aggressive realignment, as increased dorsal displacement and shortening may be compatible with satisfactory function.[15-17] Clear tolerances for this population have not yet been defined. Marked shortening of greater than 5 mm, however, weakens the wrist and substantially limits rotation, leading to poor overall outcomes. The treating surgeon must personalize the care of each patient and not rely on any specific measurements in offering treatment options.

Treatment Options: Update

Closed Treatment

A recent randomized trial reported the results of 118 patients with distal radius fractures treated with closed reduction.[25] No difference in the maintenance of reduction was detected between those treated with short arm radial gutter splints and those treated with long arm sugar tong splints. However, the short splint was better tolerated by patients.

Closed Reduction With Percutaneous Pinning

A recent Cochrane review of 13 trials involving 940 patients concluded that there is some evidence to support the use of closed reduction with percutaneous pinning, although the exact role is less clear, especially with regard to contraindications. All pinning techniques are

Table 3

Surgical Indications According to AO/ASIF Fracture Type*

	A			B			C		
Intervention	A1	A2	A3	B1	B2	B3	C1	C2	C3
Closed reduction	-	+	+	+/–	+/–	+/–	+	+	+
Closed reduction percutaneous pinning (CRPP)	-	+	+	+	+/–	-	+	+	+
Bridging external fixation	-	+/–	+/–	-	-	-	+/–	-	-
Bridging external fixation with CRPP	-	+	+	-	-	-	+	+	+
Bridging external fixation with volar locked plating	-	+	+	-	-	-	+	+	+
Nonbridging external fixation	-	++	++	-	-	-	+	+/–	-
Standard volar plating	-	+	+	-	-	++	+	+/–	-
Volar locked plating	-	+	+	-	-	+	+	+	+
Dorsal plating	-	+	+	-	++	-	+	+/–	+/–
Radial column plating	-	+	+	++	-	-	+	+/–	+/–
Fragment-specific fixation	-	+	+	+	+	+	+	+	+
Intramedullary nailing	-	+	+	-	-	-	+	-	-
Arthroscopy	-	-	-	-	+	+	+	+	+

*This classification system was chosen because it is the most commonly reported in the literature and is the most reproducible . Note that there is general agreement on treatment for type B fractures. Type A2, A3, and C1 fractures are amenable to most treatment options. This chart will change, as many more iterations with the evolution of care are anticipated.

not equal, with higher rates of complication in both the Kapandji technique and the use of biodegradable pins. One study reported excellent long-term outcomes in a series of 54 patients with closed reduction with percutaneous pinning of all but the most comminuted intra-articular fractures (AO/ASIF A2, A3, C1, and C2).[26]

External Fixation

Spanning of the wrist (bridging external fixation) is the traditional method of providing and maintaining a gentle distraction force across the radiocarpal joint through ligamentotaxis. This force can counteract the forces of compression that accompany gripping exercises, but will in most instances be inadequate to reduce and maintain depressed articular segments without adjunctive K-wire fixation. The fact that the wrist capsule is equally tensioned by the bridging frame also precludes restoration of the anatomic volar tilt of 10°, even with adjunctive intrafocal pinning. Neutral tilt, however, is satisfactory, and that is why many studies have demonstrated equivalent results compared to plating when reductions are equivalent.[27]

Nonbridging external fixation is a powerful but seldom used technique for controlling distal radial fracture fragments and allowing wrist motion. Even intra-articular fractures can be treated in this manner if the fragments are big enough to accommodate 3-mm threaded half-pins. These joysticks can be manipulated to restore volar tilt, but care must be taken to avoid overtranslation of the articular fragment if the volar cortex is unstable. This can be prevented by placing an intramedullary K-wire to block palmar translation. Both external fixation techniques may use adjunctive fixation, joystick K-wires, and metaphyseal void filling bone grafts or substitutes (**Table 3**). Patient selection is critical to avoid complications with either technique.

Two recent Cochrane reviews of more than 1,500 patients comparing external fixation to casting among different external fixation protocols did not produce compelling evidence with respect to a correct treatment modality.

In a recent retrospective study, 588 patients with unstable distal radius fractures were evaluated.[28] Fixator positioning was indicated based on fracture anatomy, with nonbridging external fixation placed if the distal bone fragments could accept the threaded half-pins. At union, patients with bridging external fixation showed a sixfold increase in dorsal malunions and a 2.5-fold increase in radial shortening. Despite the favorable results, the use of nonbridging external fixation remains infrequent.

A new system using cross K-wires and a low-profile nonbridging frame has been developed, and first clinical reports have demonstrated favorable outcomes. The

3: Upper Extremity

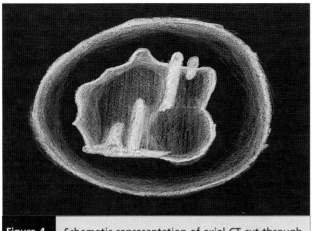

Figure 4 Schematic representation of axial CT cut through the distal radius. Note the excessive length of the screw just ulnar to the Lister tubercle. The radiodensity of the tubercle blocks visualization of the long screw on a lateral radiograph. If the screw appears to be the appropriate length, it is probably too long.

strength of this construct has been substantiated in a cadaver study that showed the cross-pin system to be comparable to volar locked plating.[29]

In general, external fixation complications are usually minor and do not affect the final outcome. Most commonly seen is pin tract infection. A recent study randomized 118 patients to compare different pin care regimens.[30] No differences between groups were identified, and the overall superficial infection rate was 19%, with 10% of patients requiring antibiotics. No serious complications or deep infections were reported.

Internal Fixation Techniques

Volar Plating

In the past decade, many clinical reports have extolled the virtues and efficacy of volar locked plating and variable axis locking screws. Clearly, the ability to confidently place screws in a buttressing plate atop severely osteoporotic bone has revolutionized the care of distal radial fractures. The concept of axial stable fixed-angle fixation with screws functioning as a raft to support the articular surface has been appealing in both the biomechanical and clinical domains. Enthusiasm for the technique has spawned commercial development of more than 30 designs with various precontours, bone fit, and screw trajectories.

Volar locked plates support the loads seen in the healing distal radial fractures. This quality was demonstrated in anatomic and mechanical fracture models of volar locked plates via cyclic loading and loading to catastrophic failure.[31] Although volar locked plates can stabilize many fractures, the most complex may require adjunctive plate fixation if the locking screws cannot reliably capture and stabilize fragments such as the radial styloid or the dorsal ulnar facet.[32]

One study evaluated the addition of a radial column plate in AO/ASIF C2 three-part fractures.[33] The authors found that the second plate enhanced the stability of the construct, as compared to volar locked plates alone. Injury films may be used to inform decision making with respect to buttressing comminuted fragments directly with a secondary plate. Ultimately, the use of a second plate may be an intraoperative decision and as such, surgeon preparation is key.

Twenty-one case series reporting more than 1,100 patients in the past 4 years support the efficacy of volar locked plates in the treatment of distal radius fractures. Comparative level I evidence is presented in **Table 4**.

As the use of volar locked plates has become widespread, the accompanying common technical errors and associated complications have become well known. Delayed extensor tendon rupture has been reported in 1.7% to 8.6% of volar locked plate fixation,[34,35] compared to 1.3% to 4.0% in dorsal plate fixation. The etiology of this complication is multifactorial and may include plate design and metallurgy, as well as the more obvious screw penetration from inaccurate measurement.

A most common complication of mismeasurement of subchondral screws occurs because of the shadowing of the Lister tubercle over the dorsal ulnar facet of the distal radius. It may appear that the most ulnar screws are quite short, even for locked screws, as it is well accepted that the longer the screw, the better the rafting potential of the subchondral facet. This has led surgeons to place longer screws, which often become the reason for the attrition of extensor tendons (**Figure 4**). When using plates with fixed angle screw trajectories, it is challenging to place the screws within 1 to 2 mm of the subchondral surface without joint penetration, especially if the articular facets are not reduced before plate application to the bone.[36] Recent cadaver studies have shown that standard AP and lateral views alone are insufficient to accurately assess for joint penetration and screw length.[36,37] One study showed fluoroscopy to have 82% sensitivity for dorsal cortex penetration of the radialmost screw and only 57% sensitivity in the ulnarmost screw.[37] Sensitivity improved with evaluator experience. Another study recommended lateral tilt radiographs to accurately evaluate joint penetration, low-angle tilt lateral view (15° to 23°) for imaging of the dorsal ulnar facet, and a more inclined lateral view for the radial styloid screw.[36]

Dorsal Plating

Plating the dorsal distal radius has always been the more intuitive of surgical approaches because the dorsal column is most often involved with comminution and displacement. Innovative dorsal plates that respected the dorsal extensor compartments were introduced but then largely abandoned because of severe tissue reaction and complications of tendon rupture and dysfunction (**Figure 5**). More recently, newer designs with better contours and less reactive metals have reduced the rate of tendon rupture. Dorsal plating for

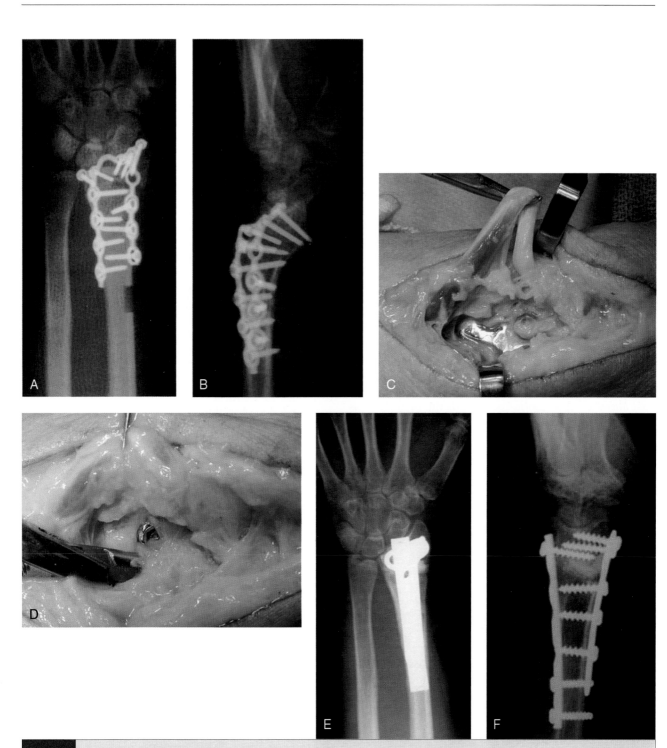

Figure 5   **A** and **B**, Radiographs showing initial treatment of an intra-articular distal radius fracture with a titanium dorsal pi plate in a 31-year-old woman. The fracture healed in a malunited position, necessitating hardware removal and a corrective osteotomy. **C** and **D**, Intraoperative photographs show profound dorsal synovitis and scar formation on plate removal. After substantial débridement, the osteotomy was performed and secured with dorsal and volar plating (**E** and **F**).

displaced distal radius fractures has delivered good to excellent results in recent case series, and this approach is still quite popular in Europe. Some bicolumnar fracture patterns may not be adequately supported by a dorsal plate alone with translation in a volar direction after the dorsal plate is applied. There are fractures that require a dorsal surgical approach such as the dorsal die punch fracture with an intact volar cortex. Also, the approach to the dorsal ulnar facet may be necessary to reduce and stabilize osteopenic fragments that cannot be held with locked screws deployed through a volar locking plate. It may also be useful when treating frac-

3: Upper Extremity

tures associated with intercarpal ligament injuries such as the transradial styloid fracture with a perilunate instability pattern requiring ligament repair.

Other Fixation Techniques

Fragment-specific fixation, intramedullary nailing, and internal bridge plating are less popular but still effective methods of treatment, especially for certain indications. Nailing is useful for the less comminuted, AO/ASIF type A and C1 fractures.[38] Fragment-specific fixation is used for more complex fractures in which smaller articular facet or periarticular shearing fractures that may not be amenable to monoblock volar or dorsal plating are encountered. These smaller plates are placed through more limited approaches with less dissection and require meticulous attention to detail but yield comparable results in experienced hands (**Table 4**).

Internal bridge plating is nothing more than a spanning external fixator placed under the skin. It is useful for markedly comminuted fractures (resulting from either high-energy injury or severe osteoporosis) and restores general alignment to union or until definitive treatment can be performed. Limited percutaneous approaches over the third metacarpal and the distal radius allow a subtendinous passage of the plate. This is especially useful for the polytrauma patient and permits early crutch ambulation.[39]

The Role of Arthroscopy

Wrist arthroscopy has become an important tool for the diagnosis and treatment of intra-articular pathology, both bony and ligamentous. The arthroscope can be used safely and effectively to directly visualize joint surfaces for articular cartilage injuries as well as associated intercarpal ligament tears and ulnocarpal injuries to the TFCC. Certain fractures are especially difficult to realign using only fluoroscopy, as it has a resolution of only 2 mm. Fractures such as dorsal die punch, radial styloid, and chauffeur can be well visualized and the reductions finely tuned with joystick K-wires or elevators. Because most fractures are now plated from the volar side, using the arthroscope to assist during the reduction and confirm its adequacy is quite useful. A recent study randomized patients with intra-articular fractures to either fluoroscopic-assisted reduction or fluoroscopic and arthroscopic reduction.[40] All fractures were stabilized with percutaneous pins. Three quarters of the arthroscopic group had associated injuries documented. At 2 years, mobility and Mayo wrist outcome scores were significantly improved in the arthroscopic group, while DASH scores were similar between the two groups.

Immediate identification of associated ligament injuries, especially in the TFCC, has led to acute direct repairs with good early and long-term results.

Wrist arthroscopy skills should be mastered before embarking on fracture reduction. Most arthroscopic systems use overhead traction for the arthroscopy and joint manipulation and ligament repair followed by the application of internal or external fixation in the usual horizontal position. However, some horizontal traction units may allow the entire procedure to be performed without a change of position. Early case series report good and excellent results with arthroscopic assisted surgery with minimal morbidity. **Figure 6** demonstrates the steps in an arthroscopically guided reduction and fixation of an intra-articular distal radius fracture.

Bone Graft

Distal radius fractures have a natural propensity to heal with a very low nonunion rate, so why consider bone grafting? High-energy mechanisms cause radii to fail in young patients, whereas elderly patients with osteopenia have a lower threshold. In both instances, the mechanisms of impaction and axial load can impact articular fragments into the metaphysis, creating a metaphyseal void after the fracture has been reduced. This void may be supported by rafting screws of a locked volar plate. However, if other fixation is elected, such as spanning external fixation, then a metaphyseal bone graft or bone filler may be used instead. By placing a metaphyseal bone graft or bone substitute, it is possible to reduce the natural tendency for subsidence and loss of radial length following removal of the fixator at bony union. There are many types of graft material, including the gold standard of iliac crest graft, which has its own morbidity. Other more common grafts include freeze-dried cancellous croutons and calcium phosphate cements. These materials support the subchondral articular facets during the healing and remodeling phases and limit subsidence.

A 2006 trial randomized the use of allograft versus iliac crest autograft, both coupled with rigid internal fixation, and found no difference in any of the measured outcome parameters at 12 months.[41] However, surgical time was shorter in the allograft group.

Treatment Summary

Despite the present enthusiasm for volar locked plating, it is important to carefully consider the patient's requirements and expectations in devising a treatment plan. Not every fracture needs fixation, and some minimally displaced osteoporotic fractures may not require a formal reduction. Fracture types should be recognized, as well as their usual collapse patterns. The surgical anatomy should be mastered, including all the approaches to the various surfaces of the distal radius that are available for plate fixation (volar, dorsal, and midaxial radial column). Modern implants are available and sized for the patient's anatomy and have both fixed and variable axis trajectories, enabling stable fixation in even the most osteopenic patient. The most frequent complications of screw penetration are avoidable with attention to detail and proper radiographs. Patient outcome does not rest solely on the reassembly of fracture fragments, but more importantly on the maintenance of a mobile and sensate hand.

Table 4

Recent Comparative Level I Trials

Comparison	N	F/u (mos.)	Outcome Measures	Results
Cast vs CRPP (Wong et al 2009, *J Hand Surg Eur*)	60	20	rad, Mayo, ROM, str, healing rate/time	K-wire had better rad, Mayo score, healing rate/time all same
Cast vs CRPP* (Zyluk and Janowski 2007, *Chir Narzadow Ruchu Ortop Pol*)	60	6	DASH, rad, ROM, str	CRPP had better DASH, rad, str
Cast vs CRPP (Azzopardi et al 2005, *J Bone Joint Surg Br*)	57	12	SF-36, rad, ROM, str, ADLs	CRPP had better rad, but no functional improvement
Cast vs BF (Kreder et al 2006, *J Orthop Trauma*)	113	24	MFA, SF-36, rad, ROM, str	No statistical difference, but "trend" for ex fix better rad, function
CRPP vs VLP* (Rozental et al 2009, *J Bone Joint Surg Am*)	45	12	DASH, rad, ROM, str	No differences
CRPP vs ORIF[+] (Leung et al 2008, *J Bone Joint Surg Am*)	144	24	G+O, G+W, K+J Arth Score	Plate had better G+W scores (esp for C2 fracture)
CRPP vs ORIF[+] (Kreder et al 2005, *J Bone Joint Surg Br*)	179	24	MA, SF-36, rad, str, VAS, ROM	CRPP had faster return to function and better outcomes
NBF vs BF (Krukhaug et al 2009, *Acta Orthop*)	75	12	DASH, rad, VAS	No differences
BF vs ORIF[+] (Xu et al 2009, *Ann Acad Med Singapore*)	35	24	G+O, G+W, rad, ROM, str	No differences
BF+K-wire vs DP (Grewal et al 2005, *J Hand Surg Am*)	62	18	DASH, rad, ROM, str	DP had higher comp rate, longer tourniquet time
BF+K-wire vs VLP (Egol et al 2008; *J Bone Joint Surg Br*)	88	12	DASH, rad, ROM, str, physical therapy sessions	No differences, but fewer reoperations for ex fix (4.5% vs 11%)
BF vs VLP* vs RCP (Wei et al 2009, *J Bone Joint Surg Am*)	46	52	DASH, rad, ROM, str	No differences
DP vs VLP (Zettl et al 2009, *Unfallchirurg*)	120	12	rad, function, satisfaction	VLP had better rad, function. No difference in subjective satisfaction
DP vs VP (Huang 2008, *Zhongguo Xiu Fu Chong Jian Wai Ke Za Zhi*)	61	16	G+W, rad, ROM	G+W, rad were the same. DP had slightly better ROM.
DLP vs VLP* (Jakubietz 2008, *J Hand Surg Eur*)	30	6	G+W, rad, VAS, str	VLP better ROM, str, VAS, G+W

* These studies showed some benefit for this treatment at 3 or 6 months, but showed no benefit at longer time points, or did not include longer time points
[+] Either volar or dorsal plate, by surgeon preference
Abbreviations: CRPP = closed reduction and percutaneous pinning, ex fix = external fixation, BF = bridging external fixation, VP = volar plating, VLP = volar locked plating, ORIF = open reduction and internal fixation, NBF = nonbridging external fixation, DP = dorsal plating, RCP = radial column plating, rad = radiographic parameters, Mayo = Mayo Wrist Score, ROM = Range of motion, str = strength measurements, DASH = Disabilities of the Arm, Shoulder, and Hand survey, SF-36 = Short-Form 36 survey, ADL = activities of daily living, MFA = musculoskeletal function assessment, G+W = Gartland and Werley point system, G+O = Green and O'Brien scoring system

Outcomes

Patient-based evaluation methods are the best way to compare modern treatment results. Studies using these methods are only now becoming available for review.

The restoration of proper anatomy through treatment is always assumed to be paramount in obtaining good patient outcomes. Simply put, bad x-rays have traditionally been thought to imply bad outcomes. However, several recent studies have shown that excellent patient outcomes can be achieved despite malunions, particularly for the elderly population.[15-17] There are only a few long-term (more than 10 years) studies that have compared posttraumatic arthrosis

with patient-based outcomes, and these do not indicate that arthritis inevitably leads to a poor outcome.[42]

Recent research has shown that pain scores tend to dominate subjective outcomes in the first 6 months after surgery, while grip strength and range of motion are important later in recovery. This suggests that regaining range of motion is most important for long-term patient satisfaction, most notably with restoration of forearm supination.

The effect of psychosocial comorbidities has also been studied, and it has been found that the DASH score correlated with depression and pain anxiety but not neurosis, whereas strength and other performance-

3: Upper Extremity

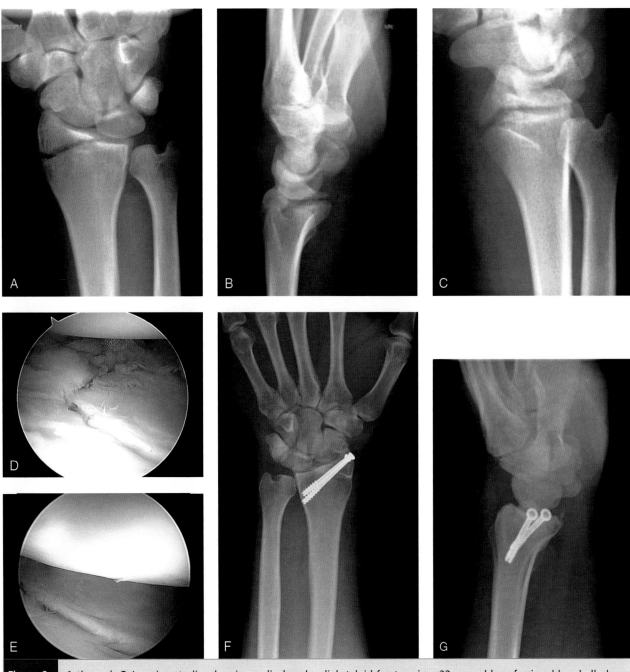

Figure 6   A through **C**, Imaging studies showing a displaced radial styloid fracture in a 22-year-old professional baseball player after a collision at home plate. A decision was made to perform arthroscopic-assisted reduction (**D** and **E**) and percutaneous fixation (**F** and **G**) with cannulated screws. Postoperative outcome was good, and the patient was able to return to spring training 2 months after surgery.

based measures were less affected by depression and other psychological factors.

Rehabilitation

Early mobilization is one of the advantages of stable internal fixation provided by modern locked plating techniques. Is this theoretical advantage realized in the rehabilitation of these patients? A 2006 Cochrane review of 15 trials involving 746 patients did not find that a

specific protocol demonstrated superior outcomes.[43] More recently, a randomized trial of 60 patients compared the effects of mobilization at 2 weeks versus a 6-week protocol in patients after volar plating for distal radius fractures.[44] The authors found no differences in range of motion, Gartland and Werley score, Mayo Wrist Score, or DASH scores. As has been previously mentioned, any associated intercarpal ligament or TFCC injuries could modify early mobilization protocols.

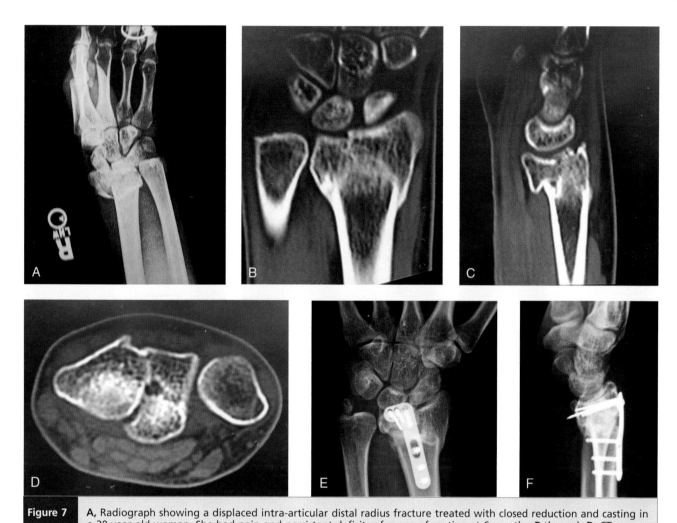

Figure 7 **A,** Radiograph showing a displaced intra-articular distal radius fracture treated with closed reduction and casting in a 20-year-old woman. She had pain and persistent deficits of range of motion at 6 months. **B** through **D,** CT scans reveal intra-articular malunion of the lunate facet causing mechanical block to supination. Dorsal intra-articular osteotomy was performed using fluoroscopic guidance. **E** and **F,** Radiographs 6 months after surgery. The patient had regained supination and was pain free.

In addition, several trials have examined the role of formal occupational or physical therapy in improving outcomes after distal radius fracture. Recent trials have looked at patients randomized to supervised physiotherapy versus a home exercise program, and no study has shown superiority in range of motion, strength, or outcome measures at 6 weeks.

Complications

Complications following distal radius fracture occur with or without surgical intervention and include tendon dysfunction and rupture, hand and wrist stiffness, and carpal tunnel syndrome. The frequency may depend on injury pattern and the elected treatment. The rates of both major and minor complications range from 7% to 44% in recent series.[34] Patient education and having full understanding of the potential for a poor outcome is a critical component of patient care.

Malunion remains the most common complication of distal radius fractures. In the elderly population,

treatment should address specific complaints, such as loss of supination. In the younger patient, gross anatomic deformity may require osteotomy and correction to realign the carpus and lessen the potential for premature arthritis, as well as to improve strength and mobility (**Figure 7**). If the patient's flexion and extension arc is good and the limitation is primarily in forearm rotation because of DRUJ incongruence, an ulnar shortening osteotomy is warranted to match the deformity and reestablish congruence.

Fortunately, nonunion and infection are rare complications, although they may be difficult to manage when present.[45] In nonunion, technical challenges exist most notably when a short end segment (less than 2 cm) is involved (**Figures 8** and **9**). Bone graft, calcium phosphate cement augmentation, combined dorsal and volar plating, and external fixation have been used separately and in combination. Some distal radius fractures are repaired with grafts and then bridge plated either to the metacarpal or the carpus. Prior to total wrist fusion,

3: Upper Extremity

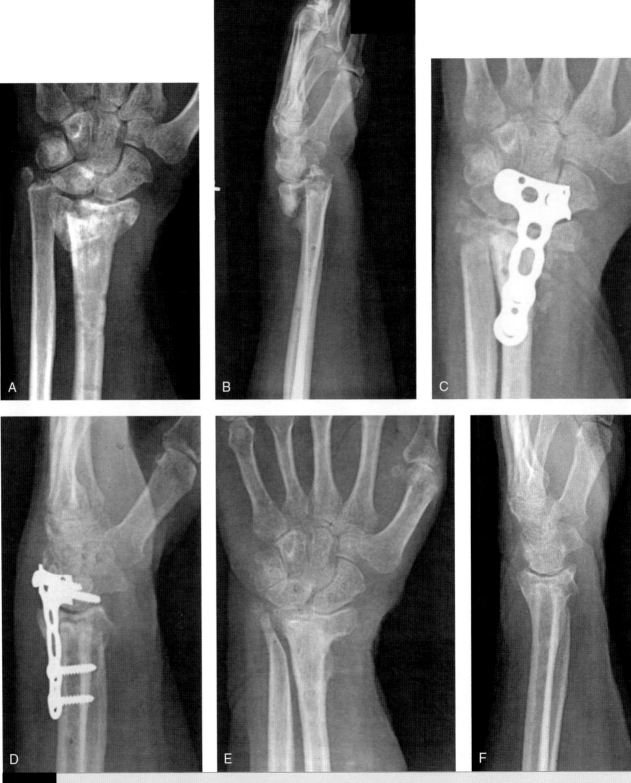

Figure 8   A 63-year-old woman with a known history of osteoporosis was treated with external fixation and percutaneous pinning. Four months postoperatively a nonunion of the distal radius was diagnosed, accompanied by pain and virtually no wrist motion. **A** and **B**, Radiographs show the extremely short end segment. Revision surgery included bridge plating to the proximal carpal row with demineralized bone matrix and allograft, as well as distal ulnar excision. **C** and **D**, Radiographs 6 months after surgery. The fracture had healed, and the patient had regained prosupination. The plate was then removed. **E** and **F**, Radiographs at 1 year.

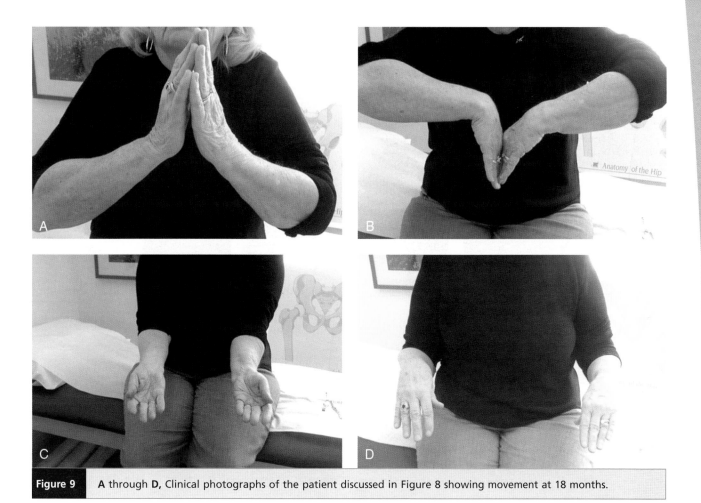

Figure 9   A through D, Clinical photographs of the patient discussed in Figure 8 showing movement at 18 months.

some of these fractures may be amenable to salvage with a distal radioscapholunate fusion.

A recent study showed the infection rate to be 7% in open distal radius fractures,[46] independent of Gustilo grade and time to débridement. Only gross contamination was a predictor of subsequent infection.

Complex regional pain syndrome (CRPS) is a common and often unrecognized complication of distal radius fractures with an incidence as high as 18%. The symptoms include hyperpathia, swelling, stiffness, and vascular changes out of proportion to the injury and treatment rendered. The incidence of CRPS does not significantly correlate to depression or other psychosocial factors. A provocative randomized trial of 416 patients compared the routine use of prophylactic vitamin C to placebo.[47] The group that received vitamin C had a significantly lower incidence of CRPS (2.4%) compared to the placebo group (10.1%).

Delayed tendon rupture continues to be an ongoing concern with both dorsal and volar plating. However, this condition may also occur with relatively nondisplaced distal radius fractures that are treated with casting. The extensor pollicis longus (EPL) tendon is the most common attritional rupture, although flexor tendon ruptures have also been reported. The EPL tendon can be adequately reconstructed with an extensor indices transfer. A more detailed discussion about tendon rupture and volar locked plating is presented in the preceding section on treatment.

Initial fracture displacement is an independent risk factor for carpal tunnel syndrome. The role of carpal tunnel release in the context of distal radius fractures remains controversial. There is no evidence to proceed with prophylactic release in patients with normal neurologic examination in whom plates are used. Patients with dense anesthesia after injury need urgent release, as do patients with a preexisting history of carpal tunnel syndrome. The obtunded patient presents a diagnostic challenge.

The surgeon must modify the surgical approach to incorporate the carpal tunnel release by using a more midline incision during both volar plating and carpal tunnel release. This approach is especially important to avoid injuring the palmar cutaneous branch of the median nerve, which lies between the typical flexor carpi radialis radial incision and the more midline carpal tunnel incision.

© 2010 American Academy of Orthopaedic Surgeons

3: Upper Extremity

The Future

Distal radius fractures are known to be an indicator of fragility fractures in the elderly, and as such, should trigger screening and treatment of osteoporosis when confirmed.[48] As osteoporosis is better understood and this public health epidemic is addressed, the severity and complexity of the geriatric distal radius fracture may diminish. However, continued high-energy injuries in the active population will lead to treatment advances including more minimally invasive techniques that reduce morbidity and improve patient outcomes. Such advances will be facilitated by large, multicenter clinical trials that can establish the high level of evidence that is necessary to influence surgeon behavior and clinical practice.

Summary

Fractures of the forearm typically occur after a traumatic event. Surgical treatment is necessary to restore proper function to the forearm. Distal radius fractures are associated with high-energy mechanisms of injury, and osteoporosis is also a predictor of susceptibility to these fractures. The rationale for surgical treatment is restoration of distal radius anatomy. The surgeon must have a knowledge of pathoanatomy, especially with regard to recognition of instability patterns, whether treating eponymous forearm injuries (Galeazzi, Monteggia) or wrist injuries (Barton, Smith). Patient outcomes and their relationship to the anatomic restoration of joint congruity and mechanics are important considerations in the treatment of these fractures.

Annotated References

1. Richard MJ, Ruch DS, Aldridge JM III: Malunions and nonunions of the forearm. *Hand Clin* 2007;23(2): 235-243.

    A review of nonunions and malunions of the forearm is presented. Nonunions require biology and stability for healing. Malunions often result in decreased range of motion and decreased grip strength. The forearm anatomy must be anatomically recreated to avoid malunion.

2. Sauder DJ, Athwal GS: Management of isolated ulnar shaft fractures. *Hand Clin* 2007;23(2):179-184.

    Isolated ulna fractures may appear benign. However, they may result in nonunion, malunion, and synostosis. Fractures displaced more than 50%, angulated more than 10 degrees, or are located in the proximal third of the ulna should be treated surgically. Stable fractures are managed well with forearm bracing.

3. Haugstvedt JR: Dislocations of the radius and ulna: Surgical anatomy and biomechanics, in Berter RA, Weiss APC, eds: *Hand Surgery*. Philadelphia, PA, Lippincott Williams and Wilkins, 2004, pp 615-644.

    The authors present a thorough discussion of the anatomy and biomechanics of radius and ulna dislocations.

4. Eglseder WA, Zadnik M: Monteggia fractures and variants: Review of distribution and nine irreducible radial head dislocations. *South Med J* 2006;99(7):723-727.

    One hundred twenty-one cases of Monteggia fractures and transolecranon fracture-dislocations were reviewed to determine the frequency of Bado types and the occurrences of irreducible radial head dislocations. The distribution of Monteggia fractures was 53 Bado type I, two Bado type II, eight Bado type III, and five Bado type IV. Nine irreducible radial head dislocations were encountered (8 in Bado type I fractures and one in Bado type IV fractures). A previously unreported cause of irreducible radial head was described of the biceps tendon.

5. Eathiraju S, Mudgal CS, Jupiter JB: Monteggia fracture-dislocations. *Hand Clin* 2007;23(2):165-177.

    The diagnosis and management of Monteggia fracture-dislocations is discussed. The fracture pattern of the ulnar fracture can influence optimal treatment. Associated radial head and coronoid fractures complicate these injury patterns and thereby alter the management and lead to worse outcomes.

6. Lindvall EM, Sagi HC: Selective screw placement in forearm compression plating: Results of 75 consecutive fractures stabilized with 4 cortices of screw fixation on either side of the fracture. *J Orthop Trauma* 2006; 20(3):157-162.

    Fifty-three patients with 75 diaphyseal forearm fractures were followed for an average of 14.6 months. All were treated with a plate three screw holes longer on each side of the fracture. The screw holes closest to and farthest from the fracture were filled. There was one atrophic nonunion in a type 2 open radius fracture. There were no hardware failures.

7. Crow BD, Mundis G, Anglen JO: Clinical results of minimal screw plate fixation of forearm fractures. *Am J Orthop* 2007;36(9):477-480.

    This is a retrospective review of 78 forearm fractures that were plated using "minimal" screw technique, less than the traditionally recommended 6 cortices of screw purchase. Nonunion or fixation failure occurred in seven fractures (five patients), producing a union rate of 91%. All nonunions were atrophic and occurred in open fractures with bone loss. No construct failed because of fixation loss caused by having too few screws.

8. Fulkerson E, Egol KA, Kubiak EN, Liporace F, Kummer FJ, Koval KJ: Fixation of diaphyseal fractures with a segmental defect: A biomechanical comparison of locked and conventional plating techniques. *J Trauma* 2006;60(4):830-835.

    A biomechanical analysis of synthetic bones simulating osteopenic ulnas evaluated bicortical locking, bicortical nonlocking, and unicortical locking screws. Bicortical locking screws withstood more cycles to failure. Plates placed farther away from bone also had more failure. Locking plates with unicortical locking screws should not be used in osteoporotic forearm fractures.

9. Martin WN, Field J, Kulkarni M: Intramedullary nailing of pathological forearm fractures. *Injury* 2002;33(6):530-532.

10. Lee YH, Lee SK, Chung MS, Baek GH, Gong HS, Kim KH: Interlocking contoured intramedullary nail fixation for selected diaphyseal fractures of the forearm in adults. *J Bone Joint Surg Am* 2008;90(9):1891-1898.

Thirty-eight interlocking nails were used in 27 adult forearm fractures. Average time to union was 14 weeks. There was one nonunion in an open ulna fracture; 81% patients had excellent results, 11% had good results, and 7% acceptable results. Supplemental immobilization was used until bridging callus was seen.

11. Ring D, Allende C, Jafarnia K, Allende BT, Jupiter JB: Ununited diaphyseal forearm fractures with segmental defects: Plate fixation and autogenous cancellous bone-grafting. *J Bone Joint Surg Am* 2004;86(11):2440-2445.

A retrospective review of 35 patients treated for forearm nonunion with plate and screw fixation with autogenous bone graft is presented. Follow-up was on average 43 months. All fractures healed within 6 months. Five patients had excellent results, 18 satisfactory results, and 11 had unsatisfactory results.

12. Chapman MW, Gordon JE, Zissimos AG: Compression-plate fixation of acute fractures of the diaphyses of the radius and ulna. *J Bone Joint Surg Am* 1989;71(2):159-169.

13. Wright RR, Schmeling GJ, Schwab JP: The necessity of acute bone grafting in diaphyseal forearm fractures: A retrospective review. *J Orthop Trauma* 1997;11(4):288-294.

14. Droll KP, Perna P, Potter J, Harniman E, Schemitsch EH, McKee MD: Outcomes following plate fixation of fractures of both bones of the forearm in adults. *J Bone Joint Surg Am* 2007;89(12):2619-2624.

Internal fixation of forearm fractures restores nearly normal anatomy and motion. However, there is a decreased grip strength, forearm strength, and wrist strength, even at 5 years after injury. Pain is the primary determinant of DASH and Short Form-36 scores.

15. Synn AJ, Makhni EC, Makhni MC, Rozental TD, Day CS: Distal radius fractures in older patients: Is anatomic reduction necessary? *Clin Orthop Relat Res* 2009;467(6):1612-1620.

The authors present a retrospective study of 53 patients older than 55 years with distal radius fractures, comparing radiographic results to functional outcome measures. They found no relationship between anatomic reduction and subjective or objective functional outcomes. Level of evidence: Diagnostic level II.

16. Grewal R, MacDermid JC: The risk of adverse outcomes in extra-articular distal radius fractures is increased with malalignment in patients of all ages but mitigated in older patients. *J Hand Surg Am* 2007;32(7):962-970.

The authors present a prospective observational study on 216 patients with extra-articular distal radius fractures. Radiographic parameters as well as patient outcome measures were assessed. They found that patients older than 65 years showed no significant relationship between malalignment and patient outcomes. Level of evidence: Prognostic level II.

17. Arora R, Gabl M, Gschwentner M, Deml C, Krappinger D, Lutz M: A comparative study of clinical and radiologic outcomes of unstable colles type distal radius fractures in patients older than 70 years: Nonoperative treatment versus volar locking plating. *J Orthop Trauma* 2009;23(4):237-242.

The authors present a retrospective study of 130 consecutive patients older than 70 years who were treated with open reduction and internal fixation (ORIF) versus cast treatment based on surgeon preference. Radiographic results were significantly better in patients with ORIF, but there was no difference in clinical outcome scores. Level of evidence: Therapeutic level III.

18. Kettler M, Kuhn V, Schieker M, Melone CP: Do we need to include osteoporosis in today's classification of distal radius fractures? *J Orthop Trauma* 2008;22(8 Suppl):S79-S82.

The effect of osteoporosis and bone mineral density on distal radius fractures is evaluated in a review article. The status of current classification systems is also discussed.

19. Zenke Y, Sakai A, Oshige T, Moritani S, Nakamura T: The effect of an associated ulnar styloid fracture on the outcome after fixation of a fracture of the distal radius. *J Bone Joint Surg Br* 2009;91(1):102-107.

One hundred eighteen consecutive patients with distal radius fracture were treated with a volar locking plate in this case series. No differences in radiologic and clinical results based on presence or type of ulnar styloid fracture were found. Level of evidence: Prognostic level IV.

20. Souer JS, Ring D, Matschke S, Audige L, Marent-Huber M, Jupiter JB; AOCID Prospective ORIF Distal Radius Study Group: Effect of an unrepaired fracture of the ulnar styloid base on outcome after plate-and-screw fixation of a distal radial fracture. *J Bone Joint Surg Am* 2009;91(4):830-838.

A retrospective comparative study was done on 76 pairs of patients with distal radius fractures with and without ulnar styloid base fractures. The authors found no difference in clinical outcomes between those with untreated styloid fractures and those without styloid fractures. Level of evidence: Therapeutic level III.

21. van Leerdam RH, Souer JS, Lindenhovius AL, Ring DC: Agreement between initial classification and subsequent reclassification of fractures of the distal radius in a prospective cohort study. *Hand* 2010;5(1):68-71.

The postinjury radiographs of 621 patients with distal radius fractures were examined in a prospective cohort study. Classification was done according to the Comprehensive Classification of Fractures by the surgeon and then a research team. Only moderate agreement of the classification of fractures was found between investigators. Level of evidence: Diagnostic level III.

3: Upper Extremity

22. Grewal R, MacDermid JC, Pope J, Chesworth BM: Baseline predictors of pain and disability one year following extra-articular distal radius fractures. *Hand* 2007;2(3):104-111.

In a prospective cohort study of 22 patients with extra-articular distal radius fractures, initial radiographs were compared with patient-based outcome scores. At 1 year, no injury characteristic was found to significantly influence patient outcomes. Level of evidence: Prognostic level I.

23. Mackenney PJ, McQueen MM, Elton R: Prediction of instability in distal radial fractures. *J Bone Joint Surg Am* 2006;88(9):1944-1951.

Four thousand patients with distal radius fractures were assessed in a prospective observational study. Demographic data, mode of injury, and radiographic parameters were all compared with radiographic alignment at 1 and 6 weeks after injury. Patient age, metaphyseal comminution, and ulnar variance were the most consistent predictors of outcome. Level of evidence: Prognostic level I.

24. Batra S, Debnath U, Kanvinde R: Can carpal malalignment predict early and late instability in nonoperatively managed distal radius fractures? *Int Orthop* 2008;32(5):685-691.

Patients with distal radius fractures were studied retrospectively and initial radiographic parameters were compared with results at 1 and 6 weeks. Prereduction axial shortening, dorsal angulation, and radiocarpal malalignment correlated with early loss of reduction at 1 week. Level of evidence: Prognostic level II.

25. Bong MR, Egol KA, Leibman M, Koval KJ: A comparison of immediate postreduction splinting constructs for controlling initial displacement of fractures of the distal radius: A prospective randomized study of long-arm versus short-arm splinting. *J Hand Surg Am* 2006;31(5):766-770.

One hundred eighteen patients with distal radius fractures were treated with either a short-arm radial gutter splint or a sugar tong splint in a randomized controlled trial. Both splints had comparable performance in maintaining initial reduction, although the short-arm splint was better tolerated by patients. Level of evidence: Prognostic level II.

26. Glickel SZ, Catalano LW, Raia FJ, Barron OA, Grabow R, Chia B: Long-term outcomes of closed reduction and percutaneous pinning for the treatment of distal radius fractures. *J Hand Surg Am* 2008;33(10):1700-1705.

Fifty-five patients with distal radius fractures treated with closed reduction and percutaneous pinning were reviewed retrospectively and followed up at an average of 59 months using radiographic assessment, objective examination, and patient-based outcome scores. These patients had an excellent range of motion and normal DASH scores. Level of evidence: Therapeutic level IV.

27. Wei DH, Raizman NM, Bottino CJ, Jobin CM, Strauch RJ, Rosenwasser MP: Unstable distal radial fractures treated with external fixation, a radial column plate, or a volar plate: A prospective randomized trial. *J Bone Joint Surg Am* 2009;91(7):1568-1577.

Forty-six patients with distal radius fractures were randomized to external fixation versus volar plate versus radial column plate. The authors found that the use of a locked volar plate led to better DASH scores in the first 3 months, but no differences between groups at 6 months and 1 year. Level of evidence: Therapeutic level I.

28. Hayes AJ, Duffy PJ, McQueen MM: Bridging and nonbridging external fixation in the treatment of unstable fractures of the distal radius: A retrospective study of 588 patients. *Acta Orthop* 2008;79(4):540-547.

A retrospective study of 588 patients comparing bridging with nonbridging external fixation is presented. Fractures with bridging external fixation had a sixfold increased risk of dorsal malunion and 2.5-fold risk of radial shortening. Level of evidence: Therapeutic level III.

29. Strauss EJ, Banerjee D, Kummer FJ, Tejwani NC: Evaluation of a novel, nonspanning external fixator for treatment of unstable extra-articular fractures of the distal radius: Biomechanical comparison with a volar locking plate. *J Trauma* 2008;64(4):975-981.

The authors present a biomechanical study comparing the stability of the CPX nonspanning external fixator with a standard volar locked plate in fresh frozen human distal radii. Both constructs were biomechanically equivalent in their experimental model.

30. Egol KA, Paksima N, Puopolo S, Klugman J, Hiebert R, Koval KJ: Treatment of external fixation pins about the wrist: A prospective, randomized trial. *J Bone Joint Surg Am* 2006;88(2):349-354.

One hundred eighteen patients with external fixators for distal radius fractures were randomized to weekly dry dressing changes, daily pin site care with washing, and treatment with chlorhexidine discs around the pins. There was no change in infection rate with treatment type. Level of evidence: Therapeutic level I.

31. Capo JT, Kinchelow T, Brooks K, Tan V, Manigrasso M, Francisco K: Biomechanical stability of four fixation constructs for distal radius fractures. *Hand* 2009;4(3):272-278.

The authors present a biomechanical study comparing dorsal nonlocked plating, volar locked plating, radial-ulnar dual-column plating, and locked intramedullary fixation and cadaver radii. They found that volar locked plates had higher stiffness, strength, and resistance to displacement in comparison with dorsal and dual column plating. Volar locked plating and intramedullary fixation achieved comparable stability.

32. Kim RY, Rosenwasser MP: Internal fixation of distal radius fractures. *Am J Orthop* 2007;36(12, Suppl 2):2-7.

This review article describes the current technology in volar plating, dorsal plating, and radial plating of distal radius fractures.

33. Grindel SI, Wang M, Gerlach M, McGrady LM, Brown S: Biomechanical comparison of fixed-angle volar plate versus fixed-angle volar plate plus fragment-specific fixation in a cadaveric distal radius fracture model. *J Hand*

Surg Am 2007;32(2):194-199.

This biomechanical study compared fixed-angle volar plating with the addition of fragment-specific fixation in cadaver distal radii. The addition of fragment-specific plating provides superior biomechanical strength and stability.

34. Arora R, Lutz M, Hennerbichler A, Krappinger D, Espen D, Gabl M: Complications following internal fixation of unstable distal radius fracture with a palmar locking-plate. *J Orthop Trauma* 2007;21(5):316-322.

One hundred fourteen patients treated with volar locked plating for distal radius fractures were examined in a prospective observational study. These patients had improved stability but there was a significant incidence of complications with volar locked plates. Level of evidence: Therapeutic level IV.

35. Al-Rashid M, Theivendran K, Craigen MA: Delayed ruptures of the extensor tendon secondary to the use of volar locking compression plates for distal radial fractures. *J Bone Joint Surg Br* 2006;88(12):1610-1612.

The authors describe the common complications of volar plating for distal radius fractures and provide three case reports of extensor tendon rupture and volar plating.

36. Soong M, Got C, Katarincic J, Akelman E: Fluoroscopic evaluation of intra-articular screw placement during locked volar plating of the distal radius: A cadaveric study. *J Hand Surg Am* 2008;33(10):1720-1723.

The authors present a biomechanical cadaver study that evaluated the ability of fluoroscopic views to assess intra-articular screw penetration using volar locked plating of distal radius fractures. They found that multiple oblique views are required to accurately evaluate screw placement.

37. Thomas AD, Greenberg JA: Use of fluoroscopy in determining screw overshoot in the dorsal distal radius: A cadaveric study. *J Hand Surg Am* 2009;34(2):258-261.

The ability of practitioners to assess dorsal cortex penetration of volar plate screws using multiple fluoroscopic images was evaluated in a biomechanical cadaver study. Evaluators with more than 3 years of experience were better at detecting incorrect screw positions, and ulnar-positioned screws were more difficult to accurately evaluate.

38. Ilyas AM, Thoder JJ: Intramedullary fixation of displaced distal radius fractures: A preliminary report. *J Hand Surg Am* 2008;33(10):1706-1715.

In a case series, 10 patients with distal radius fractures were treated with intramedullary nailing. This procedure can result in good functional outcomes but is associated with a high incidence of complications. Level of evidence: Therapeutic level IV.

39. Hanel DP, Lu TS, Weil WM: Bridge plating of distal radius fractures: The Harborview method. *Clin Orthop Relat Res* 2006;445:91-99.

The authors present a case series of 62 patients and the Harborview bridge plating technique for distal radius

fractures. Level of evidence: Therapeutic level IV.

40. Varitimidis SE, Basdekis GK, Dailiana ZH, Hantes ME, Bargiotas K, Malizos K: Treatment of intra-articular fractures of the distal radius: Fluoroscopic or arthroscopic reduction? *J Bone Joint Surg Br* 2008;90(6):778-785.

Forty patients with fluoroscopic reduction with and without arthroscopic assistance were assessed in a randomized controlled study. The authors found a relatively high incidence of TFCC tears, scapholunate interosseous ligament tears, and lunotriquetral tears. DASH scores were similar at 24 months, and Mayo wrist scores were better for the arthroscopy group. Level of evidence: Therapeutic level I.

41. Rajan GP, Fornaro J, Trentz O, Zellweger R: Cancellous allograft versus autologous bone grafting for repair of comminuted distal radius fractures: A prospective, randomized trial. *J Trauma* 2006;60(6):1322-1329.

The authors present a randomized controlled study of 90 patients in whom iliac crest bone graft and "tutoplast" bone-graft substitute were compared. The authors found comparable Demerit Point System scores at 12 months and more complications with iliac crest graft. Level of evidence: Therapeutic level I.

42. Forward DP, Davis TR, Sithole JS: Do young patients with malunited fractures of the distal radius inevitably develop symptomatic post-traumatic osteoarthritis? *J Bone Joint Surg Br* 2008;90(5):629-637.

One hundred six patients with distal radius fractures were reviewed retrospectively, with a mean follow-up of 38 years. There was radiologic evidence of osteoarthritis in 68% of patients, although DASH scores were not different from population norms. Level of evidence: Therapeutic level IV.

43. Handoll HH, Madhok R, Howe TE: Rehabilitation for distal radial fractures in adults. *Cochrane Database Syst Rev* 2006;3:CD003324.

The authors present a Cochrane meta-analysis of 15 trials involving 746 patients to examine the effects of rehabilitation on patients with distal radius fractures. There was insufficient evidence to establish the relative effectiveness of the various interventions used in rehabilitation.

44. Lozano-Calderón SA, Souer S, Mudgal C, Jupiter JB, Ring D: Wrist mobilization following volar plate fixation of fractures of the distal part of the radius. *J Bone Joint Surg Am* 2008;90(6):1297-1304.

In a randomized controlled study, 60 patients with distal radius fractures were treated with volar plate fixation. Mobilization was compared within 2 weeks or at 6 weeks. No significant differences were found with regard to Mayo wrist score, Gartland and Werley score, or DASH scores. Level of evidence: Therapeutic level I.

45. Crow SA, Chen L, Lee JH, Rosenwasser MP: Vascularized bone grafting from the base of the second metacarpal for persistent distal radius nonunion: A case report. *J Orthop Trauma* 2005;19(7):483-486.

3: Upper Extremity

In this case report, a distal radius fracture nonunion was treated with a vascularized bone graft from the base of the second metacarpal and combined with biplanar stable fixation and allogenic bone graft.

46. Glueck DA, Charoglu CP, Lawton JN: Factors associated with infection following open distal radius fractures. *Hand* 2009;4(3):330-334.

In a retrospective review of infection rates in 42 open distal radius fractures, no relationship was found between infection rate and Gustilo and Anderson type, Swanson type, or time to initial irrigation and debridement. There was a correlation between gross contamination and infection. Level of evidence: Prognostic level III.

47. Zollinger PE, Tuinebreijer WE, Breederveld RS, Kreis RW: Can vitamin C prevent complex regional pain syndrome in patients with wrist fractures? A randomized, controlled, multicenter dose-response study. *J Bone Joint Surg Am* 2007;89(7):1424-1431.

In a randomized controlled study, 416 patients with distal radius fractures were treated with three different doses of vitamin C versus placebo. Vitamin C reduces the risk of complex regional pain syndrome at 50 days. Level of evidence: Therapeutic level I.

48. Rozental TD, Makhni EC, Day CS, Bouxsein ML: Improving evaluation and treatment for osteoporosis following distal radius fractures: A prospective randomized intervention. *J Bone Joint Surg Am* 2008;90(5):953-961.

The authors present a therapeutic trial in patients with fragility fractures of the distal radius, examining the effect of the treating surgeon ordering a bone mineral density study versus sending a letter to the primary care provider. They found that rates of treatment for osteoporosis were relatively low, but that ordering a bone mineral density study improves osteoporosis treatment rates. Level of evidence: Therapeutic level I.

Chapter 21

Injuries of the Hand and Carpus

David A. Fuller, MD   John T. Capo, MD

Epidemiology

Fractures of the hand are the second most common fracture after forearm fractures, accounting for up to 20% of all fractures. Prior-incidence and demographic studies reporting on hand fractures have been limited by failure to capture entire populations. A recent study from British Columbia, Canada, attempted to capture data for an entire population over a 5-year period. The total number of hand fractures as well as age, gender, and seasonal and geographic variation is reported for this population. For the total population, the annual incidence rate for a hand fracture was 36 per 10,000; 50% were phalangeal fractures, 42% metacarpal fractures, and 8% multiple. The most common age for a hand fracture was 14 years for males and 13 years for females. Males showed a relatively greater risk of a hand fracture than females up until age 60 years, whereas females showed a greater relative risk after age 65 years. An increase in hand fractures during adolescence was likely related to increased behavioral risk factors such as participation in higher risk recreational, sports, and occupational activities.[1]

The various types of acute sports-related hand fractures were evaluated in Edinburgh, Scotland, in the adult population. Of all hand fractures, 22.4% were related to sports. Males were more commonly injured (86%). Phalangeal fractures were 54%, 33.8% were metacarpal fractures, and 12.2% were carpal fractures. The first and fifth rays were the most commonly injured, accounting for 57.3% of injuries. Football (soccer) was the most common cause of sports-related hand fractures, accounting for 35.9% of the total number. Most hand fractures (87.2%) were treated nonsurgically.[2]

The treatment of hand fractures is reported to vary widely in different regions of the world. This variability is caused by availability of resources, social factors, geographic constraints, surgeon preference and experi-

ence, and local practice patterns. Physicians are encouraged to recognize the limitations of the health care system under which they are working when making treatment decisions. Application of technologic advances and increased sophistication of treatment can add significant cost to treatment of hand fractures.[3]

A better understanding of epidemiology may enhance the ability to predict the cost and economic impact of hand fractures, and may improve efforts and prevention through public safety efforts, protective equipment, and environmental modification.

Scaphoid Fractures

The scaphoid bone is critical for proper function of the wrist because it is the link between the proximal and distal rows of the carpus. Proper and early diagnosis of scaphoid fractures is critical because this injury can present as only minor pain that may subside in a short period; it has a high chance of nonunion because of the retrograde blood supply; and nonunion results in a predictable pattern of collapse, arthrosis, and wrist pain. The mechanism of injury usually consists of a fall onto an extended hand and can be a result of low-energy or high-energy trauma.

Clinical examination includes dorsal-radial wrist swelling and tenderness in the anatomic snuffbox. Access to the snuffbox is improved with ulnar deviation of the wrist. The Watson test (palpation of the scaphoid tubercle with radial deviation of the wrist) and grind test (pain at the scaphoid with axial loading of the thumb metacarpal) may also be positive with a scaphoid fracture.

Diagnostic Imaging

Appropriate radiographs for a suspected scaphoid fracture include a true PA view, and lateral and PA views in wrist ulnar deviation (scaphoid view). This ulnar deviation posture elongates and moderately distracts the scaphoid image, thereby detecting some subtle fractures. If a scaphoid fracture is suspected but not demonstrated on initial radiographs, then the current standard of care is splinting and clinical and radiographic follow-up at 10 to 14 days. If the follow-up examination remains equivocal or if a diagnosis is desired at an earlier time, then higher level imaging studies can be

Dr. Capo or an immediate family member has received royalties from Wright Medical Technology; serves as a paid consultant for or is an employee of Wright Medical Technology and Synthes; and has received research or institutional support from Synthes and Wright Medical Technology. Neither Dr. Fuller nor any immediate family member has received anything of value from or owns stock in a commercial company or institution related directly or indirectly to the subject of this article.

3: Upper Extremity

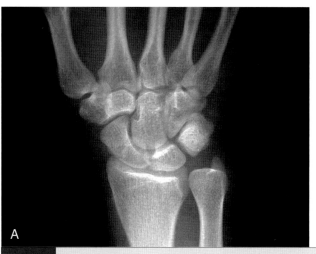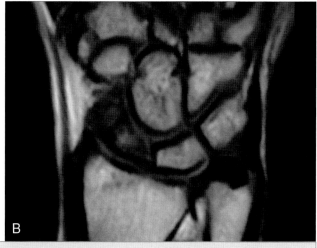

| Figure 1 | **A,** PA radiograph showing a questionable fracture in a 35-year-old woman. **B,** MRI scan taken at 5 days after injury verifying clear midwaist fracture and surrounding bone marrow edema. |

performed. Currently MRI is the best study to evaluate for occult scaphoid fractures (**Figure 1**).

The diagnostic accuracy of MRI evaluation was recently studied in a meta-analysis.[4] Twenty-two original research publications addressing the diagnostic performance characteristics of MRI for evaluation of suspected scaphoid fracture were analyzed. The average sensitivity was 98%, specificity 99%, and accuracy 96%. The prevalence-adjusted negative predictive value was 1.00, but the average prevalence-adjusted positive predictive value was 0.88. Prevalence-adjusted values were calculated using the average prevalence of true scaphoid fractures among suspected fractures of 7%, as documented in an earlier study.[5] Thus, an MRI interpreted as showing no fracture is nearly 100% reliable, but an MRI interpreted as showing a fracture indicates a true fracture only 88% of the time. Twelve percent of the time there is no fracture despite the positive findings on MRI. Some of these falsely positive results may be artifacts, normal variation, or bone bruises and often require follow-up diagnostic studies. It is therefore more likely that a fracture of the scaphoid will be diagnosed when no fracture exists than that a true fracture will be missed when using MRI for evaluation of occult fracture. This overtreatment is generally accepted so that no fractures will be missed.

In another study, 30 patients were evaluated using CT scan for suspected scaphoid fractures;[6] 13 had a confirmed nondisplaced fracture demonstrated on plain films, and 17 had no scaphoid fracture at initial presentation or on 6-week follow-up radiographs. The resulting sensitivity for detection of a nondisplaced fracture was 89%, the specificity was 91%, and the accuracy was 89%. Because of the low sensitivity, the authors of this study caution against the routine use of CT for triage of occult scaphoid fractures.

The accuracy and cost of differing imaging modalities used for evaluation of occult scaphoid fractures

was also analyzed in a 2008 study.[7] In a group of 200 patients with suspected scaphoid fractures and negative initial radiographs, 32 (16%) were subsequently found to have a true fracture. Male gender and a mechanism of injury during sporting activities were factors found to lead to a significantly higher incidence of true fracture. MRI was found to be the most accurate modality, but also the most expensive. Cost effectiveness of using MRI was also studied recently in a randomized study. Twenty-eight patients with suspected scaphoid fractures were randomized into an MRI or a non-MRI treatment protocol.[8] Of the patients without fracture, the MRI group had significantly fewer days of immobilization (3.0 versus 10; P = 0.006), and used fewer health care units (three versus five; P = 0.03) when factors such as consultation visits and physiotherapy costs were included. However, the median cost of health care in the MRI group ($594.35 Australian dollars) was slightly higher than in the control group ($428.15) ($P$ = 0.19 for the difference). When the cost of lost work and productivity was factored in, the addition of MRI became cost effective 95% of the time, when a typical laborer became 50% less productive. It was concluded that the use of MRI in the management of occult scaphoid fracture reduces the number of days of unnecessary immobilization and use of health care units. The savings in health care dollars increases as the wage level of the individual increases and decreases as the patient can do more of work-related activities with cast immobilization.

Comparison of Surgical and Nonsurgical Treatment

The most efficacious treatment of nondisplaced scaphoid waist fractures has been a highly debated topic over the past decade and is reflected in the literature by several studies.[9,10] Less invasive techniques and quicker recoveries seem to favor the surgical approach; however, unnecessary surgery may be occurring for injuries that would otherwise heal uneventfully in a nonsurgical fashion.

In a study from the Netherlands, 71 patients with nondisplaced scaphoid fractures diagnosed with radiograph, MRI, and CT were retrospectively reviewed.[9] There were 6 proximal pole, 50 waist, and 15 distal pole fractures. Of these patients, 58 or 82% demonstrated full clinical healing, and 33% had radiographic union after 6 weeks of thumb spica cast immobilization. Eleven patients required an additional 2 weeks for radiographic union and 2 required more than 12 weeks. There were no instances of nonunion. It was suggested that nonsurgical treatment should be considered for nondisplaced scaphoid fractures, as this protocol resulted in outcomes similar to those of protocols for early surgical intervention.

In a prospective, randomized study,[11] 60 patients were randomized into either a surgical or nonsurgical group for a nondisplaced waist fracture of the scaphoid. The surgical group was treated with a percutaneous screw from a volar approach, and the nonsurgical group received a short arm with the thumb free. Functional outcome including range of motion, grip, and pinch strength was improved at the early time points in the surgically treated group, but these differences equalized at 6 months. The surgical group had a quicker return to sports activity (6.4 weeks versus 15.5 weeks), and full employment (3.8 weeks versus 11.4 weeks), and a quicker union rate (9.2 weeks versus 13.9 weeks). The patients treated with surgery had a low complication rate with one prominent screw and no instances of infection or osteonecrosis. There were two patients with osteonecrosis in the cast group, three with malunion with dorsal intercalated segment instability (DISI) and one with radioscaphoid arthrosis. It was recommended that all active patients with a fracture of the waist of the scaphoid be offered percutaneous internal fixation.

In another study, 88 patients with a midwaist scaphoid fracture were randomized into two treatment arms: nonsurgical treatment with a short arm standard (thumb-free) cast or early surgical fixation through an open volar approach.[12] In the final evaluation, 71 patients were available for follow-up at a mean of 93 months (minimum of 73 months). There was no statistically significant difference in clinical outcome including range of motion and grip strength. Radiographic parameters (in 59 patients) were improved in the surgical group, with 0 of 28 in the surgical group and 5 of 31 in the cast group having an abnormal scapholunate angle. There was no screw back-out and none of the screws had to be removed. In the cast group, 10 patients had a nonunion at 12 weeks, whereas all of the fractures in the surgically treated patients healed. DISI was seen only in patients treated with a cast ($P = 0.02$).

A meta-analysis of the literature comparing surgical and nonsurgical treatment of acute nondisplaced and minimally displaced scaphoid waist fractures was published in 2009.[13] Of 111 available articles covering this topic, 12 studies were deemed as acceptable with good research methods. There were three randomized controlled trials comparing percutaneous fixation with casting, three randomized controlled trials compared open reduction and internal fixation (ORIF) with casting, two meta-analyses, a cost utility analysis, and three retrospective studies. When comparing percutaneous fixation with casting, surgical treatment resulted in a faster time to union by approximately 5 weeks and an earlier return to sports and work activities by approximately 7 weeks, with similar union rates. When comparing ORIF and cast treatment, there was no difference in the time to return to work, and function was similar over the long term. There was a significantly higher nonunion rate with cast treatment, and there was a 30% complication rate with ORIF. Manual workers are able to return to work significantly earlier after ORIF than cast treatment, producing a reduction in work disability costs. Cast treatment is more cost effective than ORIF for nonmanual workers because almost 40% are able to return to work with a cast. It was concluded that most patients can be treated in a cast with reliable and predictable results although with a potentially higher risk of nonunion. Surgical treatment should be reserved for patients who are unable to work while wearing a cast. Percutaneous treatment may offer the benefit of a faster union time and a lower complication rate than ORIF.

A cost analysis model comparing ORIF of scaphoid fractures with casting that consisted of long arm cast wear for 6 weeks followed by short arm immobilization for 4 weeks has also been published, providing an additional opinion on this controversial topic.[14] The authors included the cost of treatment by the provider and facility, along with the costs of lost income and productivity as experienced by the patient and employer. The model was tested by giving a questionnaire to medical students and determining their willingness to undergo certain treatments. Possible treatment paths were developed for a typical worker with a yearly income of $35,000. The final cost of ORIF was nearly half of the total cost of casting ($7,900 versus $13,851). The authors concluded that ORIF provides an increase in quality-adjusted life-years and earlier return to function, and that these data are a compelling case for adoption of ORIF as the standard of care for patients who are most affected by scaphoid fractures.

Surgical Treatment Methods

A recent study compared the dorsal and volar approach for percutaneous scaphoid fixation.[15] In a sequential cases series, no difference in functional outcomes or complication rate was found between the two treatment methods. All fractures healed, although there was one delayed union in the volar group. Radiographic evaluation of screw position revealed that the dorsal approach provided a screw more parallel to the long axis of the scaphoid ($P = 0.019$) and more perpendicu-

3: Upper Extremity

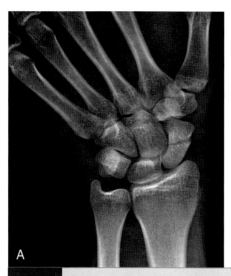
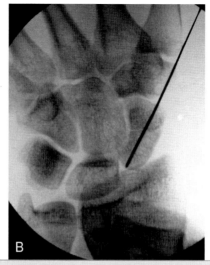
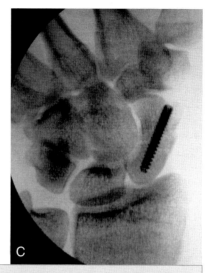

Figure 2   **A,** Preoperative ulnar deviation view demonstrating a minimally displaced scaphoid waist fracture. **B,** Intraoperative view showing proper placement of the guidewire from a volar retrograde approach. **C,** Final screw placement with proper recession of the screw's proximal and distal ends and compression of the fracture.

lar to the fracture line ($P < 0.05$). Because of this improved position of the screw, the dorsal approach can be used routinely because it provides better targeting and more precise placement. The dorsal percutaneous approach has also recently been evaluated in a cadaver model.[16] Using 40 cadavers, the guidewire for a standard dorsal percutaneous approach was placed in the center portion of the scaphoid and the surrounding soft tissues were then exposed. There were five patients with tendon injury, wherein the guidewire penetrated a wrist or finger extensor tendon. It was recommended that a small open incision and blunt dissection be used for direct viewing of the scaphoid proximal pole.

In an attempt to expand the indications for percutaneous treatment, displaced scaphoid fractures have recently been treated percutaneously using arthroscopic assistance.[17] The study included 13 patients treated from a dorsal approach and 7 from a volar retrograde approach. The fracture fragments were manipulated by percutaneously applied Kirschner wire (K-wire) joysticks and a variety of instruments. At an average follow-up of 18 months (minimum, 6 months), all fractures healed and there were no implant problems, implying that percutaneous treatment may be a viable technique for even displaced fractures.

Scaphoid Nonunions

For scaphoid nonunions without structural collapse (humpback deformity) and without clear avascular changes, percutaneous screw fixation alone has shown promising early results. Multiple authors have reported success with the percutaneous treatment of early scaphoid nonunions without collapse by using only a screw and without supplementary bone graft.[18,19] The technique can be done from a dorsal or volar approach

and can be combined with arthroscopy to confirm fragment alignment and maintenance of the cartilaginous shell of the scaphoid (**Figure 2**). The dorsal approach, with screw fixation and no bone grafting, was used in 15 patients with fibrous nonunions without sclerosis. All of the nonunions healed, and there were 12 excellent and 3 good patient outcomes.[19]

The goal in treatment of an established scaphoid nonunion with collapse is restoration of the normal anatomy and union of the fracture fragments. A volar approach with standard, nonvascularized wedge grafting from the iliac crest or distal radius still provides reliable results. For difficult nonunions, a vascularized bone graft has been suggested. The outcomes of vascularized bone grafting appear to be not as good as previously thought. An evaluation of 50 scaphoid nonunions treated with the 1-2 intercompartmental supraretinacular artery pedicle vascularized bone graft (1-2 ICSR) from the distal radius has been reported.[20] The authors report union in 34 of 50 patients (68%) at an average of 15.6 weeks. Complications occurred in 8 patients that included graft extrusion, deep infection, and failure of correction. The following risk factors were found for decreased healing: older age (30.5 versus 21.3 years), proximal pole osteonecrosis, preoperative humpback deformity, nonscrew fixation, tobacco use, and female sex. The decreased success rate compared to previous reports was attributed to a broader patient selection criteria. Small or collapsed proximal fragments, severe scapholunate dissociation, and a humpback deformity with substantial bone loss are considered contraindications to the procedure.

In an attempt to improve upon their results, some of the same authors developed a new technique for treating these difficult nonunions using a free vascularized structural graft from the medial femoral condyle.[21] A retrospective review was conducted on 22 patients with

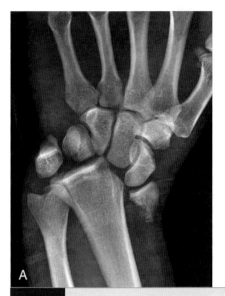
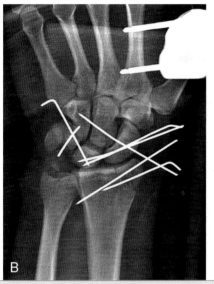
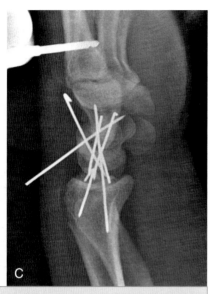

Figure 3 **A,** PA radiograph showing a transstyloid perilunate dislocation. **B** and **C,** Postoperative PA and lateral radiographs, respectively, demonstrating restoration of carpal alignment and the radial articular surface. An external fixator was used to span the wrist because of the high-energy nature of the injury.

a scaphoid waist nonunion associated with an avascular proximal pole and carpal collapse. Ten were treated with a 1-2 ICSR graft and 12 with a free vascularized medial femoral condyle graft, based on surgeon preference. Four of the 10 nonunions treated with the distal radial pedicle graft healed at a median of 19 weeks, and all 12 nonunions treated with the free medial femoral condyle graft healed at a median of 13 weeks. The rate of union and the median time to healing was significantly better for the patients treated with the medial femoral condyle graft. It was concluded that vascularized interposition bone graft from the medial femoral condyle is the preferred vascularized bone graft for the treatment of scaphoid waist nonunions with avascularity of the proximal pole and carpal collapse.

Perilunate Injuries

Perilunate dislocations are severe injuries that usually are a result of high-energy trauma to the wrist. They can be associated with acute carpal tunnel syndrome and open injuries. Proper treatment generally involves initial closed treatment and splinting followed by surgical treatment on a semielective basis if there is no skin or nerve compromise. Fixation involves a dorsal approach for reduction of the carpal bones and fixation of the intrinsic and extrinsic carpal ligaments. A volar-ulnar extensile approach is recommended to decompress the carpal tunnel and repair the volar midcarpal ligament tear. There are often osteochondral fragments that need to be repaired and excised on either the dorsal or volar sides. Fixation requires K-wire stabilization in an anatomic position, stabilizing the proximal carpal row as well as the midcarpal joint. These pins should

be left under the skin and left in place for 10 to 12 weeks. If the injury is a transscaphoid perilunate variant, a headless screw can be placed antegrade from the dorsal approach. A transradial styloid variant requires stabilization of the radius, which anchors the important radioscaphocapitate ligament (**Figure 3**).

A recent report evaluated outcomes of transscaphoid perilunate dislocations treated either early (3 days) or late (26 days) because of a delay in diagnosis.[22] In this series of only 12 patients with an average follow-up time of 45 months (range, 23 to 70 months), the authors found decreased grip strength (26 kg versus 34 kg) and decreased flexion-extension arc of motion (96° versus 130°) in the delayed treatment group. All the patients treated in the early phase returned to their previous work; however, in the group with delayed treatment only three patients returned to their previous occupation. Even with less optimal results, delayed ORIF was still recommended over a salvage procedure such as proximal row carpectomy for these challenging injuries.

Recently, authors have advocated temporary screw fixation in place of K-wires for the treatment of these difficult injuries. In a recent study,[23] nine patients treated with temporary K-wires were compared to nine patients treated with temporary screws for perilunate dislocation at an average of 44 months after fixation. All patients had a high rate of midcarpal arthritis (71%, K-wire group; 29%, screw group) and two patients in each group went on to a wrist arthrodesis. It appears in this study that neither group underwent fixation across the midcarpal joint. Final range of motion and grip strength were higher in the screw group, and final Disabilities of the Arm, Shoulder and Hand scores were higher (worse outcome) in the screw group; how-

3: Upper Extremity

ever these differences were not statistically significant. From these data, it seems that temporary screw fixation is an acceptable option for treatment of perilunate injuries that may decrease pin tract problems.

Metacarpal Fractures

Nonsurgical Treatment of Metacarpal Fractures

Conservative (nonsurgical) treatment of closed, fifth metacarpal neck fractures was studied and published in 2005 as part of the Cochrane Database of Systematic Reviews.[24] The purpose of the review was to compare functional treatment with immobilization, and to compare different periods and types of immobilization. Types of intervention ranged from full dynamic treatment with no external support to full splinting with immobilization of the wrist and metacarpophalangeal (MCP) joint. Most studies were of poor quality. Only five studies met the inclusion criteria. There was no evidence that any of the treatment modalities was statistically significantly superior. No single nonsurgical treatment regimen could be recommended as superior to another. Recovery was generally excellent whichever method of treatment was used.

Since publication of the Cochrane Review of fifth metacarpal fracture treatment, additional studies evaluating the specific question of nonsurgical treatment of fifth metacarpal neck fractures have been published. In a retrospective study published in 2005, three methods of cast immobilization were compared for treatment of extra-articular metacarpal neck fractures in 263 patients. The MCP joint was immobilized in full flexion with the interphalangeal joints either immobilized in extension or free to move; or the MCP joint was immobilized in full extension with the interphalangeal joints free to move. Immobilization was discontinued at 5 weeks. No differences were observed in the range of motion, grip strength, or fracture reduction.[25]

In a randomized, prospective study published in 2008, two methods of immobilization of fifth metacarpal neck fractures were evaluated. One cast immobilized the MCP joint in flexion with the interphalangeal joints free to move, and the other cast immobilized the MCP joint in extension with the interphalangeal joints free to move. Casts were worn for 4 weeks. No differences were observed in the two treatment groups in range of motion, grip strength, or radiographic parameters. The cast with the MCP joint in extension was found to be easier to apply and better tolerated.[26]

These two recent studies seem to support the findings of the Cochrane review that found generally excellent outcomes regardless of method of treatment. They also support the idea that the MCP joint may be placed in extension for a short period, which contradicts conventional teaching that the joint must be immobilized in flexion to prevent a joint contracture.

Surgical Treatment of Metacarpal Fractures

Various effective techniques of stabilization have evolved for treating metacarpal fractures. The least invasive surgical technique is percutaneous pinning. Intramedullary pinning is a newer technique that has shown success in simple fractures. The most invasive stabilization is internal fixation with plates and screws. Recent studies have compared some of these surgical techniques.

A 2005 study compared two surgical techniques for treating angulated fifth metacarpal neck fractures. One group was treated with antegrade, intramedullary pinning and the second group was treated with retrograde crossed pinning for the fifth metacarpal neck fracture. Based on clinical and radiologic data, antegrade intramedullary pinning was found to be superior to retrograde percutaneous crossed pinning and was recommended. Motion of the MCP joint was significantly reduced in the retrograde pinning group. This was thought to be caused by scarring and adhesions of the extensor hood. The previously described complications of intramedullary pinning of incomplete reduction, pin migration, and loss of reduction were not observed in this study.[27]

In another study evaluating the angulated fifth metacarpal neck fracture, a comparison was made between two different surgical techniques. Antegrade intramedullary pinning was compared to percutaneous transverse fixation. In the transverse pinning group, the fracture was stabilized after reduction by pinning transversely from the fifth metacarpal head into the fourth metacarpal. Both techniques were found to be effective and safe and no clinical or radiologic differences were noted. Complications of the transverse pinning technique included pin tract infection and tethering of the sagittal bands. Complications of the antegrade pinning technique included migration of the pins and perforation of the metacarpal head.[28] An example of transverse pinning is shown in **Figure 4** for a comminuted fifth metacarpal shaft fracture.

To address the complication of migration of intramedullary pins, a proximal locking mechanism has been developed and studied. A proximal locking mechanism in the pin (or nail) reportedly allows treatment of unstable fractures through a minimally invasive approach without axial collapse or loss of alignment. In a retrospective report, nonlocked nails were thought to be effective for transverse metacarpal neck or shaft fractures, but not for comminuted or spiral or rotationally unstable fractures. For the comminuted or spiral fractures, a locked intramedullary nail was recommended. The ability to lock the intramedullary nail was reported to expand the indications and effectiveness of intramedullary pinning. Complications that were noted included extensor tendon irritation on the dorsum of the hand and pin penetration into the metacarpophalangeal joint in three elderly patients.[29]

Antegrade intramedullary pinning was compared in another study with plate-screw fixation for extra-

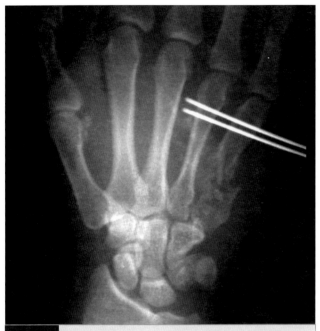

Figure 4 Transverse pinning can be a useful technique for an angulated fifth metacarpal neck fracture. In this case, transverse pinning has been used to help maintain length in a comminuted shaft fracture.

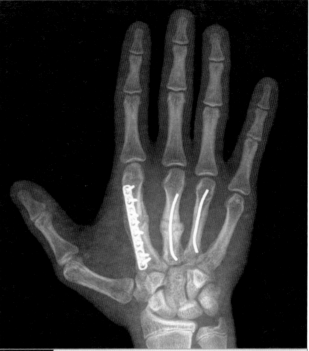

Figure 5 Both plate fixation and antegrade intramedullary nailing can be effective techniques for treatment of metacarpal shaft fractures. Complications can occur with both techniques. Antegrade intramedullary pinning can be associated with pin migration, joint penetration, and loss of alignment. This AP radiograph shows dorsal plate fixation of the index metacarpal joint and intramedullary fixation of the middle and ring metacarpal joints.

articular metacarpal fractures. There were no significant differences in the clinical outcomes between the two techniques. Surgical time was shorter in the intramedullary pin group than in the plate-screw fixation group. Loss of reduction, pin penetration into the joint, and secondary surgery for hardware removal in the operating room all had a higher incidence in the intramedullary pinning group.[30] **Figure 5** demonstrates use of both techniques for a hand with multiple metacarpal fractures.

Absorbable plates continue to hold interest in the treatment of hand fractures. In a small study (14 fractures), absorbable plates were used to treat displaced metacarpal fractures. The plates were made from an amorphic thermoplastic copolymer of 18% glycolic acid and 82% L-lactic acid. All fractures healed. However, reduction was lost in two patients, one of whom was converted to a metal plate. Keloid formation was noted as a complication, and prolonged soft-tissue swelling was observed for more than 6 weeks in three patients. Based on the loss of reduction in two patients, the authors recommended a postoperative orthosis after use of the bioabsorbable plate. The authors also noted that metal plates remain the gold standard for plate-screw fixation of metacarpal fractures.[31]

Phalangeal Fractures

Fractures of the proximal phalanx continue to challenge patients and hand surgeons alike. Both surgical

and nonsurgical techniques can have significant and disabling complications. Noninvasive techniques rarely risk adhesions but may produce malunion. Invasive techniques risk adhesions and can necessitate delayed surgery for tenolysis and hardware removal.

A recent study from Hong Kong evaluated the outcomes of 32 patients with proximal phalanx fractures treated nonsurgically with a MCP block splint followed by supervised rehabilitation. The hand-based splint flexed the MCP joint to 90° and allowed full active motion of the interphalangeal joints. The splint was used until callus was observed at about 4 to 6 weeks. Clinical and radiologic results showed 94% good or excellent results. Nonsurgical treatment was recommended based on these results.[32]

Minimally invasive surgical techniques are effective in the treatment of proximal phalanx fractures. Percutaneous pinning continues to be a favored technique for its simplicity, safety, and limitation of trauma to the gliding tendons. External fixation is also thought to be minimally invasive, and a recent study evaluated outcomes after external fixation for phalangeal fractures. Of 38 patients treated for unstable phalangeal fractures with external fixation, 76% achieved good or excellent results. Indications for operating on the phalangeal

3: Upper Extremity

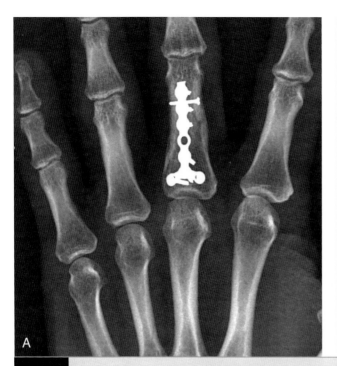
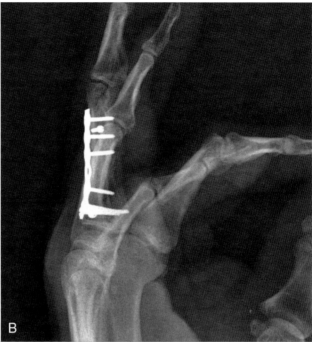

Figure 6 AP (**A**) and lateral (**B**) views of a proximal phalanx fracture treated with a low-profile dorsal plate combined with a 1.5-mm interfragmentary screw. These smaller plates and screws have less soft-tissue irritation on the adjacent extensor tendons.

fracture included: greater than 2 mm of shortening, greater than 10° of angulation, or any rotational deformity. Conversion to open technique was necessary in eight patients, the fixation technique was considered poor in seven, and tenolysis was required in one patient.[33] Another study retrospectively reviewed 51 patients with either phalangeal or metacarpal fractures treated with external fixation. Good clinical outcomes were reported overall, with a high union rate and minimal soft-tissue trauma. However worse outcomes were noted in intra-articular and open injuries.[34]

Complications of plate fixation of phalangeal fractures were recently investigated in 54 patients with 64 phalangeal fractures. One or more major complications were seen in 57% of patients. Stiffness, defined as less than 180° total active motion, was the most common complication, occurring in 22 patients. Other complications included two delayed unions, two nonunions, two infections, and complex regional pain syndrome in five patients. No differences were observed in the patients who had a dorsal tendon-splitting approach and those who had a lateral approach.[35]

The surgical approach to the proximal phalanx remains an area of active investigation. A recent biomechanical study compared a dorsal tendon-splitting approach with dorsal plating to lateral plating. In this biomechanical cadaver study, no differences were noted between the dorsal plating and the lateral plate. However, the stability was found to be greater when the soft-tissue envelope was left intact as opposed to a denuded bone specimen (**Figure 6**). This report suggested

that a laterally applied plate may provide adequate stability without violating the extensor tendon.[36] A laterally applied plate may avoid damage and subsequent scarring to the extensor mechanism.

For rotational malunion of a phalangeal fracture, the step-cut osteotomy of the metacarpal has been reintroduced as a simple and successful technique for correction. There is no consensus regarding the ideal level of osteotomy, type of osteotomy, or fixation technique for correction of the malunion. In a retrospective series of 12 patients, the Z-cut osteotomy of the metacarpal fixed exclusively with lag screws produced excellent results.[37]

Fracture-Dislocations of the Proximal Interphalangeal Joint

Recent publications continue to support the use of a dynamic distraction external fixator for comminuted fracture-dislocations of the proximal interphalangeal (PIP) joint. The dynamic external fixator can be assembled from easily available materials, typically K-wires with or without rubber bands. Some designs use rubber bands to create the distraction, other designs use the tension in a bent K-wire to distract the joint. A dynamic external fixator may be assembled from K-wires (**Figure 7**). In a 2008 study of 34 patients with unstable PIP joint fracture-dislocations and comminuted intra-articular fractures, all patients treated with dynamic distraction external fixation were able to return to

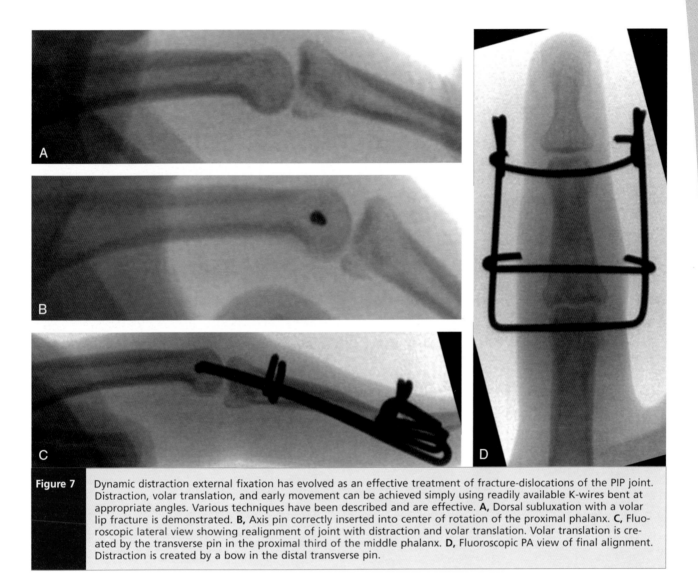

Figure 7 Dynamic distraction external fixation has evolved as an effective treatment of fracture-dislocations of the PIP joint. Distraction, volar translation, and early movement can be achieved simply using readily available K-wires bent at appropriate angles. Various techniques have been described and are effective. **A,** Dorsal subluxation with a volar lip fracture is demonstrated. **B,** Axis pin correctly inserted into center of rotation of the proximal phalanx. **C,** Fluoroscopic lateral view showing realignment of joint with distraction and volar translation. Volar translation is created by the transverse pin in the proximal third of the middle phalanx. **D,** Fluoroscopic PA view of final alignment. Distraction is created by a bow in the distal transverse pin.

prior levels of activity, and the results were comparable to those of other techniques reported in the literature. Average PIP motion was 88°. Complications included eight superficial pin tract infections.[38] In another study from 2006, 100 patients were reviewed with acute intra-articular phalangeal fractures of the hand. Most (81) of the patients had injury to the PIP joint. Average arc of motion at the PIP joint was 92° with a total active motion of 255° of the injured finger. Two main principles emphasized in this report were: (1) it is essential to obtain congruency of joint using ligamentotaxis and (2) early motion is needed to prevent joint stiffness and promote pain-free movement.[39]

An alternative approach to PIP fracture-dislocations with large comminuted fragments is the use of a hemicondylar hamate resurfacing arthroplasty. In this technique, the comminuted volar lip of the dorsally dislocated middle phalanx is reconstructed using a hemihamate osteochondral autograft. A size-matched piece of the ipsilateral hamate is transplanted to the middle phalanx to restore articular congruity and the buttress effect of the volar lip of the middle phalanx. In a cadaver study, the suitability of the graft and the lack of donor site morbidity were demonstrated. The graft provides an anatomic fit at the PIP joint, and harvesting this small portion of the fifth carpometacarpal joint did not induce any instability.[40] The technique has been proven to be clinically effective in nonreconstructable acute fracture-dislocations and chronic joint subluxation with chondral loss.[41]

Summary

Controversy continues to exist in the treatment of hand fractures. Surgical versus nonsurgical treatment continues to be debated for nondisplaced scaphoid waist fractures, angulated fractures of the metacarpal neck, and angulated fractures of the proximal phalanx. Nonsurgical techniques have historically shown success for even some angulated fractures of the hand. When skeletal deformity is unacceptable, surgical techniques can restore alignment. Surgical techniques can, however, pro-

3: Upper Extremity

duce complications such as stiffness and implant-related problems. Minimally invasive techniques may reduce stiffness. Additional research is necessary to evaluate injury prevention programs, societal costs, and newer techniques to improve functional outcomes in these difficult fractures.

Annotated References

1. Feehan LM, Sheps SB: Incidence and demographics of hand fractures in British Columbia, Canada: A population-based study. *J Hand Surg Am* 2006;31(7):1068-1074.

   Data were extracted retrospectively from a review of the British Columbia Linked Health Dataset over a 5-year period. Four million people are included in this population-based study. The epidemiology of hand fractures—excluding carpal fractures—for an entire population is described.

2. Aitken S, Court-Brown CM: The epidemiology of sports-related fractures of the hand. *Injury* 2008;39(12):1377-1383.

   Data were extracted retrospectively from a review of a hospital database over a 1-year period. The epidemiology of sports-related fractures of the hand is described.

3. Bernstein ML, Chung KC: Hand fractures and their management: An international view. *Injury* 2006;37(11):1043-1048.

   The historical development of hand fracture management is discussed. Global differences in hand fracture management are reviewed, with recommendations for resource-dependent decision making. Level of evidence: V.

4. Ring D, Lozano-Calderón S: Imaging for suspected scaphoid fracture. *J Hand Surg Am* 2008;33(6):954-957.

   The diagnostic performance characteristics of MRI, CT, bone scintigraphy, and ultrasound for evaluation of occult scaphoid fracture are described based on review of current literature. MRI is the best diagnostic test for suspected scaphoid fracture. All diagnostic tests were found to be better at excluding a fracture rather than confirming a true fracture. Level of evidence: III.

5. Hove LM: Epidemiology of scaphoid fractures in Bergen, Norway. *Scand J Plast Reconstr Surg Hand Surg* 1999;33(4):423-426.

6. Adey L, Souer JS, Lozano-Calderon S, Palmer W, Lee SG, Ring D: Computed tomography of suspected scaphoid fractures. *J Hand Surg Am* 2007;32(1):61-66.

   Eight observers reviewed CT scans of 30 patients with known or suspected scaphoid fractures. Sensitivity for detection of a nondisplaced scaphoid fracture was 89%. The authors advise caution when using CT scan to detect nondisplaced scaphoid fracture. Level of evidence: IV.

7. Jenkins PJ, Slade K, Huntley JS, Robinson CM: A comparative analysis of the accuracy, diagnostic uncertainty

   and cost of imaging modalities in suspected scaphoid fractures. *Injury* 2008;39(7):768-774.

   Two hundred consecutive patients retrospectively reviewed with radial-sided wrist pain and a suspected scaphoid fracture. Based on an economic analysis, where resources were limited, the authors concluded that clinical examination and delayed radiography appear to represent the most economic and safe option in management of suspected scaphoid fracture. Level of evidence: III.

8. Brooks S, Cicuttini FM, Lim S, Taylor D, Stuckey SL, Wluka AE: Cost effectiveness of adding magnetic resonance imaging to the usual management of suspected scaphoid fractures. *Br J Sports Med* 2005;39(2):75-79.

   The cost effectiveness of adding MRI to the usual management of suspected scaphoid fractures is discussed. This is one of the first studies to include the cost of lost productivity in the cost analysis of scaphoid fracture early diagnosis. The authors concluded that if the application of a cast decreases productivity by 50% or greater, then early diagnosis with an MRI is cost effective. Level of evidence: III.

9. Rhemrev SJ, van Leerdam RH, Ootes D, Beeres FJ, Meylaerts SA: Non-operative treatment of nondisplaced scaphoid fractures may be preferred. *Injury* 2009;40(6):638-641.

   A retrospective review of 71 patients treated nonsurgically for nondisplaced scaphoid waist fractures is presented. All fractures healed, with only two requiring immobilization longer than 12 weeks. Cast immobilization is recommended as initial treatment of nondisplaced scaphoid waist fracture. Level of evidence: IV.

10. Dias JJ, Dhukaram V, Abhinav A, Bhowal B, Wildin CJ: Clinical and radiological outcome of cast immobilisation versus surgical treatment of acute scaphoid fractures at a mean follow-up of 93 months. *J Bone Joint Surg Br* 2008;90(7):899-905.

    This important study presents the longer follow-up data for the patients presented in the 2005 study by Dias et al. No medium-term difference in function or radiologic outcome was identified in the two treatment groups at longer follow-up. Nonsurgical treatment of nondisplaced scaphoid waist fractures continues to be advocated as the initial treatment with conversion to internal fixation if no healing is observed at 8 weeks. Level of evidence: I.

11. McQueen MM, Gelbke MK, Wakefield A, Will EM, Gaebler C: Percutaneous screw fixation versus conservative treatment for fractures of the waist of the scaphoid: A prospective randomised study. *J Bone Joint Surg Br* 2008;90(1):66-71.

    In this prospective randomized study, improved alignment and healing rates with surgical treatment were demonstrated. Two patients had osteonecrosis in the cast group, three had malunion with a DISI deformity, and one had radioscaphoid arthrosis. Level of evidence: I.

12. Dias JJ, Wildin CJ, Bhowal B, Thompson JR: Should acute scaphoid fractures be fixed? A randomized controlled trial. *J Bone Joint Surg Am* 2005;87(10):2160-2168.

Eighty-eight patients were randomized to surgical and nonsurgical treatment of nondisplaced scaphoid waist fracture. This study did not demonstrate a clear overall benefit or difference in outcomes to early fixation of acute scaphoid fractures. An aggressive conservative approach was recommended whereby nonsurgical treatment is recommended initially with conversion to screw fixation if healing is not observed at 8 weeks radiographically. Early internal fixation could lead to overtreatment of a large proportion of fractures. Level of evidence: I.

13. Modi CS, Nancoo T, Powers D, Ho K, Boer R, Turner SM: Operative versus nonoperative treatment of acute undisplaced and minimally displaced scaphoid waist fractures: A systematic review. *Injury* 2009;40(3): 268-273.

A meta-analysis of the literature evaluation of surgical versus nonsurgical treatment of nondisplaced scaphoid waist fractures. Level I, II, and III studies were included. Evidence suggests that faster union and earlier return to work exist in the surgical treatment groups. Thirty percent minor complications exist in the surgical groups. Level of evidence: III.

14. Davis EN, Chung KC, Kotsis SV, Lau FH, Vijan S: A cost/utility analysis of open reduction and internal fixation versus cast immobilization for acute nondisplaced mid-waist scaphoid fractures. *Plast Reconstr Surg* 2006; 117(4):1223-1235.

A cost/utility analysis was performed using a decision-analytic model to calculate outcomes assuming the societal perspective. ORIF was found to be cost effective relative to a cast and produces a cost saving from the societal perspective. Level of evidence: III.

15. Jeon IH, Micic ID, Oh CW, Park BC, Kim PT: Percutaneous screw fixation for scaphoid fracture: A comparison between the dorsal and the volar approaches. *J Hand Surg Am* 2009;34(2):228-236, e1.

A nonrandomized, retrospective case control series of dorsal and volar screw approaches is presented. Screw position in the scaphoid was better via the dorsal approach; however, no difference in clinical outcome was observed. Level of evidence: III.

16. Weinberg AM, Pichler W, Grechenig S, Tesch NP, Heidari N, Grechenig W: The percutaneous antegrade scaphoid fracture fixation: A safe method? *Injury* 2009; 40(6):642-644.

Tendon injuries were noted in 5 of the 40 specimens wherein a percutaneous dorsal approach to scaphoid fixation was used. Extending the skin incision and using blunt dissection down to the starting point may avoid soft-tissue injuries.

17. Slade JF, Lozano-Calderón S, Merrell G, Ring D: Arthroscopic-assisted percutaneous reduction and screw fixation of displaced scaphoid fractures. *J Hand Surg Eur Vol* 2008;33(3):350-354.

This is the first study to examine the treatment of displaced scaphoid fractures with percutaneous treatment. Written by pioneers in the field of minimally invasive treatment, this technique expands the evolving indication for this treatment method. Level of evidence: IV.

18. Capo JT, Orillaza NS Jr, Slade JF III: Percutaneous management of scaphoid nonunions. *Tech Hand Up Extrem Surg* 2009;13(1):23-29.

Surgical techniques for minimally invasive scaphoid fixation are described in detail. Volar and dorsal approaches, arthroscopic assistance, and reduction maneuvers to allow percutaneous fixation are described. Level of evidence: V.

19. Slade JF III , Geissler WB, Gutow AP, Merrell GA: Percutaneous internal fixation of selected scaphoid nonunions with an arthroscopically assisted dorsal approach. *J Bone Joint Surg Am* 2003;85-A(suppl 4): 20-32.

The first report on percutaneous treatment of early scaphoid nonunions with screw fixation alone and no supplementary bone graft is presented. A union rate of 100% in 15 patients was achieved. Level of evidence: IV.

20. Chang MA, Bishop AT, Moran SL, Shin AY: The outcomes and complications of 1,2-intercompartmental supraretinacular artery pedicled vascularized bone grafting of scaphoid nonunions. *J Hand Surg Am* 2006; 31(3):387-396.

A retrospective review of 50 scaphoid nonunions treated with vascularized bone graft is presented. The study concluded that a successful outcome is not universal and depends on careful patient and fracture selection and surgical techniques. Level of evidence: IV.

21. Jones DB Jr, Bürger H, Bishop AT, Shin AY: Treatment of scaphoid waist nonunions with an avascular proximal pole and carpal collapse: A comparison of two vascularized bone grafts. *J Bone Joint Surg Am* 2008; 90(12):2616-2625.

This is a significant article describing a new technique for a distant vascularized bone graft for difficult scaphoid nonunions. Emphasis is placed on use of this technique where a structural graft is necessary for a humpback deformity. Success was obtained in all cases that used this medial femoral condyle graft. Level of evidence: IV.

22. Komurcu M, Kürklü M, Ozturan KE, Mahirogullari M, Basbozkurt M: Early and delayed treatment of dorsal transscaphoid perilunate fracture-dislocations. *J Orthop Trauma* 2008;22(8):535-540.

The authors found the injuries treated earlier had better outcomes. It was suggested that the outcomes of the delayed treatment group are better than outcomes of salvage procedures such as proximal row corpectomy and ORIF recommended even in patients presenting with delayed symptoms (< 40 days). Level of evidence: III.

23. Souer JS, Rutgers M, Andermahr J, Jupiter JB, Ring D: Perilunate fracture-dislocations of the wrist: Comparison of temporary screw versus K-wire fixation. *J Hand Surg Am* 2007;32(3):318-325.

Customarily K-wires have been used for fixation of perilunate dislocations. These authors suggest using buried screws, which seem to provide more rigid fixation and avoid pin tract problems. Level of evidence: III.

3: Upper Extremity

24. Poolman RW, Goslings JC, Lee JB, Statius Muller M, Steller EP, Struijs PA: Conservative treatment for closed fifth (small finger) metacarpal neck fractures. *Cochrane Database Syst Rev* 2005;3(3):CD003210.

    This article presents a retrospective literature review of relevant series from 1951 through 2005. All randomized and quasirandomized controlled trials were reviewed by assessing abstracts. Only five studies met inclusion criteria, including a total of 252 participants.

25. Tavassoli J, Ruland RT, Hogan CJ, Cannon DL: Three cast techniques for the treatment of extra-articular metacarpal fractures: Comparison of short-term outcomes and final fracture alignments. *J Bone Joint Surg Am* 2005;87(10):2196-2201.

    A 4-year retrospective chart review of patients at a naval hospital is presented. Three different surgeons immobilized their patients using three different techniques. No significant differences were noted. Level of evidence: III.

26. Hofmeister EP, Kim J, Shin AY: Comparison of 2 methods of immobilization of fifth metacarpal neck fractures: A prospective randomized study. *J Hand Surg Am* 2008;33(8):1362-1368.

    A randomized, prospective study comparing the effectiveness of two different positions of immobilization for fifth metacarpal neck fractures is presented. Eighty-one predominantly young active duty patients from a naval hospital were included. No differences were noted in study groups. Level of evidence: I.

27. Schädel-Höpfner M, Wild M, Windolf J, Linhart W: Antegrade intramedullary splinting or percutaneous retrograde crossed pinning for displaced neck fractures of the fifth metacarpal? *Arch Orthop Trauma Surg* 2007; 127(6):435-440.

    Thirty patients were included in this retrospective cohort study, with 15 patients in both groups. The inferior outcomes observed in the retrograde pinning technique were attributed to adhesions at the MCP joint due to the pins and scarring of the extensor hood. Level of evidence: III.

28. Wong TC, Ip FK, Yeung SH: Comparison between percutaneous transverse fixation and intramedullary K-wires in treating closed fractures of the metacarpal neck of the little finger. *J Hand Surg Br* 2006;31(1):61-65.

    Fifty-nine cases were studied in a nonrandomized, controlled clinical trial. The two techniques were found to be comparable. Level of evidence: III.

29. Orbay JL, Touhami A: The treatment of unstable metacarpal and phalangeal shaft fractures with flexible nonlocking and locking intramedullary nails. *Hand Clin* 2006;22(3):279-286.

    A retrospective review of 150 hand fractures discussing locking and nonlocking intramedullary nails for the treatment of various hand fractures is presented. Locking nails are thought to have expanded the indications for intramedullary nailing to include axially and rotationally unstable fractures. Level of evidence: IV.

30. Ozer K, Gillani S, Williams A, Peterson SL, Morgan S: Comparison of intramedullary nailing versus plate-screw fixation of extra-articular metacarpal fractures. *J Hand Surg Am* 2008;33(10):1724-1731.

    A prospective, nonrandomized study of two different treatment modalities is presented. Outcome measures reported include functional scores, radiographs, and complications. Patients with intramedullary fixation had a higher risk of tendon irritation requiring hardware removal. Intramedullary fixation is not recommended for fractures in the distal third metacarpal due to high risk of joint penetration. Level of evidence: III.

31. Dumont C, Fuchs M, Burchhardt H, Appelt D, Bohr S, Stürmer KM: Clinical results of absorbable plates for displaced metacarpal fractures. *J Hand Surg Am* 2007; 32(4):491-496.

    A case series of 12 patients with a bioabsorbable implant is presented. Failure of fixation required the authors to convert one patient to a metal plate. A recommendation was made to supplement the internal fixation with the bioabsorbable plate with an external hand orthosis. Level of evidence: IV.

32. Rajesh G, Ip WY, Chow SP, Fung BK: Dynamic treatment for proximal phalangeal fracture of the hand. *J Orthop Surg* 2007;15(2):211-215.

    Thirty-two consecutive patients are reported in a 6-year retrospective study of nonsurgical treatment of proximal phalanx fractures (regardless of geometry). Intra-articular fractures, multiple fractures, tendon injuries, infection, and pathologic fractures were exclusion criteria. No tendon adhesions, nonunion, or malunion cases were noted. Nonsurgical treatment is recommended based on 94% good and excellent results in this series. Level of evidence: IV.

33. Margić K: External fixation of closed metacarpal and phalangeal fractures of digits: A prospective study of one hundred consecutive patients. *J Hand Surg Br* 2006; 31(1):30-40.

    A prospective, nonrandomized study of 100 consecutive patients with fractures of the metacarpal and phalanges is reported. Intra-articular and extra-articular fractures were included. Good results are reported in 76% of isolated phalangeal fractures, 100% of metacarpal fractures, and 89% of multiple fractures. Level of evidence: IV.

34. Dailiana Z, Agorastakis D, Varitimidis S, Bargiotas K, Roidis N, Malizos KN: Use of a mini-external fixator for the treatment of hand fractures. *J Hand Surg Am* 2009;34(4):630-636.

    A retrospective case series of 59 fractures of the metacarpal and phalangeal bones is reported. Intra-articular and extra-articular fractures were included. Fixators were removed at a mean of 6 weeks. Best results were noted in the unstable, closed extra-articular fracture subset. Intra-articular and comminuted fractures had less successful results.

35. Kurzen P, Fusetti C, Bonaccio M, Nagy L: Complications after plate fixation of phalangeal fractures. *J Trauma* 2006;60(4):841-843.

A retrospective review of 64 phalangeal fractures in 54 patients is reported. One or more major complications were noted in 57% of patients. The most common major complication was stiffness in 22 (41%) of patients. Early motion did not prevent stiffness. Plate fixation is still recommended as efficient and reliable. Level of evidence: IV.

36. Ouellette EA, Dennis JJ, Latta LL, Milne EL, Makowski AL: The role of soft tissues in plate fixation of proximal phalanx fractures. *Clin Orthop Relat Res* 2004;418: 213-218.

    A midshaft phalangeal osteotomy model was studied in cadaver bone. Dorsally and laterally applied plates were compared. Specimens with and without soft-tissue coverage were also compared. Findings suggest that a laterally applied plate may provide as much stability as the dorsally applied plate to a phalangeal fracture.

37. Jawa A, Zucchini M, Lauri G, Jupiter J: Modified step-cut osteotomy for metacarpal and phalangeal rotational deformity. *J Hand Surg Am* 2009;34(2):335-340.

    A retrospective review of 12 patients with rotational malunion of a phalangeal fracture treated with metacarpal osteotomy is reported. A Z-cut is made in the metacarpal with removal of a dorsal wedge of bone from the central longitudinal cut to allow correction. Fixation is performed with lag screws. Rapid healing, early motion, and correction are reported. Level of evidence: IV.

38. Ruland RT, Hogan CJ, Cannon DL, Slade JF: Use of dynamic distraction external fixation for unstable fracture-dislocations of the proximal interphalangeal joint. *J Hand Surg Am* 2008;33(1):19-25.

    In a retrospective study, 34 patients with fracture-dislocation and comminuted intra-articular fractures of the proximal interphalangeal joint were treated with dynamic distraction external fixation. All patients returned to prior activity level and only superficial pin tract infections were reported. Level of evidence: IV.

39. Khan W, Fahmy N: The S-Quattro in the management of acute intraarticular phalangeal fractures of the hand. *J Hand Surg Br* 2006;31(1):79-92.

    One hundred patients were reviewed in a retrospective study of the results of intra-articular fractures treated with dynamic external fixation. Mean motion at the MCP joint was 91° (6 fractures), motion at the PIP joint was 92° (81 fractures), and motion at the distal interphalangeal joint was 82° (10 fractures). Satisfactory radiographic appearances were noted in 95% of patients. Level of evidence: IV.

40. Williams RM, Hastings H II, Kiefhaber TR: PIP fracture/dislocation treatment technique: Use of a hemihamate resurfacing arthroplasty. *Tech Hand Up Extrem Surg* 2002;6(4):185-192.

    Technical details of the hemihamate resurfacing arthroplasty are introduced for dorsal dislocations of the PIP. The hamate graft is harvested from the distal, dorsal margin of the hamate and used to reconstruct the comminuted volar lip of the middle phalanx. The hamate graft must recreate the geometry of the middle phalanx base.

41. Capo JT, Hastings H II, Choung E, Kinchelow T, Rossy W, Steinberg B: Hemicondylar hamate replacement arthroplasty for proximal interphalangeal joint fracture dislocations: An assessment of graft suitability. *J Hand Surg Am* 2008;33(5):733-739.

    Suitability of hamate grafts for hemicondylar hamate replacement is assessed in cadavers. The dorsal portion of the hamate was found to be a suitable osteochondral autograft for reconstruction of the base/volar lip of the middle phalanx in PIP joint fracture-dislocations.

Section 4

Axial Skeleton, Including Spine and Pelvis

SECTION EDITORS:

BERTON R. MOED, MD

CARLO BELLABARBA, MD

Chapter 22

Pelvic Fractures: Evaluation and Acute Management

Wade R. Smith, MD   Takashi Suzuki, MD   Paul Tornetta III, MD

Anatomy and Stability of the Pelvis

The pelvis is a ring made up of three bones: the sacrum and the two innominate bones. The innominate bones articulate with the sacrum through the sacroiliac joints and between themselves through the symphysis pubis. They are joined by important ligamentous structures. The sacroiliac joints are stabilized by the anterior sacroiliac ligament, posterior sacroiliac ligament, and interosseous ligament (the strongest ligament in the body). The pubic symphysis is reinforced by fibrocartilage and a series of thin ligaments. The pelvic floor is supported by the sacrospinous and sacrotuberous ligaments. Stability of the pelvis depends on the integrity of the posterior sacroiliac ligamentous complex. Because the pelvis is a ring structure, disruption of the pelvic ring in normal bone at one site usually requires disruption to occur in at least one more location.[1] Disruptions of the pelvic ring in two or more sites may cause biomechanical instability.[2] Biomechanical instability may provoke hemodynamic instability in the acute phase because the disrupted pelvic ring leads to damage to the many vessels adherent to the pelvic and sacral bones. The unstable pelvic ring also results in pelvis mobility, which left untreated may cause permanent disability.

The pelvis may be considered a visceral organ that contains aspects of the urinary system, reproductive system, bowel system, soft tissues, arteries, veins, nerves, and bones. Abundant blood supply from the internal iliac arteries and its branches is provided to nourish these structures. Nerves travel adjacent to the posterior pelvis, including roots (L5, S1), and the lumbosacral plexus, sciatic, femoral, obturator, pudendal, and superior gluteal nerves. The bladder, urethra, rectum, and vagina are located in close proximity to the bones. Any of these structures is susceptible to injuries when the pelvic ring is disrupted (**Figure 1**).

Mechanism of Injury

Three major force vectors can act in isolation or combination to produce pelvic fractures. A lateral compression (LC) injury leads to internal rotation of the hemipelvis and often results from side-impact motor vehicle collisions or automobile-pedestrian accidents. An anteroposterior compression (APC) injury leads to external rotation of the affected hemipelvis and can be typically caused by motorcycle collisions, mechanical crush injuries, or horseback-riding injuries. A vertical shear (VS) injury leads to cephalad displacement of the hemipelvis and usually occurs after a fall from a height. The LC injury is the most common, followed by the APC injury.

Anatomic-Mechanical Classification of Pelvic Injury

Although numerous pelvic-injury classification systems have been described, two are commonly used.[2] The Tile classification system is based on the stability and mechanism of injury, and its concept served as the foundation for the AO/Orthopaedic Trauma Association (OTA) classification.[3] Type A injuries consist of fractures that do not compromise the integrity of the pelvic ring, such as iliac wing avulsion fractures and nondisplaced fractures in more than one site. These fractures are considered stable. Type B injuries involve the pelvic ring in two or more sites and create a segment that is rotationally unstable but vertically stable due to the incomplete disruption of the posterior sacroiliac ligamentous complex. Type C injuries are both rotationally and vertically unstable due to complete disruption of the posterior ligamentous and/or bony complex. The Young-Burgess classification system is primarily based on the mechanism of injury and subdivides the force patterns according to increasing levels of energy

Dr. Smith or an immediate family member serves as a paid consultant for or is an employee of Synthes and has received research or institutional support from Synthes. Dr. Tornetta or an immediate family member has received royalties from Smith & Nephew; serves as a paid consultant for or is an employee of Smith & Nephew; and has received royalties from Lippincott Williams & Wilkins. Neither Dr. Suzuki nor any immediate family member has received anything of value from or owns stock in a commercial company or institution related directly or indirectly to the subject of this chapter.

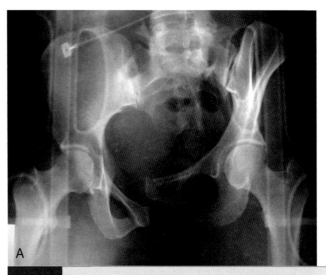

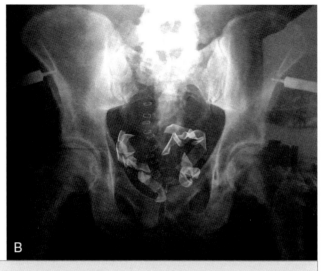

Figure 1   Radiographs of the pelvis of a 34-year-old man who sustained a pelvic fracture with hemodynamic and mechanical instability following a 50-foot fall from a height. **A**, A lateral compression–type injury on the trauma resuscitation area film is shown. The patient's systolic blood pressure was 60 mm Hg, and there were no other associated injuries. **B**, The patient was taken emergently to the operating room within 20 minutes of arrival. An AP radiograph was taken after external fixation with a C-clamp and retroperitoneal packing. The patient's blood pressure stabilized immediately. Definitive reconstruction was performed 5 days later.

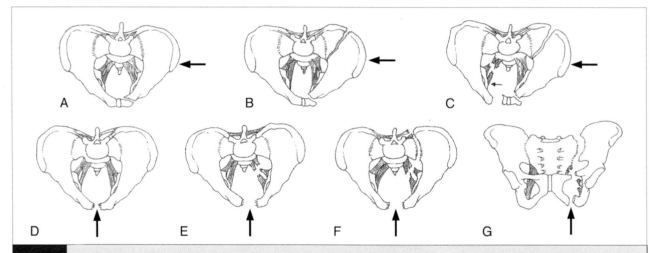

Figure 2   The Young-Burgess classification of pelvic injuries. The arrows indicate the direction of the force causing the injury. **A** through **C**, LC injuries. **D** through **F**, APC injuries. **G**, VS injury. (Reproduced from Beaty JH (ed): *Orthopaedic Knowledge Update 6*. Rosemont, IL, American Academy of Orthopaedic Surgeons, 1998, pp 427-439.)

applied to disrupt the pelvic ring and the resultant associated risk of hemodynamic instability and associated injuries (**Figure 2**). APC-I injuries have symphyseal diastasis less than 2.5 cm and no significant posterior injury. APC-II injuries are typically characterized by symphyseal diastasis greater than 2.5 cm. These injuries involve rupture of the anterior sacroiliac, sacrospinous, and sacrotuberous ligaments. APC-III injuries are defined as a vertical unstable pelvis, including complete disruption of the posterior ligamentous complex. LC-I injuries are heterogeneous[4] and consist of a spectrum of posterior compression injuries of the sacroiliac joint. The authors of a 2009 study showed that LC-I injuries may have complete sacral disruption, have significant

associated injuries, and thus require aggressive surgical management.[5] LC-II injuries accompany the rupture of the posterior sacroiliac ligament with pivotal internal rotation of the hemipelvis around the axis of the anterior sacroiliac joint. These injuries typically cause an iliac crescent fracture and/or a crush injury of the sacrum. LC-III injuries involve the findings of an LC-II injury with evidence of an APC injury to the contralateral side. Rupture of the ligaments of the pelvic floor and sacroiliac joint may coexist as in APC injuries, rendering the pelvis highly unstable mechanically. VS injuries are associated with disruption of all major ligamentous constraints and characterized by vertical displacement of the affected hemipelvis. Combined mechanism of injury is a combination of the previously mentioned forces. These anatomic-mechanical classification systems have been considered useful for predicting the presence of associated injuries, deciding if surgery is needed, and planning reduction/fixation methods. Importantly, the nomenclature is familiar to general trauma surgeons and emergency physicians, facilitating accurate and timely communication. Drawbacks to these classification systems exist, however. As discussed, the LC injuries represent a heterogeneous group of high- and low-energy fractures with various degrees of mechanical stability that may not easily be defined by current classification methodology. Additionally, these classifications usually depend upon static radiographs or CT scans taken during the initial stabilization period. Presumably, a variety of minimally displaced fractures may have had greater displacement at the time of injury, leading to potentially more soft-tissue damage and higher risk of bleeding. Once stable, often with a pelvic binder or wrap in place, these fractures may be underclassified. The correlation of associated injuries with fracture patterns appears to vary in recent studies and may be due to differing injury demographics, car safety features, or other variables.

Given the difficulty in standardizing the description of fracture patterns for the complex anatomy of the pelvis and the subjectivity of descriptions based solely on injury mechanism, the AO/OTA classification is used more frequently. The A, B, C categories for stable, rotationally unstable, and vertically unstable injuries are familiar and descriptive. The subcategory numerical delineations permit precise coding for documentation and research purposes.

Initial Evaluation and the Role of the Orthopaedic Surgeon

The cornerstones of successful initial evaluation include identification of life-threatening conditions, including the pelvic injury, and associated critical injuries. Most pelvic ring injuries are low-energy, stable injuries that may be treated nonsurgically. However, the mortality of hemodynamically unstable patients remains high and a multidisciplinary approach has repeatedly been shown to lower mortality in a variety of hospital settings throughout the world.[2,6,7] The major causes of death in these patients are early exsanguination and the late sequelae of prolonged shock and mass transfusion.[8] Thus, identification of sources of hemorrhage is critical. In all trauma patients, the Advanced Trauma Life Support (ATLS) protocol should be followed. Once the patient is determined to have a pelvic fracture and some systemic evidence of shock or impending shock, a predetermined, multidisciplinary protocol should be followed. Initial evaluation and management of life-threatening injuries are performed simultaneously.

To assess the pelvic injury, knowledge of the injury mechanism is of prime importance and should be assessed either by patient history or discussion with the prehospital provider. Some injuries can be anticipated from the direction and amount of energy behind the mechanism of injury.

Physical examination is useful to detect injuries of the pelvis, especially in the alert patient.[9] However, in severely injured or obtunded patients, physical examination is less helpful beyond identification of open wounds and obvious deformity. Deformity of the pelvis or lower extremity or limb-length discrepancy may indicate the presence of a pelvic injury but can also be caused by other fractures of the lower extremity. Additionally, manual manipulation of the pelvic ring to test mechanical instability should be avoided when radiographic evaluation is available. Stress examination has poor sensitivity, can induce further hemorrhage in the acute setting, and adds little to the initial management of the patient.[10]

A complete visual and manual examination should identify open wounds in the perineum or anterior pelvis, subcutaneous degloving injuries, blood at the urethral meatus, perineal and scrotal ecchymosis, and neurologic deficiency. Open soft-tissue injury from a pelvic fracture is most common in the perineal region. Therefore, a meticulous inspection of perianal tissues, the vaginal vault, and rectum is required, as failure of early identification of injury can lead to infectious complications. A rectal examination should be performed and the position of the prostate noted. Closed degloving injuries (Morel-Lavallée lesions) are often overlooked and undertreated, permitting bacterial colonization and subsequent deep infection of the surrounding soft tissues. Careful evaluation and débridement of the closed cavity (via open or percutaneous techniques) may reduce infection risk.[11]

All patients sustaining high-energy blunt trauma or showing evidence of hemodynamic abnormality should be assumed to have a pelvic fracture, and, consistent with ATLS protocol, a plain AP pelvic radiograph should be obtained in the emergency department. The purpose of the AP pelvic radiograph is only to determine whether the pelvis could be a source of bleeding in the hemodynamically unstable patient. CT is not a substitute for the screening AP pelvic radiograph. Inlet, outlet, or oblique pelvic radiographs are also not needed initially because these views do not assist in the immediate resuscitation decisions. In some cases, extra imaging can delay appropriate interventions to increase blood pressure. Decreased blood pressure and other obvious signs of shock may not be evident initially, especially in the physiologically young patient. Other indices of hemodynamic status that should be noted include tachycardia, increased base deficit, increased lactate level, and need for transfusion. Retroperitoneal hemorrhage should be assumed when a displaced pelvic fracture is seen on the initial AP radiograph of the pelvis. However, the appearance of retroperitoneal hemorrhage, especially on CT scan, is nonprognostic and should not be used to direct treatment steps. All pelvic fractures generate hemorrhage and no correlation exists

4: Axial Skeleton, Including Spine and Pelvis

with CT findings and outcome. A potential danger of using static CT signs of hemorrhage, to determine treatment is that stable patients may be subjected to unnecessary interventions such as angiography, whereas patients with low blood pressure and minimal signs of initial extravasation may not receive aggressive management of their injury. In all cases of displaced pelvic fracture in men, a urethral or bladder injury should be suspected. A retrograde urethrogram or cystogram should be performed prior to placement of a catheter, unless the patient is in extremis, in which case the most experienced person present should attempt a single pass of the catheter. Urethral injuries do not manifest typical physical signs, and a single cystogram for bladder injuries can produce false-negative findings.[12] The degree of displacement of the bladder on a cystogram provides some clue about the size of any associated retroperitoneal hematoma. CT scanning of the pelvis may be necessary to delineate associated intrapelvic injuries but is not necessary for appropriate initial management of a hemodynamically unstable patient with an identified pelvic ring injury on the AP pelvic examination. The CT suite is not the best resuscitation environment for unstable trauma patients, and transferring such a patient into the scanner may cause increased bleeding. Thus, CT and any additional radiographic examinations should be balanced against this risk in the hemodynamically unstable patient. The increasing use of high-speed, multislice CT may or may not change this paradigm. Currently, ATLS guidelines do not mandate CT for every patient in shock, especially if there is a positive abdominal ultrasound examination (Focused Assessment With Sonography for Trauma [FAST]) in the emergency department. These patients usually require emergent surgical intervention, and CT may delay treatment. Depending on the geography of particular institutions, the transport and setup times for scanning may be longer than that of the actual scan. Thus, the treating orthopaedic surgeon should be able to formulate a treatment plan based on the physiologic status of the patient combined with the AP pelvic radiographs.

High-energy forces are needed to disrupt the pelvic ring, and this energy is absorbed by the rest of the body as well, producing major injury to other critical organs. Up to 90% of patients with unstable pelvic fractures have associated injuries, and 50% of patients have sources of major hemorrhage other than pelvic fractures.[13] Therefore, it is important to presume that a pelvic fracture is an indicator of multiple trauma. There has not been a reliable method to estimate the amount of hemorrhage in the retroperitoneal space. Thus, determining whether the major cause of ongoing bleeding is due to pelvic fracture may often be a diagnosis of exclusion. Large transfusion requirement is not a reliable predictor of bleeding from the pelvis because other sources of bleeding may coexist. The clinical assessment of hemodynamic instability should entail rapid assessment of all sources of hemorrhage. If a pelvic fracture exists on the screening AP radiograph, no matter which pattern, then bleeding from the pelvis should be assumed to be contributing to the overall blood loss.

The immediate presence of the orthopaedic surgeon in the emergency department enhances initial evaluation and resuscitation. Orthopaedic surgeons who are familiar with pelvic fractures can identify the fracture characteristics precisely and participate in real-time decision making with the trauma surgeon regarding the most effective maneuvers for achieving hemostasis. These strategies may include closing the pelvic volume in the emergency department or surgical suite with external fixation, binders, or C-clamps, or immediate internal fixation or other maneuvers such as angiography and/or pelvic packing. If the patient's hemodynamic status stabilizes, a determination is made with the orthopaedic surgeon regarding the need for further imaging evaluation and mechanical stabilization of the pelvis. Inlet and outlet pelvic plain radiographs obtained following successful resuscitation provide important additional information regarding pelvic fracture location and ring deformity. The outlet view is achieved with a caudad-to-cephalad tilt of 40° from the AP position. The outlet view shows the degree of vertical displacement and profiles the sacrum, permitting better evaluation of some sacral fractures. The inlet radiograph is a 40° cephalad-to-caudad view that shows anterior-posterior pelvic displacement as well as crescent-type fractures of the posterior pelvis (Figure 3).

Protocols for Emergent Treatment and Resuscitation

Patients with hemodynamic instability caused by hemorrhage should be initially resuscitated with 2 L of crystalloid followed by packed red blood cells (PRBC) and fresh frozen plasma (FFP) in a 1:1 ratio and an aggressive use of pheresis platelets to maintain greater than 50,000/μL.[14,15] If massive transfusion is needed, then a 1:1:1 ratio of PRBC, FFP, and platelets is recommended. If hemodynamic instability (typically diagnosed if the systolic blood pressure remains less than 90 mm Hg) persists despite PRBC transfusion, the patient is considered a "nonresponder" who requires more advanced treatment. There is a poor correlation between the mechanical severity of the pelvic fracture pattern and the need for rapid surgical intervention.[16,17] Severe bleeding can occur in all pelvic fracture patterns; therefore, physiologic status dictates the appropriate clinical strategy for intervention to control exsanguinating hemorrhage. Currently, two fundamentally different modalities have been advocated to treat patients with displaced pelvic fractures and persistent hemodynamic instability. Angiography with sequential embolization can control major arterial bleeding, whereas pelvic packing mainly controls bleeding from veins, small diameter arteries, and fracture sites.

Pelvic angiography with therapeutic embolization is widely accepted as a safe and efficacious method for

4: Axial Skeleton, Including Spine and Pelvis

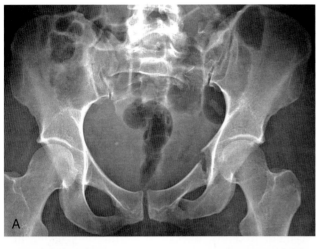

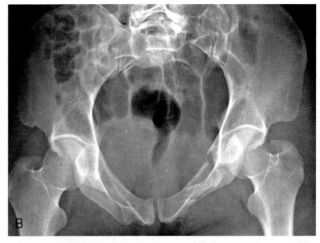

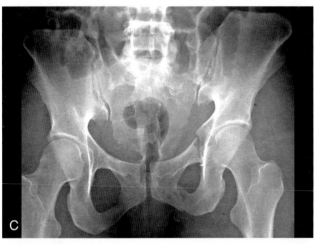

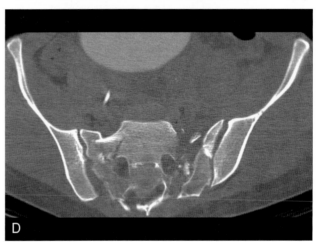

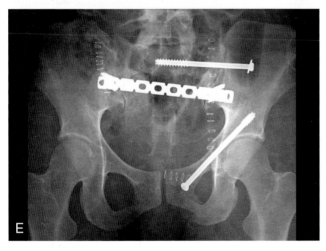

Figure 3 Inlet and outlet radiographic views and axial CT scans provide information about posterior and vertical displacement of a pelvic fracture. **A**, AP view. **B**, Inlet view. **C**, Outlet view. **D**, CT scan. **E**, Postoperative AP radiograph.

the control of arterial bleeding. Pelvic angiography consists of a nonselective injection of contrast medium just above the aortic bifurcation, followed by selective injection of the branches of the internal iliac arteries. Furthermore, branches of other arterial systems, such as the lumbar artery, median sacral artery, deep iliac circumflex artery, and corona mortis are possible sources of bleeding that may be amenable to selective catheterization. Angiographic evidence of extraluminal contrast

extravasation indicates ongoing arterial bleeding, and hemostasis is obtained by catheter embolization with gelatin sponge and/or coils. Depending on the degree of urgency and the skill of the angiographer, either selective embolization of bleeding arteries or nonselective embolization of bilateral internal iliac arteries is used. Ideally, selective embolization is preferable to minimize ischemic complications. On the other hand, nonselective embolization can provide an advantage in the unstable patient by decreasing time in the angiography suite and potentially achieving earlier hemostasis.[18]

The need for embolization is uncommon and is reported to be less than 10% in all pelvic fractures. However, angiography and subsequent embolization may be beneficial in a specific patient population to improve patient outcomes.[7] Successful embolization rates for arterial injuries have been reported to be 85% to 100%. Early pelvic angiography within 90 to 180 minutes after admission can improve mortality. Several indications for pelvic angiography to control arterial bleeding have been reported. Generally, patients who remain hemodynamically unstable after appropriate fluid resuscitation with PRBC and FFP and mechanical stabilization of the pelvis are possible candidates because hemodynamically unstable patients have a higher rate of arterial extravasation.[19] Age older than 60 years, high Revised Trauma Score, high Injury Severity Score, and female sex also have been reported to be useful predictors for arterial bleeding.[16,18,20-22] Another indication for pelvic angiography includes extravasation of contrast medium on the arterial phase of contrast-enhanced CT. CT is also useful in gauging the amount and location of pelvic hemorrhage, both of which may predict arterial injuries.[23] However, CT has a relatively low positive predictive value for the need for angiographic embolization.[24] Therefore, the decision to perform angiography should be made primarily based on clinical hemodynamics, presence of other injuries, and transfusion requirements.[24]

Several drawbacks to pelvic angiography have been reported. Allergic reaction to the contrast material, increase in serum creatinine level, or renal failure may not be noticed in severely injured patients because of concomitant hypotension, but these complications may occur and compromise patient survival. Recurrent pelvic arterial bleeding also has been shown to occur after successful embolization or after a negative initial angiography in 7.5% to 22.6% of patients.[25-27] In addition, the lack of readily available experts in angiography can limit the availability and effectiveness of emergent hemostasis. There may be considerable delays in the performance of embolization even in level I trauma centers.[28] Furthermore, angiography and embolization can be time consuming, and simultaneous treatment of other associated injuries during the procedure may be delayed. Time spent on angiography may also delay the optimal timing for lifesaving surgical interventions such as urgent laparotomy or decompressive craniotomy. Necrosis and ischemia of tissues caused by embolization of the internal iliac arteries have been reported. Some authors have reported high mortality rates in patients with gluteal muscle necrosis caused by embolization.[29] Others reported that these complications are more common when significant amounts of gelatin sponge are used in the embolization.[30] The presence of gluteal muscle necrosis creates a predisposition to infection after open reduction and internal fixation via a posterior approach to the pelvis.

Pelvic packing was developed and subsequently evolved to control the venous and bony bleeding that inevitably occurs to some degree in every pelvic fracture. Historically, it was thought that most bleeding from venous injuries arose from small- and medium-sized torn veins and would stop through clotting and tamponade. However, the ability to achieve tamponade may be lost in the presence of severe pelvic fractures because of traumatic disruption of the parapelvic fascia, and hemostasis may not be attained by the tamponade effect, despite the use of external immobilization. In particular, injury to the iliac vein and its major branch can result in a high mortality rate.[31] In these patients, time spent in angiography may be life threatening because angiography does nothing for bone and vein bleeding. Recently, direct retroperitoneal packing has been advocated to control venous bleeding and minimize the unnecessary performance of pelvic embolization.[32,33] This technique can facilitate control of retroperitoneal bleeding through a small incision that does not violate the intraperitoneal space and leaves the peritoneum intact. The total time for the packing procedure can be less than 20 minutes in expert hands, including the placement of a simple external fixation device. Blood loss during surgery is minimal. This method requires a surgeon experienced in the Pfannenstiel approach for anterior pelvis fixation. Pelvic packing also requires some form of mechanical stabilization of the pelvis, whether internal or external. Given these requirements it is advisable that an orthopaedic surgeon with expertise in pelvic external fixation is present during pelvic packing procedures to ensure appropriate technique and minimal iatrogenic soft-tissue disruption. During pelvic packing, associated injuries that contribute to mortality such as closed head injury, intra-abdominal hemorrhage, and hemothorax can be simultaneously assessed and treated with damage control techniques. Recent published series emphasize that the success of this technique is predicated upon early intervention as part of a planned approach to decreasing blood loss and limiting the need for massive resuscitation. In one series the use of pelvic packing as part of a staged protocol preceding angiography showed decreased need for transfusion and more efficient use of angiography when compared to a previous protocol without packing at the same institution. Mortality was slightly decreased.[34]

One of the disadvantages of pelvic packing is that it is a relatively invasive procedure compared to angiography, and infection at the incision site may occur. The necessity of a reoperation to remove the surgical lap packs at 24 to 48 hours is a theoretical disadvantage. However, most patients who undergo packing require multiple trips to the operating room and usually remain intubated in the intensive care unit. If pelvic packing reduces mortality in this cohort, an additional visit to the operating room is probably insignificant. Pelvic packing may also increase the incidence of abdominal compartment syndrome (ACS), which results from in-

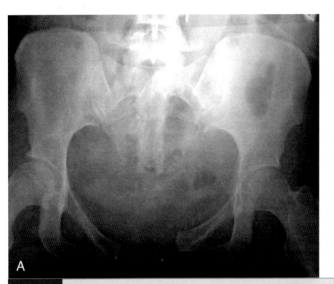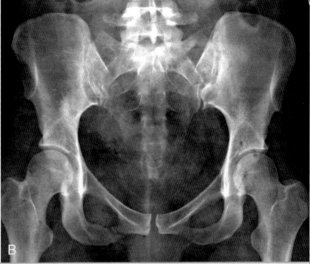

Figure 4 A circumferential sheet wrapping resulted in temporary fracture reduction and stabilization for an APC injury. Radiographs of the pelvis show the fracture preapplication (**A**) and postapplication (**B**).

creased intra-abdominal pressures due to bleeding, fluid, or space filling from packs or tumors. ACS can lead to rapid deterioration and death if left untreated. A standard method of assessing ACS is by measuring bladder pressures, which rise rapidly when intra-abdominal pressures increase past specific thresholds. Monitoring ACS via bladder pressures is unreliable in the presence of pelvic packing because of the tamponade of the bladder by the packing. Pelvic packing is likely ineffective for treatment of bleeding from large-bore arteries, especially those ruptured outside the true pelvis. Although the venous component of bleeding may be controlled, it is imperative that the use of pelvic packing does not supplant angiography in appropriate cases. Packing should be considered a quick, effective tool for diminishing venous bleeding and can usually be accomplished while the angiographic team is preparing for their procedure.[34] In this respect, pelvic packing may serve as a triage tool for angiography in that appropriately resuscitated patients with continued transfusion requirements after pelvic packing likely have a significant intrapelvic arterial injury.

Recombinant factor VIIa is a new adjunctive tool for the control of massive hemorrhage.[35] Theoretical complications such as excessive thromboembolism and systemic coagulation have not been reported in clinical use. However, factor VIIa is currently an off-label use, and its efficacy for control of hemorrhage caused by pelvic fractures remains anecdotal.[36] More studies are necessary to determine precise indications for its use in the treatment of pelvic fractures.

Pelvic packing and angiography are useful and potentially lifesaving interventions in the early management of pelvic fracture patients with hemodynamic instability. Trauma centers should have predetermined, specific protocols formulated by using available evidence-based medicine and consensus in order to maximize survival potential 365 days per year. Packing and angiography address different aspects of pelvic bleeding that often occur in unison. Therefore, protocols should stress immediate identification of the injury and balanced, aggressive resuscitation with blood products. Because almost all arterial bleeding is accompanied by venous bleeding, mechanical stabilization followed by pelvic packing can be used for those patients who do not respond to a threshold of blood transfusion. Mortality curves associated with pelvic bleeding suggest that after 2 to 4 units of RBC transfusion, mortality increases significantly.[8] In patients with ongoing instability despite packing, the likelihood of arterial bleeding is high, and angioembolization should be used. Many centers prefer angiography prior to packing. In either case, the principle is that these modalities are complementary and should play a role in controlling venous and arterial bleeding.[37]

Pelvic Binders and Sheets

Historically, military antishock trousers were advocated to achieve direct compression and immobilization of the pelvic ring and lower extremity via pneumatic pressure. However, it has been reported that military antishock trousers are associated with inherent complications, such as lower extremity ischemia/reperfusion syndrome, development of compartment syndrome, and skin necrosis. Instead, simple devices such as bed sheets have been tied around the pelvis, placed between the iliac crest and greater trochanter, to apply pressure with internal rotation of the legs. Sheeting facilitates closing the pelvis in open-book pelvic injuries but avoids lower extremity ischemia. Circumferential pelvic sheets are advantageous because of their ease of application, relative safety, cost-effectiveness, and noninvasive character (**Figure 4**). Recently, commercial pelvic binders have been devised that permit tension adjust-

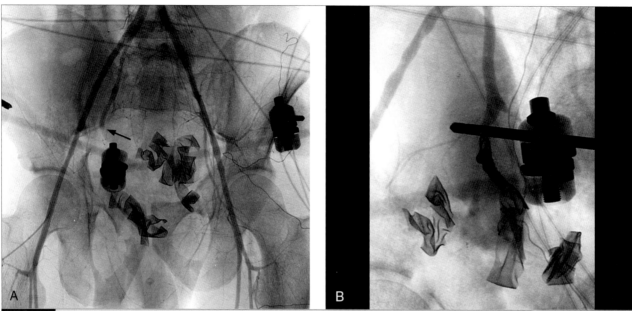

Figure 5 A sequential approach including external fixation, pelvic packing, and angiographic embolization showed successful management of hemodynamically unstable patients with pelvic fracture. **A,** Temporary stabilization of hemodynamics was obtained following external fixation and pelvic packing. Angiography revealed arterial occlusion that was the potential source of future bleeding. **B,** Embolization with coils was performed to achieve definitive cessation of arterial hemorrhage under the relatively stabilized condition of the patient.

ment to approximately 180 N.[38] These sheets or binders also partially reduce the fracture, minimize the movement of the fracture site during transport, and provide pain relief for patients.[39] The application of a pelvic binder should be considered as early as possible. However, it should be recognized that they may be effective only in cases of external rotation of the pelvis. Placement for short periods of time is unlikely to cause complications and may be beneficial. Therefore, in the decision-making process, the orthopaedic surgeon should err on the side of overuse.

Potential complications of external wraps include the development of pressure ulcerations, skin necrosis, or slough, particularly when left on for more than 6 hours.[40] Another disadvantage is that these devices may compromise access for laparotomy or pelvic packing as well as prevent monitoring of the skin around the pelvis. Sheet wrapping and pelvic binders are less rigid than external fixators, and fracture reduction and restoration of bone contact is tenuous except in cases of simple open-book injuries. There are a limited number of efficacy series, and some recent studies have shown conflicting conclusions regarding mortality and blood transfusion requirements following the use of binders.[41] A recent literature review concluded that binders appear to be reasonably effective, although there is only level IV and V evidence.[42] Binders can be associated with skin complications if placed too tightly or for too long, and thus they should be used with caution and are not a substitute for overall proper management. Pelvic binders or sheets should be considered as temporary measures bridging toward more rigid stabilization. If the binder

appears to be effective and longer application is needed, other definitive means such as external fixation or internal fixation should be planned (**Figure 5**).

Open Pelvic Fractures
The mortality rate in patients with open pelvic fractures is as high as 50% because of loss of the self-tamponade effect in the acute phase and pelvic sepsis in the late phase.[43,44] Mortality is particularly high with severe soft-tissue injuries that often involve the rectum or genital tracts.[43] Emergency management of open pelvic fractures includes control of any torrential external bleeding by packing and direct pressure, mechanical stabilization to prevent further soft-tissue damage, aggressive irrigation and débridement of open wounds, and selective use of fecal diversion. Angiography should be considered after these measures if there is ongoing hemodynamic instability and/or active visible bleeding (**Figure 6**). Fecal diversion should be used for patients with extensive open perianal wounds and should be considered initially in all open pelvic fractures. Patients who have an open rectal wound also require fecal diversion with early sphincter repair and local open wound management. Vaginal lacerations require prompt repair.[44] The orthopaedic surgeon should be present when possible to help place diverting colostomies and bladder catheters in locations that will not compromise subsequent pelvic reconstruction surgery.

Biomechanics of Temporary Fixation
Temporary fixation that reduces the displaced fracture allows the hemostatic pathway to control bleeding

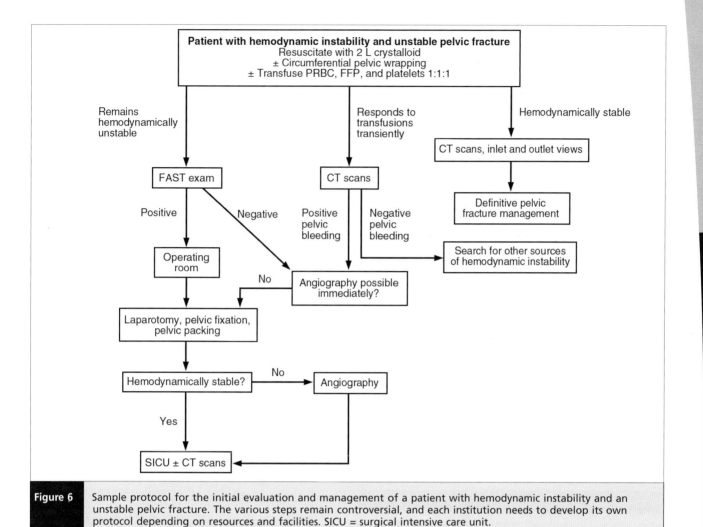

Figure 6 Sample protocol for the initial evaluation and management of a patient with hemodynamic instability and an unstable pelvic fracture. The various steps remain controversial, and each institution needs to develop its own protocol depending on resources and facilities. SICU = surgical intensive care unit.

from raw bony surfaces. External fixation can be performed either by placing the pins in the iliac crest under direct palpation without fluoroscopy or placing the pins in the supra-acetabular region of the innominate bones with fluoroscopy. Biomechanical studies show that supra-acetabular pin placement has greater rigidity and pullout strength. However, for the patient in shock and undergoing resuscitation, iliac crest placement is quicker and requires less equipment.

Experimental studies have shown that external fixation provides only a small volume change within the true pelvis even if applied to open-book pelvic fractures. Thus, an external fixator is thought to contribute to hemostasis primarily by decreasing bony motion at the fracture site, reopposing the cancellous bone surface, and allowing stable clot formation as well as maintaining a reduced pelvic volume. Disadvantages of external fixators are that they do not provide posterior stability and can potentially increase pelvic deformity and increase posterior displacement in a pelvis with a vertically unstable fracture configuration.[45] Skeletal traction of the affected side to control vertical instability may be necessary to reduce and maintain the unsta-

ble hemipelvis. External fixation plus longitudinal traction is an effective and accepted damage control modality in these cases.

Pelvic C-clamps can be placed either anteriorly or posteriorly on the pelvis, or on the greater trochanters (**Figure 7**). The insertion site on the greater trochanter is easy to access; however, the reduction force is not strong and almost similar to that of a pelvic binder or external fixation. The pins of the anteriorly placed C-clamp are located in the lateral and supra-acetabular area, where neurovascular complications are relatively uncommon, and the placement can be performed without fluoroscopic control. The anteriorly placed C-clamp is useful especially for Young-Burgess APC-2 type (OTA 61-B1,2) injuries.[46] The posterior placement can provide direct reduction and stabilization of the posterior pelvic fracture and can be effective in case of complete disruption of the posterior ring. Because the clamp can be rotated cephalad and caudad, access to the abdomen and perineum is not limited. Posterior placement is not applicable in iliac fractures and transiliac fracture-dislocations. Also, pelvic penetration or misplacement through the greater sciatic notch causing iatrogenic nerve and vascular injuries has been re-

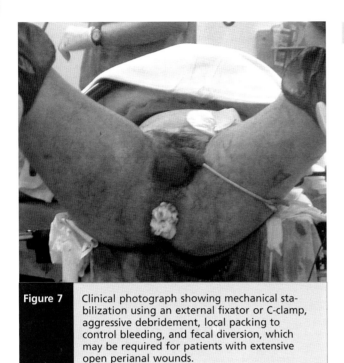

Figure 7 Clinical photograph showing mechanical stabilization using an external fixator or C-clamp, aggressive debridement, local packing to control bleeding, and fecal diversion, which may be required for patients with extensive open perianal wounds.

ported. Therefore, C-clamps should be applied by an experienced surgeon after careful evaluation of radiographs, and, if possible, with the aid of fluoroscopy in the case of posterior placement.

Summary

Pelvic fractures encompass a broad spectrum of injury from low-energy ramus fractures to high-energy dissociations of the pelvic ring. Although minimally displaced injuries can often be treated nonsurgically with expectant management, higher energy and more displaced injuries can result in severe disability unless optimally treated.

Unstable patients with pelvic fractures continue to present significant challenges in acute management. Successful treatment of pelvic fracture bleeding is best accomplished by a multidisciplinary team approach involving orthopaedic surgeons. Angiography and subsequent embolization can provide effective control of ongoing hemorrhage caused by arterial bleeding, if immediately available. Although its use is currently not widespread, pelvic packing is useful for hemodynamically unstable patients as part of a combined approach in conjunction with pelvic angiography. Standardized protocols should be adopted at any institution treating these severely injured patients in order to facilitate effective assessment and treatment. Ongoing quality assessments and further efforts to understand and minimize bleeding in the acute phase will improve the outcome for pelvic fracture patients.

Annotated References

1. Chenoweth DR, Cruickshank B, Gertzbein SD, Goldfarb P, Janosick J: A clinical and experimental investigation of occult injuries of the pelvic ring. *Injury* 1980;12: 59-65.

2. Olson SA, Burgess A: Classification and initial management of patients with unstable pelvic ring injuries. *Instr Course Lect* 2005;54:383-393.

   The authors discuss current methods of evaluating, assessing, and treating unstable pelvic ring injuries. They recommended that surgeons first determine whether patients have hemodynamic instability and identify the source of the hemorrhage. Then patients should be assessed for stabilization of pelvic ring. Level of evidence: V.

3. Marsh JL, Slongo TF, Agel J, et al: Fracture and dislocation classification compendium, 2007: Orthopaedic Trauma Association classification, database and outcomes committee. *J Orthop Trauma* 2007;21:S1-S133.

   The authors provide an updated revision of the original classification published in 1996.

4. Khoury A, Kreder H, Skrinskas T, Hardisty M, Tile M, Whyne CM: Lateral compression fracture of the pelvis represents a heterogeneous group of complex 3D patterns of displacement. *Injury* 2008;39:893-902.

   CT data from 60 patients with unilateral LC fractures were obtained. Fracture morphometry was perfomed using three-dimensional visualization software. Fractures initially diagnosed as LC actually represent a spectrum of displacement patterns, ranging from a minimally displaced hemipelvis to complex combinations of displacements. Fractures were grouped based on pattern of rotation and translation into five distinct groups. Three-dimensional analysis of displacement patterns demonstrated a complexity in LC fractures that may explain the variations seen in outcomes associated with this injury.

5. Lefaivre KA, Padelecki JR, Starr AJ: What constitutes a Young and Burgess lateral compression-I (OTA 61-B2) pelvic ring disruption? A description of computed tomography-based fracture anatomy and associated injuries. *J Orthop Trauma* 2009;23:L16-L21.

   The authors describe characteristics of LC-I pelvic fractures from a retrospective cohort from a trauma registry. They identified 100 consecutive fractures with 98 sacral fractures. Of these, 50 (50%) were Denis type I, 41 (41.8%) Denis type II and 7 (7.1%) Denis type III. Higher Denis types were more likely to result in complete sacral fractures.

6. Biffl WL, Smith WR, Moore EE, et al: Evolution of a multidisciplinary clinical pathway for the management of unstable patients with pelvic fractures. *Ann Surg* 2001;233(6):843-850.

7. Balogh Z, Caldwell E, Heetveld M, et al: Institutional practice guidelines on management of pelvic fracture-related hemodynamic instability: Do they make a difference? *J Trauma* 2005;58(4):778-782.

The authors developed evidence-based institutional guidelines and compared the outcomes before and after their implementation. The guidelines included abdominal clearance with diagnostic peritoneal aspiration/lavage or Focused Assessment With Sonography for Trauma, pelvic binding, pelvic angiography, and minimally invasive fixation of the pelvis in a timely fashion. Mortality rates decreased significantly with adherence to the guidelines. Level of evidence: III.

8. Smith W, Williams A, Agudelo J, et al: Early predictors of mortality in hemodynamically unstable pelvis fractures. *J Orthop Trauma* 2007;21(1):31-37.

The authors conducted a retrospective study of 187 hemodynamically unstable patients. It was noted that blood transfusion, Injury Severity Score, Revised Trauma Score, and age older than 60 years were significant predictors of mortality. Death within 24 hours was most often caused by acute blood loss, whereas death after 24 hours was most often caused by multiple organ failure. Level of evidence: V.

9. McCormick JP, Morgan SJ, Smith WR: Clinical effectiveness of the physical examination in diagnosis of posterior pelvic ring injuries. *J Orthop Trauma* 2003;17(4):257-261.

10. Shlamovitz GZ, Mower WR, Bergman J, et al: How (un)useful is the pelvic ring stability examination in diagnosing mechanically unstable pelvic fractures in blunt trauma patients? *J Trauma* 2009;66(3):815-820.

The authors assessed the sensitivity and specificity of manual examination for detection of mechanically unstable pelvic fractures by reviewing 1,502 blunt trauma patients. They concluded that the presence of either pelvic deformity or an unstable pelvic ring on physical examination had poor sensitivity. Level of evidence: III.

11. Tseng S, Tornetta P III: Percutaneous management of Morel-Lavallee lesions. *J Bone Joint Surg Am* 2006;88(1):92-96.

The authors reported on 19 patients with a Morel-Lavallée lesion who were managed with percutaneous drainage and débridement within 3 days after the injury. No deep infection occurred after internal fixation of the pelvic and acetabular fractures. They concluded that early percutaneous management of Morel-Lavallée lesions was safe and effective. Level of evidence: IV.

12. Ziran BH, Chamberlin E, Shuler FD, Shah M: Delays and difficulties in the diagnosis of lower urologic injuries in the context of pelvic fractures. *J Trauma* 2005;58(3):533-537.

This article describes the characteristics of 43 pelvic fracture patients with concomitant urologic injuries. The findings showed that 23% of all bladder and urethral disruptions were missed at initial evaluation. Bladder ruptures were missed because of errors in cystography, and urethral tears were missed because suggestive physical finding were absent. Level of evidence: IV.

13. Papadopoulos IN, Kanakaris N, Bonovas S, et al: Auditing 655 fatalities with pelvic fractures by autopsy as a basis to evaluate trauma care. *J Am Coll Surg* 2006;203(1):30-43.

In this study based on autopsy-evaluated circumstances of 655 deaths of patients with pelvic fractures, the authors showed that nearly half of the patients had a potential cause of major hemorrhage other than pelvic fractures. Level of evidence: III.

14. Sperry JL, Ochoa JB, Gunn SR, et al: An FFP:PRBC transfusion ratio >/=1:1.5 is associated with a lower risk of mortality after massive transfusion. *J Trauma* 2008; 65(5):986-993.

The authors conducted a multicenter cohort study evaluating clinical outcomes in 415 blunt trauma patients with hemorrhagic shock. It was noted that patients who received transfusion products in a greater than 1:1.5 FFP:PRBC ratio versus a less than 1:1.5 ratio had significant less blood transfusion requirements and lower mortality at 24 hours. Level of evidence: III.

15. Zink KA, Sambasivan CN, Holcomb JB, Chisholm G, Schreiber MA: A high ratio of plasma and platelets to packed red blood cells in the first 6 hours of massive transfusion improves outcomes in a large multicenter study. *Am J Surg* 2009;197(5):565-570.

The authors present a retrospective study of the transfusion ratios in the first 6 hours in 466 massive transfusion trauma patients. A higher ratio of FFP:PRBC and platelets: PRBC led to improved 6-hour mortality. They concluded that early administration of FFP and platelets is critical to improve the outcomes. Level of evidence: III.

16. Sarin EL, Moore JB, Moore EE, et al: Pelvic fracture pattern does not always predict the need for urgent embolization. *J Trauma* 2005;58(5):973-977.

The authors analyzed 283 pelvic fractures for evidence of a relationship between major ligamentous disruption and the need for angiographic embolization. They concluded that the pelvic fracture pattern did not consistently correlate with the patient's need for urgent embolization. Level of evidence: III.

17. Elzik ME, Dirschl DR, Dahners LE: Hemorrhage in pelvic fractures does not correlate with fracture length. *J Trauma* 2008;65(2):436-441.

The authors analyzed the relationship between fracture types and hematocrit change in 72 isolated pelvic fracture patients. No significant correlations were found between change in hematocrit and length of fracture lines. They concluded that pelvic hemorrhage could not be reliably predicted based on AP radiograph assessments. Level of evidence: III.

18. Velmahos GC, Toutouzas KG, Vassiliu P, et al: A prospective study on the safety and efficacy of angiographic embolization for pelvic and visceral injuries. *J Trauma* 2002;53(2):303-308.

19. Miller PR, Moore PS, Mansell E, Meredith JW, Chang MC: External fixation or arteriogram in bleeding pelvic fracture: Initial therapy guided by markers of arterial hemorrhage. *J Trauma* 2003;54(3):437-443.

20. Kimbrell BJ, Velmahos GC, Chan LS, Demetriades D: Angiographic embolization for pelvic fractures in older patients. *Arch Surg* 2004;139(7):728-733.

4: Axial Skeleton, Including Spine and Pelvis

The authors present an observational study of 92 patients who underwent angiography. They concluded that an age of 60 years or older was the independent factor of the need for angiographic embolization. Level of evidence: III.

21. Salim A, Teixeira PG, DuBose J, et al: Predictors of positive angiography in pelvic fractures: A prospective study. *J Am Coll Surg* 2008;207(5):656-662.

   The authors conducted a prospective observational study of 137 patients who had angiography for hemodynamic instability, fracture pattern, or CT demonstrating a large pelvic hematoma. Presence of sacroiliac joint disruption, female sex, and duration of hypotension could reliably predict patients who had contrast extravasation by angiography. Level of evidence: III.

22. Starr AJ, Griffin DR, Reinert CM, et al: Pelvic ring disruptions: Prediction of associated injuries, transfusion requirement, pelvic arteriography, complications, and mortality. *J Orthop Trauma* 2002;16(8):553-561.

23. Blackmore CC, Jurkovich GJ, Linnau KF, Cummings P, Hoffer EK, Rivara FP: Assessment of volume of hemorrhage and outcome from pelvic fracture. *Arch Surg* 2003;138(5):504-509.

24. Brasel KJ, Pham K, Yang H, Christensen R, Weigelt JA: Significance of contrast extravasation in patients with pelvic fracture. *J Trauma* 2007;62(5):1149-1152.

   The authors reviewed 42 patients who showed contrast extravasation on CT scans. Seventeen of the patients actually required angiographic embolization. They concluded that contrast extravasation is a marker of severe injury but does not mandate angiography. Level of evidence: III.

25. Gourlay D, Hoffer E, Routt M, Bulger E: Pelvic angiography for recurrent traumatic pelvic arterial hemorrhage. *J Trauma* 2005;59(5):1168-1174.

   The authors describe a subset of patients requiring repeat pelvic angiogram in which 68% of the patients were identified as having a new bleeding site. They concluded that although angiographic control of pelvic arterial injuries is successful, recurrent pelvic arterial hemorrhage can occur. Level of evidence: IV.

26. Shapiro M, McDonald AA, Knight D, Johannigman JA, Cuschieri J: The role of repeat angiography in the management of pelvic fractures. *J Trauma* 2005;58(2):227-231.

   The authors performed a retrospective study of 31 patients who underwent angiographic embolizaton. Seven (22.6%) patients required repeat angiography. Continued or recurrent hypotension, absence of intra-abdominal injury, and persistent base deficit were predictive of need for angiography. Level of evidence: III.

27. Fang JF, Shih LY, Wong YC, Lin BC, Hsu YP: Repeat transcatheter arterial embolization for the management of pelvic arterial hemorrhage. *J Trauma* 2009;66(2):429-435.

   The authors reported on a retrospective review of 140 patients who had angiographic embolization. Repeat angiography was performed in 18.6% of patients. Initial hemoglobin level lower than 7.5 g/dL and more than 6 units of blood transfusion were predictors for repeat angiographic embolization. Level of evidence: III.

28. Gänsslen A, Giannoudis P, Pape HC: Hemorrhage in pelvic fracture: Who needs angiography? *Curr Opin Crit Care* 2003;9(6):515-523.

29. Suzuki T, Shindo M, Kataoka Y, et al: Clinical characteristics of pelvic fracture patients with gluteal necrosis resulting from transcatheter arterial embolization. *Arch Orthop Trauma Surg* 2005;125(7):448-452.

   The authors reviewed 165 patients treated with nonselective angiographic embolization of bilateral internal iliac arteries, of whom 12 patients had gluteal necrosis. They concluded that patients with clear-border low density area on CT, skin necrosis centered on the buttock, and delayed appearance of a skin lesion would be highly indicative of the necrosis caused by embolization. Level of evidence: IV.

30. Yasumura K, Ikegami K, Kamohara T, Nohara Y: High incidence of ischemic necrosis of the gluteal muscle after transcatheter angiographic embolization for severe pelvic fracture. *J Trauma* 2005;58(5):985-990.

   The authors reported a small subset of patients who underwent MRI of the pelvis following bilateral massive angiographic embolization. All six patients demonstrated ischemic damage of the gluteal muscle on MRI, and five of them showed macroscopic muscle necrosis during open reduction of the pelvic fractures. Level of evidence: IV.

31. Kataoka Y, Maekawa K, Nishimaki H, Yamamoto S, Soma K: Iliac vein injuries in hemodynamically unstable patients with pelvic fracture caused by blunt trauma. *J Trauma* 2005;58(4):704-710.

   The authors reviewed 72 patients with unstable pelvic fractures who presented with shock. Following successful angiographic embolization, 11 patients who had persistent hemodynamic instability underwent venography of the iliac veins. Of these patients, 9 showed significant venous extravasation, and 7 of the 9 patients died due to exsanguination. Level of evidence: IV.

32. Cothren CC, Osborn PM, Moore EE, Morgan SJ, Johnson JL, Smith WR: Preperitonal pelvic packing for hemodynamically unstable pelvic fractures: A paradigm shift. *J Trauma* 2007;62(4):834-842.

   The authors developed protocols including early intervention of external fixation and preperitoneal pelvic packing. During their study period, 28 patients with pelvic fractures underwent packing, and no deaths as a result of acute blood loss were observed. They concluded that packing was a rapid method for controlling pelvic fracture-related hemorrhage. Level of evidence: IV.

33. Tötterman A, Madsen JE, Skaga NO, Røise O: Extraperitoneal pelvic packing: A salvage procedure to control massive traumatic pelvic hemorrhage. *J Trauma* 2007;62(4):843-852.

The authors present their experiences of extraperitoneal pelvic packing to control massive pelvic bleeding. In total, 18 patients underwent the packing, and 72.2% of patients survived. Only one of the nonsurvivors died of exsanguination. They concluded that pelvic packing might be lifesaving in patients with severe pelvic injuries. Level of evidence: IV.

34. Osborn PM, Smith WR, Moore EE, et al: Direct retroperitoneal pelvic packing versus pelvic angiography: A comparison of two management protocols for haemodynamically unstable pelvic fractures. *Injury* 2009; 40(1):54-60.

The authors compared patients treated with pelvic angiography with ones treated with pelvic packing. The packing group underwent surgical packing at a mean of 45 minutes, and the angiography group at a mean of 130 minutes. The packing group demonstrated a significant decrease in blood transfusions over the 24 hours postintervention. Level of evidence: III.

35. Boffard KD, Riou B, Warren B, et al: Recombinant factor VIIa as adjunctive therapy for bleeding control in severely injured trauma patients: Two parallel randomized, placebo-controlled, double-blind clinical trials. *J Trauma* 2005;59(1):8-18.

The authors conducted two randomized, placebo-controlled, double-blind trials (blunt trauma and penetrating trauma) evaluating the efficacy and safety of factor VIIa. In 143 blunt trauma patients, red blood cell transfusion was significantly reduced with factor VIIa. Adverse events were evenly distributed between the two groups. Level of evidence: I.

36. Raobaikady R, Redman J, Ball JA, Maloney G, Grounds RM: Use of activated recombinant coagulation factor VII in patients undergoing reconstruction surgery for traumatic fracture of pelvis or pelvis and acetabulum: A double-blind, randomized, placebo-controlled trial. *Br J Anaesth* 2005;94(5):586-591.

The authors conducted a double-blind, randomized, placebo-controlled trial of use of factor VIIa for 48 patients undergoing pelvic reconstruction surgery. The blood loss during operations was not significantly different between two groups. They concluded that the prophylactic use of factor VIIa did not decrease the volume of perioperative blood loss in pelvic surgery. Level of evidence: I.

37. Suzuki T, Smith WR, Moore EE: Pelvic packing or angiography: Competitive or complementary? *Injury* 2009;40:343-353.

This article details recent evidence and data regarding pelvic resuscitation, packing, and angiography. The authors make a point that the various modalities should be viewed as part of a complementary treatment approach. Specific protocols and details in management are described.

38. Bottlang M, Krieg JC, Mohr M, Simpson TS, Madey SM: Emergent management of pelvic ring fractures with use of circumferential compression. *J Bone Joint Surg Am* 2002;84(suppl 2):43-47.

39. Krieg JC, Mohr M, Ellis TJ, Simpson TS, Madey SM, Bottlang M: Emergent stabilization of pelvic ring injuries by controlled circumferential compression: A clinical trial. *J Trauma* 2005;59(3):659-664.

In this prospective clinical trial, the authors evaluated 16 patients with pelvic ring injuries. In patients with external rotation injuries, a pelvic circumferential compression device significantly reduced pelvic displacement. In patients with internal rotation injuries, the device did not cause significant overcompression. Level of evidence: III.

40. Jowett AJ, Bowyer GW: Pressure characteristics of pelvic binders. *Injury* 2007;38(1):118-121.

In this experimental study of 10 healthy volunteers, the authors reported the pressures developed at the bony prominences when a pelvic binder was applied. The pressures between the pelvic binder and the skin were all greater than the pressure recommended at interfaces to avoid the development of pressure sores. Level of evidence: IV.

41. Ghaemmaghami V, Sperry J, Gunst M, et al: Effects of early use of external pelvic compression on transfusion requirements and mortality in pelvic fractures. *Am J Surg* 2007;194(6):720-723.

The authors present the results of a retrospective study evaluating the efficacy of pelvic binder in 118 patients compared with historical controls. In patients with the pelvic binder, there was no effect on mortality, need for pelvic angioembolization, or 24-hour transfusions. The authors concluded that the pelvic binders may have limited use in control of hemorrhage. Level of evidence: III.

42. Spanjersberg WR, Krops SP, Schep NWL, et al: Effectiveness and complications of pelvic circumferential compression devices in patients with unstable pelvic fractures: A systematic review of literature. *Injury* 2009; 40:1031-1035.

The authors provide a comprehensive review of the literature regarding sheets, binders, beanbags, and other temporary fixation devices. They conclude that although no clear prospective study exists defining the comparative efficacy of differing stabilization strategies, pelvic compression devices are inexpensive and useful. Complications can occur, however, and placement of these devices should be accompanied by careful observation and appropriate timing of removal.

43. Dente CJ, Feliciano DV, Rozycki GS, et al: The outcome of open pelvic fractures in the modern era. *Am J Surg* 2005;190(6):830-835.

In this study, 44 patients were identified as having open pelvic fractures. The overall mortality rate was 45%. The risk factors for overall mortality included vertical shear pattern of injury, Revised Trauma Score, transfusion requirements, and Injury Severity Score. Level of evidence: IV.

44. Grotz MR, Allami MK, Harwood P, Pape HC, Krettek C, Giannoudis PV: Open pelvic fractures: Epidemiology, current concepts of management and outcome. *Injury* 2005;36(1):1-13.

The authors discuss current management of open pelvic fractures. They recommend that repeated, meticulous wound irrigation and débridement, administration of broad-spectrum antibiotics, and selective fecal diversion are undertaken to minimize the risk of sepsis and reduce mortality. Level of evidence: V.

45. Dickson KF, Matta JM: Skeletal deformity after anterior external fixation of the pelvis. *J Orthop Trauma* 2009;23(5):327-332.

The authors present 11 transferred patients who had emergent application of an anterior external fixator by the referring orthopaedist. They compared radiographs before and after the placement of external fixation. It was noted that all patients displayed either posterior cephalad translation or posterior diastasis of more than 1 cm. Level of evidence: IV.

46. Richard MJ, Tornetta P III: Emergent management of APC-2 pelvic ring injuries with an anteriorly placed C-clamp. *J Orthop Trauma* 2009;23(5):322-326.

The authors conducted a prospective cohort study of anterior placement of pelvic C-clamps to control APC-2 type injuries. Twenty-four patients were emergently managed with C-clamps, and the symphyseal separation was reduced to less than 2 cm in all cases. They concluded that the C-clamps could be placed anteriorly with a short application time in a variety of patient care areas. Level of evidence: IV.

Pelvic Fractures: Definitive Treatment and Expected Outcomes

H. Claude Sagi, MD   Matthew Jimenez, MD, FACS

Introduction

The primary goal in the treatment of pelvic ring fractures is prevention of malunion. Nonunion is an infrequent occurrence secondary to the rich vascular supply to all regions of the pelvic ring. Malposition of one hemipelvis relative to the other can result in any or all of the following conditions, and surgery is indicated to prevent or mitigate the likelihood of their occurrence: leg length inequality and mechanical low back pain, sitting imbalance, dyspareunia, and bowel and bladder dysfunction. With purely ligamentous injuries (for example, symphyseal disruptions and sacroiliac [SI] joint dislocations), persistent "instability" and chronic pain in addition to malunion must also be considered as possible sequelae of a pelvic ring injury. However, it is difficult to identify those injuries that exhibit sufficient ligamentous instability to warrant surgical stabilization.

With complete instability of the posterior ring (posterior SI ligamentous disruption or nonimpacted displaced sacral fractures), anterior fixation alone is inadequate for maintaining reduction and restoring stability to the pelvic ring. In addition, with instability of the posterior ring and cephalad displacement, posterior fixation should be supplemented with some form of anterior stabilization (open reduction and internal fixation [ORIF] or external fixation).[1] Although the pubic symphysis supplies only 10% to 15% of the stability to the intact pelvic ring,[2] it is critical in restoring the normal loading response and stability to the unstable hemipelvis.[3]

Dr. Sagi or an immediate family member is a member of a speakers' bureau or has made paid presentations on behalf of Stryker, Synthes, and Smith & Nephew; is a paid consultant for or an employee of Stryker, Synthes, and Smith & Nephew; has received research or institutional support from Stryker, Synthes, and Smith & Nephew; and is a board member, owner, officer, or committee member for the American Academy of Orthopaedic Surgeons, the Orthopaedic Trauma Association, and the foundation for Orthopaedic Trauma. Dr. Jimenez or an immediate family member is a board member, owner, officer, or committee member of the Illinois Association of Orthopaedic Surgeons.

Definitive Radiographic Evidence of Injury

Diagnosing and defining pelvic ring instability, particularly as a precursor for indicating surgical intervention, is not always straightforward. Certainly, the extremes of a nondisplaced crack in the ramus or the vertical instability of a completely detached hemipelvis do not present much of a clinical dilemma. However, with regard to the pelvic ring, there exists a large spectrum of poorly stratified or defined injuries that could, depending on the clinical scenario and patient, be either stable or unstable.

Pelvic ring injuries can be classified according to anatomic and mechanistic schema. However, it is also useful to compartmentalize pelvic ring injuries into a basic scheme that may better define the need for surgical reduction and fixation. It is important to categorize the pelvic ring injury as involving bony and/or ligamentous structures, and the anterior and/or posterior pelvic ring.

Bony injuries have a tendency to heal more predictably with biomechanical properties that equal the pre-injury state in terms of strength and stability. Ligamentous injuries heal with scar tissue formation, less predictability, and the potential for residual instability. For these reasons, certain bony injuries are more likely to be treated successfully with nonsurgical intervention and simple protected weight bearing.

Additionally, it tends to be easier for the surgeon to have confidence that a given bony injury is stable or unstable based on a static radiograph. Impacted fractures without gaps in good bone quality tend to have at least some inherent stability. The same principle, however, does not hold true for a ligamentous injury to the pelvic ring, which can appear relatively benign on a static film but under stress examination discloses significant instability. There is some evidence in the literature supporting the notion that bony pelvic injuries have better outcomes compared to ligamentous injuries.

Based on early cadaver work, it is known that diastasis of the symphysis of greater than 2.5 cm implies that the sacrospinous, sacrotuberous, and anterior SI ligaments have been compromised and, importantly, that the posterior SI ligaments are intact.[2] Clearly,

---

though, this value cannot be applied to patients of varying ages, sexes, and pelvic diameters. Additionally, the human pelvic tissues are elastic and a certain amount of recoil (or a pelvic binder/sheet) may hide occult instability. For these reasons, some surgeons may elect to perform stress examination of the pelvic ring to help disclose any potential occult instability for ligamentous injuries. It is important to remember, however, that although some surgeons may advocate stress examination of the pelvic ring, formal well-defined parameters for "normal" and "abnormal" motion of one hemipelvis relative to the other have not yet been established.

Force transmission from the lower extremities to the trunk occurs via the pelvis: from the ischial tuberosities to the SI joints, then to the axial skeleton during sitting, and from the acetabulae to the SI joints, then to the axial skeleton during standing. During single-leg stance, the symphysis has a tendency to open and shear, whereas during double-leg stance it has a tendency to close. In all situations, the posterior ring (sciatic buttress, SI joint, sacral alae) is pivotal in this force transmission and is therefore considered to be the key element that requires as close to anatomic reconstruction as possible.

Based on a few clinical analyses on outcomes of pelvic injuries in the literature, combined (axial and coronal planes) displacement of the posterior pelvic ring greater than 1 cm potentially correlates with a worse clinical outcome (to be discussed later). Based on the mechanics of force transmission and the importance of this combined displacement, the posterior ring injury tends to be what drives the decision to operate in most cases. With injuries to the posterior ring, the anterior injury is often reduced and stabilized to simply augment and protect the posterior reconstruction. Indications for surgical treatment of an anterior ring injury in isolation are uncommon and dictated more by the existence of or potential for visceral (primarily bladder) injury.

The presentation of the patient on the ward can at times help determine the degree of injury. A patient who can roll around and sit up in bed is unlikely to have a grossly unstable pelvic fracture, and nonsurgical treatment is warranted. However, the patient who complains of severe low back or buttock pain with log-rolling in bed for hygienic purposes is more likely to have an unstable pelvic ring.

Nonsurgical Treatment of Pelvic Ring Injuries

Nonsurgical treatment of pelvic ring injuries is reserved for those situations where the anatomy and stability of the pelvic ring are maintained to a sufficient degree so as not to result in the consequences of malunion as previously outlined. In addition, nonsurgical treatment is indicated when the physiologic condition of the patient is compromised to such a degree that the consequences of malunion are preferable to the risks of major complications from surgical intervention.

In general terms, the following injuries can be considered stable and the patient offered a trial of nonsurgical care: nondisplaced or minimally displaced ramus fractures, symphyseal disruptions with less than 2.5 cm of widening (Young-Burgess anterior posterior compression-1 injury), impacted sacral fractures (Young-Burgess lateral compression-1 injury) without cephalad displacement or excessive internal rotation of the hemipelvis that may result in impingement upon the bladder, dyspareunia, or sitting imbalance (not quantified in the literature).

Patients with stable pelvic ring injuries often have minimal discomfort and are able to mobilize in 1 to 2 days. Patients with occult instability of seemingly benign pelvic ring injuries may have difficulty with simple movements such as rolling in bed. Some authors[4] advocate the use of single-leg stance or "flamingo" views for diagnosing occult instability of the pelvic ring. However, in the acute setting, these views have limited applicability because of patient discomfort. Examination under anesthesia with dynamic intraoperative stress fluoroscopic views may be indicated in some patients in whom occult ligamentous instability of the pelvic ring is suspected. With the patient supine, the pelvis is stressed using external rotation, internal rotation, and push-pull maneuvers on the lower extremities while taking AP, inlet, and outlet projections. No change in pelvic relationships can be interpreted as a stable pelvic ring. However, the normal ranges of motion of the pelvic ring under stress examination are not well defined. The consequences of malunion can significantly affect function and quality of life for patients. Therefore, a course of nonsurgical care must be undertaken only in compliant patients who can be followed closely with serial physical and radiographic examinations to detect any early displacement

Anterior Pelvic Ring Injuries

The main indications for surgical treatment of anterior pelvic ring injuries include symphyseal dislocations demonstrating greater than 2.5 cm of diastasis on either static or dynamic (examination under anesthesia) imaging and to augment posterior fixation in vertically displaced unstable pelvic ring injuries. The correction of pelvic ring deformity, such as with a locked (overlapping) symphysis, and the relief of pain and immobility associated with fracture of the anterior ring injury constitute additional indications.

External Fixation of the Anterior Pelvic Ring

With regard to controlling external rotation of the hemipelvis with an anterior posterior compression-type injury susceptible to external rotation forces, biomechanical studies[1,2] have shown no significant clinically beneficial difference between anterior external or internal fixation of the pelvis. In other words, internal fixation, particularly with two plates, has been shown to be su-

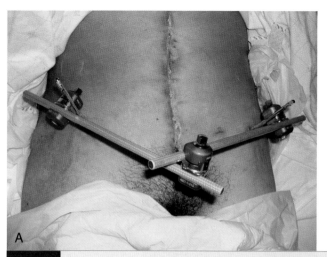
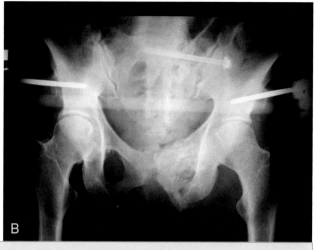

Figure 1 A, Clinical photograph of a supra-acetabular fixator placed low enough to provide access to the abdomen. **B**, AP radiograph of a supra-acetabular external fixator. (Courtesy of H. Claude Sagi, MD, Tampa, FL.)

perior to resisting rotational forces with vertical loading. The load at which failure (as defined by greater than 1 cm of displacement) occurs exceeded that of what is normally experienced by the pelvis for all constructs including external fixation frames. However, anterior internal fixation is significantly superior to external fixation in resisting vertical displacement of the hemipelvis.[2] It has also been shown that there is significant improvement in pelvic ring stability when posterior fixation constructs are augmented with some form of anterior fixation in vertical shear injury patterns.[1,3]

Additionally, the use of anterior inferior distraction external fixation to reduce lateral compression injuries has been described. Provided that there is no residual sagittal plane rotational deformity, the frame can be left in place for 6 to 8 weeks to maintain the reduction while the patient resumes mobilization.[5]

Although external fixators are relatively easy to apply, reports of pin site complications, interference with abdominal access, poor ergonomics, inability to maintain accurate reductions, and bladder entrapment have limited their use in modern pelvic reconstructions.[6] Currently, anterior pelvic external fixation is used predominantly for definitive stabilization of the anterior pelvis when ORIF is precluded by the clinical situation of the patient (for example, contaminated anterior abdominal incisions and bladder ruptures).

Two techniques for application of anterior pelvic external fixators are currently used: Schanz pins placed into the iliac crest and wing,[7,8] or Schanz pins placed into the supra-acetabular bone at the anterior inferior iliac spine directed toward the sciatic buttress[9] (**Figure 1**). Five-millimeter Schanz pins for both constructs have been shown to be significantly stronger than 4-mm pins.[10] Recent biomechanical studies have demonstrated that the supra-acetabular frame is equal in stiffness to the iliac crest frame for resisting flexion and extension; however, it is stiffer in resisting internal and external rotation and out-of-plane loading.[11]

Currently, there are no scientific data to support the use of one plate-screw configuration over another for fixation of the pubic symphysis. Some authors believe that two-hole plates are advantageous because they allow some degree of "physiologic" motion to occur at the symphysis.[12] However, one study has shown a higher rate of fixation failure and pelvic malunion with two-hole plating, recommending a plating configuration that has at least two points of fixation on either side of the symphysis.[13] Dual plating and multiplanar plates have not been found to offer improved stability over single uniplanar symphyseal plates in biomechanical studies.[14] The use of a locked screw-plate construct to augment fixation is another option in osteoporotic bone, but there are no published clinical or biomechanical studies endorsing this technique. The current preferred method consists of a four- or six-hole symphyseal plate with at least two 3.5-mm or 4.5-mm cortical screws on each side of the symphysis.

ORIF of Ramus Fractures

Ramus fractures, unlike symphyseal disruptions, are bony injuries with a surrounding periosteal sleeve that will enhance stability in minimally displaced fractures and provide more predictable bony healing. Because of these factors, many ramus fractures can be treated nonsurgically. However, for widely displaced fracture-dislocations of the pelvic ring with considerable soft-tissue damage and instability (particularly very unstable vertical shear injuries), ORIF of a ramus fracture with a plate and screw construct may be indicated to augment posterior fixation and improve upon the reduction and stability of the reconstructed pelvic ring.[15]

The use of intramedullary screws is another option for stabilization of ramus fractures that may permit percutaneous application where indicated.[16] However, a closed or careful percutaneous reduction must be possible to allow passage of the screw through the narrow

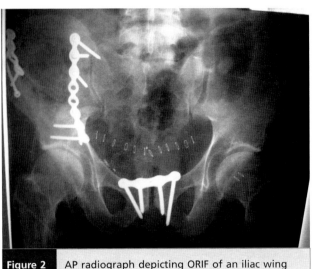

| Figure 2 | AP radiograph depicting ORIF of an iliac wing fracture. (Courtesy of H. Claude Sagi, MD, Tampa, FL.) |

| Figure 3 | AP radiograph depicting ORIF of a large crescent fracture without the need for ilio-sacral screws. (Courtesy of H. Claude Sagi, MD, Tampa, FL.) |

corridor provided by the superior ramus. Ramus screws are also an option for fixation after formal open reduction of the ramus if there is minimal comminution at the fracture site. The choice for antegrade or retrograde medullary fixation of a ramus fracture may depend on the location of the fracture. Based on the patient's anatomy and diameter of the medullary canal, an antegrade anterior column screw may be technically easier to apply with superior fixation for laterally located fractures. Conversely, more medial fractures may be better treated with a retrograde screw, again depending on the anatomy. One study, however, found a higher failure rate with elderly patients, in particular with fractures medial to the lateral border of the obturator foramen.[16]

Posterior Pelvic Ring Injuries

The primary indications for surgical treatment of posterior pelvic ring injuries include displaced iliac wing fractures that traverse the crest and greater sciatic notch or sacroiliac joint (crescent fractures) and Orthopaedic Trauma Association 61-C type injuries, with disruption of the posterior SI ligaments resulting in multiplanar instability of the SI joint and nonimpacted, comminuted, displaced sacral fractures. Other indications include any posterior ring injury that has demonstrated or has the propensity for cephalad (vertical) displacement and U-shaped sacral fractures with spinal-pelvic dissociation.

Iliac Wing Fractures and Fracture-Dislocations (Crescent Fractures)

Iliac wing fractures can be reduced and stabilized with either an anterior or posterior approach, depending on the location of the fracture. A single pelvic reconstruction plate or lag screw along the crest, supplemented

with a second reconstruction plate or lag screw at the level of the pelvic brim (anterior approach), or sciatic buttress (posterior approach) will usually suffice in neutralizing deforming forces until healing has occurred[17] (Figure 2).

Iliac wing fractures are more often associated with open wounds than other pelvic ring injuries, and may be associated with entrapped bowel.[18] Careful examination of the wound and CT scan are imperative. Early reconstruction of the ilium and serial débridements with open packing and delayed closure is the recommended approach for treatment of these injuries.[17,18]

The iliac wing fracture may enter the SI joint, resulting in partial dislocation of the SI joint and disruption of some or all of the SI ligaments: the so-called crescent fracture.[19] The crescent fragment is of variable size, containing the posterior superior iliac spine and posterior inferior iliac spine and remains attached to the sacrum via the posterior and (depending on the fracture location) the intraosseous SI ligaments. The anterior SI ligaments are disrupted along with displacement of the iliac wing fracture fragment.

For crescent fractures that involve only a small portion of the SI joint and have a large crescent fragment maintaining attachment to uninjured posterior and intraosseous ligaments, the treatment parallels that for an iliac wing fracture. Stable fixation of the iliac wing to this crescent fragment with intact ligaments will provide adequate and stable fixation to maintain reduction of the posterior ring until healing occurs. Supplemental iliosacral screws should not be needed (Figure 3). Standard fixation involves a superiorly placed pelvic reconstruction plate along the iliac crest with supplemental lag screws from the posterior inferior iliac spine into the sciatic buttress just above the greater notch. As the crescent fragment becomes smaller, this injury approaches an SI dislocation, and consideration must be given to supplemental fixation with SI screws or plates.[19]

SI Joint Dislocations

The SI joint can be treated using either an anterior or posterior approach.[20,21] Longitudinal traction is the single most important maneuver to use, and it is important to position the patient on the table (whether prone or supine) in such a way that the hemipelvis can be easily manipulated and adequate longitudinal traction can be applied. In situations where significant amounts of traction are required, the patient can be rigidly fixed to the operating room table using some form of table-skeletal fixation[22] to prevent distal migration of the patient and tilting of the pelvis (Figure 4).

With the joint satisfactorily reduced, stable fixation can be applied using iliosacral lag screws, transiliac bars/screws, or anterior SI plating if the reduction has been performed from anterior. Although biomechanical studies[23] have not shown significant superiority of either iliosacral screw fixation, transiliac fixation, or anterior SI plating, iliosacral screws can be applied in either the prone or supine position, and in open or percutaneous situations of severe soft-tissue damage when closed reduction is possible. For these reasons, iliosacral screws are the most commonly used form of fixation for the unstable SI joint.[24] Tension band plating and anterior SI plating are more commonly used to aid in reduction or to supplement iliosacral screw fixation in very unstable fracture patterns with poor iliosacral screw fixation.

Technical Considerations for Iliosacral Screw Fixation

An experienced surgeon, excellent intraoperative fluoroscopic imaging, and thorough knowledge of pelvic anatomy, including radiographic and surface landmarks, are necessary to prevent complications with iliosacral screw fixation[25-27] Three clear radiographic projections are necessary for the safe and accurate placement of iliosacral screws: the lateral sacrum, the pelvic inlet, and the pelvic outlet (Figure 5).

Although surgical navigation systems have enjoyed a rapid increase in popularity and utility with spinal pedicle screws and total joint arthroplasty, they have not enjoyed the same popularity with pelvic surgery. This is in part because of the inherent difficulties in fiducial positioning and obtaining image quality sufficient for tracking and navigation. However, there have been several preliminary reports examining the placement of iliosacral screws in cadaver pelves demonstrating improved or equal accuracy with a substantial decrease in radiation exposure to the surgeon.[28] Currently these systems, whether based on optical or electromagnetic guidance, still add considerable time to the procedure and should not be used in place of experience and knowledge of three-dimensional pelvic anatomy.

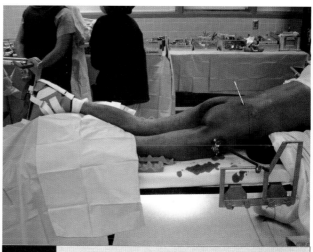

Figure 4 Clinical photograph depicting the use of table-skeletal fixation with the patient in the prone position and traction being applied. (Courtesy of H. Claude Sagi, MD, Tampa, FL.)

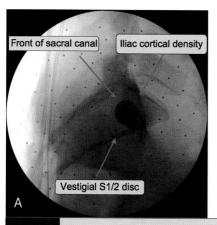
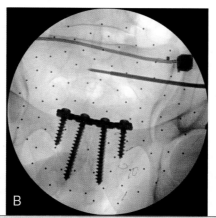
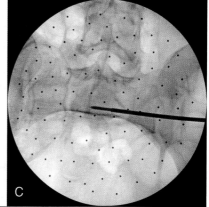

Figure 5 Intraoperative lateral (**A**), outlet (**B**), and inlet (**C**) projections with landmarks for iliosacral screw placement. (Courtesy of H. Claude Sagi, MD, Tampa, FL.)

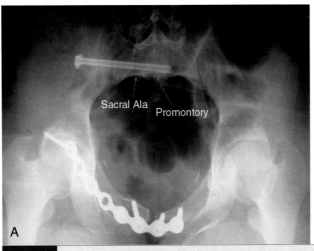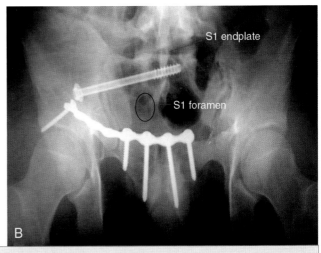

Figure 6 Correct iliosacral screw placement for stabilization of SI joint dislocation as pictured on the inlet (**A**) and outlet (**B**) views. (Courtesy of H. Claude Sagi, MD, Tampa, FL.)

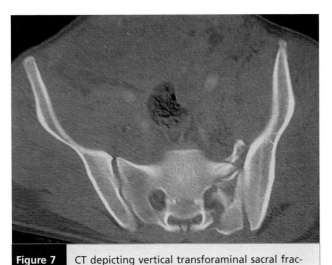

Figure 7 CT depicting vertical transforaminal sacral fracture. (Courtesy of H. Claude Sagi, MD, Tampa, FL.)

Partially threaded cannulated screws with diameters of 6.5 mm, 7.3 mm, or 8.0 mm have all been used to stabilize SI joint dislocations. There are no studies citing the superiority of one diameter over the other. Screw placement into the contralateral ala is suboptimal because this places the contralateral L5 nerve root at risk, and decreased bone density results in poor screw purchase. Therefore, long thread lengths with the tip of the screw in the sacral body and promontory offer the greatest resistance to screw pull-out.[27,29] The SI screw should be directed superiorly and anteriorly to avoid the S1 nerve root tunnel[30] (**Figure 6**). A second iliosacral screw can be placed into S1 or S2 if purchase of the first SI screw is thought to be suboptimal or considerable instability of the pelvic ring exists.[31] Additionally, improved purchase and fixation can be achieved with a transsacral screw placed into the contralateral ilium.[32] Careful scrutiny of the preoperative CT scan is imperative to ensure the patient's anatomy will permit placement of this screw. Currently available data from biomechanical studies suggest increased stability with a second iliosacral screw for SI dislocations, with a second screw into the S2 vertebral body being superior to a second screw into S1.[33] The final consideration for iliosacral screw placement must include an evaluation for sacral dysmorphism and segmentation anomalies of the lumbosacral junction. Significant variability in the relationship between lumbosacral nerve roots and bony anatomy exists, particularly with segmentation anomalies. These peculiarities in sacral anatomy have been well described and need to be recognized prior to placement of iliosacral screws.[26]

Vertical Sacral Fractures

Depending on the injury pattern, sacral fractures can be regarded as a pelvic ring injury, spinal injury, or both. Longitudinal or vertical sacral fractures result in disruption of the posterior pelvic ring. These fractures have been classified into three zones: lateral to the sacral foramina, through the foramina, and medial to the foramina[34] (**Figure 7**). U-shaped sacral fractures (bilateral longitudinal transforaminal fractures joined by a transverse fracture line) result in disruption of the spinal-pelvic junction (**Figure 8**). Additionally, sacral fractures can result in varying degrees of neurologic deficit ranging from unilateral peripheral nerve root injuries in the case of vertical shear fracture patterns,[34] to cauda equina lesions in the case of transverse or U-shaped fractures.[35] Reduction and stabilization techniques and decision algorithms largely depend on which of the aforementioned clinical scenarios exist.

The main indications for surgical treatment of sacral fractures include anterior and posterior pelvic ring disruption with vertical or cephalad instability in the case of a vertical shear sacral fracture, nonimpacted and/or comminuted sacral alar fractures with external rotation deformity of the hemipelvis, and U-shaped sacral frac-

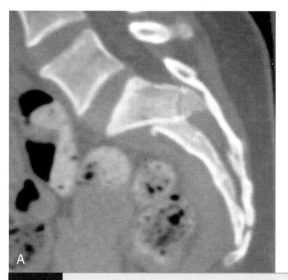
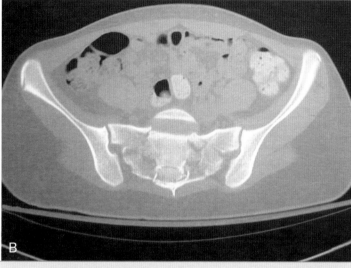

Figure 8 **A,** Sagittal CT depicting U-shaped sacral fracture with spinal-pelvic dissociation. Note occlusion of sacral spinal canal on axial cut (**B**). (Courtesy of H. Claude Sagi, MD, Tampa, FL.)

tures with spinal-pelvic dissociation, cauda equina syndrome, or excessive sacral kyphosis.[35,36] Most longitudinal sacral fractures that arise from lateral compression injuries and result in impaction of the sacral ala are inherently stable and will not require surgical stabilization. However, impacted sacral fractures from lateral compression injuries with excessive internal rotation and pelvic deformity can become disimpacted and unstable when the anterior ring is reduced. In this situation, the posterior ring will require internal fixation.

Reduction of displaced and unstable longitudinal sacral fractures, like SI joint dislocations, relies heavily on longitudinal traction and patient positioning.[36] Once the correct length is achieved, it is imperative that any residual fracture gap is reduced to avoid delayed union or nonunion.[36] Anatomic reduction is also important for improving fracture stability and increasing the diameter of the safe corridor for iliosacral screw placement.[37] Stabilization of most sacral fracture reductions is usually accomplished with one or two iliosacral screws. Placement of an iliosacral screw for stabilization of sacral fractures differs slightly from the technique used for stabilization of SI joint dislocations in that the screw trajectory should be as perpendicular as possible to the fracture plane (not SI joint) to achieve optimal reduction and stability. Some authors advocate the use of a transsacral screw that completely crosses the sacrum and gains purchase in the contralateral ilium[32] There are no published biomechanical studies demonstrating superiority of transsacral screws over standard iliosacral screws. Currently, the literature is not clear on the additional benefit provided by a second iliosacral screw in the case of comminuted vertical sacral fractures.[33,38] However, if a second screw can be safely placed into either S1 or S2, most surgeons would agree to proceed with this supplemental technique in the case of a displaced, unstable sacral fracture.

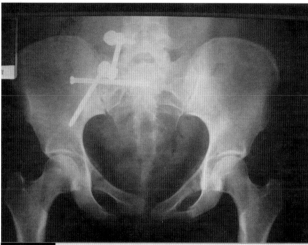

Figure 9 AP radiograph depicting a typical spinal-pelvic construct using the concept of triangular osteosynthesis. (Courtesy of H. Claude Sagi, MD, Tampa, FL.)

Vertical sacral fractures associated with severe comminution, osteoporotic bone, or disruption of the L5/S1 facet joint treated with iliosacral screws alone have been associated with a higher failure rate in some series,[39] and consideration should be given to proceed with some form of spinal-pelvic construct such as triangular osteosynthesis to augment the iliosacral screw fixation. These constructs have been shown to be superior both biomechanically and clinically to SI screws alone for maintaining reduction in comminuted sacral fractures[40,41] (**Figure 9**). Spinal-pelvic constructs involve the use of lumbar spinal pedicle screws attached to iliac screws directed from the posterior superior iliac spine to the anterior inferior iliac spine to resist vertical shear deforming forces through comminuted sacral fractures.

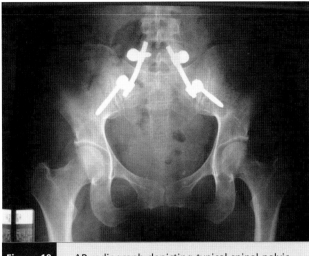

Figure 10   AP radiograph depicting typical spinal pelvic construct for stabilization of a U-shaped sacral fracture (spinal-pelvic dissociation). (Courtesy of H. Claude Sagi, MD, Tampa, FL.)

The reported benefits of spinal-pelvic constructs, also termed triangular osteosynthesis, are that they provide improved stability with a lower rate of hardware failure and loss of reduction. Patients are able to fully weight bear within a few weeks of surgery.[40,41] Prominent and symptomatic fixation, delayed union and nonunion, and lumbosacral scoliosis are the most commonly encountered conditions unless careful attention is paid during reduction and implantation. Spinal-pelvic constructs usually need to be removed after the fracture is healed in 6 to 9 months.[36,41]

Sacral nerve root decompression may be necessary in two circumstances with vertical sacral fractures: sacral nerve root radiculopathy with a preoperative CT scan demonstrating a fragment of bone in the nerve root foramen, or a neurologically intact patient with a preoperative CT scan showing a fragment of bone in the foramen that may injure the nerve root with the reduction maneuver. If sacral nerve root decompression is necessary, it can be performed directly through the fracture by gently opening the fracture with a laminar spreader; a sacral laminectomy is generally not required.[36]

U-Shaped Sacral Fractures: Spinal-Pelvic Dissociation

These injuries tend to occur through the vestigial disk spaces between the sacral bodies and result in kyphosis and posterior translation of the upper sacral (and lumbar) spinal segments.[42] These fractures (**Figure 8**) are easily overlooked on standard AP pelvic radiographs and axial CT scans. Therefore, sagittal and coronal CT reconstructions are often critical in identifying this injury pattern. Although some trauma surgeons have advocated in situ bilateral SI screw fixation alone for impacted, stable injuries without significant kyphosis or neurologic deficit,[43] U-shaped sacral fractures with

spinal-pelvic dissociation commonly require reduction, decompression, and some form of bilateral posterior lumbopelvic fixation construct to control kyphotic deformity and allow early mobilization of the patient (**Figure 10**).[35] Iliosacral screws are not generally neccessary, and an L5 to sacral fusion may or may not be performed depending on the integrity of the L5/S1 facet joints.[35,36] The presence of cauda equina syndrome mandates sacral laminectomy and decompression with removal of bone in the anterior aspect of the sacral spinal canal.

Sequence of Treating Combined Anterior and Posterior Pelvic Ring Injuries

Considerable discussion surrounds the strategy for obtaining an anterior versus posterior reduction in the case of complete instability of the hemipelvis. The classic teaching for an injury such as a complete SI dislocation associated with a symphyseal disruption has been to perform ORIF of the more biomechanically critical posterior ring injury first, followed by ORIF of the anterior ring injury. This rationale is based on the assumptions that an anatomic reduction of the posterior ring is necessary for a good outcome, and an anatomic reduction of the posterior ring will be impeded by a (mal)reduced and rigidly fixed anterior ring. Proponents of an initial anterior reduction believe that reducing the anterior ring first will help with reduction of the posterior ring, permitting closed manipulative indirect reduction and percutaneous fixation. In reality both philosophies have validity. Some patients will have soft-tissue wounds or a precarious physiologic status that will preclude a formal posterior open reduction or prone positioning; these patients may benefit from the "anterior first" strategy that will impose less surgical morbidity. In essence, however, the surgeon needs to use the techniques with which the best reduction with the least morbidity can be achieved.

Perioperative Care and Postoperative Rehabilitation

Drains, Soft Tissues, and Bowels

Medium- to large-sized drains may be used anteriorly in the retropubic space and the internal iliac fossa, and posteriorly in the subgluteal space if the gluteus is elevated from the ilium. Sutures are generally left in place for 2 to 3 weeks. Postoperative ileus is common and needs to be managed with careful advancement of dietary intake. Aggressive postoperative bowel regimens are necessary and should be part of the postoperative protocol.

Patients with internal degloving soft tissue injuries, or Morel-Lavallée lesions, merit close attention. Some surgeons advocate that serial drainage, débridement, and vacuum-assisted closure of the wound should precede formal ORIF, whereas others believe that percutaneous drainage and lavage are all that are required.[44,45]

In any case, the soft tissues should be allowed to recover before any formal open reduction and extensive surgical dissection are undertaken. If a large degloving lesion exists, complete full-thickness necrosis and slough may result in the need for débridement and soft tissue reconstruction in the central portion of the injury to cover exposed bone and/or fixation. Prudence and experience is required to know when it is safe to proceed with formal open treatment of the associated pelvic fracture. On occasion, a suboptimal closed reduction and percutaneous fixation will have to be accepted in lieu of an extensive open approach to prevent disastrous soft-tissue complications.

Mobilization and Weight Bearing

When systemic issues and physiologic status allow, patients should be mobilized as soon as possible. This helps with pulmonary toilet and bowel/bladder function. Any pelvic ring injury that is associated with complete disruption of the posterior ring (vertical shear injuries, complete dislocation of the SI joint, crescent fractures) should be mobilized with touch-down or no weight bearing for 10 to 12 weeks (fractures generally for shorter durations and dislocations for longer durations), at which point full weight bearing may be permitted. Incomplete posterior ring disruptions such as stable impacted lateral compression injuries or anterior posterior compression 1 and 2 injuries can typically be allowed full weight bearing as tolerated by the patient. However, careful radiographic follow-up is necessary within 1 week of mobilization to ensure that occult instability has not been missed.

Deep Venous Thrombosis/Pulmonary Embolism Prophylaxis

Prophylaxis of venous thromboembolism is a controversial topic that remains a major source of debate. From the available data, it appears that some form of prophylaxis should be started within 12 to 24 hours of pelvic fracture. This can be in the form of low molecular weight heparins or unfractionated heparins given subcutaneously.[46] Intermittent pneumatic compressive devices applied to the calves or feet have been shown to help decrease the incidence of venous thrombus formation and should be used in all patients whose condition tolerates their application. Screening with duplex Doppler, contrast venography, and magnetic resonance venography has not been shown to be efficacious in patients with pelvic fractures.[47,48]

For those patients with contraindications to anticoagulation, consideration should be given to placement of an inferior vena cava filter (IVCF). Modern IVCF placement is associated with a low complication rate, and usually involves placement of a retrievable filter that should be removed within 3 months, depending on the manufacturer and clinical situation. However, few patients have the filter removed, and the incidence of postphlebitic syndrome can be as high as 70%. IVCFs, while reducing the incidence of pulmonary embolism (PE), have not been shown to improve survival or affect the incidence of fatal PE.[49]

Discharge anticoagulation again has no scientific basis or established standard of care. The risk factors that need to be considered in the decision to send a patient home on anticoagulation medication are: ambulatory status, age older than 40 years, body mass index greater than 30, female sex, use of birth control, deep venous thrombosis (DVT) or PE, and smoking. If a patient is young, healthy, and ambulatory with no other independent risk factors for DVT/PE, then consideration can be made for no discharge anticoagulation medication, provided that appropriate in-hospital anticoagulation has been implemented and after careful discussion with the patient and documentation in the medical chart. All other patients should be discharged on some form of anticoagulation (low molecular weight heparin or warfarin) for 4 to 6 weeks. Aspirin and elastic stockings are considered inadequate discharge thromboprophylaxis for trauma patients.[50]

Complications Associated With the Management of Pelvic Fractures

Surgery for pelvic fracture reduction and fixation can be associated with large blood losses and fluid shifts, periods of hypotension, and prolonged anesthetics use and operating room times, all of which contribute significantly to the increased potential for complications.

Intraoperative Hemorrhage

Intraoperative vascular injury is potentially life threatening and needs to be managed expeditiously. Injury to vessels such as the superior gluteal artery/vein, obturator artery/vein, corona mortis, and external iliac artery/vein can occur with fracture reduction and insertion of fixation. Unless the blood vessel injury is easily identified and can be separated from the associated neurologic structures, the wound should be packed and closed, and angiographic embolization performed to address the offending vessel.

Constant uncontrollable venous bleeding secondary to coagulopathy, hypothermia, or massive transfusion can lead to significant blood loss. Focusing on achieving a difficult reduction while ignoring the patient's physiologic status and blood loss is always a risk, and it is imperative that the surgeon and anesthesiologist stay in close communication throughout the case regarding body temperature, blood loss volume, urine output, and blood gas results. If the patient's physiologic status deteriorates before the pelvis is reduced and stabilized, the wound needs to be packed and closed, and the patient transferred to the intensive care unit for resuscitation and stabilization, with plans to return to the operating room when the patient has recovered sufficiently.

Inability to Achieve Adequate Fixation

Inadequate anterior pelvic plate fixation (usually associated with extensive comminution or osteoporosis) can be augmented with either multiplanar symphyseal plates, locked plate-screw constructs, or a supplemental anterior pelvic external fixator. There are no data in the current literature to guide the surgeon in this respect, and he or she must depend on clinical acumen to decide which supplement would be best indicated for that particular scenario.

Addressing inadequate posterior pelvic fixation usually entails the addition of supplemental fixation techniques to the construct. One iliosacral screw can be supplemented with a second or third iliosacral screw into S1 and S2. Poor-quality purchase in the S1 promontory may necessitate converting to a transsacral screw. If fracture comminution and sacral anatomy preclude multiple iliosacral screw placements, a spinal pelvic construct may be needed. As a final effort, transiliac bars or plates can be used to augment poor posterior pelvic ring fixation.

Postoperative Wound Infection and Dehiscence

If the patient presents with prolonged (more than 3 to 5 days) wound drainage and/or erythema, fever, and elevated white blood cell count in the early postoperative period (first 2 to 3 weeks), a return trip to the operating room is necessary for wound débridement and irrigation to prevent osteomyelitis and infected internal fixation. Depending on the intraoperative findings, multiple repeat débridements and antibiotic-impregnated polymethylmethacrylate beads may be necessary, followed by culture-specific intravenous antibiotics for up to 6 weeks (after consultation with infectious disease specialists).

If the suspected infection appears later during the course of the healing process and the prospect of an established, deep infection or abscess around the fixation and bone is present, careful workup and management are necessary. Preoperative blood work for white blood cell counts, erythrocyte sedimentation rate, and C-reactive protein levels, while not necessarily useful for confirming infection, are useful for following the patient's response to surgical and medical therapies. A preoperative CT scan of the pelvis and abdomen with contrast is helpful for assessing abscess formation, location, and depth, as well as the extent of fracture healing. As a general rule, it is not considered a good idea to treat a deep pelvic infection around internal fixation with percutaneous drainage and antibiotic therapy alone unless the patient is too physiologically frail because of age and/or comorbidity to withstand an open procedure. Depending on the extent of infection and fixation/bone involvement, the surgeon should consider multiple débridements, removal of fixation (if the fracture is healed), and placement of antibiotic beads.

Newly Recognized Postoperative Neurologic Deficits

Displaced posterior pelvis fractures and dislocations are not infrequently associated with subtle neurologic injuries that may not manifest until sometime during the postoperative period. If a patient is known to be neurologically intact preoperatively, and then demonstrates a deficit postoperatively, a postoperative CT scan is needed to assess the sacral canal and foraminal anatomy. MRI is generally not useful secondary to the image distortion created from the internal fixation. At times a postmyelogram CT scan will be needed to fully assess the nerve roots. The following scenarios are possible: a misplaced screw is injuring a nerve root; a fragment of bone or overreduction of the fracture is impinging on the nerve root; or there is no nerve root impingement and the deficit is the result of fracture manipulation.

Nerve impingement from a bony fragment or misplaced fixation can be treated nonsurgically depending on the presenting deficit and symptoms. A patient with radiculitis only and no motor deficit can be managed with observation and medications such as steroids or gabapentin to control neurogenic pain. However, if radicular pain does not decrease or motor deficit is present, then consideration should be given to revision of the fixation or removal of the bone fragment. New neurologic deficits without radiographic evidence of nerve root impingement are managed with observation, pain medicines, physical therapy, splinting, and tendon transfers as needed, depending on the severity of the deficit and muscle groups involved.

Postoperative Loss of Fixation and Reduction

Pelvic malunion can be an extremely debilitating condition. Pelvic obliquity, sitting imbalance, limb-length discrepancy, and low back pain with disability are the usual sequelae. Internal rotation and adduction of the hemipelvis can lead to pain while sitting, dyspareunia, and constipation. For these reasons, frequent follow-up radiographs are important in the early postoperative period, and acting on loss of reduction early is essential in preventing late deformity and disability.

Outcome Studies for Pelvic Fractures

Many clinicians have documented the high prevalence of poor functional outcome and chronic pain in patients with vertically unstable pelvic fractures treated nonsurgically. Improved short-term patient outcome with early stabilization of the pelvic fracture and mobilization of the patient, as well as numerous reports citing improved outcome with anatomic reduction of the posterior ring, have continued to provide the impetus to develop more rigid and stable fixation constructs.[51,52]

Some outcome studies[53,54] support the position that the long-term functional results are improved if reduction with less than 1 cm of combined displacement of the posterior ring is obtained, especially with pure dislocations of the sacroiliac complex. Fractures of the posterior ring tend to fare better functionally than dislocations that rely on scar formation and ligamentous healing, presumably because bone healing can restore initial strength and stability.[55] However, one study has found that patients with pure dislocations of the SI joint that healed with a solid bony ankylosis did not demonstrate improved outcome over those without bony ankylosis of the joint.[53]

Males frequently report erectile dysfunction, and females frequently report dyspareunia, urinary difficulty, and pregnancy-related issues with an increase in the need for cesarean section.[56,57] Outcome after pelvic fracture is associated with significantly higher mortality in the elderly: 12.3% versus 2.3% in the younger age groups, despite equal need for transfusion and similar injury patterns. This is largely because of the decreased physiologic reserve and higher incidence of cardiovascular disease.[58]

The poor outcomes are likely multifactorial.[59] Associated neurologic, visceral, and urogenital injuries with dyspareunia, sexual dysfunction, and incontinence occur in a substantial proportion of patients. In addition, extensive soft-tissue damage and associated long-bone and extremity fractures complicate functionality. Finally, outcome studies after fixation of pelvic injuries are difficult to interpret because of poor follow-up, heterogeneity of the injury pattern, associated visceral and neurologic injury, and the lack of a reliable outcome measure for pelvic ring injuries.

Debate continues regarding the definition of adequate reduction of the pelvic ring and how malreduction affects functional outcome, if at all.[60] Fewer than 50% of patients with severe pelvic fractures return to their previous level of function and work status, and most sustain persistent impairment in both the physical and mental components of the Short Form-36 questionnaire.[61]

Summary

Pelvic fractures encompass a wide spectrum of injury patterns, associated visceral and neurologic injuries, and outcomes. Complex anatomy, prolonged surgery, and associated multisystem injuries make for difficult surgical conditions and require thorough knowledge and considerable experience and clinical acumen to prevent the potentially significant and devastating complications that accompany these injuries.

Annotated References

1. Stocks GW, Gabel GT, Noble PC, Hanson GW, Tullos HS: Anterior and posterior internal fixation of vertical shear fractures of the pelvis. *J Orthop Res* 1991;9(2):237-245.

2. Vrahas M, Hern TC, Diangelo D, Kellam J, Tile M: Ligamentous contributions to pelvic stability. *Orthopedics* 1995;18(3):271-274.

3. Sagi HC, Ordway NR, DiPasquale T: Biomechanical analysis of fixation for vertically unstable sacroiliac dislocations with iliosacral screws and symphyseal plating. *J Orthop Trauma* 2004;18(3):138-143.

   The authors examined the effects of various iliosacral screw configurations with and without symphyseal plating on SI motion and hemipelvis stability in the vertically unstable pelvic model. They found that anterior symphyseal plating for the vertically unstable hemipelvis significantly increases the stability of the fixation construct and restores the normal response of the hemipelvis to axial loading. A significant benefit to supplementary iliosacral screws in addition to a properly placed S1 iliosacral screw was not shown.

4. Siegel J, Templeman DC, Tornetta P III: Single-leg-stance radiographs in the diagnosis of pelvic instability. *J Bone Joint Surg Am* 2008;90(10):2119-2125.

   The authors evaluated single-leg-stance radiographs in the diagnosis of pelvic instability in a consecutive series of patients presenting with pelvic pain. Each patient was evaluated with supine anteroposterior, inlet, and outlet pelvic radiographs; a standing anteroposterior pelvic radiograph; and two single-leg-standing pelvic radiographs. A positive finding was defined as 0.5 cm or greater of vertical translation measured at the symphyseal bodies between the two single-leg-stance radiographs. The authors found that standing anteroposterior and single-leg-stance pelvic radiographs aid in the diagnosis of pelvic instability more effectively than do the standard three radiographs of the pelvis made in the supine position or a standing anteroposterior radiograph of the pelvis alone.

5. Bellabarba C, Ricci WM, Bolhofner BR: Distraction external fixation in lateral compression pelvic fractures. *J Orthop Trauma* 2006;20(suppl 1):S7-S14.

   The authors evaluated closed reduction and placement of a two-pin supra-acetabular external fixator, followed by immediate weight bearing, in the treatment of displaced vertically stable lateral compression pelvic fractures. They found that the treatment of type B lateral compression injuries of the pelvic ring with anterior distraction external fixation is a highly effective yet relatively simple and minimally invasive treatment method.

6. Mason WT, Khan SN, James CL, Chesser TJ, Ward AJ: Complications of temporary and definitive external fixation of pelvic ring injuries. *Injury* 2005;36(5):599-604.

   The authors reviewed 100 patients with both temporary (mean 8 days) and definitive (mean 60 days) pelvic external fixation. Pin tract infection was predictably the most common complication occurring in 50% of definitive and 13% of temporary frames. Septic and aseptic pin loosening was the main cause for frame or pin revision.

7. Kellam JF: The role of external fixation in pelvic disruptions. *Clin Orthop Relat Res* 1989;241:66-82.

8. Tucker MC, Nork SE, Simonian PT, Routt ML Jr: Simple anterior pelvic external fixation. *J Trauma* 2000; 49(6):989-994.

9. Gänsslen A, Pohlemann T, Krettek C: A simple supraacetabular external fixation for pelvic ring fractures. *Oper Orthop Traumatol* 2005;17(3):296-312.

   The authors used bilateral percutaneous insertion of Schanz screws into the supra-acetabular area of iliac bone. Closed reduction and stabilization of the pelvic ring by compression and application of a connecting rod under image intensification was performed. There were no secondary displacements of the anterior or posterior pelvic ring in types B and C injuries. There was one pseudarthrosis of the pubic and ischial rami requiring surgical treatment. It was concluded that simple supra-acetabular external fixation is safe and efficacious.

10. Brown TD, Stone JP, Schuster JH, Mears DC: External fixation of unstable pelvic ring fractures: Comparative rigidity of some current frame configurations. *Med Biol Eng Comput* 1982;20(6):727-733.

11. Archdeacon MT, Arebi S, Le TT, Wirth R, Kebel R, Thakore M: Orthogonal pin construct versus parallel uniplanar pin constructs for pelvic external fixation: A biomechanical assessment of stiffness and strength. *J Orthop Trauma* 2009;23(2):100-105.

    The authors compared the structural stiffness of an orthogonal pelvic external fixator pin construct with two different parallel external fixator pin constructs in a simulated bone model. The orthogonal pelvic external fixator pin construct produced a significantly stiffer construct for in-plane loading (flexion/extension moment) compared with either parallel pin construct; however, a parallel supra-acetabular pin construct was stiffer for out-of-plane loading.

12. Webb LX, Gristina AG, Wilson JR, Rhyne AL, Meredith JH, Hansen ST Jr: Two-hole plate fixation for traumatic symphysis pubis diastasis. *J Trauma* 1988;28(6): 813-817.

13. Sagi HC, Papp S: Comparative radiographic and clinical outcome of two-hole and multi-hole symphyseal plating. *J Orthop Trauma* 2008;22(6):373-378.

    The authors reported on the radiographic and clinical outcome of symphyseal plating techniques, with specific attention to the incidence of implant failure, reoperation secondary to implant complication, and ability to maintain reduction of the pelvic ring. Symphyseal plating: (1) group THP, a two-hole plate; (2) group MHP, a multi-hole plate (minimum two holes/screws on either side of the symphysis). They showed that the two-hole symphyseal plating technique group had a higher implant failure rate, and more important, a significantly higher rate of pelvic malunion. On the basis of these findings, multihole plating of unstable pubic symphyseal disruptions was recommended.

14. Simonian PT, Schwappach JR, Routt ML Jr, Agnew SG, Harrington RM, Tencer AF: Evaluation of new plate designs for symphysis pubis internal fixation. *J Trauma* 1996;41(3):498-502.

15. Matta JM: Indications for anterior fixation of pelvic fractures. *Clin Orthop Relat Res* 1996;329:88-96.

16. Starr AJ, Nakatani T, Reinert CM, Cederberg K: Superior pubic ramus fractures fixed with percutaneous screws: What predicts fixation failure? *J Orthop Trauma* 2008;22(2):81-87.

    The authors retrospectively reviewed the early complications of percutaneous screw fixation of superior pubic ramus fractures and a new classification scheme for superior pubic ramus fractures. Superior pubic ramus fractures were classified according to a new scheme, the Nakatani system, which categorizes superior ramus fractures according to location with respect to the obturator foramen. The most common mechanism of reduction loss was a collapse of the pubic ramus over the screw, with recurrence of an internal rotation deformity of the injured hemipelvis. The prevalence of loss of reduction after percutaneous screw fixation of pubic ramus fractures was 15%. Loss of reduction is more common in elderly and female patients and in patients whose ramus screws are placed in a retrograde fashion. Also, loss of reduction appears to be more common in fractures medial to the lateral border of the obturator foramen.

17. Switzer JA, Nork SE, Routt ML Jr: Comminuted fractures of the iliac wing. *J Orthop Trauma* 2000;14(4): 270-276.

18. Emery KH: Lap belt iliac wing fracture: A predictor of bowel injury in children. *Pediatr Radiol* 2002;32(12): 892-895.

19. Borrelli J Jr, Koval KJ, Helfet DL: The crescent fracture: A posterior fracture dislocation of the sacroiliac joint. *J Orthop Trauma* 1996;10(3):165-170.

20. Simpson LA, Waddell JP, Leighton RK, Kellam JF, Tile M: Anterior approach and stabilization of the disrupted sacroiliac joint. *J Trauma* 1987;27(12):1332-1339.

21. Moed BR, Karges DE: Techniques for reduction and fixation of pelvic ring disruptions through the posterior approach. *Clin Orthop Relat Res* 1996;329:102-114.

22. Matta JM, Yerasimides JG: Table-skeletal fixation as an adjunct to pelvic ring reduction. *J Orthop Trauma* 2007;21(9):647-656.

    The reduction of displaced pelvic ring injuries remains a technical challenge, especially when treatment is delayed. The authors present a pelvic frame to provide a means of external skeletal fixation, rigidly stabilizing the intact hemipelvis to the operating room table. The fractured and displaced fragments are then manipulated around the securely fixed uninjured hemipelvis, allowing the application of more directions and magnitudes of force for reduction maneuvers than allowed by the traditional means of pelvic reduction.

23. Yinger K, Scalise J, Olson SA, Bay BK, Finkemeier CG: Biomechanical comparison of posterior pelvic ring fixation. *J Orthop Trauma* 2003;17(7):481-487.

24. Keating JF, Werier J, Blachut P, Broekhuyse H, Meek RN, O'Brien PJ: Early fixation of the vertically unstable pelvis: The role of iliosacral screw fixation of the posterior lesion. *J Orthop Trauma* 1999;13(2):107-113.

25. Collinge C, Coons D, Aschenbrenner J: Risks to the superior gluteal neurovascular bundle during percutaneous iliosacral screw insertion: An anatomical cadaver study. *J Orthop Trauma* 2005;19(2):96-101.

The authors assessed the risks of injury and proximity of percutaneously inserted iliosacral screws to the superior gluteal nerve and vessels using a cadaver model. The branching pattern of the superior gluteal nerve and vessels after they exit the greater sciatic notch demonstrated considerable variation, but was generally consistent with prior descriptions in most cases. Ten of 58 (18%) iliosacral screws caused injury to the superior branch of the superior gluteal nerve and vessels; 8 neurovascular bundles were impaled and 2 others were partly entrapped between the screw head and the ilium. The authors found that the deep superior branch of the superior gluteal nerve and vessels is at significant risk during the percutaneous placement of iliosacral screws, even when placed correctly and soft tissue protecting cannulas are used.

26. Routt ML Jr, Simonian PT, Agnew SG, Mann FA: Radiographic recognition of the sacral alar slope for optimal placement of iliosacral screws: A cadaveric and clinical study. *J Orthop Trauma* 1996;10(3):171-177.

27. Carlson DA, Scheid DK, Maar DC, Baele JR, Kaehr DM: Safe placement of S1 and S2 iliosacral screws: The "vestibule" concept. *J Orthop Trauma* 2000;14(4):264-269.

28. Collinge C, Coons D, Tornetta P, Aschenbrenner J: Standard multiplanar fluoroscopy versus a fluoroscopically based navigation system for the percutaneous insertion of iliosacral screws: A cadaver model. *J Orthop Trauma* 2005;19(4):254-258.

The authors compared the safety and efficiency of standard multiplanar fluoroscopy and virtual fluoroscopy for use in the percutaneous insertion of iliosacral screws. They found that most of the percutaneous iliosacral screws were safely inserted using both techniques, and total surgical times were similar using both methods. As virtual fluoroscopy continues to evolve, improved efficiency in operating room times may be expected. Currently, the most beneficial aspect of using virtual fluoroscopy during the insertion of percutaneous iliosacral screws appears to be significantly decreased use of fluoroscopy when compared with standard fluoroscopy.

29. Kraemer W, Hearn T, Tile M, Powell J: The effect of thread length and location on extraction strengths of iliosacral lag screws. *Injury* 1994;25(1):5-9.

30. Sagi HC, Lindvall EM: Inadvertent intraforaminal iliosacral screw placement despite apparent appropriate positioning on intraoperative fluoroscopy. *J Orthop Trauma* 2005;19(2):130-133.

The authors reported on a case of an intraforaminal ili-
osacral screw placed percutaneously with aid of C-arm using inlet, outlet, and lateral views of the pelvis. The iliosacral screw was placed above the S1 foramen on the outlet view, into the middle of S1 via the ala on the inlet view, and below the cortical shadow of the ala on the lateral view. Because of the tangential nature of the S1 foramen, slight posterior placement of the screw into the S1 body and not into the promontory resulted in violation of the foramen despite it being above the cortical shadow on the outlet view.

31. Moed BR, Geer BL: S2 iliosacral screw fixation for disruptions of the posterior pelvic ring: A report of 49 cases. *J Orthop Trauma* 2006;20(6):378-383.

A retrospective analysis was done to evaluate the clinical safety and efficacy of using S2 iliosacral screws for pelvic fracture fixation. Forty-nine patients were treated with S2 iliosacral screws. There were 9 bilateral injuries with a total of 53 S2 screws inserted. There were no intraoperative iatrogenic nerve injuries. However, postoperative loss of reduction requiring revision surgery occurred in two patients with osteopenia. One was associated with injury to the S1 nerve root, which had full return of function within 1 year. Satisfactory screw position was documented on postoperative CT in all cases. The authors concluded that S2 iliosacral screw fixation is a safe and effective technique. However, it should be used with caution in patients with suspected pelvic osteopenia.

32. Beaulé PE, Antoniades J, Matta JM: Trans-sacral fixation for failed posterior fixation of the pelvic ring. *Arch Orthop Trauma Surg* 2006;126(1):49-52.

This report describes early experience with the surgical technique for transsacral fixation (fixation from one iliac wing to the other traversing the body of S1). The authors' initial experience with transsacral fixation has proven to be effective in solving the most difficult problems in posterior pelvic ring fixation. Its use is reserved for nonunion/malunion of the pelvic ring, and sacral fractures.

33. van Zwienen CM, van den Bosch EW, Snijders CJ, Kleinrensink GJ, van Vugt AB: Biomechanical comparison of sacroiliac screw techniques for unstable pelvic ring fractures. *J Orthop Trauma* 2004;18(9):589-595.

The authors conducted a randomized comparative study on embalmed human pelves to determine the stiffness and strength of various sacroiliac screw fixations in sacral fractures with one of the following methods: one sacroiliac screw in the vertebral body of S1, two screws convergingly in S1, or one screw in S1 and one in S2. Significant differences were found for the load to failure and rotation stiffness between the techniques with two screws and a single screw in S1. The techniques using two screws showed no differences.

34. Denis F, Davis S, Comfort T: Sacral fractures: An important problem. Retrospective analysis of 236 cases. *Clin Orthop Relat Res* 1988;227:67-81.

35. Schildhauer TA, Bellabarba C, Nork SE, Barei DP, Routt ML Jr, Chapman JR: Decompression and lumbopelvic fixation for sacral fracture-dislocations with

4: Axial Skeleton, Including Spine and Pelvis

spino-pelvic dissociation. *J Orthop Trauma* 2006;20(7): 447-457.

The authors reported on the results of sacral decompression and lumbopelvic fixation in neurologically impaired patients with highly displaced, comminuted sacral fracture-dislocations resulting in spino-pelvic dissociation. They found that lumbopelvic fixation provided reliable fracture stability and allowed consistent fracture union without loss of alignment. Neurologic outcome was, in part, influenced by completeness of injury and presence of sacral root disruption.

36. Sagi HC: Technical aspects and recommended treatment algorithms in triangular osteosynthesis and spinopelvic fixation for vertical shear transforaminal sacral fractures. *J Orthop Trauma* 2009;23(5):354-360.

The author describes the relatively new technique of triangular osteosynthesis and spinal-pelvic constructs that are used to avoid loss of reduction for treating vertically unstable pelvic ring injuries associated with comminuted transforaminal sacral fractures.

37. Reilly MC, Bono CM, Litkouhi B, Sirkin M, Behrens FF: The effect of sacral fracture malreduction on the safe placement of iliosacral screws. *J Orthop Trauma* 2003;17(2):88-94.

38. Simonian PT, Routt C Jr, Harrington RM, Tencer AF: Internal fixation for the transforaminal sacral fracture. *Clin Orthop Relat Res* 1996;323:202-209.

39. Griffin DR, Starr AJ, Reinert CM, Jones AL, Whitlock S: Vertically unstable pelvic fractures fixed with percutaneous iliosacral screws: Does posterior injury pattern predict fixation failure? *J Orthop Trauma* 2003;17(6): 399-405.

40. Schildhauer TA, Ledoux WR, Chapman JR, Henley MB, Tencer AF, Routt ML Jr: Triangular osteosynthesis and iliosacral screw fixation for unstable sacral fractures: A cadaveric and biomechanical evaluation under cyclic loads. *J Orthop Trauma* 2003;17(1):22-31.

41. Sagi HC, Militano U, Caron T, Lindvall E: A comprehensive analysis with minimum 1-year follow-up of vertically unstable transforaminal sacral fractures treated with triangular osteosynthesis. *J Orthop Trauma* 2009; 23(5):313-319.

The authors analyzed the radiographic, clinical, and functional results of triangular osteosynthesis constructs for the treatment of vertically unstable comminuted transforaminal sacral fractures. They found that triangular osteosynthesis fixation is a reliable form of fixation that allows early full weight bearing at 6 weeks while preventing loss of reduction in comminuted vertical shear transforaminal sacral fractures. However, the 1-year follow-up shows a substantial rate of potential technical problems and complications. Of primary concern were the asymmetric L5 tilting with L5-S1 facet joint distraction and the need for a second surgery in all patients to remove painful fixation. The authors recommended selective use of this technique for comminuted transforaminal sacral fractures in situations only where reliable iliosacral or transsacral screw fixation is not obtainable.

42. Strange-Vognsen HH, Lebech A: An unusual type of fracture in the upper sacrum. *J Orthop Trauma* 1991; 5(2):200-203.

43. Nork SE, Jones CB, Harding SP, Mirza SK, Routt ML Jr: Percutaneous stabilization of U-shaped sacral fractures using iliosacral screws: Technique and early results. *J Orthop Trauma* 2001;15(4):238-246.

44. Labler L, Trentz O: The use of vacuum assisted closure (VAC) in soft tissue injuries after high energy pelvic trauma. *Langenbecks Arch Surg* 2007;392(5):601-609.

The authors used a vacuum-assisted closure in soft-tissue defects after high-energy pelvic trauma. Because high-energy trauma causing severe soft-tissue injuries requires multiple surgical débridements to prevent high morbidity and mortality rates, it was concluded that the application of vacuum-assisted closure as temporary coverage of large tissue defects in pelvic regions supports wound conditioning and facilitates the definitive wound closure.

45. Tseng S, Tornetta P III: Percutaneous management of Morel-Lavallée lesions. *J Bone Joint Surg Am* 2006; 88(1):92-96.

The authors reviewed the use of percutaneous drainage for the initial management of Morel-Lavallée soft-tissue degloving lesions. They concluded that early percutaneous drainage with débridement, irrigation, and suction drainage for the treatment of Morel-Lavallée lesions appears to be safe and effective. Percutaneous procedures for pelvic fixation were well tolerated by the small number of patients in this series, and open procedures appeared to be safe when performed in a delayed fashion.

46. Slobogean GP, Lefaivre KA, Nicolaou S, O'Brien PJ: A systematic review of thromboprophylaxis for pelvic and acetabular fractures. *J Orthop Trauma* 2009;23(5):379-384.

The authors performed a systematic review to evaluate the effectiveness of thromboprophylactic strategies to prevent DVT or PE after pelvic or acetabular fractures. Most studies were observational designs with minimal control data for comparison. Their review showed that clinicians have limited data to guide their prophylactic decisions. Well-designed clinical trials to prevent and detect venous thromboembolism in pelvic and acetabular trauma are still needed.

47. Stannard JP, Singhania AK, Lopez-Ben RR, et al: Deep-vein thrombosis in high-energy skeletal trauma despite thromboprophylaxis. *J Bone Joint Surg Br* 2005;87(7): 965-968.

The authors report the incidence and location of DVT in 312 patients who had sustained high-energy skeletal trauma. The DVTs were investigated using magnetic resonance venography and duplex ultrasound. When compared with magnetic resonance venography, ultrasound had a false-negative rate of 77% in diagnosing pelvic DVT. Its value in the pelvis was limited, although it was more accurate than magnetic resonance venography in diagnosing clots in the lower limbs. Additional screening may be needed to detect pelvic DVT in patients with pelvic or acetabular fractures.

48. Borer DS, Starr AJ, Reinert CM, et al: The effect of screening for deep vein thrombosis on the prevalence of pulmonary embolism in patients with fractures of the pelvis or acetabulum: A review of 973 patients. *J Orthop Trauma* 2005;19(2):92-95.

The authors compared the prevalence of pulmonary embolism without screening for DVT to a screening protocol for pelvic and acetabular fractures. They found that discontinuation of screening for the diagnosis of deep vein thrombosis did not change the rate of PE.

49. PREPIC Study Group: Eight-year follow-up of patients with permanent vena cava filters in the prevention of pulmonary embolism: The PREPIC (Prevention du Risque d'Embolie Pulmonaire par Interruption Cave) randomized study. *Circulation* 2005;112(3):416-422.

The authors found that in a randomized trial in patients with proximal DVT, permanent vena cava filters reduced the incidence of pulmonary embolism but increased that of DVT at 2 years. They performed an 8-year follow-up to assess their long-term effect. At 8 years, vena cava filters reduced the risk of pulmonary embolism but increased that of DVT and had no effect on survival. They concluded that vena cava filter use may be beneficial in patients at high risk of pulmonary embolism, but systematic use in the general population with venous thromboembolism is not recommended.

50. Geerts WH, Pineo GF, Heit JA, et al: Prevention of venous thromboembolism: The Seventh ACCP Conference on Antithrombotic and Thrombolytic Therapy. *Chest* 2004;126(suppl 3):S338-S400.

This article discusses the prevention of venous thromboembolism (VTE) and is part of the Seventh American College of Chest Physicians Conference on Antithrombotic and Thrombolytic Therapy; several key recommendations are presented.

51. Kabak S, Halici M, Tuncel M, Avsarogullari L, Baktir A, Basturk M: Functional outcome of open reduction and internal fixation for completely unstable pelvic ring fractures (type C): A report of 40 cases. *J Orthop Trauma* 2003;17(8):555-562.

52. Latenser BA, Gentilello LM, Tarver AA, Thalgott JS, Batdorf JW: Improved outcome with early fixation of skeletally unstable pelvic fractures. *J Trauma* 1991; 31(1):28-31.

53. Mullis BH, Sagi HC: Minimum 1-year follow-up for patients with vertical shear sacroiliac joint dislocations treated with iliosacral screws: Does joint ankylosis or anatomic reduction contribute to functional outcome? *J Orthop Trauma* 2008;22(5):293-298.

The authors prospectively analyzed a homogenous group of trauma patients with pure SI joint dislocations treated with iliosacral screws, with specific attention to functional outcome and its correlation with the presence or absence of SI joint ankylosis and quality of reduction. They found that in the treatment of vertically displaced pure SI joint dislocations, an anatomic reduction (whether closed or open), followed by iliosacral screw fixation should be the goal, because this appears to be the only predictor of a more favorable functional outcome in patients with this injury. Complete SI joint ankylosis appears to have no effect, either positive or negative, on functional outcome in these patients.

54. Tornetta P III, Matta JM: Outcome of operatively treated unstable posterior pelvic ring disruptions. *Clin Orthop Relat Res* 1996;329:186-193.

55. Cole JD, Blum DA, Ansel LJ: Outcome after fixation of unstable posterior pelvic ring injuries. *Clin Orthop Relat Res* 1996;329:160-179.

56. Lowe MA, Mason JT, Luna GK, Maier RV, Copass MK, Berger RE: Risk factors for urethral injuries in men with traumatic pelvic fractures. *J Urol* 1988;140(3): 506-507.

57. Copeland CE, Bosse MJ, McCarthy ML, et al: Effect of trauma and pelvic fracture on female genitourinary, sexual, and reproductive function. *J Orthop Trauma* 1997; 11(2):73-81.

58. O'Brien DP, Luchette FA, Pereira SJ, et al: Pelvic fracture in the elderly is associated with increased mortality. *Surgery* 2002;132(4):710-714.

59. Gustavo Parreira J, Coimbra R, Rasslan S, Oliveira A, Fregoneze M, Mercadante M: The role of associated injuries on outcome of blunt trauma patients sustaining pelvic fractures. *Injury* 2000;31(9):677-682.

60. Nepola JV, Trenhaile SW, Miranda MA, Butterfield SL, Fredericks DC, Riemer BL: Vertical shear injuries: Is there a relationship between residual displacement and functional outcome? *J Trauma* 1999;46(6):1024-1029.

61. Oliver CW, Twaddle B, Agel J, Routt ML Jr: Outcome after pelvic ring fractures: Evaluation using the medical outcomes short form SF-36. *Injury* 1996;27(9):635-641.

4. Axial Skeleton, Including Spine and Pelvis

Chapter 24

Acetabular Fractures: Acute Evaluation

Jaimo Ahn, MD, PhD   Mark C. Reilly, MD · Dean G. Lorich, MD   David L. Helfet, MD

Anatomic Considerations

The acetabulum is a complex bony and soft-tissue structure whose anatomy is a reflection of the functional mechanics of the hip joint and must be understood before proper evaluation can be performed. In addition, during proper preoperative planning (if warranted) and reconstruction, special attention must be paid to spatial bony relationships, as their reestablishment is critical in functional restoration of the hip joint, weight transfer, and gait mechanics.

The acetabular surface is covered with a horseshoe-shaped area of articular cartilage (with a recessed inferocentral cotyloid fossa) that covers slightly less than half of the femoral head. In a nondysplastic form, it is essentially semispheroid in shape with an infero-anterior notch and a mean lateral inclination of 40° to 48° and anteversion of 18° to 21°.[1,2]

The overall bony structure of the acetabulum is composed of the pubis, ischium, and ilium, the three embryologic components of the innominate bone that fuse in skeletal maturity and contribute predominantly to an anterior column, posterior column, and roof/sciatic buttress, respectively (**Figure 1, A**). Conceptually, the

longer anterior column and shorter posterior column intersect in a lambda configuration ("inverted Y") to support the acetabular roof (major weight-bearing surface, **Figure 1, B**), which is then connected to the sacrum through a sciatic buttress (**Figure 1, C**).

The posterior column is composed of the quadrilateral surface internally; the posterior wall and dome, subcotyloid groove (obturator externus tendon), and ischial tuberosity laterally; and the greater and lesser sciatic notches separated by the ischial spine posteriorly. The anterior column consists of the anterior ilium (including the gluteus medius tubercle and incorporating the anterosuperior and anteroinferior iliac spine), a portion of the acetabulum (the anterior wall and anterior dome), and a portion of the pubis (iliopectineal eminence, lateral superior pubic ramus).

The bony acetabulum has a rich extraosseous anastomotic network of vessels. Understanding this vascular anatomy is important for the acute management of the hemodynamically unstable patient as well as surgical treatment. The iliolumbar, superior gluteal, inferior gluteal, and obturator arteries primarily provide most of the blood supply to the acetabulum and columns (**Figure 1, D and E**). The internal pudendal, fourth lumbar, sciatic, and medial femoral circumflex arteries may also provide a secondary blood supply to the anastomoses. In addition, recent studies suggest the importance of maintaining terminal vessels that enter the acetabulum from the posterior and posterolateral aspect of the capsule.[3] Although another study demonstrated maintenance of intraosseous blood flow (albeit reduced compared to baseline) following periacetabular osteotomy,[4] the relationship between the extraosseous arterial network and intraosseous blood supply has not been clearly delineated. As such, the implications of injury patterns on blood flow to specific portions of the acetabulum are not well understood.

The pattern of injury to the bony acetabulum is dependent on the position of the femur and femoral head and the force vector transmitted through the hip joint as well as the magnitude of the force itself. Letournel and Judet described the importance of hip position (rotation, adduction, and so on) on the pattern of injury (**Figure 2**). Most often the hip is flexed with a posterior directed axial force through the femur (such as during a

Dr. Ahn or an immediate family member serves as a board member, owner, officer, or committee member of the Foundation for Orthopedic Trauma and American Physician Scientists Association; and has received research or institutional support from the Orthopaedic Trauma Association. Dr. Reilly or an immediate family member serves as a board member, owner, officer, or committee member of the AO Foundation; is a member of a speakers bureau or has made paid presentations on behalf of Synthes and Smith & Nephew; and has received research or institutional support from EBI, Musculoskeletal Transplant Foundation, Smith & Nephew, Stryker, and Synthes. Dr. Helfet or an immediate family member serves as a board member, owner, officer, or committee member of the Orthopaedic Trauma Association; has received research or institutional support from Synthes; is a member of the Board of Directors of Synthes; and has stock or stock options held in Synthes. Neither Dr. Lorich nor an immediate family member has received anything of value from or owns stock in a commercial company or institution related directly or indirectly to the subject of this chapter.

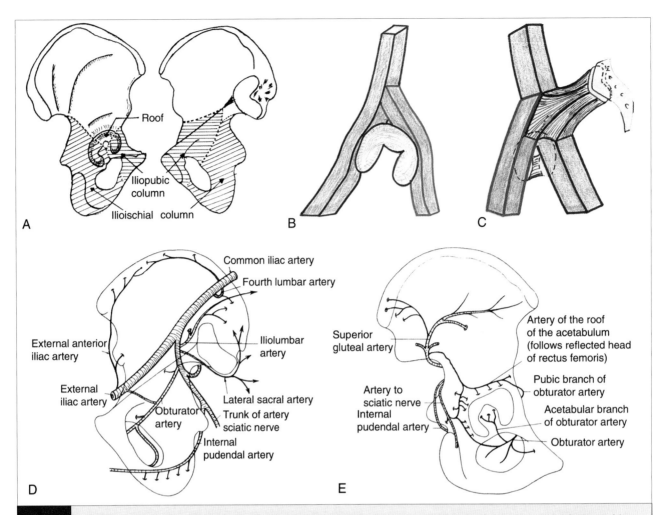

Figure 1 Anatomy of the acetabulum. The acetabulum is composed of the three elements of the innominate bone: pubis, ischium, and ilium, which contribute predominantly to the anterior column, posterior column, and roof/sciatic buttress, respectively (**A**). The two columns support the roof in a lambda configuration (**B**) and are connected to the sacrum through a buttress (**C**). A rich internal (**D**) and external (**E**) anastomotic network provides vascular support for the acetabulum. (Reproduced with permission from Letournel E, Judet R, eds: *Fractures of the Acetabulum*, ed 2. New York, NY, Springer-Verlag, 1981, pp 18-24.)

motor vehicle crash) leading to the most commonly encountered posterior wall fracture. In contrast, in falls from a standing height in the elderly, the force is transmitted medially through the greater trochanter without hip flexion, resulting in injury to the anterior column and quadrilateral plate.[5] Greater forces can result in associated dislocations of the femoral head (posterior or central for the examples given).

Epidemiology and Associated Injuries

A recent British prospective study gathering data from 1988 to 2003 described the incidence of acetabular fractures as being 3 patients per 100,000 per year.[6] The study period was divided into thirds, and no significant change in overall incidence over time was noted. Other studies from the 1990s provided conflicting data re-

garding changes in overall incidence of these injuries: although one study suggested a decreased incidence of injury because of seat-belt policies,[7] another indicated an increase due to motorcycle helmet laws.[8] In the British study, there were 351 acetabular fractures in a population with a mean age of 50 years (range, 16 to 98 years). There was an increase in age over time from 46.8 years to 53.7 years, perhaps reflecting the increasing aging population as well as a bimodal distribution pattern (younger patients with high-energy trauma and older patients with low-energy trauma). No study has clearly documented an increasing incidence in acetabular fractures among older age groups, despite anecdotal references to this trend. There was, however, a significant shift in gender. In the first third of the study, 25% of patients were female; in the last third, 40% were female. Consistent with previous studies, motor vehicle crash was the most common mechanism of injury, fol-

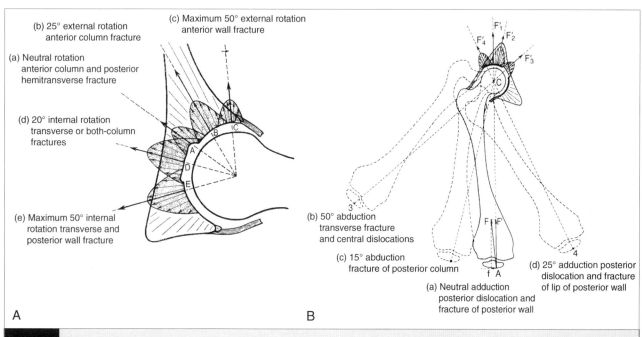

(b) 25° external rotation anterior column fracture

(c) Maximum 50° external rotation anterior wall fracture

(a) Neutral rotation anterior column and posterior hemitransverse fracture

(d) 20° internal rotation transverse or both-column fractures

(e) Maximum 50° internal rotation transverse and posterior wall fracture

A

(b) 50° abduction transverse fracture and central dislocations

(c) 15° abduction fracture of posterior column

(a) Neutral adduction posterior dislocation and fracture of posterior wall

(d) 25° adduction posterior dislocation and fracture of lip of posterior wall

B

Figure 2 The rotational position (**A**) and coronal position (**B**) of the femur predicts the injury patterns seen clinically. (Reproduced with permission from Letournel E, Judet R, eds: *Fractures of the Acetabulum*, ed 2. New York, NY, Springer-Verlag, 1981, pp 24-25.)

lowed remotely by pedestrian-motor vehicle crash and fall from a height. Notably, low-energy falls (from less than 10 feet) increased from 17% to 38% during the study. The injury severity of patients also appeared to decrease, with mean Injury Severity Score (ISS) decreasing from 16 to 10 and mortality decreasing ninefold over the duration of the study. The specific numbers and percentages from this study may not be reflected in other studies because of regional differences (for example, another US study[9] showed a motor vehicle crash rate of 80%, versus 38% in the British study), but the changes (or lack thereof) reported from a longitudinal study reporting true incidence over time are instructive.[6]

Since Letournel and Judet's original concepts, it has been well established that acetabular fractures are commonly associated with other significant injuries.[10] A recent study examined 323 acetabular fractures over 4 years and found injury to the lower extremities to be the most commonly associated (36%), followed by injuries to the lungs, retroperitoneum, upper extremities (20% to 30% each), spine, brain, liver, spleen, bladder, and vascular system (between 5% and 20% each).[9] Lateral loads were associated with retroperitoneal hematomas and splenic, hepatic, vascular, renal, and bladder injuries when compared to posteriorly directed loads. Another study found that blood loss was not randomly distributed among acetabular fracture patterns—transverse, associated both-column, and anterior column posterior hemitransverse patterns required the greatest number of transfusions for resuscitation

(13.0 units, 8.8 units, and 6.4 units of packed red blood cells, respectively).[11] These three patterns also required transfusion in 50% or more of patients. In addition, there have been further descriptions regarding various local or regional conditions associated with acetabular fractures. Soft-tissue injury such as closed degloving (or Morel-Lavallée lesion) about the greater trochanter, although rare (less than 2% in one series of more than 1,000 acetabular fractures),[12] continues to be an unsolved problem that can lead to wound breakdown and deep infections. Based on the rationale that these injuries involve devascularization of the local area and can harbor bacteria even without violation of the integument, one report has advocated for percutaneous treatment of the degloving injuries with underlying fractures rather than open treatment.[12] Of six surgical acetabular fractures with Morel-Lavallée lesions (all treated with percutaneous drainage, débridement, irrigation, and suction drainage), one required open surgical débridement due to persistent drainage, and none developed long-term sequelae including deep infection.[12] Despite continuing investigations, the best management of these lesions—be it method of débridement, antibiotic treatment, or timing of fixation surgery—remains unclear.

Acetabular fractures can be associated with a dislocation or fracture of the femoral head. The largest recent series showed that approximately 30% of displaced acetabular fractures had a concomitant dislocation of the femoral head.[10] With timely reduction and fixation, the fractures involving dislocation had out-

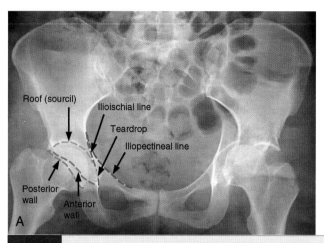

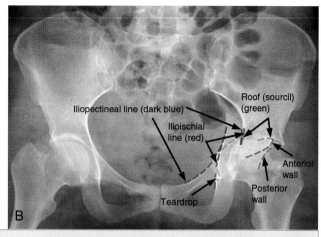

Figure 3 AP pelvis radiographs show a left acetabular fracture including radiographic landmarks on the fractured and unfractured sides (**A** and **B**). Six landmarks to be examined include the iliopectineal line (anterior column), ilioischial line (posterior column), anterior wall, posterior wall, sourcil ("eyebrow" roof), teardrop (obturator canal, cotyloid fossa, quadrilateral plate).

comes similar to those without dislocation (71% versus 78% good to excellent results). The true prevalence of femoral head fractures in the setting of an acetabular fracture (Pipkin type IV) is unknown. Only small series have been reported, with a recent report showing a good Merle d'Aubigné-Postel score of 15.6 (out of 18) and one documented osteonecrosis of the femoral head among 12 patients treated with surgical fixation through a trochanteric flip osteotomy.[13]

Another associated injury in the setting of acetabular fractures is sciatic nerve palsy. Letournel and Judet reported a 12.2% rate (115 of 940) in their series, which they attributed primarily to posterior or central dislocation of the femoral head. A recent report showed that the nerve can be entrapped in the fracture itself with resolution of symptoms following neuroplasty and transposition out of the fracture site at time of fixation.[14]

Radiologic Evaluation

Radiologic evaluation of acetabular fractures typically involves the use of AP and oblique (Judet) pelvic plain radiography and CT. There have been continued discussions regarding the utility of obtaining specific oblique views and the various uses of CT (reconstructed radiographs, three-dimensional [3D] reconstructions, and image-guided surgical planning).

Standard plain radiographic imaging consists of an AP pelvic view with the patient supine and the image centered on the symphysis pubis (**Figure 3,** *A*). Letournel and Judet described six radiographic lines that represent an anatomic element or confluence of anatomic structures (**Figure 3,** *A*). Two additional 45° oblique (Judet) views are obtained. The obturator oblique view is a 45° view angled toward the injured side (**Figure 4,** *A,* middle image, in which the ipsilateral obturator fo-

ramen is maximally seen) and allows for less obstructed assessment of the anterior column and posterior wall. The iliac oblique view is a 45° view angled away from the injured side (**Figure 4,** *A,* right image, in which the ipsilateral iliac wing is maximally seen), more clearly showing the posterior column and anterior wall. Because the image cassette must be perpendicular to the x-ray beam (and therefore requires rotation of the patient, as shown in **Figure 4,** *B*), it can be difficult to obtain these views during initial trauma workup. There is evidence that the oblique views do not improve reliability of fracture classification per se,[15] but rather that a systematic approach (using the six-landmark system) and reader experience improve the ability to read the AP views alone. Whereas a high percentage of injuries can be identified and classified based on careful evaluation of the AP image, the oblique images provide additional information regarding the morphology of the injury.

Although the almost-routine use of CT scanning in initial trauma workups has further questioned the need for additional plain radiographic views, many surgeons still prefer the use of Judet views to assess overall length, alignment, and rotation of the injury and for preoperative planning. Recent use of CT technology has allowed for the reconstruction of plain radiographic views ("ghost" views) from CT data (**Figure 4,** *C*); in one study these images were shown to be equivalent for fracture pattern recognition, image clarity, information provided, and overall satisfaction of the reviewers.[16] However, further studies are needed to validate the clinical usefulness of this methodology.

The two-dimensional CT scan remains an essential tool in the detailed assessment and treatment of acetabular fractures (**Figure 5**). Recent studies have validated older literature on the utility of CT scans in providing greater injury detail when compared to plain radiographs—details such as intra-articular loose bodies, im-

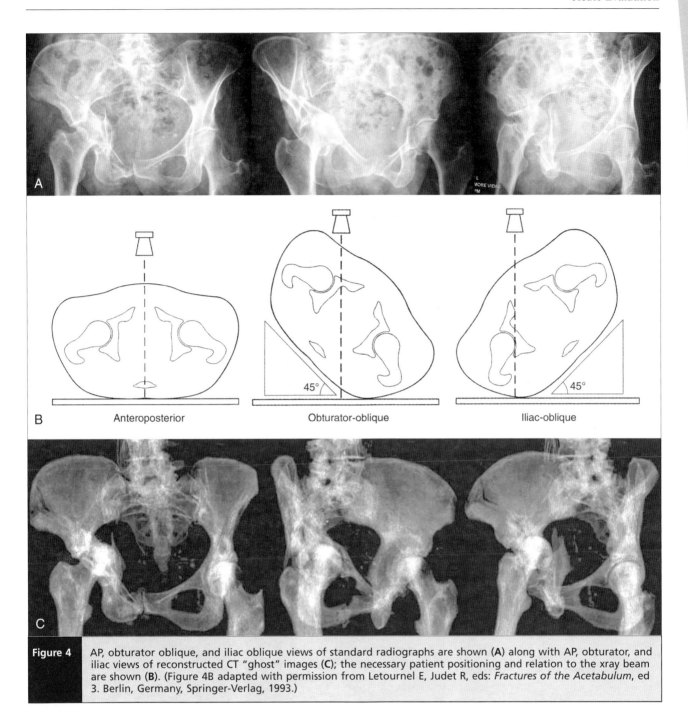

Figure 4   AP, obturator oblique, and iliac oblique views of standard radiographs are shown (**A**) along with AP, obturator, and iliac views of reconstructed CT "ghost" images (**C**); the necessary patient positioning and relation to the xray beam are shown (**B**). (Figure 4B adapted with permission from Letournel E, Judet R, eds: *Fractures of the Acetabulum*, ed 3. Berlin, Germany, Springer-Verlag, 1993.)

paction, step-offs, or gaps are better delineated[17]—especially for those not well acquainted with acetabular trauma.[18] Similarly, a study from the radiology literature showed that 3D reconstructed images (**Figure 6**) may provide more useful information than helical CT images, which in turn provide more information than conventional tomography.[19]

The fine detail and the multiaxial nature of data obtained from CT scans—for example, providing accurate measurement of posterior wall size and involvement—have also allowed for the use of these studies in the assessment of stability and the possible need for surgical fixation. One study compared three different methods of measuring the extent of posterior wall involvement using two-dimensional CT and found one to be most predictive of stability (**Figure 7**) on stress-fluoroscopic examination; however, the authors note that none of the CT-based methods was highly predictive of stability.[20] Further study on a larger group of patients may allow for the development of a highly predictive model to predict stability based on injury scans. The continued increase in computing power has allowed for the consideration of virtual 3D surgical planning (including fracture reduction and hardware placement) for acetabular fractures.[21] The utility of such an approach is currently unknown but merits further investigation.

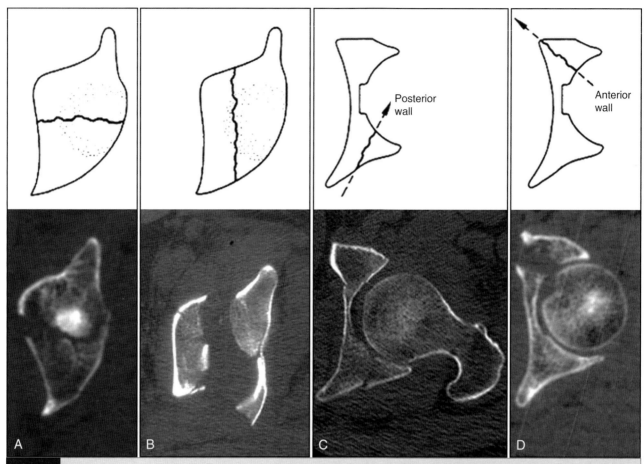

Figure 5 CT images have the ability to show the plane of a column fracture (**A**), transverse fracture (**B**), and a wall fracture (**C** and **D**). (Adapted with permission from Letournel E, Judet R: Radiology of the normal acetabulum, in Letournel E, Judet R, eds: *Fractures of the Acetabulum*, ed 3. New York, NY, Springer-Verlag, 1993, p 61.)

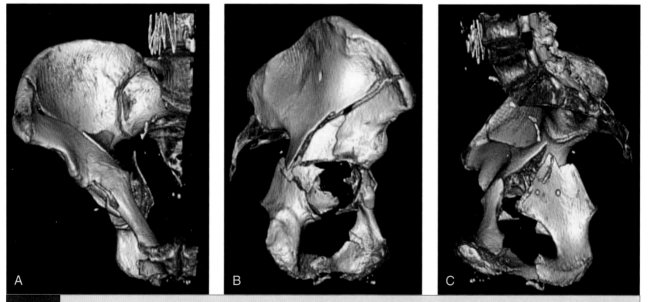

Figure 6 Three-dimensional CT reconstructions show topographic detail of an associated both-column acetabular fracture with the femoral head subtracted from the front (**A**), outside (**B**), and inside (**C**).

Classification

The classification system of Letournel and Judet, the most useful and widely accepted systematic description of acetabular fractures, was originally proposed in 1961 and was derived from an analysis of the plain radiographs of 75 cases and an understanding of the radiographic landmarks determined from study of the dry innominate bone. The classification was modified and improved by Letournel but has remained essentially unchanged since its inception. Alphanumeric classification systems have been proposed but have not altered the basic structure of the original classification system and hence have not been accepted.

The classification system has been tested numerous times for interobserver and intraobserver reliability.[15,18,22-24] The most widely accepted analysis compared three different groups of reviewers with different levels of experience with acetabular fracture treatment. The classification was found to have substantial reliability when determined by plain radiographs alone. The addition of axial CT did not improve this reliability.[18] Although other studies have reported an improvement in examiners' reliability with the addition of the 3D CT scan, in none of these articles did the interobserver or intraobserver reliability exceed that of experienced acetabular fracture surgeons interpreting the plain radiographs alone.[15,22-24]

The 10 fracture patterns in the Letournel-Judet classification are divided into 5 elementary and 5 associated fracture patterns. The elementary fractures are defined as those that separate a portion of an anatomic column or the column in its entirety from the intact innominate bone. These include the posterior wall fracture, the posterior column fracture, the anterior wall fracture, and the anterior column fracture. The transverse fracture is included in this group because of the purity of its fracture pattern and the resultant single displaced fragment, despite the involvement of both the

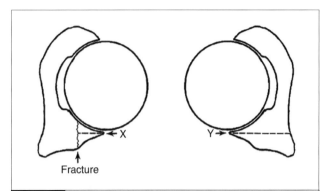

| Figure 7 | Stability of a posterior wall fracture may be predicted based on calculating the ratio of the measured medial to lateral fracture depth (X) to the depth of the normal uninjured side (Y). (Reproduced with permission from Moed BR, Ajibade DA, Israel H: Computed tomography as a predictor of hip stability status in posterior wall fractures of the acetabulum. *J Orthop Trauma* 2009;23:7-15.) |

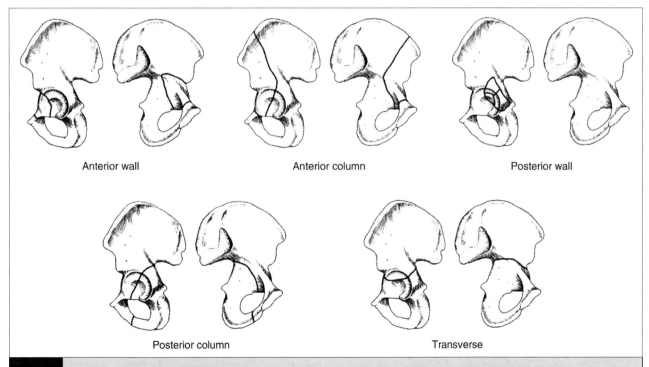

| Figure 8 | The five elementary acetabular fracture patterns in the Letournel-Judet classification. (Adapted with permission from Letournel E, Judet R, eds: *Fractures of the Acetabulum*, ed 3. Berlin, Germany, Springer-Verlag, 1993.) |

4: Axial Skeleton, Including Spine and Pelvis

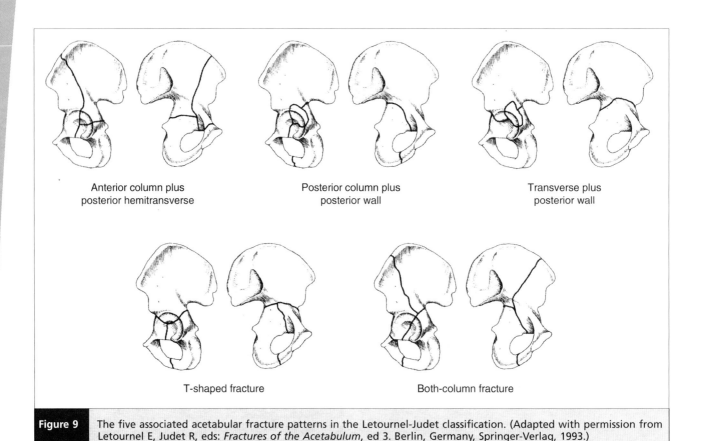

| Figure 9 | The five associated acetabular fracture patterns in the Letournel-Judet classification. (Adapted with permission from Letournel E, Judet R, eds: *Fractures of the Acetabulum*, ed 3. Berlin, Germany, Springer-Verlag, 1993.) |

anterior and posterior columns of the acetabulum (**Figure 8**).

The associated fracture patterns are combinations that involve at least two of the elementary fracture patterns. These are the associated posterior column and posterior wall fracture, the associated transverse and posterior wall fracture, the associated anterior column or wall with posterior hemitransverse fracture, the associated both-column fracture, and the T-shaped fracture (**Figure 9**).

Variants of these fracture patterns exist, as do transitional forms, but in general they can fit into the classification by following the guidelines set forth by Letournel and Judet. The classification guides the surgeon in understanding the nuances of the fracture anatomy and helps in the selection of the most appropriate surgical approach with which to treat the fracture.

Elementary Fracture Patterns

Fractures of the posterior wall of the acetabulum are the most common fracture pattern and separate a portion of the posterior rim with a variable amount of retroacetabular surface. The fracture may be single or multifragmentary and may be associated with articular impaction and/or incarcerated fragments within the hip joint. The posterior wall fracture is initially identified on the AP radiograph as a disruption or absence of the posterior rim shadow with or without femoral head

subluxation. The obturator oblique radiograph confirms the diagnosis and better demonstrates the number and size of the posterior wall fracture fragments. Thorough evaluation of the CT scan will better highlight any articular impaction and free osteochondral fragments that are often associated with this fracture pattern.

The posterior column fracture detaches the entire caudal portion of the posterior articular surface, retroacetabular surface, and posterior border of the innominate bone. On the AP radiograph, medial displacement of the ilioischial line is noted and loss of congruity with the roof is not unusual. The relationship between the ilioischial line and the teardrop is disrupted in most instances unless a large portion of the quadrilateral surface remains intact to the posterior column fragment. In this instance, the ilioischial line and teardrop may displace together. The fracture is best seen on the iliac oblique view, where the entire fracture line can be seen from the apex of the greater sciatic notch, propagating across the posterior articular surface, entering the roof of the obturator canal, and fracturing the ischial ramus.

The anterior wall fracture detaches the central portion of the anterior column along with a fragment of the anterior articular rim. The anterior rim shadow and the iliopectineal line on the AP radiograph will show displacement in two locations, but all posterior landmarks will remain intact. A variable-sized portion of the quadrilateral surface may be detached with the anterior wall, and this may result in an apparent "thinning" or duplication of the ilioischial line, but some portion of the line will remain intact. Femoral head subluxation is commonly seen, and the femoral head will be noted to follow the anterior wall fragment, particularly visible on the obturator oblique radiograph.

Anterior column fractures detach the anterior border of the innominate bone and are subclassified by the location at which they exit superiorly. High anterior column fractures exit the iliac crest, best appreciated on the iliac oblique radiograph. On the AP radiograph, the iliopectineal line is displaced and the femoral head and roof (or portion of the roof) are moved cranially and medially. An associated fracture of the ischial ramus is seen and is generally more anterior in the high or intermediate fracture patterns and more posterior in the lower fractures.

Transverse fractures divide the acetabulum into two fragments: the intact roof and the displaced ischiopubic fragment. The obturator ring remains intact. Transverse fractures are subdivided according to where the transverse fracture line crosses the articular surface. Transtectal fractures cross the weight-bearing dome of the acetabulum. Juxtatectal fractures cross the articular surface at the level of the top of the cotyloid fossa. Infratectal fractures cross the cotyloid fossa. The typical displacement of the fracture involves a rotation of the ischiopubic fragment about the symphysis pubis, resulting in a proximal and medial displacement of the fragment. The femoral head often follows the displacement of the ischiopubic fragment.

Associated Fracture Patterns

The associated posterior column plus posterior wall fracture combines the typical displacements of the radiographic landmarks on the AP and iliac oblique views that are seen with the typical posterior column fracture with the displaced posterior wall fragment best seen on the obturator oblique view. The femoral head is frequently dislocated cranially and posteriorly away from the acetabular roof on presentation, and the posterior column fragment (ischioacetabular fragment) follows the displacement of the femoral head. The posterior wall fragment remains with the femoral head while dislocated but typically stays in a displaced position once the femoral head is reduced.

The association of the transverse and posterior wall fractures combines the typical radiographic features of the transverse fracture with those of the posterior wall fracture. As with the elementary patterns, the transverse component may be transtectal, juxtatectal, or infratectal, and the posterior wall component may be single or multifragmentary and associated with marginal impaction. Dislocation of the femoral head is common in these fractures and the dislocation may be either posteriorly through the wall defect or the head may follow the ischiopubic segment medially and dislocate away from the acetabular roof through the transverse frac-

ture. The T-shaped fracture involves a transverse fracture with an associated inferior vertical fracture line across the quadrilateral surface, cotyloid fossa, and ischial ramus. However, it may also extend posteriorly (exiting through the ischium) or anteriorly (exiting near the pubic body). The caudal ischiopubic segment created by the transverse fracture component is divided into a posterior (ischial) and anterior (pubic) articular segment. Depending on the relative degree of displacement between the fragments, the relationship of the ilioischial line, iliopectineal line, and teardrop will change.

The associated anterior wall or column with posterior hemitransverse fractures comprises a heterogeneous group of fractures in which the main feature of the fracture is a typical anterior wall or column fracture. This is associated with a transverse posterior column fracture that is typically lower and less displaced than the anterior fracture moiety.

The associated both-column fracture is defined as a fracture in which all portions of the acetabular articular surface are detached. No portion of the articular surface remains intact to the ilium. The intact iliac fragment includes the posterosuperior iliac spine and sacroiliac joint and typically terminates in a caudal "spur sign" seen most prominently on the obturator oblique view. This sign is pathognomonic of the associated both-column fracture because this spur can only be seen when all fragments of the articular surface are displaced medially and cranially away from the intact ilium. It is important to distinguish the associated both-column fracture from fracture patterns that involve both anatomic columns. The transverse, transverse plus posterior wall, T-shaped, and anterior plus posterior hemitransverse fracture all involve both the anterior and posterior columns, but all have some portion of the acetabular articular surface that remains intact to the ilium.

Emergent Treatment

Although acetabular fractures are generally the result of high-energy mechanisms, the incidence of life- or limb-threatening complications associated with the fracture generally is low. That does not preclude a thorough evaluation of the trauma patient according to Advanced Trauma Life Support guidelines, as associated injuries to the patient are not uncommon. Hemodynamic instability may be encountered in patients with acetabular fractures but is infrequently caused by a vascular injury associated with the fracture. If other sources of hemodynamic instability have been excluded, angiographic evaluation may be indicated, particularly with fractures that violate the greater sciatic notch or the obturator canal.[11] Open fractures of the acetabulum are rare, but a thorough examination of the integument about the hip is mandatory, including an examination of the perineum and genitalia. Acetabular fractures may also be seen in association with bowel or bladder injuries, and communication and coordination of surgical procedures with the general surgical trauma surgeons will help to maximize outcomes after such devastating injuries while preventing compromise of subsequent fracture reconstruction. Thorough neurologic examination is mandatory to identify any preoperative nerve dysfunction that has occurred as a result of the trauma.

Subluxation of the femoral head is frequently seen, and the femoral head may wear against a fracture edge or intra-articular osteochondral fragment. Although skeletal traction would not be expected to produce a complete reduction of a displaced acetabular fracture, there remains a role for it when the femoral head articular surface is at risk for ongoing damage during the preoperative evaluation and preparation of the patient for surgery. Dislocation of the femoral head in association with acetabular fracture must be identified by a careful evaluation of the radiographic studies because the resting position of the leg will often not be the typical position seen after an isolated dislocation.

Posttraumatic and postoperative thromboembolism is a significant problem in acetabular fracture patients. Proximal deep venous thrombosis was identified using magnetic resonance venography in 34% of acetabular fracture patients but has been reported to be as high as 61% in patients with pelvic fractures.[25,26] Therefore, some form of mechanical or chemical prophylaxis is recommended to decrease the risk of thromboembolic complications. One study indicated that mechanical prophylaxis with foot pumps at the time of hospital admission and the addition of enoxaparin 5 days after admission was a successful strategy for prophylaxis against venous thromboembolic disease following serious musculoskeletal injury.[27] Despite the use of prophylactic treatment, however, the prevalence of posttraumatic and postoperative thromboembolism is approximately 11%.[27-29] The value of screening using Doppler ultrasound or magnetic resonance venography remains controversial.[28] Limited information is available to clinicians to guide their treatment decisions. In a meta-analysis, 1,760 patients in 11 studies were reviewed but no conclusions were made because of the heterogeneity within the studies. The recommendation was for well-designed clinical trials to evaluate both the detection and prevention of thromboembolic disease after pelvic and acetabular fracture.[30]

The placement of prophylactic vena caval filters is controversial but may be indicated in selected high-risk patients.[28,29,31] In patients with known preoperative deep venous thrombosis, the placement of a vena caval filter has been shown to be associated with a low rate of recurrent deep venous thrombosis and postthrombotic syndrome. In a study of 102 patients with caval filters for pelvic or acetabular surgery with an average follow-up of 4 years, no patient was readmitted for thromboembolic disease.[32]

Summary

The complete evaluation of the patient with an acute traumatic acetabular injury requires both an assessment of the patient's overall physiologic and pathologic status through a trauma evaluation and of the specific injury pattern to the hip based on an understanding of normal anatomy. Goals of treatment will include restoration of the columnar support, articular congruity, and inclination/version of the acetabulum through eventual bony and soft-tissue healing (with or without surgical fixation). The mechanisms responsible for and injuries associated with particular fracture patterns may change with time and may differ from patient population to population. Therefore, a high level of clinical vigilance is required as is the collection and dissemination of injury data. Radiologic evaluation including standard radiographic views and CT scans is required. The utility of 3D reconstructions, virtual surgical planning, and intraoperative navigation requires further investigation before these methods can be incorporated into standard practice.

The evaluation of the patient with an acetabular fracture includes a thorough evaluation of the integument, along with neurologic and vascular status of the limb. Radiographic evaluation with the standard three plain radiographs enables proper classification of the fracture. Accurately classifying the fracture by the system of Letournel and Judet increases the surgeon's understanding of the fracture pattern and aids in the correct selection of the surgical approach that will maximize the opportunities for anatomic reduction and fixation of the fracture. Thromboembolic prophylaxis remains an important adjunct in the treatment of trauma patients with pelvic and acetabular injuries.

Acknowledgments

The authors acknowledge Gregory R. Saboeiro, MD, Chief of Interventional Radiology at the Hospital for Special Surgery, for his technical knowledge and expert assistance with preparation of computer-reconstructed radiographs and three-dimensional CT reconstruction images.

Annotated References

1. Krebs V, Incavo SJ, Shields WH: The anatomy of the acetabulum: What is normal? *Clin Orthop Relat Res* 2009;467(4):868-875.

   Data regarding the topology of the normal acetabulum have been limited. This study measured angles and distances between landmarks and created a topographic characterization of normal acetabuli using 100 cadaver specimens.

2. Letournel E, Judet R: *Fractures of the Acetabulum*, ed 2. Berlin: Springer-Verlag, 1993.

3. Kalhor M, Beck M, Huff TW, Ganz R: Capsular and pericapsular contributions to acetabular and femoral head perfusion. *J Bone Joint Surg Am* 2009;91(2):409-418.

   Silicone injection studies in 20 cadaver specimens showed that posterior and posterolateral capsular and pericapsular vessels contribute to the blood supply of the acetabulum.

4. Hempfing A, Leunig M, Nötzli HP, Beck M, Ganz R: Acetabular blood flow during Bernese periacetabular osteotomy: An intraoperative study using laser Doppler flowmetry. *J Orthop Res* 2003;21(6):1145-1150.

5. Pagenkopf E, Grose A, Partal G, Helfet DL: Acetabular fractures in the elderly: Treatment recommendations. *HSS J* 2006;2(2):161-171.

   The authors consider their experience and a nonsystematic review of the literature to offer an algorithm to address the acetabular fracture in the elderly. Key considerations in the algorithm include preinjury status of the patient, anticipated surgical stress and time relative to the patient's health, and reconstructable anatomy of the injury. Level of evidence: V.

6. Laird A, Keating JF: Acetabular fractures: A 16-year prospective epidemiological study. *J Bone Joint Surg Br* 2005;87(7):969-973.

   The authors report the results of a 16-year epidemiologic study involving more than 600,000 total patients, 351 with acetabular fractures. They report demographics, injury patterns, and outcomes. They note an overall decrease in Injury Severity Score, mortality, length of hospital stay, and incidence of posttraumatic osteoarthritis over time. Level of evidence: I.

7. al-Qahtani S, O'Connor G: Acetabular fractures before and after the introduction of seatbelt legislation. *Can J Surg* 1996;39(4):317-320.

8. Dakin GJ, Eberhardt AW, Alonso JE, Stannard JP, Mann KA: Acetabular fracture patterns: Associations with motor vehicle crash information. *J Trauma* 1999;47(6):1063-1071.

9. Porter SE, Schroeder AC, Dzugan SS, Graves ML, Zhang L, Russell GV: Acetabular fracture patterns and their associated injuries. *J Orthop Trauma* 2008;22(3):165-170.

   A retrospective review of 323 acetabular injuries in a prospectively collected database is reported. Injury characteristics reported in relation to direction of load (lateral or posterior) suggest a higher rate of nonorthopaedic injuries from lateral loads. Level of evidence: II.

10. Matta JM: Fractures of the acetabulum: Accuracy of reduction and clinical results in patients managed operatively within three weeks after the injury. *J Bone Joint Surg Am* 1996;78(11):1632-1645.

11. Magnussen RA, Tressler MA, Obremskey WT, Kregor PJ: Predicting blood loss in isolated pelvic and acetabular high-energy trauma. *J Orthop Trauma* 2007;21(9):603-607.

    A retrospective review of 382 pelvic and acetabular injuries examined the relationship between injury pattern and blood transfusion requirements and noted a positive relationship with high-energy injuries for the pelvis and anterior column and T type for the acetabulum. Level of evidence: III.

12. Tseng S, Tornetta P III: Percutaneous management of Morel-Lavallée lesions. *J Bone Joint Surg Am* 2006;88(1):92-96.

    In this proof-of-concept paper, 19 patients with Morel-Lavallée lesions with surgical pelvic and acetabular injuries were treated with percutaneous débridement, irrigation, and suction drainage before definitive management. Subsequent development of deep infection or wound breakdown occurred in none of the patients. Level of evidence: IV.

13. Solberg BD, Moon CN, Franco DP: Use of a trochanteric flip osteotomy improves outcomes in Pipkin IV fractures. *Clin Orthop Relat Res* 2009;467(4):929-933.

    This retrospective case series reports the results of 12 patients with combined femoral head and acetabular fractures treated through a trochanteric flip osteotomy approach. The benefits of using such an approach are described, and good clinical outcomes are compared to those previously reported in the literature. Level of evidence: IV.

14. Dunbar RP Jr, Gardner MJ, Cunningham B, Routt ML Jr: Sciatic nerve entrapment in associated both-column acetabular fractures: A report of 2 cases and review of the literature. *J Orthop Trauma* 2009;23:80-83.

    This case report provides two examples of patients with associated both-column acetabular injuries in which the sciatic nerve was trapped within the posterior portion of the fracture. Neuroplasty at the time of fracture fixation improved patient symptoms.

15. Petrisor BA, Bhandari M, Orr RD, Mandel S, Kwok DC, Schemitsch EH: Improving reliability in the classification of fractures of the acetabulum. *Arch Orthop Trauma Surg* 2003;123(5):228-233.

16. Borrelli J Jr, Peelle M, McFarland E, Evanoff B, Ricci WM: Computer-reconstructed radiographs are as good as plain radiographs for assessment of acetabular fractures. *Am J Orthop* 2008;37(9):455-459.

    Using 11 retrospectively identified patients with displaced acetabular fractures and 5 independent readers, this study suggests that radiographs constructed from CTs are as informative, if not more, than standard radiographs in the assessment of acetabular injuries. Level of evidence: III.

17. Borrelli J Jr, Ricci WM, Steger-May K, Totty WG, Goldfarb C: Postoperative radiographic assessment of acetabular fractures: A comparison of plain radiographs and CT scans. *J Orthop Trauma* 2005;19(5):299-304.

4: Axial Skeleton, Including Spine and Pelvis

Analysis of 15 postoperative patients with acetabular injuries provides evidence that CT scans are superior to radiographs in detecting residual gaps and step-offs when compared to standard radiography. Level of evidence: II.

18. Beaulé PE, Dorey FJ, Matta JM: Letournel classification for acetabular fractures: Assessment of interobserver and intraobserver reliability. *J Bone Joint Surg Am* 2003;85(9):1704-1709.

19. Kickuth R, Laufer U, Hartung G, Gruening C, Stueckle C, Kirchner J: 3D CT versus axial helical CT versus conventional tomography in the classification of acetabular fractures: A ROC analysis. *Clin Radiol* 2002;57(2): 140-145.

20. Moed BR, Ajibade DA, Israel H: Computed tomography as a predictor of hip stability status in posterior wall fractures of the acetabulum. *J Orthop Trauma* 2009;23(1):7-15.

Thirty-three consecutive patients with isolated posterior wall fractures were evaluated with dynamic fluoroscopic stress testing for fracture instability. Using this as a gold standard, investigators examined the ability of three different methods using static CT images to predict instability. Using a ratio of medial to lateral fracture depth relative to the uninjured acetabular depth was most predictive. Level of evidence: I.

21. Citak M, Gardner MJ, Kendoff D, et al: Virtual 3D planning of acetabular fracture reduction. *J Orthop Res* 2008;26(4):547-552.

Using 10 surgeons and 4 acetabular fracture models, this study explores the potential ability of virtual 3D operative planning to improve reduction accuracy and efficiency. Level of evidence: IV.

22. Ohashi K, El-Khoury GY, Abu-Zahra KW, Berbaum KS: Interobserver agreement for Letournel acetabular fracture classification with multidetector CT: Are standard Judet radiographs necessary? *Radiology* 2006; 241(2):386-391.

Musculoskeletal radiologists demonstrated improved interobserver agreement after review of 3D CT scans when compared with plain radiographs alone. Interobserver agreement with CT scans was kappa = 0.7.

23. Prevezas N, Antypas G, Louverdis D, Konstas A, Papasotiriou A, Sbonias G: Proposed guidelines for increasing the reliability and validity of Letournel classification system. *Injury* 2009;40(10):1098-1103.

Orthopaedic surgeons significantly improved their accuracy of classifying acetabular fractures with the use of an algorithm. This effect was most pronounced in less experienced surgeons. Level of evidence: I.

24. Visutipol B, Chobtangsin P, Ketmalasiri B, Pattarabanjird N, Varodompun N: Evaluation of Letournel and Judet classification of acetabular fracture with plain radiographs and three-dimensional computerized tomographic scan. *J Orthop Surg* 2000;8(1):33-37.

25. Geerts WH, Code KI, Jay RM, Chen E, Szalai JP: A prospective study of venous thromboembolism after major trauma. *N Engl J Med* 1994;331(24):1601-1606.

26. Rubel IF, Potter H, Barie P, Kloen P, Helfet DL: Magnetic resonance venography to evaluate deep venous thrombosis in patients with pelvic and acetabular trauma. *J Trauma* 2001;51(3):622.

27. Stannard JP, Lopez-Ben RR, Volgas DA, et al: Prophylaxis against deep-vein thrombosis following trauma: A prospective, randomized comparison of mechanical and pharmacologic prophylaxis. *J Bone Joint Surg Am* 2006;88(2):261-266.

Two hundred twenty-four patients were randomized prospectively into two groups. Early mechanical prophylaxis with introduction of enoxaparin at 5 days after injury resulted in a reduction in large/occlusive deep venous thrombosis over that seen with enoxaparin alone. Level of evidence: I.

28. Borer DS, Starr AJ, Reinert CM, et al: The effect of screening for deep vein thrombosis on the prevalence of pulmonary embolism in patients with fractures of the pelvis or acetabulum: A review of 973 patients. *J Orthop Trauma* 2005;19(2):92-95.

Four hundred eighty-six consecutive patients screened for deep venous thrombosis with ultrasound and magnetic resonance venography were compared to 487 consecutive patients in whom no screening was used. Discontinuation of the screening protocol did not affect the rate of pulmonary embolus (1.7% overall, 0.3% fatal). Level of evidence: II.

29. Stannard JP, Singhania AK, Lopez-Ben RR, et al: Deep-vein thrombosis in high-energy skeletal trauma despite thromboprophylaxis. *J Bone Joint Surg Br* 2005;87(7): 965-968.

Both ultrasound and magnetic resonance venography were reported to have high false negative rates in this study of 312 trauma patients. Despite prophylaxis, the rate of venous thromboembolic disease was 11.5%. Level of evidence: II.

30. Slobogean GP, Lefaivre KA, Nicolaou S, O'Brien PJ: A systematic review of thromboprophylaxis for pelvic and acetabular fractures. *J Orthop Trauma* 2009;23(5): 379-384.

Review of 1760 subjects in 11 studies attempted to identify the efficacy of mechanical compression devices, inferior vena caval filters, low molecular weight heparin, ultrasound, and magnetic resonance venography screening. The authors concluded that limited data were available for decision-making in thromboembolic prophylaxis in pelvic fracture patients.

31. Rogers FB, Shackford SR, Ricci MA, Huber BM, Atkins T: Prophylactic vena cava filter insertion in selected high-risk orthopaedic trauma patients. *J Orthop Trauma* 1997;11(4):267-272.

32. Toro JB, Gardner MJ, Hierholzer C, et al: Long-term consequences of pelvic trauma patients with thromboembolic disease treated with inferior vena caval filters. *J Trauma* 2008;65(1):25-29.

One hundred two patients treated with inferior vena caval filters for deep venous thrombosis before acetabular fracture treatment were followed for an average of 4 years. No patients were readmitted for recurrent deep venous thrombosis or pulmonary embolism. Seven patients had some evidence of swelling or postthrombotic syndrome. Level of evidence: II.

4: Axial Skeleton, Including Spine and Pelvis

Chapter 25

Acetabular Fractures: Definitive Treatment and Expected Outcomes

Milton L. Routt Jr, MD   Animesh Agarwal, MD

Indications for Surgical Management

Choosing and applying the appropriate management plan for a patient with an acetabular fracture can be daunting. The overall goals are to achieve a functional and pain-free hip joint. Numerous factors related to the patient, specific fracture details, treatment facility, and treating physician must be considered as the plan is formulated.

Important patient-related factors that influence outcome include age, functional status, bone quality, body habitus, and medical comorbidities. Most acetabular fractures occur in young adults, but children and patients age 65 years and older also sustain them. Children with acetabulum fractures involving open triradiate physes warrant special care and follow-up, because posttraumatic physeal bars can cause hip dysplasia if left untreated.[1] In patients age 65 years and older, bone quality impacts not only the fracture patterns and details, but also the strength and durability of the surgical repair[2,3] (Figure 1). Poor bone quality is associated with more significant fracture impaction to both the acetabulum[4] and the femoral head[5] in all age groups. These acetabular impaction fractures complicate accurate reduction and also require bone grafting or other support techniques to maintain fracture reduction until bony union.[6,7] One such support technique is to use small subchondral screws to hold impacted osteochondral fragments in place after elevation and reduction beneath larger fixation constructs.[8] No reliable fracture repair treatment options exist at this time for associated femoral head impaction fractures.

Dr. Agarwal or an immediate family member is a board member, owner, officer, or committee member for the American Academy of Orthopaedic Surgeons, the Orthopaedic Trauma Association, the Orthopaedic Research Society, the Mid-American Orthopaedic Association, and the Alamo Orthopaedic Society; serves as a paid consultant for or is an employee of Synthes, Smith & Nephew, Medtronic, and AcryMed; and has received research or institutional support from DePuy, Smith & Nephew, Stryker, Synthes, and Wyeth. Neither Dr. Routt nor any immediate family member has received anything of value from or own stock in an commercial company or institution related directly or indirectly to the subject of this chapter.

Modern populations are not only living longer but are becoming more obese. As a result, obesity has become an important issue relating not only to overall patient care and wellness, but also to its impact on specific injuries such as acetabular fractures. Obese patients with acetabular fractures are much more difficult to accurately and routinely image before, during, and after surgery. Specialized CT scanners and fluoroscopy units are needed to penetrate the additional soft tissue depths. Obesity also causes surgery-related difficulties that usually require specialized equipment. Such equipment would include sturdier operating tables and larger and longer retractors and clamps, as well as additional length devices such as drills and screwdrivers. Obese patients also require additional surgical assistants to provide sufficient retraction during the operation, have worsened reduction quality, and their perioperative complications are known to be worse than those of nonobese patients.[9,10]

Medical comorbidities and other important related issues are also carefully considered as management decisions are made in patients with acetabular fractures. Similarly in polytraumatized patients, the numerous injuries are prioritized and management of the acetabulum occurs as soon as the patient's condition permits, without unnecessary delay. In particular, those patients with irreducible, grossly unstable, or significantly incongruent hip joints warrant more urgent surgical treatment. The treating physician must assess whether the patient's overall medical condition is optimized. Important questions to ask as the operating surgeon are: (1) Does the medical condition allow for general anesthesia, appropriate positioning, and perhaps extensive surgical repair and blood loss? (2) Does the medical condition allow for nonsurgical management such as prolonged bed rest with or without traction? (3) Do religious beliefs such as refusing blood transfusions complicate or restrict routine care options? Patients with extensive comorbidities or polytrauma require a multidisciplinary approach to the preoperative evaluation that may include trauma surgery, internal medicine, anesthesia, and neurosurgery. An incorrect decision regarding if or when to operate can doom the patient to a poor clinical outcome (Figure 2).

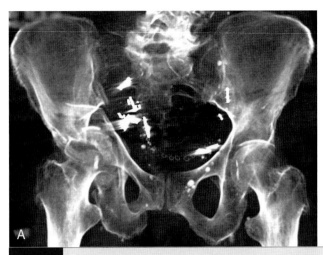
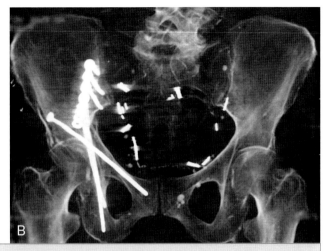

Figure 1 A and B, Radiographs of the pelvis of an 80-year-old woman who fell from standing while closing her car door. Her past surgical history was significant for prior abdominal procedures, and her medical problem list included hypertension. A, Displaced, associated, both-column acetabular fracture. Three days after injury she was medically optimized and underwent uneventful open reduction and internal fixation using the lateral and middle surgical intervals of the ilioinguinal exposure along with percutaneously inserted screw support of the anterior column fracture component (B). Secure and stable fixation was achieved routinely despite poor bone quality.

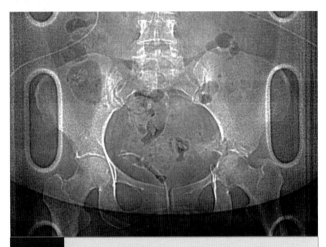

Figure 2 Radiograph of the pelvis of a 58-year-old morbidly obese woman who was injured in an automobile accident and sustained a displaced, unstable, and comminuted acetabular fracture. She had significant medical comorbidities that precluded safe surgical intervention. Her fracture was managed with skeletal traction for 8 weeks until fracture callus was noted on her plain pelvic radiographs. Her early clinical result only 6 months after injury was poor because of hip pain and other orthopaedic injuries. In retrospect, acetabular surgical management would have allowed earlier mobility and possibly improved hip function.

Once patient-related factors are considered, fracture specifics are evaluated next. Most surgeons use Letournel and Judet's classification of five elementary and five associated acetabular fracture patterns based on their two-column concept, which relies on anteroposterior and oblique plain pelvic films and two-dimensional pel-

vic CT scans to demonstrate the fracture details (see chapter 24). As discussed in chapter 24, modern CT scanning allows the radiology technician to reconstruct entire images of the pelvis. However, these reconstructed oblique images from gathered computer data do not reflect fracture instability as clearly as routine oblique plain films, because the patient remains supine during CT scanning rather than being positioned onto his or her side as during plain imaging (**Figure 3**). Closed treatment is recommended for unhealthy patients (for example, those unable to withstand anesthesia, volumetric changes due to potential blood loss, or other such conditions) and for stable fracture patterns that spare the weight-bearing dome. Roof arc angle measurement is one way to assess the integrity of the acetabular dome and coverage of the femoral head. Large roof arc angles signify an intact acetabular roof and correlate with improved clinical results.[11,12] The simplest form of closed treatment of acetabular fractures consists of a period of protected weight bearing on the injured hip. If the fracture is unstable but the patient is not healthy enough for surgical intervention, then skeletal traction is used to maintain the reduction while early healing progresses for the initial 6 to 8 weeks after injury. Closed management with or without traction mandates frequent serial pelvic radiographs to ensure normal healing and rule out unexpected early fracture displacement. The fracture stability can be evaluated objectively using an examination of the injured hip under anesthesia and fluoroscopy.[13]

Surgical management is selected when closed techniques fail, if the hip is unstable due to the fracture, when the reduction is incongruent, when significant intra-articular loose bodies are present,[14] when the fracture is displaced 1 to 2 mm through the weight-bearing dome either in gap or step deformity, when sciatic

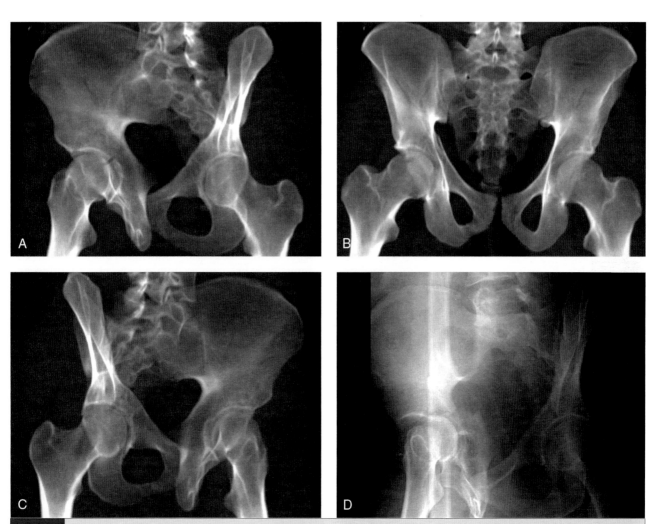

Figure 3 Pelvic images reconstructed from CT data may mask instability because the patient remains supine as the CT information is obtained. **A to C,** Pelvic radiographs reconstructed from pelvic CT scan data obtained from a supine patient. The images represent AP and Judet oblique projections and demonstrate the right-sided acetabular fracture. Although the fracture is identified, the reconstructed images do not reveal any information regarding fracture instability. **D,** This iliac oblique plain film was obtained by rolling the patient on his right side. The fracture instability is easily seen as the femur dislocates from the dome as it follows the unstable caudal segment of this previously minimally displaced acetabular fracture.

nerve function is decreased after closed reduction, and when the fracture is open.[15] If surgical management is indicated, the treating facility, the surgeon, and surgical team should be experienced and have the special equipment necessary to perform an accurate open reduction along with stable internal fixation. Many hospitals have dedicated surgical teams of anesthetists, nurses, assistants, and radiology technicians assigned to acetabular surgeries to optimize consistent and efficient care delivery. Special reduction clamps, intraoperative imaging, malleable plates, and long fixation screws are some of the required items. Blood salvage systems have been used; however, their routine use is not recommended because they are not cost-effective.[16] Skilled consultants, such as a vascular, general, or urologic surgeon, should be available during acetabular surgery if needed to repair an injured deep pelvic vessel[17] or help reconstruct the injured inguinal floor at closure or repair an associated bladder injury.

Surgical Approaches

The surgical exposure is selected after careful preoperative planning. Generally, the approach is dictated by the location of the major fracture displacement. The appropriate exposure allows the surgeon to visualize the fracture, clean the fracture surfaces, safely manipulate and accurately reduce the fracture fragments, and then apply definitive stable fixation. The mainstay surgical exposures for acetabular surgery include the Kocher-Langenbeck, ilioinguinal, and the extended iliofemoral. Other surgical exposures have been described and include the modified extended iliofemoral,[18] combined exposures,[19] and extensile triradiate,[20] among others.[21,22] The Kocher-Langenbeck exposure, if performed with the patient positioned prone, provides direct surgical access to the posterior column, posterior wall, and quadrilateral surface through the greater sciatic notch. With the patient positioned laterally, the surgeon is able to manipulate the hip more freely but the quadrilateral surface access is limited. The lateral position also frustrates accurate reduction of certain fracture patterns such as the transverse because of the weight of the limb accentuating the fracture displacement. Some patients, particularly those who are obese, are difficult to safely secure on the operating table in the lateral position. Some surgeons advocate a fracture table to provide sustained traction as needed. Fracture tables are expensive, and their manipulation during surgery requires an experienced, unscrubbed assistant. Complications directly related to the fracture table include pudendal nerve palsy, scrotal and perineal necrosis, and compartment syndrome of the leg. Recently, several authors have reported the additional use of a digastric trochanteric flip osteotomy to aid exposure to the dome of the acetabulum with or without the use of the surgical dislocation. This exposure is performed with the patient positioned laterally with all the potential positional problems as previously described, but a greater trochanteric osteotomy is added. The osteotomy allows the hip abductors to be retracted, potentially with less tension of the superior gluteal neurovascular bundle. The femoral head can be surgically dislocated, which should improve reduction quality. Nonunion and symptomatic implants related to the osteotomy are potential risks.[23-25]

The ilioinguinal exposure is usually performed with the patient in the supine position and the injured lower extremity included in the surgical field for manipulation as needed. A perhaps less invasive ilioinguinal approach has also been described, where only the lateral window and symphyseal exposure is performed. Longer follow-up and more extensive experience with this exposure will be helpful.[26] Many surgeons use the extended Pfannenstiel exposure as an additional surgical interval for the ilioinguinal exposure.[27,28] The ilioinguinal exposure provides direct surgical access to the internal iliac fossa, anterior sacroiliac joint, pelvic brim, anterior wall, and pubic ramus while the extended Pfannenstiel adds direct surgical access to bilateral superior pubic rami, the symphysis pubis, and the quadrilateral surface. The extended Pfannenstiel exposure is accomplished by incising the midline rectus abdominus raphe, and then incompletely tenotomizing the ipsilateral rectus abdominus insertion.[29] The ipsilateral rectus abdominus muscle is retracted anterolaterally, the bladder is retracted posteriorly, and then the periosteum of the superior pubic ramus is incised and elevated in continuity along the pelvic brim. The obturator neurovascular bundle is visualized and protected, and communicating vessels between it and the iliac or epigastric system are ligated. The obturator internus muscle is el-

evated from the quadrilateral surface to complete the surgical dissection. This additional interval facilitates improved fracture access and thereby reduction and plating of the quadrilateral surface (**Figure 4**).

Fracture Fixation

Fixation of acetabular fractures has remained relatively unchanged, with the utilization of 3.5-mm pelvic reconstruction malleable plates and long length screws. Standard fixation still uses the principles of lag screw fixation across fracture planes with buttressing or neutralization by the plates. The use of the extended Pfannenstiel approach has also allowed these plating methods to be extended to the quadrilateral surface.[30] Regardless of the fixation method, it is important to reduce marginal articular impaction and stabilize the fragments. These osteochondral pieces can often require small subchondral screw depending on the level at which these fragments occur.[6] Contoured spring-hook plates are occasionally needed to stabilize small and peripheral posterior wall fragments that are not amenable to routine screw and plate fixation.[31] Unfortunately in these posterior wall fractures, despite what is thought to be anatomic reduction and adequate fixation, hip joint loading has not returned to normal.[32] The use of artificial bone substitutes to supplement fixation constructs in acetabular fractures has been studied[33] in hopes of alleviating this issue. Use of a calcium phosphate cement has shown some promising results in partially restoring the joint loading closer to that of the normal hip.[34] Locked pelvic reconstruction plates have also been described. Biomechanical evaluation has shown these constructs to be as strong as traditional methods of interfragmentary screw fixation with conventional plating.[35] Locked plates, however, have screw holes that command the direction of the screw insertions. These locked implants therefore do not allow the surgeon to direct the screws into appropriate locations to optimize stability.

Percutaneous Techniques

As experience with acetabular fracture management has increased and intraoperative imaging techniques have improved,[36] percutaneous fixation after closed or percutaneous manipulative reduction has become possible for certain fracture patterns.[37,38] Utilization of percutaneous methods should be undertaken with a complete understanding of the relevant anatomy[39,40] and risks[38] associated with such procedures, and they should be performed by those with experience.[41] The indications for percutaneous acetabular surgery include minimally displaced yet unstable fractures, minimally displaced acetabular fracture as a component of an associated unstable pelvic ring disruption, minimally displaced fracture in a patient with a spinal cord injury, acetabular fracture with associated soft tissue trauma that prevents standard safe open techniques, and minimally displaced yet symptomatic insufficiency acetabular fractures. Whether the approach is percutaneous or

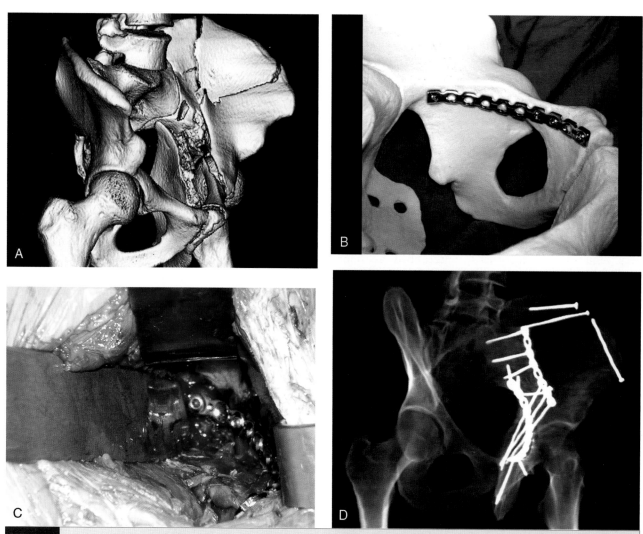

Figure 4   **A**, The three-dimensional pelvic CT shows the displacements of this associated both-column acetabular fracture. The posterior column component's surface anatomy and its displacement pattern are perfect for intrapelvic plating to maintain the reduction. **B**, The pelvic model demonstrates the surface application site of an intrapelvic reconstruction plate to support the quadrilateral surface and pubic ramus fragments of an acetabular fracture. **C**, The clinical intraoperative photograph reveals the retractors on the left rectus abdominis muscle, bladder, and iliac vessels and iliopsoas muscle. **D**, Radiograph shows that an ilioinguinal exposure along with the extended Pfannenstiel exposure was used to reduce and stabilize the fracture. An intrapelvic plate was applied along with other fixation devices.

open, the goal remains anatomic reduction.[41] Percutaneous fixation techniques are based on the two-column concept of Judet and Letournel. Long and large screws are inserted into the anterior and/or posterior columns to stabilize the column fracture components.[42] Percutaneous fixation surgery is not recommended for acetabular wall patterns. The outcomes of percutaneous fixation techniques in acetabular fractures remain unknown (**Figure 5**).

Acute Total Hip Arthroplasty

Total hip replacement for certain acetabular fractures has been described with mixed clinical results.[43,44] This treatment is usually reserved for older patients,[2,45,46] es-

pecially those with underlying and symptomatic hip arthritis along with acetabular fracture.[47] No studies directly compare open reduction and internal fixation versus acute total hip replacement in the treatment of acetabular fractures in this geriatric population. The acetabular fracture instability and comminution can complicate achieving a stable acetabular cup component with resultant loosening. The associated soft-tissue injuries related to the traumatic fracture-dislocation may account for high dislocation rates after hip arthroplasty for acetabular fracture.[43] Initial open reduction and internal fixation of the arthritic hip with an acetabular fracture allows for routine fracture union, and can then be followed with eventual hip replacement as the symptoms mandate.[48]

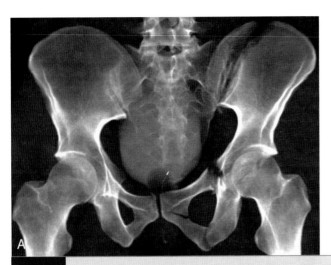
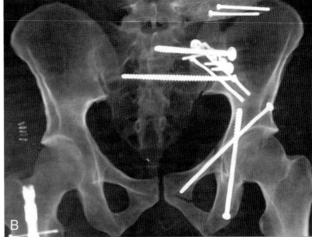

Figure 5 Imaging studies of the pelvis of a 22-year-old man who sustained numerous injuries after a motorcycle crash. **A,** Pelvic ring disruption and left-sided acetabular fracture. The patient also had an extensive traumatic open and contaminated wound on his left proximal thigh and underwent urgent anterior pelvic external fixation and right-sided femoral medullary nailing, along with irrigation and débridement of the left thigh wound and open packing. **B,** Open reduction and internal fixation of the left posterior iliac fracture-dislocation was done 2 days after injury with the patient in the prone position. The posterior pelvic open reduction produced an indirect acetabular reduction. In view of the traumatic open thigh wound, the left acetabular fracture was stabilized percutaneously using anterior and posterior column lag screws. The lag screws improved the acetabular fracture reduction as they were tightened. Healing was uneventful and without pelvic-related complaints.

Complications

Numerous complications are associated with acetabular fractures and their management.[49] Deep venous thrombosis is not uncommon. Fracture displacement, especially in the inguinal area, may cause iliac venous flow disturbance or injury and resultant clot formation. Bed rest and inactivity are also significant risk factors. Surgeons understand that retraction on the iliac vessels during the ilioinguinal exposure could also be responsible for flow abnormalities[17] as well as potential injury. Hip flexion relaxes the local soft tissues and facilitates inguinal retraction. Unless contraindicated due to associated injuries or other conditions, pharmacologic and mechanical DVT prophylaxis is recommended in patients with acetabular fractures,[50-52] but routine screening is not.[50,51,53] Vena caval filters are used for patients at risk for pulmonary embolus.[52] Temporary filters have been developed recently to avoid chronic complications.

Surgical technical complications occur for a variety of reasons ranging from poor preoperative planning, incomplete reduction, unstable fixation, and misplaced implants. Planning the proper exposure necessary to adequately reduce and stabilize the fracture is based on the fracture specifics. Improper planning and poor surgical technique can lead to inadequate fixation, which has been shown to be a cause of acetabular nonunions.[54] The overall prevalence of nonunion is low (2%).[49]

Excessive retraction during surgery injures muscle tissue, and, more important, may cause local nerve and/or vascular injury. For ilioinguinal exposures, the lateral femoral cutaneous nerve is at risk due to excessive retraction through the lateral iliac interval; the obturator nerve is at risk during medial retraction through the Stoppa interval; the femoral nerve[55] and iliac vessels[17] are at risk during retraction through the middle vascular interval; and the fifth lumbar nerve root can be injured due to retraction along the sacroiliac joint and lateral sacral alar area through the lateral iliac interval, as well as deep retraction through the Stoppa interval. In Kocher-Langenbeck exposures, the sciatic[56] as well as the superior and inferior gluteal nerves are at risk due to excessive or sustained retraction.

Prior to acetabular surgery, the perineum and rectal areas should be thoroughly cleansed and then isolated from the anticipated surgical field. These acetabular surgical wounds are typically located in the zone of injury and therefore add surgical insult to these previously traumatized tissues.[57] Necrotic fat and muscle tissues are débrided thoroughly, and the wound closed in layers to eliminate the resultant dead space. Deep wound infections may cause septic arthritis.

Ectopic bone formation is associated with acetabular surgery and occurs more extensively and frequently in patients with craniocerebral trauma and extensive exposures. Prophylactic measures vary and include simple débridement of dead muscle at surgery,[58] low-dose focal irradiation,[59] and medications such as indomethacin. Significant ectopic bone obstructs hip motion or can cause progressive nerve injury. The hip survivability is directly linked to chondral viability and thereby hip motion. Patients with acetabular fractures and significant ectopic bone warrant early surgical excision (**Fig-**

ure 6). Acetabular fractures are different from hip arthroplasty in that the fracture repair and cartilage surfaces benefit from motion. Symptomatic ectopic bone that either restricts hip motion or affects sciatic nerve function after acetabular fracture repair should be excised soon after diagnosis rather than after ectopic bone maturation. This may occur as soon as 8 weeks after open reduction and internal fixation.

Expected Outcomes

Reports on the outcomes of acetabular fractures are difficult to interpret because of the lack of an acetabular fracture-specific outcome score.[60] Traditionally, most studies use various scores[61] to report outcomes such as the Merle D'Aubigne,[6] Harris Hip score, or Musculoskeletal Functional Assessment, among others. Recently, scores have been created specifically for use in the assessment of acetabular fracture outcomes, a modified Harris Hip score and the roof arc score.[11,62] The roof arc score has been shown to correlate well with clinical outcome at 2 years postoperatively.[11]

Because of the diversity of acetabular fracture types, it is also difficult and perhaps incorrect to consider them as a single type of injury. More authors have started to report on acetabular-fracture-specific types, which will help in the understanding of these difficult injuries. The most reported acetabular fracture type is the posterior wall fracture, which has been shown to be deceptive in terms of its outcomes despite the general misconception regarding the ease of treatment of such injuries.[3,61,63,64] Other isolated reports have included transverse fractures[65] or posterior column fractures, with or without posterior wall fractures. Despite the heterogeneity of studies in the literature, several factors hold true for improved outcomes in all acetabular fractures: (1) anatomic reductions,[11,65-67] (2) early surgery (elementary, less than 15 days; associated, 5 to 10 days),[68] (3) lack of femoral head damage,[67] and (4) lack of comminution.[3] Unfortunately, posttraumatic arthritis (15% to 25%)[3,7,66] and osteonecrosis (less than 10%)[67] still occur and can cause disability.

In addition to functional scores, other modalities have been used to report outcomes.[69,70] One study to compare an anterior approach to a posterior approach in the treatment of acetabular fractures showed no difference in gait changes, muscle strength, or Musculoskeletal Function Assessment scores.[69] Decreased muscle strength has been shown to correlate with worse function.[70] The routine use of postoperative CT scan to evaluate the reduction is at the surgeon's discretion.[71]

Summary

Successful acetabular fracture management remains challenging. Treatment is based on numerous details specific to the patient and injury. Closed management is chosen for stable fractures with minimal displacement. Open anatomic reduction and internal fixation of dis-

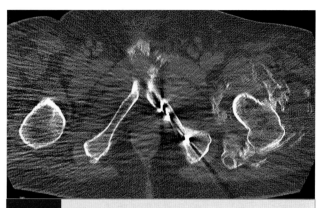

Figure 6 This pelvic axial CT image demonstrates significant ectopic bone formation surrounding the pubis, left hip, and left sciatic nerve 4 months after injury. The patient noted progressive hip stiffness approximately 8 weeks after operation. Ten weeks after surgery, the patient reported decreased sensory and motor function of his previously normal left sciatic nerve that was confirmed on physical examination. This CT scan revealed the sciatic nerve to be surrounded by ectopic bone at this and contiguous levels. He underwent sciatic neuroplasty and ectopic bone removal 2 days later. His nerve function recovered almost completely and his hip motion was restored. Indomethacin was administered orally for 6 weeks after the excision.

placed acetabular fractures remains the mainstay of treatment. Early surgical intervention with an anatomic reduction and stable fixation of displaced or unstable fractures performed by an experienced team and avoiding complications will optimize outcome.

Annotated References

1. Karunakar MA, Goulet JA, Mueller KL, Bedi A, Le TT: Operative treatment of unstable pediatric pelvis and acetabular fractures. *J Pediatr Orthop* 2005;25(1):34-38.

   The surgical management of pediatric acetabular fractures has been controversial. The authors report their series of surgically treated acetabular fractures in children. Displaced fractures benefit from operative stabilization in this group as well.

2. Vanderschot P: Treatment options of pelvic and acetabular fractures in patients with osteoporotic bone. *Injury* 2007;38(4):497-508.

   The article provides an overview of the treatment of acetabular fractures in patients with osteoporotic bone. These options include conservative methods, minimally invasive procedures, open reduction and fixation, and primary total hip arthroplasty. The goal remains early mobilization of these patients.

3. Kreder HJ, Rozen N, Borkhoff CM, et al: Determinants of functional outcome after simple and complex acetabular fractures involving the posterior wall. *J Bone Joint Surg Br* 2006;88(6):776-782.

These authors identify factors that are associated with adverse outcomes in patients with acetabular fractures (elementary and associated patterns) involving the posterior wall. Despite obtaining an anatomic reduction, function was not restored. The development of arthritis was related to the existence of marginal impaction and a residual displacement of > 2 mm. Approximately 54% of patients who were older than 50 and had both findings ended up with a total hip arthroplasty. The authors suggest the consideration of open reduction and internal fixation and total hip arthroplasty in this group of patients.

4. Anglen JO, Burd TA, Hendricks KJ, Harrison P: The "Gull Sign": A harbinger of failure for internal fixation of geriatric acetabular fractures. *J Orthop Trauma* 2003;17(9):625-634.

5. Matta JM: Fractures of the acetabulum: Accuracy of reduction and clinical results in patients managed operatively within three weeks after the injury. *J Bone Joint Surg Am* 1996;78(11):1632-1645.

6. Giannoudis PV, Nikolaou VS: Surgical techniques—How do I do it? Open reduction and internal fixation of posterior wall fractures of the acetabulum. *Injury* 2008;39(10):1113-1118.

The surgical management of the posterior wall acetabular fracture is reviewed. Details are provided regarding the patient's positioning and draping, surgical approach, osteosynthesis, and wound closure.

7. Petsatodis G, Antonarakos P, Chalidis B, Papadopoulos P, Christoforidis J, Pournaras J: Surgically treated acetabular fractures via a single posterior approach with a follow-up of 2-10 years. *Injury* 2007;38(3):334-343.

This study reports the outcome of a small number (50) of all acetabular fractures treated over a 10-year period via a posterior (Kocher-Langebeck) approach with or without a trochanteric osteotomy as needed. The mean follow-up was 5.8 years (2 to 10 years). There were 38 patients with good to excellent clinical results, fair in 5, and poor in 7. The radiologic results were good to excellent in 36 patients, fair in 5, and poor in 9. There were 5 patients with grade III and IV Brooker heterotopic ossification. There were 12 patients with posttraumatic osteoarthritis of the hip joint.

8. Giannoudis PV, Tzioupis C, Moed BR: Two-level reconstruction of comminuted posterior-wall fractures of the acetabulum. *J Bone Joint Surg Br* 2007;89(4):503-509.

Comminuted posterior wall acetabular fractures can be problematic in terms of fixation. A two-level reconstruction technique is described and outcomes reported. The technique uses subchondral miniscrews to stabilize the comminuted marginal acetabular fragments as a first step. This is followed by standard fixation with lag screws and a buttress plate to the main posterior fragment. This was performed on 29 consecutive patients with acute comminuted displaced posterior-wall fractures of the acetabulum. All hips were graded as anatomic. The clinical outcome was good to excellent in 93% of patients. Poor results were in older patients (> 55 years).

9. Karunakar MA, Shah SN, Jerabek S: Body mass index as a predictor of complications after operative treatment of acetabular fractures. *J Bone Joint Surg Am* 2005; 87(7):1498-1502.

This retrospective study looks at the body mass index (BMI) of 169 consecutive patients in whom an acetabular fracture had been treated with open reduction and internal fixation at a level-1 trauma center. Outcomes were evaluated to determine whether BMI was predictive of complications. The BMI was found to have a significant relationship with estimated blood loss, and incidence of wound infection, and deep venous thrombosis. Patients with a BMI > 30 were much more likely than patients of normal weight (BMI of < 25) to have complications. The findings were more pronounced in patients with a BMI > 40.

10. Porter SE, Russell GV, Dews RC, Qin Z, Woodall J Jr , Graves ML: Complications of acetabular fracture surgery in morbidly obese patients. *J Orthop Trauma* 2008;22(9):589-594.

The complications in a group of morbidly obese patients that underwent open reduction and internal fixation for their acetabular fractures are compared to a "nonobese" group. The morbidly obese group had significantly longer surgery times, length of hospital stay, and wound complications. Overall they had 2.6 times increased risk of having a complication.

11. Øvre S, Madsen JE, Røise O: Acetabular fracture displacement, roof arc angles and 2 years outcome. *Injury* 2008;39(8):922-931.

Correlation between a roof arc score and clinical outcome in a group of patients treated with open reduction and internal fixation for an acetabular fracture is reported. A fracture involving the dome, expressed as a roof arc score, was found to be more important than a residual step at 2 years. If an anatomic reduction was performed, this effect of location disappeared. Any fracture diastases resulted in a poor functional outcome.

12. Chuckpaiwong B, Suwanwong P, Harnroongroj T: Roof-arc angle and weight-bearing area of the acetabulum. *Injury* 2009;40(10):1064-1066.

A displaced fracture through the weight-bearing dome is an indication for surgery. Cadaveric specimens underwent simulated transverse transtectal fractures followed by radiographic examination. Roof arc measurements were taken and guidelines for operative intervention are given.

13. Moed BR, Ajibade DA, Israel H: Computed tomography as a predictor of hip stability status in posterior wall fractures of the acetabulum. *J Orthop Trauma* 2009;23(1):7-15.

Dynamic fluoroscopic stress testing under general anesthesia was done for a group of patients with posterior wall fractures. The results were compared to their CT scans based on traditional criteria. The most reliable determination for hip stability was examination under anesthesia.

14. Pascarella R, Maresca A, Reggiani LM, Boriani S: Intra-articular fragments in acetabular fracture-dislocation. *Orthopedics* 2009;32(6):402.

The authors describe their experience with acetabular fracture-dislocations. Of 127 cases over a 10-year period, 45 had incarcerated fragments. The importance and need for surgical intervention to remove such loose bodies is reviewed.

15. Tornetta P III: Displaced acetabular fractures: Indications for operative and nonoperative management. *J Am Acad Orthop Surg* 2001;9(1):18-28.

16. Scannell BP, Loeffler BJ, Bosse MJ, Kellam JF, Sims SH: Efficacy of intraoperative red blood cell salvage and autotransfusion in the treatment of acetabular fractures. *J Orthop Trauma* 2009;23(5):340-345.

   The efficacy of cell saver usage during open reduction and internal fixation of acetabular fractures is reported in this retrospective study. Out of 186 cases, the cell saver was used in 32% with an average volume of 345 mL of blood autotransfused. There were no differences in the rates or volumes of intraoperative and postoperative blood transfusions between the two groups. The routine use of cell saver in acetabular surgery could not be recommended.

17. Langford JR, Trokhan S, Strauss E: External iliac artery thrombosis after open reduction of an acetabular fracture: A case report. *J Orthop Trauma* 2008;22(1):59-62.

   Thrombosis of the external iliac artery following open reduction and internal fixation of an anterior column fracture via an ilioinguinal approach is reported. The presence of a pulse does not rule out such injuries, and a heightened awareness of subtle differences, side-to-side, in postoperative pulses may reveal occult injuries.

18. Stöckle U, Hoffmann R, Südkamp NP, Reindl R, Haas NP: Treatment of complex acetabular fractures through a modified extended iliofemoral approach. *J Orthop Trauma* 2002;16(4):220-230.

19. Harris AM, Althausen P, Kellam JF, Bosse MJ: Simultaneous anterior and posterior approaches for complex acetabular fractures. *J Orthop Trauma* 2008;22(7):494-497.

   The use of simultaneous Kocher-Langenbeck and iliofemoral approaches in the treatment of associated fracture patterns of the acetabulum are described. This dual approach is useful when both columns are involved with or without a posterior wall component.

20. Kinik H, Armangil M: Extensile triradiate approach in the management of combined acetabular fractures. *Arch Orthop Trauma Surg* 2004;124(7):476-482.

   The authors report on the use of the triradiate approach in a group of patients with associated acetabular fractures. A total of 48 fractures underwent open reduction and internal fixation through this approach. The reduction was graded as excellent in 68%. Good to excellent outcomes were reported in 80% of patients. The incidence of nondisabling heterotopic ossification was 16%.

21. Hirvensalo E, Lindahl J, Kiljunen V: Modified and new approaches for pelvic and acetabular surgery. *Injury* 2007;38(4):431-441.

   A variety of alternative approaches for the fixation of acetabular fractures is described. The outcomes of these new operative techniques in 120 consecutive patients with fractures of the pelvic ring and 164 patients with acetabular fractures are reported.

22. Lefaivre KA, Starr AJ, Reinert CM: A modified anterior exposure to the acetabulum for treatment of difficult anterior acetabular fractures. *J Orthop Trauma* 2009; 23(5):370-378.

   A modification of a traditional Smith-Peterson approach is described. Osteotomies are performed to provide extensile exposure to the anterior column of the acetabulum.

23. Naranje S, Shamshery P, Yadav CS, Gupta V, Nag HL: Digastric trochanteric flip osteotomy and surgical dislocation of hip in the management of acetabular fractures. *Arch Orthop Trauma Surg* 2010;130(1):93-101.

   The efficacy and safety of the digastric trochanteric flip osteotomy in the management of acetabular fractures is reported. Good to excellent outcomes with low morbidity can be expected with this approach.

24. Hadjicostas PT, Thielemann FW: The use of trochanteric slide osteotomy in the treatment of displaced acetabular fractures. *Injury* 2008;39(8):907-913.

   The authors describe their use of a single straight lateral incision centered over the greater trochanter, a trochanteric osteotomy, and dislocation of the femoral head in the treatment of acetabular fractures. The osteotomy allows for exposure of the entire acetabulum and the femoral head.

25. Ellis TJ, Beck M: Trochanteric osteotomy for acetabular fractures and proximal femur fractures. *Orthop Clin North Am* 2004;35(4):457-461.

   This article reviews the indications of using the trochanteric osteotomy combined with the Kocher-Langenbeck in the treatment of acetabular fractures and other fractures around the hip joint. This allows for direct visualization of the joint without the risk for osteonecrosis of the femoral head.

26. Wolf H, Wieland T, Pajenda G, Vécsei V, Mousavi M: Minimally invasive ilioinguinal approach to the acetabulum. *Injury* 2007;38(10):1170-1176.

   The classic ilioinguinal approach is a gold standard in acetabular surgery. The authors developed a modification, a minimally invasive method that entails a median lower abdominal approach with extraperitoneal dissection and exposure of the pubic symphysis. The second incision is lateral, next to the iliac crest. This allows an easy, safe, and quick exposure of the anterior iliac ring, as well as easy access to the posterior column and wall toward the sacroiliac joint. The iliac vessels and nerves are thereby protected, and no preparation of neurovascular structures is required. The technique was applied in 23 clinical cases and compared with the classic ilioinguinal approach in 9 similar cases over the same period.

27. Ponsen KJ, Joosse P, Schigt A, Goslings JC, Goslings CJ, Luitse JS: Internal fracture fixation using the Stoppa ap-

proach in pelvic ring and acetabular fractures: Technical aspects and operative results. *J Trauma* 2006;61(3):662-667.

The Stoppa approach has been used in the treatment of acetabular fractures. This is a retrospective review of a group of patients treated for pelvic or acetabular fractures via a Stoppa approach. Anatomic reduction was achieved in 95% using this approach.

28. Karunakar MA, Le TT, Bosse MJ: The modified ilioinguinal approach. *J Orthop Trauma* 2004;18(6):379-383.

The authors describe a modified ilioinguinal approach for acetabular fractures in which an ilioinguinal approach is combined with the Stoppa approach.

29. Heineck J, Rammelt S, Grass R, Schneiders W, Amlang M: Transsection of the rectus abdominis muscle in the treatment of acetabular fractures: Operative technique and outcome in 21 patients. *Acta Orthop* 2008;79(2):225-229.

The ilioinguinal approach may not provide full exposure for reduction and stabilization of some associated acetabular fractures. To gain additional exposure, the authors describe a medial extension of the approach by transverse splitting of the rectus abdominis muscle. This allows increased exposure of the dorsal column and the medial acetabular wall.

30. Qureshi AA, Archdeacon MT, Jenkins MA, Infante A, DiPasquale T, Bolhofner BR: Infrapectineal plating for acetabular fractures: A technical adjunct to internal fixation. *J Orthop Trauma* 2004;18(3):175-178.

A technique describing use of a medial buttress plate along the quadrilateral plate as an adjunct to internal fixation is presented. The approach is either through an ilioinguinal approach or a modified Stoppa approach. This aids in resisting medial secondary redisplacement.

31. Ebraheim NA, Patil V, Liu J, Sanford CG Jr, Haman SP: Reconstruction of comminuted posterior wall fractures using the buttress technique: A review of 32 fractures. *Int Orthop* 2007;31(5):671-675.

The authors report the results of using a buttress technique to reconstruct comminuted posterior wall fractures. The reduction was anatomic in 88%. The clinical outcome was good to excellent in 74%.

32. Olson SA, Bay BK, Hamel A: Biomechanics of the hip joint and the effects of fracture of the acetabulum. *Clin Orthop Relat Res* 1997;339:92-104.

33. Moed BR, Willson Carr SE, Craig JG, Watson JT: Calcium sulfate used as bone graft substitute in acetabular fracture fixation. *Clin Orthop Relat Res* 2003;410:303-309.

34. Olson SA, Kadrmas MW, Hernandez JD, Glisson RR, West JL: Augmentation of posterior wall acetabular fracture fixation using calcium-phosphate cement: A biomechanical analysis. *J Orthop Trauma* 2007;21(9):608-616.

The use of calcium phosphate cement as an adjunct to internal fixation for posterior wall acetabular fracture is described. The goal was to assess whether joint loading parameters could be restored to the intact condition in a cadaver model. Hips were loaded under 4 conditions: (1) intact; (2) posterior wall osteotomy without fixation; (3) standard open reduction and internal fixation; and (4) open reduction and internal fixation with calcium phosphate cement as a "grout." Fragment motion data were then obtained. Calcium phosphate cement significantly decreased fragment micromotion. The addition of calcium phosphate cement also resulted in a partial restoration of joint loading parameters closer to the intact state.

35. Mehin R, Jones B, Zhu Q, Broekhuyse H: A biomechanical study of conventional acetabular internal fracture fixation versus locking plate fixation. *Can J Surg* 2009;52(3):221-228.

This biomechanical cadaver study compares the use of locked plating versus conventional plating in the fixation of transverse acetabular fractures. The locking plate construct was found to be as strong as the conventional plate plus interfragmentary lag screw construct.

36. Stöckle U, Schaser K, König B: Image guidance in pelvic and acetabular surgery—Expectations, success and limitations. *Injury* 2007;38(4):450-462.

This article reviews the indications for use of image guided surgical techniques in the treatment of pelvic and acetabular fractures.

37. Mouhsine E, Garofalo R, Borens O, et al: Percutaneous retrograde screwing for stabilisation of acetabular fractures. *Injury* 2005;36(11):1330-1336.

A consecutive series of minimally or nondisplaced geriatric acetabular fractures were treated with a retrograde percutaneous screw. Two retrograde cannulated cancellous 7.3-mm screws were placed to stabilize both the anterior and posterior columns. The technique was shown to be safe for this fracture pattern while allowing early mobilization.

38. Starr AJ, Jones AL, Reinert CM, Borer DS: Preliminary results and complications following limited open reduction and percutaneous screw fixation of displaced fractures of the acetabulum. *Injury* 2001;32(suppl 1):SA45-SA50.

39. Sen M, Harvey EJ, Steinitz D, Guy P, Reindl R: Anatomical risks of using supra-acetabular screws in percutaneous internal fixation of the acetabulum and pelvis. *Am J Orthop* 2005;34(2):94-96.

This cadaver study describes anatomic risks associated with placement of percutaneous screws in acetabular fractures. There is considerable risk for injury to the lateral femoral cutaneous nerve at the level of the pelvic brim.

40. Attias N, Lindsey RW, Starr AJ, Borer D, Bridges K, Hipp JA: The use of a virtual three-dimensional model to evaluate the intraosseous space available for percutaneous screw fixation of acetabular fractures. *J Bone Joint Surg Br* 2005;87(11):1520-1523.

Three-dimensional reconstruction models were created from CT scans obtained from patients with acetabular fractures. The goal was to assess the intraosseous space available in the anterior column, the posterior column, and across the dome of the acetabulum for implant placement. The authors suggest that virtual three-dimensional reconstructions might be helpful in preoperative planning.

41. Rommens PM: Is there a role for percutaneous pelvic and acetabular reconstruction? *Injury* 2007;38(4):463-477.

    The author looks at the utility of percutaneous techniques for pelvic and acetabular fractures with an emphasis on maintaining the goals required for fixation of such injuries. The primary goal in the treatment of acetabular fractures is to restore anatomy. Open reduction and internal fixation still remains the standard of care in the treatment of displaced pelvic and acetabular fractures. Percutaneous techniques should be limited to the experienced surgeon.

42. Ebraheim NA, Xu R, Biyani A, Benedetti JA: Anatomic basis of lag screw placement in the anterior column of the acetabulum. *Clin Orthop Relat Res* 1997;339:200-205.

43. Sermon A, Broos P, Vanderschot P: Total hip replacement for acetabular fractures: Results in 121 patients operated between 1983 and 2003. *Injury* 2008;39(8):914-921.

    This study compares the results of acute total hip arthroplasty (THA) for acetabular fractures versus late THA after failed or nonsurgical treatment of acetabular fractures. The "acute" THA patients were older and had fewer revisions (8% versus 22%) than the late reconstruction group.

44. Mears DC, Velyvis JH: Acute total hip arthroplasty for selected displaced acetabular fractures: Two to twelve-year results. *J Bone Joint Surg Am* 2002;84(1):1-9.

45. Boraiah S, Ragsdale M, Achor T, Zelicof S, Asprinio DE: Open reduction internal fixation and primary total hip arthroplasty of selected acetabular fractures. *J Orthop Trauma* 2009;23(4):243-248.

    In this retrospective review, the authors report their results in a group of patients age 55 to 86 years (mean age, 71 years) who underwent combined open reduction and internal fixation and acute total hip arthroplasty for a displaced acetabular fracture. Successful outcomes can be achieved in a properly selected group.

46. Mouhsine E, Garofalo R, Borens O, Blanc CH, Wettstein M, Leyvraz PF: Cable fixation and early total hip arthroplasty in the treatment of acetabular fractures in elderly patients. *J Arthroplasty* 2004;19(3):344-348.

    A group of 18 elderly patients (mean age, 76 years) with acetabular fractures were treated with acute total hip arthroplasty and supplemented with cable fixation. All but one had a good outcome at a mean follow-up time of 3 years. No loosening was reported with complete healing of the fracture.

47. Pagenkopf E, Grose A, Partal G, Helfet DL: Acetabular fractures in the elderly: Treatment recommendations. *HSS J* 2006;2(2):161-171.

    This review article outlines treatment recommendations in the elderly with acetabular fractures. Patterns in which an anatomic reduction can be achieved should be treated with open reduction and internal fixation. Those in whom early posttraumatic arthritis is likely should be treated with both open reduction and internal fixation and total hip arthroplasty. A treatment algorithm is provided.

48. Ranawat A, Zelken J, Helfet D, Buly R: Total hip arthroplasty for posttraumatic arthritis after acetabular fracture. *J Arthroplasty* 2009;24(5):759-767.

    Successful hip replacement can be achieved for posttraumatic arthritis. Historically, the outcomes for THA for posttraumatic arthritis after acetabular fracture have been inferior when compared to primary nontraumatic THA. The authors report their results in a series of patients with a 79%, 5-year survival rate. There was a 97% survival rate for patients with aseptic acetabular loosening as the endpoint.

49. Pavelka T, Houcek P: Complications associated with the surgical treatment of acetabular fractures. *Acta Chir Orthop Traumatol Cech* 2009;76(3):186-193.

    This article reviews the complications associated with surgical fixation of acetabular fractures in their series of 251 patients. The complications are divided into three categories: intraoperative, early postoperative, and late postoperative. Intraoperative complications include vascular injuries (2%), damage to the sciatic nerve (5%), incomplete reduction (13%), and nonunion (2%). Early postoperative complications include revision surgery secondary to infection, hematoma, and hardware failure. Late complications reported were osteonecrosis (7%), posttraumatic arthritis (17%), heterotopic ossification (Brooker III and IV; 7%) and late infection (0.5%).

50. Slobogean GP, Lefaivre KA, Nicolaou S, O'Brien PJ: A systematic review of thromboprophylaxis for pelvic and acetabular fractures. *J Orthop Trauma* 2009;23(5):379-384.

    This is a meta-analysis reviewing the literature on current recommendations and strategies in deep venous thrombosis prevention. Although many surgeons prescribe some form of deep venous thrombosis prophylaxis, the literature is lacking in terms of clinical guidance as to the best prophylactic management.

51. Steele N, Dodenhoff RM, Ward AJ, Morse MH: Thromboprophylaxis in pelvic and acetabular trauma surgery: The role of early treatment with low-molecular-weight heparin. *J Bone Joint Surg Br* 2005;87(2):209-212.

    The use of low molecular weight heparin is assessed in the management of patients with pelvic and acetabular fractures.

52. Morgan SJ, Jeray KJ, Phieffer LS, Grigsby JH, Bosse MJ, Kellam JF: Attitudes of orthopaedic trauma surgeons regarding current controversies in the management of pelvic and acetabular fractures. *J Orthop Trauma* 2001;15(7):526-532.

4: Axial Skeleton, Including Spine and Pelvis

53. Borer DS, Starr AJ, Reinert CM, et al: The effect of screening for deep vein thrombosis on the prevalence of pulmonary embolism in patients with fractures of the pelvis or acetabulum: A review of 973 patients. *J Orthop Trauma* 2005;19(2):92-95.

This study looks at the utilization and effect of screening for deep venous thrombosis on the incidence of pulmonary embolism. Discontinuation of a screening protocol did not affect the rate of pulmonary embolism. Routine screening was not justified.

54. Mohanty K, Taha W, Powell JN: Non-union of acetabular fractures. *Injury* 2004;35(8):787-790.

This retrospective study reports seven cases of acetabular nonunions. Most were in transverse patterns and related to unstable fixation.

55. Gruson KI, Moed BR: Injury of the femoral nerve associated with acetabular fracture. *J Bone Joint Surg Am* 2003;85-A(3):428-431.

56. Issack PS, Helfet DL: Sciatic nerve injury associated with acetabular fractures. *HSS J* 2009;5(1):12-18.

This is a review of the causes of sciatic nerve palsy related to acetabular fractures. The natural history regarding recovery is discussed. Methods for preventing injury include attention to intraoperative limb positioning, retractor placement, and instrumentation use. Use of somatosensory-evoked potentials and spontaneous electromyography may help minimize iatrogenic nerve injury during surgical repair.

57. Hak DJ, Olson SA, Matta JM: Diagnosis and management of closed internal degloving injuries associated with pelvic and acetabular fractures: The Morel-Lavallée lesion. *J Trauma* 1997;42(6):1046-1051.

58. Rath EM, Russell GV Jr, Washington WJ, Routt ML Jr: Gluteus minimus necrotic muscle debridement diminishes heterotopic ossification after acetabular fracture fixation. *Injury* 2002;33(9):751-756.

59. Haas ML, Kennedy AS, Copeland CC, Ames JW, Scarboro M, Slawson RG: Utility of radiation in the prevention of heterotopic ossification following repair of traumatic acetabular fracture. *Int J Radiat Oncol Biol Phys* 1999;45(2):461-466.

60. Øvre S, Sandvik L, Madsen JE, Røise O: Comparison of distribution, agreement and correlation between the original and modified Merle d'Aubigné-Postel Score and the Harris Hip Score after acetabular fracture treatment: Moderate agreement, high ceiling effect and excellent correlation in 450 patients. *Acta Orthop* 2005; 76(6):796-802.

Three main outcomes scores in the treatment of acetabular fractures are compared to assess the agreement and correlation in evaluating functional outcomes. Although the overall correlation was found to be excellent, the kappa agreements were only moderate. Because the scores were skewed in distribution with considerable ceiling effects, the clinical use of such scores is questioned.

61. Moed BR, McMichael JC: Outcomes of posterior wall fractures of the acetabulum. *J Bone Joint Surg Am* 2007;89(6):1170-1176.

This study reports the functional outcome of a group of patients (46) with posterior wall acetabular fractures treated with open reduction and internal fixation. Both the Musculoskeletal Function Assessment and the Merle d'Aubigne score were performed and the outcome information evaluated. The mean follow-up was five years (range 2-14 years). Despite the mean Merle d'Aubigne score being 17, which indicates overall good-to-excellent clinical results, the mean total Musculoskeletal Function Assessment score was significantly worse (23.17) than the normative mean (9.26). It appears that many patients after a posterior wall acetabular fracture continue to have residual functional deficits.

62. Øvre S, Sandvik L, Madsen JE, Roise O: Modification of the Harris Hip Score in acetabular fracture treatment. *Injury* 2007;38(3):344-349.

A modification of the Harris Hip Score is presented. It was then used in the evaluation of acetabular fracture treatment. The modified score improved the discrimination, and thus differences in treatment outcome of acetabular fractures will be easier to detect.

63. Moed BR, McMichael JC: Outcomes of posterior wall fractures of the acetabulum: Surgical technique. *J Bone Joint Surg Am* 2008;90(suppl 2, pt 1):87-107.

The author's surgical technique for fixation of posterior wall acetabular fractures is described.

64. Moed BR: Improving results in posterior wall acetabular fracture surgery. *J Trauma* 2007;62(suppl 6)S63.

The author relates his experience with the outcomes of posterior wall acetabular fractures.

65. Oh CW, Kim PT, Park BC, et al: Results after operative treatment of transverse acetabular fractures. *J Orthop Sci* 2006;11(5):478-484.

This study reports the outcome of a small number of transverse acetabular fractures, with or without posterior wall fractures, treated with open reduction and internal fixation. Anatomic reduction of the fracture yielded a higher satisfactory result. Comminution of the transverse fracture was prognostic of poor results.

66. Bhandari M, Matta J, Ferguson T, Matthys G: Predictors of clinical and radiological outcome in patients with fractures of the acetabulum and concomitant posterior dislocation of the hip. *J Bone Joint Surg Br* 2006; 88(12):1618-1624.

This study identifies variables that are associated with the clinical and radiologic outcomes following posterior dislocation of the hip in patients with acetabular fractures. The quality of the fracture reduction was the only significant predictor of radiologic grade, clinical function, and the development of posttraumatic arthritis.

67. Giannoudis PV, Grotz MR, Papakostidis C, Dinopoulos H: Operative treatment of displaced fractures of the acetabulum: A meta-analysis. *J Bone Joint Surg Br* 2005; 87(1):2-9.

In this article, the authors perform a meta-analysis of the literature regarding the treatment of acetabular fractures. A summary of complications and outcomes is reported.

68. Madhu R, Kotnis R, Al-Mousawi A, et al: Outcome of surgery for reconstruction of fractures of the acetabulum: The time dependent effect of delay. *J Bone Joint Surg Br* 2006;88(9):1197-1203.

This study focuses on the radiologic and functional outcomes of acetabular fractures treated with open reduction and internal fixation (ORIF) and its relation to time to surgery. The ability to obtain anatomic reduction significantly decreased if ORIF was performed after 15 days (elementary patterns) and after 5 days (associated patterns). Similarly, the odds of obtaining excellent/good outcomes decreased significantly when ORIF was performed after 15 days (elementary patterns) and 10 days (associated patterns). Time to surgery was found to be a significant predictor of both the radiologic and functional outcomes for fractures of the acetabulum.

69. Engsberg JR, Steger-May K, Anglen JO, Borrelli J Jr: An analysis of gait changes and functional outcome in patients surgically treated for displaced acetabular fractures. *J Orthop Trauma* 2009;23(5):346-353.

Functional outcomes to include evaluation of gait and muscle strength are reported in a group of patients with acetabular fractures treated with open reduction and internal fixation via an anterior ilioinguinal approach and compared to those treated with a posterior approach.

Musculoskeletal Function Assessment scores did not differ significantly between the two groups. Both groups had similar alterations in their gait, muscle strength, and functional outcome. This finding suggests that gait changes are related to factors other than surgical approach.

70. Borrelli J Jr, Ricci WM, Anglen JO, Gregush R, Engsberg J: Muscle strength recovery and its effects on outcome after open reduction and internal fixation of acetabular fractures. *J Orthop Trauma* 2006;20(6):388-395.

This study assesses the functional outcome and muscle strength recovery in patients treated for an acetabular fracture via an anterior approach. Muscle strength was decreased when compared with that of the nonoperated side. The decreased muscle strength correlated with patients reporting worsening function. Hip range of motion was not statistically different between the two sides.

71. Borrelli J Jr, Ricci WM, Steger-May K, Totty WG, Goldfarb C: Postoperative radiographic assessment of acetabular fractures: A comparison of plain radiographs and CT scans. *J Orthop Trauma* 2005;19(5):299-304.

Postoperative radiographic assessments between CT and plain radiography were compared. The authors believe that CT provides the best information regarding articular reductions postoperatively.

4: Axial Skeleton, Including Spine and Pelvis

Chapter 26

Spinal Cord Injury: Pathophysiology and Current Treatment Strategies

Mitchel Harris, MD, FACS   Andrew J. Schoenfeld, MD

Introduction

The devastating effects and dismal prognosis of traumatic spinal cord injuries were recognized by physicians in the Ancient Period (3000 BC to 500 AD), although the first surgical intervention for these injuries would not be proposed until much later.[1] Nonetheless, surgery could not be regularly applied in these situations until the late 19th century and, even then, the pathophysiologic basis for the condition was not understood, rendering most treatments ineffective.

The annual incidence of spinal cord injury in North America currently ranges from 25 to 93 per million individuals.[2-5] Although the incidence of these conditions appears to have decreased over the past two decades, injury to the spinal cord results in an enormous social burden because of lost productivity and the costs of treatment and rehabilitation.[2,6] Despite dramatic advances in recent years, a tremendous effort is still under way to understand the pathophysiology, the benefits of surgical intervention, and the role of evolving therapies.

Pathophysiology

Damage to the spinal cord following trauma occurs via two distinct pathways: primary and secondary injury.[7] Primary injury to the spinal cord results from the traumatic mechanism itself. Kinetic energy transferred to the spinal cord during the traumatic event causes disruption of the microvasculature, axonal injury, and cell membrane damage. These insults are compounded by the compressive-contusive injury that occurs from the displaced vertebral fragments and gross instability associated with ligamentous disruption.[8] The immediate

trauma, as well as the sustained compression, leads to compromise of the blood supply through intraparenchymal hemorrhage, damage to the blood-brain barrier, vasospasm, and thrombosis. These factors culminate in local ischemia that causes further tissue edema and secondary cell death.[7-12] When the spinal cord is completely transected (**Figure 1**), local pathology consists of axonal disruption, cell death, and hemorrhage.

In most clinical situations, the primary injury triggers a complex pathophysiologic process that leads to further

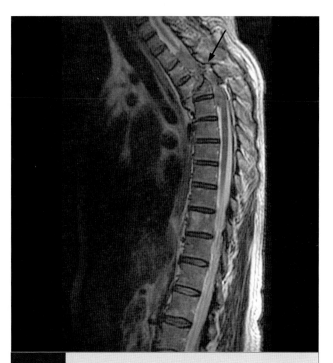

Figure 1   Parasagittal T2-weighted MRI of the thoracic spine in a 64-year-old woman who was thrown from a horse. Radiographic evaluation revealed a fracture-dislocation at the T3-T4 level with complete transection of the cord (*arrow*). The patient presented to the hospital with a complete loss of function below the level of injury (American Spinal Injury Association grade A).

Dr. Harris or an immediate family member has received research or institutional support from AO, DePuy, Medtronic Sofamor Danek, Synthes, and OMeGA. Dr. Schoenfeld and immediate family members have no financial interests to disclose.

Table 1

Stages of Spinal Cord Injury With Targeted Interventions

Stage (Time Period)	Pathophysiology	Targeted Intervention
Primary Injury (0 h)	Damage to the cord from transfer of kinetic energy, compression, or contusion	Prevention
Immediate phase (0-2 h)	Hemorrhage, cord edema, cell death, and release of cytokines and glutamate	Spinal immobilization/realignment, maintenance of cord perfusion, decompression, high-dose steroids, hypothermia
Early acute phase (2-48 h)	Free-radical production, height of neurotoxicity	Spinal realignment, decompression, high-dose steroids, hypothermia, minocycline, riluzole, erythropoietin, autologous macrophage implantation
Subacute phase (2 days–2 weeks)	Phagocytic removal of debris, astrocytes begin forming gliotic scar	Autologous macrophage implantation
Intermediate phase (2 weeks–6 months)	Growth and maturation of gliotic scar, axonal regeneration if possible	Schwann cell transplantation, olfactory ensheathing cell transplantation, bone marrow transplantation
Chronic phase (6 months–2 years)	Wallerian degeneration, final scar maturation and cystic degeneration of the cord	Schwann cell transplantation, olfactory ensheathing cell transplantation, future applications of gene therapy and stem cell–based therapy

damage within, and beyond, the original zone of injury. This so-called secondary injury has been postulated to last as long as 1 to 2 years following the initial trauma, and is divided into five distinct phases (**Table 1**).

The immediate phase generally lasts for the first 2 hours after injury and is characterized by cord edema and hemorrhage within the gray and white matter. Swelling and vascular disruption lead to local ischemia and the death of neurons and glial cells. Axonal swelling contributes to the disruption of action potentials.[11] Damage to cell membranes, as well as cell death, results in the massive release of matrix metalloproteinases and cytokines such as interleukin (IL)-1, IL-6, and tumor necrosis factor–α.[7,9,10] Lipid peroxidation and free-radical production amplify local cytotoxicity, as do the extracellular release of glutamate and the activation of N-methyl-D-aspartate receptors. Additionally, local hypoxia sensitizes neurons and glial cells to the presence of glutamate, which induces cell death through prolonged excitation. The release of proinflammatory cytokines from damaged neurons leads to the migration of microglial cells into the zone of injury, heralding the end of the immediate phase.

The early acute phase lasts from 2 to 48 hours following initial injury and consists of continued hemorrhage, further edema, and inflammation. The production of free radicals and immune- as well as glutamate-mediated neurotoxicity reaches its peak during this interval.[7,11]

The early acute phase is quickly followed by the subacute phase, which can last up to 2 weeks after injury and is characterized by the phagocytic removal of debris from the zone of injury. Additionally, peripheral astrocytes undergo hypertrophy during this phase and extend cytoplasmic processes into the injured regions.

The astrocytic processes are integral to the formation of gliotic scar, which reestablishes the blood-brain barrier and restores ionic homeostasis. This scar not only prevents further infiltration of macrophages and neutrophils, but also leads to the resolution of tissue edema.[7,13] Paradoxically, astrocytic scar also inhibits effective axonal regeneration.[13]

The intermediate phase lasts for the first 6 months after injury and is characterized by continued axonal regeneration wherever possible, as well as growth and maturation of the gliotic scar.[7,12]

The chronic phase starts 6 months after injury and can last for 1 to 2 years. The process of wallerian degeneration occurs extensively during this period and is accompanied by final scar maturation, cystic degeneration, and potential syrinx formation.[7,14] The spinal cord lesion will fully mature within 2 years after injury, with cystic cavitation and myelomalacia characterizing the final appearance.

Early Treatment Principles

The goals of treatment in the patient with acute spinal cord injury include the prevention of further injury as well as the inhibition of pathways that lead to secondary cord injury.[15] Initial treatment of the patient follows Advanced Trauma Life Support protocols, as advocated by the American College of Surgeons,[4-6,8] with airway and circulatory management taking precedence. Emergent management at the scene of the accident includes placing the patient on a backboard in a neutral spine position and using provisional cervical stabilization. While the spine is protected, life-threatening injuries are identified and treated first.

Early treatment seeks to limit further disruption of the spinal cord and can possibly preserve function one or two segments below the level of injury. This becomes especially important in the cervical spine, where restoration of function at even one level can drastically alter a patient's potential for independent function (Table 2). For example, maintenance of C7 motor function enables a patient to transfer and use a wheelchair without assistance.

In the acute resuscitation phase, early recognition of neurogenic shock is paramount. Diaphragmatic paralysis from a high cervical spine injury can lead to impaired breathing, whereas neurogenic shock may mask the presence of hypovolemic shock. In this acute traumatic setting, maintaining blood pressure is vital to preserve the necessary perfusion and oxygen supply to the spinal cord. In addition to local ischemia and vascular disruption, injury to the cord leads to dysregulation of local blood flow (loss of autoregulation).[9] Therefore, in this pathologic setting, the spinal cord becomes increasingly reliant on systemic arterial pressure. Studies have demonstrated that maintaining the mean blood pressure above 85 mm Hg improves neurologic outcomes.[16] The initial management of hypotension in the spine trauma patient includes aggressive intravascular fluid resuscitation, blood replacement, and the discriminate use of vasopressors in the setting of neurogenic shock.

After the patient has been adequately resuscitated and life-threatening issues have been identified and stabilized, a comprehensive physical examination is performed as part of the Advanced Trauma Life Support secondary survey. This examination will identify a spinal cord injury and indicate whether such a lesion is complete or incomplete. With complete spinal cord injuries, there is no motor or sensory function below the damaged segment, including the absence of perianal sensation. With incomplete lesions, some sensation or motor function is preserved below the level of injury, or in the perineum and remainder of the sacral root distribution. Complete radiographic imaging of the spine is necessary to characterize the extent of the injury. In most trauma centers, CT has replaced plain radiography as the screening modality of choice. MRI is useful to characterize ligamentous or other soft-tissue disruption within the spinal column and to identify the extent of injury to the spinal cord and the prognosis for recovery. Once a fracture or dislocation has been identified, complete imaging of the spine is warranted because the presence of an additional noncontiguous spinal injury has been documented to occur in approximately 15% of patients.[4,5,7,8]

Once a spinal cord injury has been diagnosed in an unstable spinal column, treatment includes realignment of the spinal column, surgical decompression, and stabilization. The administration of high-dose methylprednisolone has become increasingly controversial. The safest and most effective means of initial cervical immobilization includes the application of a cervical or-

Table 2

Level of Spinal Cord Injury Correlated With Functional Capacity

Level of Injury	Functional Capacity
C1-3	Respirator dependent
C4	Wheelchair with chin or tongue control
C5	Electric wheelchair; assisted transfers
C6	Electric wheelchair; independent transfers; Patient may drive
C7	Manual wheelchair
C8-L1	Manual wheelchair
L2	KAFO; limited household ambulation
L3-L4	AFO; community ambulation
L5	AFO; independent ambulation
S1	Limited bowel and bladder function

KAFO = knee-ankle-foot orthosis; AFO = ankle-foot orthosis.

thosis and firm taping of the forehead to the backboard at the scene of injury. In the emergency department, once a cervical dislocation or malaligned and unstable injury pattern is identified, traction should be applied using Gardner-Wells tongs or a halo ring to realign the injured segments. Some authors have advocated for prereduction MRI to identify herniated intervertebral disks in the cervical spine.[17] However, in the alert, nonintoxicated patient, substantial research has documented the safe use of traction-assisted reduction of dislocations.[18,19]

Status of High-Dose Methylprednisolone Therapy

Since publication of the results of the National Acute Spinal Cord Injury Studies (NASCIS) II and III in the 1990s, administration of high-dose methylprednisolone within 3 hours of injury has become widely accepted in the acute management of patients with spinal cord injuries and neurologic deficits.[20,21] If administered during the acute phase of secondary injury, methylprednisolone was thought to be a potent neuroprotective agent that helped stabilize cell membranes, maintain cord perfusion, enhance axonal transmission, and inhibit lipid peroxidation.[20,21]

However, several problems have been identified with the methodology of the NASCIS trials. As a result, the appropriateness of administration of high-dose steroids in patients with acute spinal cord injury has been strongly challenged.[22-26] Specifically, the stratification that resulted in significant findings in the NASCIS trials occurred only in post-hoc analysis, as initial results

4: Axial Skeleton, Including Spine and Pelvis

were inconclusive.[22,25] Furthermore, the neurologic improvement documented in the trials was of little clinical relevance, and the raw data from the study have only recently been released to the public for independent analysis.[25]

Similarly positive clinical results with the use of high-dose methylprednisolone in spinal cord injury have not been reproduced in subsequent investigations performed by researchers outside of the NASCIS group.[26,27] For example, in a review of 412 patients with traumatic incomplete cervical spinal cord injuries, researchers found that high-dose steroid administration had no impact on neurologic recovery.[26] Younger age and the presence of an incomplete lesion were the only factors found to positively influence the prognosis for neurologic recovery.[26]

The use of high-dose methylprednisolone has been associated with adverse effects, such as an increased risk of pneumonia, sepsis, and the potential for death from respiratory failure. Acute corticosteroid myopathy has also been reported, and it is possible that improvements documented in the NASCIS trials may have been related to recovery from acute corticosteroid myopathy rather than from any neuroprotection afforded by the steroids.[28]

A recent survey of spine surgeons documented that, while many continue to use the NASCIS steroid protocol, most do not believe in its efficacy.[12] The most common justification for steroid administration was fear of medicolegal ramifications. Similar findings were presented in a study from Canada, where the administration of steroids following acute spinal cord injury is no longer considered the standard of care.[29]

In 2002 the American Association of Neurological Surgeons–Congress of Neurological Surgeons Joint Section of Disorders of the Spine and Peripheral Nerves Guidelines Committee amended its stance on the steroid protocol to reflect the fact that such therapy should be considered only a treatment option rather than the standard of care.[25,30] Moreover, the committee stressed that "[t]he evidence suggesting harmful side effects [of high-dose steroid administration] is more consistent than suggestions of 'clinical benefit.'"[30]

Timing of Surgical Intervention

There is a general consensus that most patients with incomplete spinal cord injury benefit from surgical decompression and stabilization. Persistent compression of the injured spinal cord represents a potentially reversible form of secondary injury that should respond positively to decompression.[31-34] A great deal of controversy remains, however, in terms of the optimal timing of surgery. Proponents of early surgical intervention cite the potential for a worsening neurologic deficit in the setting of increased spinal cord edema and structural instability.[35] Others maintain that the potential for neurologic complications is higher in the acutely in-

jured patient taken to surgery before medical optimization. Furthermore, many think that the presence of spinal cord edema increases the risk of additional iatrogenic compromise to the cord during emergent decompressions.[31,34,35] Such a sentiment may be supported by evidence documenting an increase in intrathecal pressure and decreased spinal cord perfusion during surgical decompression.[36]

Currently, the main obstacle to a universally accepted guideline is the lack of level I evidence in support of emergent decompression.[31] In one study, neurologic and functional outcomes were prospectively examined in patients with spinal cord injuries treated surgically within 72 hours and were compared with those of patients who underwent surgery more than 5 days following injury.[35] Group comparison demonstrated no significant functional difference in American Spinal Injury Association (ASIA) grade or motor function. This report has been criticized by some, however, who believe that surgery within 72 hours does not constitute an "emergent" intervention. Nonetheless, other studies have been unable to document the influence of early surgery on neurologic outcome.[26]

Support for surgery within 24 hours of spinal cord injury is largely derived from studies performed using animal models.[15,37,38] To date, the findings in animal models have not been readily translated to clinical experience with human patients. Although some prospective series have documented significantly improved neurologic outcomes in patients receiving surgery within 8 to 12 hours,[32,39] similar results have not been encountered within the larger body of spine literature, and surgical intervention within this narrow time frame is not always feasible.[31,32,40] In a systematic review of the literature from 1966 to 2000, investigators reported that patients who received surgery within 24 hours of spinal cord injury had better outcomes than those operated on after 24 hours, or those treated nonsurgically.[40] Analysis of these data, however, revealed that only findings for patients with incomplete neurologic deficits were reliable. Given the methodologic limitations of this meta-analysis, the authors were able to conclude only that early surgical decompression is a viable option for most patients with spinal cord injury.[40]

Similarly, a more recent attempt to synthesize evidence-based recommendations from the available literature resulted in the conclusion that "[w]hile early surgery is a valid practice option, there is no definite evidence supporting its application over later surgical intervention, or even non-operative management."[31] Level II evidence does support the efficacy and safety of early surgical decompression, especially in the event of acute neurologic deterioration following spinal cord injury. Additionally, level II evidence supports emergent closed reduction for patients with bilateral facet dislocations and spinal cord injury.[31] Nonetheless, no standard of care regarding the timing of surgical intervention can be substantiated using evidence-based guidelines, and it is noteworthy that 24 hours is still considered well beyond the time that secondary injury pathways have been initiated[31] (**Table 1**).

Although high-quality scientific evidence is lacking in regard to the optimal timing for surgical intervention following spinal cord injury, a large multicenter prospective observational study was initiated by the Surgical Treatment of Acute Spinal Cord Injury Study group in 2003.[41] The goal of this investigation is to document outcomes in 450 patients receiving surgery within 24 hours versus more than 24 hours after their spinal cord injuries. A minimum 2-year follow-up for all patients is planned. Early data suggest a benefit to decompression within 24 hours of injury.[41] Final outcomes from this trial should become available within the next few years. Once released, these findings may well represent the best evidence regarding the impact of early surgical intervention for spinal cord injury recovery.

Status of Spinal Cord Injury Research

Current spinal cord injury research largely focuses on neuroprotection and engineered regeneration. Neuroprotective research seeks to limit the adverse effects of secondary injury pathways, whereas regenerative strategies attempt to augment the spinal cord's healing ability following injury.

Although many neuroprotective efforts have met with success in basic science studies as well as animal models, similar results have not been seen in human trials.[7,9,25] For example, monosialotetrahexosyl ganglioside showed a great deal of promise in animal trials and a small pilot study in humans. Yet, in a large prospective multicenter study, the drug had no effect on outcome following spinal cord injury.[9,25] Similar disappointing results in human trials have been reported for the glutamate antagonist gacyclidine (GK-II), the calcium channel blocker nimodipine, and the opioid antagonist naloxone.[20,41]

Researchers still hold out substantial hope for other drugs already approved for clinical use in human patients, including minocycline, riluzole, and erythropoietin. Although the Food and Drug Administration has approved these medications for use in areas outside of spinal cord injury, experimental studies have demonstrated a neuroprotective potential for all three. Clinical trials regarding the use of these medications in spinal cord injury are still in progress, with results likely to become available within the next 5 to 10 years.

Another effort focuses on the use of incubated autologous macrophages as adjuvants to alter the inflammatory response to cord injury and influence healing. The rationale behind this treatment is that the different regenerative capacities between cells in the central and peripheral nervous systems rest in the macrocytic response within those environments. Investigators hope that macrophages transplanted from the peripheral nervous system to the spinal cord can more rapidly clear myelin debris, stimulate nerve growth, and limit the deleterious effects of secondary cord injury. Results of a prospective trial were published in 2005 and documented improvement in ASIA grade from A to C in three of eight patients.[42] Unfortunately, because of financial considerations, a phase II trial for this intervention was suspended in 2006 and is yet to resume.[41]

Research into neuroprotection through the use of systemic and epidural hypothermia received a flurry of media attention after it was recently used on a professional football player after a spinal cord injury.[7,43-45] Hypothermia is hypothesized to limit the extent of secondary injury through a reduction of edema, inflammatory cell infiltration, cellular apoptosis, metabolic rate, and oxidative stress.[43,44] Animal models have reported some promising results in this arena but, as of 2008, no clinical evidence existed to support a beneficial role for hypothermia in human patients.[44] A recent investigation reported the safe administration of systemic hypothermia in 14 patients with acute, complete spinal cord injuries.[45] Long-term outcomes from this ongoing trial have yet to be reported, however.

Advances in cell culture techniques, cell transplantation, and tissue engineering have also broadened horizons aimed at regenerating neurologic tissue within the damaged spinal cord. Many bench-top and animal studies are currently investigating the potential for gene therapy, cell-based remyelination, and stem cells (neural, adult, as well as embryonic) to play a future role in the treatment of spinal cord injuries.[7,9,25,41] Because many of these trials have not proceeded beyond the laboratory, they are beyond the scope of this chapter. Of the many proposed regenerative therapies, only Schwann cells, olfactory ensheathing cells, and bone marrow–derived mesenchymal stem cells have been used in humans.[7,41]

Schwann cells perform myelinating functions within the peripheral nervous system and have been found to support the axonal regeneration of neurons in the central nervous system.[46] These cells have also been found to integrate within the parenchyma of the cord and serve as a potential matrix for neurologic regeneration. A case report has documented the use of sural nerve grafts in a 24-year-old man who was wheelchair bound, with ASIA grade C paraplegia and neurogenic bowel and bladder.[47] At 30 months after surgery, the patient had improved to an ASIA grade D and was able to ambulate with a walker. Although this is the only case currently reported in the literature, a formal clinical trial investigating Schwann cell transplantation is in the early phases of development.[41]

Olfactory ensheathing cells are specialized cells that assist in the transfer of new axons from cells within the peripheral nervous system to the central nervous system.[7,9,41] The unique ability of these cells to escort peripheral nerve axons into the central nervous system has made them attractive targets for facilitating peripheral nerve regeneration techniques in the spinal cord, or for stimulating cord repair de novo.

The use of olfactory ensheathing cells for spinal cord

injury achieved considerable success in animal models before investigations using human patients commenced.[48] Clinical studies using such cells have met with equivocal results. One study in three patients with complete spinal cord injuries showed no demonstrable improvement at 1-year follow-up.[49] Another study in seven individuals with complete spinal cord injuries reported improvements to ASIA grade C for two patients.[50] Both patients had return of bladder sensation, and one reportedly regained anal sphincter control. Although results presented in this work are encouraging, these unusual findings have not undergone independent verification.[41]

Chinese surgeons have reported considerable success in more than 300 patients with complete spinal cord injury treated with olfactory ensheathing cell transplantation.[51] However, an examination of the research protocols by American investigators, including interviews with seven participants, documented significant disparities in terms of the Chinese study's methodology as well as reported outcomes.[51] Specifically, independent observation by the American group failed to reveal any clinically significant improvements.

Of all the clinical neuroregenerative investigations, those involving mesenchymal and hematopoietic stem cells derived from human bone marrow have had the most success. In the right environment, stem cells obtained from human bone marrow have been found to differentiate into neural cells.[7] One clinical trial investigated outcomes in 20 individuals who received transplants of unmanipulated autologous bone marrow following complete spinal cord injury.[52] Five of seven patients treated within 30 days of their spinal cord injury were found to have improved motor and sensory function within 1 year of bone marrow implantation.

A similar investigation was performed in 35 patients with complete spinal cord injury.[53] These individuals were treated with autologous bone marrow stem cells combined with a granulocyte macrophage-colony stimulating factor. At an average of 10 months after surgery, improved neurologic function was documented in 30% of patients receiving the transplantation within 8 weeks of their spinal cord injury. Results from both of these studies suggest that mesenchymal stem cells derived from human bone marrow have the greatest potential to improve outcomes when they are administered during the acute period following spinal cord injury.

Summary

Spinal cord injuries are devastating conditions that have challenged physicians since the Ancient Period. Although great strides have been made in regard to characterizing the pathophysiology behind this condition, the ability to positively affect outcomes remains quite limited. Questions persist regarding the effect of surgical as well as pharmacologic interventions on functional restoration, particularly in patients with complete spinal cord injuries.

Numerous novel treatment strategies exist on the horizon, but most are in their infancy and have no demonstrable scientific data to support their use. The enthusiasm for these new therapies must be tempered with a judicious evaluation of the science supporting their application. Only rigorous prospective, randomized, multicenter trials can provide definitive evidence for new treatment strategies. Many such investigations are under way, however, and the next decade will undoubtedly prove to be an exciting time for those treating patients with spinal cord injuries.

Annotated References

1. Lifshutz J, Colohan A: A brief history of therapy for traumatic spinal cord injury. *Neurosurg Focus* 2004; 16(1):E5.

   An excellent historical review of surgical developments in the treatment of spinal cord injury from the Ancient Period to the 21st century is presented.

2. Price C, Makintubee S, Herndon W, Istre GR: Epidemiology of traumatic spinal cord injury and acute hospitalization and rehabilitation charges for spinal cord injuries in Oklahoma, 1988-1990. *Am J Epidemiol* 1994; 139(1):37-47.

3. Surkin J, Gilbert BJ, Harkey HL III, Sniezek J, Currier M: Spinal cord injury in Mississippi: Findings and evaluation, 1992-1994. *Spine* 2000;25(6):716-721.

4. Burke DA, Linden RD, Zhang YP, Maiste AC, Shields CB: Incidence rates and populations at risk for spinal cord injury: A regional study. *Spinal Cord* 2001; 39(5):274-278.

5. Saunders LL, Selassie AW, Hill EG, et al: Traumatic spinal cord injury mortality, 1981-1998. *J Trauma* 2009; 66(1):184-190.

   A retrospective analysis of data collected from the South Carolina Traumatic Spinal Cord Injury surveillance system is presented. The rate of spinal cord injury was 27.4 per million, with older patients, cervical injury, higher Frankel grade, and black race associated with greater mortality. Level of evidence: IV.

6. DeVivo MJ: Causes and costs of spinal cord injury in the United States. *Spinal Cord* 1997;35(12):809-813.

7. Rowland JW, Hawryluk GW, Kwon B, Fehlings MG: Current status of acute spinal cord injury pathophysiology and emerging therapies: Promise on the horizon. *Neurosurg Focus* 2008;25(5):E2.

   A systematic review of the pathophysiology behind spinal cord injury and potential implications for innovative treatment strategies for regeneration and repair is presented. Level of evidence: V.

8. Sekhon LH, Fehlings MG: Epidemiology, demographics, and pathophysiology of acute spinal cord injury. *Spine* 2001;26(24, suppl):S2-S12.

9. Kwon BK, Fisher CG, Dvorak MF, Tetzlaff W: Strategies to promote neural repair and regeneration after spinal cord injury. *Spine* 2005;30(17, suppl):S3-S13.

   The authors present a literature review with a focus on emerging neuroprotective and axonal regenerative therapies. They conclude that results of novel therapeutic agents in human trials are very limited, and larger peer-reviewed trials are necessary. Level of evidence: V.

10. Dusart I, Schwab ME: Secondary cell death and the inflammatory reaction after dorsal hemisection of the rat spinal cord. *Eur J Neurosci* 1994;6(5):712-724.

11. Donnelly DJ, Popovich PG: Inflammation and its role in neuroprotection, axonal regeneration and functional recovery after spinal cord injury. *Exp Neurol* 2008;209(2):378-388.

   A review of the pathophysiology of spinal cord injury with special attention to the roles inflammatory markers play in spinal cord injury and healing is presented. Level of evidence: V.

12. Eck JC, Nachtigall D, Humphreys SC, Hodges SD: Questionnaire survey of spine surgeons on the use of methylprednisolone for acute spinal cord injury. *Spine* 2006;31(9):E250-E253.

   A survey of spine surgeons documenting use of steroid protocol in acute spinal cord injury is presented. Ninety percent reported that they used the steroid protocol, but only 24% indicated that it improved clinical outcome. The plurality responded that steroid use was driven by medicolegal issues. Level of evidence: V.

13. Herrmann JE, Imura T, Song B, et al: STAT3 is a critical regulator of astrogliosis and scar formation after spinal cord injury. *J Neurosci* 2008;28(28):7231-7243.

   The authors performed investigations using knockout of STAT3 from astrocytes in mice. The results of this animal study show that STAT3 molecular signaling is critical to astrogliosis and that astrocytic scar formation inhibits spread of inflammatory cells and decreases lesion volume.

14. Beattie MS, Hermann GE, Rogers RC, Bresnahan JC: Cell death in models of spinal cord injury. *Prog Brain Res* 2002;137:37-47.

15. Rabinowitz RS, Eck JC, Harper CM Jr, et al: Urgent surgical decompression compared to methylprednisolone for the treatment of acute spinal cord injury: A randomized prospective study in beagle dogs. *Spine* 2008;33(21):2260-2268.

   In a randomized prospective study, the value of steroids, surgical decompression, or a combination of both for the treatment of spinal cord injury in a dog model were compared. Surgical decompression within 6 hours of injury led to better neurologic outcome than steroid administration alone.

16. Vale FL, Burns J, Jackson AB, Hadley MN: Combined medical and surgical treatment after acute spinal cord injury: Results of a prospective pilot study to assess the merits of aggressive medical resuscitation and blood pressure management. *J Neurosurg* 1997;87(2):239-246.

17. Eismont FJ, Arena MJ, Green BA: Extrusion of an intervertebral disc associated with traumatic subluxation or dislocation of cervical facets: Case report. *J Bone Joint Surg Am* 1991;73(10):1555-1560.

18. Vaccaro AR, Falatyn SP, Flanders AE, Balderston RA, Northrup BE, Cotler JM: Magnetic resonance evaluation of the intervertebral disc, spinal ligaments, and spinal cord before and after closed traction reduction of cervical spine dislocations. *Spine* 1999;24(12):1210-1217.

19. Lee AS, MacLean JC, Newton DA: Rapid traction for reduction of cervical spine dislocations. *J Bone Joint Surg Br* 1994;76(3):352-356.

20. Bracken MB, Shepard MJ, Collins WF, et al: A randomized, controlled trial of methylprednisolone or naloxone in the treatment of acute spinal-cord injury: Results of the Second National Acute Spinal Cord Injury Study. *N Engl J Med* 1990;322(20):1405-1411.

21. Bracken MB, Shepard MJ, Holford TR, et al: Administration of methylprednisolone for 24 or 48 hours or tirilazad mesylate for 48 hours in the treatment of acute spinal cord injury: Results of the Third National Acute Spinal Cord Injury Randomized Controlled Trial. National Acute Spinal Cord Injury Study. *JAMA* 1997;277(20):1597-1604.

22. Hurlbert RJ: Methylprednisolone for acute spinal cord injury: An inappropriate standard of care. *J Neurosurg* 2000;93(1, suppl):1-7.

23. Hurlbert RJ: The role of steroids in acute spinal cord injury: An evidence-based analysis. *Spine* 2001;26(24, suppl):S39-S46.

24. Hugenholtz H, Cass DE, Dvorak MF, et al: High-dose methylprednisolone for acute closed spinal cord injury: only a treatment option. *Can J Neurol Sci* 2002;29(3):227-235.

25. Hurlbert RJ: Strategies of medical intervention in the management of acute spinal cord injury. *Spine* 2006;31(11, suppl):S16-S21.

   The authors present a literature review from 1996 to 2006 addressing clinical advancements in the medical treatment of spinal cord injury. Currently there are no pharmacologic strategies of proven benefit. Steroids continue to be given primarily out of fear of litigation. Level of evidence: V.

26. Pollard ME, Apple DF: Factors associated with improved neurologic outcomes in patients with incomplete tetraplegia. *Spine* 2003;28(1):33-39.

4: Axial Skeleton, Including Spine and Pelvis

27. Pointillart V, Petitjean ME, Wiart L, et al: Pharmacological therapy of spinal cord injury during the acute phase. *Spinal Cord* 2000;38(2):71-76.

28. Qian T, Guo X, Levi AD, Vanni S, Shebert RT, Sipski ML: High-dose methylprednisolone may cause myopathy in acute spinal cord injury patients. *Spinal Cord* 2005;43(4):199-203.

    In a small prospective series, evidence for acute corticosteroid myopathy was examined among patients with spinal cord injury who received high-dose methylprednisolone. Muscle biopsies and electromyogram results for patients who received steroids showed evidence of acute corticosteroid myopathy. Level of evidence: II.

29. Hurlbert RJ, Moulton R: Why do you prescribe methylprednisolone for acute spinal cord injury? A Canadian perspective and a position statement. *Can J Neurol Sci* 2002;29(3):236-239.

30. Hadley MN, Walters BC, Grabb PA, et al: Guidelines for the management of acute cervical spine and spinal cord injuries. *Clin Neurosurg* 2002;49:407-498.

31. Fehlings MG, Perrin RG: The timing of surgical intervention in the treatment of spinal cord injury: A systematic review of recent clinical evidence. *Spine* 2006; 31(11, suppl):S28-S35.

    In a literature search from 1966 to 2005, the effect of surgical decompression on neurologic outcome after spinal cord injury was investigated. There is level II evidence supporting early surgical decompression as a safe and effective treatment. There is no conclusive evidence demonstrating a benefit over conservative management, however. Level of evidence: II.

32. Papadopoulos SM, Selden NR, Quint DJ, Patel N, Gillespie B, Grube S: Immediate spinal cord decompression for cervical spinal cord injury: Feasibility and outcome. *J Trauma* 2002;52(2):323-332.

33. Delamarter RB, Sherman J, Carr JB: Pathophysiology of spinal cord injury: Recovery after immediate and delayed decompression. *J Bone Joint Surg Am* 1995;77(7): 1042-1049.

34. Fehlings MG, Sekhon LH, Tator C: The role and timing of decompression in acute spinal cord injury: What do we know? What should we do? *Spine* 2001;26(24, suppl):S101-S110.

35. Vaccaro AR, Daugherty RJ, Sheehan TP, et al: Neurologic outcome of early versus late surgery for cervical spinal cord injury. *Spine* 1997;22(22):2609-2613.

36. Kwon BK, Curt A, Belanger LM, et al: Intrathecal pressure monitoring and cerebrospinal fluid drainage in acute spinal cord injury: A prospective randomized trial. *J Neurosurg Spine* 2009;10(3):181-193.

    A randomized prospective study of 22 patients treated with intrathecal pressure monitoring and cerebrospinal fluid drainage after acute spinal cord injury is presented. Surgical decompression resulted in increased intrathecal pressure and decreased spinal cord perfusion that extended into the postoperative period. Level of evidence: IV.

37. Shields CB, Zhang YP, Shields LB, Han Y, Burke DA, Mayer NW: The therapeutic window for spinal cord decompression in a rat spinal cord injury model. *J Neurosurg Spine* 2005;3(4):302-307.

    Research was conducted to determine the effect of surgical decompression on functional recovery in a rat spinal cord injury model. Improved motor function was appreciated in those rats that received surgical decompression at 6 and 12 hours postinjury when compared to those undergoing surgery at 24 hours.

38. Ouyang H, Galle B, Li J, Nauman E, Shi R: Critical roles of decompression in functional recovery of ex vivo spinal cord white matter. *J Neurosurg Spine* 2009;10(2): 161-170.

    An investigation using ex vivo guinea pig spine tissue attempted to determine the effect of severity and duration of compression on spinal cord function. Results demonstrated that spinal cord electrical conductivity was inversely correlated to the duration and severity of spinal cord compression.

39. Cengiz SL, Kalkan E, Bayir A, Ilik K, Basefer A: Timing of thoracolomber spine stabilization in trauma patients; impact on neurological outcome and clinical course: A real prospective (rct) randomized controlled study. *Arch Orthop Trauma Surg* 2008;128(9):959-966.

    Outcomes in 27 patients treated for acute thoracolumbar spine injury with neurologic deficit were examined in a prospective series. Neurologic outcome was increased and intensive care unit stay, as well as the rate of systemic complications, was reduced among patients who received surgery within 8 hours of injury. Level of evidence: II.

40. La Rosa G, Conti A, Cardali S, Cacciola F, Tomasello F: Does early decompression improve neurological outcome of spinal cord injured patients? Appraisal of the literature using a meta-analytical approach. *Spinal Cord* 2004;42(9):503-512.

    The authors present a systematic review investigating neurologic outcomes for patients receiving surgery within 24 hours compared to those receiving late surgery, or nonsurgical management. Surgery within 24 hours resulted in better outcomes. Only data regarding patients with incomplete neurologic injury were found to be reliable. Level of evidence: III.

41. Hawryluk GW, Rowland J, Kwon BK, Fehlings MG: Protection and repair of the injured spinal cord: A review of completed, ongoing, and planned clinical trials for acute spinal cord injury. *Neurosurg Focus* 2008; 25(5):E14.

    Recently completed and ongoing human clinical trials for the treatment of spinal cord injury were reviewed. Ten randomized controlled trials have been completed, with mostly negative results. Ongoing trials hold promise for substantial advances in treatment over the next decade. Level of evidence: V.

42. Knoller N, Auerbach G, Fulga V, et al: Clinical experience using incubated autologous macrophages as a treatment for complete spinal cord injury: Phase I study results. *J Neurosurg Spine* 2005;3(3):173-181.

A prospective nonrandomized trial of eight patients treated with incubated autologous macrophages for complete spinal cord injury is presented. Three of eight patients improved to ASIA grade C function at 12-month follow-up. Two patients demonstrated clear improvement in spinal cord integrity on MRI. Level of evidence: IV.

43. Erecinska M, Thoresen M, Silver IA: Effects of hypothermia on energy metabolism in mammalian central nervous system. *J Cereb Blood Flow Metab* 2003;23(5):513-530.

44. Kwon BK, Mann C, Sohn HM, et al; NASS Section on Biologics: Hypothermia for spinal cord injury. *Spine J* 2008;8(6):859-874.

The authors present a literature review from 1940 to the present on the use of hypothermia in spinal cord injury. Animal studies of acute traumatic spinal cord injury have not demonstrated neuroprotective benefits for hypothermia, and there is little scientific evidence in support of its use in human patients. Level of evidence: V.

45. Levi AD, Green BA, Wang MY, et al: Clinical application of modest hypothermia after spinal cord injury. *J Neurotrauma* 2009;26(3):407-415.

Fourteen patients treated with systemic hypothermia for acute complete spinal cord injury were studied prospectively. Excellent correlation was achieved between intravascular and intrathecal temperatures. This study represents the largest modern series and documents safe hypothermia. Level of evidence: IV.

46. Cheng H, Cao Y, Olson L: Spinal cord repair in adult paraplegic rats: Partial restoration of hind limb function. *Science* 1996;273(5274):510-513.

47. Cheng H, Liao KK, Liao SF, Chuang TY, Shih YH: Spinal cord repair with acidic fibroblast growth factor as a treatment for a patient with chronic paraplegia. *Spine* 2004;29(14):E284-E288.

A case report documents the use of four sural nerve grafts in a 24-year-old patient with ASIA grade C paraplegia. At 30 months after surgery the patient demonstrated significant motor recovery and improved to an ASIA grade D. Level of evidence: V.

48. Ramón-Cueto A, Cordero MI, Santos-Benito FF, Avila J: Functional recovery of paraplegic rats and motor axon regeneration in their spinal cords by olfactory ensheathing glia. *Neuron* 2000;25(2):425-435.

49. Féron F, Perry C, Cochrane J, et al: Autologous olfactory ensheathing cell transplantation in human spinal cord injury. *Brain* 2005;128(Pt 12):2951-2960.

The safety of olfactory ensheathing cell transplantation in three patients with complete spinal cord injuries was investigated. Results at 1 year showed that there were no indications that the procedure was unsafe. None of the patients demonstrated neurologic improvement. Level of evidence: IV.

50. Lima C, Pratas-Vital J, Escada P, Hasse-Ferreira A, Capucho C, Peduzzi JD: Olfactory mucosa autografts in human spinal cord injury: A pilot clinical study. *J Spinal Cord Med* 2006;29(3):191-203.

A pilot study involving seven patients who received olfactory ensheathing cell transplantation after suffering ASIA grade A spinal cord injury was performed. At 18- month follow-up, two patients had improved to ASIA grade C with return of bladder sensation, and anal sphincter control in one individual. Level of evidence: IV.

51. Dobkin BH, Curt A, Guest J: Cellular transplants in China: Observational study from the largest human experiment in chronic spinal cord injury. *Neurorehabil Neural Repair* 2006;20(1):5-13.

An American observational study of seven participants from a large series of Chinese patients receiving olfactory ensheathing cell transplantation was performed. Researchers found several issues with the Chinese study's methodology. Complications were high and no clinically significant sensorimotor or autonomic improvements were identified. Level of evidence: IV.

52. Syková E, Homola A, Mazanec R, et al: Autologous bone marrow transplantation in patients with subacute and chronic spinal cord injury. *Cell Transplant* 2006;15(8-9):675-687.

A prospective study of 20 patients with complete spinal cord injury treated with autologous bone marrow transplantation is presented. Patients were followed for 1 year postoperatively. Those who received treatment within 30 days of spinal cord injury were more likely to exhibit improved sensorimotor outcomes. Level of evidence: II.

53. Yoon SH, Shim YS, Park YH, et al: Complete spinal cord injury treatment using autologous bone marrow cell transplantation and bone marrow stimulation with granulocyte macrophage-colony stimulating factor: Phase I/II clinical trial. *Stem Cells* 2007;25(8):2066-2073.

Thirty-five patients with complete spinal cord injury treated with bone marrow stem cell transplantation were studied. At an average of 10 months after surgery, no adverse events were noted, and 30% of those patients treated within 8 weeks of injury regained some neurologic function. Level of evidence: II.

4. Axial Skeleton, Including Spine and Pelvis

Chapter 27

Upper Cervical Spine Injury: Occiput to C2

John C. France, MD

4: Axial Skeleton, Including Spine and Pelvis

Introduction

The anatomy of the upper cervical spine (occiput to C2) is unique in comparison to the subaxial spine (C3-7). As a result of these anatomic differences, the fracture patterns cannot be easily characterized under a single classification system and must be considered individually according to location of the injury. Additionally, this area of the spine is frequently overlooked when screening for spine injuries after trauma. Therefore, it is important to review the evaluation and treatment of the more common fracture patterns of the upper cervical spine.

Occipital Condyle Fractures

Occipital condyle fractures are now more commonly identified because of the increased use of helical CT as the primary screening tool for cervical clearance in the trauma patient.[1] Once these injuries are identified, it is important to recognize the potential for an unstable occipitocervical dissociation. Any incongruity of the occipitocervical joints, severe anterior soft-tissue swelling in the upper cervical region, neurologic deficit that involves the cranial nerves, or an altered relationship between the clivus and the tip of the odontoid would suggest the presence of occipitocervical dissociation. If some question exists as to the integrity of the upper cervical ligaments, then MRI is warranted.

The Anderson and Montesano classification of occipital condyle fractures, based on the mechanism of injury, is the one most commonly used. Type I injuries are impaction fractures of the condyle secondary to an axial load. Type II injuries are essentially basilar skull fractures that extend through the condyle and communicate with the foramen magnum. Type III injuries are avulsion fractures of the condyle from the alar ligaments (**Figure 1**). A distinction between a unilateral injury and

Dr. France or an immediate family member serves as a board member, owner, officer, or committee member of AO Spine North America; and has received research or institutional support from Medtronic Sofamor Danek and Synthes.

a bilateral injury would also contribute to determining the degree of stability. The type III injury raises the greatest concern for occipitocervical instability because of associated compromise of the alar ligament.

When occipital condyle injuries are unilateral with no evidence of a greater injury such as occipitocervical dissociation, treatment consists of hard collar immobilization for 6 to 12 weeks.[2] Type III injuries are the most likely to indicate a more unstable injury, and nonsurgical treatment should be undertaken cautiously. At the completion of treatment, a lateral flexion-extension radiograph, centered on the upper cervical spine or base of the skull to avoid parallax and provide the most accurate images, should be used to confirm stability.

Occipitocervical Dissociation

The occipitocervical or craniocervical dissociation is an injury that warrants greater discussion. Once thought to be nearly universally fatal, this injury is now encountered with greater frequency in survivors of high-energy trauma, probably because of improved extraction, pre-hospital immobilization and resuscitation techniques, more efficient transportation, and improved imaging techniques. If this injury is undetected, the risk of progressive deficit and even death is high. This injury is easily missed during screening, so it must be specifically searched for on CT scans.[3]

Craniocervical dislocations have been classified according to the direction of the dislocation with anterior dislocations being most common, although posterior and vertical dislocations also occur. However, classification based on the direction of displacement is faulty, in that these injuries are so highly unstable that the direction of displacement on any static film depends more on forces being applied to the head relative to the neck at the time of the imaging study than on any inherent injury characteristic. This injury is thought to be approximately twice as common in children as in adults, possibly because of smaller occipital condyles, a more horizontal or shallow occipitoatlantal joint line, and larger head relative to the body.

On the screening cervical CT scan, the base of the skull must be included in the axial images, as well as

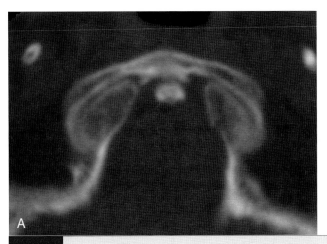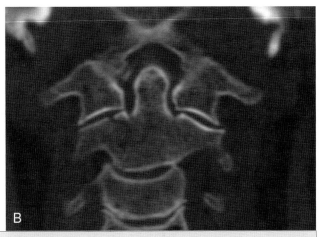

Figure 1 An axial (**A**) and coronal (**B**) CT image of a type III occipital condyle fracture.

the sagittal and coronal reconstructions. One of the most easily detectable signs of occipitocervical dissociation is the presence of severe soft-tissue swelling, often representing hemorrhage, anterior to the C1 and C2 vertebrae. Although the presence of soft-tissue swelling does not mean that an injury is absolutely present, it is seldom absent in the presence of an occipitocervical dissociation (unlike the subaxial cervical spine, where the absence of anterior soft-tissue swelling by no means excludes significant injury). Other important radiographic diagnostic parameters include the Powers ratio, the "Rule of Twelve," and the dens-basion relationship. These various radiographic lines were established primarily because of the inability to more directly assess congruity of the occipitocervical junction on standard radiographs, and are now becoming historically significant with the increasing use of CT, during which joint subluxation can be more directly assessed. The Powers ratio[4] assesses the ratio of two distances measured between four points: the distance between the basion and the posterior arch of C1 is measured in relation to the distance between the opisthion and the anterior arch of C1. A ratio greater than one is significant for an anterior atlantoccipital dislocation. Ratios less than one are normal except in posterior occipitoatlantal dislocations, associated fractures of the odontoid process or ring of C1, and congenital abnormalities of the foramen magnum. It should be noted that in purely distractive injuries, the ratio may remain normal despite the presence of a highly unstable injury. This is the main reason that the "Rule of Twelve," or Harris lines, are superior to the Powers ratio. This measurement uses three landmarks: the basion, the rostral tip of the odontoid, and the posterior axial line (cephalad extension of the posterior cortical margin of the body of the axis). Two distances are measured: the basion-posterior axial line interval and the basion-dens interval. Both distances should be less than 12 mm in individuals with a normal cervical spine who are older than 13 years.[5] A more direct approach involves simply assessing the

dens-basion relationship. In a normal cervical spine with the head in neutral, the tip of the odontoid should be in vertical alignment with the basion within a distance of 4 to 5 mm.[6,7] The Wackenheim line runs along the posterior aspect of the clivus and should pass the tip of the odontoid and abut the posterior edge of the tip.[8] On CT, the occipital condyle should be perfectly congruent with the C1 superior articular surface, and any incongruity is indicative of this injury pattern.

MRI can be used to better visualize the soft-tissue components such as the alar ligaments.[9,10] Soft-tissue swelling anteriorly is also a hallmark of MRI findings for these injuries. Additionally the tectorial membrane may be lifted off the clivus or even disrupted (**Figure 2**).

Once such an injury is identified, the cervical spine should be immediately immobilized and traction should be avoided. The treatment of occipitocervical dissociation is a posterior occipitocervical fusion, the caudal extent of which is dictated by associated fractures, bone quality, and other factors that affect bony attachment points such as vertebral artery anatomy.[11] If surgical stabilization is going to be delayed at all, then halo vest immobilization and spine precautions are prudent.

C1 Fractures

Fractures of the C1 ring are commonly associated with other upper cervical fractures, so the identification of a C1 ring injury should prompt a search for those fractures. Likewise, the presence of a C1 fracture can influence the surgical stabilization options of other upper cervical fractures, so these fractures should be kept in mind when planning surgery. With isolated C1 ring or atlas fractures, neurologic deficits are relatively rare because of the extra space within the spinal canal at that level and the tendency for these injuries to displace outwardly, away from the spinal cord.

Jefferson, whose name is usually associated with the bursting type of atlas fracture, described an anatomic

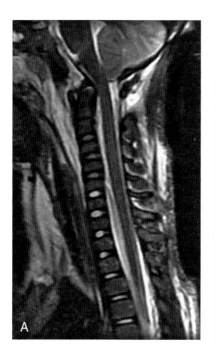

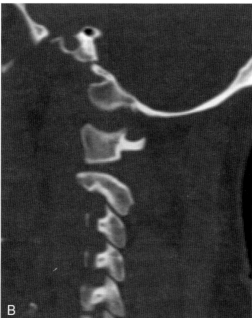

Figure 2 **A,** The midline sagittal T2 MRI demonstrates anterior soft-tissue swelling, the tectorial membrane elevated off the clivus, and malalignment of the tip of the odontoid relative to the Wackenheim line (a line drawn along the posterior slope of the clivus that should abut the posterior edge of the odontoid tip). **B,** A T2 sagittal MRI that is more lateral at the occipitocervical joint shows incongruity of the joint characteristic of occipitocervical dissociation.

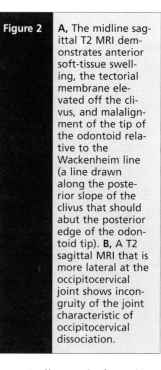

4: Axial Skeleton, Including Spine and Pelvis

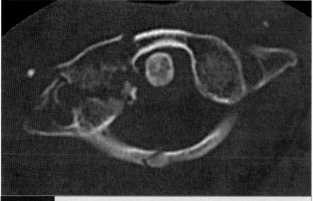

Figure 3 An axial CT image of a type 3 comminuted lateral mass fracture of the C1 ring. This type of injury can be problematic as the lateral mass displaces outward and the occipital condyle settles down onto the superior articular surface of C2.

classification system[12] that included posterior arch fractures, anterior arch fractures, lateral mass fractures, and transverse process fractures. This classification was later expanded[13] to include six subtypes based on CT imaging. A seventh subtype has been added.[14]

1. Burst fractures (type 1), usually the result of an axial load on the lateral masses of C1, are forced apart to produce either three- or four-part fractures. In the pediatric population, the separation can occur through the anterior synchondrosis and persistent posterior synchondrosis or posterior arch fracture.[15] Recent biomechanical testing suggests that this pattern is the result of a high-energy injury and that the remaining patterns of

injury that follow numerically result from low-energy mechanisms.[16] Treatment is dependent on the severity of displacement, which is measured as the lateral offset between the lateral edge of the C1 lateral mass and the lateral edge of the C2 lateral mass. Left- and right-sided offsets that add up to 7 mm of displacement or greater are thought to represent disruption of the transverse atlantal ligament, which is considered an indication for surgical stabilization. Long-term outcomes following treatment of this fracture demonstrate function below normative data, with the worst being those fractures with 7-mm offsets.[17]

2. Posterior arch fractures (type 2) result from cervical hyperextension and are important to recognize, because in more than 50% of cases, they are associated with other fractures such as odontoid fractures, traumatic spondylolisthesis of the axis, or occipital condyle fractures.[13,18-20] The presence of additional injuries may alter the treatment plan and outcomes, although when posterior C1 arch fractures occur in isolation, nonsurgical treatment is recommended.

3. Comminuted fractures (type 3) represent 22% of C1 ring injuries and are defined anatomically by combined unilateral transverse ligament avulsion with an ipsilateral anterior and/or posterior arch fracture (**Figure 3**). They result from combined forces: axial compression and lateral flexion. More aggressive treatment is often warranted with these injuries because they are the most likely to result in nonunion, torticollis deformity, and a poor functional outcome.[21]

4. Anterior arch fractures (type 4) occur with failure of the anterior arch while abutting the dens during hyperextension.[22,23] Associated disruption of the posterior longitudinal ligament (PLL) (tectorial membrane) can lead to instability with this variant.[24] In the absence of associated atlanto-occipital instability, the treatment is nonsurgical.

5. Lateral mass fractures (type 5) are generally the result of combined axial loading and lateral compression. If the fracture is severe enough, the occipital condyle can settle onto the lateral mass of C2, creating a cock-robin deformity.

6. Transverse process fractures (type 6) may be unilateral or bilateral, resulting from an avulsion with lateral bending. These are usually considered benign injuries when in isolation.

7. Inferior tubercle avulsion fractures (type 7) are thought to be an avulsion injury of the longus colli muscle caused by hyperextension of the neck. Nonsurgical treatment is recommended.

Based on the above classification, fracture types 2, 4, 6, and 7, when they occur as isolated injuries, are typically treated nonsurgically in a hard collar for 6 weeks, followed by an open mouth AP (odontoid) radiograph and lateral flexion-extension radiographs to ensure the absence of instability. In fracture types 1, 3, and 5, nonsurgical treatment can still be considered if the displacement is minimal and a hard collar or halo vest is used, depending on the concern for progressive displacement. If the patient has significant displacement or deformity, for example, the occipital condyle is settled caudally onto the C2 superior articulation, surgical treatment is recommended. Lateral mass fractures can be repaired with direct osteosynthesis by applying compression between the lateral pillars of C1 using lateral mass screws with a transverse rod, but this method has not yet been extensively studied. More commonly, the fracture is reduced with traction and C1-2 transarticular screws, or a C1-2 screw and rod construct is used. Alternatively, a posterior occipital-C2 fusion can be used to span the injury if the C1 lateral mass is highly comminuted.

C1-2 Instability

Atlantoaxial instability as a true acute traumatic event is rare and is usually fatal, but more commonly such an instability is identified incidentally following a traumatic event. The causes of preexisting C1-2 instability are numerous and include rheumatoid arthritis, dwarfing syndromes, connective tissue disorders, os odontoidium, neoplastic process, Griesel syndrome, and congenital malformations. Once identified, these conditions need to be addressed and atlantoaxial arthrodesis

considered, but a thorough discussion of these conditions is beyond the scope of this chapter.

An acute traumatic instability can result from transverse ligament disruption, creating instability in the sagittal plane or in the form of rotary instability, with the latter being more common in children. Generally, the pediatric rotary subluxations, when traumatic, are the result of low energy mechanisms, and thus are easily reduced in occipitomandibular sling traction followed by treatment in a soft collar for comfort. In the recalcitrant or recurrent patient, more aggressive options can be considered. Rotary subluxations are rare in the adult, but the possibility of this injury is occasionally considered by the radiologist on initial imaging. With the use of multiplanar reformatted CT, the anatomy can usually be clarified but if any question remains, a rotational CT with axial cuts through the C1-2 articulation while the patient rotates from left to right is the diagnostic imaging method of choice.

Also rare but slightly more common would be an acute traumatic disruption of the transverse ligament causing C1-2 instability. If suspected from a static image, this injury can be identified using lateral flexion-extension views with the understanding that the normal atlanto-dens interval should be 3 mm or less in an adult (5 mm in a child younger than 10 years). Sometimes the acute nature of the instability is in question, and an MRI can offer clarification by showing edema or specific ligament disruption. If an MRI is ordered for this purpose, the radiologist should be contacted directly so the MRI can be formatted to offer enough detail of the upper cervical ligaments. Once this injury identified, the mainstay of treatment is a posterior C1-2 arthrodesis, because ligament healing is unlikely. Fusion will help prevent long-term instability, although a recent review indicates there may be room for more conservative options such as 3 months of halo vest immobilization in children.[25] It should be noted that craniocervical dissociation can occur through the atlantoaxial joint rather than the occipitocervical joints. Similar to occipitocervical dissociations, craniocervical dissociation is treated with a posterior arthrodesis.

Odontoid Fractures

In recent years, odontoid fractures have received the most attention of upper cervical fractures as a group, with particular emphasis on the elderly. It is clear that an odontoid fracture in a patient older than 65 years is fraught with complications regardless of the selected treatment. As techniques for upper cervical fixation have improved and gain wider popularity, there has been a trend away from nonsurgical treatment toward surgical stabilization. In particular, nonsurgical management with halo vest immobilization has been highly scrutinized.[26,27]

Most of the controversy has focused on type II fractures, which run through the base of the odontoid process. The type III fracture pattern, which extends into the body of C2, has greater intrinsic stability and a larger bony surface area for healing; therefore, nonunion and late instability are of less concern. Most type III fractures can be treated using simple hard collar immobilization with an anticipated satisfactory radiographic and clinical result. If the initial displacement of a type III fracture is significant and requires reduction, the alignment can usually be maintained with halo vest immobilization or a surgical option would be reasonable. This is a less common scenario in fractures in elderly patients and is underrepresented in the literature.

The abundance of literature in recent years has centered on the type II fracture pattern because the intrinsic instability and small bony surface area increases the likelihood of nonunion. Risk factors for nonunion are reasonably established and include initial displacement greater than 6 mm, posterior displacement, delay in diagnosis, failure to maintain reduction, and age older than 65 years.

For younger patients, an odontoid fracture is usually a high-energy injury. If associated injuries exist and the patient has experienced multitrauma, surgical stabilization is preferred to aid mobilization and nursing care. In the isolated injury, both surgical and nonsurgical treatment can both be considered and should be discussed with the patient. If nonsurgical treatment is selected, then halo vest immobilization can be expected to yield a greater union rate and would be chosen over a hard collar. Surgical treatment should be given strong consideration if the initial fracture displacement is greater than 6 mm or the patient has risk factors such as a history of smoking or diabetes that may interfere with bony union. In addition, if the halo vest fails to maintain reduction, surgical management can offer better stability. Anterior screw fixation is preferred in this patient group because the strong bone diminishes the risk of loss of fixation, avoids having to risk displacement while turning prone, and has the potential to preserve neck rotation. The limits to anterior screw fixation that would make posterior C1-2 fusion a better choice include a barrel chest body habitus that precludes the ability to achieve the desired screw trajectory, a comminuted fracture pattern (type IIa), and a reverse obliquity fracture pattern in which the fracture line parallels the screw trajectory such that compression across the fracture cannot be effectively achieved without causing the fracture to displace.

In contrast to the young patient with odontoid fracture, treatment in the elderly remains controversial. In recent years, nonsurgical treatment with the halo vest has come under significant criticism for this group of patients. There has been a trend toward more surgical treatment and use of a hard collar when nonsurgical treatment is selected. Unlike in younger patients, preexisting comorbidities and functional status play the most important roles in the elderly. An odontoid fracture in an elderly person is similar to hip fracture in that it is an insufficiency fracture sustained from a low-energy

mechanism and is often a sign of general failing health. As a result, early morbidity and mortality with any form of treatment are significant.[28] A stable fibrous union may be acceptable in elderly patients, depending on age and overall health (bony union is necessary in the younger patient). The risks associated with fibrous union are late pain and sudden or gradual onset of myelopathy, but these conditions are lower commonly seen in the elderly. For the patient with very low physical demands or a nursing home patient, a hard collar may be adequate treatment, accepting that a nonunion will probably ensue. For the nondisplaced fracture in a moderately or higher functioning patient, the risk of a nonunion from nonsurgical treatment is less with the halo vest; thus, halo vest immobilization is an option.[29] Potential early and late complications are associated with halo vest wear. During early treatment, dysphagia, respiratory distress, and gait instability can be problematic. Dysphagia can be minimized by keeping the head in a neutral position (avoiding hyperextension or flexion) and using aspiration precautions initially. The respiratory distress also can be minimized with aspiration precautions as well as aggressive immediate mobilization. The use of a walker for stability is important as the patient first begins to ambulate, but can gradually be weaned, depending on patient factors. If these early complications appear insurmountable, then a switch to surgical treatment is easily justified. The late complications of the halo vest include loss of alignment and pin tract infection. In the event of loss of alignment, a reduction could be considered but again this would also justify surgery. Pin tract infection is usually the result of loosening and therefore is seen in the later stages of treatment. It can be managed with cautious retightening, change of pin location, or early halo removal depending on the time frame and severity of the infection as well as the perceived degree of fracture healing and stability. For the patient with a displaced fracture, especially greater than 6 mm, surgical treatment is more heavily favored. Again, the two options are anterior screw direct osteosynthesis and posterior C1-2 arthrodesis. The risk of loss of fixation from poor-quality bone is higher in elderly patients and tends to occur more frequently with anterior screws, because the bone in the C2 body is the weakest. Additionally, recent studies have shown a high rate of postoperative dysphagia severe enough to require a feeding tube and result in aspiration pneumonia. These complications prolong the hospital stay and occur at a frequency high enough to make anterior fixation less attractive in the elderly population.[30] The posterior bone at C1 and C2 is stronger, so loss of fixation is relatively infrequent, and bony union occurs at a high rate following posterior C1-2 arthrodesis. Therefore, many surgeons prefer the posterior C1-2 arthrodesis when surgical management is selected[31] (**Figure 4**). The improvements in posterior upper cervical fixation with C2 lateral mass, C2 intralaminar (**Figure 5**), and C2 pedicle screws have made this approach safer with respect to potential in-

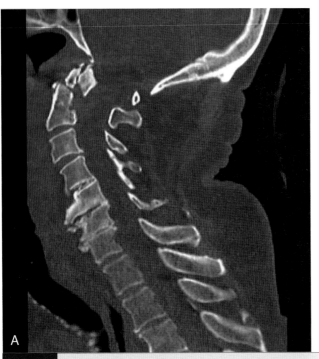
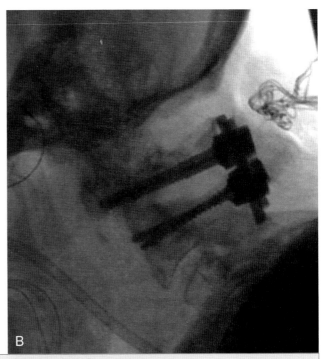

Figure 4 A posteriorly displaced odontoid fracture in a highly functional 87-year-old man (**A**), treated with a posterior C1-2 arthrodesis using C1 lateral mass and C2 pedicle screws (**B**).

Figure 5 An axial CT showing the path of C2 intralaminar screws, which are useful in patients with small C2 pedicles or vertebral artery anatomy that poses a risk forarterial injury with the insertion of C1-2 transarticular or C2 pedicle screws. The preoperative CT must be assessed to ensure there is enough room between the cortices to accommodate the screw.

jury to the vertebral arteries, further improving the appeal of the posterior procedure.

Despite careful review of the current studies available, it remains difficult to make definitive recommendations for the treatment of odontoid fracture in elderly patients.[32-34] The risk factors for nonunion discussed earlier, when present, would make surgical treatment favorable, but for the nondisplaced or minimally displaced fracture, the patient's preinjury functional status, comorbidities, and the desires of the patient as well as those of the family, must be taken into account when formulating a treatment plan.

Hangman's Fractures

The diagnosis and treatment of C2 traumatic spondylolisthesis, also known as hangman's fracture, has not changed significantly in recent years.[35] For the type I, nondisplaced fracture, a hard collar is generally adequate. For type II, displaced fractures, reduction can be obtained through halo traction and then maintained with the halo vest. Care should be taken to identify the type IIa fracture, which is characterized by significant angulation in the absence of translation (**Figure 6**), because traction can easily cause overdistraction. The type IIa fracture has historically been treated with extension into a reduced position and halo vest immobilization.[36] However, surgical intervention in the form of anterior C2-3 interbody arthrodesis or posterior C2-3 or C1-3 arthrodesis has become the more common treatment of these unstable three-column flexion-

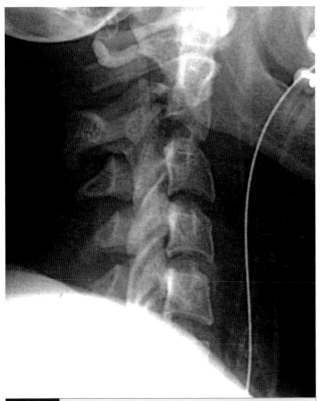

Figure 6 | A lateral radiograph of the cervical spine of a type IIa hangman's fracture. Notice the significant angulation at the C2-3 disk space with lack of translation, which is the radiographic hallmark.

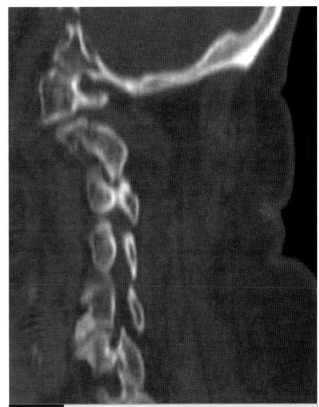

Figure 7 | A lateral cervical radiograph of a type III hangman's fracture with C2-3 bilateral facet dislocation.

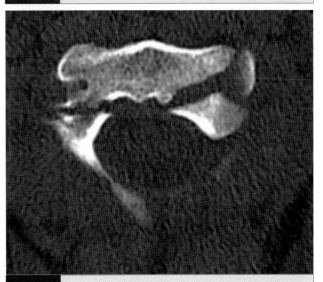

Figure 8 | An axial CT image of a variant of hangman's fracture that may be at greater risk for neurologic deterioration.

distraction injuries with discoligamentous disruption. In recent years there has been a move away from halo vest treatment toward surgical intervention for more typical type II fractures with either posterior direct screw osteosynthesis, posterior C1-3 spanning arthrodesis versus C2-3 posterior arthrodesis using C2 screws across the pars interarticularis fracture, or an anterior C2-3 fusion.[37] Each of these techniques can result in a biomechanically sound stabilization.[38] The type III fracture includes bilateral C2-3 facet dislocation associated most commonly with a type I pars interarticularis fracture pattern (**Figure 7**). Type III fractures require open posterior reduction of the facets with C2-3 posterior fusion. Although the pars fracture could then be treated nonsurgically as would a type I, most surgeon currently perform either C1-3 or a C2-3 posterior fusion, which includes C2 screws across the pars fractures (direct osteosynthesis).

Although most hangman's fractures occur through the pars, there is a variant that involves the posterior aspect of the vertebral body (**Figure 8**). This is an important distinction and should be recognized because of the greater potential for neurologic injury. In the typical hangman's fracture, the vertebral body displaces away from the posterior bony arch, increasing the effective anterior-posterior space available for the spinal cord. In the atypical hangman's fracture variant, however, the posterior aspect of the vertebral body remains with the posterior elements as the anterior portion of the vertebral body displaces forward with C1, effectively narrowing the space available for the spinal cord and placing the cord at greater risk. For this reason, other than type III fractures, atypical hangman's fractures are the

4: Axial Skeleton, Including Spine and Pelvis

only other type in which neurologic deficits are frequently encountered. When the latter fracture pattern is identified, greater consideration should be given to operative stabilization.

Summary

Upper cervical fractures represent a unique subset of spine fractures that must be considered independently with regard to diagnosis and treatment options. The increased use of helical reformatted CT scanning as the primary cervical spine screening tool for trauma has identified more of these fractures, but careful attention must be paid to identifying specific injuries that would otherwise be commonly missed. The greatest advances over the past 5 years have been in improved instrumentation techniques such as the use of C1 lateral mass screws, C2 pedicle screws, and C2 laminar screws that provide greater stability, increased safety, and a wider variety of options for safe instrumentation of the variable upper cervical anatomy. With these new fixation methods, the use of more rigid external fixation such as the halo vest has come into question, especially in elderly patients with odontoid fractures.

Annotated References

1. Aulino JM, Tutt LK, Kaye JJ, Smith PW, Morris JA Jr: Occipital condyle fractures: Clinical presentation and imaging findings in 76 patients. *Emerg Radiol* 2005; 11(6):342-347.

   Seventy-six patients with occipital condyle fractures were identified retrospectively from a trauma database. Sixty of these patients had plain radiographs and none of the occipital condyle fractures could be identified on these films, emphasizing the importance of multiplanar reformatted CT imaging as a trauma screening tool.

2. Maserati MB, Stephens B, Zohny Z, et al: Occipital condyle fractures: Clinical decision rule and surgical management. *J Neurosurg Spine* 2009;11(4):388-395.

   One hundred patients were identified from a level I trauma center database with occipital condyle fractures for an incidence of 0.4%. Two patients presented with occipitocervical malalignment and two had associated upper cervical fractures that warranted immediate occipitocervical arhrodesis. Otherwise they were all treated with hard collar immobilization. None of the 96 patients treated nonsurgically experienced late instability or neurologic deterioration.

3. Bellabarba C, Mirza SK, West GA, et al: Diagnosis and treatment of craniocervical dislocation in a series of 17 consecutive survivors during an 8-year period. *J Neurosurg Spine* 2006;4(6):429-440.

   Seventeen patients over an 8-year period with craniocervical dissociation were reviewed. A delay in diagnosis was common and put the patient at risk for neurologic deterioration.

4. Powers B, Miller MD, Kramer RS, Martinez S, Gehweiler JA Jr: Traumatic anterior atlanto-occipital dislocation. *Neurosurgery* 1979;4(1):12-17.

5. Harris JH Jr, Carson GC, Wagner LK, Kerr N: Radiologic diagnosis of traumatic occipitovertebral dissociation: 2. Comparison of three methods of detecting occipitovertebral relationships on lateral radiographs of supine subjects. *AJR Am J Roentgenol* 1994;162(4): 887-892.

6. Wholey MH, Bruwer AJ, Baker HL Jr: The lateral roentgenogram of the neck; with comments on the atlanto-odontoid-basion relationship. *Radiology* 1958; 71(3):350-356.

7. Botelho RV, de Souza Palma AM, Abgussen CM, Fontoura EA: Traumatic vertical atlantoaxial instability: The risk associated with skull traction. Case report and literature review. *Eur Spine J* 2000;9(5):430-433.

8. Chirossel JP, Passagia JG, Gay E, Palombi O: Management of craniocervical junction dislocation. *Childs Nerv Syst* 2000;16(10-11):697-701.

9. Ben-Galim PJ, Sibai TA, Hipp JA, Heggeness MH, Reitman CA: Internal decapitation: Survival after head to neck dissociation injuries. *Spine* 2008;33(16):1744-1749.

   A retrospective review of 6 patients with occipitocervical dissociation is presented, emphasizing the value of MRI in detecting and characterizing the soft-tissue damage (the main component of this injury pattern).

10. Willauschus WG, Kladny B, Beyer WF, Glückert K, Arnold H, Scheithauer R: Lesions of the alar ligaments. In vivo and in vitro studies with magnetic resonance imaging. *Spine* 1995;20(23):2493-2498.

11. Vaccaro AR, Lim MR, Lee JY: Indications for surgery and stabilization techniques of the occipito-cervical junction. *Injury* 2005;36(suppl 2):B44-B53.

    A thorough review of indications for posterior occipitocervical fusion and techniques that can be used is presented, with advantages and disadvantages for each technique.

12. Jefferson G: Fracture of the atlas vertebra: Report of four cases and a review of those previously recorded. *Br J Surg* 1920;7:407-422.

13. Segal LS, Grimm JO, Stauffer ES: Non-union of fractures of the atlas. *J Bone Joint Surg Am* 1987;69(9): 1423-1434.

14. Levine AM, Edwards CC: Traumatic lesions of the occipitoatlantoaxial complex. *Clin Orthop Relat Res* 1989;239:53-68.

15. AuYong N, Piatt J Jr: Jefferson fractures of the immature spine. Report of 3 cases. *J Neurosurg Pediatr* 2009; 3(1):15-19.

The authors discuss a small cases series of three children with atlas burst-type fractures through the anterior synchondrosis presenting with pain, torticoli, and muscle spasm following a trauma. Care must be taken to recognize the difference between the normal synchodrosis and one that is disrupted.

16. Gebauer M, Goetzen N, Barvencik F, et al : Biomechanical analysis of atlas fractures: A study on 40 human atlas specimens. *Spine* 2008;33(7):766-770.

    Axial loads were applied to 40 cadaver atlas specimens at either a slow fixed rate of speed (0.5 mm/s) or a high rate of speed (300 mm/s), and the only type of fracture produced at the high rate of speed was the three- or four-part Jefferson fractures, whereas the low rate of applied load produced a variety of all of the other fracture types.

17. Dvorak MF, Johnson MG, Boyd M, Johnson G, Kwon BK, Fisher CG: Long-term health-related quality of life outcomes following Jefferson-type burst fractures of the atlas. *J Neurosurg Spine* 2005;2(4):411-417.

    Thirty-four Jefferson fractures were identified retrospectively from a trauma database and administered the Short Form-36 form and American Academy of Orthopaedic Surgeons/North American Spine Society outcome measure at a mean 75-month follow-up. It did not appear that this group of patients returned to preinjury status or normative levels, and those with greater than 7 mm of lateral mass offset did the worst.

18. Esses S, Langer F, Gross A: Fracture of the atlas associated with fracture of the odontoid process. *Injury* 1981; 12(4):310-312.

19. Levine AM, Edwards CC: Treatment of injuries in the C1-C2 complex. *Orthop Clin North Am* 1986;17(1): 31-44.

20. Lipson SJ: Fractures of the atlas associated with fractures of the odontoid process and transverse ligament ruptures. *J Bone Joint Surg Am* 1977;59(7):940-943.

21. Bransford R, Falicov A, Nguyen Q, Chapman J: Unilateral C-1 lateral mass sagittal split fracture: An unstable Jefferson fracture variant. *J Neurosurg Spine* 2009; 10(5):466-473.

    Six patients with displaced unilateral atlas split type fractures were identified from a total of 56 patients with C1 ring fractures in a trauma database. These patients were treated with traction reduction and posterior occipital cervical fusion.

22. Landells CD, Van Peteghem PK: Fractures of the atlas: Classification, treatment and morbidity. *Spine* 1988; 13(5):450-452.

23. Spence KF Jr, Decker S, Sell KW: Bursting atlantal fracture associated with rupture of the transverse ligament. *J Bone Joint Surg Am* 1970;52(3):543-549.

24. Lee C, Woodring JH: Unstable Jefferson variant atlas fractures: An unrecognized cervical injury. *AJNR Am J Neuroradiol* 1991;12(6):1105-1110.

25. Rahimi SY, Stevens EA, Yeh DJ, Flannery AM, Choudhri HF, Lee MR: Treatment of atlantoaxial instability in pediatric patients. *Neurosurg Focus* 2003;15(6):ECP1.

    A retrospective review of 23 pediatric patients with atlantoaxial instability from a variety of trauma causes as well as some nontraumatic causes is presented. Nonsurgical treatment was used in 60.9% with good long-term outcomes.

26. Majercik S, Tashjian RZ, Biffl WL, Harrington DT, Cioffi WG: Halo vest immobilization in the elderly: A death sentence? *J Trauma* 2005;59(2):350-356.

    A retrospective review of 129 patients older than 65 years and 289 patients age 18 to 65 years with cervical spine fractures is presented. The mortality for the elderly group treated in the halo vest was 40%, which was higher than that for patients treated with surgery or a hard collar.

27. Tashjian RZ, Majercik S, Biffl WL, Palumbo MA, Cioffi WG: Halo-vest immobilization increases early morbidity and mortality in elderly odontoid fractures. *J Trauma* 2006;60(1):199-203.

    Seventy-eight elderly patients with cervical spine fractures were reviewed. The reported mortality for those treated with the halo vest was 40% compared to 20% for those who were not treated with a halo vest, and the major complication rates for the halo vest group was 66% compared to 36% in those not treated with a halo vest.

28. Smith HE, Kerr SM, Maltenfort M, et al: Early complications of surgical versus conservative treatment of isolated type II odontoid fractures in octogenarians: A retrospective cohort study. *J Spinal Disord Tech* 2008; 21(8):535-539.

    A multicenter, retrospective review of 72 patients older than 80 years who were neurologically intact with type II odontoid fractures. Thirty-two were treated surgically and 40 nonsurgically. The early morbidity and mortality was high in both groups regardless of treatment but the mortality, morbidity, and length of stay were all statistically higher in the surgical group.

29. Platzer P, Thalhammer G, Sarahrudi K, et al: Nonoperative management of odontoid fractures using a halothoracic vest. *Neurosurgery* 2007;61(3):522-529.

    A review of 90 patients, average age 69 years, with type II odontoid fractures treated with the halo vest is presented. The 84% rate of healing and 75 of 90 patients returning to preinjury functional status were factors supportive of the halo vest as a treatment option.

30. Dailey AT, Hart D, Finn MA, Schmidt MH, Apfelbaum RI: Anterior fixation of odontoid fractures in an elderly population. *J Neurosurg Spine* 2010;12(1):1-8.

    Fifty-seven patients older than 75 years treated with anterior odontoid screw fixation were studied. Fracture union using one screw was 56% and 96% for two screws, supporting two screws in the elderly to increase union rates. However, the incidence of aspiration pneumonia was 19%, and 25% of patients required a postoperative feeding tube.

4: Axial Skeleton, Including Spine and Pelvis

31. Frangen TM, Zilkens C, Muhr G, Schinkel C: Odontoid fractures in the elderly: Dorsal C1/C2 fusion is superior to halo-vest immobilization. *J Trauma* 2007;63(1):83-89.

Twenty-seven patients age 63 to 98 years with type II odontoid fractures were treated with posterior C1-2 fusion. Early mortality was 22.2% (six patients). All but one patient had a stable union, there was one revision for hardware displacement, and all patients reported no or minimal pain.

32. Nourbakhsh A, Shi R, Vannemreddy P, Nanda A: Operative versus nonoperative management of acute odontoid Type II fractures: A meta-analysis. *J Neurosurg Spine* 2009;11(6):651-658.

A meta-analysis of available literature comparing surgical and nonsurgical treatment of odontoid fractures is presented.

33. Shears E, Armitstead CP: Surgical versus conservative management for odontoid fractures. *Cochrane Database Syst Rev* 2008;4:CD005078.

A Cochrane review comparing surgical and nonsurgical treatment of odontoid fractures is presented.

34. Ochoa G: Surgical management of odontoid fractures. *Injury* 2005;36(suppl 2):B54-B64.

A systematic, evidence-based review of the treatment of all types and ages of odontoid fractures is presented.

35. Li XF, Dai LY, Lu H, Chen XD: A systematic review of the management of hangman's fractures. *Eur Spine J* 2006;15(3):257-269.

A systematic review of the treatment of hangman's fractures is presented. The use of hard collars is supported for type I and some type II fractures, but the authors note that rigid external immobilization or surgery is used for more unstable types II, IIa, and III fractures.

36. Vaccaro AR, Madigan L, Bauerle WB, Blescia A, Cotler JM: Early halo immobilization of displaced traumatic spondylolisthesis of the axis. *Spine* 2002;27(20):2229-2233.

37. Ying Z, Wen Y, Xinwei W, et al : Anterior cervical discectomy and fusion for unstable traumatic spondylolisthesis of the axis. *Spine* 2008;33(3):255-258.

A retrospective review of 30 consecutive anterior C2-3 fusions for traumatic spondylolisthesis of the axis is presented. Fusion was achieved with mainteinance of alignment in all cases.

38. Chittiboina P, Wylen E, Ogden A, Mukherjee DP, Vannemreddy P, Nanda A: Traumatic spondylolisthesis of the axis: A biomechanical comparison of clinically relevant anterior and posterior fusion techniques. *J Neurosurg Spine* 2009;11(4):379-387.

A cadaver study re-creating the instability pattern of C2 traumatic spondylolisthesis, then using either posterior screw-rod C1-3 or anterior plate C2-3 instrumentation to restore stability is presented. Both techniques reestablished stability to at least that of the intact specimens and in some instances greater than that of the intact specimen.

Chapter 28

Lower Cervical Spine Injuries

Daniel T. Altman, MD   Robert M. Greenleaf, MD

Introduction

Although subaxial cervical spine injuries (C3 to C7) are relatively uncommon, occurring in only 2% to 3% of blunt trauma patients,[1] they remain the focus of ardent study and debate, given the potential for catastrophic spinal cord injury. Patient morbidity after head and neck trauma is common given the subaxial cervical spine's relative mobility and proximity to vital neurovascular structures. During initial evaluation of the traumatized patient, a cervical injury must be assumed present until definitively ruled out by a combination of history, physical examination, and imaging when necessary. This process of cervical spine "clearance" may vary across institutions as some general guidelines are agreed upon but no concrete protocols established. If an injury is detected, prevention of neurologic deterioration and assurance of spinal stability is crucial. Controversy exists regarding how best to achieve these goals. The areas of greatest controversy and ongoing research, which are the focus of this chapter, include classification systems; the spinal clearance protocol; reduction, imaging, and surgical care of fracture/dislocations; optimal fixation of the unstable cervical spine; timing of surgery; and vertebral artery injuries.

Anatomy

The unique anatomy of the cervical spine, which affords it a wide range of motion, is consequently what predisposes it to injury and instability. Unlike the atlas and axis, the vertebrae of C3-7 are relatively similar in their anatomy and physiology. Longitudinal ligamentous structures, particularly the anterior and posterior longitudinal ligaments (ALL and PLL), ligamentum flavum), and interspinous and supraspinous ligaments serve as restraints on excessive flexion and extension. The ligamentum flavum and the posterior ligamentous complex, along with the facet capsules, are particularly important posterior structures that serve as a tension

band during flexion. Damage to the integrity of these soft-tissue constraints may predispose to chronic pain, kyphosis, and neurologic deterioration.[2] Injuries to these structures are a useful marker for instability. The overall structure of the lower cervical spine is simplified using the concept of an anterior column including the ALL, intervertebral disk/vertebral body, and PLL; and posterior column consisting of the spinal canal, facets and posterior arch, and interspinous ligaments. The facet joints link the posterior elements and are angled approximately 30° in the sagittal plane relative to the transverse plane in a shinglelike pattern.

The vertebral artery enters the transverse foramen within the transverse process of C6 and travels cranially through the atlas, lying anterior to the exiting nerve roots. According to CT and cadaver studies, the artery lies progressively farther from the midline in more caudal areas of the spine, ranging from a distance of approximately 13 mm from the midline more rostrally to approximately 18 mm from midline at C7.[3] The artery is at risk during anterior and posterior approaches to the spine; during posterior hardware placement; and during spinal injuries with vertebral distraction, subluxation, or dislocation or with fractures through the transverse foramen.

Spinal Clearance

Early clearance and discontinuation of the cervical collar is important to avoid associated morbidity, including increased intracranial pressure, pneumonia and deep venous thrombosis, poor feeding, impaired ventilation, decreased or delayed mobilization because of suspicion of cervical injury, and skin ulceration. Delay in collar removal is the greatest risk factor for cervical ulceration.[4]

Initial Evaluation

Subaxial cervical spine trauma offers one of the most precarious situations for the examiner, particularly in obtunded patients. Occult injuries are difficult to detect but may have disastrous ramifications if left undetected. Evaluation begins with obtaining a detailed history to gain insight into the mechanism of injury and level of energy, as well as patient comorbidities, presence of intoxicants, and level of function at the scene of

Dr. Altman or an immediate family member has received research or institutional support from Synthes. Neither Dr. Greenleaf nor an immediate family member has received anything of value from or owns stock in a commercial company or institution related directly or indirectly to the subject of this chapter.

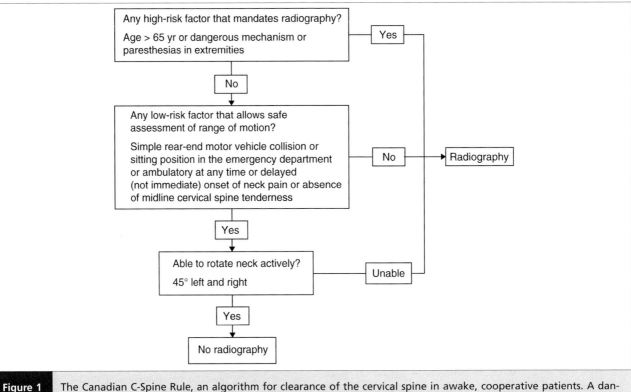

Figure 1 The Canadian C-Spine Rule, an algorithm for clearance of the cervical spine in awake, cooperative patients. A dangerous mechanism is considered to be a fall from an elevation of 3 feet or greater or 5 stairs; an axial load to the head (such as during diving); a motor vehicle collision at high speed (greater than 100 km/h) or with rollover or ejection; a collision involving a motorized recreational vehicle; or a bicycle collision. A simple rear-end motor vehicle collision excludes being pushed into oncoming traffic, being hit by a bus or a large truck, rollover, and being hit by a high-speed vehicle. (Reproduced with permission from Stiell IG, Clement CM, McKnight RD, et al: The Canadian C-Spine Rule versus the NEXUS Low-Risk Criteria in patients with trauma. *N Engl J Med* 2003;349: 2510-2518.)

the accident. Physical examination and initial treatment should follow Advanced Trauma Life Support guidelines. While gentle in-line traction is manually applied to stabilize the neck, the collar should be carefully removed (and subsequently replaced) to palpate the neck for deformity, spinous process splaying, or any other sign of trauma. The entire head should be examined for signs of craniofacial trauma, which may suggest a mechanism of injury. A cervical collar should remain in place throughout the initial evaluation except when critical interventions about the neck are necessary, such as tracheostomy placement or evaluation of penetrating wounds. When such life-saving interventions are required, the collar is removed and in-line traction is maintained.[5]

Imaging

"Clearance" of the cervical spine implies that the evaluator can confidently assume that the spine is unaffected and that continued immobilization or protection is unnecessary.[6] A common scenario where spine clearance is necessary involves the awake, cooperative patient in the acute setting. A protocol combining history and physical examination along with plain radiography has historically been used for clearance. However, the

Canadian C-Spine Rule (CCR) (**Figure 1**) and the National Emergency X-Radiography Utilization Study (NEXUS) Low-Risk Criteria (**Table 1**) are two management guidelines aimed at reducing the unnecessary use of radiography in the spine clearance process. The CCR is slightly more complex but is more sensitive in ruling out injury when directly compared to NEXUS.[7]

Spinal clearance of patients failing any of the above criteria continues to be an area of significant controversy. Adequate imaging becomes paramount in spinal clearance. The most common reason for a missed diagnosis is insufficient imaging.[8] Plain radiography is being used less as a primary radiographic screening tool because of its low sensitivity and the improved efficiency of immediately obtaining other more sensitive studies. Flexion-extension radiographs to rule out occult ligamentous injury have historically been advocated in specific circumstances[9,10] and are still accepted by the Eastern Association for the Surgery of Trauma (EAST) as a viable method of ruling out spinal instability in the nonobtunded patient with cervical pain and no neurologic deficits.[11] Critics of dynamic fluoroscopy[6,12-16] cite the inability of trauma patients to comply, the need for an attending surgeon or physician to perform the maneuvers, poor or inconsistent visualization of

Table 1

NEXUS Low-Risk Criteria* Guideline for cervical spine clearance in awake, cooperative patient. Patients with suspected cervical spine trauma should undergo radiographic evaluation of the cervical spine unless all five criteria are met.

Cervical spine radiography is indicated for patients with trauma unless they meet all of the following criteria:

No posterior midline cervical-spine tenderness*

No evidence of intoxication†

A normal level of alertness‡

No focal neurologic deficit,§ and

No painful distracting injuries.¶

* Midline posterior bony cervical-spine tenderness is present if the patient reports pain on palpation of the posterior midline neck from the nuchal ridge to the prominence of the first thoracic vertebra, or if the patient evinces pain with direct palpation of any cervical spinous process.

† Patients should be considered intoxicated if they have either of the following: a recent history provided by the patient or an observer of intoxication or intoxicating ingestion, or evidence of intoxication on physical examination such as an odor of alcohol, slurred speech, ataxia, dysmetria, or other cerebellar findings, or any behavior consistent with intoxication. Patients may also be considered to be intoxicated if tests of bodily secretions are positive for alcohol or drugs that affect the level of alertness.

‡ An altered level of alertness can include any of the following: Glasgow Coma Scale score of 14 or less; disorientation to person, place, time, or events; an inability to remember three objects at five minutes; a delayed or inappropriate response to external stimuli; or other findings.

§ A focal neurologic deficit is any focal neurologic finding on motor or sensory examination.

¶ No precise definition of a painful distracting injury is possible. This category includes any condition thought by the clinician to be producing pain sufficient to distract the patient from a second (neck) injury. Such injuries may include, but are not limited to, any long-bone fracture; a visceral injury requiring surgical consultation; a large laceration, degloving injury, or crush injury; large burns; or any other injury causing acute functional impairment. Physicians may also classify any injury as distracting if it is thought to have the potential to impair the patient's ability to appreciate other injuries.

(Reproduced with permission from Stiell IG, Clement CM, McKnight RD, et al: The Canadian C-Spine Rule versus the NEXUS Low-Risk Criteria in patients with trauma. *N Engl J Med* 2003;349:2510-2518.)

the skull base and cervicothoracic junction, and one report of iatrogenic quadriplegia during the maneuver.[10]

CT imaging has improved considerably with the advent of faster multislice models. New CT scanners produce extraordinarily detailed images in a matter of seconds, making their use invaluable in the evaluation of acutely injured patients. Although CT scans are more expensive and require more advanced technology and operational skills, CT may ultimately be more cost effective given the high incidence of injuries missed on plain radiographs and subsequently identified with CT.[17-20] Trauma centers are increasingly using CT as first-line imaging in trauma patients who cannot be cleared by history and examination alone.[11] MRI of

discoligamentous structures and other soft tissues, particularly the spinal cord itself, is a useful complement to CT, which has lower sensitivity for soft-tissue injuries.[21] Soft-tissue injuries seen on MRI correspond well with intraoperative findings.[22]

There is general agreement that CT is the gold standard for assessing bony pathology, whereas MRI will identify ligamentous injuries missed on CT. Controversy remains regarding whether the discoligamentous injuries identified by MRI significantly help in assessing for instability and ultimately become a factor in treatment. Those advocating against routine use of MRI cite high costs, inconvenience of transport and long test duration, delay in clearance, and inability to gain clinically useful information.[23-25] Others consider MRI necessary for ruling out instability and guiding treatment decisions, including immobilization requirements and need for surgery.[26-28] Moreover, the primary challenge with the use of MRI as a means of establishing cervical spine stability lies in attempting to correlate the identified soft-tissue injuries to the degree of cervical instability. Protocols for cervical spine clearance vary among institutions; a suggested protocol is illustrated in **Figure 2**.

Lower Cervical Spine Injuries

Injury Classification

The American Spinal Injury Association, which assigns a specific functional grade and score to patients with spinal cord injury, remains widely accepted and has been shown to have good interobserver reliability.[29] Application and documentation of the American Spinal Injury Association classification system from initial evaluation throughout the course of treatment and rehabilitation is important to help determine the course of recovery and the effect of interventions.

Specific to the subaxial cervical spine, a widely used classification system was proposed in 1982 by Allen and Ferguson. This is a mechanism-based system using only static radiographs.[30] Although easy to use and reproducible, this and similar classifications[31] fail to consider ligamentous stability and neurologic injury. The more recent Subaxial Cervical Spine Injury Classification System (SLIC) attempts to overcome the shortcomings of earlier systems by taking fracture morphology, discoligamentous injury, and neurologic injury into account.[32] Within these three components, subclasses based on injury severity are identified and assigned a point score (**Table 2**). This point score is used to help guide treatment and predict outcome. Injuries with a score of less than 4 can typically be treated nonsurgically whereas a score of five or more typically indicates the need for surgical intervention. A score of 4 is intermediate and requires individualized assessment of patient and surgeon factors.[33]

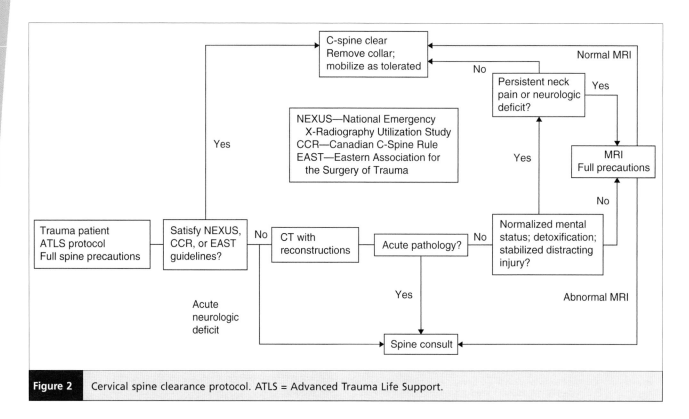

Figure 2 Cervical spine clearance protocol. ATLS = Advanced Trauma Life Support.

Management of Lower Cervical Spine Injuries

Basic Care

In patients with suspected cervical spine injury, strict immobilization with a proper fitting cervical collar is maintained unless the collar is removed to palpate the spine or examine neck or head injuries. It is imperative that a meticulous neurologic examination be performed on initial evaluation to accurately identify and document sensory, motor, and reflex findings as well as gross abnormalities or tenderness on palpation. Subsequent serial examinations will identify progressive neurologic deficits, one of the few acute spinal conditions that may necessitate emergent intervention. In obtunded or uncooperative patients in whom the physical examination is unreliable, treatment decisions rely more on history and mechanism of injury along with radiographic findings.

Reduction of Fracture/Dislocations

Realignment of subaxial spine fracture/dislocations should be achieved as early as possible. However, the timing of reduction in relation to neuroimaging and whether reduction should be performed closed or open in the operating room remain controversial. The risk of causing iatrogenic spinal cord injury during reduction by displacing tissue, such as bone or disk, posteriorly into the spinal canal stems largely from case reports in a heterogeneous group of patients under varying clinical circumstances.[32,34,35] The extremely low risk of spinal cord injury with closed reduction must be weighed

against the need to correct the pressure/deformity on neural tissue caused by the injury and the low likelihood that MRI will provide clinically useful information. In many trauma centers a significant delay in reduction is incurred when obtaining an MRI. Basic science studies have shown that neurologic recovery after injury is directly related to the duration of external compression on the spinal cord.[36] However, clinical confirmation of animal studies suggesting a relationship between timing of decompression and improved neurologic outcome has not been definitively obtained. A recent cohort review showed that timing of reduction did not have a significant impact on long-term outcome. Younger patients with lesser degrees of neurologic injury tend to achieve the best neurologic recovery after a traumatic facet dislocation.[37] It is generally agreed that reduction by trained personnel can safely proceed before MRI in the alert, awake patient with no distracting injury or intoxication regardless of neurologic status.[38,39] There are no reports of permanent neurologic deterioration caused by a herniated disk after closed reduction in the cooperative patient. Further, reduction should occur without delay in any patient with a known complete or high-grade incomplete injury, because immediate reduction poses little additional risk while offering the potential benefits of early neural element realignment/decompression. Researchers recently reported a series of patients with facet dislocations reduced with concurrent MRI. At no time during the reduction did any herniated disk material, even if present before reduction, cause anterior impingement of the cord. Further, overall canal dimensions never decreased

Table 2

SLIC Point System. Injuries are assigned points based on the scale below. An injury with a point total of less than 4 can typically be treated nonsurgically while injuries accruing 5 or more points typically require surgical intervention.

	Points
Morphology	
No abnormality	0
Compression	1
Burst	+1 = 2
Distraction (eg, facet perch, hyperextension)	3
Rotation/translation (eg, facet dislocation, unstable teardrop or advanced staged flexion compression injury)	4
Discoligamentous complex (DLC)	
Intact	0
Indeterminate (eg, isolated interspinous widening, MRI signal change only)	1
Disrupted (eg, widening of disk space, facet perch or dislocation)	2
Neurologic status	
Intact	0
Root injury	1
Complete cord injury	2
Incomplete cord injury	3
Continuous cord compression in setting of neurodeficit (neuromodifier)	+1

(Reproduced with permission from Vaccaro AR, Hulbert RJ, Patel AA, et al: Spine Trauma Study Group: The subaxial cervical spine injury classification system: A novel approach to recognize the importance of morphology, neurology, and integrity of the disco-ligamentous complex. *Spine* 2007;32:2365-2374.)

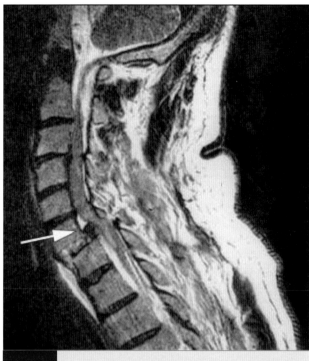

Figure 3   Sagittal T2-weighted MRI demonstrating a large disk fragment behind the body of C6 (*arrow*) in a patient with a facet dislocation. This fragment may be driven posteriorly into the cord during closed reduction; therefore, an anterior approach and diskectomy is necessary prior to reduction. (Reproduced from Kwon BK, Vaccaro AR, Grauer JN, Fisher CG, Dvorak MF: Subaxial cervical spine trauma *J Am Acad Orthop Surg* 2006;14:78-89.)

during the reduction.[40] A similar in vivo study in healthy volunteers showed that cervical traction up to 15 kg significantly increased the area of the neural foramen, decompressing the exiting nerve roots.[41]

The most controversial scenario is the uncooperative or obtunded patient in whom a baseline neurologic examination is not available. A survey of the Spine Trauma Study Group regarding treatment after being presented with similar clinical vignettes resulted in vast disagreement.[42] Those advocating prereduction MRI cited the presence of disk material behind the cephalad vertebral body as an indication to proceed with open reduction.[42] However, interpretation of the MRI is rarely if ever clear-cut, and instead is subjective with no consensus regarding a critical size of disk material or even if disk can be accurately differentiated from hematoma.[43] Currently there is no consensus regarding optimal treatment. It is generally recommended that an un-

cooperative or obtunded patient should receive a prereduction MRI to evaluate the neural elements and search for any potentially offending soft-tissue or bony structures because of the inability to monitor for clinical clues that may help prevent neurologic injury. However, this recommendation is by no means universally agreed upon.

After deciding to proceed with a reduction maneuver, controversy also exists regarding open versus closed reduction. Immediate closed reduction before MRI, assuming trained personnel and monitoring capabilities, is generally indicated in any cooperative patient regardless of neurologic status. Open reduction and decompression is indicated after failed closed reduction (**Figure 3**). Indirect anterior reduction and plate fixation for facet dislocations is gaining popularity and may be particularly valuable when a prereduction MRI shows a large disk herniation behind the cephalad body.[44]

Nonsurgical Care

Common forms of nonsurgical treatment include activity modification alone, soft collars, rigid collars such as Aspen or Miami J collars, cervicothoracic orthoses, and halo vests. Injuries appropriate for nonsurgical treatment include predominantly bony injuries with minimal ligamentous injury and no neurologic compromise. Soft collars offer minimal support and should be reserved for simple muscle strains or stable fractures in elderly patients who may be less able to tolerate a rigid collar or halo. Halo vests cause complications in more than half of patients older than 65 years, including pin-site infections or loosening, respiratory complications, and poor feeding and hygiene.[45]

Surgical Treatment

The inherent instability of the lower cervical spine often makes surgical fixation necessary. Long-term quality of life evaluations are fueling current trends toward surgical treatment of many injuries once thought amenable to nonsurgical treatment. Surgery for lower cervical spine injuries is indicated to prevent progressive deformity or neurologic deterioration or to relieve any nerve root or cord compression. Determining which injuries would benefit from surgery, particularly in the acute setting, is at times difficult.

This difficulty in determining the need for stabilization has been obstructed by the lack of an evidence-based predictive classification system. The SLIC system described earlier provides the most comprehensive subjective analysis to date helping to determine which patients need surgical intervention. The surgeon must next decide which approach and method of fixation are most appropriate to the specific injury.

Anterior Surgery

The anterior Smith-Robinson approach is familiar to most spine surgeons. This approach is associated with low infection rates, convenient supine positioning, and typically less postoperative pain and stiffness compared to posterior approaches. However, the standard anterior approach limits exposure to only a few cervical levels, presents considerable limitations in reaching extreme upper and lower levels while placing more vital structures at risk, and remains associated with a risk of dysphagia and hoarseness.

Biomechanical in vitro evaluation shows that anterior cervical fusion with a wedged graft and a locked plate can confer stability to the cervical spine equal to that of the intact spine after simultaneous anterior and posterior ligamentous disruption.[46] In biomechanical cadaver models of bilateral facet dislocations and burst fractures, anterior fixation alone provides stability equivalent to the intact spine but less than posterior fixation alone or combined anterior and posterior fixation.[47] Whether this increased stability translates into improved fusion rates, less hardware failure, and better patient outcomes remains unknown. An increasing number of both prospective and retrospective human studies with Allen and Ferguson stages I and II flexion/distraction injuries show anterior fixation alone results in good clinical and radiographic outcomes.[48,49] High failure rates of anterior instrumentation alone may oc-

cur with more severe flexion/distraction injuries categorized as Allen and Ferguson stage III/IV.[50]

Anterior subaxial surgery for trauma should achieve three objectives: decompression, reconstruction, and stabilization.

Decompression

Anterior surgery facilitates direct removal of bone or disk material compressing neural elements. In cervical burst fractures, retropulsed bone fragments are removed via corpectomy. Diskectomy removes traumatic disk herniations or disk material seen on MRI that could compress the cord if driven posteriorly by the displaced vertebral body during reduction.

Anterior Column Reconstruction

Reconstruction after diskectomy may be achieved with polyethyletherketone spacers, allograft, titanium cages, or iliac crest bone graft (ICBG). Corpectomy of one or more vertebrae may be reconstructed with ICBG, fibular strut allograft, or titanium cages (fixed or expandable.) Because of the morbidity associated with ICBG harvest and the relative equivalency of other techniques, ICBG usage is becoming less prevalent.

Anterior Stabilization

Anterior midline plating is routinely used to stabilize anterior column reconstructive efforts. Anterior dynamic plating may seem attractive as a means of providing increased load sharing and, theoretically, higher fusion rates. However, in trauma situations, rigid locked plating is still preferred for preventing progressive kyphosis. Although fusion rates are similar between locked and dynamic plating in the nontraumatic setting, there is no conclusive evidence to support the use of dynamic plating in acute trauma.[51]

Posterior Surgery

The posterior approach to lower cervical spine injuries is a straightforward and convenient means for accessing all spine levels. The posterior approach is associated with increased infection rates, pain, stiffness, and the risks of prone positioning. Posterior fixation can be achieved using wiring techniques, lateral mass screw/plates, or lateral mass or pedicle screws/rods constructs. Wiring, though less costly, provides inferior rigidity and cannot be used with posterior arch injury or deformity. Posterior plating has lost popularity in favor of screw/rod constructs because the fixed screw hole location in the plate can hinder optimal screw positioning and because screw-rod constructs offer a more rigid fixed-angle construct.[52] Pedicle screw fixation has shown superior fixation compared to lateral mass screws at all levels.[53,54] However, pedicle screw placement is more technically demanding and places local neurovascular structures at higher risk, especially with traumatized or deformed anatomy.[53] A large meta-analysis suggests that accuracy of pedicle screw placement may be increased from 90% to 95% with naviga-

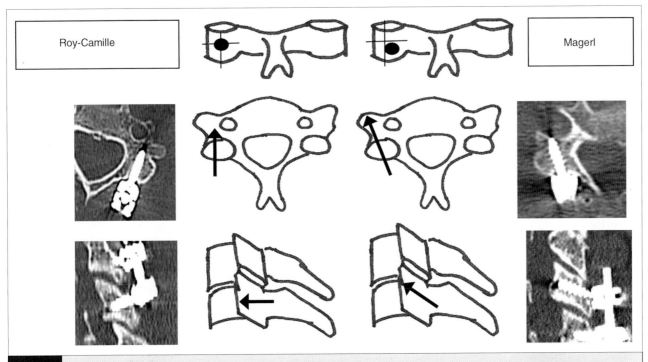

Figure 4 Modifications of the Roy-Camille technique. Magerl and others modified the Roy-Camille technique for posterior lateral mass screw insertion by using a more inferomedial starting point and aiming 15° to 30° superolaterally. The two center columns of diagrams illustrate differences in screw starting point (*black dots*) and trajectory (*arrows*) of the two techniques.

tional assistance such as two-dimensional fluoroscopy or three-dimensional imaging such as CT guidance.[55]

Lateral mass screw fixation of C3-7 has undergone subtle changes since Roy-Camille's original description. Subsequent modifications to this technique, particularly Magerl's technique, mainly involve a more medial and/or inferior starting point allowing for a more superolateral screw trajectory[52] (**Figure 4**). When compared to Roy-Camille's method, these techniques allow for greater screw length, greater pullout strength, and less facet joint disruption.[52,56] Screw lengths can be assessed on preoperative sagittal CT and in general are greater in males and at levels C3-6, and show minimal correlation with anthropometric measurements including stature, body weight, and neck length.[56]

Combined Anterior and Posterior Surgery

Improvements in instrumentation techniques have decreased the need for combined approaches in patients with subaxial trauma. Circumstances that should be considered when combining anterior and posterior surgery are those in which the patient has pathologic bone, ankylosing spondylitis, or unstable fracture-dislocations, or when stabilization is needed at the cervicothoracic junction. The initial approach is often dictated by the specific injury or patient comorbidities. For example, in severe fracture-dislocations in which there is anterior cord compromise from bone or disk material, the anterior approach should usually be performed first.

Treatment of Specific Injuries

Most subaxial cervical spine injuries can be classified morphologically as compression or burst, distraction, or translational or rotational injuries.

Compression-Burst Fractures

These axial load injuries without vertebral translation or discoligamentous injury may or may not be associated with neurologic deficit. If retropulsed bone causing cord compression and neurologic deficits is present, then an anterior decompressive corpectomy and strut graft/plate stabilization is used. Neurologically intact patients with minimally displaced compression or burst fractures can be offered nonsurgical treatment with external immobilization. They should be followed closely for progressive deformity or deterioration. Nondisplaced lateral mass fractures without any signs of translation of one vertebral body on the next result from lateral compression and can be treated nonsurgically.

Distraction Injuries

These injuries may occur from hyperextension in the spondylotic spine resulting in avulsion fractures of anterior osteophytes and anterior disk space widening, or as the result of hyperflexion leading to facet subluxation. Distraction injuries have in common some degree of discoligamentous disruption. If there is an associated fracture with a subluxation, these injuries become translational injuries. A unilateral or bilateral sublux-

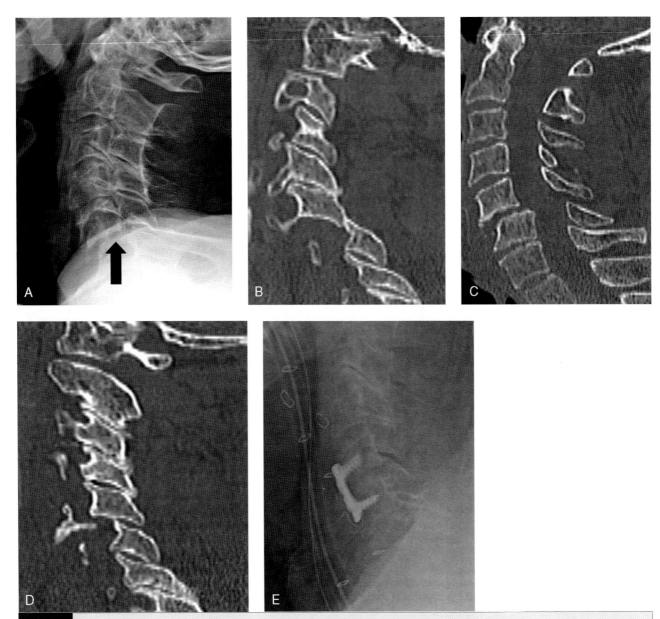

Figure 5 Unilateral facet dislocation. **A,** Lateral radiograph showing anterolisthesis of C5 on C6 (*arrow*). **B,** Parasagittal CT of jumped C5 facet without evidence of fracture. **C,** Midsagittal CT with approximately 25% C5 vertebral body subluxation. **D,** Contralateral parasagittal CT shows mild C5-6 facet joint subluxation. **E,** The patient was awake and neurologically intact, so a closed reduction was followed by a C5-6 anterior cervical diskectomy and fusion with plate instrumentation.

ation or perched facet is a common flexion/distraction injury that infers damage to the posterior stabilizing ligaments and facet capsule. In the alert and cooperative patient, immediate closed reduction may be attempted followed by MRI. The MRI results, combined with neurologic status, will determine the surgical approach. Treatment can proceed with either posterior reduction and instrumented fusion or anterior reduction, decompression, and fusion. If closed reduction is attempted and unsuccessful, a preoperative MRI should be obtained. In the obtunded patient, MRI should precede reduction attempts. If it is determined that there is

a risk of displacing bone or disk material posteriorly into the cord, then anterior decompression, open reduction, and fusion are indicated. In rare circumstances, if an open anterior approach fails, a posterior open reduction is necessary with both anterior and posterior fusion.

Translation/Rotation

This pattern is characterized by horizontal displacement of one vertebral body on another, implying disruption to both anterior and posterior stabilizing structures. Included are unilateral and bilateral facet

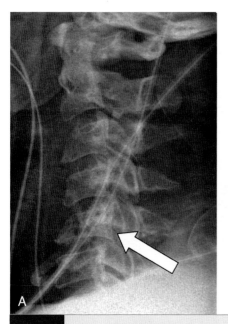
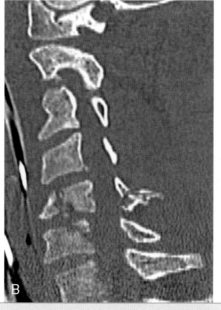
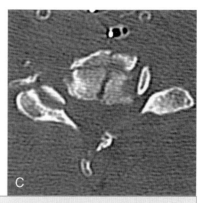

4: Axial Skeleton, Including Spine and Pelvis

Figure 6 **A,** Lateral radiograph showing a C5 burst fracture with posterior vertebral body translation into the spinal canal (*arrow*). **B,** Sagittal CT scan demonstrating a C5 quadrangular fracture. This is a fracture/dislocation with translation and concomitant posterior element involvement. **C,** Axial CT shows a classic coronal shear with a sagittal split through the remaining posterior vertebral body.

dislocations or fracture-dislocations (**Figure 5**), fracture separation of the lateral mass, and vertebral flexion teardrop fractures (also known as burst fracture-dislocations). Unilateral or bilateral facet fracture-dislocation/subluxations are unstable vertebral translational or rotational injuries with inevitable discoligamentous injury and often neurologic injury. Initial treatment should proceed with appropriately timed reduction and MRI. The concomitant bony integrity of the anterior and middle column is an important determinant of surgical treatment. Simple end plate or compression fractures need not be addressed anteriorly and may be stabilized with either approach.

Teardrop Fracture

Also known as a quadrangular fracture, these translational burst fracture/dislocations are unstable and frequently associated with cord injury. Classically, there is a large sagittal shear fragment and a coronal split posteriorly through the remaining vertebral body (**Figure 6**). Anterior and posterior discoligamentous injury is typical, resulting in retropulsion of the remaining posterior vertebral body and various posterior column fractures. In-line traction to decompress the spinal cord and MRI are recommended. Because of anterior compressive injury with instability combined with posterior instability, these injuries typically require 360° of fusion, with anterior corpectomy and interbody reconstruction followed by posterior stabilization. Teardrop fractures should be differentiated from simple avulsion teardrop fractures, which are anteroinferior vertebral body fractures from extension injuries.

Lateral Mass Separations

Displaced lateral mass separations, or floating lateral mass injuries, imply fractures through the pedicle and lamina (**Figure 7**). These injuries are often associated with nerve root injury and have worse outcomes with conservative treatment compared to other isolated lateral mass fractures. The floating lateral mass is highly unstable and may lead to translational or rotational instability of the two adjacent motion segments. This unstable segment should be spanned with either a two-level anterior cervical diskectomy and fusion or three-level posterior instrumentation.[57]

Associated Injuries and Conditions

Central Cord Syndrome

Growth of an active, elderly population with hyperextension injuries in spondylotic cervical spines has led to an increase in central cord syndrome seen acutely in trauma centers. Treatment is largely dictated by neurologic status. If the physical examination indicates that neurologic status is stable or improving, nonsurgical treatment with external immobilization is recommended. If there is persistent cord compression upon examination, surgical decompression is appropriate. The surgical approach is dictated by alignment and the number of levels involved. Laminectomy or laminoplasty can be performed with multilevel compression in a normal or lordotic spine, whereas kyphotic deformity requires an anterior approach and either multiple diskectomies or corpectomy with grafting.

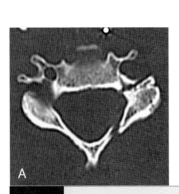
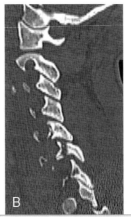
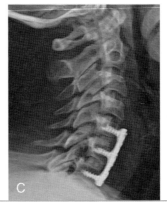
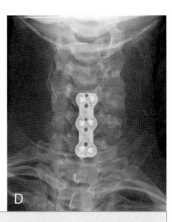

| Figure 7 | Lateral mass separation. **A**, Axial CT showing fractures through the ipsilateral pedicle and lamina of C6, creating a floating lateral mass. **B**, Sagittal CT showing a vertically oriented fracture at the lateral mass/pedicle junction and subluxation of the C6-7 facet joint. **C** and **D**, Postoperative lateral and AP radiographs showing two-level anterior cervical diskectomy and fusion with plating. |

Vertebral Artery Injury

A potential complication associated with lower cervical spine injuries and an area of controversy is vertebral artery injury. The reported incidence is as high as 19%, resulting from nonpenetrating cervical spine trauma.[58] No consensus exists regarding who should be screened for vertebral artery injury or what screening method is most cost-effective. Angiography is the gold standard imaging study but is invasive and carries a small risk of stroke, whereas CT angiogram and magnetic resonance angiography are increasingly popular noninvasive methods. Irreversible vertebral arterial injuries are more common in distraction injuries versus compression injuries and in fractures extending into the transverse foramen.[59,60] Of the fractures extending into the transverse foramen, comminution and fractures at consecutive spinal levels are associated with higher risks for vertebral artery injury and should be imaged.[60] The American Association of Neurological Surgeons 2001 (www.aans.org/shared_pdfs/TraumaGuideline.pdf) clinical guidelines state that insufficient evidence exists to support standards or guidelines for either the diagnosis or treatment of these injuries. Anticoagulation treatment was recommended in patients with evidence of a posterior fossa stroke. There are few data guiding the optimal medical treatment of patients with traumatic vertebral artery injury but no signs of ischemia.

Ankylosing Spondylitis

Ankylosing spondylitis is a systemic inflammatory condition leading to a rigid, kyphotic, osteoporotic cervical spine. The ankylosing spondylitis spine has a long, brittle lever arm, often unable to withstand low energy forces. This results in extension-type fractures that commonly occur through the disk space because of incomplete ossification of the nucleus pulposus[61] (**Figure 8**). A 35% mortality rate is associated with cervical fractures in the patient with ankylosing spondylitis.[62]

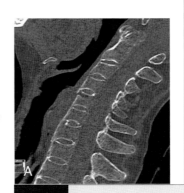
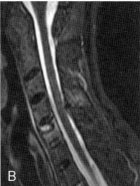

| Figure 8 | Three-column hyperextension injury in a patient with ankylosing spondylitis. A, Fracture near the C4-5 disk space with extension posteriorly. B, Short-tau inversion recovery MRI showing prevertebral and C4-5 disk space edema, edema in the posterior elements, and a posterior epidural hematoma. |

Care should be taken to immobilize the spine as close as possible to the patient's native kyphotic position, because in-line traction or application of a hard collar will typically result in relative extension and could cause catastrophic injury. A high level of suspicion for noncontiguous spine injury should be maintained and imaging of the entire spine should be done. Surgery may be complicated by increased epidural bleeding, osteoporotic bone, and long fused segments with deformity.[63] Posterior pedicle or lateral mass screw/rod fixation should be attempted several levels above and below the injury.[64,65]

Timing of Surgery

The timing of surgical treatment of lower cervical spine injuries remains controversial. With incomplete injuries, urgent reduction is important either before or after obtaining an MRI. Worsening neurologic deficit is an indication for emergent decompression. Animal studies have shown that early decompression (30 minutes to 6 hours) improved neurologic outcomes.[36,66] It was again demonstrated in animal studies that decompression by 6 hours improved outcomes, regardless of whether or not steroids were administered.[67] However, discordance exists between animal and human studies because it typically is not feasible to decompress an acute spinal cord injury in less than 6 hours from injury and certainly not by 30 minutes. Human studies reflect this disparity, as most categorize "early" decompression to be less than 24 to 72 hours. Numerous studies comparing decompression before and after 72 hours found no significant difference in long-term outcome[68,69] Decompression by 24 hours was found to benefit neurologic recovery in patients with incomplete injury.[70] A recent meta-analysis also suggests that decompression within 24 hours benefits patients with incomplete cord injuries, especially those with progressive deficits, and can be done safely with low risk of iatrogenic injury. Further, it suggests that duration of intensive care unit stay and associated medical complications are reduced with early decompression.[71] A retrospective study also showed decreased length of hospital stay with early (less than 48 hours) surgical fixation of spinal injury but also noted a significantly increased mortality in this subgroup.[72] No human study has shown early decompression to alter outcomes in patients with complete spinal cord injury.

Summary

Cervical spine injury must be suspected in high-energy trauma, especially to the head and neck region. CT scans are increasingly being used as the primary screening modality. However, identification of fractures or malalignment alone may not assess discoligamentous injuries or ultimate stability. Classification of these injuries is still varied and nonstandardized.

Management of lower cervical spine injuries is based on proper identification and understanding of biomechanics as well as neurologic status. Early closed reduction of fracture-dislocations in the awake, cooperative patient is supported by the literature. Newer instrumentation such as anterior locking plates and cages has allowed more anterior stabilizing procedures. Severe fracture patterns or translational injuries are still best managed with circumferential fusion.

Annotated References

1. Lowery DW, Wald MM, Browne BJ, et al: Epidemiology of cervical spine injury victims. *Ann Emerg Med* 2001;38(1):12-16.

2. Albert TJ, Vacarro A: Postlaminectomy kyphosis. *Spine* 1998;23(24):2738-2745.

3. Heary RF, Albert TJ, Ludwig SC, et al: Surgical anatomy of the vertebral arteries. *Spine* 1996;21(18):2074-2080.

4. Ackland HM, Cooper DJ, Cooper JD, Malham GM, Kossmann T: Factors predicting cervical collar-related decubitus ulceration in major trauma patients. *Spine* 2007;32(4):423-428.

   The authors performed a retrospective review of 299 level 1 trauma patients, with 29 patients (9.7%) developing an ulceration. Clinically significant predictors of ulceration were intensive care unit admission, mechanical ventilation, need for cervical MRI, and time to cervical spine clearance. Level of evidence: IV.

5. Medzon R, Rothenhaus T, Bono CM, Grindlinger G, Rathlev NK: Stability of cervical spine fractures after gunshot wounds to the head and neck. *Spine* 2005; 30(20):2274-2279.

   A restrospective chart review of 81 patients suffering gunshot wounds to the neck area is presented. An effort was made to predict risk factors for unstable spine injuries necessitating stricter immobilization. Neurologically intact patients have a lower rate of fracture than those presenting with a spinal cord injury or altered mental status. Level of evidence: IV.

6. Shen HX, Li M: Cervical spine clearance in obtunded patients after severe polytrauma. *Chin J Traumatol* 2009;12(3):157-161.

   The authors discuss controversies in cervical spine clearance in obtunded trauma patients. They recommend increased utilization of advanced imaging techniques such as CT and MRI and provide an algorithmic approach. Level of evidence: IV.

7. Stiell IG, Clement CM, McKnight RD, et al: The Canadian C-spine rule versus the NEXUS low-risk criteria in patients with trauma. *N Engl J Med* 2003;349(26): 2510-2518.

8. Levi AD, Hurlbert RJ, Anderson P, et al: Neurologic deterioration secondary to unrecognized spinal instability following trauma—a multicenter study. *Spine* 2006; 31(4):451-458.

   The authors present a multicenter retrospective review identifying 24 patients suffering neurologic deterioration after a missed unstable cervical spine injury. The most common reason for the missed injury was insufficient imaging studies (58.3%), whereas only 33.3% were a result of misread radiographs or 8.3% poor quality radiographs. Older age and high-energy mechanism of injury were also risk factors for missed neurologic injury. Level of evidence: IV.

9. Davis JW, Kaups KL, Cunningham MA, et al: Routine evaluation of the cervical spine in head-injured patients with dynamic fluoroscopy: A reappraisal. *J Trauma* 2001;50(6):1044-1047.

10. Sees DW, Rodriguez Cruz LR, Flaherty SF, Ciceri DP: The use of bedside fluoroscopy to evaluate the cervical spine in obtunded trauma patients. *J Trauma* 1998; 45(4):768-771.

11. Como JJ, Diaz JJ, Dunham CM, et al: Practice management guidelines for identification of cervical spine injuries following trauma: Update from the eastern association for the surgery of trauma practice management guidelines committee. *J Trauma* 2009;67(3):651-659.

    This article discusses changes in practice since the publication of the previous cervical spine injury guidelines.

12. Anekstein Y, Jeroukhimov I, Bar-Ziv Y, et al: The use of dynamic CT surview for cervical spine clearance in comatose trauma patients: A pilot prospective study. *Injury* 2008;39(3):339-346.

    The authors sought to use multiple CT surviews, or "scout films," in the CT scanner in flexion and extension to serve as dynamic imaging to help rule out instability. They also suggest that if the occipitocervical or cervicothoracic junction is still not adequately visualized, sagittal reconstruction CT cuts of this area can be conveniently obtained. Level of evidence: II.

13. Anglen J, Metzler M, Bunn P, Griffiths H: Flexion and extension views are not cost-effective in a cervical spine clearance protocol for obtunded trauma patients. *J Trauma* 2002;52(1):54-59.

14. Bolinger B, Shartz M, Marion D: Bedside fluoroscopic flexion and extension cervical spine radiographs for clearance of the cervical spine in comatose trauma patients. *J Trauma* 2004;56(1):132-136.

    The authors compared flexion-extension views to CT in 56 comatose trauma patients. Flexion-extension radiographs allowed adequate visualization of the entire cervical spine in only 4% of patients, leading to the recommendation against dynamic radiographs in comatose patients. Level of evidence: IV.

15. Padayachee L, Cooper DJ, Irons S, et al: Cervical spine clearance in unconscious traumatic brain injury patients: Dynamic flexion-extension fluoroscopy versus computed tomography with three-dimensional reconstruction. *J Trauma* 2006;60(2):341-345.

    The authors present a retrospective review comparing results of dynamic fluoroscopy versus CT with reconstructions in 276 trauma patients. Dynamic flexion-extension radiographic studies with fluoroscopy delayed cervical spine clearance and were almost always reported as normal. In a cervical spine clearance protocol for unconscious traumatic brain injury patients, dynamic flexion-extension radiographic studies with fluoroscopy did not identify any patients with cervical fracture or instability not already identified by plain radiographs and fine-cut CT (C0 to T2) with three-dimensional reconstructions. Level of evidence: IV.

16. Sliker CW, Mirvis SE, Shanmuganathan K: Assessing cervical spine stability in obtunded blunt trauma patients: Review of medical literature. *Radiology* 2005; 234(3):733-739.

    A literature review of dynamic fluoroscopy and MRI in obtunded trauma patients is presented. The authors state that the current medical literature provide no clear evidence of the superiority of either MRI or dynamic fluoroscopy in the diagnosis of unstable ligamentous injury, although other relative advantages of MR imaging indicate that it is preferred for assessing cervical spine stability in obtunded blunt trauma patients. Level of evidence: II.

17. Daffner RH: Helical CT of the cervical spine for trauma patients: A time study. *AJR Am J Roentgenol* 2001; 177(3):677-679.

18. Grogan EL, Morris JA Jr, Dittus RS, et al: Cervical spine evaluation in urban trauma centers: Lowering institutional costs and complications through helical CT scan. *J Am Coll Surg* 2005;200(2):160-165.

    A cost-minimization study was performed using decision analysis examining helical CT scan versus radiographic evaluation of the c-spine. Parameter estimates were obtained from the literature for probability of c-spine injury, probability of paralysis after missed injury, plain film sensitivity and specificity, CT scan sensitivity and specificity, and settlement cost of missed injuries resulting in paralysis. Level of evidence: II.

19. Rybicki F, Nawfel RD, Judy PF, et al: Skin and thyroid dosimetry in cervical spine screening: Two methods for evaluation and a comparison between a helical CT and radiographic trauma series. *AJR Am J Roentgenol* 2002;179(4):933-937.

20. McCulloch PT, France J, Jones DL, et al: Helical computed tomography alone compared with plain radiographs with adjunct computed tomography to evaluate the cervical spine after high-energy trauma. *J Bone Joint Surg Am* 2005;87(11):2388-2394.

    The authors performed a prospective evaluation comparing both plain radiographs (three views) and CT in 407 trauma patients, 58 of whom ultimately had injuries. No injuries were detected on radiographs. Level of evidence: I.

21. Diaz JJ Jr, Aulino JM, Collier B, et al: The early work-up for isolated ligamentous injury of the cervical spine: Does computed tomography scan have a role? *J Trauma* 2005;59(4):897-903.

    A prospective consecutive series in trauma patients undergoing plain radiographs, helical CT, and MRI is presented. CT is the most sensitive, specific, and cost-effective modality for screening the cervical spine bony injuries, but is inferior to MRI screening for cervical ligamentous injury. The indications for MRI include abnormalities on CT, neurologic deficits, cervical pain or tenderness on examination, or the inability to clear the cervical spine in the obtunded patient. Level of evidence: II.

22. Goradia D, Linnau KF, Cohen WA, Mirza S, Hallam DK, Blackmore CC: Correlation of MR imaging findings with intraoperative findings after cervical spine trauma. *AJNR Am J Neuroradiol* 2007;28(2):209-215.

    Intraoperative findings in 31 consecutive patients with

subaxial cervical spine injuries are compared to preoperative MR findings. Level of evidence: IV.

23. Horn EM, Lekovic GP, Feiz-Erfan I, Sonntag VK, Theodore N: Cervical magnetic resonance imaging abnormalities not predictive of cervical spine instability in traumatically injured patients: Invited submission from the Joint Section Meeting on Disorders of the Spine and Peripheral Nerves, March 2004. *J Neurosurg Spine* 2004;1(1):39-42.

This retrospective review identifies 70 patients with abnormal MRI after normal plain radiograph and CT studies. No instability requiring treatment was detected only by MRI. Level of evidence: IV.

24. Hogan GJ, Mirvis SE, Shanmuganathan K, Scalea TM: Exclusion of unstable cervical spine injury in obtunded patients with blunt trauma: Is MR imaging needed when multi-detector row CT findings are normal? *Radiology* 2005;237(1):106-113.

The authors compared CT and MRI findings in 366 obtunded trauma patients and determined that a negative multidetector row CT had 100% negative predictive value. Level of evidence: II.

25. Como JJ, Thompson MA, Anderson JS, et al: Is magnetic resonance imaging essential in clearing the cervical spine in obtunded patients with blunt trauma? *J Trauma* 2007;63(3):544-549.

Prospective evaluation following 115 level 1, obtunded, blunt trauma patients who underwent both CT and MRI: 5.2% additional injuries not detcted on the CT were detected on MRI. However, none of these findings changed the patient management while an estimated $250,000 was spent performing MRI. Level of evidence: II.

26. Stassen NA, Williams VA, Gestring ML, Cheng JD, Bankey PE: Magnetic resonance imaging in combination with helical computed tomography provides a safe and efficient method of cervical spine clearance in the obtunded trauma patient. *J Trauma* 2006;60(1):171-177.

The authors present a prospective study evaluating safety and efficacy of an institutional guideline in obtunded trauma patients using CT as initial screening followed by MRI at 72 hours if still obtunded. The authors concluded that CT alone misses a statistically significant number of c-spine injuries. Level of evidence: II.

27. Sarani B, Waring S, Sonnad SS, Schwab CW: Magnetic resonance imaging is a useful adjunct in the evaluation of the cervical spine of injured patients. *J Trauma* 2007; 63(3):637-640.

The authors present a retrospective review of 53 obtunded trauma patients undergoing both CT and MRI. The frequency of injury missed by CT and consequent treatment changes is evaluated. In the unexaminable cohort, MRI detected an injury in 5 of 46 patients whose CT scan disclosed nothing abnormal; 4 of these injuries were ligamentous and were treated by cervical collar immobilization. Level of evidence: IV.

28. Menaker J, Philp A, Boswell S, Scalea TM: Computed tomography alone for cervical spine clearance in the unreliable patient—are we there yet? *J Trauma* 2008; 64(4):898-903.

A retrospective review of 203 obtunded patients receiving both a normal CT and MRI is presented. New findings on the MR after CT changed management in 7.9% of patients. Level of evidence: IV.

29. Savic G, Bergström EM, Frankel HL, Jamous MA, Jones PW: Inter-rater reliability of motor and sensory examinations performed according to American Spinal Injury Association standards. *Spinal Cord* 2007;45(6): 444-451.

The authors examine interrater reliability of motor and sensory examinations performed according to American Spinal Injury Association standards.

30. Allen BL Jr, Ferguson RL, Lehmann TR, O'Brien RP: A mechanistic classification of closed, indirect fractures and dislocations of the lower cervical spine. *Spine* 1982; 7(1):1-27.

31. Harris JH, Edeiken-Monroe B, Kopansiky DR: A practical classification of acute cervical spine injuries. *Orthop Clin North Am* 1986;17(1):15-30.

32. Ludwig SC, Vaccaro AR, Balderston RA, Cotler JM: Immediate quadriparesis after manipulation for bilateral cervical facet subluxation: A case report. *J Bone Joint Surg Am* 1997;79(4):587-590.

33. Vaccaro AR, Hulbert RJ, Patel AA, et al; Spine Trauma Study Group: The subaxial cervical spine injury classification system: A novel approach to recognize the importance of morphology, neurology, and integrity of the disco-ligamentous complex. *Spine* 2007;32(21):2365-2374.

The authors present a novel classification system grading and assigning points to injury morphology, discoligamentous stability, and neurologic status. The point total is used to guide treatment. Comparisons are made to existing classification systems. Level of evidence: IV.

34. Eismont FJ, Arena MJ, Green BA: Extrusion of an intervertebral disc associated with traumatic subluxation or dislocation of cervical facets: Case report. *J Bone Joint Surg Am* 1991;73(10):1555-1560.

35. Wimberley DW, Vaccaro AR, Goyal N, et al: Acute quadriplegia following closed traction reduction of a cervical facet dislocation in the setting of ossification of the posterior longitudinal ligament: Case report. *Spine* 2005;30(15):E433-E438.

This case report highlights the advantages and shows some safety concerns regarding immediate, closed traction reduction of cervical facet dislocation with real-time neural monitoring in an awake, alert, oriented, and appropriately selected patient before MRI studies in the setting of preexisting central stenosis from ossification of the posterior longitudinal ligament. Level of evidence: IV.

36. Delamarter RB, Sherman J, Carr JB: Pathophysiology of

spinal cord injury: Recovery after immediate and delayed decompression. *J Bone Joint Surg Am* 1995;77(7): 1042-1049.

37. Greg Anderson D, Voets C, Ropiak R, et al: Analysis of patient variables affecting neurologic outcome after traumatic cervical facet dislocation. *Spine J* 2004;4(5): 506-512.

A retrospective study of 45 patients sustaining traumatic cervical facet dislocation is presented. Using improvement (American Spinal Injury Association) motor score as the primary outcome measure, patient data were used to construct a statistical model designed to analyze the contribution of variables such as age, gender, time to reduction of the spine and initial motor score to neurologic improvement. In addition, the effect of variable interaction was studied.

38. Grant GA, Mirza SK, Chapman JR, et al: Risk of early closed reduction in cervical spine subluxation injuries. *J Neurosurg* 1999;90(suppl 1)13-18.

39. Vaccaro AR, Falatyn SP, Flanders AE, Balderston RA, Northrup BE, Cotler JM: Magnetic resonance evaluation of the intervertebral disc, spinal ligaments, and spinal cord before and after closed traction reduction of cervical spine dislocations. *Spine* 1999;24(12):1210-1217.

40. Darsaut TE, Ashforth R, Bhargava R, et al: A pilot study of magnetic resonance imaging-guided closed reduction of cervical spine fractures. *Spine* 2006;31(18): 2085-2090.

In a prospective study of 17 patients with fracture-dislocations of the subaxial cervical spine, the fractures were reduced under MRI guidance. The incidence of posteriorly herniated disk material was noted, and the diameter of the spinal canal at the injured level was recorded before and after traction.

41. Liu J, Ebraheim NA, Sanford CG Jr, et al: Quantitative changes in the cervical neural foramen resulting from axial traction: In vivo imaging study. *Spine J* 2008;8(4): 619-623.

An apparatus was created to apply traction to 15 healthy volunteers and measure via MRI increases in foraminal area with 0, 5, 10, and 15 kg.

42. Grauer JN, Vaccaro AR, Lee JY, et al: The timing and influence of MRI on the management of patients with cervical facet dislocations remains highly variable: A survey of members of the Spine Trauma Study Group. *J Spinal Disord Tech* 2009;22(2):96-99.

A questionnaire study in which clinical vignettes, plain radiographs, CT scans, and eventually MRIs of 10 cases of cervical facet dislocation were presented to 25 fellowship trained spine surgeons is discussed. Participants were analyzed as to their next step in diagnosis or treatment. Level of evidence: V.

43. Lee JY, Nassr A, Eck JC, Vaccaro AR: Controversies in the treatment of cervical spine dislocations. *Spine J* 2009;9(5):418-423.

A case series of cervical spine dislocations and a review of the literature is presented regarding the major controversial aspects of the treatment of cervical spine dislocations. Level of evidence: IV.

44. Reindl R, Ouellet J, Harvey EJ, Berry G, Arlet V: Anterior reduction for cervical spine dislocation. *Spine* 2006; 31(6):648-652.

In a retrospective review, eight patients failing closed facet reduction were assessed for rate of successful reduction and stabilization using only the anterior surgical approach; and complications and long-term clinical and radiologic outcome. Level of evidence: IV.

45. Taitsman LA, Altman DT, Hecht AC, Pedlow FX: Complications of cervical halo-vest orthoses in elderly patients. *Orthopedics* 2008;31(5):446.

A retrospective review of 75 halo patients older than 65 years at two level 1 trauma centers is presented. Fifty-five percent of patients experienced at least one complication, with 29% experiencing pin-site complications, 23% respiratory complications, and 8% early mortality. Level of evidence: III.

46. Paxinos O, Ghanayem AJ, Zindrick MR, et al: Anterior cervical discectomy and fusion with a locked plate and wedged graft effectively stabilizes flexion-distraction stage-3 injury in the lower cervical spine: A biomechanical study. *Spine* 2009;34:E9-E15.

Eight specimens were used in an in vitro cadaver study. Range of motion was studied with all structures intact, after ACDF with posterior ligamentous structures intact, and after ACDF with release of all posterior ligamentous structures. There was no significant increase in the range of motion of ACDF plus all ligament released specimens versus control specimens.

47. Kim SM, Lim TJ, Kim DH, et al: A biomechanical comparison of three surgical approaches in bilateral subaxial cervical facet dislocation. *J Neurosurg Spine* 2004;1: 108-115.

Cadavers were used to compare fixation with anterior cervical diskectomy and plating alone versus anterior plating combined with posterior wiring or transpedicular screw-rod constructs. The anterior plating with posterior screw-rod construct was most rigid. Anterior plating alone was more rigid than the intact cadaver, suggesting that this method provides adequate fixation. Level of evidence: III.

48. Dvorak MF, Fisher CG, Aarabi B, et al: Clinical outcomes of 90 isolated unilateral facet fractures, subluxations, and dislocations treated surgically and nonoperatively. *Spine* 2007;32(26):3007-3013.

A retrospective outcomes study evaluated unilateral facet injury data, radiographs, and outcomes (North American Spine Society Cervical Follow-up Questionnaire and Short Form-36) in 90 patients collected from members of the Spine Trauma Study Group. After more than 1 year follow-up, there was more disability in the nonsurgical patients, despite relatively simpler injury patterns.

49. Kwon BK, Fisher CG, Boyd MC, et al: A prospective randomized controlled trial of anterior compared with posterior stabilization for unilateral facet injuries of the cervical spine. *J Neurosurg Spine* 2007;7(1):1-12.

The authors present a randomized prospective study of 42 patients with unilateral facet injuries undergoing ACDF with plating versus posterior fusion and instrumentation. This trial provided level 1 evidence that both the anterior and posterior fixation approaches appear to be valid treatment options. Although statistical significance was not reached in the primary outcome measure, some secondary outcome measures favored anterior fixation and others favored posterior treatment of unilateral facet injuries.

50. Henriques T, Olerud C, Bergman A, Jónsson H Jr: Distractive flexion injuries of the subaxial cervical spine treated with anterior plate alone. *J Spinal Disord Tech* 2004;17(1):1-7.

The authors studied 36 consecutive patients with distractive flexion injuries treated with anterior plate fixation. This method provided adequate stability in stage 1 and 2 injuries but failed in 7 of 13 stage 3 injuries. Level of evidence: IV.

51. Ghahreman A, Rao PJ, Ferch RD: Dynamic plates in anterior cervical fusion surgery: Graft settling and cervical alignment. *Spine* 2009;34(15):1567-1571.

The authors present a retrospective cohort of 55 patients after ACDF using the dynamic plating system. Early settling and loss of lordosis was seen with fusion rates similar to those of locked plating. Level of evidence: III.

52. Wu JC, Huang WC, Chen YC, Shih YH, Cheng H: Stabilization of subaxial cervical spines by lateral mass screw fixation with modified Magerl's technique. *Surg Neurol* 2008;70(suppl 1):25-33.

In a retrospective review of 115 patients receiving modified lateral mass screw placement and rod constructs, fusion occurred in 99%, with no neurovascular injuries or improper screw placements. The most common screw length was 16 mm. Level of evidence: II.

53. Jones EL, Heller JG, Silcox DH, Hutton WC: Cervical pedicle screws versus lateral mass screws: Anatomic feasibility and biomechanical comparison. *Spine* 1997;22(9):977-982.

54. Rhee JM, Kraiwattanapong C, Hutton WC: A comparison of pedicle and lateral mass screw construct stiffnesses at the cervicothoracic junction: A biomechanical study. *Spine* 2005;30(21):E636-E640.

In a cadaver study, the authors compared C7 pedicle screw fixation to lateral mass screw fixation with and without supplemental wiring. C7 pedicle screws provided more rigid fixation than any lateral mass/wiring construct and combined C6-7 lateral mass fixation. Level of evidence: II.

55. Kosmopoulos V, Schizas C: Pedicle screw placement accuracy: A meta-analysis. *Spine* 2007;32(3):E111-E120.

During a meta-analysis of pedicle screw accuracy litera-ture (all levels), an overall accuracy of 91% was calculated. Accuracy without the aid of navigation was 90.3% and 95.2% in the navigation-assisted subgroup. The authors did not discuss specific methods of assisted navigation. Level of evidence: III.

56. Stemper BD, Marawar SV, Yoganandan N, Shender BS, Rao RD: Quantitative anatomy of subaxial cervical lateral mass: An analysis of safe screw lengths for Roy-Camille and Magerl techniques. *Spine* 2008;33(8):893-897.

Bicortical screw lengths were bilaterally measured at each spinal level from C3-C7 in 98 young volunteers using CT reconstructions through the lateral masses obtained in the plane of the screw in Roy-Camille and Magerl techniques. The authors suggest that significant variations exist at each subaxial level and recommend the surgeon determine screw lengths for fixation at each level using preoperative sagittal oblique CT scans. Level of evidence: II.

57. Lee SH, Sung JK: Unilateral lateral mass-facet fractures with rotational instability: New classification and a review of 39 cases treated conservatively and with single segment anterior fusion. *J Trauma* 2009;66(3):758-767.

The authors performed a retrospective review of 39 patients with lateral mass or facet joint fractures. Surgical treatment was superior over nonsurgical with single level ACDF. Separation type often required two-level anterior fusion or posterior pedicle screw fixation. Level of evidence: IV.

58. Giacobetti FB, Vaccaro AR, Bos-Giacobetti MA, et al: Vertebral artery occlusion associated with cervical spine trauma: A prospective analysis. *Spine* 1997;22(2):188-192.

59. Taneichi H, Suda K, Kajino T, Kaneda K: Traumatically induced vertebral artery occlusion associated with cervical spine injuries: Prospective study using magnetic resonance angiography. *Spine* 2005;30(17):1955-1962.

The incidence of traumatically induced vertebral artery occlusion was 17.2%. The potential for blood flow restoration was higher in compressive injuries (secondary to vasospasm rather than dissection) than in distractive injuries. Vertebral artery occlusion was rarely symptomatic. Level of evidence: II.

60. Oetgen ME, Lawrence BD, Yue JJ: Does the morphology of foramen transversarium fractures predict vertebral artery injuries? *Spine* 2008;33(25):E957-E961.

A retrospective review found patients presenting with multilevel foramen transversarium fractures and foramen transversarium fracture comminution to be at significantly increased risk for vertebral artery injury. The study suggested that patients with these fracture patterns should undergo further evaluation with vertebral artery imaging. Level of evidence: II.

61. Graham B, Van Peteghem PK: Fractures of the spine in ankylosing spondylitis: Diagnosis, treatment, and complications. *Spine* 1989;14(8):803-807.

62. Murray GC, Persellin RH: Cervical fracture complicating ankylosing spondylitis: A report of eight cases and review of the literature. *Am J Med* 1981;70(5):1033-1041.

63. Samartzis D, Anderson DG, Shen FH: Multiple and simultaneous spine fractures in ankylosing spondylitis: Case report. *Spine* 2005;30(23):E711-E715.

    The authors present a literature review and case report of a patient with ankylosing spondylitis fracturing adjacent to preexisting internal spine instrumentation.

64. Cornefjord M, Alemany M, Olerud C: Posterior fixation of subaxial cervical spine fractures in patients with ankylosing spondylitis. *Eur Spine J* 2005;14(4):401-408.

    This retrospective review shows optimal rates of healing with long screw-rod fixation systems that allow using both pedicle screws and lateral mass screws. Level of evidence: IV.

65. Caron T, Bransford RJ, Nguyen QT, et al: Spine fractures in patients with ankylosing spinal disorders. *Spine* 2010;35(11):E458-E464.

66. Carlson GD, Gorden CD, Oliff HS, Pillai JJ, LaManna JC: Sustained spinal cord compression: Part I. Time-dependent effect on long-term pathophysiology. *J Bone Joint Surg Am* 2003;85(1):86-94.

67. Rabinowitz RS, Eck JC, Harper CM Jr, et al: Urgent surgical decompression compared to methylprednisolone for the treatment of acute spinal cord injury: A randomized prospective study in beagle dogs. *Spine* 2008;33(21):2260-2268.

    Spinal cord compression was induced in three groups of six beagles. Three different treatments included decompression at 6 hours with steroids, decompression at 6 hours with saline only, and steroids only. The dogs that underwent decompression did better than the steroids-only group, with no significant difference in outcome between the two decompression groups. Level of evidence: II.

68. Vaccaro AR, Daugherty RJ, Sheehan TP, et al: Neurologic outcome of early versus late surgery for cervical spinal cord injury. *Spine* 1997;22(22):2609-2613.

69. Sapkas GS, Papadakis SA: Neurological outcome following early versus delayed lower cervical spine surgery. *J Orthop Surg* 2007;15(2):183-186.

    In a retrospective review, 29 patients were divided into early (less than 72 hours) or late (more than 72 hours) surgery. There was no statistically significant difference in final neurologic outcomes in patients having early as opposed to delayed surgery. Level of evidence: IV.

70. La Rosa G, Conti A, Cardali S, Cacciola F, Tomasello F: Does early decompression improve neurological outcome of spinal cord injured patients? Appraisal of the literature using a meta-analytical approach. *Spinal Cord* 2004;42(9):503-512.

    The authors performed a meta-analysis and concluded that early decompression of patients with incomplete spinal cord injuries resulted in significant clinical improvement over conservative or late treatment. Level of evidence: III.

71. Fehlings MG, Perrin RG: The timing of surgical intervention in the treatment of spinal cord injury: A systematic review of recent clinical evidence. *Spine* 2006;31(suppl 11):S28-S35.

    This evidence-based literature review recommends urgent decompression of bilateral locked facets in a patient with incomplete tetraplegia or in a patient with spinal cord injury with neurologic deterioration. There is emerging evidence that surgery within 24 hours is safe, assuming hemodynamic stability, and may reduce length of intensive care unit stay and reduce postinjury medical complications. Level of evidence: II.

72. Kerwin AJ, Frykberg ER, Schinco MA, et al: The effect of early surgical treatment of traumatic spine injuries on patient mortality. *J Trauma* 2007;63(6):1308-1313.

    The authors present a retrospective review of 361 patients requiring surgical fixation. At final follow-up there was a significantly higher mortality rate seen in patients undergoing surgery in less than 48 hours but also a shorter hospital stay.

Chapter 29

Thoracolumbar Trauma

Richard J. Bransford, MD   Robert A. Morgan, MD

4: Axial Skeleton, Including Spine and Pelvis

Classification

Numerous classification systems are currently in use, with considerable controversy as to which is ideal and which lends itself to better intraobserver agreement and efficacy. A few of the more commonly accepted classification systems include the morphologic description of Denis, the mechanistic classification of Allen and Ferguson, and the AO classification.

Introduced in 2005, the thoracolumbar injury classification and severity score (TLICS) is primarily a scoring system designed to help determine whether nonsurgical or surgical treatment should be performed, based on three general injury characteristics: bony morphology, integrity of the posterior ligamentous complex, and neurologic status. This is the first system to consider the neurologic status of the patient as it pertains to management of the injury. A score of 5 or greater suggests surgical management; a score of 3 or less suggests a conservative approach; and a score of 4 could be treated either way, with other factors contributing to the decision (**Table 1**).

This system has undergone testing and comparisons to other classifications and is gaining popularity. A recent study concluded that, as a management tool, the TLICS seems to be an acceptably reliable system when compared with the Denis and AO systems. A basic level of knowledge and familiarity is necessary for the application of the system at reliable levels.[1] This classification has also demonstrated good interobserver and intraobserver reliability, based on a 2006 study that demonstrated an interrater reliability assessed by generalized kappa coefficients of 0.33 for injury mechanism, 0.91 for neurologic status, 0.35 for posterior ligamentous complex status with 0.29 for TLICS total and 0.52

Dr. Bransford or an immediate family member is a member of a speaker's bureau or has made paid presentations on behalf of AO and Synthes; is a paid consultant to or is an employee of Synthes; and has received research or institutional support from AO, Biomet, Pfizer, Wright Medical Technology, DePuy, Spinevision, Stryker, and Synthes. Dr. Morgan or an immediate family member has received research or institutional support from Synthes and DePuy; and has received nonincome support (such as equipment or services), commercially derived honoraria, or other non–research-related funding (such as paid travel) from Medtronic Sofamor Danek.

for treatment recommendation.[2] Surgeons agreed with the TLICS recommendation 96.4% of the time. Intrarater kappa coefficients were 0.57 for injury mechanism, 0.93 for neurologic status, 0.48 for posterior ligamentous complex status, 0.46 for TLICS total, and 0.62 for treatment recommendation. The authors concluded that TLICS is reliable and compares favorably to other contemporary thoracolumbar fracture classification systems.[2] The Denis and AO classifications have demonstrated only moderate reliability and repeatability. The AO classification was fairly reproducible, with an average kappa of 0.48 for the agreement regarding the assignment of the three primary types and an average kappa coefficient of 0.54 for the agreement regarding the nine subtypes. The average kappa coefficient for the agreement regarding the assignment of the four Denis fracture types was 0.61, and it was 0.17 for agreement regarding the 16 subtypes.[3] Thus, the TLICS adds a new dimension to previous classifications, focusing on neurologic injury and the posterior ligamentous complex, and appears to be a useful guide in helping to direct treatment.

Role of Bracing

Historically, braces have been a mainstay in the management of all types of thoracolumbar fractures, either as a stand-alone treatment or as an adjunct to surgical management. Braces range from simple corsets to Jewett type hyperextension braces, soft overlap braces, and rigid thoracolumbosacral orthoses with or without thigh and/or cervical extensions. Interestingly, there are numerous articles on the various bracing types and the utility of each from a biomechanical standpoint for different locations within the spine; however, the real efficacy and utility of such postural aids has not been well proven in comparative studies. Increasingly, the question has been raised as to whether braces really have any impact on the natural history of thoracolumbar fractures as an isolated management choice or as an aid to surgical stabilization.

With progressively more severe injuries, clinicians are more likely to want to provide some type of support for pain control and to prevent further deformity. In a retrospective study of 178 patients, two methods for treating patients with compression as great as 30% were compared: early ambulation with and without

Table 1

Thoracolumbar Injury Classification and Severity Score

	Points
Injury morphology	
No abnormality	0
Compression	1
Burst	+1 = 2
Translational injury	3
Distraction injury	4
Integrity of posterior ligamentous complex	
intact	0
Indeterminate (eg, isolated interspinous widening, MRI signal change only)	2
Disrupted (eg, widening of disk space, facet perch or dislocation)	3
Neurologic status	
Intact	0
Root injury	1
Complete spinal cord injury	2
Incomplete spinal cord injury	3
Cauda equina injury	3

Injuries are assigned points based on the scale above. An injury with a point total of less than 4 can typically be treated nonsurgically while injuries accruing 5 or more points typically require surgical intervention.Injuries with scores of 4 can be treated surgically or nonsurgically based on patient- and surgeon- related factors. (Reproduced with permission from Vaccaro AR, et al: A new classification of thoracolumbar injuries: The importance of injury morphology, the integrity of the posterior ligamentous complex, and neurologic status. *Spine* 2005;15;30: 2325-2333.)

lumbar orthosis. Results showed that although demographic variables, type of injury, and cause of injury were similar between the groups, neither treatment emerged as superior.[4] A similar study in 124 patients also demonstrated a lack of improvement with braces compared to no brace.[5]

Although final data are still being collected and analyzed, there are currently prospective randomized trials comparing braces to no brace in nonsurgically managed thoracolumbar fractures. Early data suggest no efficacy of bracing and no change in any measurable parameters suggestive of a benefit to bracing.

A recent systematic review used an electronic search strategy with extensive headings to identify studies that compared bracing and nonbracing therapies.[6] No systematic reviews or randomized controlled trials were found. Seven retrospective series studying the role of braces in fractures were identified. None of these studies showed bracing to have an effect. Because of poor methodologic quality, no best-evidence synthesis could be performed. The authors concluded that, in the present literature, there is no evidence for the effectiveness of bracing in patients with traumatic thoracolumbar fractures. The lack of high-quality studies prevents relevant conclusions from being drawn.[6]

There is also no evidence that braces provide any additional benefit as an adjunct to surgery. A biomechanical study assessing the role of Boston overlap braces, reclination braces, and lumbotrain harnesses examined the effect of the braces on the loads of internal spinal fixation devices with several positions and activities, including sitting, standing, walking, bending forward, and lifting an extended leg in a supine position.[7] The authors found that none of the braces markedly reduced the loads on the fixators. Frequently, even higher fixator loads were measured when wearing a brace or harness. It was concluded that bracing did not seem helpful after surgical stabilization of the lumbar spine.[7] Given the current systems that are largely based on pedicle screws, the biomechanics of internal fixation are significantly better than previous generational systems. The effectiveness and necessity of postsurgical bracing must therefore be carefully considered.

The cost and possible complications of braces must also be carefully assessed. There are innate complications associated with braces, including the risk of pressure sores, skin breakdown and chafing, and peripheral nerve compression (particularly the lateral femoral cutaneous nerve as it crosses the iliac crest). These seemingly benign issues must not be overlooked or neglected and may be significant issues in an already traumatized patient.

There are no conclusive studies demonstrating any measurable benefit to the utility of braces in the setting of stable fractures or as an adjunct to surgical stabilization. Braces carry an added expense and a risk of real, though usually minor, complications. Braces may have a role with respect to pain control, but clinicians should carefully consider the use of braces and their impact, if any, on overall fracture alignment weighed against the costs and risks.

Timing of Surgical Stabilization

There are numerous factors that affect the timing of surgical stabilization, including impact on neurologic recovery, impact on early rehabilitation, pulmonary issues, and convenience and lifestyle choices of the treating team.

A recent study of timing of spine fracture fixation as defined by analysis of the National Trauma Data Bank used histogram analysis to assess how many days after injury initial surgical fixation was performed.[8] Patients were stratified based on early surgical treatment (within 72 hours) or late treatment (more than 72 hours) after injury. Patients in the early group were matched to a cohort from the late group with similar age, Injury Severity Score (ISS), and Glasgow Coma Scale values. Outcome data included hospital length of stay, intensive care unit length of stay, ventilator days, charges, incidence of complications, and mortality. Of

16,812 patients who underwent surgical fixation, 59% completed treatment within 3 days of injury. There was no significant difference in the presence of spinal cord injury (SCI) between the early and late groups, with SCI present in 51% of the early group and 48% in the late group, with a *p* value of 0.3735. Complications were significantly higher in the late group (30% versus 17.5%, with a *P* value of < 0.0001). However, mortality was similar in both groups (2% versus 1.9%, with a *P* value of > 0.05). The conclusion of this study was that most patients with spine fractures underwent surgical fixation within 3 days and that these patients had fewer complications and required less resources. There was no difference in mortality and neurologic recovery.

With a late group defined as greater than 3 days and an earlier group defined as less than 3 days, the acute phase for stabilization of spine procedures also must be determined. Early surgery for thoracic injury with SCI has been correlated with lower morbidity, hospital length of stay, and intensive care unit length of stay. A 2004 study looked at a damage control paradigm for spine trauma and how damage control principles can be applied to polytraumatized patients with spine injuries, to patients with isolated spine injuries, and to those with spine injuries with and without neurologic impairment.[9] In an earlier study, urgent surgical stabilization of spinal fractures in polytrauma patients was examined in a prospective longitudinal study to determine the relative safety of very early surgical stabilization.[10] The population consisted of 27 patients with severe polytrauma and an ISS greater than 25. The results of surgery performed within 24 hours of injury, which constituted an urgent care group, were compared with those of surgery performed between 24 and 72 hours of injury, which constituted an early group. The findings in the two groups were similar in terms of demographics and injury characteristics. Neurologic injury was common with 63% having some neurologic injury and 26% of these patients suffering either a complete SCI or cauda equina injury. Specific indications for urgent surgery included progressive neurologic deficit, polytrauma, and chest and pulmonary contusions. In patients who underwent posterior thoracic spinal stabilization, no significant difference between urgent or early surgical groups were found in terms of length of stay, intraoperative blood loss, rate of perioperative complications, morbidity rate, or mortality rate. The authors concluded that urgent stabilization within 24 hours was at least as safe as delaying surgery more than 24 hours. In this study, however, neurologic recovery was looked at as an end point, and patients who underwent surgery within 24 hours had a higher rate of neurologic recovery than those undergoing more delayed surgery, with a mean Frankel grade improvement of 1.1 compared with 0.57.

A retrospective chart review published in 2001 looked at spinal fracture fixation following blunt trauma involving cervical, thoracic, and lumbar fractures with and without SCI. The study showed that early spine fixation within 3 days was safe in polytrauma patients and preferred in thoracic injured patients due to reduced pneumonia rates.[11]

Although the physiologic benefits of early surgery are well documented, the rates of neurologic improvement from early surgery are less clear. A recent study showed no correlation between timing of surgical decompression and motor improvement in the setting of conus medullaris injury, specifically looking at blunt traumatic injuries between T12 and L1.[12] A systematic review of neurologic and clinical outcomes evaluated the effects of the timing of thoracic and lumbar fracture fixation.[13] The effect of having a ready trauma team, including experienced spine surgeons, has been demonstrated in several studies, with most studies showing decreased complications with early surgery. No statistical difference was found between the timing of thoracolumbar surgery and complications,[14] with implant loosening reported in 4.5% of patients and failure of fixation in 6.8%.[15] Similarly, a 2005 study showed a trend toward increased mortality in the early surgery patients and recommended an individualized treatment strategy for hemodynamic optimization before surgery.[16]

One study noted that resuscitation of these patients typically involves high-volume crystalloid with limited amounts of blood products and a resultant respiratory failure rate of 11.5% of patients in surgery within 72 hours versus 37% in surgery 72 hours or more after injury.[17] Resuscitation strategies are critically important for early surgery in the spine injured patient, and the high incidence of respiratory failure and pneumonia in these patients may be related to the resuscitation strategy, which may blunt the positive effects of early surgery.

Special categories include the spinal cord injured patient, the polytraumatized patient, and the patient with a mechanically unstable spine who is neurologically intact. Patients should be operated on when medically stable, with normal coagulation parameters, peak airway pressures of less than 40 cm of water in the prone position, a normal perfusion status as represented by base deficit not greater than 2 and normal serum lactate, and adequate hemoglobin and hemodynamic parameters to support spinal cord perfusion. It is imperative, particularly in the spinal cord injured patient, that there be no period of hypotension, because this could lead to a spinal cord infarction that could render permanent a potentially recoverable lesion.

The issue of adequate resuscitation is not only important with regard to preservation of spinal cord function, but also to minimizing the morbidity and mortality associated with both the injury and with early surgical intervention, when clinically indicated. A recent evidence-based review of the literature on the timing of stabilization of thoracolumbar fractures[18] concluded that stabilization of thoracic spine fractures within 72 hours is safe, and appears to result in decreased respiratory morbidity and length of intensive care unit and hospital stay. There is not enough evidence to determine the effect of the timing of stabiliza-

4: Axial Skeleton, Including Spine and Pelvis

tion on mortality in thoracolumbar fractures. A slightly higher mortality rate was reported in 2007 in patients treated within 48 hours compared with those treated later, 5.6% versus 0%.[19] This difference was primarily seen in patients with an ISS greater than 25. In a 2005 study using overlapping data with the 2007 study, patients were compared using a 72-hour cutoff and stratified by the presence or absence of SCI.[16] There were no deaths in those with SCI. Among those without SCI, two patients (11%) died in the early group, and no patients died in the late group. The sample size for this analysis included only 18 and 26 patients in the early and late groups, respectively. Because of their findings and the concern that early surgery may be associated with higher mortality, the authors investigated the relationship between timing of surgery and mortality in greater detail by reviewing 871 patients from a national trauma database. They found no difference in mortality in two groups of ISS and Glasgow Coma Scale-matched patients whose spine fractures had been stabilized before and after 72 hours.[16]

These issues underscore the importance of adequate resuscitation in spine trauma patients, particularly with regard to the concern for occult hypoperfusion as denoted by a lactic acid level greater than 2.5 in the absence of clinical signs of shock.[20] In light of the resuscitation strategy, which has been called into question in more recent literature, particularly regarding the use of blood and blood products in critically ill patients with combat-related injuries, the resuscitation strategy on the acutely injured spine patient must be attended to closely.[17] Similarly underscoring this discussion was the 2008 study in which exclusion criteria for early surgery included patients with an abnormal biochemical profile.[21] This study showed that patients in the early group had a significantly shorter hospital and intensive care unit stay and lesser systemic complications such as pneumonia, and also exhibited better neurologic improvement than the late surgery group. This was a small study comparing surgery within 8 hours after SCI in 12 patients, to surgery performed between 3 and 15 days, with 15 patients included in this category. The authors concluded that very early surgery might improve neurologic recovery and decrease hospitalization time and systemic complications in patients with thoracolumbar SCIs; thus early stabilization of thoracolumbar spine fractures within 8 hours after trauma is recommended to be favorable in patients who are hemodynamically normal. However, the applicability of these conclusions to the multiply injured patient is in serious question by the exclusion of multiply injured patients. The effect of early stabilization is underscored by a 2006 study in which surgical stabilization performed more than 2 days after admission was an independent risk factor for respiratory failure following operative stabilization of thoracic and lumbar spine fractures.[22]

Early surgery seems to positively influence cost, pulmonary disease, and rehabilitation in patients with tho-

racolumbar spine fractures, although controversy exists as to whether early versus late surgery has any impact on neurologic recovery in patients with SCI. However, it is imperative that traumatized patients be adequately resuscitated before surgical intervention.

Osteoporotic Fractures

More than 700,000 vertebral compression fractures are diagnosed each year in the United States.[23] The prevalence of vertebral compression fractures in women older than 50 years is estimated at 26%[24] and increases to 80% in patients older than 80 years.[25] The main causes of vertebral compression fracture are primary osteoporosis in 85% of patients and malignancy in the remaining 15%.[26] Clinical symptoms include back pain, limited spinal mobility, height loss, deformity, and disability. These symptoms diminish physical efficiency and adversely affect the quality of life. In addition, both symptomatic and asymptomatic fractures are linked to increased disease and mortality rate. Nonsurgical management of vertebral compression fracture includes medical therapy with nonsteroidal anti-inflammatory drugs and opioids as well as brace or cast immobilization. The efficacy of surgical management, including vertebroplasty and kyphoplasty, has more recently been called into question.

A series of recent studies published in the *New England Journal of Medicine* studied the efficacy of vertebroplasty in treating osteoporotic vertebral fractures. The first study was a multicenter randomized, double-blind, placebo-controlled trial in which participants with one or two painful osteoporotic vertebral fractures that were less than 12 months old and unhealed (as confirmed by MRI) were randomly assigned to undergo vertebroplasty or a sham procedure.[27] A total of 78 participants were enrolled, and 71 completed the 6-month follow-up. Vertebroplasty did not result in a significant advantage in any measured outcome at any time. There were, however, significant reductions in overall pain in both study groups at each follow-up assessment. Similar improvements were seen in both groups with respect to pain at night and at rest, physical functioning, quality of life, and perceived improvement. A multicenter trial, published simultaneously, involved 131 patients with one to three painful osteoporotic vertebral compression fractures who were randomly assigned to receive either vertebroplasty or a simulated procedure without cement. At 1 month there was no significant difference between the vertebroplasty group and the control group in either the Roland Morris disability questionnaire or the pain rating. Both groups had immediate improvement in disability and pain scores after the intervention. Although the two groups did not differ significantly on any secondary outcome measure at 1 month, there was a trend toward a higher rate of clinically meaningful improvement in pain in the vertebroplasty group. Meaningful improvement in pain was defined as a 30% decrease from baseline and was achieved in 64% of the vertebroplasty group versus 48% in the control group, ($P = 0.06$). In this study, patients were allowed to cross over to the other study group after 1 month, a fact that clouds some of the suggested outcomes. At 3 months there was a significantly higher crossover rate in the control group than in the vertebroplasty group. There was one serious adverse event in each group. The authors concluded that improvements in pain and pain-related disability were similar with vertebroplasty and the control group.

However, the treatment of severe osteoporotic spinal fractures, particularly those with neurologic deficits, has not been addressed by these studies. Open or percutaneous kyphoplasty following surgical reduction and instrumentation can be useful for anterior column reconstruction while avoiding the morbidity or blood loss associated with a formal anterior column reconstruction.

In a prospective case series of patients with vertebral compression fractures associated with spinal cord or radicular deficits, the use of cement in an open fashion to provide anterior column support for short segment instrumentation of fractures was evaluated.[28] All 16 patients in this series had a laminectomy. The neurologic status of all 16 patients improved, with 14 experiencing complete recovery and 2 with enough neurologic recovery to resume walking. There was a significant improvement in kyphotic angle from a mean of 14° preoperatively to 5° postoperatively. Cement leakage occurred in two patients without clinical sequelae, once into the intervertebral disk and once laterally.[28]

Although the benefits of percutaneous vertebroplasty in osteoporotic vertebral compression fractures have been questioned,[27,29] complications of this procedure remain well defined. A 23% incidence of pulmonary cement emboli was reportedly detected in the distal to third-order pulmonary arteries in 78 percutaneous vertebroplasties.[30] This underscores the importance of demonstrating superiority of any intervention over nonsurgical management to balance the risk-benefit ratio. In a recent uncontrolled, prospective study,[23] visual analog scale values in patients with symptoms lasting longer than 2 months were 8.7 before vertebroplasty, 1.1 at 1 week after vertebroplasty, and 1.5 at 1 year. Of particular note, among the 90 of 285 patients who were either bedridden or restricted to a wheelchair before vertebroplasty, none remained in this state after vertebroplasty. There was a 4.8% incidence of polymethylmethacrylate leakage within the disk and paravertebral veins; there were no symptoms and no intervention was required. No major complications were reported. All P values were less than 0.001, between preprocedure and postprocedure scores.

A recent evidence-based review of the literature reviewed all articles published between 1980 and 2008 with reported outcomes of either vertebroplasty or kyphoplasty for osteoporotic or tumor-associated vertebral compression fractures.[31] The level of evidence was rated in grades of recommendation for the North American Spine Society guidelines supporting the use of vertebroplasty or kyphoplasty for the treatment of vertebral compression fractures. There were 74 vertebroplasty studies and 35 kyphoplasty studies for the treatment of osteoporotic vertebral compression fractures. Compared with optimal medical management for osteoporotic vertebral compression fractures, there was good evidence that vertebroplasty provided superior pain control within the first 2 weeks of intervention; fair evidence that vertebroplasty results in less analgesic use, less disability, and greater improvement in general health within the first 3 months after intervention; fair evidence that vertebroplasty provided a similar degree of pain control and physical function 2 years after intervention; and fair evidence that kyphoplasty resulted in greater improvement in daily activity, physical function, and pain relief 6 months after intervention. It was recommended that high-quality randomized trials with 2-year follow-up were needed to confirm these favorable results. It was further concluded that the reported incidence of symptomatic procedure-related morbidity for both vertebroplasty and kyphoplasty is very low.

A more recent study showed that 30 consecutive patients receiving percutaneous vertebroplasty within a mean of 7.7 months of injury (range of 2.2 to 39 months), showed an immediate significant and lasting reduction in their average and worst back pain at 3-year follow-up.[32] Comparison of the prevertebroplasty and postvertebroplasty scores on the various SF-36 domains showed a significant increase in six of eight domains in both summary scores. Asymptomatic leakage of cement was found in 47 of 58 (81%) of treated vertebrae. Two minor complications occurred, including an asymptomatic pulmonary cement embolism and a cement spur along a needle track. The spur was removed immediately, resulting in postoperative hematoma pain that resolved within 2 days. It was recommended that compression fractures, characterized by a single attack of intense back pain and short duration, be treated nonsurgically because they can be expected to heal within 4 to 8 weeks. The remaining 20% of symptomatic osteoporotic vertebral compression fractures tend to heal spontaneously only after 45 to 60 weeks and benefited significantly from percutaneous vertebroplasty.

Another recent study on the comparison of percutaneous vertebroplasty with nonsurgical management of patients with painful, acute, or subacute osteoporotic vertebral fractures concluded that most patients with subacute or acute painful osteoporotic compression fractures in the spine will recover after a few months of nonsurgical management.[33] In this prospective study of 50 patients, it was noted that reduction in pain from initial visit to 3-month follow-up was comparable in the two groups. This study confirms the conclusion made in another 2009 study,[32] that Lyritis type I fractures do not significantly benefit from vertebroplasty. Moreover, it was demonstrated that two adjacent fractures occurred in the vertebroplasty group, whereas

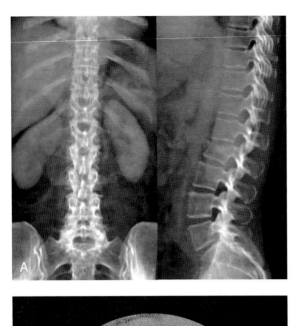

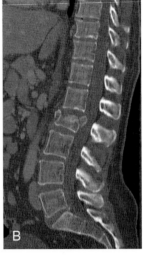

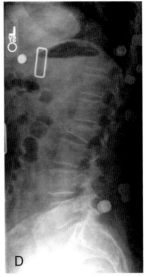

Figure 1 Imaging studies showing L2 three-column burst fracture with no neurologic deficits in a 57-year-old woman injured in a high-speed motor vehicle crash. **A,** AP (left) and lateral (right) reformatted images of the injury with the patient in supine position. **B,** Sagittal CT image demonstrating approximately 50% loss of vertebral body height. **C,** Axial CT image demonstrating approximately 50% canal compromise with retropulsed fragment at typical location between the pedicles of the injured vertebra. **D,** Upright lateral radiograph with thoracolumbosacral orthosis in place. Acceptable alignment with approximately 4° of focal kyphosis is demonatrated. The patient went on to uneventful healing, weaning from the brace with minimal to no pain, and return to preinjury employment.

none were found in the nonsurgically managed group, raising the possibility that adjacent fracture risk is elevated in the vertebroplasty group without significant benefit of intervention.[33]

There continues to be discrepant evidence with respect to vertebroplasty and kyphoplasty as they pertain to osteoporotic fractures. Recent articles have introduced a new level of skepticism among practitioners and the public despite the conclusions of the 2009 meta-analysis of the large body of literature.[31] Further well-designed studies are necessary to fully ascertain which patients are ideal candidates for either vertebroplasty or kyphoplasty.

Burst Fractures Without Neurologic Deficits

A major issue with respect to management of burst fractures is accurate definitions and appropriate classification. By definition, a burst fracture should be primarily an axial load injury and must be differentiated from a flexion injury (either a flexion-distraction type injury or a Chance injury), an extension injury, or a translational injury (dislocation); the latter three injuries are generally more biomechanically unstable because of the bending moment and shear and thus more likely to require surgical intervention for a successful outcome. Most if not all burst fractures without neurologic deficits ought to be successfully treated nonsurgically (**Figure 1**); however, other injury patterns must be accurately ruled out with the assurance that the injury assessed is truly an axial load burst fracture. If the new TLICS is used, a neurologically intact patient with a burst fracture would attain a score of 2, with 0 points assigned for intact neurologic status, 0 points for intact posterior ligamentous complex, and 2 points for injury morphology.[34] The main issues that must be carefully assessed include integrity of the posterior ligamentous complex (PLC) and documentation of absence of neurologic deficit.

It is the responsibility of the treating physician to rule out a PLC injury. Clinical signs of PLC disruption include posterior tenderness, a palpable step-off or gap, and/or significant posterior edema. Radiographic signs on CT and plain radiographs include horizontal fractures through the posterior elements, widening of the facet joints, or widening between the spinous processes. MRI with short-tau inversion recovery sequences can be helpful for ruling out indeterminate injuries to the PLC.[35-37] Kyphosis greater than 25° to 30° or height loss greater than 50% have previously been emphasized as surgical indications, and their true significance is that kyphosis or loss of vertebral body height to that extent likely represents disruption of the PLC and therefore a flexion-distraction injury. Thus, these parameters ought to be used as markers to consider injuries other than a neurologically intact burst fracture; however, as stand-alone guides, they have minimal bearing on management.

It has been suggested that canal compromise greater than 50% is an indication for surgical management. However, this traditional indication has no bearing on stability or neurologic status, particularly in the elderly patient with osteoporosis. Severity of neurologic deficit does not appear to correlate with the amount of residual canal stenosis, but is more likely influenced by the extent of instantaneous canal compromise that occurs at the time of injury. A study assessing canal remodeling in 115 patients found a mean canal clearance ranging from 49% to 72% postoperatively and 87% at final follow-up, suggesting tremendous remodeling potential. Moreover, canals with greater initial compromise demonstrated greater remodeling.[38] Thus, canal compromise should have no bearing on the decision to proceed with surgery. The neurologic status of the patient should be the key determinant.

Nonsurgical management of burst fractures can involve no bracing and early mobilization, prolonged bed rest, custom orthoses, or hyperextension casting, depending on the severity of the injury, associated injuries, goals, and other factors. Each patient should have upright AP and lateral radiographs to assess baseline alignment and ensure that there is no missed ligamentous injury or subtle instability. The kyphotic angle and vertebral height should be compared to that seen on the initial CT scan or plain radiographs. Typically, patients with a PLC injury will have incapacitating pain with mobilization beyond that expected with a burst fracture. In patients with stable injuries, braces, if used, are typically worn for 3 months. It is imperative to counsel these patients with respect to signs of conus medullaris or cauda equina syndromes.

Clear treatment recommendations do not exist primarily because of inconsistent injury description and classification, which makes interpretation of published data difficult. The available literature suggests successful results in patients with burst fractures treated conservatively. The problem is not in the management of burst fractures but rather in the certainty that the injury truly is a burst fracture and not a missed flexion-distraction type of injury. One study that followed 42 patients for up to 55 years found that kyphosis after burst fracture, which averaged 17° to 26°, did not correlate with the level of pain. No patient had a neurologic deterioration. Eighty-eight percent of patients were able to return to work and resume their preinjury occupations.[39]

Another retrospective study of 38 patients with burst fractures found an increase in kyphosis ranging from 20° to 24° over an average of 4 years. There was no correlation between kyphosis and canal compromise or clinical outcome. 76% of patients returned to their preinjury occupations.[40] Another study followed 60 consecutive patients for 42 months and found a progression of kyphosis from 6° to 8°, with 91% having a satisfactory outcome.[41]

Comparative studies of surgical and nonsurgical management of burst fractures show no substantial differences in outcomes, other than more complications in surgically treated patients. A recent study compared 25 cases treated without surgery with 38 cases treated surgically and found that at 5-year follow-up there was no significant difference in the mean visual analog scale and Roland Morris Disability Questionnaire scores between the surgically and nonsurgically treated groups. Functional outcome also appears to be equally favorable 5 years after surgical or nonsurgical treatment of AO type A3 burst fractures.[42] A prospective study compared 47 nonsurgically treated patients with 33 patients surgically treated with short segment fixation and found mean outcome scores better in the surgically treated group at 3 months but no difference at 6 months and 2 years. Final kyphosis also was not significantly different.[43] The only prospective, randomized study followed 47 patients with burst fractures. There was no statistical difference in kyphosis, pain, or functional outcome in those treated surgically compared to those treated nonsurgically.[44] A recent Cochrane review comparing surgically and nonsurgically treated burst fractures concluded that there was no statistically significant difference in pain and function-related outcomes, rates of return to work, radiographic findings, or average length of hospitalization at final follow-up. The degree of kyphosis or the percentage of correction lost did not correlate with any clinical symptoms at the time of the final follow-up. Average costs related to hospitalization and treatment in the surgical group appeared to be more than in the nonsurgical group. There was no statistically significant difference in the functional outcome 2 years or more after therapy between surgical and nonsurgical treatment of thoracolumbar burst fractures without neurologic deficit.[45]

No level I studies assess management of burst fractures, but the studies available support that neurologically intact patients with burst fractures can be successfully treated without surgery. Much of the controversy arises from a failure to appropriately classify and thus understand the pathologic entity being discussed.

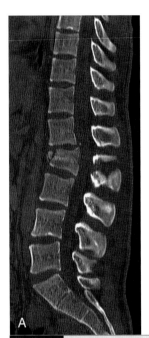
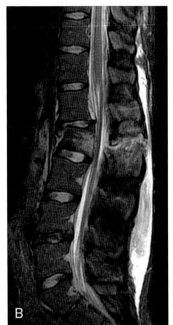
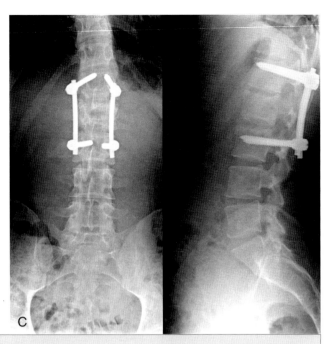

Figure 2 Imaging studies from a 17-year-old boy who presented with no neurologic deficits after an ice cave collapsed on top of him. **A,** Midsagittal CT reformat demonstrating posterior element widening and anterior vertebral body compression. **B,** MRI demonstrating disruption of the posterior ligamentous complex and soft-tissue hemorrhage. **C,** Upright AP (left) and lateral (right) images 1 year after surgery demonstrating short segment pedicle fixation and restoration of alignment. The patient returned to unrestricted activity, including competitive soccer and running.

Flexion-Distraction Injuries

With a flexion-distraction injury, a significant flexion moment causes disruption of the PLC. These are innately unstable injuries due to the loss of the posterior tension band, which must generally be restored through surgical intervention to prevent kyphosis (**Figure 2**). By convention, flexion-distraction injuries are distinguished from fracture-dislocations by the absence of translation or transverse plane rotation. Flexion-distraction injuries have a fulcrum located within the anterior column and typically present radiographically with compression of the vertebral body that may be interpreted as a simple compression fracture. Flexion-distraction injuries are differentiated from Chance injuries wherein the fulcrum is anterior to the vertebral body, and the anterior column fails in tension and not compression. In general, these two distinct yet similar injury patterns are treated according to identical principles and can be discussed together as flexion-distraction injuries. It is imperative that an abdominal visceral injury be ruled out with both of these injuries. In a recent retrospective study of 153 patients with flexion-distraction injuries, 30% had significant intra-abdominal injuries.[46] This finding has also been noted in previous studies.[47]

Surgical management is generally recommended other than with purely bony injuries, in which a hyperextension cast or brace may be equally successful. Posterior compressive, usually short segment instrumentation and fusion, is the recommended treatment of most

flexion-distraction injuries, with the primary goal of correcting the kyphosis and restoring the posterior tension band. There have been relatively few studies investigating flexion-distraction injuries. One retrospective study assessing 17 patients, of which 82% were treated nonsurgically, found that only 65% returned to preinjury activities. The authors concluded that surgical management is recommended and that early recognition of the constellation of injuries involving the spine and abdomen associated with the use of the lap belt is imperative.[47] Another small study of 16 patients treated surgically with short segment posterior fixation found that 87% had little or no pain at follow-up.[48] A more recent retrospective study of 26 patients with flexion-distraction injuries who were treated surgically found that average kyphosis improved from 9.5° to 5.4° and pain was absent or mild in 91% of patients.[49]

There is a subset of flexion-distraction injuries that may be referred to as unstable burst fractures, in which there may be significant height loss or comminution of the vertebral body with fracture involving the posterior cortex and retropulsion of fracture fragments. In these cases, a combined anterior and posterior approach may be indicated, with the goal of restoring the tension band posteriorly and of restoring height and decompressing the canal anteriorly. Failure of instrumentation has been reported with anterior fixation alone, which is biomechanically unfavorable in this injury type and is generally not recommended.

Flexion-distraction injuries have a 25% rate of neurologic injury and a 30% likelihood of intra-abdominal injury. Good outcomes can be expected with short-segment posterior instrumentation to restore the disrupted tension band and maintain physiologic alignment. Rarely these injuries will require an anterior approach for decompression or anterior column support.

Minimally Invasive Techniques: Is There a Role?

Spine surgery has seen a recent trend toward minimally invasive techniques for procedures ranging from diskectomies to interbody fusions to scoliosis corrections. There has likewise been a growing interest in the use of minimally invasive techniques for spine trauma as well. The definition of minimally invasive spine surgery (MISS) is a controversial topic, so for the purpose of this discussion, it is defined as percutaneous instrumentation with or without formal arthrodesis.

Many advocates of MISS suggest placement of percutaneous pedicle screws and rods as an alternative to bracing in the management of otherwise stable injuries. It has been suggested that temporary, percutaneous stabilization without fusion is less cumbersome to patients with stable injuries. Internal fixation serves as an internal brace to help minimize pain and prevent further deformity while the fracture heals. In a recent study involving percutaneous stabilization of 64 fractures, consisting of 57 AO type A injuries, 4 type B injuries and type 3 C injuries, the authors specifically state that "minimally invasive percutaneous fixation in the treatment of thoracolumbar and lumbar spine fractures represents a good alternative option to conservative treatment" suggesting that this treatment can be used in place of brace management or bed rest.[50] Certainly the potential benefit of such a procedure for the indications suggested must be carefully weighed against factors such as cost and potential complications.

Other authors have advocated that MISS can be used in certain fracture types as an alternative to traditional open instrumentation in neurologically intact patients who do not require decompression of the neural elements. A recent study compared 10 patients with burst fractures treated with MISS to 10 patients treated with conventional open techniques and found no major differences in wound complications or operative time. MISS is recommended in "cases that do not require excessive force to reduce the fracture."[51] An additional study comparing 11 open with 10 MISS patients with AO type A fractures and 5-year follow-up concluded that blood loss was significantly lower among those patients who had minimally invasive surgery. The operating time, the time of x-ray exposure, and the loss of correction were identical in both groups.[52]

Others have proposed minimally invasive techniques for anterior decompressions and instrumentation. One study compared 174 consecutive patients who had corpectomies, anterior column reconstruction, and anterior instrumentation done through a thoracoscopic approach to 197 consecutive patients treated with traditional open procedures. The incidence of vascular injury and neurologic deterioration was higher with MISS technique than with open surgery. The MISS group had one case each of aortic injury, splenic contusion, neurologic deterioration, cerebrospinal fluid leak, and severe wound infection for an overall major complication rate of 1.3%. The authors concluded that a complete anterior thoracoscopically assisted reconstruction of thoracic and thoracolumbar fractures can be safely and effectively accomplished, thereby reducing the pain and morbidity associated with conventional thoracotomy and thoracolumbar approaches.[53]

Many factors need to be assessed regarding the indications and utility of MISS in the trauma scenario. Another important factor that must be considered is the potentially steep learning curve associated with the implementation of a new technique. It is generally agreed upon that the ideal candidate for MISS instrumentation is the patient with either a bony Chance fracture, bony flexion-distraction injury, or fracture seen with a preexisting ankylosing spine condition. The advantage in bony Chance fractures or bony flexion-distraction injuries is that a formal arthrodesis is not necessary because the instrumentation provides bony apposition and creates an environment for primary healing of the fracture. In ankylosing spine conditions such as ankylosing spondylitis or diffuse idiopathic skeletal hyperostosis, because the disease process promotes bone formation, formal arthrodesis may not be indicated. Regardless of whether MISS is used to treat fractures in patients with ankylosing spine conditions, it is important to understand that short segment fixation is not indicated, and the same principles described for open treatment with regard to the need for long instrumentation constructs with multiple points of fixation need to be adhered to.[54] There are currently no well-designed prospective studies with respect to MISS in the management of thoracolumbar spine trauma. Most studies to date are retrospective cohort studies. Higher quality research is required to determine the utility, efficacy, and safety of MISS in the treatment of thoracolumbar injuries and to help guide the future of MISS in the realm of spine trauma.

Summary

Although there are many ways to treat varying thoracolumbar injury patterns, several treatment principles and goals need to be maintained. The TLICS classification system is an aid to help systematically evaluate an injury and is the first system to take into consideration the neurologic status of a patient in determining whether surgical or nonsurgical treatment should be used. Significant controversy remains as to the optimal management of many fracture patterns. Surgical stabilization is generally indicated in patients with an incompetent posterior ligamentous complex. In patients with true burst injuries who are neurologically intact, there is no indication for surgical treatment. The role of bracing in the treatment of fractures has not been shown to provide any long-term benefit and is increasingly being questioned. Minimally invasive techniques are gaining in popularity in the treatment of fractures; however, indications and rationale still lack scientific evidence. In patients with unstable injuries, adequate resuscitation is imperative. Early surgery is beneficial from a cost and morbidity standpoint, but there is no evidence that early surgery has any effect on mortality or neurologic outcome.

Annotated References

1. Lenarz CJ, Place HM, Lenke LG, Alander DH, Oliver D: Comparative reliability of 3 thoracolumbar fracture classification systems. *J Spinal Disord Tech* 2009;22(6): 422-427.

   Twenty-one spine clinicians took a prospective look at 97 fractures and compared the AO, Denis, and TLICS classifications. It was concluded that as a management tool, the TLICS seems to be an acceptably reliable system when compared with the Denis and AO systems.

2. Vaccaro AR, Baron EM, Sanfilippo J, et al: Reliability of a novel classification system for thoracolumbar injuries: The Thoracolumbar Injury Severity Score. *Spine* 2006;31(suppl 11):S62-S69.

   In this prospective study, 5 spine surgeons rated 71 clinical cases of thoracolumbar spinal injuries using the TLICS and then re-rated the cases in a different order 1 month later. It was concluded that the TLICS has good reliability and compares favorably to other contemporary thoracolumbar fracture classification systems.

3. Wood KB, Khanna G, Vaccaro AR, Arnold PM, Harris MB, Mehbod AA: Assessment of two thoracolumbar fracture classification systems as used by multiple surgeons. *J Bone Joint Surg Am* 2005;87(7):1423-1429.

   Nineteen raters classified 31 fractures and concluded that both the Denis and the AO system for the classification of spine fractures had only moderate reliability and repeatability.

4. Ohana N, Sheinis D, Rath E, Sasson A, Atar D: Is there a need for lumbar orthosis in mild compression fractures of the thoracolumbar spine?: A retrospective study comparing the radiographic results between early ambulation with and without lumbar orthosis. *J Spinal Disord* 2000;13(4):305-308.

5. Weitzman G: Treatment of stable thoracolumbar spine compression fractures by early ambulation. *Clin Orthop Relat Res* 1971;76:116-122.

6. Giele BM, Wiertsema SH, Beelen A, et al: No evidence for the effectiveness of bracing in patients with thoracolumbar fractures. *Acta Orthop* 2009;80(2):226-232.

   The authors perform an electronic search strategy iden-

   tifying brace and nonbrace therapies in traumatic injuries. Seven studies were identified and the authors conclude that there is no evidence for the effectiveness of bracing in patients with thoracolumbar fractures.

7. Rohlmann A, Bergmann G, Graichen F, Neff G: Braces do not reduce loads on internal spinal fixation devices. *Clin Biomech* 1999;14(2):97-102.

8. Kerwin AJ, Griffen MM, Tepas JJ III, Schinco MA, Devin T, Frykberg ER: Best practice determination of timing of spinal fracture fixation as defined by analysis of the National Trauma Data Bank. *J Trauma* 2008; 65(4):824-830.

   The authors assess 16,812 patients in the National Trauma Data Bank who have undergone surgery for spine fractures. Most undergo surgery within 3 days, and these patients had fewer complications and required less resources.

9. Kossmann T, Trease L, Freedman I, Malham G: Damage control surgery for spine trauma. *Injury* 2004;35(7): 661-670.

10. McLain RF, Benson DR: Urgent surgical stabilization of spinal fractures in polytrauma patients. *Spine* 1999; 24(16):1646-1654.

11. Croce MA, Fabian TC, Waddle-Smith L, Maxwell RA: Identification of early predictors for post-traumatic pneumonia. *Am Surg* 2001;67(2):105-110.

12. Rahimi-Movaghar V, Vaccaro AR, Mohammadi M: Efficacy of surgical decompression in regard to motor recovery in the setting of conus medullaris injury. *J Spinal Cord Med* 2006;29(1):32-38.

    The authors reviewed 24 patients with traumatic conus injuries between T12 and L1 and followed the patients for neurologic improvement. They found no correlation between the timing of surgical decompression and motor improvement.

13. Rutges JP, Oner FC, Leenen LP: Timing of thoracic and lumbar fracture fixation in spinal injuries: A systematic review of neurological and clinical outcome. *Eur Spine J* 2007;16(5):579-587.

    A systematic review of 10 articles demonstrated fewer complications, shorter hospital stays, and shorter intensive care unit stays with early fracture fixation. The effect of early treatment on neurologic outcome remains unclear.

14. Dai LY, Yao WF, Cui YM, Zhou Q: Thoracolumbar fractures in patients with multiple injuries: Diagnosis and treatment—A review of 147 cases. *J Trauma* 2004; 56(2):348-355.

    One hundred forty-seven consecutive patients with acute thoracolumbosacral fractures and multiple trauma were retrospectively reviewed. Appropriate timing of thoracolumbar fracture fixation in patients with multiple injuries should not be dependent on a rigid protocol.

15. Gaebler C, Maier R, Kutscha-Lissberg F, Mrkonjic L, Vècsei V: Results of spinal cord decompression and thoracolumbar pedicle stabilisation in relation to the time of operation. *Spinal Cord* 1999;37(1):33-39.

16. Kerwin AJ, Frykberg ER, Schinco MA, Griffen MM, Murphy T, Tepas JJ: The effect of early spine fixation on non-neurologic outcome. *J Trauma* 2005;58(1):15-21.

    The authors retrospectively reviewed 1,741 patients with spine fractures and concluded that reasonable compliance with an early spinal fracture fixation protocol produced some improvements in nonneurologic outcome. Early spine stabilization reduced hospital length of stay in all patients. The timing of this procedure should be individualized to allow patients with the most severe physiologic derangements to be optimized preoperatively.

17. Chipman JG, Deuser WE, Beilman GJ: Early surgery for thoracolumbar spine injuries decreases complications. *J Trauma* 2004;56(1):52-57.

    A retrospective review of 146 patients with thoracolumbar spine injuries concluded that early surgery in severely injured patients with thoracolumbar spine trauma was associated with fewer complications and shorter hospital and intensive care unit stays, required less ventilator support for noninfectious reasons, and did not increase neurologic deficits.

18. Bellabarba C, Fisher C, Chapman JR, Dettori JR, Norvell DC: Does early fracture fixation of thoracolumbar spine fractures decrease morbidity or mortality? *Spine* 2010;35(9S):S138-S145.

    A systematic review of the literature from 1990 to 2008 identified nine appropriate articles that suggest that ideally patients with unstable thoracic fractures should undergo early (less than 72 hours after injury) stabilization to reduce morbidity and, possibly, mortality.

19. Kerwin AJ, Frykberg ER, Schinco MA, et al: The effect of early surgical treatment of traumatic spine injuries on patient mortality. *J Trauma* 2007;63(6):1308-1313.

    A review of 361 patients showed that spinal fixation within 48 hours of fracture appeared to increase mortality. Incomplete resuscitation before surgery may have contributed to this result.

20. Crowl AC, Young JS, Kahler DM, Claridge JA, Chrzanowski DS, Pomphrey M: Occult hypoperfusion is associated with increased morbidity in patients undergoing early femur fracture fixation. *J Trauma* 2000; 48(2):260-267.

21. Cengiz SL, Kalkan E, Bayir A, Ilik K, Basefer A: Timing of thoracolumbar spine stabilization in trauma patients; impact on neurological outcome and clinical course: A real prospective (rct) randomized controlled study. *Arch Orthop Trauma Surg* 2008;128(9):959-966.

    The authors review 27 patients with neurologic deficits and thoracolumbar fractures. Their results led them to conclude that early surgery may improve neurologic recovery and decrease hospitalization time and additional

systemic complications. A major limitation of this study is that multiply injured patients were excluded.

22. McHenry TP, Mirza SK, Wang J, et al: Risk factors for respiratory failure following operative stabilization of thoracic and lumbar spine fractures. *J Bone Joint Surg Am* 2006;88(5):997-1005.

    The authors carry out a retrospective cohort study in 1,032 patients with thoracolumbar fractures. They conclude that early surgical stabilization may decrease the risk of respiratory failure in multiply injured patients.

23. Masala S, Mammucari M, Angelopoulos G, et al: Percutaneous vertebroplasty in the management of vertebral osteoporotic fractures: Short-term, mid-term and long-term follow-up of 285 patients. *Skeletal Radiol* 2009; 38(9):863-869.

    After reviewing 285 patients, the authors conclude that vertebroplasty is a safe and useful treatment of osteoporotic fractures and produces enduring pain reduction while improving patients' mobility and decreasing the need for analgesic drugs.

24. Silverman SL: The clinical consequences of vertebral compression fracture. *Bone* 1992;13(suppl 2):S27-S31.

25. Melton LJ III, Kan SH, Frye MA, Wahner HW, O'Fallon WM, Riggs BL: Epidemiology of vertebral fractures in women. *Am J Epidemiol* 1989;129(5):1000-1011.

26. Watts NB: Osteoporotic vertebral fractures. *Neurosurg Focus* 2001;10(4):E12.

27. Buchbinder R, Osborne RH, Ebeling PR, et al: A randomized trial of vertebroplasty for painful osteoporotic vertebral fractures. *N Engl J Med* 2009;361(6):557-568.

    Seventy-eight patients were enrolled in a randomized, double-blind study. The authors found no beneficial effect of vertebroplasty compared with a sham procedure in patients with painful osteoporotic fractures.

28. Fuentes S, Blondel B, Metellus P, Adetchessi T, Gaudart J, Dufour H: Open kyphoplasty for management of severe osteoporotic spinal fractures. *Neurosurgery* 2009; 64(5, suppl 2):350-354.

    A prospective study of 16 patients undergoing open kyphoplasty and decompression for osteoporotic fractures with neurologic disorders led the authors to conclude that this technique gives successful results and is a good alternative in elderly patients with comorbidities.

29. Kallmes DF, Comstock BA, Heagerty PJ, et al: A randomized trial of vertebroplasty for osteoporotic spinal fractures. *N Engl J Med* 2009;361(6):569-579.

    The authors carry out a prospective, multicenter study on 131 patients with painful, osteoporotic fractures. They conclude that inprovements in pain and disability in patients treated with vertebroplasty are similar to improvements in a control group.

30. Kim YJ, Lee JW, Park KW, et al: Pulmonary cement embolism after percutaneous vertebroplasty in osteoporotic vertebral compression fractures: Incidence, characteristics, and risk factors. *Radiology* 2009;251(1): 250-259.

The authors prospectively evaluate 75 patients with osteoporotic compression fractures treated with percutaneous vertebroplasty. Pulmonary cement was detected in 23% of vertebroplasty sessions and was related to leakage into the inferior vena cava.

31. McGirt MJ, Parker SL, Wolinsky JP, Witham TF, Bydon A, Gokaslan ZL: Vertebroplasty and kyphoplasty for the treatment of vertebral compression fractures: An evidence-based review of the literature. *Spine J* 2009; 9(6):501-508.

The authors review 127 studies with vertebroplasty and kyphoplasty. They conclude that although evidence suggests that physical disability, general health, and pain relief are better with vertebroplasty and kyphoplasty than those with medical management, high-quality studies are needed to confirm these findings.

32. Muijs SP, Nieuwenhuijse MJ, Van Erkel AR, Dijkstra PD: Percutaneous vertebroplasty for the treatment of osteoporotic vertebral compression fractures: Evaluation after 36 months. *J Bone Joint Surg Br* 2009;91(3): 379-384.

The authors prospectively review 30 consecutive patients who underwent percutaneous vertebroplasty for osteoporotic fractures. Eighty-one percent of patients had asymptomatic leakage. They found that percutaneous vertebroplasty resulted in an immediate, significant, and lasting reduction in back pain and overall improvement in physical and mental health.

33. Rousing R, Andersen MO, Jespersen SM, Thomsen K, Lauritsen J: Percutaneous vertebroplasty compared to conservative treatment in patients with painful acute or subacute osteoporotic vertebral fractures: Three-months follow-up in a clinical randomized study. *Spine* 2009; 34(13):1349-1354.

A prospective randomized study comparing vertebroplasty versus conservative treatment was carried out on 50 patients with osteoporotic fractures. Clinical outcomes were similar between the two groups, and the authors concluded that most patients will recover after a few months of nonsurgical treatment.

34. Vaccaro AR, Lehman RA Jr, Hurlbert RJ, et al: A new classification of thoracolumbar injuries: The importance of injury morphology, the integrity of the posterior ligamentous complex, and neurologic status. *Spine* 2005; 30(20):2325-2333.

The authors propose a thoracolumbar injury classification and injury severity score based on three major variables: The mechanism of injury determined by radiographic appearance, the integrity of the posterior ligamentous complex, and the neurologic status of the patient.

35. Brightman RP, Miller CA, Rea GL, Chakeres DW, Hunt WE: Magnetic resonance imaging of trauma to the thoracic and lumbar spine: The importance of the posterior longitudinal ligament. *Spine* 1992;17(5):541-550.

36. Oner FC, Ramos LM, Simmermacher RK, et al: Classification of thoracic and lumbar spine fractures: Problems of reproducibility. A study of 53 patients using CT and MRI. *Eur Spine J* 2002;11(3):235-245.

37. Oner FC, van Gils AP, Faber JA, Dhert WJ, Verbout AJ: Some complications of common treatment schemes of thoracolumbar spine fractures can be predicted with magnetic resonance imaging: Prospective study of 53 patients with 71 fractures. *Spine* 2002;27(6):629-636.

38. Wessberg P, Wang Y, Irstam L, Nordwall A: The effect of surgery and remodelling on spinal canal measurements after thoracolumbar burst fractures. *Eur Spine J* 2001;10(1):55-63.

39. Weinstein JN, Collalto P, Lehmann TR: Thoracolumbar "burst" fractures treated conservatively: A long-term follow-up. *Spine* 1988;13(1):33-38.

40. Shen WJ, Shen YS: Nonsurgical treatment of three-column thoracolumbar junction burst fractures without neurologic deficit. *Spine* 1999;24(4):412-415.

41. Dendrinos GK, Halikias JG, Krallis PN, Asimakopoulos A: Factors influencing neurological recovery in burst thoracolumbar fractures. *Acta Orthop Belg* 1995;61(3): 226-234.

42. Post RB, van der Sluis CK, Leferink VJ, ten Duis HJ: Long-term functional outcome after type A3 spinal fractures: Operative versus non-operative treatment. *Acta Orthop Belg* 2009;75(3):389-395.

The authors retrospectively studied the long-term (5 years) functional outcome after surgical (38 cases) and nonsurgical (25 cases) treatment of type A3 spinal fractures without neurologic deficit and concluded that functional outcome was equally good 5 years after surgical versus nonsurgical treatment of type A3 burst fractures.

43. Shen WJ, Liu TJ, Shen YS: Nonoperative treatment versus posterior fixation for thoracolumbar junction burst fractures without neurologic deficit. *Spine* 2001;26(9): 1038-1045.

44. Wood K, Buttermann G, Mehbod A, et al: Operative compared with nonoperative treatment of a thoracolumbar burst fracture without neurological deficit: A prospective, randomized study. *J Bone Joint Surg Am* 2003;85(5):773-781.

45. Yi L, Jingping B, Gele J, Baoleri X, Taixiang W: Operative versus non-operative treatment for thoracolumbar burst fractures without neurological deficit. *Cochrane Database Syst Rev* 2006;4:CD005079.

The authors perform a Cochrane review comparing surgical with nonsurgical treatment of thoracolumbar burst fractures without neurologic deficits. They acknowledged significant deficiencies in the quality of the available literature, while concluding that there was no statistically significant difference in the functional outcome 2 years or more after surgical versus nonsurgical treatment of thoracolumbar burst fractures without neurologic deficit.

46. Chapman JR, Agel J, Jurkovich GJ, Bellabarba C: Thoracolumbar flexion-distraction injuries: Associated morbidity and neurological outcomes. *Spine* 2008;33(6): 648-657.

    The authors assess abdominal comorbidities, missed injuries, and complications associated with thoracolumbar flexion-distraction injuries in 153 patients. They found a 25% incidence of spinal cord injury and a 30% incidence of intra-abdominal injuries.

47. LeGay DA, Petrie DP, Alexander DI: Flexion-distraction injuries of the lumbar spine and associated abdominal trauma. *J Trauma* 1990;30(4):436-444.

48. Triantafyllou SJ, Gertzbein SD: Flexion distraction injuries of the thoracolumbar spine: A review. *Orthopedics* 1992;15(3):357-364.

49. Razak M, Mahmud MM, Hyzan MY, Omar A: Short segment posterior instrumentation, reduction and fusion of unstable thoracolumbar burst fractures—a review of 26 cases. *Med J Malaysia* 2000;55(suppl C):9-13.

50. Palmisani M, Gasbarrini A, Brodano GB, et al: Minimally invasive percutaneous fixation in the treatment of thoracic and lumbar spine fractures. *Eur Spine J* 2009; 18(suppl 1):71-74.

    The authors assess 51 patients with 64 fractures of the thoracolumbar and lumbar spine undergoing surgical treatment by percutaneous transpedicular fixation and stabilization with minimally invasive technique.

51. Merom L, Raz N, Hamud C, Weisz I, Hanani A: Minimally invasive burst fracture fixation in the thoracolumbar region. *Orthopedics* 2009;32(4):pii: orthosupersite.com/view.asp?rID=38353.

    The authors compare 10 patients treated with percutaneous instrumentation with 10 patients treated with traditional open instrumentation.

52. Wild MH, Glees M, Plieschnegger C, Wenda K: Five-year follow-up examination after purely minimally invasive posterior stabilization of thoracolumbar fractures: A comparison of minimally invasive percutaneously and conventionally open treated patients. *Arch Orthop Trauma Surg* 2007;127(5):335-343.

    The authors compare 11 patients treated with conventional open treatment and 10 patients treated with minimally invasive techniques.

53. Khoo LT, Beisse R, Potulski M: Thoracoscopic-assisted treatment of thoracic and lumbar fractures: A series of 371 consecutive cases. *Neurosurgery* 2002;51(suppl 5): S104-S117.

54. Caron T, Bransford RJ, Nguyen QT, Agel J, Chapman JR, Bellabarba C: Spine fractures in patients with ankylosing spinal disorders. *Spine* 2010;35(11):E458-E464.

    A retrospective review of 122 spine fractures in 112 consecutive patients with ankylosing spondylitis and diffuse idiopathic skeletal hyperostosis concluded that patients with spine fractures and ankylosing conditions are at high risk for complications and death. Multilevel posterior segmental instrumentation allows effective fracture healing.

4: Axial Skeleton, Including Spine and Pelvis

Chapter 30

Low Lumbar Burst and Lumbosacral Fractures

Hossein Elgafy, MD, MCh, FRCS Ed, FRCSC   Troy Caron, DO

4: Axial Skeleton, Including Spine and Pelvis

Low Lumbar Fractures

Because of the different biomechanical and neuroanatomic properties in the thoracic and lumbar regions of the spine, low lumbar fractures should be considered as distinct from fractures in the remainder of the lumbar and thoracic spine. The low lumbar spine is generally defined as involving the L3–L5 levels, whereas most of the current literature reporting on burst fractures pertains to the thoracolumbar region (T10–L2). The L2 vertebra is above the apex of the lordotic curve of the spine and therefore, when injured, has more of a tendency toward kyphotic deformity.[1] The L3 vertebra is a transitional vertebra between the thoracolumbar region and the low lumbar region, which is positioned at the apex of the lumbar lordosis.

Low lumbar fractures make up less than 4% of all fractures of the spine[2,3] As a result, the current literature regarding these fractures is sparse. Many of the studies that have evaluated these fractures involve a small number of patients treated in many different ways.[1-19]

Anatomy

The normal lumbar spine has 30° to 60° of lordosis and is more mobile than the thoracic spine, particularly in flexion and extension. This is due primarily to the sagittal orientation of the facets as well as the absence of rib attachments. The lumbar laminae progressively increase in width and decrease in height from L2 to L5. The size and medial angulation of the pedicles also increase from L2 to L5.[20]

The anatomic characteristics of the low lumbar spine distinguish fractures in this region from those in the thoracolumbar region. The low lumbar spine is, in large part, located below the level of the pelvic brim and is protected by the iliolumbar ligaments. As a result, the typical fracture pattern in this region is differ-

Dr. Elgafy or an immediate family member has received research or institutional support from Synthes. Neither Dr. Caron nor any immediate family member has received anything of value from or owns stock in a commercial company or institution related directly or indirectly to the subject of this chapter.

ent from that seen in the thoracolumbar spine. The space available for neurologic structures is greater as well, and canal contents consist entirely of lumbar roots, which results in a lower likelihood of neurologic injury.

Characteristics

Low lumbar burst fractures typically occur in younger patients, with more than 50% occurring in patients younger than 20 years. The typical amount of canal compromise is 47%. The mean loss of height is approximately 25%.[3,4,20]

There are many differences between low lumbar and thoracolumbar burst fractures (**Table 1**). Because the thoracolumbar spine is a transition zone between the stiff thoracic spine and a more mobile lumbar spine, it is a high stress area that is more prone to injury. The thoracolumbar region is posterior to the weight-bearing axis of the spine and is therefore more prone to kyphotic deformity. Alternatively, the low lumbar spine is lordotic and positioned anterior to the weight-bearing axis of the spine. Therefore, the forces acting on the spine in this region cause more of an axial load and less of a flexion moment, resulting in less loss of height and degree of kyphosis than with similar fractures in the thoracolumbar region.[3,20] The typical burst fracture pattern at L4 or L5 consists of a comminuted superior end plate and cephalad portion of the vertebral body and an inferior sagittal split. There is typically considerable canal compromise and the posterior elements are usually fractured. The combination of a sagittal split in the posterior elements associated with neurologic deficits raises the probability of a dural laceration or even nerve root entrapment within the lamina fracture.[4,20] If surgical intervention is undertaken in these circumstances, the surgeon should be aware of the potential for nerve root entrapment when performing a decompression procedure. Any attempt at decompression and dural repair should be done before reduction maneuver, because additional neurologic compromise can occur during reduction.[20,21]

At the L1 level the conus medullaris occupies 50% of the canal, whereas below this the cauda equina comprises approximately one third of the contents of the neural canal. Injuries to the low lumbar spine, unlike

Table 1		
Difference Between Low Lumbar Fractures and Thoracolumbar Fractures		
	Low Lumbar (L3-L5)	**Thoracolumbar (T10-L2)**
Anatomy	Protected by iliolumbar ligaments and their location below pelvic brim	High stress transition zone
Sagittal alignment	Lordotic	Kyphotic
Sagittal alignment postinjury	Average 8° kyphosis (23° relative kyphosis)	Average 21° kyphosis
Fracture pattern	Proximal comminution, inferior split, minimal kyphosis	Posterior superior retropulsion, significant kyphosis
Neurologic injury	Cauda equina and nerve roots occupy one third of canal, more likely to recover	Spinal cord and conus occupy 50% of canal, less likely to recover
Treatment	Controversial, more likely nonsurgical	Controversial, more likely surgical

those of other regions of the spine, do not involve the spinal cord. The cauda equina is much more resilient, and peripheral nerve root injuries have more potential for spontaneous recovery. There have been several reports of up to 90% canal compromise in this region without neurologic deficit.[8] Neurologic compromise or issues pertaining to canal compromise are therefore less likely to dictate the need for surgical intervention in low lumbar burst fractures than in their thoracolumbar counterparts.

Treatment

The goals of treatment of low lumbar fractures are to preserve sagittal balance, conserve motion segments, and decompress the neural elements when indicated. Complications associated with hook and rod surgical fixation methods of the past have included high rates of iatrogenic flat back, pseudarthrosis, and hook dislodgement. The advent of pedicle screw fixation has decreased the likelihood of these complications, and has consequently yielded improved results.[3]

Nonsurgical Treatment

Most low lumbar burst fractures can be treated nonsurgically. If bracing is the selected treatment method, it is important to note that the typical thoracolumbosacral orthosis (TLSO) will cause a fulcrum effect and lead to more motion at the fractured level. A leg extension (hip TLSO) is therefore mandatory when using a brace for low lumbar fractures. It is recommended that an upright radiograph be obtained before the patient is mobilized, because there is up to a 25% incidence of change in the fracture alignment in the upright position, which may cause the method of treatment to be reconsidered.

Indications for Surgical Treatment

The indications for surgery of the low lumbar spine have yet to be well defined. Even in the presence of neurologic injury, surgical indications are not absolute; several reports have described patients who have recovered neurologic function when treated nonsur-

gically.[1,2,4,6-9,13,14,16] The amount of canal compromise is also an unknown variable, because up to 90% canal compromise has been reported in the absence of neurologic deficit. The degree of kyphosis is also an unknown variable, particularly because the tendency for these fractures to develop progressive kyphotic deformities is considerably lower than in the thoracolumbar region, but the presence of absolute kyphosis across the injury level has been cited as grounds for surgical intervention. A major obstacle has been that studies investigating indications for surgery have not used rigorous objective criteria and have not been well controlled. Keeping these significant limitations in mind, these studies have suggested 50% canal compromise, 50% loss of height, and the presence of neurologic deficit as indications for surgical intervention. The use of either loss of height or degree of canal compromise as isolated criteria for surgical intervention should be cautioned, given that these variables in isolation may be relatively meaningless to the patient's clinical outcome. In addition to the previously mentioned criteria, one study separated patients with single root injuries from those with multiple root injuries and recommended surgical intervention for patients with multiple nerve root injuries (**Table 2**).

In a 2005 study,[22] the Thoracolumbar Injury Classification and Severity Score (TLICS) was introduced as an attempt to facilitate appropriate surgical versus nonsurgical treatment recommendations by predicting spinal stability, future deformity, and progressive neurologic compromise in a given fracture type. If this classification were applied to low lumbar burst fractures, surgery would generally be indicated in patients with injury to the posterior ligamentous complex and patients with neurologic deficits.

Outcomes

Because low lumbar fractures are uncommon, there are no large prospective studies from which to determine the best form of treatment. Nonsurgical treatment appears to be appropriate in most situations. In the absence of a randomized controlled study, it is difficult to

Table 2

Different Studies Involving Low Lumbar Burst Fractures

Name/year	No. of Patients	Level treated	Indication for Surgery	Treatment (No. of patients)	Comments
Levine and Edwards 1988[4]	22	L4, L5		Nonsurgical or distraction rod (22), pedicle fixation (8)	Improved fusion rates, preservation of motion segments, early mobilization with pedicle fixation
An et al 1991[6]	31	L3-L5		Nonsurgical (6), Harrington rod (7), Luque rods (11), plates (6), anterior strut graft (1)	Back pain more persistent in patient with long fusion and loss of lordosis
An et al 1992[7]	20	L3-L5	Neurologic injury, severity of injury, patient choice	Nonsurgical (7), non-instrumented fusion (1). Instrumented fusion: Harrington (5), Luque segmental (2), pedicle screw (5)	Improved sagittal correction with surgery, less back pain in nonsurgical group
Chan et al 1993[11]	20	L2-L5 (without neurologic deficit)		Nonsurgical (20)	Neurologic loss and symptomatic kyphosis are uncommon
Mick et al 1993[16]	11	L5	50% canal compromise (relative indication)	Nonsurgical (5), pedicle screws (6)	Nonsurgical treatment successful with minimal canal compromise, surgical treatment successful when canal compromise is large, decompression helpful with neurologic deficit
Huang et al 1995[14]	14	L3-L5	Anterior: incomplete neurologic injury, > 50% canal encroachment, > 50% loss of vertebral height. Posterior: significant lamina fracture, L5 fracture	Anterior locking plate (7), pedicle screw (7)	Anterior plate had no failures, posterior construct had two screws break
Andreychik et al 1996[8]	55	L2-L5		Nonsurgical (30), long posterior (8), pedicle screw (8), anterior and posterior (6), anterior (3)	Nonsurgical treatment recommended for neurologically intact or single nerve root injury. Surgery if multiple nerve roots injured
Seybold et al 1999[1]	42	L3-L5		Nonsurgical (20), pedicle screw (10), anterior fusion (3), combined (2), hook and rod long (7)	Neurologic recovery occurred in all groups, functional outcome between groups no different. Reoperation rate, 41%
Benzel and Ball 2000[9]	6	L4, L5		S2 hooks, laminar wires in distraction method	All but one patient improved neurologically, only one patient progressed into kyphosis after surgery
Dai 2002[13]	54 (21 burst)	L3-L5		Nonsurgical (26), Luque or Harrington rods (8), pedicle screw (18), 12 also had anterior procedure	Surgery should be performed with severe spinal stenosis or kyphotic deformity
Butler et al 2007[2]	14	L5 (without neurologic deficit)	> 50% canal comp > 15° kyphosis > 50% loss anterior body height	Nonsurgical (10), pedicle fixation (4)	Better clinical outcome and better maintenance of correction with nonsurgical treatment

4. Axial Skeleton, Including Spine and Pelvis

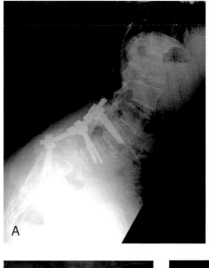
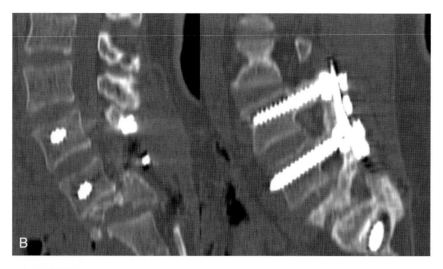
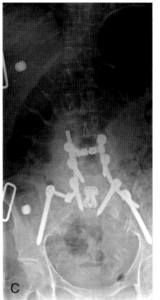
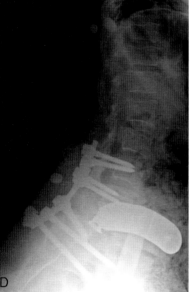

Figure 1   A 49-year-old woman presented with low back pain, right foot drop, and lumbar flat back after L4-S1 laminectomy and instrumentation for L5 burst fracture. Plain radiograph and CT sagittal reformation views (**A** and **B**) show lumbar flat back secondary to focal L4-S1 kyphosis, pseudarthrosis, loose S1 screws, and retropulsed fragment from L5 vertebral body. The patient was treated with staged back and front procedures that involved L3-ilium instrumentation and posterolateral fusion and second stage L5 corpectomy and cage insertion (**C** and **D**). The patient regained her sagittal balance, and her back pain has improved.

compare surgical treatment to nonsurgical treatment in that a selection bias probably exists that associates surgical treatment with more severely injured patients. This problem is further compounded by the fact that the studies investigating surgical treatment often involve different surgical techniques and types of instrumentation, including Luque rods, Harrington rods, pedicle screw instrumentation, anterior fusions, posterior fusions, and combined anterior and posterior fusions. However, it is clear from the current literature that long instrumentation, particularly with distracting forces that place the lumbar spine into kyphosis and create an iatrogenic flat back, have poor outcomes. If surgical fixation is undertaken in this part of the spine, care should be taken to minimize the number of fused motion segments and to restore lumbar lordosis, regardless of the approach used.

Although it seems logical that correcting sagittal imbalance in the lumbar spine would improve long-term outcomes with regard to back pain (**Figure 1**), unlike for patients with kyphotic deformity and degenerative scoliosis, current spine trauma literature does not support this contention.

Future Treatments

Minimally invasive techniques have been used for degenerative spine problems for several years. Recently, these techniques have been applied to the treatment of burst fractures. A case report has described the use of L4-S1 minimally invasive instrumentation as an internal brace in a noncompliant patient with an L5 burst fracture, with subsequent removal of hardware after fracture healing.[5]

Lumbosacral Trauma

The sacrum, located between the two iliac wings, is essentially the structure that joins the spine to the lower extremities through the sacroiliac joints. The upper three vertebrae form the articular facet of the sacroiliac joint. The lower two sacral vertebrae and the coccyx are nonarticular, and supply the attachments for the sacrotuberous and sacrospinous ligaments. The sacrum and its surrounding ligaments form the integral foundation for the structural integrity of the lumbar spine and the posterior pelvic ring. In a metabolically healthy individual, high-energy injury mechanisms are required for structural disruption of this area.[23]

Pathomechanics of Sacral Fractures

Sacral fractures may be vertical, transverse, or complex with vertical and transverse components, the so-called H or U fractures. There is an important distinction between an isolated transverse sacral fracture, which is usually caudal to the sacroiliac joints and does not compromise pelvic ring stability, and the vertical fractures, which do affect pelvic ring stability. Isolated transverse fractures usually occur as the result of direct trauma, such as a fall onto the buttocks. Vertical fractures may be caused by lateral compression, in turn causing impaction of the cancellous bone of the sacrum, by tension failure from an "open book" pelvic injury or by a shear mechanism. High-energy fractures, especially those that result from falls from a height, may involve bilateral vertical fractures joined by one or more horizontal fracture lines, the so-called H or U fracture pattern. The transverse fracture component of these complex sacral fractures usually involves the upper sacral segments. The injury pattern, known as spinopelvic dissociation, results in two primary fracture fragments, one consisting of the spine and central sacral fragment and the other the pelvis and peripheral sacral fragment. Although uncommon, sacral fracture-dislocations that result in spinopelvic dissociation with neurologic impairment occur almost exclusively in polytraumatized patients. If left untreated, either intentionally or in the common scenario of a missed diagnosis, painful deformity or progressive neurologic dysfunction may occur. Late corrective surgery is more complex and generally associated with worse outcomes.[23,24]

In a postmortem study of 42 individuals with posterior pelvic ring disruptions, the incidence and anatomic basis of lumbosacral nerve injuries was studied.[25] A total of 40 lumbosacral nerve injuries were identified in 20 of the autopsies. Traction injuries comprised 53%, and root disruption was noted in 38%. Compression injuries, the most amenable to surgical intervention, were present in only 20% of the nerve injuries.

Classification

Based on a series of 236 sacral fractures, a simplified anatomic classification was formulated that correlates fracture location with the incidence of neurologic injury.[24] This classification divides the sacrum into three zones (**Figure 2**). Zone I or alar zone fractures remain lateral to the neuroforamina throughout their course. Zone II or foraminal zone fractures are located in the

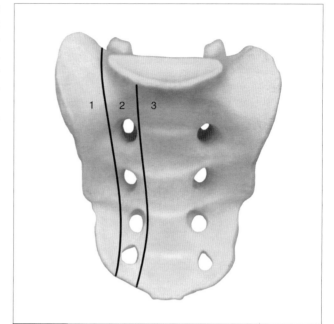

Figure 2   Three-zone sacral classification by Denis. (Reproduced with permission from Bellabarba C, Schildhauer T, Vaccaro A, et al: Complications associated with surgical stabilization of high-grade sacral fracture dislocations with spino-pelvic instability. *Spine* 2006;31(suppl 11):80-88).

transition area between the sacral ala and body and involve one or more neuroforamina while remaining lateral to the spinal canal. Zone III or central zone fractures involve the spinal canal. The key relationship is that the incidence of neurologic injury increases as fractures are more centrally located. Accordingly, zone I fractures had a 5.9% incidence of neurologic injury, primarily to the L5 nerve root as it coursed over the ala. Zone II fractures had a 28.4% incidence of associated neurologic injury occurring as a result of either foraminal displacement and resulting impingement on the exiting nerve root or the "traumatic far-out syndrome" in which the L5 nerve root is caught between the L5 transverse process and the displaced sacral ala. Zone III fractures had a 56.7% incidence of neurologic injury due to injury at the level of the spinal canal, with 76.1% of these individuals having bowel, bladder, and sexual dysfunction. Subsequently, 44 cases of sacral fracture according to the Denis classification system were studied.[26] A 34% incidence of neurologic injury was found overall. Six of 25 patients (24%) with zone I injuries had L5 and/or S1 nerve root injuries. Two of seven zone II injuries similarly had L5 and S1 deficits. No patients with zone I or II injuries had bowel or bladder dysfunction. Three of five patients with zone III injuries had neurologic injury, two with bladder dysfunction. These findings were used as a basis for a classification of neurologic injury from sacral fractures (**Table 3**). It was also noted that significant neurologic deficit is rare in transverse sacral fractures below the S-4 level.

Because of the high potential for neurologic injury as well as spinal column instability, sacral body (Denis zone III) fractures have been specifically investigated. Early case reports often characterized the injury pattern as solely a transverse fracture, possibly because of imaging limitations. CT demonstrates that most transverse fractures of the upper sacrum have complex fracture patterns. Most of these injuries are now understood to consist of a transverse fracture of the sacrum with associated longitudinal or "vertical" injury components, usually in the form of bilateral transforaminal fractures that extend rostrally to the lumbosacral junction, the so-called U fracture. Variations in fracture line propagation include the H, Y, and lambda fracture patterns. Thirteen patients with transverse sacral fractures, 11 as a result of attempted suicide by jumping, were reviewed.[23] The fractures were classified as type 1, flexion deformity of upper sacrum (angulation alone); type 2, flexion deformity with posterior displacement of the upper sacrum on the lower sacrum (angulation and posterior translation); and type 3, anterior displacement of the upper sacrum without angulation (anterior translation alone). Based on cadaver studies it was hypothesized that types 1 and 2 were caused by impact with the lumbar spine in the flexed position, whereas type 3 fractures were caused by impact with the lumbar spine and hips in extension. In a subsequent study of a case of comminution of the upper sacrum without significant angulation or translation, the type 4 injury was reported, which was believed to be an axial loading injury resulting from a neutral lumbosacral spine position at the point of impact[27] (Figure 3).

Even in the absence of a transverse fracture line, sacral fractures can result in spinal column instability. Variations of longitudinal sacral fractures through the S1 and S2 neuroforamina that result in L5-S1 motion segment instability due to associated L5-S1 facet joint disruption have been described.[28] Injuries with the fracture line lateral to the S1 articular process are not associated with instability of the lumbosacral articulation because the L5-S1 articulation remains continuous with the stable fracture component of the sacrum. A fracture that extends into or medial to the S1 articular process, however, may disrupt the associated facet joint and potentially destabilize the lumbosacral junction. Fractures medial to the facet joint are typically vertically stable. Fractures that involve or course lateral to the facet joint are typically vertically unstable. Complete displacement of the facet joint can lead to a locked facet joint, making sacral fracture reduction difficult with closed methods alone. Facet disruption may also cause posttraumatic arthrosis and late lumbosacral pain.

Indications for Treatment

The indications to treat sacral fractures and lumbosacral dissociation are based on the stability of the

Table 3

The Gibbons Classification of Neurologic Injury

Type	Neurologic deficit
1	None
2	Paresthesias only
3	Lower extremity motor deficit
4	Bowel/bladder dysfunction

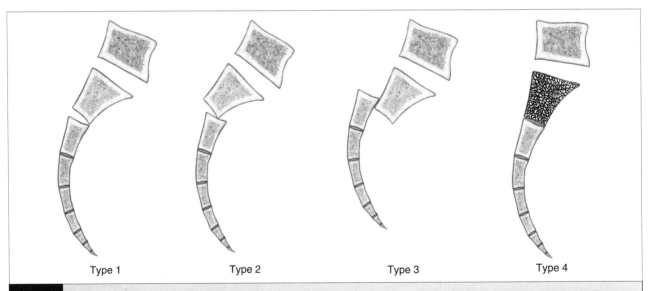

Type 1   Type 2   Type 3   Type 4

Figure 3 Subclassification of Denis zone III fractures according to sagittal plane alignment by Roy-Camille et al, and Strange-Vognsen and Lebech. (Reproduced with permission from Bellabarba C, Schildhauer T, Vaccaro A, et al: Complications associated with surgical stabilization of high-grade sacral fracture dislocations with spino-pelvic instability. *Spine* 2006;31(suppl 11):80-88.)

Table 4

Biomechanical Studies Comparing Different Fixation Constructs

Name/ Year	Constructs	Results
Leighton et al 1991[33]	Sacroiliac screw fixation versus four-hole anterior sacroiliac joint plate	No difference in loading to failure with loads of 1,000 N.
Pohlemann et al 1993[34]	Sacral bars versus internal spine fixator (bolts into the sacral ala cross-connected versus local osteosynthesis	Sacral bars had the highest load to failure, with internal fixator being the least. No significant differences in displacements were noted between fixation methods at loads of 900 N to 1,200 N.
Simonain et al 1996[35]	One versus two iliac screws versus tension band plating versus transiliac bars	No differences between stiffness of any type of the fixation used at loads of approximately 200 N.
Comstock et al 1996[36]	Anterior sacroiliac joint plating versus sacral bar fixation versus two iliosacral screws versus two iliosacral screws with sacral bars	Two iliosacral screws alone and two iliosacral screws combined with two sacral bars provided the stiffest fixation; sacral bars alone were the least stiff fixation with loads of 1,400 N.
Schildhauer et al 2003[32]	Triangular osteosynthesis versus standard iliosacral screw osteosynthesis	Triangular osteosynthesis for unstable transforaminal sacral fractures provided significantly greater immediate postoperative stability than the iliosacral screw fixation.

fracture and neurologic involvement. Displaced fractures generally require a stabilization procedure. The exceptions to this are fractures associated with a lateral compression type mechanism. Patients who have a neurologic injury with bone fragments compressing a nerve root will likely require a decompressive procedure with a stabilization procedure.

Neurologic improvement after sacral fractures with spinopelvic instability patterns has been reported to approach 80%, regardless of surgical or nonsurgical management. However, the wide variability in injury types, degree of improvement, and outcome criteria have lessened the significance and reliability of reported recovery rates. Several case series have described better neurologic outcome with surgical treatment, particularly in patients with bowel and bladder impairment. However, these studies have significant limitations with regard to cohort size, selection bias, objective evaluation of neurologic status, and documentation of the type and severity of neural encroachment in nonsurgically treated patients, consistency in the type and timing of surgical intervention, evaluation of the adequacy of decompression, and the influence of persistent pelvic instability. Furthermore, these studies often grouped widely heterogeneous Denis zone I-III injuries collectively as a single group.[26,29,30]

Unlike cauda equina syndrome caused by acute lumbar disk herniation where urgent decompression within 24 to 48 hours is generally advocated, the timing of sacral root decompression for fracture has not been studied specifically. Because of the highly dissimilar injury mechanism and patient populations, it is unlikely that the recommendations for surgical intervention in patients with cauda equina resulting from lumbar disk herniation can be extrapolated to patients with sacral

fractures. Potential benefits of early surgical intervention include patient mobilization and early decompression of compromised neural elements. These benefits must be weighed against increased risks of hemodynamic instability, severe blood loss, and wound infection in the physiologically compromised sacral fracture population. Indications for emergent surgical intervention include deteriorating neurologic status, dorsal soft-tissue compromise from displaced fractures, and the presence of an open fracture. It appears that most patients can otherwise be effectively treated surgically within a 48-hour to 2-week window. Prolonged delay in patients with canal encroachment and concordant neurologic deficit, however, may negatively influence neurologic recovery.[24,31]

Treatment Options

Treatment of high-energy displaced sacral fractures has traditionally been nonsurgical by default because of the absence of cogent surgical treatment alternatives. Until recently, surgical treatment offered limited, if any, capacity for fracture reduction and effective stabilization. However, currently available posterior internal fixation options for sacral fractures include a spectrum of percutaneous and open techniques such as iliosacral screws, iliac bars, small fragment posterior plate fixation, and lumbopelvic adaptations of the Galveston-type rod constructs. The literature regarding comparative biomechanical testing of posterior pelvic ring fixation techniques showed few differences between these forms of fixation. However, each of these investigations used a different loading condition and different methods to assess fixation stiffness[32-36] (Table 4).

Highly displaced multiplanar sacral fracture-dislocations that result in spinopelvic dissociation and

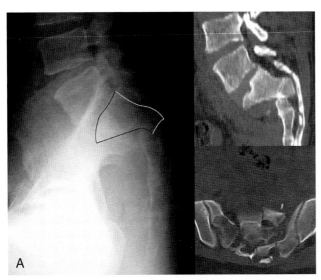

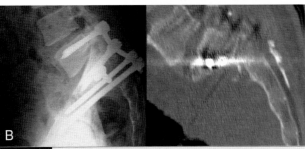

Figure 4	Radiographic studies of a 25-year-old involved in a motor vehicle crash who sustained a Roy-Camille type 2 sacral U-fracture with cauda equina injury. **A,** Lateral radiograph, sagittal CT reformation, and axial CT view show comminuted bilateral transforaminal and transverse sacral fractures with severe kyphosis and canal compromise. **B,** Postoperative lateral radiograph and sagittal CT reformation after L5-S3 laminectomy and lumbopelvic fixation show improved sacral kyphosis and decompression of the sacral canal. (Reproduced with permission from Schildhauer T, Bellabarba C, Nork S, et al: Decompression and lumbopelvic fixation for sacral fracture-dislocations with spino-pelvic dissociation. *J Orthop Trauma* 2006;20:447-457.)

with aggressive neural decompression, while permitting early mobilization without supplemental bracing (**Figure 4**). Iliosacral screws offer an elegant percutaneous method of posterior pelvic ring fixation but are limited by requiring a virtually anatomic reduction and the absence of anatomic variants, or either poor bone quality or extensive comminution of the sacrum. Furthermore, percutaneous iliosacral screw fixation provides little or no load-bearing capacity to a compromised lumbopelvic junction.[37,38]

Lumbopelvic fixation is designed to counteract the commonly misunderstood resulting pattern of instability. Securing the lumbosacral spine to the iliac wings with segmental spinal fixation neutralizes the deforming forces by gaining solid fixation in both major components of the fracture. This method of fixation is particularly valuable because sacral anatomic constraints have made stable fracture fixation difficult to achieve with more traditional plate and screw constructs. Biomechanical analysis has confirmed that segmental lumbopelvic instrumentation, a method derived from the Galveston technique of anchoring spine constructs caudally to the ilium, is among the most stable methods of posterior pelvic fixation. This technique is particularly well suited to the treatment of sacral fractures because it unloads the area of injury by mimicking the normal load transfer from the acetabulae across the sacroiliac joints to the lumbar spine. This configuration allows for comprehensive decompression of sacral neural elements and open reduction of sacral fractures, while permitting early mobilization and weight bearing without the need for cumbersome external braces.[32,38,39]

Summary

Low lumbar burst fractures are uncommon injuries that behave differently than typical thoracolumbar burst fractures. With the advent of pedicle screw fixation, surgical options for these injuries, when necessary, have improved. However, most patients with these injuries can be treated nonsurgically if neurologically intact, regardless of the extent of bony retropulsion and canal compromise. Surgical indications remain unclear, with newer scoring systems suggesting surgical intervention in the presence of neurologic deficits or disruption of the posterior osseoligamentous tension band. Because low lumbar burst fractures are uncommon injuries, multicenter prospective studies would likely be required to determine the most effective treatment of these injuries.

Sacral fractures are commonly seen in multiply injured patients as a result of high-energy mechanisms. Patients are usually physiologically compromised, and a large number of them are intubated in intensive care units, which usually makes neurologic assessment difficult and incomplete. A careful assessment of pelvic radiographs and CT is essential to better understand the personality of this injury and guide the decisions regarding the best form of management. The literature

cauda equina deficits are poorly understood and continue to pose diagnostic and treatment challenges. Because they are generally composed of a transverse sacral fracture component with associated bilateral longitudinal fracture components, these fractures result in dissociation of the spine and upper central sacral segment from the pelvis and peripheral sacral fragments, giving rise to the term "spinopelvic dissociation." The relative paucity of these injuries and the polytraumatized nature of this widely heterogeneous patient population have resulted in few investigations upon which to base treatment algorithms. The emergence of segmental spinal fixation techniques that can incorporate the iliac wings has allowed an opportunity to achieve reduction and stabilization of fracture-dislocations involving the lumbosacral region, along that neurologic injuries from sacral fractures usually improve with or without surgical treatment. However, in part based on studies demonstrating objective evidence of neurologic recovery in up to 83% of patients treated by surgical decompression and stabilization, surgical decompression is recommended. The timing of surgery is debatable, but one must confirm that these multiply injured patients are cleared by the general surgery team and deemed stable enough to undergo surgery.

Annotated References

1. Seybold EA, Sweeney CA, Fredrickson BE, Warhold LG, Bernini PM: Functional outcome of low lumbar burst fractures: A multicenter review of operative and nonoperative treatment of L3-L5. *Spine* 1999;24(20):2154-2161.

2. Butler JS, Fitzpatrick P, Ni Mhaolain AM, Synnott K, O'Byrne JM: The management and functional outcome of isolated burst fractures of the fifth lumbar vertebra. *Spine* 2007;32(4):443-447.

   This is a retrospective review of 14 L5 burst fractures, of which 10 were treated nonsurgically and 4 surgically. Clinical and radiographic criteria were reviewed. The authors strongly recommend nonsurgical treatment of this injury.

3. Levine AM: The surgical treatment of low lumbar fractures. *Semin Spine Surg* 1990;2:41-53.

4. Levine AM, Edwards CC: Low lumbar burst fractures: Reduction and stabilization using the modular spine fixation system. *Orthopedics* 1988;11(10):1427-1432.

5. Sahin S, Resnick DK: Minimally incisional stabilization of unstable L5 burst fracture. *J Spinal Disord Tech* 2005;18(5):455-457.

   A case report of treating a noncompliant patient with an L5 burst fracture is presented. Minimally invasive L4–S1 screw fixation was used. The hardware was removed at 4 months and at 6 months the patient was doing well.

6. An HS, Vaccaro A, Cotler JM, Lin S: Low lumbar burst fractures: Comparison among body cast, Harrington rod, Luque rod, and Steffee plate. *Spine* 1991;16(suppl 8):S440-S444.

7. An HS, Simpson JM, Ebraheim NA, Jackson WT, Moore J, O'Malley NP: Low lumbar burst fractures: Comparison between conservative and surgical treatments. *Orthopedics* 1992;15(3):367-373.

8. Andreychik DA, Alander DH, Senica KM, Stauffer ES: Burst fractures of the second through fifth lumbar vertebrae: Clinical and radiographic results. *J Bone Joint Surg Am* 1996;78(8):1156-1166.

9. Benzel EC, Ball PA: Management of low lumbar frac-
tures by dorsal decompression, fusion, and lumbosacral laminar distraction fixation. *J Neurosurg* 2000;92(suppl 2):142-148.

10. Boucher M, Bhandari M, Kwok D: Health-related quality of life after short segment instrumentation of lumbar burst fractures. *J Spinal Disord* 2001;14(5):417-426.

11. Chan DP, Seng NK, Kaan KT: Nonoperative treatment in burst fractures of the lumbar spine (L2-L5) without neurologic deficits. *Spine* 1993;18(3):320-325.

12. Court-Brown CM, Gertzbein SD: The management of burst fractures of the fifth lumbar vertebra. *Spine* 1987;12(3):308-312.

13. Dai LD: Low lumbar spinal fractures: Management options. *Injury* 2002;33(7):579-582.

14. Huang TJ, Chen JY, Shih HN, Chen YJ, Hsu RW: Surgical indications in low lumbar burst fractures: Experiences with Anterior Locking Plate System and the reduction-fixation system. *J Trauma* 1995;39(5):910-914.

15. Knight RQ, Stornelli DP, Chan DP, Devanny JR, Jackson KV: Comparison of operative versus nonoperative treatment of lumbar burst fractures. *Clin Orthop Relat Res* 1993;293:112-121.

16. Mick CA, Carl A, Sachs B, Hresko MT, Pfeifer BA: Burst fractures of the fifth lumbar vertebra. *Spine* 1993;18(13):1878-1884.

17. Miyakoshi N, Abe E, Shimada Y, Hongo M, Chiba M, Sato K: Anterior decompression with single segmental spinal interbody fusion for lumbar burst fracture. *Spine* 1999;24(1):67-73.

18. Slosar PJ Jr, Patwardhan AG, Lorenz M, Havey R, Sartori M: Instability of the lumbar burst fracture and limitations of transpedicular instrumentation. *Spine* 1995;20(13):1452-1461.

19. Strømsøe K, Hem ES, Aunan E: Unstable vertebral fractures in the lower third of the spine treated with closed reduction and transpedicular posterior fixation: A retrospective analysis of 82 fractures in 78 patients. *Eur Spine J* 1997;6(4):239-244.

20. Levine AM: Low lumbar fractures, in Browner BD, Levine AM, Jupiter JB, Trafton PG, Krettek C, eds: *Skeletal Trauma*, ed 4. Philadelphia, PA, Saunders, 2009, pp 979-1017.

   Low lumbar fractures are discussed in detail.

21. Ozturk C, Ersozlu S, Aydinli U: Importance of greenstick lamina fractures in low lumbar burst fractures. *Int Orthop* 2006;30(4):295-298.

   Greenstick lamina fractures occur mostly in the L2-L4 area in 7 (25%) of 28 burst fractures. All patients with the lamina fracture underwent open book laminectomy, replacement of roots within dura, and primary dural repair before instrumentation. All patients with neurolgic deficit improved.

22. Vaccaro AR, Lehman RA Jr , Hurlbert RJ, et al: A new classification of thoracolumbar injuries: The importance of injury morphology, the integrity of the posterior ligamentous complex, and neurologic status. *Spine* 2005; 30(20):2325-2333.

  This article describes a new thoracolumbar fracture classification system that is easy to use and assigns point values to injury morphology, integrity of posterior ligamentous complex, and neurologic injury. The point value determines the treatment course.

23. Roy-Camille R, Saillant G, Gagna G, Mazel C: Transverse fracture of the upper sacrum: Suicidal jumper's fracture. *Spine* 1985;10(9):838-845.

24. Denis F, Davis S, Comfort T: Sacral fractures: An important problem. Retrospective analysis of 236 cases. *Clin Orthop Relat Res* 1988;227:67-81.

25. Huittinen VM: Lumbo-sacral nerve injury in fracture of the pelvis: A postmortem radiographic and pathoanatomical study. *Acta Chir Scand* 1972;429:3-43.

26. Gibbons KJ, Soloniuk DS, Razack N: Neurological injury and patterns of sacral fractures. *J Neurosurg* 1990; 72(6):889-893.

27. Strange-Vognsen HH, Lebech A: An unusual type of fracture in the upper sacrum. *J Orthop Trauma* 1991; 5(2):200-203.

28. Isler B: Lumbosacral lesions associated with pelvic ring injuries. *J Orthop Trauma* 1990;4(1):1-6.

29. Bellabarba C, Schildhauer TA, Vaccaro AR, Chapman JR: Complications associated with surgical stabilization of high-grade sacral fracture dislocations with spinopelvic instability. *Spine* 2006;31(suppl 11):S80-S88.

  This is a retrospective review of 19 consecutive patients with sacral fracture-dislocations and cauda equina syndrome that were treated with neural decompression and lumbopelvic fixation. During the index surgical intervention, 14 of 19 patients (74%) had either a traumatic dural tear or nerve root avulsion. Major complications involved fracture of the connecting rods in 6 of 19 (31%) patients and wound healing disturbances in 5/19 (26%). The authors concluded that rigid segmental lumbopelvic stabilization allowed reliable fracture reduction and permitted early mobilization and neurologic improvement in a large number of patients.

30. Schildhauer TA, Bellabarba C, Nork SE, Barei DP, Routt ML Jr, Chapman JR: Decompression and lumbopelvic fixation for sacral fracture-dislocations with spino-pelvic dissociation. *J Orthop Trauma* 2006;20(7): 447-457.

  A retrospective clinical study of 19 patients with highly displaced, comminuted, irreducible Roy-Camille type 2-4 sacral fractures with spinopelvic instability patterns and cauda equina deficits is presented. Sacral fractures healed in all 18 patients without loss of reduction. Average sacral kyphosis improved from 43° to 21°. Fifteen patients (83%) had full or partial recovery of bowel and bladder deficits. Wound infection (16%) was the most common complication. Complete recovery of cauda equina function was more likely in patients with continuity of all sacral roots and incomplete deficits. Although not statistically significant, recovery of bowel and bladder function specifically was more closely associated with absence of any sacral root discontinuity than with completeness of the injury.

31. Zelle BA, Gruen GS, Hunt T, Speth SR: Sacral fractures with neurological injury: Is early decompression beneficial? *Int Orthop* 2004;28(4):244-251.

  The authors studied 177 patients with displaced sacral fractures over a 6-year period. Those who underwent surgical decompression had a significantly better neurologic improvement and physical function than those who were treated without surgical decompression.

32. Schildhauer TA, Ledoux WR, Chapman JR, Henley MB, Tencer AF, Routt ML Jr: Triangular osteosynthesis and iliosacral screw fixation for unstable sacral fractures: A cadaveric and biomechanical evaluation under cyclic loads. *J Orthop Trauma* 2003;17(1):22-31.

33. Leighton RK, Waddell JP, Bray TJ, et al: Biomechanical testing of new and old fixation devices for vertical shear fractures of the pelvis. *J Orthop Trauma* 1991;5(3):313-317.

34. Pohlemann T, Angst M, Schneider E, Ganz R, Tscherne H: Fixation of transforaminal sacrum fractures: A biomechanical study. *J Orthop Trauma* 1993;7(2):107-117.

35. Simonain PT, Routt C Jr, Harrington RM, Tencer AF: Internal fixation for the transforaminal sacral fracture. *Clin Orthop Relat Res* 1996;323:202-209.

36. Comstock CP, van der Meulen MC, Goodman SB: Biomechanical comparison of posterior internal fixation techniques for unstable pelvic fractures. *J Orthop Trauma* 1996;10(8):517-522.

37. Hunt N, Jennings A, Smith M: Current management of U-shaped sacral fractures or spino-pelvic dissociation. *Injury* 2002;33(2):123-126.

38. Schildhauer TA, Josten CH, Muhr G: Triangular osteosynthesis for unstable sacral fractures. *Orthop Traumatol* 2001;9:24-38.

39. Schildhauer TA, McCulloch P, Chapman JR, Mann FA: Anatomic and radiographic considerations for placement of transiliac screws in lumbopelvic fixations. *J Spinal Disord Tech* 2002;15(3):199-205.

Section 5

Lower Extremity

SECTION EDITORS:

KEVIN J. PUGH, MD

MICHAEL D. STOVER, MD

Chapter 31

Hip Dislocations and Femoral Head and Neck Fractures

Kenneth A. Egol, MD   Ross Leighton, MD, FRCS(C), FACS   Alun Evans, MSc, FRCS   Michael D. Stover, MD

Hip Dislocations

Epidemiology

The hip joint is inherently stable; dislocation requires significant force. Stability of the hip comes mainly from its skeletal architecture, with some contributions from the capsule, labrum, and ligamentum teres. Simple hip dislocation requires disruption to all of these soft-tissue structures. However, in dislocations with associated femoral head fractures, the ligamentum teres may remain attached to the femoral head if the fracture exits above the fovea. Simple hip dislocations usually result from high-energy injuries, such as a motor vehicle crash, fall from a height, or industrial accident. Sciatic nerve injury is present in 10% to 20% of posterior dislocations. Up to 50% of patients sustain other concomitant fractures at the time of the hip dislocation.

Dr. Egol or an immediate family member serves as a board member, owner, officer, or committee member of Orthopaedic Trauma Association Research Committee; serves as an unpaid consultant to Exactech; has received research or institutional support from Biomet, Smith & Nephew, Stryker, and Synthes; and has stock or stock options held in Johnson & Johnson and Surgix Inc. Dr. Leighton or an immediate family member serves as a board member, owner, officer, or committee member of Canadian Orthopaedic Association and Orthopaedic Trauma Association; has received royalties from Zimmer and AO; is a member of a speakers' bureau or has made paid presentations on behalf of AO, Biomet, DePuy, Johnson & Johnson, Etex, and Smith & Nephew; serves as a paid consultant to or is an employee of Etex, DePuy, Johnson & Johnson, and Smith & Nephew; has received research or institutional support from AO, the Canadian Orthopaedic Foundation, DePuy, Johnson & Johnson, Etex, Medtronic, Smith & Nephew, and Zimmer; and has received nonincome support (such as equipment or services), commercially derived honoraria, or other non-research–related funding (such as paid travel) from the Canadian Orthopaedic Foundation. Dr. Stover or an immediate family member serves as a board member, owner, officer, or committee member of Association of Bone and Joint Surgeons and Orthopaedic Trauma Association. Neither Dr. Evans nor any immediate family member has received anything of value from or owns stock in a commercial company or institution related directly or indirectly to the subject of this chapter.

Anterior Dislocations

Anterior dislocations comprise 10% to 15% of traumatic hip dislocations. These injuries result from forced external rotation and abduction of the hip. The degree of hip flexion determines whether a superior or inferior type of anterior hip dislocation occurs, with inferior (obturator) dislocation resulting from simultaneous abduction and external rotation with the hip in flexion. Superior (iliac or pubic) dislocation is the result of simultaneous abduction, external rotation, and hip extension.

Posterior Dislocations

Posterior dislocations are five to six times more frequent than anterior hip dislocations and most commonly result from trauma to the flexed knee (for example, a dashboard injury) with the hip in varying degrees of flexion. If the hip is in the neutral or slightly adducted position at the time of impact, a dislocation without acetabular fracture will likely occur. If the hip is in slight abduction, an associated fracture of the posterior wall of the acetabulum usually occurs.

Clinical Evaluation

A complete evaluation of a patient with a hip dislocation is essential because of the high-energy nature of these injuries. Concomitant intra-abdominal, chest, and other musculoskeletal injuries, such as acetabular, pelvic, or spine fractures, or fractures of the ipsilateral extremity are common. Patients presenting with dislocations of the hip typically are unable to move the lower extremity and experience severe discomfort. A careful neurovascular examination is essential. Sciatic nerve injury may occur, and the peroneal portion of the nerve is typically more affected. Rarely, injury to the femoral artery, vein, or nerve may occur as a result of an anterior dislocation.

Radiographic Evaluation

An AP radiograph of the pelvis is essential, as well as a cross-table lateral view of the affected hip. On the AP view of the pelvis, the femoral heads should appear similar in size and the joint spaces should be symmetric throughout. With the hip reduced, the Shenton line

5: Lower Extremity

should be smooth and continuous. The relative appearance of the greater and lesser trochanters may indicate pathologic internal or external rotation of the hip. The adducted or abducted position of the femoral shaft also should be noted. Evaluation of the femoral neck is essential to rule out the presence of a femoral neck fracture before any manipulative reduction. A cross-table lateral view of the affected hip may help distinguish a posterior from an anterior dislocation, serve as an orthogonal view for evaluation of the proximal femur and acetabulum, and can be obtained without manipulation of the extremity.

Use of 45° oblique (Judet) views of the hip may be helpful to ascertain the presence of osteochondral fragments, the integrity of the acetabulum, and the congruence of the joint spaces. Femoral head fractures or impaction may also be seen. Concentric reduction of the hip on plain radiographs does not preclude the presence of loose bodies within the hip joint.[1] If closed reduction is not possible and an open reduction is planned, CT should be performed to detect the presence of intra-articular fragments and to rule out associated femoral head, neck, and acetabular fractures. Even after successful closed reduction, CT will help identify loose bodies and areas of articular impaction. The role of MRI in the evaluation of hip dislocations has recently been further clarified; it may prove useful in the evaluation of the integrity of the labrum, presence of chondral injury, and vascularity of the femoral head.[2]

Treatment
Urgent reduction of the dislocated hip is necessary to minimize the risk of osteonecrosis of the femoral head. Closed reduction under anesthesia (or deep sedation with muscle relaxation) is usually successful, but there are specific circumstances when open reduction is necessary, including instances in which there is an associated fracture of the proximal femur or an incarcerated fragment. The long-term prognosis worsens if reduction (closed or open) is delayed more than 12 hours. Following successful closed reduction, associated acetabular or femoral head fractures can be treated in the subacute phase.

Closed Reduction
Regardless of the direction of the dislocation, reduction of the hip can be attempted with in-line traction with the patient lying supine. The preferred method is to perform a closed reduction using general anesthesia, but if this is not feasible, reduction under conscious sedation is possible if adequate muscle relaxation can be achieved.

Open Reduction
Absolute indications for urgent open reduction of a dislocated hip include a dislocation irreducible by closed means, an ipsilateral femoral neck fracture (displaced or nondisplaced), or a delayed presentation of dislocation. Urgent open reduction may be indicated if an os-teochondral fragment of the acetabulum or femoral head prevents closed reduction or reduction results in a markedly nonconcentric joint. A standard posterolateral hip approach (Kocher-Langenbeck) will allow exploration of the sciatic nerve, removal of incarcerated fragments, treatment of major posterior labral disruptions or instability, and repair of posterior acetabular fractures. An anterior (Smith-Petersen) approach is recommended for isolated femoral head fractures and irreducible anterior hip dislocations. An anterior approach for a simple posterior dislocation is typically not recommended. Alternatively, the anterolateral (Watson-Jones) approach can be used for most anterior dislocations and combined fractures of both femoral head and neck. A direct lateral (Hardinge) approach will allow exposure anteriorly and posteriorly through the same incision. In the case of an ipsilateral displaced or nondisplaced femoral neck fracture, closed reduction of the hip should not be attempted. The hip fracture should be provisionally stabilized through an anterior or lateral approach. A gentle reduction of the dislocation is then performed, followed by definitive fixation of the femoral neck.

Management after closed or open reduction of hip dislocation ranges from short periods of bed rest to various durations of skeletal traction. No correlation exists between early weight bearing and osteonecrosis. Therefore, partial weight bearing is advised. If reduction is concentric and stable, a short period of bed rest is followed by protected weight bearing for 4 to 6 weeks. If the reduction is concentric but unstable, meaning redislocation on examination under anesthesia, then surgical intervention should be considered.

Arthroscopic Evaluation Following Hip Dislocation
Arthroscopy is becoming widely accepted as a treatment modality for various hip conditions including femoroacetabular impingement, labral pathology, and presence of loose bodies. Recently, hip arthroscopy has been performed following traumatic hip dislocation.[3] Diagnostic arthroscopy is performed through anterior and anterolateral portals with the patient supine. Incomplete capsular integrity must be assumed until 3 months after injury; thus, if undertaken acutely, low pressure irrigation or "dry" arthroscopy should be used.[4] Arthroscopic evaluations following hip dislocation reveal several pathologic conditions, including labral and loose bodies in almost all patients, as well as capsular injuries, chondral injuries of the femoral head and acetabulum, ligamentum teres tears, and acetabular rim fractures in many.[5] In the setting of acute trauma about the hip, the long-term significance of these findings is still unknown. Although no treatment recommendations have been established regarding arthroscopic management of acute hip dislocations, removal of encountered loose bodies should be performed to limited third body wear in the joint.

Prognosis After Hip Dislocation

The outcome following hip dislocation ranges from an essentially normal hip to a severely painful and degenerated joint. Most authors report good or excellent outcomes in 70% to 80% of simple posterior dislocations. When posterior dislocations are associated with a femoral head or acetabular fracture, however, the associated fractures generally dictate the outcome. Anterior dislocations of the hip are noted to have a higher incidence of associated femoral head injuries (transchondral or impaction types). The only patients with excellent results in most series are those without an associated femoral head injury. According to one study of eight American football players with traumatic hip dislocations, those without MRI evidence of osteonecrosis at 6 weeks reportedly returned to activities,[6] but data do not yet support the routine use of MRI as a prognostic tool in this population.

Complications

Osteonecrosis is observed in 5% to 40% of hip dislocations, with increased risk associated with increased time to reduction (more than 6 to 24 hours). In some cases, osteonecrosis may result from the initial injury; nevertheless, the need to obtain an expeditious reduction should be considered a priority.

Posttraumatic osteoarthritis is the most frequent long-term complication of hip dislocations. The incidence is dramatically higher when dislocations are associated with acetabular fractures or transchondral fractures of the femoral head. Recurrent dislocation is rare (less than 2%), although patients with decreased femoral anteversion may be at increased risk for recurrent posterior dislocation. Those with increased femoral anteversion may be more prone to recurrent anterior dislocations. Sciatic nerve injury occurs in 10% to 20% of hip dislocations and is associated with longer time to reduction following posterior hip dislocation.[7] Heterotopic ossification occurs in 2% of patients.

Femoral Head Fractures

Femoral head fractures occur in 7% to 16% of hip dislocations and are associated almost exclusively with posterior dislocation of the hip, although case reports have described the fracture without dislocation or in association with anterior dislocation.[8] With the associated dislocation, urgent relocation of the hip is essential to limit vascular injury to the femoral head. Fractures of the acetabulum or proximal femur occur frequently enough that an AP pelvis radiograph is necessary following hip dislocation and should be carefully evaluated for associated injuries before reduction.

Classification

Fractures of the femoral head are most commonly discussed with reference to the Pipkin classification, which is based on the fracture location and associated injuries affecting the hip.[9] In type I injuries, the fracture is below the fovea, separating the fractured fragment from the ligamentum teres and keeping the weight-bearing portion of the femoral head intact. Type II fractures extend above the fovea and into the weight-bearing portion of the femoral head, frequently maintaining attachment of the fractured fragment to the ligament. In type III and IV injuries, the femoral head fracture is associated with a fracture of the femoral neck or acetabulum, respectively. Although the Pipkin classification provides a system on which treatment can be based, it does not indicate severity of injury or predict prognosis. It also does not differentiate the size or location of the femoral head fracture in types III and IV, or the location or type of associated acetabulum fracture.

Initial Treatment

Reduction of the hip in the presence of a femoral head fracture should proceed with care, because nondisplaced or unrecognized femoral neck fractures can occur or secondarily displace with reduction maneuvers. Recently, the physical examination, plain radiography, and prereduction CT findings in irreducible femoral head fracture-dislocations without fractures of the posterior wall were described.[10] These irreducible injuries occurred in less than 10% of femoral head fracture-dislocations. Physical examination revealed a significant leg length inequality and slight flexion of the hip without the typical rotation deformity of the leg that occurs with uncomplicated hip dislocation. All patients had a suprafoveal femoral head fracture and posterior-superior dislocations of the hip with the femoral head intimately opposed to the supra-acetabular ilium. The injuries were irreducible and were treated by open reduction from an anterior Smith-Petersen approach. Surgeons should be aware of this specific fracture pattern.

Evaluation

Femoral head fractures usually involve the anterior and medial surface of the femoral head. An AP pelvis radiograph following reduction is mandatory to confirm repositioning of the dislocated femoral head and the associated fracture fragment within the acetabulum and to evaluate for a congruent reduction. A CT scan with two-dimensional reconstructions is mandatory following reduction because it is the only way to adequately evaluate the fracture reduction and the presence of residual intra-articular fragments.

Treatment

Suprafoveal femoral head fractures (Pipkin type II) with any residual displacement after reduction are commonly considered for surgical reduction and fixation because they involve the weight-bearing portion of the femoral head. Any residual displacement of such fractures could potentially increase focal joint reactive forces and acetabular wear, resulting in arthrosis. The degree of cranial femoral head involvement and the amount of residual displacement that necessitates treatment has not been characterized. Similarly, residual displacement of infrafoveal fractures (Pipkin type I) or the resection of femoral head fragments has resulted in malunion or instability and joint dysfunction requiring treatment.[11] In general, a hip that is stable with anatomic reduction of a femoral head fragment without a large suprafoveal extension or minimal displacement of a subfoveal fracture can be treated without surgery.

Choice of Surgical Approach

Both anterior and posterior surgical approaches have been used for reduction and fixation of femoral head fractures. The benefits of the posterior approach are its familiarity and the presumed advantage of operating on the side of the soft-tissue pathology resulting from the posterior dislocation. The posterior approach also allows repair of associated posterior acetabulum fractures. However, the femoral head fracture, which almost always involves an anterior medial fragment, is difficult to visualize and stabilize from a posterior approach. The anterior approach to the hip sacrifices little femoral head vascularity. The anterior approach and a technique for reduction of locked or irreducible femoral head dislocations without acetabulum fracture has been described.[10] The improved visualization of the femoral head afforded by the anterior approach has been shown to improve reductions.[12] However, access to posterior wall acetabular fractures is limited from the anterior approach. In the setting of combined injuries to the femoral head and posterior acetabulum, the digastric trochanteric osteotomy provides safe exposure of both fractures.[13-16]

The role of arthroscopy in the management of femoral head fractures has yet to be defined, although arthroscopic reduction and fixation with headless screws has been reported.[17] This approach should only be used by those with advanced experience in hip arthroscopy techniques.

Fixation Technique

Appropriate surgical reduction of suprafoveal fractures may require release of the ligamentum teres. The remaining femoral head commonly has peripheral areas of bone and cartilage impaction adjacent to the fracture bed, and small irregular cartilage flaps may be present on either side of the fracture. Release of the ligamentum teres, with cleaning and débridement of the zone of injury, may still result in focal marginal areas that are reduced imperfectly. Most authors recommend multiple points of compressive fixation of the femoral head fragment, typically with smaller implants placed outside of the weight-bearing area of the femoral head when possible. Screws that are 1.5 to 2.4 mm in diameter have smaller, flat heads that can be countersunk below the articular cartilage. Titanium or bioabsorbable implants have not caused difficulties with fixation or joint irritation in small series and allow MRI evaluation of the femoral head during posttraumatic treatment.[18]

Unusual Circumstances

Persistent Dislocation of the Femoral Head Fragment

The displaced fragment initially dislocates and remains posteriorly displaced following relocation of the head. Retrieval and fixation may require access to both sides of the joint and can be simultaneously achieved with a digastric osteotomy.

Pipkin Type III Injuries

Treatment of these injuries is emergent, and priority should be given to the femoral neck fracture. If nondisplaced, provisional stabilization of the femoral neck fracture should be performed before proceeding with open reduction of the proximal head-neck fragment. If the femoral head fragment is displaced, surgery to carefully access the femoral head while maintaining its soft-tissue attachments during reduction will be necessary followed by reduction and stabilization of the head to the neck fragment. Most series of fracture-dislocations include very few type III injuries and document universally poor results following attempts at femoral head salvage. Consideration should be given to primary arthroplasty in an older patient.

Femoral Head Fractures Associated With Acetabulum Fractures Other Than the Posterior Wall

This uncommon injury requires evaluation of the individual injury components to provide for optimal treatment. Residual displacement of the femoral head may interfere with reduction of the acetabulum. Often optimal reduction of both cannot be achieved through a single approach. Staged reconstruction of the femoral head and acetabulum through separate approaches may be indicated.

Outcomes

Most studies have focused on complications of injury and/or treatment following femoral head fracture-dislocations. Osteonecrosis has been reported to occur in 0% to 23% of cases. In a small series, prolonged time to open relocation (more than 8 hours) in an irreducible dislocation was associated with femoral head necrosis.[10]

A recent study summarized the impact of the surgical approach used to treat femoral head fractures on the incidence of osteonecrosis and heterotopic ossification.[16] Heterotopic ossification was less frequent after use of the digastric (flip) trochanteric osteotomy than after both anterior and posterior approaches. Osteonecrosis was most common following the posterior approach and least common after the anterior approach.

Long-term outcome studies are lacking for femoral head injuries, with most failures reported due to osteonecrosis and the need for conversion to total hip arthroplasty (THA) for this complication. Short-term studies report good to excellent results in 70% to 80% of cases, with better results reported in Pipkin type I fractures. Fractures treated nonsurgically or with fragment removal demonstrated less arthosis,[19] which prob-

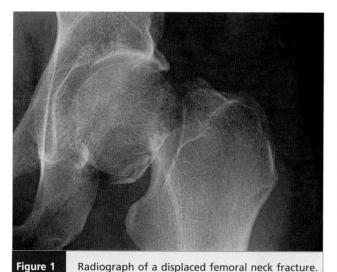

Figure 1   Radiograph of a displaced femoral neck fracture.

ably reflects a selection bias because the less severe injuries are treated nonsurgically. One study concluded that the size and location of the fractured fragment influences the outcome and that exact anatomic reconstruction, especially of the weight-bearing part, is absolutely necessary.[20] Associated fractures also influence outcome, with most poor outcomes in the absence of osteonecrosis attributable to the associated hip injury. However, a recent report of digastric osteotomy in Pipkin type IV fractures demonstrated good to excellent results in more than 80% of cases, which is comparable to those after isolated femoral head fracture.[15] This suggests that some of the poor results of the past were due to inadequate understanding of the injury and lack of an appropriate surgical approach to repair the associated fractures anatomically while maintaining blood supply to the femoral head.

Fractures of the Neck of the Femur

Hip fractures are devastating injuries that most often affect elderly patients and have a tremendous impact on their health (**Figure 1**). More than 250,000 hip fractures occur in the United States each year, and this number is projected to double by the year 2050 as the population ages. The incidence of hip fractures and dislocations also is increasing among young patients who sustain high-energy trauma. The development of regional trauma centers has concentrated these types of injuries, making their frequency much more apparent.[21] The combination of a growing elderly population and a rising incidence of high-energy traumatic injuries make a thorough understanding of hip fractures and dislocations essential.[22] Despite advances in the treatment of femoral neck fractures, these fractures can still be referred to as the unsolved fracture. The average age at occurrence of a femoral neck fracture is 77 years for

women and 72 years for men. The fracture rate doubles for each decade of life after the fifth decade.

Clinical Significance of Vascular Anatomy

Femoral head circulation arises from three sources: intraosseous cervical vessels that cross the marrow spaces; the artery of the ligamentum teres (medial epiphyseal vessels); and, chiefly, the retinacular vessels, which are branches of the extracapsular arterial ring that run along the femoral neck beneath the synovium (**Figure 2**). When a femoral neck fracture occurs, the intraosseous cervical vessels are disrupted; femoral head nutrition is then dependent on any remaining retinacular vessels and functioning vessels in the ligamentum teres. For some time, it has been recognized that the femoral head is either partially or totally avascular (in most cases) after displaced femoral neck fractures. Revascularization occurs through the remaining blood supply by the process of creeping substitution. Therefore, every attempt should be made to protect the remaining vascular supply to the femoral head after fracture. Many physicians believe that traction to the affected leg prevents further injury to the joint capsule and its vessels. There is a possibility that increased pressure within the hip joint will damage the already tenuous circulation.[23,24] Ly and Swiontkowski[23] recommend aspirating the hip if surgery is delayed more than a few hours and suggest a decompressive capsulotomy at the time of internal fixation. Late segmental collapse occurs only when the fracture has healed, and is associated with revascularization of the femoral head (**Figure 3**).

Etiologic Factors

Femoral neck fractures are uncommon in young patients with normal bone and in older patients of races in which osteoporosis is uncommon, such as African Americans. The ratio of the incidence of intertrochanteric to femoral neck fracture increases with age in both white and black women. In men, the ratio of intertrochanteric to femoral neck fractures is stable across all ages for both races. The average age of patients with femoral neck fractures is 3 years younger than that of those with intertrochanteric fractures, both of which occur most commonly in the eighth decade. The risk of hip fractures increases exponentially with age in both men and women.[25]

In the elderly patients, femoral neck fractures should be considered to occur through pathologic bone secondary to either osteomalacia or osteoporosis. By 65 years of age, 50% of women have bone mineral content below fracture threshold, and by 85 years of age, 100% of women have a bone mineral content below this threshold.[26]

Not only does osteoporosis play a role in the etiology of femoral neck fractures (**Figure 4**), it also plays an important role in their treatment. Osteoporotic bone leads to more marked comminution of the posterior cortex and to decreased quality and stability of internal fixation. Osteoporosis increases the failure rate of inter-

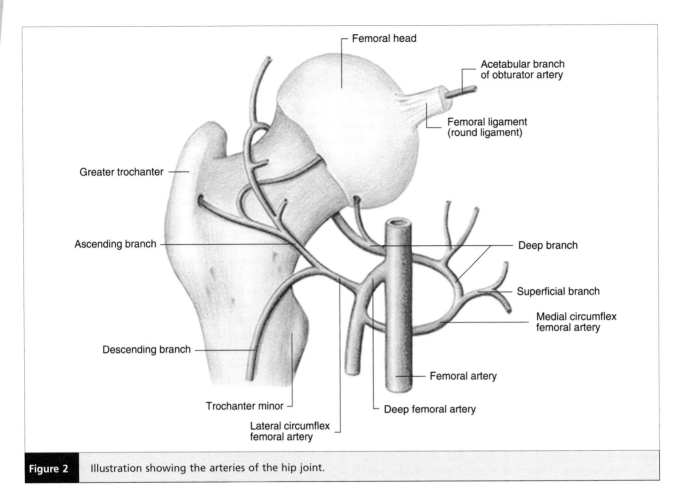

Femoral head

Acetabular branch
of obturator artery

Femoral ligament
(round ligament)

Greater trochanter

Ascending branch

Deep branch

Superficial branch

Medial circumflex
femoral artery

Descending branch

Femoral artery

Trochanter minor

Deep femoral artery

Lateral circumflex
femoral artery

Figure 2 Illustration showing the arteries of the hip joint.

nal fixation and nonunion following surgical repair of a hip fracture.[27]

In patients younger than 60 years, significant energy is required to fracture the femoral neck (**Figure 5**). Fractures typically occur because of force applied along the shaft of the femur with or without a rotational component. The increased energy involved leads to more marked soft-tissue injury and fracture comminution, which give rise to the increased incidence of failure in the treatment of these fractures in young adults.[21]

Classification

There are several ways to classify femoral neck fractures, including classifying these injuries based on patient characteristics such as age, premorbid activity levels, and bone quality. A second method is to classify femoral neck fractures based on fracture characteristics. The three common classifications of femoral neck fractures are those based on (1) anatomic location of the fracture (Garden classification, **Figure 6**), (2) direction of the fracture angle (Pauwels classification), and (3) displacement of the fracture fragments.[28,29]

Diagnosis

Stress Fractures and Impacted Fractures

Patients with stress fractures and those with impacted fractures may report only a slight pain in the groin or

pain referred along the medial side of the thigh and knee. They may walk with a limp (antalgic gait) and may delay seeking medical evaluation.

Physical examination reveals no obvious clinical deformity, minor discomfort with active or passive hip range of motion, and muscle spasm at extremes of motion. Percussion over the greater trochanter is particularly painful. Failure to recognize nondisplaced stress fractures or impacted fractures may result in future fracture displacement. Missed diagnoses or this type of displacement can be minimized if all patients reporting groin or thigh pain after an injury, or those exposed to physical stress (for example, military recruits or joggers), are assumed to have a femoral neck fracture until proven otherwise. If the initial radiographs are normal but pain persists, a femoral neck fracture should be suspected. When the fracture is not shown on plain radiographs, an MRI or bone scan may be required to diagnose these fractures. Because bone scans must be delayed up to 72 hours in older patients with osteopenia to ensure an accurate diagnosis, MRI is now considered the imaging modality of choice in diagnosing femoral neck fractures (**Figure 7**). According to a recent study, MRI obtained on the first day after injury can show findings consistent with an acute fracture.[30] Therefore, a patient arriving at the hospital with a suspected but unconfirmed fracture involving the femoral

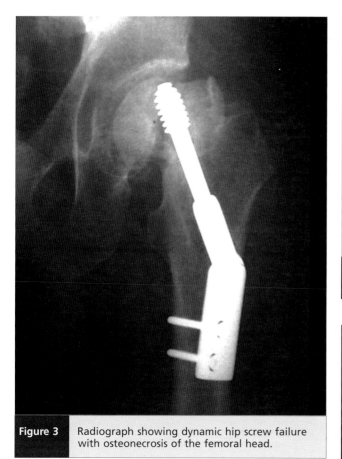

Figure 3 Radiograph showing dynamic hip screw failure with osteonecrosis of the femoral head.

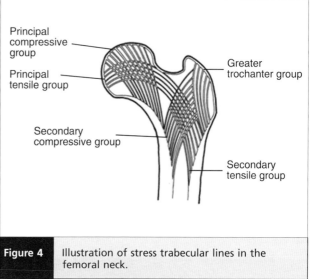

Figure 4 Illustration of stress trabecular lines in the femoral neck.

Principal compressive group

Principal tensile group

Greater trochanter group

Secondary compressive group

Secondary tensile group

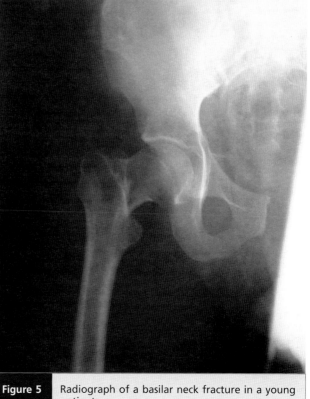

Figure 5 Radiograph of a basilar neck fracture in a young patient.

neck should receive an MRI acutely to determine if the femoral neck is fractured. An identified femoral neck fracture allows for early decision making regarding treatment, whereas the absence of such a fracture allows for early mobilization and discharge.

Displaced Fractures

Patients with displaced intracapsular fractures may have pain in the entire hip region. They usually lie with the leg in external rotation and abduction and have evident shortening of the limb. Skin traction and/or foam boot traction has not been shown to aid in pain relief but may reduce further displacement of the fracture and protect the capsular vessels. A Cochrane review reported that there was no superior method of treating pain in displaced fractures; however, further studies were recommended because no studies to date have been adequately powered to make a proper determination on the benefits of traction.[31]

Displaced fractures are confirmed by routine radiographs. Radiographic evaluation of the fracture type, the degree of posterior comminution, and the presence or absence of osteoporosis is essential before selecting the treatment regimen. The routine radiographic evaluation of a patient with a hip fracture should include a true AP view with the maximum degree of internal rotation possible, as well as a cross table lateral radiograph, which will limit motion through the fracture site during positioning.

Treatment

There are several options for treating femoral neck fractures, including traditional solid screws, cannulated screws, a hip screw and side plate, monoblock (Austin-Moore) arthroplasty, modular hemiarthroplasty, or total hip replacement. The options for a given patient de-

5: Lower Extremity

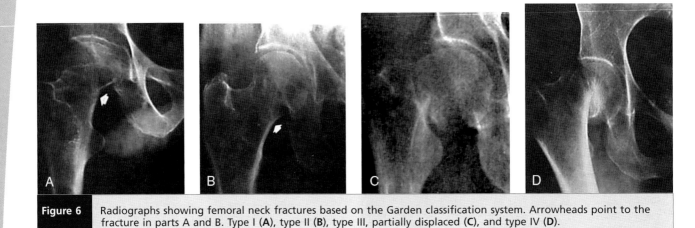

Figure 6 Radiographs showing femoral neck fractures based on the Garden classification system. Arrowheads point to the fracture in parts A and B. Type I (**A**), type II (**B**), type III, partially displaced (**C**), and type IV (**D**).

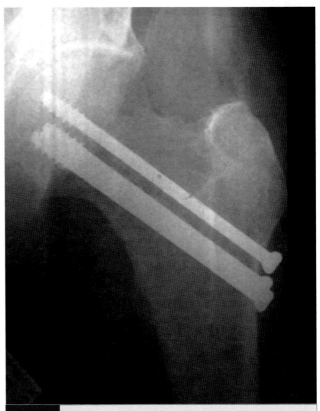

Figure 7 MRI scan of an acute fracture (arrow) of a left femoral neck.

Figure 8 Three parallel screws are used to treat a Garden type II injury. One screw runs along the calcar, one along the posterior cortex of the neck, and one anteriorly to improve stability.

pend on the patient's age, health, and functional demands, as well as the specific type of fracture present.

Although the choice of whether to use internal fixation or some form of arthroplasty is controversial for the older patient, most agree that in a patient younger than 60 years, open reduction and internal fixation should be attempted if a timely and adequate reduction can be achieved. Screw fixation with three parallel screws is considered the treatment of choice (**Figure 8**), although sliding hip screws may be used and may have particular benefit in certain fractures such as those that are more vertical in orientation.[32] Highly functional patients older than 60 years with sufficient bone density can also be treated with reduction and fixation.[33]

Nondisplaced Fractures (Garden Types I and II)

In patients older than 60 years, a nondisplaced or a stable valgus-impacted fracture should be stabilized with internal fixation. Fixation should be performed at the

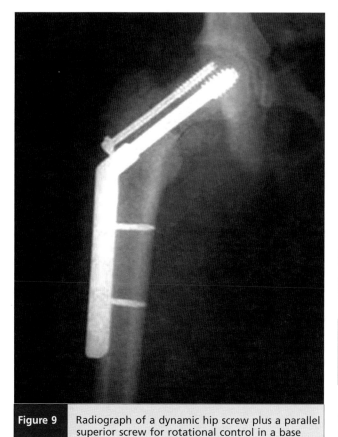

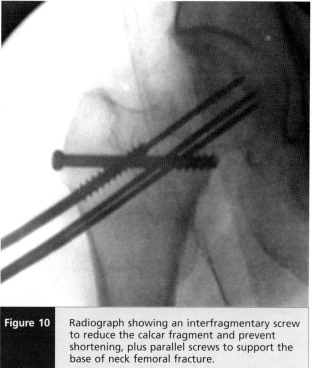

Figure 10 Radiograph showing an interfragmentary screw to reduce the calcar fragment and prevent shortening, plus parallel screws to support the base of neck femoral fracture.

Figure 9 Radiograph of a dynamic hip screw plus a parallel superior screw for rotational control in a base of neck femoral fracture in a young patient.

earliest opportunity, ideally within 24 hours. In adults younger than 60 years with a nondisplaced fracture, expeditious treatment should include internal fixation with parallel screws.[34] In comminuted, basicervical, or more vertical fractures, a sliding hip screw with a derotation screw may offer biomechanical advantages[29,35] (**Figure 9**).

Displaced Femoral Neck Fractures

Numerous randomized controlled trials have compared internal fixation to hemiarthroplasty for displaced femoral neck fractures in elderly patients.[34,36-38] The advantages of internal fixation include decreased blood loss, decreased surgical time, lower transfusion requirements, decreased length of hospital stay, and early improved mortality in debilitated patients. Disadvantages are discussed later in this chapter.

Open Reduction

If the fracture has not been acceptably reduced after one to two attempts at closed reduction, consideration should be given to performing an open reduction. Open reduction decreases the incidence of both nonunion and aseptic necrosis compared with an inadequate closed reduction. Therefore, if closed reduction proves inadequate, open reduction and internal fixation under di-

rect vision should be considered if the patient is not a candidate for prosthetic hemiarthroplasty.

Open reduction can be performed through an anterior or anterolateral approach. A threaded pin can be placed in the femoral head and used as a joystick to rotate the head and facilitate reduction. The preferred technique for screw fixation is to position the screws in an inverted triangular configuration. The first screw runs along the calcar to compress the fracture and prevent inferior displacement of the femoral head. The second screw is placed posteriorly along the neck of the femur, with the shaft of the screw as close as possible to the posterior cortex of the femoral neck to prevent the femoral head from drifting posteriorly. Stability is achieved by the screw contact with the posterior cortex. A final screw would be placed anteriorly along the midaxis of the neck to provide additional support. The inverted triangle configuration may reduce the chance of a fracture occurring at the level of the lesser trochanter. Oakey et al[39] reported that more force to failure is required for subtrochanteric fracture with this configuration. Some surgeons report the triangle configuration is stronger and better able to resist deformation compared with parallel screws in a vertical line. Three or four screws have been used successfully in both nondisplaced and displaced fractures. A fourth screw, if added, should be placed along the posterior cortex of the neck and would be indicated to support gross posterior comminution.[40] Young patients with a vertically oriented femoral neck fracture may benefit from the addition of a transversely directed compression calcar screw (**Figure 10**). It is important to initiate

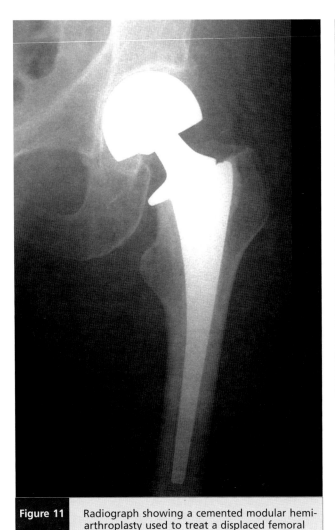

Figure 11 Radiograph showing a cemented modular hemiarthroplasty used to treat a displaced femoral neck fracture.

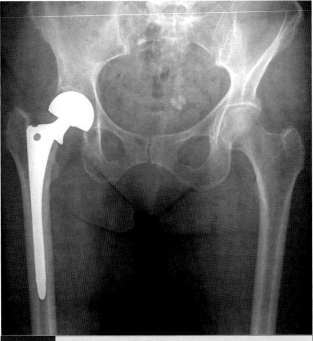

Figure 12 Radiograph showing a fully porous uncemented bipolar arthroplasty.

the screw fixation above the level of the lesser trochanter.[41] A hip screw and side plate may be the device of choice for fractures that extend to the base of the femoral neck.[35]

Arthroplasty for Displaced Femoral Neck Fractures in Elderly Patients

Because of frequent complications (such as nonunion, malunion, osteonecrosis, and shortening of the limb) and the need for reoperation after internal fixation of the femoral neck, most elderly patients with a displaced femoral neck fracture are treated with some form of femoral head replacement.[40] Modern modular prostheses, whether cemented or uncemented,[42] should be used to allow adjustment and restoration of offset and lengthening and tensioning of the hip girdle muscles (Figure 11). In patients with a thick femoral cortex and an intramedullary canal measurement of 15 mm or less, a fully porous uncemented femoral stem can be considered[43,44] (Figure 12). The surgical approach to either hemiarthroplasty or THA can be either anterolateral (Hardinge approach) or posterolateral. Anterior ap-

proaches have a theoretic advantage in this patient population regarding the risk of posterior dislocation, which may be mitigated by maintaining an intact posterior capsule. There appears to be a slightly higher long-term chance of abductor weakness and Trendelenburg gait after use of the anterolateral approach. The authors of a recent study noted a slight increase in time and blood loss with the lateral approach (Hardinge), when compared with the posterior approach. There was no difference in length of hospital stay, dislocation, or the rate of mortality with either approach, with the conclusion that the favored approach should be the one with which the surgeon is most comfortable.[34]

The main indications for hip replacement[45] appear to be (1) displaced fractures in patients older than 60 years (Garden types III and IV); (2) antecedent osteoarthritis (symptomatic); (3) inflammatory disease involving the hip joint; (4) poor surgical risk and subsequent reduced life span; and (5) poor bone quality. Modular hemiarthroplasty has been the workhorse for displaced femoral neck fractures over the past decade. In most cases, it is inserted as a cemented femoral stem with neck length, offset, and acetabular adjustments. It can be used with a fixed head (unipolar) or a bipolar head and provides a relatively easy conversion to a THA if required in the future. It is therefore the ideal implant for most patients with displaced subcapital neck fracture who are community ambulators.[38] Comparative studies have shown that bipolar and unipolar arthroplasty are equivalent in outcome.[46] The main differences in these two implants appear to be cost. The remaining indication for a monoblock hemiarthroplasty

(Austin-Moore type) would be in nonambulatory or minimally ambulatory, low-demand patients—the patient profile for which the implant was originally designed.[47]

THA is increasingly used in older patients with higher functional demands. THA is not associated with the high incidence of complications seen after internal fixation of subcapital fractures and the acetabular erosion and migration seen after a hemiarthroplasty. With proper patient selection, THA provides excellent outcomes that are more durable and predictable than those after hemiarthroplasty or internal fixation.[36,47-50] THA may reduce overall costs of treating femoral neck fractures because of the improved long-term survival after THA and decreased need for reoperation[48] (**Figure 13**). Disadvantages of THA are the greater magnitude of surgery and increased blood loss. The major concern regarding the use of THA in elderly patients with a femoral neck fracture is the increased risk of dislocation, which in many studies approaches 10% or more. The position and offset of the prosthesis are important variables influencing the risk of dislocation regardless of the approach. Use of a modular component to ensure restoration of the hip abductor moment arm reduces the risk of dislocation.[51] The use of a cementless implant could reduce perioperative cardiovascular risk;[52] however, if there is poor bone quality or increased canal size (for example, larger than 15 mm), a cemented implant should be used and has been considered the standard of care.

THA has commonly been performed to salvage complications of femoral neck fractures such as nonunion and aseptic necrosis. It has also been used extensively to manage failed endoprostheses inserted primarily for femoral neck fractures. The short-term results of THA for nonunion, aseptic necrosis, and failure of internal fixation of femoral neck fractures have been uniformly good. However, there are no agreed-upon guidelines for the use of THA in the management of acute femoral neck fractures. A reasonable indication would be a very active patient older than 70 years with a displaced fracture (**Figure 14**). According to a 2006 study,[37] THA is recommended in suitably active and cooperative patients, as well as patients with the following conditions: (1) femoral neck fractures with associated hip disease (such as Paget disease); (2) ipsilateral hip advanced osteoarthrosis; (3) significant symptomatic contralateral hip disease; (4) femoral neck fracture and poor bone quality in older patients (in which case internal fixation historically has a high potential for failure); and (5) required revision of failed open reduction and internal fixation (**Figure 15**).

Traumatic Femoral Neck Fractures in Young Adults

Adults younger than 60 years with femoral neck fractures are considered as a separate group because these patient usually have normal bone and the fractures are distinctly uncommon. The bone in the femoral neck is very hard, and considerable trauma is required for it to fracture.[21] The fracture pattern in young patients with

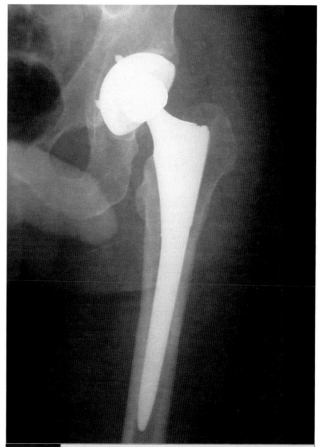

| Figure 13 | Radiograph of a cementless THA, which offers a viable alternative to a hemiarthroplasty. |

femoral neck fractures secondary to high-velocity trauma does not fit either the Garden or Pauwels classifications. The typical fracture in this patient population is a high-angle shear-type fracture that extends to near the lesser trochanter. The high incidence of aseptic necrosis and nonunion reported in the management of these fractures is distinctly different from that seen in elderly patients (**Figure 16**). Open reduction and internal fixation with or without bone graft can be used to treat a nonunion with an acceptable Pauwels angle. Aseptic necrosis is more likely to be symptomatic in younger patients.[29,53] Reconstructive procedures such as THAs are more likely to fail in young patients.[29]

Late Diagnosis of Femoral Neck Fractures

Occasionally, patients present with neglected fractures.[54] If the fracture remains nondisplaced, stabilization with screw fixation is appropriate. If the fracture is displaced in a young patient, then anatomic reduction and stable fixation of the fracture should be attempted. Valgus-producing osteotomy with a blade plate device remains a viable reconstructive technique in late presentation of a femoral neck fracture.[55,56]

If a late presentation occurs after nailing of a femoral shaft fracture, reduction and pinning of the femoral

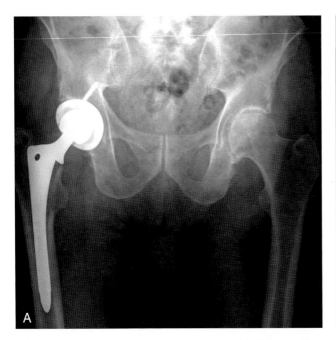

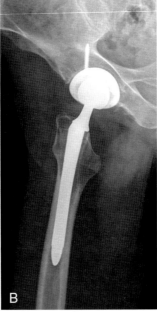

Figure 14   AP (A) and lateral (B) radiographic views of a fully porous THA used to treat an elderly but active patient with a displaced femoral neck fracture.

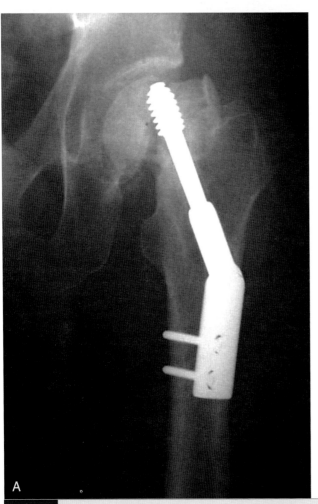

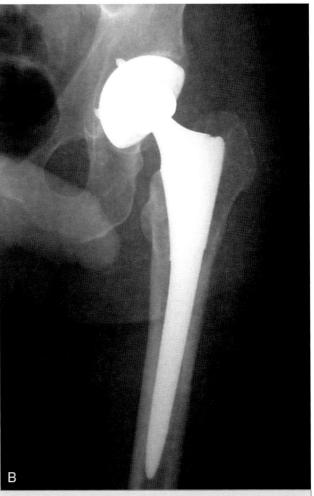

Figure 15   Radiographs of failed fixation of a femoral neck fracture with a dynamic hip screw (A) and revision to a THA (B).

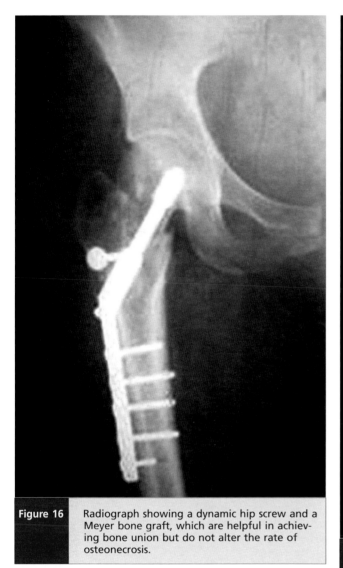

Figure 16 Radiograph showing a dynamic hip screw and a Meyer bone graft, which are helpful in achieving bone union but do not alter the rate of osteonecrosis.

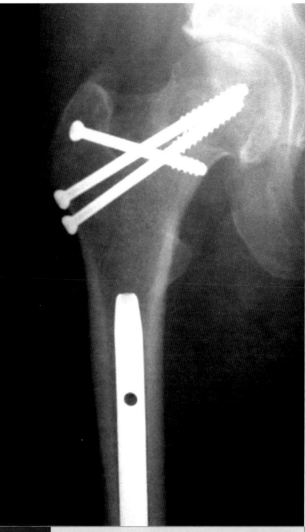

Figure 17 Radiograph showing a healed base of femoral neck fracture with an associated femoral shaft fracture.

neck around the nail is the usual treatment. If the femoral nail interferes with reduction, it should be removed. The neck is then reduced and a cephalomedullary nail, a retrograde nail with separate fixation of the neck with a hip screw and side plate or multiple screws (**Figure 17**), or screws placed around a conventional nail will provide fixation of both fractures. Stability of the femoral neck is of primary concern.[56]

Outcome of Femoral Neck Fractures

Factors predictive of outcome after hip fracture are dependent on the definition of "outcome," specifically the outcome of the patient versus the outcome of the fracture.[57] Traditionally, outcome has focused on the result of the fracture (that is, union, osteonecrosis). In the current cost-sensitive environment, a more comprehensive definition of outcome after hip fracture is the restoration of function (that is, ambulation, self-care, and social reintegration).[57] Up to 60% of patients with hip fractures may require institutionalized care. Avoiding nursing home placement and restoring independence in

a home environment are important outcomes. Three negative predictors of return to ambulation have been identified: (1) age older than 60 years; (2) dementia; and (3) male sex.

The premorbid ability to ambulate is a positive predictor for return to a prefracture living situation. Ambulation at the time of hospital discharge correlates with return to home living. Return to a home environment also depends on the patient's functional status and living environment before injury.[58] The use of a comprehensive interdisciplinary care program for elderly patients with hip fractures has been reported.[59] The interdisciplinary team consists of a surgeon, a general medical officer, a physical therapist, an occupational therapist, a nutritionist, and a social worker. Comparatively, patients treated with a multidisciplinary program had fewer postoperative complications, fewer intensive care unit transfers, and a significantly improved ambulatory status at the time of

5: Lower Extremity

hospital discharge. In addition, fewer of these patients were discharged to a nursing home. These results support the use of a multidisciplinary approach to improve the hospital care of elderly patients with hip fractures.

Summary

Hip dislocations and femoral head and neck fractures are challenging injuries in all patients. In elderly patients, femoral head and neck fractures are usually treated with hemiarthroplasty or THA, depending on the personality of the fracture and the patient. A hip dislocation without a posterior wall fracture is usually stable and can be treated by closed reduction. A hip dislocation with an associated posterior wall fracture usually requires open reduction and internal fixation of the wall injury to achieve adequate stability. Fixation of a femoral neck fracture in a patient younger than 60 years should occur within 24 hours of injury to allow for an optimal outcome.

Annotated References

1. Foulk DM, Mullis BH: Hip dislocation: Evaluation and management. *J Am Acad Orthop Surg* 2010;18(4):199-209.

   This review article describes simple hip dislocations, acetabular fractures, and fracture-dislocations around the hip, as well as their diagnosis and management.

2. Clegg TE, Roberts CS, Greene JW, Prather BA: Hip dislocations: Epidemiology, treatment, and outcomes. *Injury* 2010;41(4):329-334.

   This review article focuses on traumatic dislocations of the hip and describes the epidemiology, treatment, and outcomes of simple and complex hip dislocations. Algorithms are presented to facilitate the diagnosis and management of hip dislocations.

3. Mullis BH, Dahners LB: Hip arthroscopy to remove loose bodies after traumatic dislocation. *J Orthop Trauma* 2006;20(1):22-26.

   This retrospective study reviews 36 patients at a level 1 trauma center who sustained traumatic hip injuries and were treated nonsurgically. All 36 patients underwent hip arthroscopy following a traumatic hip dislocation or small acetabular wall fracture. Preoperative radiographs and CT scans were compared to surgical findings. The results showed that most patients (92%) who sustained traumatic hip dislocation or acetabular wall fractures had intra-articular loose bodies. After closed treatment of hip dislocations or wall fractures, surgeons should have a high level of suspicion for intra-articular loose bodies despite negative findings on pelvic radiographs.

4. Yamamoto Y, Ide T, Ono T, Hamada Y: Usefulness of arthroscopic surgery in hip trauma cases. *Arthroscopy* 2003;19(3):269-273.

5. Philippon MJ, Kuppersmith DA, Wolff AB, Briggs KK: Arthroscopic findings following traumatic hip dislocation in 14 professional athletes. *Arthroscopy* 2009; 25(2):169-174.

   This retrospective study reviews 14 professional athletes who sustained a traumatic hip dislocation during competitive play. The purpose of the study was to evaluate intra-articular hip pathology in this cohort of patients who were treated by a single surgeon using hip arthroscopy. Results showed that all patients had sustained a labral tear following traumatic hip dislocation, which was diagnosed on hip arthroscopy. Other intra-articular hip pathology diagnosed with surgery included intra-articular loose bodies, and femoral head and acetabular chondral lesions. Treatment of intra-articular hip pathology allows early restoration of function in this cohort of active patients.

6. Moorman CT III, Warren RF, Hershman EB, et al: Traumatic posterior hip subluxation in American football. *J Bone Joint Surg Am* 2003;85(7):1190-1196.

7. Hillyard RF, Fox J: Sciatic nerve injuries associated with traumatic posterior hip dislocations. *Am J Emerg Med* 2003;21(7):545-548.

8. Kim KI, Koo KH, Sharma R, Park HB, Hwang SC: Concomitant fractures of the femoral head and neck without hip dislocation. *Clin Orthop Relat Res* 2001; 391:247-250.

9. Pipkin G: Treatment of grade IV fracture-dislocation of the hip. *J Bone Joint Surg Am* 1957;39(5):1027-1042.

10. Mehta S, Routt ML Jr: Irreducible fracture-dislocations of the femoral head without posterior wall acetabular fractures. *J Orthop Trauma* 2008;22(10):686-692.

    The authors provide a retrospective review of cases in a prospective trauma database to define the unique clinical and radiographic features, surgical treatment, and complications of irreducible fracture-dislocations of the femoral head without posterior wall acetabular fractures.

11. Yoon TR, Chung JY, Jung ST, Seo HY: Malunion of femoral head fractures treated by partial ostectomy: Three case reports. *J Orthop Trauma* 2003;17(6):447-450.

12. Stannard JP, Harris HW, Volgas DA, Alonso JE: Functional outcome of patients with femoral head fractures associated with hip dislocations. *Clin Orthop Relat Res* 2000;377:44-56.

13. Gardner MJ, Suk M, Pearle A, Buly RL, Helfet DL, Lorich DG: Surgical dislocation of the hip for fractures of the femoral head. *J Orthop Trauma* 2005;19(5):334-342.

    The authors describe a technique of surgical dislocation to access acetabular fractures and deformities of the proximal femur instead of using an anterior approach.

14. Henle P, Kloen P, Siebenrock KA: Femoral head injuries: Which treatment strategy can be recommended? *Injury* 2007;38(4):478-488.

    A report of one center's experience using a trochanteric flip (digastric) osteotomy for femoral head fractures is presented.

15. Ansari A, Day AC, Franco DP: Letter to the editor: Use of a trochanteric flip osteotomy improves outcomes in Pipkin IV fractures. *Clin Orthop Relat Res* 2010;468: 906-907.

    The authors provide their letter supporting the use and describing the technique of trochanteric flip osteotomy for Pipkin type IV fractures.

16. Guo JJ, Tang N, Yang HL, Qin L, Leung KS: Impact of surgical approach on postoperative heterotopic ossification and avascular necrosis in femoral head fractures: A systematic review. *Int Orthop* 2010;34(3):319-322.

    A systematic review of 10 studies found that the trochanteric flip approach appears to lower the risk of heterotopic ossification and osteonecrosis.

17. Matsuda DK: A rare fracture, an even rarer treatment: The arthroscopic reduction and internal fixation of an isolated femoral head fracture. *Arthroscopy* 2009;25(4): 408-412.

    The author describes a case report of arthroscopic reduction and internal fixation to treat an isolated femoral head fracture.

18. Prokop A, Helling HJ, Hahn U, Udomkaewkanjana C, Rehm KE: Biodegradable implants for Pipkin fractures. *Clin Orthop Relat Res* 2005;432:226-233.

    A prospective cohort of nine patients treated with biodegradable implants for Pipkin fractures were followed for an average of 54.2 months. Results indicated that Pipkin fractures can be fixed successfully with biodegradable polylactide pins.

19. Yoon TR, Rowe SM, Chung JY, Song EK, Jung ST, Anwar IB: Clinical and radiographic outcome of femoral head fractures: 30 patients followed for 3-10 years. *Acta Orthop Scand* 2001;72(4):348-353.

20. Lederer S, Tauber M, Karpik S, Bogner R, Auffarth A, Resch H: Fractures of the femoral head: A multicenter study. *Unfallchirurg* 2007;110(6):513-520.

    A multicenter study follow-up on 46 patients with Pipkin fractures is presented by the authors. They found that the size and location of the fracture fragment affects the outcome and that an exact reconstruction of the femoral head is necessary.

21. Haidukewych GJ, Rothwell WS, Jacofsky DJ, Torchia ME, Berry DJ: Operative treatment of femoral neck fractures in patients between the ages of fifteen and fifty years. *J Bone Joint Surg Am* 2004;86(8):1711-1716.

    The authors reviewed 83 femoral neck fractures in 82 patients treated with internal fixation and reported the 10-year survival rate of the femoral head was 85%. Osteonecrosis was the main reason for conversion to THA.

22. Johnell O, Kanis JA: An estimate of the worldwide prevalence, mortality and disability associated with hip fracture. *Osteoporos Int* 2004;15:897-902.

    The authors estimate the global burden of osteoporosis based on hip fractures in different socioeconomic regions of the world.

23. Ly TV, Swiontkowski MF: Treatment of femoral neck fractures in young adults. *J Bone Joint Surg Am* 2008; 90(10):2254-2266.

    This article based on an instructional course lecture reviews anatomy, diagnosis, and treatment options for fractures in young adults.

24. Bonnaire F, Schaefer DJ, Kuner EH: Hemarthrosis and hip joint pressure in femoral neck fractures. *Clin Orthop Relat Res* 1998;353:148-155.

25. Miyamoto RG, Kaplan KM, Levine BR, Egol KA, Zuckerman JD: Surgical management of hip fractures: An evidence-based review of the literature. I: Femoral neck fractures. *J Am Acad Orthop Surg* 2008;16(10): 596-607.

    An evidence-based review of the current literature found minimal differences among implants used for internal fixation of displaced fractures. Outcomes following THA appear to be superior to those of internal fixation in certain patients.

26. Heijckmann AC, Huijberts MS, Geusens P, de Vries J, Menheere PP, Wolffenbuttel BH: Hip bone mineral density, bone turnover and risk of fracture in patients on long-term suppressive L-thyroxine therapy for differentiated thyroid carcinoma. *Eur J Endocrinol* 2005; 153(1):23-29.

    A cross-sectional study of 59 patients treated with L-thyroxine suppressive therapy found that low doses of the drug do not appear to increase the risk of low bone mass developing or increase the prevalence of vertebral fractures.

27. Heetveld MJ, Raaymakers EL, van Eck-Smit BL, van Walsum AD, Luitse JS: Internal fixation for displaced fractures of the femoral neck. Does bone density affect clinical outcome? *J Bone Joint Surg Br* 2005;87(3):367-373.

    The results of a meta-analysis show that the clinical outcome of internal fixation for displaced fractures of the femoral neck does not depend on bone density.

28. Zlowodzki M, Bhandari M, Keel M, Hanson BP, Schemitsch E: Perception of Garden's classification for femoral neck fractures: An international survey of 298 orthopaedic trauma surgeons. *Arch Orthop Trauma Surg* 2005;125(7):503-505.

    An international survey found that only 39% surgeons were able to distinguish all four types of Garden fractures. However, 96% of the surgeons could differentiate between nondisplaced and displaced fractures.

29. Liporace F, Gaines R, Collinge C, Haidukewych GJ: Results of internal fixation of Pauwels type-3 vertical femoral neck fractures. *J Bone Joint Surg Am* 2008;90(8): 1654-1659.

5: Lower Extremity

Cannulated screws had a higher nonunion rate than fixed-angle devices, but the result was not statistically significant.

30. Frihagen F, Nordsletten L, Tariq R, Madsen JE: MRI diagnosis of occult hip fractures. *Acta Orthop* 2005; 76(4):524-530.

    The authors present the results of a prospective study of 100 consecutive patients with clinical suspicion of hip fracture and negative or equivocal conventional radiographs. MRI was found to be useful in diagnosing occult fractures with good interobserver reliability.

31. Parker MJ, Handoll HH: Preoperative traction for fractures of the proximal femur in adults. *Cochrane Database Syst Rev* 2006;19(3):CD000168.

    A systematic review of randomized trials found no benefit to the preoperative use of traction prior to hip fracture surgery, but recommended further high-quality studies to confirm or refute the absence of benefits.

32. Bhandari M, Tornetta P III, Hanson B, Swiontkowski MF: Optimal internal fixation for femoral neck fractures: Multiple screws or sliding hip screws? *J Orthop Trauma* 2009;23(6):403-407.

    Results of a meta-analysis, literature review, and survey indicated a possible benefit for a sliding hip screw over multiple cancellous screws in reducing the need for revision surgery in patients with femoral neck fractures. However, the indirect nature of the comparison from the meta-analysis of arthroplasty versus internal fixation, and the small sample sizes, methodologic limitations, and nonsignificant pooled estimate from the direct comparisons, leaves the issue in doubt.

33. Kakar S, Tornetta P III, Schemitsch EH, et al; International Hip Fracture Research Collaborative: Technical considerations in the operative management of femoral neck fractures in elderly patients: A multinational survey. *J Trauma* 2007;63(3):641-646.

    A multinational survey of orthopaedic traumatologists conducted by mail and Internet showed a lack of consensus in the management of displaced femoral neck fractures and disparities in the technical aspects of fixation and perioperative care.

34. Parker MJ, White A, Boyle A: Fixation versus hemiarthroplasty for undisplaced intracapsular hip fractures. *Injury* 2008;39(7):791-795.

    The authors compare age, sex, and comorbidity matched cohorts of 346 patients who had their nondisplaced intracapsular hip fracture treated using cannulated screws with a group of 346 patients who had a displaced intracapsular fracture treated using a hemiarthroplasty.

35. Farooq MA, Orkazai SH, Okusanya O, Devitt AT: Intracapsular fractures of the femoral neck in younger patients. *Ir J Med Sci* 2005;174(4):42-45.

    The authors evaluate the results of internal fixation of femoral neck fractures in patients between 20 and 60 years, and determine reasons for failure. The study emphasizes the importance of timely surgery and adequate reduction of displaced femoral neck fractures in younger patients.

36. Macaulay W, Nellans KW, Garvin KL, Iorio R, Healy WL, Rosenwasser MP; other members of the DFACTO Consortium: Prospective randomized clinical trial comparing hemiarthroplasty to total hip arthroplasty in the treatment of displaced femoral neck fractures: Winner of the Dorr Award. *J Arthroplasty* 2008;23(6, Suppl 1): 2-8.

    Forty patients were evaluated in this study. At 24 months, the patients treated with THA had significantly better outcome scores than the hemiarthroplasty patients and no greater incidence of complications.

37. Rogmark C, Johnell O: Primary arthroplasty is better than internal fixation of displaced femoral neck fractures: A meta-analysis of 14 randomized studies with 2,289 patients. *Acta Orthop* 2006;77(3):359-367.

    In this study, the authors reported that primary arthroplasty had fewer complications and reoperations than internal fixation. Mortality rates were the same.

38. Wang J, Jiang B, Marshall RJ, Zhang P: Arthroplasty or internal fixation for displaced femoral neck fractures: Which is the optimal alternative for elderly patients? A meta-analysis. *Int Orthop* 2009;33(5):1179-1187.

    A meta-analysis of 20 randomized controlled trials showed that compared with internal fixation, arthroplasty led to significantly fewer surgical complications and reduced the incidence of reoperation. However, arthroplasty was associated with a greater risk of deep wound infection, longer surgical time, and greater surgical blood loss. There was no difference in pain at 1-year follow-up.

39. Oakey JW, Stover MD, Summers HD, Sartori M, Havey RM, Patwardhan AG: Does screw configuration affect subtrochanteric fracture after femoral neck fixation? *Clin Orthop Relat Res* 2006;443:302-306.

    A biomechanical human cadaver study reported that an apex-distal screw configuration tolerated higher loads than an apex-proximal configuration.

40. Schemitsch E, Bhandari M: Femoral neck fractures: Controversies and evidence. *J Orthop Trauma* 2009; 23(6):385.

    This is an editorial that outlines the need for an evidence-based approach to treating hip fractures.

41. Stiasny J, Dragan S, Kulej M, Martynkiewicz J, Płochowski J, Dragan SL: Comparison analysis of the operative treatment results of the femoral neck fractures using side-plate and compression screw and cannulated AO screws. *Ortop Traumatol Rehabil* 2008;10(4):350-361.

    In a study of 112 patients with femoral neck fractures, compression screw and side-plate fixation resulted in better performance than AO screws with respect to stabilization and early mobilization.

42. Figved W, Opland V, Frihagen F, Jervidalo T, Madsen JE, Nordsletten L: Cemented versus uncemented hemi-

arthroplasty for displaced femoral neck fractures. *Clin Orthop Relat Res* 2009;467(9):2426-2435.

In a randomized controlled trial, both cemented and uncemented hemiarthroplasties had good results.

43. Ahn J, Man LX, Park S, Sodl JF, Esterhai JL: Systematic review of cemented and uncemented hemiarthroplasty outcomes for femoral neck fractures. *Clin Orthop Relat Res* 2008;466(10):2513-2518.

A meta-analysis shows few statistical differences between cemented and uncemented techniques based on reported outcome measurements.

44. Macaulay W, Pagnotto MR, Iorio R, Mont MA, Saleh KJ: Displaced femoral neck fractures in the elderly: Hemiarthroplasty versus total hip arthroplasty. *J Am Acad Orthop Surg* 2006;14(5):287-293.

The choice of internal fixation, unipolar hemiarthroplasty, bipolar hemiarthroplasty, or THA to treat displaced femoral neck fractures in elderly patients should be based on the patient's mental status, living arrangement, level of independence and activity, and bone and joint quality.

45. Dai Z, Li Y, Jiang D. Meta-analysis comparing arthroplasty with internal fixation for displaced femoral neck fracture in the elderly. *J Surg Res* 2009, April 23. [Epub ahead of print]

This meta-analysis shows that there is an evidence base to support arthroplasty over internal fixation as a primary treatment of displaced femoral neck fractures in the elderly.

46. Bhattacharyya T, Koval KJ: Unipolar versus bipolar hemiarthroplasty for femoral neck fractures: Is there a difference? *J Orthop Trauma* 2009;23(6):426-427.

The authors show equivalent functional outcomes at 1 to 3 years follow-up for unipolar and bipolar hemiarthroplasties.

47. Tannast M, Mack PW, Klaeser B, Siebenrock KA: Hip dislocation and femoral neck fracture: Decision-making for head preservation. *Injury* 2009;40(10):1118-1124.

The authors review the timing and the approach for the terrible combination of a femoral neck fracture with associated femoral head dislocation. In the young patient everything possible should be done to preserve the native femoral head.

48. Sayana MK, Lakshmanan P, Peehal JP, Wynn-Jones C, Maffulli N, Maffuli N: Total hip replacement for acute femoral neck fracture: A survey of National Joint Registries. *Acta Orthop Belg* 2008;74(1):54-58.

A comparison of national joint registries found that in Sweden, THA is performed for the management of a femoral neck fracture six times more often than in England and Wales, four times more often than in Australia, and twice as often as in Canada.

49. Schmidt AH, Leighton R, Parvizi J, Sems A, Berry DJ: Optimal arthroplasty for femoral neck fractures: Is total hip arthroplasty the answer? *J Orthop Trauma* 2009; 23(6):428-433.

The authors review the recent literature regarding the results of THAs in patients with a displaced fracture of the femoral neck. THA may have a larger role in the treatment of displaced femoral neck fractures than it had in past years.

50. Gjertsen JE, Vinje T, Lie SA, et al: Patient satisfaction, pain, and quality of life 4 months after displaced femoral neck fractures: A comparison of 663 fractures treated with internal fixation and 906 with bipolar hemiarthroplasty reported to the Norwegian Hip Fracture Register. *Acta Orthop* 2008;79(5):594-601.

A study of data from the Norwegian Hip Fracture Register compared satisfaction, pain, and quality of life 4 months after surgery in patients older than 70 years with a displaced femoral neck fracture treated with internal fixation or with bipolar hemiarthroplasty. The findings suggest that elderly patients with displaced femoral neck fractures should be treated with arthroplasty.

51. Patel PD, Potts A, Froimson MI: The dislocating hip arthroplasty: Prevention and treatment. *J Arthroplasty* 2007;22(4 suppl 1):86-89.

The authors present an excellent review article with a good algorithm for treating a dislocated hip arthroplasty. The article provides a large amount of data prior to 2007.

52. Parvizi J, Ereth MH, Lewallen DG: Thirty-day mortality following hip arthroplasty for acute fracture. *J Bone Joint Surg Am* 2004;86(9):1983-1988.

A retrospective review of 7,774 patients treated with THA for an acute hip fracture is presented. The 30-day mortality rate was significantly higher for patients who had been treated with a cemented implant, female patients, elderly patients, those with cardiorespiratory comorbidities, and patients with intertrochanteric fractures.

53. Bhandari M, Devereaux PJ, Tornetta P III, et al: Operative management of displaced femoral neck fractures in elderly patients: An international survey. *J Bone Joint Surg Am* 2005;87(9):2122-2130.

An international survey found surgeons prefer internal fixation for younger patients and arthroplasty for older patients to treat femoral neck fractures. They disagree on the management of patients between 60 and 80 years of age with a displaced fracture, and active patients with a Garden type III fracture. Surgeons also disagree on the optimal implant for internal fixation or arthroplasty.

54. Roshan A, Ram S: The neglected femoral neck fracture in young adults: Review of a challenging problem. *Clin Med Res* 2008;6(1):33-39.

This review of current literature discusses the various treatment options and compares the published long-term results of neglected femoral neck fractures in young adults. The authors found that bone grafting with internal fixation is a reliable method with good long-term outcomes.

55. Zlowodzki M, Jönsson A, Paulke R, Kregor PJ, Bhandari M: Shortening after femoral neck fracture fixation: Is there a solution? *Clin Orthop Relat Res* 2007;461: 213-218.

5: Lower Extremity

When using parallel screws for treating femoral neck fractures, shortening of the femoral neck can occur. A plate with multiple nonparallel lag screws that can be locked into the plate may be a solution. However, the findings in this study are based on the opinions of surgeons, which may not be confirmed by scientific evidence.

56. Tsai CH, Hsu HC, Fong YC, Lin CJ, Chen YH, Hsu CJ: Treatment for ipsilateral fractures of femoral neck and shaft. *Injury* 2009;40(7):778-782.

A retrospective study comparing treatments of ipsilateral femoral neck and shaft injuries showed that an antegrade nail with screw fixation is not a recommended treatment method.

57. Frihagen F, Grotle M, Madsen JE, Wyller TB, Mowinckel P, Nordsletten L: Outcome after femoral neck fractures: A comparison of Harris Hip Score, Eq-5d and Barthel Index. *Injury* 2008;39(10):1147-1156.

The objective of this study was to evaluate the discriminatory ability and responsiveness of the Harris Hip Score, the Barthel Index, and the Eq-5d in an unselected population of patients with displaced femoral neck fractures. The Harris Hip Score performed the best.

58. Mendonça TM, Silva CH, Canto RS, Morales NdeM, Pinto RdeM, Morales RdeR: Evaluation of the health-related quality of life in elderly patients according to the type of hip fracture: Femoral neck or trochanteric. *Clinics* 2008;63(5):607-612.

The Health-Related Quality of Life scores were compared according to fracture type, undisplaced versus displaced femoral neck fractures, and stable versus unstable trochanteric fractures. The mental and physical quality of life of elderly patients with a hip fracture is severely impaired 1 month after fracture, with partial recovery by the end of the fourth month. The negative impact on the Health-Related Quality of Life score did not differ significantly according to fracture type.

59. Zuckerman JD, Skovron ML, Koval KJ, Aharonoff G, Frankel VH: Postoperative complications and mortality associated with operative delay in older patients who have a fracture of the hip. *J Bone Joint Surg Am* 1995;77(10):1551-1556.

Chapter 32

Fractures of the Proximal Femur

Mark A. Lee, MD   Edward J. Harvey, MD, MSc, FRCSC

Introduction

The management of extracapsular proximal femur fractures is of burgeoning importance because of the rapidly aging demographic profile of most developed countries. Most of these fractures are adequately treated with traditional methods of orthopaedic surgery, such as the sliding hip screw or cephalomedullary nail. The frequency of complications along with new treatment modalities and approaches are being more clearly defined for specific subgroups of these fractures. These include severely comminuted fractures, high-energy fractures in patients younger than 50 years, and fractures in elderly patients. Yet, despite these well-defined needs related to specific conditions, the mere introduction of newer implants and techniques, even for use with more simple fractures, has a tendency to influence surgical practice. Over the past 5 years, the main objective of many of the published research papers in this area has been in validating these new instrumentation systems. Many of these devices have yet to show clear advantage over other more commonly available and less expensive implants. It is yet to be determined (by properly designed clinical trials) where these new devices will fit in the surgeon's armamentarium.

Intertrochanteric Hip Fractures

Diagnosis and Classification

Plain radiographs are the primary means of diagnosing proximal femur fractures. Typically, the limb shortens and rotates as a consequence of these injuries so that standard AP and lateral projections of the hip do not adequately show the bony anatomy. Recently, it was

Dr. Lee or an immediate family member is a member of a speakers' bureau or has made paid presentations on behalf of Synthes and Zimmer; and has received research or institutional support from Synthes and Zimmer. Dr. Harvey or an immediate family member serves as a board member, owner, officer, or committee member of Canadian Orthopaedic Association, Federation des Medecins Specialists du Quebec, and Orthopaedic Trauma Association; and has received research or institutional support from Canadian Institutes of Health Research (CIHR), Stryker, Smith & Nephew, Synthes, Zimmer, DePuy, Kyphon, and Medtronic Sofamor Danek.

shown that an internal rotation and traction view not only improves sensitivity for diagnosis, but actually changes the choice of implant (especially for junior surgeons) by helping to distinguish the true position of the fracture line.[1] When plain radiographs are nondiagnostic, MRI and CT are two sensitive methods for diagnosing proximal femur fractures.

Several classification schemes have been used to describe proximal femur fractures. Varying results have been reported regarding interobserver and intraobserver reliability among these classification groups. Several authors simply refer to these fractures as either stable or unstable. However, even these terms require definition, and there is yet to be any validation of whether surgeons can reliably differentiate a stable from an unstable fracture. Recently, several studies compared classification systems. In a 2005 study comparing the AO/Orthopaedic Trauma Association (OTA), Evans, Kyle, and Boyd groupings, the authors found that the AO/OTA first level classifications (A,B,C) were the most reliable.[2] The authors of a 2007 study sought to determine if increasing rater experience would improve the reliability of classification of proximal femur fractures.[3] It was concluded that the AO/OTA classification was of most use to the general population of surgeons. More experienced surgeons successfully used the AO/OTA classification, but experience was a detriment when using the Evans classification system. Interestingly, based on a subanalysis of this study, it appears that surgeons cannot define if a fracture is stable with a high degree of reliability. The Evidence-Based Orthopaedic Trauma Working Group examined the literature to determine the effect of therapy on AO/OTA 31-A3 fractures and found that these fractures were not consistently categorized correctly and that treatment recommendations could not be made.[4] Better ways to classify these fractures on plain radiographs are certainly needed, and ideally any classification scheme will correlate with a logical treatment protocol.

Basic Science

The biomechanics of proximal femur fractures continues to be an area of active research, particularly with the number of new implants that are appearing on the market. Implants about the hip have been redesigned in an attempt to improve outcomes by facilitating mini-

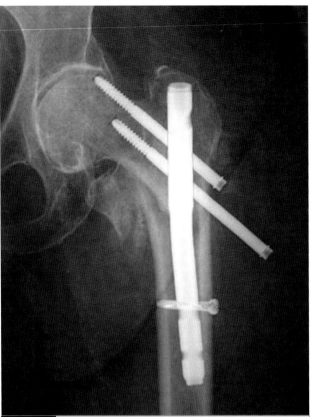

Figure 1 Radiograph showing the Z-effect, a recognized complication in which the inferior lag screw migrates laterally and the superior lag screw migrates medially during loading. (Courtesy of Kenneth A. Egol, MD, New York, NY, and Kenneth J. Koval, MD, Lebanon, NH.)

tures with intramedullary implants containing two femoral head screws is the "Z-effect," in which the superior screw migrates medially while the inferior screw backs out (**Figure 1**). Reproduction of this complication was attempted experimentally using simulated bones of varying densities to determine a biomechanical explanation.[6] Backing out of the inferior screw occurred when there was a mismatch in compressive bone strength of the femoral head and neck, whereas medial penetration of the superior screw only occurred in the specimens with low density in the femoral head. It was suggested that medial migration of the head screw also occurs in single-screw intramedullary devices. Five implants were tested under similar conditions to determine which devices allowed migration.[7] There was no significant difference between the implants, and all implants allowed some amount of migration of the screw into the femoral head (a phenomenon not observed in screw-side plate devices). This same phenomenon also has been observed in clinical studies; a routine 2- to 3-mm penetration of the femoral head lag screw toward the hip joint has been observed.[8] Five hip implants were evaluated in an attempt to examine different constructs for fixation of ipsilateral intertrochanteric and femoral shaft fractures.[9] No differences in proximal femoral failure were noted among the various devices.

Sliding hip screws are commonly used for intertrochanteric hip fixation. Two such devices designed for minimally invasive insertion were compared in cadaver femurs.[10] Unstable four-part fractures were created and fixed with a minimally invasive screw system or percutaneous compression plate. Significant differences were detected after cyclical loading between plate systems with respect to sliding of the lag screw. However, no statistically significant difference was noted in three-dimensional displacement and load to failure between these two devices. Neither of these implants has been compared to a conventional, short, side-plate sliding hip screw inserted in a minimally invasive manner, so it is unknown whether these devices confer any benefit over conventional sliding hip screw systems. Another recent advance in fracture fixation has been the introduction of locking implants. The use of a locking side plate in relation to increased load to failure was studied.[11] A simulated hip screw with a standard side plate was compared to one with a side plate using fixed-angle locking screws holding the plate to synthetic, osteoporotic bone. The mean number of cycles to failure for the locking plate construct was 2.6 times greater than for the standard screw construct ($P = 0.016$).

Several clinical papers have been published over the past decade assessing the biomechanics and clinical outcomes of dual sliding screw percutaneous compression plates (PCCP). A PCCP (which has two compression screws through the proximal plate) and a standard dynamic hip screw (DHS)-like implant with an additional derotation screw were compared.[12] Specimens fixed with the PCCP showed higher displacements in varus during a low-force loading scenario (200 and

mal access surgery, to improve fixation by adding locking capability to either the plate or cephalomedullary part of the implant, to lessen complications and poor outcomes associated with the use of early generation, short, intramedullary nails for these fractures, or in an attempt to differentiate an implant from its competitors.

New features among the latest generation of implants for the treatment of proximal femur fractures include intramedullary nails with helical blades for the femoral neck and head to reduce bone loss and to allow a smaller slot in the proximal nail; dual cephalomedullary locking screws that engage in the head to prevent migration; sliding hip screws with locking screws through the side plate; and locking plates. One study compared an intramedullary nail incorporating a helical blade to a standard cephalomedullary nail and single femoral head lag screw.[5] After cyclic loading at multiple force levels there was significantly more inferior femoral head displacement, permanent fracture site opening, and inferior displacement in the nail with the traditional femoral head screw. The final loads to failure were not significantly different. A rarely reported complication of the fixation of intertrochanteric frac-

400 N). A similar tendency was observed for higher loads. The PCCP allowed more external rotation of the proximal fragment ($P = 0.019$). Load to failure revealed no statistical difference between the two implants. Although both implants have been used in clinical practice, this outcome may be a consideration in the treatment of unstable intertrochanteric fractures with inferior comminution in osteoporotic patients.

During repair of the proximal femur with a sliding hip screw, central placement of the lag screw within the femoral head, as quantified by a tip-apex distance (TAD) of less than 25 mm, has been considered to be an important criterion for successful fixation. A biomechanical study from Korea examined the failure rate for DHS placement, comparing anterior to posterior placement in the neck (group 1) with posterior to anterior placement (group 2).[13] Both groups represent implant positions often seen in clinical practice, with only a variance of 4 mm from straight lateral at the insertion site and 6 mm within the head. Theoretically, both groups have a TAD of 25 mm or less, within the acceptable range. In this study, breakage of the anterior cortex of the lateral wall occurred in five of the eight cases in group 1 and none in group 2 ($P = 0.026$). The authors of this study concluded that fracture of the anterior cortices threatens the integrity of the lateral wall of the greater trochanter and therefore the outcome.

Treatment

Several recent studies examined the clinical and radiographic outcomes of various implant devices for intertrochanteric fractures. Many of the studies were statistically underpowered, and it is difficult to interpret the clinical relevance of the results because many times the only outcomes that differ are those related to surgical measures such as surgery time, blood loss, and postoperative pain. For the following discussion, articles reporting comparative studies are reviewed.

A recent randomized prospective study compared the gamma trochanteric nail and the ACE trochanteric nail (DePuy, Warsaw, IN) for treating elderly patients with intertrochanteric femur fractures.[14] Fifty-six patients were treated with the gamma nail, and 56 were treated with the ACE trochanteric nail. Surgery time, fluoroscopy time, units of blood transfused, and complications were recorded. A mobility score was used to assess both preinjury and postoperative mobility status. There was no statistically significant difference between the two groups with regard to the studied parameters. There was no mechanical failure of the implants despite early patient mobilization. Both of these trochanteric nails provided effective methods of treatment of intertrochanteric fractures in elderly patients. A cephalomedullary nail placed through the piriformis fossa was compared to one using a trochanteric starting point in 34 consecutive patients (ages 18 to 50 years) with high-energy proximal femur fractures.[15] No difference was found between the two devices with regard to incision length, duration of surgery, blood loss, ability to achieve reduction, ease of use, union rate, complication rate, or outcome.

With respect to sliding hip screws, identical implants inserted using different surgical approaches were compared in a study of 102 patients with intertrochanteric fractures treated with either a minimally invasive DHS or a conventional DHS.[16] The hip score, union rate, healing time, adequacy of reduction, and proportion of cases with adequate screw position was not significantly different between the two groups. The authors concluded that either method is effective, simple, and safe. The minimally invasive technique, in comparison with the conventional technique, was associated with smaller wound size, lower pain level, and less blood loss. The length of the hospital stay and total analgesic use were decreased. In another randomized study, the 1-year outcome of the PCCP was compared to DHS-like implants in 104 patients.[17] The pain score and ability to bear weight were significantly better in the PCCP group at 6 weeks after surgery. Analysis of the radiographs in a proportion of the patients showed a reduced amount of medial displacement in the PCCP group (two patients, 4%) compared with the other group (10 patients, 18.9%). The PCCP arm of the study was associated with reduced intraoperative blood loss, less postoperative pain, and a reduced incidence of fracture collapse. Finally, the PCCP was compared with the traditional DHS in a meta-analysis.[18] The authors believed that there was a decreased trend in overall mortality in the PCCP group. Similar trends favoring the PCCP technique were seen with the other outcomes. It should be noted that these various implants have not been adequately compared in randomized trials, and it is not known whether demonstrated benefits of the percutaneous devices are implant-related or if similar results could be achieved by using standard sliding hip screw inserted in a percutaneous fashion.

Several studies have compared sliding hip screws to intramedullary devices. In one study, the treatment of young patients with a DHS-like device was associated with more shortening than if nails were used.[19] A variable-angle DHS-plate and the gamma nail were compared for the treatment of intertrochanteric hip fractures.[20] A prospective cohort of elderly patients was followed, and no statistically significant difference (intraoperative, radiographic, or clinical) was found between the two groups of patients, except for shortening. The plate system had much more shortening than the nail, particularly in unstable and comminuted fracture patterns. Plate systems may be less useful in comminuted fracture patterns. A prospective trial compared the Holland nail with the DHS in the treatment of intertrochanteric fractures of the hip.[21] Ninety-two patients were treated with a Holland nail and 98 with a DHS. There were no revisions in the Holland nail group, whereas the DHS group had two revisions. It was concluded that the DHS could be implanted more quickly with less radiation exposure than the nail. However, the resultant blood loss and need for transfu-

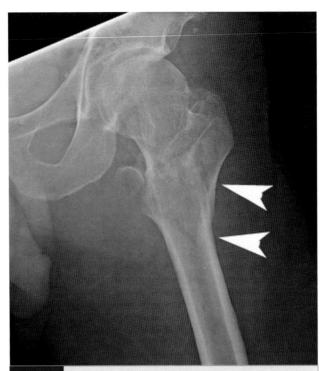

Figure 2 Radiograph showing a typical severely comminuted fracture with a subtrochanteric extension. Lateral wall comminution (*top arrowhead*) with the lower extension (*bottom arrowhead*) to exit where a lag screw inserts through the femur makes it difficult to use a side-plate device without some additional superior plate to decrease medial migration of the femoral shaft. Intramedullary nails decrease the amount of migration possible by becoming a medullary block to femoral neck lateralization.

sion is greater. The Holland nail may allow patients to mobilize faster. Ninety-three patients who were treated for an intertrochanteric fracture with either a DHS or the short trochanteric nail were retrospectively reviewed.[22] This latter implant is a redesign of an older implant (Gamma nail; Stryker, Kalamazoo, MI) with less lateral bend, a smaller nail diameter, and fewer distal locking screws. Ninety-four percent of the patients in the DHS group healed without complication, and 89% of the patients in the trochanteric nail group healed without complication. There was one late fracture at the tip of the nail, three cases of lag screw cutout, and one nonunion. This study suggests that the trochanteric nail is a reasonable alternative to the sliding hip screw when used for intertrochanteric fractures, although it may be associated with higher complication rates. In a prospective cohort study, 30 patients treated with the trochanteric fixation nail (TFN) were compared with 30 patients treated with a DHS.[8] No intraoperative or perioperative complications occurred with the new nail device. Surgery time was 10 minutes shorter with the TFN. No Trendelenburg gait was reported in either group. No femur fractures or distal locking difficulties occurred in the TFN group, a major

problem when short nails were used. More TFN patients returned to prefracture ambulation 6 months after surgery compared with DHS patients ($P = 0.09$). Compared to historic results reported for short nails, this study reported a significantly reduced complication rate. Other studies have found the same type of results for this nail.[23] The ability of the TFN to stabilize intertrochanteric hip fractures was studied radiographically.[24] After adjustments were made for magnification and rotation in almost 100 cases, blade migration and telescoping of the blade along its axis were measured. Mean telescoping was 4.3 mm in the unstable group, compared with 2.6 mm in the stable group ($P < 0.05$). Blade migration within the femoral head averaged 2.2 mm overall, with no difference between stable and unstable fractures. For both telescoping and blade migrations, no significant change occurred after the 6-week time point in the stable or unstable group. Nail length, age, and sex did not have a significant effect on either blade migration or telescoping implant position change. More telescoping occurred in unstable compared with stable fractures, but this averaged 4 mm and did not affect stable fixation or fracture healing. The subtle migration (approximately 2 mm) of the tip of the blade within the femoral head that occurred in all fractures is an important consideration in deciding the ideal implant position for this type of device. Because of the possibility of medial migration of femoral head screws observed with cephalomedullary nails, insertion of the femoral head fixation as near the subchondral surface as is commonly done with the DHS may not be desirable. The TAD measurement used in DHS surgery has not been formally studied with intramedullary devices, and the same criteria for fixation should probably not be adapted as a standard for cephalomedullary implants until further work has been accomplished.

Recent studies have highlighted the importance of maintaining the integrity of the lateral wall of the greater trochanter when using a sliding hip screw[25] (Figure 2). A postoperative fracture of the lateral femoral wall was found to be the main predictor for reoperation after an intertrochanteric fracture.[25] Intertrochanteric fractures should be classified according to the integrity of the lateral femoral wall, especially in randomized trials comparing fracture implants.

External fixation continues to be an option in the mortally ill patient.[26] In one study of 56 elderly, high-risk patients, external fixation was associated with short surgery time, no need for blood transfusion, and a short hospitalization.[26] Union was obtained in all patients after 6 months. There was no significant difference between the functional status before the injury and at follow-up after 12 months. No deep pin tract or wound infections occurred, but not surprisingly a superficial skin reaction was seen in 39.3% of patients. The mortality rate was 20.4% at 12 months, which compares favorably with other types of treatment in this patient population.

Arthroplasty is typically used as a salvage procedure for failed intertrochanteric fractures, and there seems to be little indication for its use as a primary clinical therapy. The authors of a 2005 study reviewed their experience with primary hip arthroplasty in 34 consecutive patients with intertrochanteric fractures; 5 had hemiarthroplasty and 29 were treated with total hip arthroplasty.[27] Five patients (all with total hip arthroplasties) required subsequent surgeries: four for dislocation and one for sepsis. In this series there was a 15% complication rate and a high mortality rate at 12-year follow-up. Dislocation was significantly higher than in other studies of primary total hip arthroplasty for degenerative disease. In a retrospective case-control study, the effectiveness of internal fixation versus cone hemiarthroplasty for the treatment of unstable intertrochanteric fractures was evaluated.[28] At final follow-up, 32 hemiarthroplasty patients and 38 internal fixation patients had no significant differences in hospital stay, surgery time, or receipt of blood transfusions. Clinical outcomes were similar. There were no dislocations in the hemiarthroplasty group. Based on the reported results, it appears that primary arthroplasty cannot be recommended at this time as the optimal surgical option for intertrochanteric fractures.

Outcomes Analysis

With the explosion of new nail devices for intertrochanteric hip fractures, there was a demonstrable change in utilization patterns among orthopaedic surgeons. Although published in 2008, data from 2000 to 2002 were examined for nail usage.[29] The mean adjusted intramedullary nailing rate per 100 Medicare patients with an intertrochanteric fracture increased nationally from 7.84 in 2000 to 16.98 in 2002. In 2000, surgeons in 16 states used an intramedullary nail for fewer than 1 of every 20 Medicare patients with an intertrochanteric fracture. By 2002, surgeons in only two states used an intramedullary nail for fewer than 1 of every 20 patients with an intertrochanteric fracture, and in eight states they used an intramedullary nail in more than 1 of every 4 patients with an intertrochanteric fracture. This shift was reflected in a dramatic change in practice patterns for orthopaedic surgeons taking part 2 of the American Board of Orthopaedic Surgery examinations.[30] Intramedullary nail fixation rates increased from 3% in 1999 to 67% in 2006. Regional variation was substantial. Overall, patients treated with plate fixation had slightly less pain and deformity in comparison with those treated with intramedullary nailing, with no significant identified differences in terms of function or satisfaction. Patients managed with intramedullary nailing had more procedure-related complications, particularly bone fracture. In a 2008 study, 43,659 Medicare beneficiaries 65 years or older who sustained intertrochanteric femur fractures between 1999 and 2001 were analyzed.[31] Two fracture implant groupings, intramedullary nail and sliding hip screw, were identified. Patients

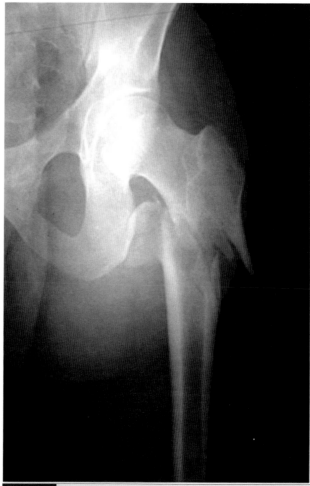

Figure 3 Radiograph showing a classic reverse obliquity fracture with proximal medial to distal lateral fracture line.

treated with an intramedullary nail had higher rates of revision surgery during the first year than those treated with a sliding hip screw (7.2% intramedullary nail versus 5.5% sliding hip screw). Mortality rates at 30 days (14.2% intramedullary nail versus 15.8% sliding hip screw) and 1 year (30.7% intramedullary nail versus 32.5% sliding hip screw) were similar. Adjusted secondary outcome measures showed significant increases in the intramedullary nail group relative to the sliding hip screw group for index hospital length of stay, days of rehabilitation services in the first 6 months after discharge, and total expenditures for doctor and hospital services. The Cochrane group also analyzed evidence comparing the nail and sliding hip screw.[32] Given the lower complication rate of the sliding hip screw in comparison with intramedullary nails, they concluded that the sliding hip screw appears superior for trochanteric fractures. They also cautioned that further studies are required to determine if different types of intramedullary nails produce similar results, or if intramedullary nails have advantages for selected fracture types.

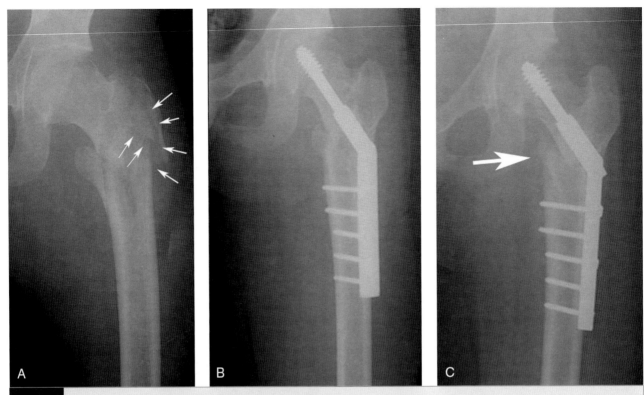

Figure 4 Radiograph showing extensive comminution (**A**) illustrates the area of lateral wall that is not intact (*arrows*). Initial radiograph (**B**) shows it is possible to obtain a reduction, but early migration (**C**) is the danger because the femoral neck no longer is reduced at the calcar (*arrow*) and the shaft is medialized in relation to the neck. The neck has only stopped migrating when it rests on the side plate. This patient is left with a significant leg length abnormality.

Reverse Oblique Fractures and Fractures With Subtrochanteric Extension

The reverse oblique fractures and peritrochanteric fractures with subtrochanteric extension are considered transitional fracture types between intertrochanteric patterns and subtrochanteric fractures. Essential features of these fracture patterns are the classic proximal medial to distal lateral fracture line (**Figure 3**) or the extensively comminuted intertrochanteric region (**Figure 2**). As in all proximal femoral fractures, these fractures can be seen in both young and old patient populations.

The key to treating these fractures is pattern identification. Correctly identifying the unstable patterns steers the surgeon away from the use of sliding hip screw devices that are unsuitable secondary to the fracture location and configuration and that typically lead to unacceptable shortening (**Figure 4**). A traction radiograph may be helpful for clarifying the fracture line obliquity and pattern and may aid in preventing a missed diagnosis.[33]

The current recommendation for implant choice for these specific fracture patterns is a fixed-angle plate-screw construct or a fixed-angle cephalomedullary implant. Because the implant must withstand significant loads with fracture malreduction or with associated comminution, and because intramedullary rods offer optimal stability under these conditions,[34] intramedullary rods have become increasingly popular. Additionally, contemporary studies have suggested a higher reoperation rate for implant failure with fixed-angle plates versus intramedullary implants.[35] However, these results may be biased because many traditional plate applications were performed with open techniques versus a biologic, soft-tissue sparing approach in which healing is more rapid and implant fatigue less important. At this point, either device is likely appropriate for these fracture types provided a minimally invasive, soft-tissue sparing approach is used and fracture reduction is adequate with sufficient hardware to maintain the reduction.

Subtrochanteric Femur Fractures

These fractures are functionally distinct from intertrochanteric fractures, although they still exhibit a bimodal age distribution. The technical challenges associated with repairing subtrochanteric fractures are related to the unique anatomic features of this region, typically defined as the region from the lesser trochanter to a level 5 cm distal.

Two critical characteristics of this fracture pattern must be appreciated before undertaking internal fixa-

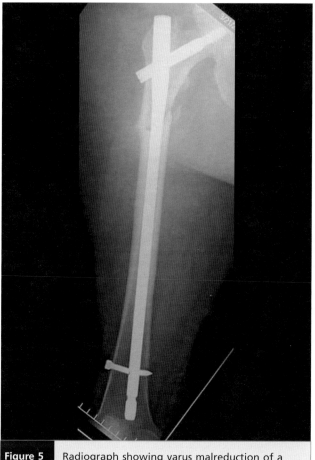

Figure 5 Radiograph showing varus malreduction of a subtrochanteric fracture fixed with a cephalomedullary nail. Resultant subsidence at the fracture site has resulted in a broken locking screw distally.

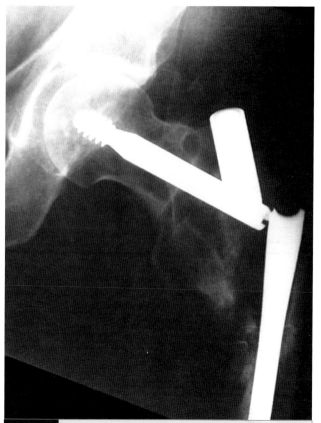

Figure 6 Radiograph showing a broken cephalomedullary implant after fatigue failure in a slow-healing fracture. This was a classic failure point for implants with large screws. The large implant fenestration needed for screw passage increased the chances of stress failure at the thin remaining walls.

tion in this region. First are the strong muscular attachments to the fracture fragments that result in predictable displacement of the fracture fragments. Specifically, the proximal fragment flexes and abducts because of the pull of the iliopsoas and the abduction force applied by the gluteus medius, whereas the action of the adductors tends to produce shortening and medialization of the shaft segment. These displacements are common regardless of the degree of comminution and must be addressed by specific reduction maneuvers. Without appropriate attention to these deforming forces, nonunions secondary to proximal fragment malreduction are common (**Figure 5**). Second, the physiologic forces during weight bearing in this region are some of the highest seen in the human skeleton, with extreme lateral tensile forces and medial compressive loads during weight bearing and stance. These forces are problematic in the setting of malreduction and comminution when cortical contact and compression are not possible; in these settings the implant is exposed to increased mechanical stress, and fatigue failures are common (**Figure 6**). Classic biomechanics have clarified the variability in bending and torsional strength of various devices,[34,36]

usually favoring an intramedullary implant. Yet, these studies fail to consider intermediate fracture patterns (that is, those in which some cortical contact is achieved), reduction accuracy, and rate of healing related to newer biologically optimal techniques. Recent biomechanical evaluations have verified higher implant stresses in subtrochanteric fractures, accentuating the importance of accurate reduction and compression when possible.[37]

Classification and Diagnosis

Historically, the Russell-Taylor classification was used to identify fracture types and aid in implant choice for subtrochanteric femur fractures and was based on involvement of the piriformis fossa and the lesser trochanter. This system was initially helpful in choosing between intramedullary fixation (when the piriformis fossa was intact) and lateral fixed-angle plate devices (when the piriformis fossa was disrupted). However, this classification had more applicablity when interlocking options were limited to single oblique proximal to distal locks or traditional parallel high-angle interlocking screws into the femoral neck and head (recon-

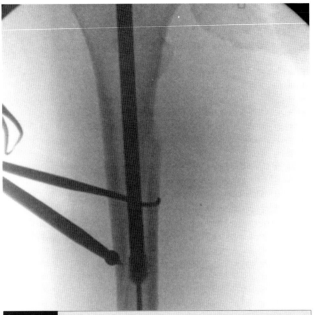

Figure 7 | Intraoperative radiograph showing the bone hook and spiked pusher used to hold fracture reduction during reaming.

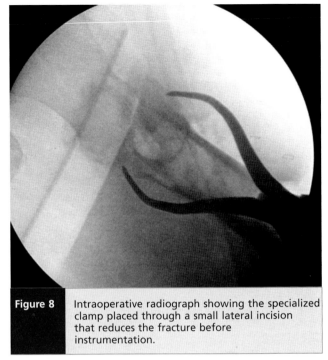

Figure 8 | Intraoperative radiograph showing the specialized clamp placed through a small lateral incision that reduces the fracture before instrumentation.

struction nail interlocks) and when most nail designs were based on piriformis start sites.

Currently, trochanteric-entry, off-axis intramedullary devices have emerged with the option for interlocked screws or compression screws into the femoral head; thus, piriformis involvement no longer precludes intramedullary fixation techniques. Additionally, piriformis, on-axis intramedullary devices now offer a myriad of interlock positions and trajectories, so that the status of the lesser trochanter is less significant. Because of the change in implant proximal fixation options and start sites, the AO/OTA classification may ultimately be more useful in planning the surgical approach and technique.

Treatment

Classic biomechanical studies suggest that intramedullary implants can withstand loads greater than three times body weight.[36] These studies are based on worst-case scenario testing configurations with segmental bone loss. If cortical contact with acceptable reduction can be achieved, especially along the medial calcar, the stability achieved between plates and nails is similar under physiologic loads.

Trochanteric insertion cephalomedullary nails are growing in popularity for subtrochanteric fractures and provide a durable, stable implant in comminuted fractures, with results comparable to those reported with piriformis insertion nailing.[15] Ongoing studies have evaluated abduction function and gait following fixation, and early results are favorable.

Intramedullary nailing for subtrochanteric fractures requires specialized techniques, and traditional closed

nailing is rarely adequate to obtain an optimal reduction. Frequently, percutaneous incisions anteriorly and laterally around the proximal fracture segment are performed to allow placement of sharp pushing instruments, bone hooks, or other tools to achieve and maintain proximal segment alignment[38] (Figures 7 and 8). One author described good outcomes in 24 of 60 cases using a cephalomedullary nailing technique that was "open," with no increase in the infection rate.[39] Systematic analysis of the morbidity of these small incisions has yet to be performed, but similar techniques in the tibia have not shown increased rates of infection or wound complications.[40]

Occasionally, even more invasive techniques are required to achieve reduction. Cerclage techniques have traditionally been maligned as detrimental secondary to the medial dissection required to position these wires, even though the cerclage technique can effectively reduce oblique subtrochanteric patterns. The cerclage application technique may be significant in terms of the amount of soft-tissue disruption, and differences may exist between braided cables and standard wires. Further published studies may assist in understanding the benefits and drawbacks of cerclage reduction techniques. Current recommendations are to not use cerclage wires for fixation of femur fractures in general. Unreduced proximal femur fractures are usually the result of an inappropriate starting point.

In isolated subtrochanteric femur fractures, lateral positioning—either free leg or in traction on a fracture table—may simplify both reduction and start site localization for intramedullary nailing. A slightly more anterior and medial (4 mm lateral to the piriformis fossa) starting point aids the maintenance of reduction of the

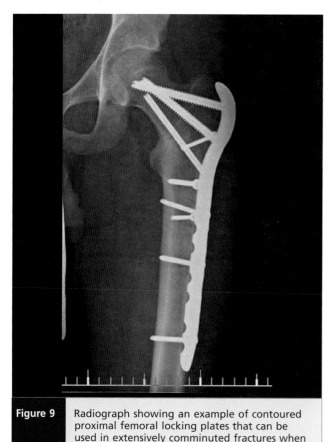

Figure 9 Radiograph showing an example of contoured proximal femoral locking plates that can be used in extensively comminuted fractures when the surgeon is uncomfortable with using a nail but the lateral wall comminution is too severe for a conventional plating technique.

and retain the ability to insert the implant percutaneously. Nonanatomically contoured implants (distal femoral locking plates) have been used in the proximal femur to take advantage of locking screw technology and have been effective.[46] New precontoured proximal femoral locking plates have been introduced by several companies (**Figure 9**) and have been useful in treating proximal femoral fractures in some centers.[47] A recent biomechanical analysis in a subtrochanteric gap model showed equivalent stability between a proximal femoral locking plate and a traditional angled blade plate. A straight large fragment locking plate with locking screws was also shown to provide inadequate stability.[48] Therefore, a surgeon may select open plating or percutaneous reduction and plating with a locking system as a viable option for simple subtrochanteric fractures. Further reports of clinical experiences and outcomes with this plate will assist in validating these biomechanical studies and assist in appropriate implant selection in clinical settings.

Outcomes

Good and excellent functional outcomes have been reported with the use of cephalomedullary nails and with extramedullary techniques for subtrochanteric fractures.[15,33,44-47,49-52] The outcomes are more likely related to adequacy of reduction and maintenance of local biology than to implant type. Unique complications exist with both techniques, including a higher secondary procedure rate with plate fixation[35,53] and risk of distal cortical perforation with intramedullary nailing, especially in older patients.[54]

Summary

Extracapsular femur fractures continue to be clinically challenging. There remain some subgroups of these fractures—severely comminuted fractures, high-energy fractures in young patients, and fractures in elderly patients—that continue to challenge the newest implant technology and fixation techniques. New implants in some ways have made fracture care simpler. Many of these devices have yet to show clear advantage over other more common and cheaper implants. Implant options and techniques have evolved to include minimally invasive plating options. Intramedullary techniques, particularly for subtrochanteric fractures, provide reproducibly good results, and options for entry site have expanded indications for fractures that involve the piriformis fossa. Good outcomes can be expected with adequate reduction and with approaches that respect and maintain the local fracture biology. Specific complications continue to exist with either plating or nailing techniques. Surgeons should be guided by their comprehension of the fracture type, the biologic milieu, and their comfort level with the chosen implant.

major fragments. Hip flexion will aid in reduction of the proximal segment, and abduction is easily neutralized with gentle lateral manipulation. In larger patients, the lateral position also aids in open surgical approaches with the soft-tissue envelope falling away because of gravity; therefore, less retraction is required.

Although intramedullary devices remain a mainstay of treatment, there is sustained interest in biologically friendly, minimally invasive plating techniques with both traditional and newer locked fixed-angle plate constructs.[41,42] Dynamic condylar screw devices can be inserted using a minimally invasive technique, and the results for comminuted subtrochanteric femoral fractures are favorable.[43-45] Proper planning and experience with these techniques is required to achieve good functional outcomes and to master the significant learning curve. With this technique, preserving the vascularity of the medial fragments can lead to rapid callus formation and early union.

Locking implants have also been evaluated for their use in minimally invasive approaches to subtrochanteric fixation. Although the dynamic condylar screw devices can be placed percutaneously, there has been long-standing concern for this implant because of the amount of bone sacrificed in the femoral head. Locking implants solve this bone loss issue in the femoral head

5: Lower Extremity

Annotated References

1. Koval KJ, Oh CK, Egol KA: Does a traction-internal rotation radiograph help to better evaluate fractures of the proximal femur? *Bull NYU Hosp Jt Dis* 2008;66(2): 102-106.

   The routine addition of a traction-internal rotation radiograph increased the ability to accurately classify proximal femur fractures by junior residents in the authors' department. This has a direct impact on accurate surgical planning and implant choice.

2. Jin WJ, Dai LY, Cui YM, Zhou Q, Jiang LS, Lu H: Reliability of classification systems for intertrochanteric fractures of the proximal femur in experienced orthopaedic surgeons. *Injury* 2005;36(7):858-861.

   This study suggests that the AO classification system can be used more reliably to measure intertrochanteric fractures of the proximal femur than Evans, Kyle, and Boyd classification systems.

3. Fung W, Jonsson A, Buhren V, Bhandari M: Classifying intertrochanteric fractures of the proximal femur: Does experience matter? *Med Princ Pract* 2007;16(3):198-202.

   The AO/OTA classification is more useful than the Evans/Jensen classification. The findings suggest that surgeons' perceptions about stability vary to a significant extent.

4. Kregor PJ, Obremskey WT, Kreder HJ, Swiontkowski MF: Unstable pertrochanteric femoral fractures. *J Orthop Trauma* 2005;19(1):63-66.

5. Strauss E, Frank J, Lee J, Kummer FJ, Tejwani N: Helical blade versus sliding hip screw for treatment of unstable intertrochanteric hip fractures: A biomechanical evaluation. *Injury* 2006;37(10):984-989.

   This study showed that fixation of the femoral head with a helical blade was biomechanically superior to fixation with a standard sliding hip screw in a cadaver model of an unstable intertrochanteric hip fracture.

6. Strauss EJ, Kummer FJ, Koval KJ, Egol KA: The "Z-effect" phenomenon defined: A laboratory study. *J Orthop Res* 2007;25(12):1568-1573.

   The Z-effect phenomenon is a potential complication of two lag screw intramedullary nail designs used for fixation of intertrochanteric hip fractures, in which the inferior lag screw migrates laterally and the superior lag screw migrates medially during physiologic loading.

7. Weil YA, Gardner MJ, Mikhail G, Pierson G, Helfet DL, Lorich DG: Medial migration of intramedullary hip fixation devices: A biomechanical analysis. *Arch Orthop Trauma Surg* 2008;128(2):227-234.

   All five implants studied showed medial migration to a similar distance. The TFN required the highest number of cycles and the intramedullary hip screw the lowest, although this difference did not reach statistical significance ($P = 0.07$). Changing the pivot point for the medial calcar did not significantly alter the results.

8. Bienkowski P, Reindl R, Berry GK, Iakoub E, Harvey EJ: A new intramedullary nail device for the treatment of intertrochanteric hip fractures: Perioperative experience. *J Trauma* 2006;61(6):1458-1462.

   The rate of femoral fractures for short femoral nails was decreased compared with historic controls. Improved early mobilization was noted in the TFN group.

9. McConnell A, Zdero R, Syed K, Peskun C, Schemitsch E: The biomechanics of ipsilateral intertrochanteric and femoral shaft fractures: A comparison of 5 fracture fixation techniques. *J Orthop Trauma* 2008;22(8):517-524.

   All constructs showed no statistical differences with the exception of the long intramedullary hip screw, which provided the least torsional stiffness. However, the current in vitro model did not simulate fracture healing or support offered by soft tissues, both of which would affect the stiffness and load-to-failure levels reached.

10. Ropars M, Mitton D, Skalli W: Minimally invasive screw plates for surgery of unstable intertrochanteric femoral fractures: A biomechanical comparative study. *Clin Biomech* 2008;23(8):1012-1017.

    PCCP and the minimally invasive screw system appear to be mechanical devices that may improve clinical outcomes and reduce the risk of comorbidities associated with unstable trochanteric fractures without increased risk of mechanical failure.

11. Jewell DP, Gheduzzi S, Mitchell MS, Miles AW: Locking plates increase the strength of dynamic hip screws. *Injury* 2008;39(2):209-212.

    A dynamic hip screw with fixed-angle locking screws may reduce the risk of DHS failure.

12. Krischak GD, Augat P, Beck A, et al: Biomechanical comparison of two side plate fixation techniques in an unstable intertrochanteric osteotomy model: Sliding Hip Screw and Percutaneous Compression Plate. *Clin Biomech* 2007;22(10):1112-1118.

    The PCCP as a double-axis fixation device with a sliding capability allows higher displacements in the varus direction and also in external rotation at 800 N loading compared with the sliding hip screw as a single-axis fixation device combined with an additional derotation screw. Although both implants are successfully used in clinical practice, this difference should be considered in treatment of unstable intertrochanteric fractures with inferior comminution in osteoporotic patients.

13. Park SY, Park J, Rhee DJ, Yoon HK, Yang KH: Anterior or posterior obliquity of the lag screw in the lateral view: Does it affect the sliding characteristics on unstable trochanteric fractures? *Injury* 2007;38(7):785-791.

    The authors used a model of 31-A2 fractures in artificial femurs. When the lag screw was inserted with an anterior-to-posterior vector within the neck and the head of the femur, the results were worse.

14. Efstathopoulos NE, Nikolaou VS, Lazarettos JT: Intramedullary fixation of intertrochanteric hip fractures:

A comparison of two implant designs. *Int Orthop* 2007;
31(1):71-76.

Both the trochanteric gamma nail and ACE trochanteric nail provide effective methods of treatment of intertrochanteric fractures in elderly patients.

15. Starr AJ, Hay MT, Reinert CM, Borer DS, Christensen KC: Cephalomedullary nails in the treatment of high-energy proximal femur fractures in young patients: A prospective, randomized comparison of trochanteric versus piriformis fossa entry portal. *J Orthop Trauma* 2006;20(4):240-246.

Both devices yield predictably good results in these difficult fractures. No difference between the two devices with regard to incision length, duration of surgery, blood loss, reduction, ease of use, union rate, complication rate, or outcome was found.

16. Lee YS, Huang HL, Lo TY, Huang CR: Dynamic hip screw in the treatment of intertrochanteric fractures: A comparison of two fixation methods. *Int Orthop* 2007; 31(5):683-688.

The minimally invasive DHS technique was associated with smaller wound size, lower pain level, and lower blood loss compared with the conventional technique. Hospital stay and total analgesic use were decreased, benefiting the patient and reducing hospital cost.

17. Peyser A, Weil YA, Brocke L, et al: A prospective, randomised study comparing the percutaneous compression plate and the compression hip screw for the treatment of intertrochanteric fractures of the hip. *J Bone Joint Surg Br* 2007;89(9):1210-1217.

The authors randomized 104 patients to one of two surgical treatment arms comparing the percutaneous compression plate and the compression hip screw for treating intertrochanteric fractures of the hip. The PCCP group had a better outcome with respect to reduced blood loss, postoperative pain, and less postoperative collapse of the fracture (perhaps the only relevant finding).

18. Panesar SS, Mirza S, Bharadwaj G, Woolf V, Ravikumar R, Athanasiou T: The percutaneous compression plate versus the dynamic hip screw: A meta-analysis. *Acta Orthop Belg* 2008;74(1):38-48.

There was a decreased trend in overall mortality in the PCCP group. Similar trends favoring the PCCP technique were seen with the other outcomes.

19. Platzer P, Thalhammer G, Wozasek GE, Vécsei V: Femoral shortening after surgical treatment of trochanteric fractures in nongeriatric patients. *J Trauma* 2008;64(4): 982-989.

Femoral shortening after surgical treatment of pertrochanteric and intertrochanteric fractures was found to be a common clinical finding in nongeriatric patients. Nearly half of these patients had a lower limb-length inequality after fracture fixation. The degree of the shortening was rather low and depended mainly on the fracture type. Comparing the two different implants used for surgical treatment, a cephalomedullary nail was more successful in preventing limb-length discrepancy in unstable fracture types than dynamic hip screw.

20. Tarantino U, Oliva F, Impagliazzo A, et al: A comparative prospective study of dynamic variable angle hip screw and Gamma nail in intertrochanteric hip fractures. *Disabil Rehabil* 2005;27(18-19):1157-1165.

The dynamic screw plate allows effective management of intertrochanteric fractures of the femur. In less comminuted fractures, a compression hip screw may be a faster and safer surgical solution. In comminuted fractures, surgical difficulties may increase in parallel to fracture complexity.

21. Little NJ, Verma V, Fernando C, Elliott DS, Khaleel A: A prospective trial comparing the Holland nail with the dynamic hip screw in the treatment of intertrochanteric fractures of the hip. *J Bone Joint Surg Br* 2008;90(8): 1073-1078.

The authors conclude that the DHS can be implanted more quickly and with less exposure to radiation than the Holland nail. However, the resultant blood loss and need for transfusion was greater. The Holland nail allowed patients to mobilize faster and to a greater extent.

22. Crawford CH, Malkani AL, Cordray S, Roberts CS, Sligar W: The trochanteric nail versus the sliding hip screw for intertrochanteric hip fractures: A review of 93 cases. *J Trauma* 2006;60(2):325-328.

This study suggests that the trochanteric nail is a reasonable alternative to the sliding hip screw when used for intertrochanteric fractures, although it may be associated with higher complication rates.

23. Gill JB, Jensen L, Chin PC, Rafiei P, Reddy K, Schutt RC Jr: Intertrochanteric hip fractures treated with the trochanteric fixation nail and sliding hip screw. *J Surg Orthop Adv* 2007;16(2):62-66.

The TFN procedure required shorter surgical times and was used in more complex fracture patterns. The sliding hip screw group had fewer blood transfusions. The sliding hip screw group had a higher complication rate of 19.6%, versus an 11.4% rate in the TFN group. The TFN is an appropriate and acceptable treatment method for intertrochanteric hip fractures.

24. Gardner MJ, Briggs SM, Kopjar B, Helfet DL, Lorich DG: Radiographic outcomes of intertrochanteric hip fractures treated with the trochanteric fixation nail. *Injury* 2007;38(10):1189-1196.

Subtle migration of the tip of the blade within the femoral head occurred in all fractures, but this did not preclude maintenance of reduction and fracture healing and was not predicted by fracture type, reduction quality, age, or sex. More telescoping occurred in unstable compared with stable fractures. All position changes occurred within the first 6 weeks postoperatively.

25. Palm H, Jacobsen S, Sonne-Holm S, Gebuhr P; Hip Fracture Study Group: Integrity of the lateral femoral wall in intertrochanteric hip fractures: An important predictor of a reoperation. *J Bone Joint Surg Am* 2007; 89(3):470-475.

Patients with preoperative or intraoperative fracture of the lateral femoral wall are not treated adequately with a sliding compression hip-screw device, and intertro-

5: Lower Extremity

a sliding compression hip-screw device, and intertrochanteric fractures should therefore be classified according to the integrity of the lateral femoral wall, especially in randomized trials comparing fracture implants.

26. Kazakos K, Lyras DN, Verettas D, Galanis V, Psillakis I, Xarchas K: External fixation of intertrochanteric fractures in elderly high-risk patients. *Acta Orthop Belg* 2007;73(1):44-48.

The Citieffe/Ch-N (Citieffe, Bologna, Italy) external fixation device can be used successfully for the treatment of elderly high-risk patients with intertrochanteric fractures.

27. Berend KR, Hanna J, Smith TM, Mallory TH, Lombardi AV: Acute hip arthroplasty for the treatment of intertrochanteric fractures in the elderly. *J Surg Orthop Adv* 2005;14(4):185-189.

The study results do not support routine use of arthroplasty in treatment of intertrochanteric hip fractures in the elderly.

28. Kayali C, Agus H, Ozluk S, Sanli C: Treatment for unstable intertrochanteric fractures in elderly patients: Internal fixation versus cone hemiarthroplasty. *J Orthop Surg* 2006;14(3):240-244.

Cone hemiarthroplasty can be an alternative treatment of unstable intertrochanteric fractures in elderly patients to achieve earlier mobilization.

29. Forte ML, Virnig BA, Kane RL, et al: Geographic variation in device use for intertrochanteric hip fractures. *J Bone Joint Surg Am* 2008;90(4):691-699.

There was substantial geographic variation by states in the use of intramedullary nailing from 2000 through 2002, which was largely unexplained by patient-related factors.

30. Anglen JO, Weinstein JN; American Board of Orthopaedic Surgery Research Committee: Nail or plate fixation of intertrochanteric hip fractures: Changing pattern of practice. A review of the American Board of Orthopaedic Surgery Database. *J Bone Joint Surg Am* 2008; 90(4):700-707.

From 1999 to 2006, a dramatic change in surgeon preference for the fixation device used for the treatment of intertrochanteric fractures has occurred among young orthopaedic surgeons. This change has occurred despite a lack of evidence in the literature supporting the change and in the face of the potential for more complications.

31. Aros B, Tosteson AN, Gottlieb DJ, Koval KJ: Is a sliding hip screw or IM nail the preferred implant for intertrochanteric fracture fixation? *Clin Orthop Relat Res* 2008;466(11):2827-2832.

This study was performed to determine whether patients who sustain an intertrochanteric fracture have better outcomes when stabilized using a sliding hip screw or an intramedullary nail. The cohort consisted of 43,659 patients. Patients treated with an intramedullary nail had higher rates of revision surgery during the first year than those treated with a sliding hip screw. Mortality rates at 30 days and 1 year were similar. Adjusted secondary outcome measures showed significant increases in the intramedullary nail group relative to the sliding hip screw group for index hospital length of stay, days of rehabilitation services in the first 6 months after discharge, and total expenditures for doctor and hospital services.

32. Parker MJ, Handoll HH: Gamma and other cephalocondylic intramedullary nails versus extramedullary implants for extracapsular hip fractures in adults. *Cochrane Database Syst Rev* 2008;3:CD000093.

Given the lower complication rate of the sliding hip screw in comparison with intramedullary nails, the sliding hip screws appears superior for treating trochanteric fractures.

33. Celebi L, Can M, Muratli HH, Yagmurlu MF, Yuksel HY, Bicimoğlu A: Indirect reduction and biological internal fixation of comminuted subtrochanteric fractures of the femur. *Injury* 2006;37(8):740-750.

Indirect reduction and biologic internal fixation yield acceptable results in comminuted fractures. These good results can be attributed to early weight bearing with rapid solid callus formation and early union, which are particularly advantageous in comminuted subtrochanteric fractures, avoiding the implant failure that is not uncommon in these fractures.

34. Tencer AF, Johnson KD, Johnston DW, Gill K: A biomechanical comparison of various methods of stabilization of subtrochanteric fractures of the femur. *J Orthop Res* 1984;2(3):297-305.

35. Sadowski C, Lübbeke A, Saudan M, Riand N, Stern R, Hoffmeyer P: Treatment of reverse oblique and transverse intertrochanteric fractures with use of an intramedullary nail or a 95 degrees screw-plate: A prospective, randomized study. *J Bone Joint Surg Am* 2002; 84(3):372-381.

36. Kraemer WJ, Hearn TC, Powell JN, Mahomed N: Fixation of segmental subtrochanteric fractures: A biomechanical study. *Clin Orthop Relat Res* 1996;332:71-79.

37. Eberle S, Gerber C, von Oldenburg G, et al: Type of hip fracture determines load share in intramedullary osteosynthesis. *Clin Orthop Relat Res* 2009;467(8):1972-1980.

The authors used a finite element model with some biomechanical correlation to determine load share in intramedullary osteosynthesis. Intramedullary implants seemed to stabilize unstable hip fractures with almost the same amount of stiffness as seen in stable fractures; however, the implants bear a higher load share, resulting in higher stresses in the implant.

38. Ramakrishnan M, Prasad SS, Parkinson RW, Kaye JC: Management of subtrochanteric femoral fractures and metastases using long proximal femoral nail. *Injury* 2004;35(2):184-190.

The authors reported that early results showed the Long Proximal Femoral Nail (Synthes, Europe) was a reliable and safe method of proximal femoral fracture fixation. The authors also concluded that cerclage wiring was safe.

39. Shukla S, Johnston P, Ahmad MA, Wynn-Jones H, Patel AD, Walton NP: Outcome of traumatic subtrochanteric femoral fractures fixed using cephalo-medullary nails. *Injury* 2007;38(11):1286-1293.

    The authors advocate the use of open reduction if necessary to avoid varus malreduction and other complications, particularly because open reduction was not associated with a higher complication rate in this series. The study supports the use of cephalomedullary nailing for subtrochanteric fractures with a union rate of 95%.

40. Tang P, Gates C, Hawes J, Vogt M, Prayson MJ: Does open reduction increase the chance of infection during intramedullary nailing of closed tibial shaft fractures? *J Orthop Trauma* 2006;20(5):317-322.

    This study found that the rate of infection for open versus closed reductions during intramedullary nailing of closed tibial shaft fractures was higher but not statistically different. Careful use of open reduction techniques during intramedullary nailing of closed tibia fractures may have a minimal risk of infection, which is offset by aiding reduction and healing (theoretically).

41. Kinast C, Bolhofner BR, Mast JW, Ganz R: Subtrochanteric fractures of the femur: Results of treatment with the 95 degrees condylar blade-plate. *Clin Orthop Relat Res* 1989;238:122-130.

42. Bolhofner BR, Carmen B, Clifford P: The results of open reduction and internal fixation of distal femur fractures using a biologic (indirect) reduction technique. *J Orthop Trauma* 1996;10(6):372-377.

43. Vaidya SV, Dholakia DB, Chatterjee A: The use of a dynamic condylar screw and biological reduction techniques for subtrochanteric femur fracture. *Injury* 2003;34(2):123-128.

44. Rohilla R, Singh R, Magu NK, Siwach RC, Sangwan SS: Mini-incision dynamic condylar screw fixation for comminuted subtrochanteric hip fractures. *J Orthop Surg* 2008;16(2):150-155.

    Results of indirect reduction and mini-incision dynamic condylar screw fixation for comminuted subtrochanteric femoral fractures are favorable. Preservation of vascularity of the medial fragments may lead to rapid callus formation and early union, and avoid implant failure and secondary bone grafting.

45. Lee PC, Hsieh PH, Yu SW, Shiao CW, Kao HK, Wu CC: Biologic plating versus intramedullary nailing for comminuted subtrochanteric fractures in young adults: A prospective, randomized study of 66 cases. *J Trauma* 2007;63(6):1283-1291.

    The dynamic condylar screw proved to be a feasible fixation device for comminuted subtrochanteric fractures in young patients. The authors concluded that results indicated that intramedullary nailing showed no advantages over biologic plating.

46. Oh CW, Kim JJ, Byun YS, et al: Minimally invasive plate osteosynthesis of subtrochanteric femur fractures with a locking plate: A prospective series of 20 fractures. *Arch Orthop Trauma Surg* 2009;129(12):1659-1665.

    The minimally invasive plate osteosynthesis technique with a locking plate provides an alternative method for fixing subtrochanteric femur fractures, when intramedullary nailing is inappropriate. This technique provides stable fixation, with a high union rate and a minimal complication rate.

47. Hasenboehler EA, Agudelo JF, Morgan SJ, Smith WR, Hak DJ, Stahel PF: Treatment of complex proximal femoral fractures with the proximal femur locking compression plate. *Orthopedics* 2007;30(8):618-623.

    The authors report on the surgical technique and an early clinical case using the proximal femur locking compression plate. They believe that the proximal femur locking compression plate represents a feasible alternative for treating unstable intertrochanteric and subtrochanteric fractures.

48. Crist BD, Khalafi A, Hazelwood SJ, Lee MA: A biomechanical comparison of locked plate fixation with percutaneous insertion capability versus the angled blade plate in a subtrochanteric fracture gap model. *J Orthop Trauma* 2009;23(9):622-627.

    The authors examined the conventional blade plate with the newer proximal femur locking compression plate. Their data showed that the proximal femur locking compression plate with a "kickstand" screw provides more axial stiffness, less torsional stiffness, and equivalent irreversible deformation to cyclic axial loading when compared with the blade plate.

49. Robinson CM, Houshian S, Khan LA: Trochanteric-entry long cephalomedullary nailing of subtrochanteric fractures caused by low-energy trauma. *J Bone Joint Surg Am* 2005;87(10):2217-2226.

    Subtrochanteric fractures caused by low-energy trauma are similar to other proximal femoral fractures, with a high mortality rate during the first year after the injury. Trochanteric-entry cephalomedullary nails are associated with an acceptable rate of perioperative complications and favorable functional outcomes.

50. Borens O, Wettstein M, Kombot C, Chevalley F, Mouhsine E, Garofalo R: Long gamma nail in the treatment of subtrochanteric fractures. *Arch Orthop Trauma Surg* 2004;124(7):443-447.

    The minimally invasive technique and simple application of the long gamma nail lead to a low percentage of complications in these difficult fractures after a relatively short learning curve. The biomechanical properties of this implant allow early mobilization and partial weight-bearing even in patients with advanced osteoporosis.

51. Papakostidis C, Grotz MR, Papadokostakis G, Dimitriou R, Giannoudis PV: Femoral biologic plate fixation. *Clin Orthop Relat Res* 2006;450:193-202.

    The high union rate, low infection rate (2%), and occa-

5: Lower Extremity

sional need for bone graft indicate biologic plate fixation is a viable alternative to modern nailing techniques, particularly in patients with polytrauma.

52. Yoo MC, Cho YJ, Kim KI, Khairuddin M, Chun YS: Treatment of unstable peritrochanteric femoral fractures using a 95 degrees angled blade plate. *J Orthop Trauma* 2005;19(10):687-692.

Thirty-nine consecutive patients with peritrochanteric femoral fractures were followed for a minimum of 12 months. There were 29 subtrochanteric fractures and 10 intertrochanteric fractures (reverse obliquity pattern) for which the compression hip screw could not be used. A 95° angled blade plate can be a useful alternative fixation device for the treatment of unstable peritrochanteric femoral fractures.

53. Rahme DM, Harris IA: Intramedullary nailing versus fixed angle blade plating for subtrochanteric femoral fractures: A prospective randomised controlled trial. *J Orthop Surg* 2007;15(3):278-281.

Patients were randomized for treatment with either intramedullary nailing or a fixed-angle blade plate. Internal fixation using a fixed-angle blade plate for subtrochanteric femoral fractures had higher implant failure and revision rates compared with closed intramedullary nailing.

54. Ostrum RF, Levy MS: Penetration of the distal femoral anterior cortex during intramedullary nailing for subtrochanteric fractures: A report of three cases. *J Orthop Trauma* 2005;19(9):656-660.

It appears that the difference in the femoral anteroposterior bow between the bone and the implant is a contributing factor to distal femoral anterior cortex penetration in intramedullary nailing of subtrochanteric fractures.

Chapter 33

Fractures of the Femoral Diaphysis

William M. Ricci, MD   Gary S. Gruen, MD   Hobie Summers, MD   Peter A. Siska, MD

Evaluation of the Patient With a Femoral Shaft Fracture

Physical Examination

Evaluation of patients with a femoral shaft fracture begins with the procedures recommended by the Advanced Trauma Life Support training program (American College of Surgeons), directed at protecting the airway and ensuring adequate breathing and circulation. Although children and geriatric patients may sustain femoral shaft fractures after low-energy mechanisms, most are the result of high-energy injury, and many have associated injuries. Obvious deformities related to long bone fractures may be temporarily stabilized with a traction splint or skeletal traction pin, so the overall well-being of the patient may be adequately assessed and resuscitation efforts maximized. A thorough examination is mandatory to detect neurologic deficits as well as potential vascular injuries sustained during the traumatic event. A motor and sensory examination distal to the knee and the status of pedal pulses should be well documented. If pulses are absent on presentation, realignment of the limb with traction or splinting may reestablish blood flow. The ankle-brachial index (ABI) should be determined if pulses are difficult to palpate or asymmetric. An ABI below 0.9 is indicative of a vascular injury, and further evaluation is required.[1,2] Upon completion of the primary survey and

Dr. Ricci or an immediate family member serves as a board member, owner, officer, or committee member of Orthopaedic Trauma Association; has received royalties from Smith & Nephew and Wright Medical Technology; is a member of a speakers' bureau or has made paid presentations on behalf of AO, Wright Medical Technology, Synthes, and Smith & Nephew; serves as a paid consultant to or is an employee of Wright Medical Technology and Smith & Nephew; and has received research or institutional support from AONA, Synthes, Smith & Nephew, Foundation for Orthopaedic Trauma, Axial Biotech, Biomet, Breg, Cerapedics, K2M, Medtronic, Midwest Stone Institute, Stryker, Synthes Spine, Wright Medical Technology, and Wyeth. Dr. Gruen or an immediate family member serves as a paid consultant to or is an employee of Smith & Nephew. Dr. Summers or an immediate family member is a member of a speakers' bureau or has made paid presentations on behalf of Synthes; and has received research or institutional support from Synthes. Dr. Siska or an immediate family member has received research or institutional support from Synthes.

initiation of resuscitation, a secondary survey of all extremities, the pelvis, and the spine should be performed to identify associated injuries.

Radiographic Examination

Good-quality AP and lateral radiographs of the injured femur are mandatory and can be obtained in the trauma room using portable techniques. Providing assistance to the radiology technicians will ensure satisfactory imaging and improve patient comfort. Radiographic determination of the fracture pattern and location assists with preoperative planning. The joint above and below the fracture must be evaluated to identify associated injuries of the femoral neck, distal femur, and proximal tibia. Noncontiguous fractures of the femoral neck, shaft, and distal articular surface are rare but have been described.[3]

An associated femoral neck fracture occurs in up to 10% of femoral shaft fractures caused by blunt trauma. Approximately 30% (20% to 50%) of these fractures are missed on initial evaluation.[4] A protocol to identify associated fractures of the femoral neck has been proposed.[5] The recommended protocol consists of a dedicated internal rotation AP radiograph of the hip, a fine cut (2-mm) CT scan through the femoral neck, and an intraoperative fluoroscopic lateral radiograph of the hip, as well as postoperative AP and lateral radiographs of the proximal femur before awakening the patient. The delay in diagnosis was reduced 91% by using this protocol in 268 consecutive injuries.

Classification

In the Winquist-Hansen classification of femoral shaft fractures[6] (**Figure 1**), type I fractures have a small area of comminution, with more than 75% of the diameter of the bone in continuity following intramedullary (IM) stabilization. Type II fractures have increased comminution, but at least 50% of the diameter remains intact. Type III fractures have less than 50% cortical contact. Type IV fractures have no abutment of the cortices at the level of the fracture to prevent shortening. Type I and type II fractures are thought to be axially stable, whereas type III and type IV fractures are thought to be both axially and rotationally unstable. Rotational stability for less comminuted fractures is determined by the amount of comminution and obliquity of the fracture, with more transverse fracture patterns being less rotationally stable. Despite this framework for

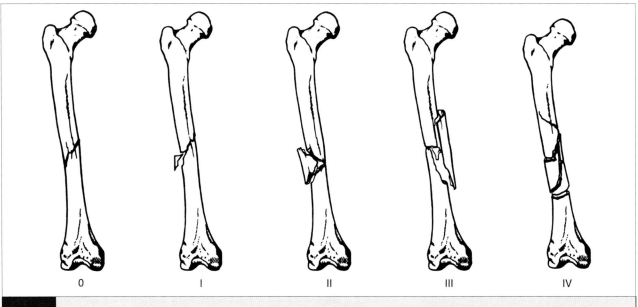

0   I   II   III   IV

Figure 1 | Winquist-Hansen classification of femoral shaft fractures. (Reproduced from Poss R, ed: *Orthopaedic Knowledge Update 3*. Park Ridge, IL, American Academy of Orthopaedic Surgeons, 1990, pp 513-527.)

predicting stability, virtually all femoral fractures treated with IM nailing undergo static interlocking fixation along with progressive early weight bearing as tolerated.

The Orthopaedic Trauma Association (OTA) classification is also commonly used for comparative investigations[7] (**Figure 2**). Fractures of the femoral shaft are designated as type 32. Type 32A fractures are simple (without comminution), type 32B are comminuted but maintain some degree of cortical continuity between the proximal and distal shaft fragments, and type 32C fractures have loss of continuity between the proximal and distal fragments. Further subtypes represent increasing fracture complexity.

Another important descriptor of femur fractures is the location of the fracture along the length of the shaft, usually described as the proximal, middle, or distal third. There is some overlap between subtrochanteric fractures and proximal-third shaft fractures. Fractures within 5 cm of the lesser trochanter can be considered to be in the subtrochanteric region.

Treatment of Femoral Shaft Fractures

Timing of Surgical Management

It has been more than 20 years since a prospective randomized study supported early rather than delayed stabilization of femoral fractures was published.[8] In the decades since, there continues to be significant controversy and research directed at determining the optimum timing and technique of surgical management of femoral shaft fractures. A complete discussion of the pathophysiology of trauma and damage control orthopaedics is presented in chapters 12 and 16.

Provisional Stabilization Techniques

Provisional External Fixation

External fixation, as applied to patients with femoral shaft fractures, is most commonly used as temporary treatment in a damage control scenario or if there is such severe contamination that definitive fixation cannot safely be accomplished as a primary procedure (see chapter 16). External fixation provides a form of portable traction allowing reasonably comfortable patient transfer and positioning for pulmonary toilette and ease of nursing care. As a provisional form of skeletal stabilization, the external fixator provides enough stability to minimize further fat embolization from the fracture site. In general, the external fixator is applied as a uniplanar device with two half pins in each major fracture fragment. In distal fracture variants, it is acceptable to span the knee joint for placement of half pins. Conversion from external fixation to an IM nail has been shown to be safe when performed within 2 weeks of initial external fixation, in the absence of pin site infection.[9,10] Should the patient's condition require prolonged external fixation or should a pin site infection develop, it is possible to remove the external fixator, débride the pin sites, and stabilize the fracture with use of skeletal traction before performing the definitive IM nailing.

Traction

In the past, skeletal traction has been used as the definitive treatment modality for femoral diaphyseal fractures. However, it has several disadvantages, including prolonged immobilization with risk of decubiti, pneumonia, cardiac complications, urinary tract infection, axial and rotational malunion, knee stiffness, and increased hospital cost. In certain instances, traction is still used to

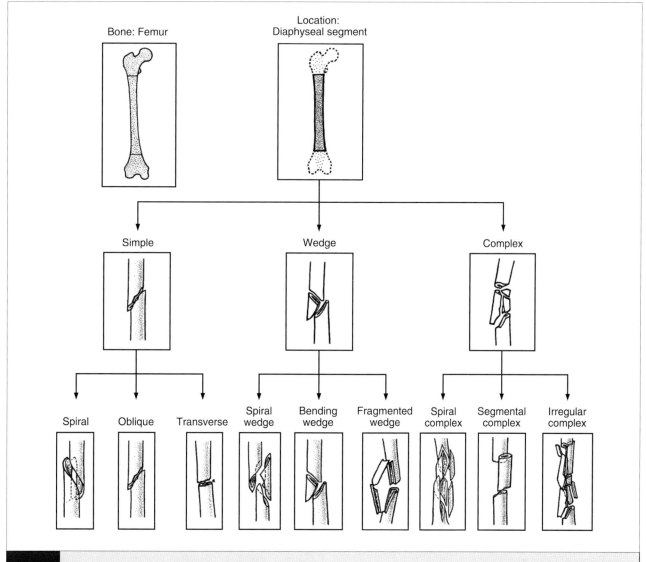

| **Figure 2** | The OTA classification of femoral shaft fractures. (Reproduced with permission from Marsh JL, Slongo TF, Agel J, et al: Fracture and Dislocation Classification Compendium, 2007: Orthopaedic Trauma Association Classification, Database and Outcomes Committee. *J Orthop Trauma* 2007;21:10.) |

treat femoral fractures in children. In adults, traction is recommended as a temporary measure before surgical treatment, especially when delay is expected, or in patients who are unable to undergo surgery.

Damage Control Nailing

Recently, the concept of damage control nailing has been proposed.[11] In critically injured patients who are deemed too ill to tolerate reamed IM nailing, the use of an unreamed retrograde IM nail is an alternative to external fixation. The primary goal is rapid fracture stabilization to allow for resuscitation and patient care with ease of transport, patient positioning, and pulmonary toilette without exacerbation of the existing lung or intracranial injury. To facilitate the performance of damage control nailing in an expedient manner, preoperative communication is paramount. This includes re-

viewing steps with the operating room staff so the procedure is performed in a stepwise manner without unnecessary pauses, as well as coordination with the anesthesia team and general and neurosurgical teams if simultaneous procedures are performed. Another potential advantage of this technique includes the decreased risk of pin site contamination or the need for pin site care for an external fixator. However, given the inferior biomechanical characteristics of a smaller diameter unreamed nail, adequately resuscitated patients may be taken back to the operating room for an exchange of the unreamed nail for a statically locked, reamed IM nail. Another potential disadvantage of damage control nailing compared with external fixation is that embolization still occurs with insertion of an unreamed nail.

IM Nailing

There are several starting points for nailing from which the surgeon may choose, such as the piriformis fossa, greater trochanter, or intercondylar (retrograde) points. There is little evidence to support the superiority of any one starting point over another; each has advantages and disadvantages. When modern techniques are used, union rates can be expected to be nearly equal for the various methods.[12-14] The relatively low union rates seen in early series of retrograde nailing probably are related to the use of a nonreamed technique and the relatively small diameter nails compared to the diameter of the femoral canal. Retrograde nailing using modern techniques that include reaming, snug-fitting nails, and interlocking screws are associated with union rates similar to those of antegrade nailing.

Other outcomes, potential complications, and technical considerations that are patient- and surgeon-specific differentiate the methods. Residual pain, functional deficits, and malalignment may differ between methods, but their effect on overall outcomes is difficult to distinguish. For instance, when comparing antegrade and retrograde femoral nailing, more symptoms related to the knee have been found with retrograde nailing, and more hip-related symptoms with antegrade nailing.[12,13] When considering antegrade nailing through the piriformis fossa in comparison with nailing through the greater trochanter, the associated soft-tissue injury is different. Piriformis nailing causes more injury to the external rotators, whereas trochanteric nailing potentially damages the gluteus medius insertion.[15,16] The relative functional consequences of these differences are unclear. It has been shown, however, that after antegrade nailing there is a significant negative effect on hip kinematics and kinetics, and this effect is time dependent.[17] The portion of the deficit related to the nailing procedure and that related to the injury remains unknown. Fracture alignment after IM nailing is primarily related to surgeon technique and secondarily may be related to the chosen starting point. Control and therefore alignment of distal fractures may be more easily accomplished with a retrograde technique and for proximal fractures with an antegrade technique.[18]

Antegrade Nailing Via a Piriformis Fossa Starting Point

The main advantage of a piriformis fossa starting point is its colinear alignment with the long axis of the femoral shaft. This reduces risk of iatrogenic fracture comminution and varus malalignment compared with off-axis starting points such as the trochanteric entry portal. Disadvantages of a piriformis starting point include relative technical difficulty obtaining such a starting point compared to retrograde and trochanteric portals, especially in patients who are obese.[19] The piriformis starting point is also very sensitive to anterior-posterior translation, with anterior positioning being associated with extreme hoop stresses and increased risk of iatrogenic bursting of the proximal segment.[20] The trochanteric portal, given its more cancellous nature, is more

forgiving with regard to generation of hoop stress[20] such that a relatively anterior starting point in the trochanteric region is acceptable. When proximal fractures extend to the piriformis fossa, this entry site can lead to further comminution and, therefore, should be avoided.

Antegrade Nailing Via a Trochanteric Starting Point

Antegrade femoral nailing through the tip of the greater trochanter was the original technique. With the patient in the supine position, the subcutaneous location of the greater trochanter provides a technically easier starting point for IM nailing than the piriformis fossa, especially in obese patients.[19,21] The major pitfalls with this off-axis starting point are the potential for varus malalignment and iatrogenic fracture comminution that can occur when this starting point is combined with nails designed for piriformis insertion (that is, without trochanteric proximal bend). Implants specifically designed for trochanteric insertion usually have a slight proximal lateral bend of approximately 4° to 5°. Use of these nails combined with a modified insertion technique have been shown to essentially eliminate varus deformity and iatrogenic comminution.[22,23] The lateral proximal bend, as it engages the proximal fragment, tilts the proximal fragment out of varus. However, it is critical that the starting point not be too lateral. The tip of the greater trochanter is not necessarily the proper landmark for the starting point. The alignment of the tip of the greater trochanter, relative to the long axis of the femoral shaft, varies substantially.[24] Therefore, the proper starting point for trochanteric nailing is just lateral to the long axis of the femur. Depending on the individual patient's anatomy, this point can vary from just medial to just lateral to the tip of the greater trochanter.[25] On the lateral view, the starting point for trochanteric nailing is colinear with the long axis of the femur.

The potential for iatrogenic comminution with trochanteric nailing is related to a medially directed insertion angle. The proximal trochanteric bend does not help avoid this complication because the distal portion of the nail contacts the medial femoral cortex before the trochanteric bend, engaging bone. A proper starting point, one that is not too lateral, is the primary step to avoid such iatrogenic comminution. A subtle, but important, modification of standard nailing technique can also help avoid iatrogenic comminution. This modification leverages the nail's anterior bow. Rotating the nail 90° upon insertion, directing the anterior bow of the nail apex medially, directs the tip of the nail centrally. After the nail crosses the fracture, it is derotated gradually with successive mallet blows. Recent reports of trochanteric femoral nailing that uses modern implants and modern techniques found reduced complication rates and similar results, as also seen with piriformis nailing.[22,23]

Positioning for Antegrade Nailing

Supine positioning on a fracture table with traction applied through the foot secured in a boot is a common

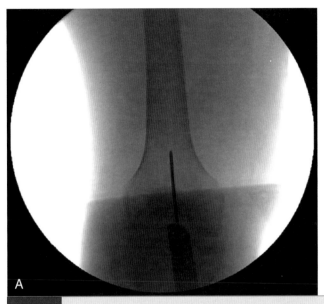
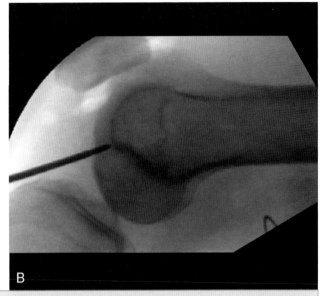

Figure 3 AP (**A**) and lateral (**B**) fluoroscopic views showing the proper starting point and trajectory (colinear with the long axis of the femur) for retrograde nailing. (Courtesy of William M. Ricci, MD, St. Louis, MO.)

method for antegrade nailing. Skeletal traction is usually not required. The noninjured leg can be in the hemilithotomy position, widely abducted or scissored. The choice largely depends on surgeon preference and the capabilities of the selected operating table. It should be noted that elevated calf compartment pressures can be generated with the hemilithotomy position, especially if the limb in question has associated injuries or the femoral nailing procedure is prolonged.[26] The well leg should be carefully monitored to avoid the development of compartment syndrome. Antegrade nailing without traction on a radiolucent table can reduce operative time, and because of better access to the contralateral limb, can reduce the incidence of rotational malalignment.[26] The lateral decubitus position offers improved access to the piriformis fossa but can be associated with difficulty imaging the proximal fracture fragment. Regardless of the position selected, AP and lateral fluoroscopic views of the entire femur are required.

Retrograde Starting Point

Retrograde nailing has evolved as a viable alternative to antegrade nailing. Proper technique includes an insertion site in the intracondylar notch at the apex of the Blumensatt line, which is approximately 1 cm anterior to the posterior cruciate ligament origin. Using this starting point, the trajectory for nail insertion should be colinear with the long axis of the femur in both the AP and lateral planes (**Figure 3**). The distal end of the nail must be buried beneath the subchondral bone to avoid injury to the patella during knee flexion. At least two distal interlocks should be used to minimize the risk for secondary telescoping of the nail into the knee joint, which can also occur after fracture of the distal

interlocking screws associated with comminuted, axially unstable fracture patterns.[13] A nail length that allows proximal interlocking above the lesser trochanter minimizes risk of injury to the femoral neurovascular structures and avoids subtrochanteric stress risers.

Knee stiffness and septic arthritis have not been shown to be significant complications after retrograde nailing. Retrograde nailing has the added benefit of helping provide improved fracture alignment of distal shaft fractures,[18] decreased operating room time, and decreased blood loss.[19] Retrograde nailing is favored in clinical situations in which proximal access to the femur for antegrade nailing is either difficult (for example, obesity, bilateral femur fracture) or not desired (for example, ipsilateral pelvic or hip fracture, ipsilateral tibia fracture, pregnancy). In some centers, retrograde nailing has become the preferred method for femoral nailing.

Reaming

Whether to use a reamed or unreamed technique has been a topic of persistent debate. There has been concern about the systemic effects of reaming on polytrauma patients, especially those with pulmonary injury. Reaming has been shown to increase IM and pulmonary artery pressures and to be associated with fat embolization in animal models.[27] However, several studies have demonstrated only limited and transient effects of emboli on the development of adult respiratory distress syndrome and further systemic compromise.[28,29] The degree of fat embolization associated with reamed nailing has been shown to be similar or only marginally greater than that associated with unreamed nailing, with fat extravasation being greatest during nail insertion and not necessarily dependent on the increase in IM pressure. Modern reaming technique calls for minimal reaming (0.5 to 1 mm) beyond the occurrence of isthmal cortical chatter. The proper nail diameter for a snug fit is therefore 1 to 1.5 mm smaller than the largest reamer used, which also correlates with the isthmal diameter. Such undersizing of the nail diminishes risks of iatrogenic bursting of the femoral canal caused by mismatch of femoral and nail bows. Other strategies to avoid thermal necrosis and excessive fat embolization include use of modern deeply fluted reamer designs and sharp reamers. The optimal reaming speed remains unknown. Slower reaming generates less heat but more emboli than faster reaming and remains the standard choice for most power reamer attachments.[30] Despite the theoretical detriments of reaming on fracture healing, multiple clinical studies demonstrate beneficial effects of reaming on union rates,[28,31] primarily because of increased cortical support for the nail and therefore stability of the fracture, a beneficial inflammatory response caused by reaming, and the deposition of local bone graft at the fracture site.

Plating

Plate fixation of acute femoral shaft fractures is reserved for the pediatric population and for adults in situations where IM nailing is either impossible or undesirable. Indications include ipsilateral femoral neck and shaft fractures, extremely small IM canals, associated vascular injury, and most commonly those with periprosthetic fractures about IM implants.[32-34] Still, plating results can be satisfactory with modern surgical techniques that respect soft-tissue integrity.[35] Submuscular techniques continue to revolutionize trauma care and provide another alternative for femur fracture fixation. These techniques applied to the femur have been popularized in pediatric femur fractures, but also can be used in the adult population.[36,37] Attention to careful dissection, plate placement, and particularly fracture reduction is critical, as the advantages of minimally invasive techniques can come at the expense of quality fracture reduction.[38] Plating femoral shaft fractures, therefore, represents a good option for patients with femoral neck fractures, periprosthetic fractures, or associated injuries about the knee.

Special Circumstances

Bilateral Femoral Shaft Fractures

Bilateral femoral shaft fractures deserve special mention because patients with these injuries have a higher rate of mortality than those with unilateral fractures. One study found that those with bilateral fractures had a mortality rate twice that of those with a unilateral fracture (25.9% versus 11.7%).[39] The associated Injury Severity Score (ISS) was also higher for patients with bilateral injuries (30.2) than for those with a single femur fracture (24.5). These data include patients who did not survive long enough to undergo surgical fixation. In another study that identified patients who survived to undergo reamed nailing of their fractures, the mortality rates were even more disparate: 1.5% (ISS, 16.5) for unilateral fractures; and 5.6% (ISS, 20.2) for bilateral fractures.[40] Both studies demonstrate the severity of injury sustained in patients with bilateral femoral shaft fractures.

Ipsilateral Tibial and Femoral Shaft Fractures

Ipsilateral femoral and tibial shaft fractures have been termed floating knee injuries. They typically occur in the polytrauma patient as the result of severe high-energy mechanisms such as motor vehicle and motorcycle crashes, as well as pedestrian-auto accidents. A high rate of head, solid organ, and multiple extremity injuries in patients with a floating knee pattern has been documented.[41,42] The most common related injuries include pelvis fractures and contralateral femur fractures. Vascular injuries are also more prevalent when compared to isolated femur and tibial shaft fractures, occurring in more than 20% of patients in some series. Likewise, ligamentous injuries to the knee occur more commonly in floating knee injuries than with isolated femoral shaft fractures (53% versus 27%). The incidence of open fractures is increased with the floating knee injury, but the tibia is still the location of the more common open fracture. Serial vascular examinations as well as a ligamentous examination after fracture fixation is paramount.

The Fraser classification of ipsilateral fractures of the femur and tibia groups these injuries into extra-articular and intra-articular sites.[43] Type I fractures are extra-articular. Type II fractures are classified according to the intra-articular injury: type IIA injuries are characterized by a tibial plateau fracture and ipsilateral femoral shaft fracture; type IIB injuries have an intra-articular distal femur fracture and ipsilateral tibial shaft fracture; and type IIC injuries have intra-articular fractures of both the tibial plateau and distal femur. The Fraser classification is prognostic, and patients with type I injuries have a better functional outcome compared with type II injuries. It also has been shown that the severity of soft-tissue injury over the tibia is a prognostic factor for functional outcome.[42,44]

Treatment methods for type I floating knee injuries have included antegrade femoral nailing along with tibial nailing. However, more recently the commonly accepted treatment has become retrograde femoral nailing along with antegrade tibial nailing through the same surgical approach. Good results similar to those found after high-energy isolated injury have been obtained with this method. A series of 20 patients were treated with a single percutaneous approach through a 4-cm medial parapatellar tendon incision.[45] An alternative approach is through a transpatellar tendon incision that splits the tendon longitudinally and provides direct access to the femoral and tibial starting points without need for retraction of the tendon. The authors reported

88% good-to-excellent results. No patients had knee pain, and all patients except one had full knee motion (the remaining patient obtained 115° of knee flexion). An advantage of this technique is the ease of operating room set-up and supine patient positioning for both the femur and the tibia without the need to transfer to and from a fracture table. Additionally, it is recommended that the femoral shaft fracture be fixed first, for two reasons. The first is that should the patient decompensate during the procedure, the femur will have been stabilized so that the patient will be able to be transported without the need for traction, and the tibia can be treated in a splint until the patient is fit for further surgery. The second reason is that fixing the femur will allow the surgeon to obtain sufficient knee flexion to access the proximal tibia for the tibial nail starting point.

Ipsilateral Femoral Neck and Shaft Fractures

Ipsilateral fractures of the femoral neck and shaft occur in up to 10% of femoral shaft fractures. Often, these fractures occur in younger patients as a result of high-energy trauma and are frequently missed. A specific protocol should be followed for identifying these injuries, as discussed at the beginning of this chapter. Those with a vertical femoral neck fracture (high Pauwels angle) are at increased risk of femoral neck nonunion. However, the most common fracture pattern is basicervical, and corresponding osteonecrosis rates are low.

Many fixation methods have been used for this fracture pattern, including antegrade femoral nailing of the shaft with cancellous screws placed anterior to the nail for fixation of the femoral neck fracture; a "reconstruction nail" with proximal interlocking screws passing through the proximal nail segment and into the femoral head as fixation for the femoral neck fracture (with or without additional cancellous lag screws); a variety of plate combinations ranging from a hip screw with a long side plate to a hip screw with a short side plate and a separate plate for the femoral shaft fracture; and retrograde IM nailing for the femoral shaft fracture along with cancellous screws, a hip screw with short side plate, or a proximal femoral locking plate to address the femoral neck component.[4] No recent series demonstrates superiority of one method. Most centers repair the femoral shaft fracture with a retrograde IM nail and the femoral neck fracture with a hip screw and a short side plate, with priority given to the femoral neck fracture.

Open Fractures

Open fractures of the femur are much less common (5% to 20%) than of the tibia. Because of the presence of a large protective soft-tissue envelope about the femur, open fractures are often associated with significant soft-tissue trauma. Small skin wounds can disguise significant deep muscle and periosteal injury. All open fractures of the femoral shaft should be treated in a timely fashion as directed by the patient's medical status and the availability of appropriate resources. Several studies have shown that the timing to initial débridement of open fractures does not significantly affect infection risk, and the most significant factor determining risk of deep infection is the severity of the open injury.[46,47] Wounds should be extended for evaluation of the deep soft tissues, and all nonviable soft tissues and bone should be débrided. Serial débridements at 24- to 48-hour intervals are traditionally recommended for higher grade or highly contaminated open injuries. Although closure of contaminated wounds should be avoided, whether clean wounds should be left open or closed between serial débridements is controversial because concerns for nosocomial infection provide a theoretic basis for closure between surgical débridements. Immediate IM nailing of open femoral shaft fractures is indicated except for the most severe cases, especially those with grossly contaminated canals. Provisional external fixation for open fractures is useful when repeat irrigation and débridement of a contaminated IM canal is necessary. IM nailing can be performed once the canal has been sufficiently cleansed. Intravenous antibiotics should be initiated upon presentation and continued until definitive wound closure. Routine wound culture is not indicated.[48]

Gunshot Fractures

A thorough neurologic and vascular examination is mandatory for patients with penetrating injury mechanisms such as gunshot fractures. Vascular studies (for example, arteriograms or CT angiography) are typically indicated in patients with abnormal examinations and in those with a bullet pathway in close proximity to major vascular structures. Fractures of the femur as a result of gunshot wounds are technically open fractures. However, they can be treated as closed injuries when they are caused by low-energy civilian firearms (less than 2,000 ft/s).[14,49] Local wound care is performed for the entrance and exit wounds, with débridement at the level of the skin and subcutaneous tissues. The deeper tissues do not require formal irrigation and débridement. Definitive fracture treatment is then performed, most often with reamed, locked, IM nailing as is done for closed fractures. For low-velocity gunshot wounds, antibiotic prophylaxis beyond 24 hours after surgery is not recommended. Exceptions to this rule include high-velocity military grade bullets (greater than 2,000 ft/s) or shotgun wounds at a close range. These injuries transfer a greater amount of kinetic energy to the extremity and thus cause a greater degree of injury and devitalization of the soft tissues and bone. In these instances, treatment should be similar to that of other high-grade open injuries, and débridement of all nonviable tissues is mandatory.[49] In cases of more severe grade IIIC injuries, plate fixation or external fixation may be considered. Successful limb salvage is most dependent on the associated vascular injury, while long-term disability is most dependent on associated neurologic injury. A low incidence of shortening, angular deformity, complication, and infection rates was found following the treatment of 74 gunshot diaphyseal fractures with a retrograde IM nail.[50]

Obese Patients

It has been estimated that 54% of adults in the United States are overweight or obese. Furthermore, the percentage of adults who are obese is increasing at a fast pace. Thus, orthopaedic surgeons will be required to care for an increasing percentage of obese patients, creating a unique set of challenges. Specific to femoral shaft fractures, patient positioning, implant choice, ability to obtain the starting point for an antegrade nail, and ability to obtain adequate intraoperative fluoroscopic views are the central issues. In particular, obtaining a piriformis starting point is made difficult by an obese body habitus, especially when nailing in the supine position.

A prospective multicenter nonrandomized study of 151 patients with femoral shaft fractures was performed to determine the results of IM nailing in obese patients (BMI > 30) compared with nonobese patients (BMI ≤ 30).[19] When antegrade nailing was used (piriformis or trochanteric starting point) the obese group had a 52% increase in operating room time and a 79% greater radiation exposure. With the use of retrograde nailing, there was a similar operating room time between the obese group and the nonobese group, as well as a similar fluoroscopy time. When comparing antegrade nailing with retrograde nailing within the obese group, there was a 40% greater operating room time as well as a threefold increase in fluoroscopy time with the use of antegrade nailing. Healing rates and complications were similar between the obese and nonobese groups. At baseline, the two groups had similar functional scores. Postoperatively, obese patients tended to recover more slowly and more incompletely than nonobese patients.

Vascular and Nerve Injuries

Femoral shaft fractures associated with either vascular or nerve injury are relatively uncommon (< 1%) and are usually associated with penetrating trauma. The algorithm for management of fractures with associated vascular injury traditionally includes bony stabilization, either definitive or provisional, regaining adequate length, before neurovascular repair. The most expeditious stabilization method is usually external fixation, which can be safely converted to definitive IM nailing within 2 weeks.[10] Another expeditious alternative is retrograde nailing with interlocking deferred until after neurovascular repair.[11] Deferring any skeletal stabilization until after vascular repair can reduce ischemia time and the need for fasciotomy. Recent clinical evidence indicates that this sequence can be applied safely without disruption of the vascular repair during definitive fracture treatment.[51]

Compartment Syndrome

Compartment syndrome associated with femoral shaft fracture is uncommon. A heightened index of suspicion should accompany injuries with a crushing mechanism, prolonged compression, vascular injury, systemic hypotension, and coagulopathy. When a clinical diagnosis is made, fasciotomy should be performed emergently. Compartment pressure measurements can be used as an adjunct to clinical diagnosis, especially in obtunded patients.

Complications

Malalignment

Fractures of the middle third of the shaft have a very low incidence of angular malalignment (2%), whereas fractures of the proximal and distal thirds of the shaft are at higher risk of malalignment (30% and 10%, respectively). Antegrade nailing can facilitate improved reduction for proximal fractures and retrograde nailing for distal fractures.[18] Rotational malalignment, in particular, is difficult to detect intraoperatively, especially in segmental or comminuted fractures. Malrotation is one of the more common complications following femoral shaft fracture IM nailing. It is estimated that 20% to 30% of femoral shaft fractures are malrotated more than 15°.[52] Moreover, it is estimated that more than half of all patients exhibit at least a 10° malrotation compared to the unaffected side.[53] Malrotation can have cosmetic and functional implications and often leads to litigation. Traditionally, the general appearance of the extremity, with the patella pointed anteriorly, skin folds, and soft-tissue tension has been used as an intra-operative indicator of adequate rotation reduction, but recently this method has been discredited. Several other intraoperative techniques have been described for assessment and correction of rotational alignment during femoral shaft fracture IM nailing. An image intensifier has been used to adjust for the affected limb's femoral neck anteversion, thus correcting for rotational deformity.[54,55] One of these described methods, which requires images of the unaffected hip before the surgical procedure to assess native femoral anteversion, adds an average of 15 minutes of operating room time but was shown to reduce malrotation to a mean of 5°.[55] That such utilization of the opposite extremity as an internal control yielded superior results in reduction of rotational deformity was recently verified.[56] The lesser trochanteric shape sign, which uses the shape of the lesser trochanter under image intensification to assess for rotational deformity in femur fractures, has been described in several studies.[57,58] The lesser trochanteric shape sign has been shown to have similar efficacy in preventing rotational deformity as the femoral anteversion method.[57] Both methods require a normal contralateral limb. The cortical step sign, or incongruity of cortical widths on either side of a femur fracture, is reported as a useful adjunct in assisting rotation reduction and has been recently studied.[58,59] It has been shown that the medial cortical step sign is most useful in the proximal and middle sections of the femur where circumferential differences in cortical width vary the most.[59] This sign, however, cannot detect whether a rotational malreduction is due to internal or external rotation.

All patients should be evaluated for rotational symmetry compared to the uninjured limb before leaving the operating suite. When symmetry is in doubt, objective methods of assessing malrotation postoperatively most commonly include CT.[52,53,55,60]

Delayed Union or Nonunion

The rate of nonunion reported after nailing of femoral shaft fractures, regardless of starting point, is usually less than 10%.[6,13,22] In the presence of nonunion, deep infection should be considered and ruled out before surgical repair is begun. The treatment of nonunion ranges from dynamization to exchange nailing to plate fixation with bone grafting, and it varies based on the situation. Dynamization can be useful for distracted fractures. However, no large series exist evaluating the efficacy of this strategy, and success rates vary from 50% to 90%. Fractures with bony defects, atrophic characteristics, or failed dynamizations may benefit from reaming and exchange nailing or open grafting and repair. Results for exchange nailing of femoral shaft fractures show good, but not outstanding, union rates that range from 76% to 96%.[61,62] Recalcitrant nonunions may deserve an evaluation for underlying metabolic disturbances[63] and can be successfully managed with bone grafting and plating.[64]

Infection

Large series of femoral shaft fractures treated with IM nails report low infection rates ranging from 1% to 4%.[51] Infections can be categorized as early (less than 3 months) or chronic, and both usually are associated with nonunited fractures. Early infections, such as those associated with open fracture wounds, can typically be treated with nail retention, serial débridement, and organism-specific intravenous antibiotics. If the early infection cannot be controlled, then nail removal is indicated. External fixation or antibiotic cement nails, created over a metal wire or other substrate, can provide stability during treatment.[65] The cement nail offers more limited mechanical support but fills the dead space in the medullary canal and delivers high concentrations of local antibiotics. Chronic infections or infected nonunions are treated based on the principles of osteomyelitis management. Generally, the nail is removed, the canal is reamed for débridement purposes, and nonviable bone from the fracture margin is resected. Intravenous and potentially local antibiotics in the form of cement beads or a cement spacer are typically administered for at least 6 weeks. Definitive reconstruction is delayed until the infection is controlled. The progress of the infection is monitored through close clinical observation and routine laboratory values (complete blood count, erythrocyte sedimentation rate, C-reactive protein level). Host factors such as smoking or malnutrition should be addressed. If concern for infection remains at the time of reconstruction, frozen tissue sections can be taken intraoperatively. More than 10 white blood cells per high-power field is suggestive of persistent infection.

Functional Disability

Although IM nailing is the gold standard for treatment of diaphyseal femur fractures, patients can report residual functional deficits following fracture fixation. Reduced strength of both the hip abductors and hip extensors and altered gait pattern have recently been demonstrated after antegrade femoral nailing.[17,66] Also, functional outcome scores have been found to be persistently reduced relative to baseline 1 year after antegrade nailing.[23] These findings support the need for prolonged muscle strengthening therapy protocols. Heterotopic ossification and prominent implants increase the incidence of these complications. Thorough irrigation of the surgical wound and the use of tissue protectors may reduce the risk of heterotopic ossification. Whenever possible, the fixation devices should be countersunk beneath bone to minimize related pain and muscle dysfunction. Injury to the patellofemoral articulation can be avoided with retrograde nailing by countersinking the nail beneath the articular surface. Retrograde nails should be locked with at least two distal interlocking bolts, especially for axially unstable fractures, to avoid migration of the nail into the knee joint.

Other Complications

Use of the hemilithotomy position for antegrade femoral nailing increases compartment pressures in the well leg. Prolonged use of this position should be undertaken with caution to avoid contralateral leg compartment syndrome, especially in patients with injury to the contralateral limb. Excessive and prolonged traction against a perineal post should be avoided to minimize the risk of pudendal and sciatic nerve injury from compression and stretch, respectively.

Summary

The gold standard definitive treatment method for most fractures of the femoral shaft is IM nailing. However, circumstances exist in which other methods, such as plating or external fixation, represent more appropriate modalities. IM nailing of diaphyseal femur fractures provides a stable fixation construct that can be applied using indirect reduction techniques and that yields high union rates and low complication rates if vigilance is maintained during preoperative planning, the surgical procedure, and the postoperative period. The piriformis fossa, greater trochanter, and retrograde starting points each have relative advantages, disadvantages, and indications. Therefore, this decision should be made based on individual patient and fracture characteristics and surgeon experience. Specifically, associated patient medical comorbidities, the patient's body habitus, and associated injuries should be considered when choosing the technique of stabilization. The timing of femoral IM nailing, as well as the use of reaming, must be tailored to each individual clinical situation to avoid systemic complications. All of these considerations are critical to optimizing patient outcomes and minimizing complications.

Annotated References

1. Johansen K, Lynch K, Paun M, Copass M: Non-invasive vascular tests reliably exclude occult arterial trauma in injured extremities. *J Trauma* 1991;31(4):515-519.

2. Mills WJ, Barei DP, McNair P: The value of the ankle-brachial index for diagnosing arterial injury after knee dislocation: A prospective study. *J Trauma* 2004;56(6): 1261-1265.

   The authors present a prospective study on 38 patients with knee dislocations. The ABI was used to evaluate the potential for vascular injury for all patients. All patients with an ABI greater than 0.9 did not have a vascular injury, whereas those with an ABI less than 0.9 did have a vascular injury. The authors concluded that the ABI is a noninvasive, effective way to determine the presence or absence of a vascular injury in patients with knee dislocations.

3. Barei DP, Schildhauer TA, Nork SE: Noncontiguous fractures of the femoral neck, femoral shaft, and distal femur. *J Trauma* 2003;55(1):80-86.

4. Watson JT, Moed BR: Ipsilateral femoral neck and shaft fractures: Complications and their treatment. *Clin Orthop Relat Res* 2002;399:78-86.

5. Tornetta P III, Kain MS, Creevy WR: Diagnosis of femoral neck fractures in patients with a femoral shaft fracture: Improvement with a standard protocol. *J Bone Joint Surg Am* 2007;89(1):39-43.

   The authors created a protocol for diagnosis of femoral neck fractures in patients with femoral shaft fractures. The protocol consisted of preoperative dedicated hip radiographs, a 2-mm fine cut CT scan through the femoral neck, and an intraoperative lateral fluoroscopic radiograph. Postoperative hip radiographs were obtained before leaving the operating room. In 254 patients who were followed for at least 2 months, 16 were identified as having a femoral neck fracture using this protocol. Thirteen femoral neck fractures were identified before the patient entered the operating room, and 12 were identified with the fine cut CT scan. One fracture was identified intraoperatively. There was one iatrogenic fracture and one delayed diagnosis of a fracture. This protocol reduced the delay in diagnosis of an associated femoral neck fracture by 91% compared

   with the year before initiation of this protocol. Level of evidence: II.

6. Winquist RA, Hansen ST, Clawson DK: Closed intramedullary nailing of femoral fractures. *J Bone Joint Surg Am* 1984;66:529-539.

7. Marsh JL, Slongo TF, Agel J, et al: Fracture and Dislocation Classification Compendium, 2007: Orthopaedic Trauma Association Classification, Database and Outcomes Committee. *J Orthop Trauma* 2007;21:10.

   The OTA classification is republished in this new classification compendium.

8. Bone LB, Johnson KD, Weigelt J, Scheinberg R: Early versus delayed stabilization of femoral fractures: A prospective randomized study. *J Bone Joint Surg Am* 1989; 71(3):336-340.

9. Bhandari M, Zlowodzki M, Tornetta P III, Schmidt A, Templeman DC: Intramedullary nailing following external fixation in femoral and tibial shaft fractures. *J Orthop Trauma* 2005;19(2):140-144.

   A meta-analysis of 22 studies regarding conversion of external fixation to intramedullary nailing is presented. There was one level II study (a randomized controlled trial with methodologic limitations) whereas the remaining were case series (level IV evidence). For femur fractures, the authors report infection rates of 3.6% for intramedullary nailing following temporary external fixation, with union rates averaging 98%. Intramedullary nailing as a reconstructive procedure following failed external fixation had an infection rate of 40%. For tibial fractures, infection rates averaged 9% while union rates averaged 90%. Length of external fixation less than or equal to 28 days reduced the risk of infection by 83%. Casting did not decrease the risk of infection but did increase the rate of nonunion.

10. Harwood PJ, Giannoudis PV, Probst C, Krettek C, Pape HC: The risk of local infective complications after damage control procedures for femoral shaft fracture. *J Orthop Trauma* 2006;20(3):181-189.

    The authors present a retrospective case series including patients with an ISS above 20 and a femoral shaft fracture. The objective was to determine the rates of infection between damage control orthopaedics (initial external fixation converted to intramedullary nail) and primary intramedullary nail fixation. A total of 173 patients with 192 fractures were included; 111 fractures were treated with damage control orthopaedics and 81 by primary intramedullary nail fixation. Although there was a significantly increased risk of pin site contamination when conversion was performed after the external fixator had been in place longer than 2 weeks, there was no difference in the rates of deep infection between the two groups.

11. Higgins TF, Horwitz DS: Damage control nailing. *J Orthop Trauma* 2007;21(7):477-484.

    The authors discuss a case series of six closed femoral diaphyseal fractures in five polytrauma patients in whom unreamed retrograde intramedullary nails were used for initial fracture stability. Four out of five patients returned to the operating room for placement of additional locking screws and/or exchange to a reamed, larger diameter nail. All six fractures went on to union within 4 months of the final procedure.

12. Ostrum RF, Agarwal A, Lakatos R, Poka A: Prospective comparison of retrograde and antegrade femoral intramedullary nailing. *J Orthop Trauma* 2000;14(7):496-501.

13. Ricci WM, Bellabarba C, Evanoff B, Herscovici D, Di-Pasquale T, Sanders R: Retrograde versus antegrade nailing of femoral shaft fractures. *J Orthop Trauma* 2001;15(3):161-169.

14. Tornetta P III, Tiburzi D: Antegrade or retrograde reamed femoral nailing: A prospective, randomised trial. *J Bone Joint Surg Br* 2000;82(5):652-654.

15. Dora C, Leunig M, Beck M, Rothenfluh D, Ganz R: Entry point soft tissue damage in antegrade femoral nailing: A cadaver study. *J Orthop Trauma* 2001;15(7):488-493.

16. McConnell T, Tornetta P III, Benson E, Manuel J: Gluteus medius tendon injury during reaming for gamma nail insertion. *Clin Orthop Relat Res* 2003;407:199-202.

17. Archdeacon M, Ford KR, Wyrick J, et al: A prospective functional outcome and motion analysis evaluation of the hip abductors after femur fracture and antegrade nailing. *J Orthop Trauma* 2008;22(1):3-9.

    Eight patients with isolated femur fractures treated with antegrade nailing were studied with dynamic gait analysis. Patients demonstrated significant negative hip kinematics and kinetics, depending on time from surgery.

18. Ricci WM, Bellabarba C, Lewis R, et al: Angular malalignment after intramedullary nailing of femoral shaft fractures. *J Orthop Trauma* 2001;15(2):90-95.

19. Tucker MC, Schwappach JR, Leighton RK, Coupe K, Ricci WM: Results of femoral intramedullary nailing in patients who are obese versus those who are not obese: A prospective multicenter comparison study. *J Orthop Trauma* 2007;21(8):523-529.

    In this prospective, multicenter, nonrandomized study of 151 patients with femoral shaft fractures, the results of intramedullary nailing in obese patients was compared with that of nonobese patients. Antegrade nailing in the obese group was associated with a significantly greater operating room time and radiation exposure. Retrograde nailing was associated with similar operating room time and radiation exposure in obese and nonobese patients. Healing rates and complications were similar between the two groups.

20. Johnson KD, Tencer AF, Sherman MC: Biomechanical factors affecting fracture stability and femoral bursting in closed intramedullary nailing of femoral shaft fractures, with illustrative case presentations. *J Orthop Trauma* 1987;1(1):1-11.

21. Ostrum RF: A greater trochanteric insertion site for femoral intramedullary nailing in lipomatous patients. *Orthopaedics* 1996;19:337-340.

22. Ricci WM, Devinney S, Haidukewych G, Herscovici D, Sanders R: Trochanteric nail insertion for the treatment of femoral shaft fractures. *J Orthop Trauma* 2005;19(8):511-517.

    In a prospective clinical trial, 61 consecutive patients with femoral shaft fractures were treated with the Trigen Trochanteric Antegrade Nail inserted through a greater trochanteric starting point. The study demonstrated that antegrade nailing of femoral shaft fractures with a nail specifically designed for trochanteric insertion provides high union rates (60 of 61) and low complication rates (no angular malunion and no iatrogenic fractures).

23. Ricci WM, Schwappach J, Tucker M, et al: Trochanteric versus piriformis entry portal for the treatment of femoral shaft fractures. *J Orthop Trauma* 2006;20(10):663-667.

    The authors present a prospective cohort study of 108 patients with femoral shaft fractures treated with either the Trigen Trochanteric Antegrade Nail through a greater trochanteric starting point or a Trigen nail through the piriformis fossa. Similar results were found for the two groups with regard to union, complications, and function. The trochanteric starting point was associated with less fluoroscopy time and less operating room time in patients who were obese.

24. Antonelli L: Closed intramedullary nailing of diaphyseal fractures of the femur: Problems related to anatomical variations of the greater trochanter. *Ital J Orthop Traumatol* 1989;15(1):67-74.

25. Ostrum RF, Marcantonio A, Marburger R: A critical analysis of the eccentric starting point for trochanteric intramedullary femoral nailing. *J Orthop Trauma* 2005;19(10):681-686.

    The authors performed a cadaver study evaluating the optimal trochanteric starting point for antegrade nailing of reverse oblique femur fractures. A starting point lateral to the tip of the trochanter led to varus malalignment for all of the five nails tested. A starting point at or just medial to the tip of the greater trochanter was recommended.

26. Tan V, Pepe MD, Glaser DL, Seldes RM, Heppenstall RB, Esterhai JL Jr: Well-leg compartment pressures during hemilithotomy position for fracture fixation. *J Orthop Trauma* 2000;14(3):157-161.

27. Kröpfl A, Davies J, Berger U, Hertz H, Schlag G: Intramedullary pressure and bone marrow fat extravasation in reamed and unreamed femoral nailing. *J Orthop Res* 1999;17(2):261-268.

28. Bhandari M, Guyatt GH, Tong D, Adili A, Shaughnessy SG: Reamed versus nonreamed intramedullary nailing of lower extremity long bone fractures: A systematic overview and meta-analysis. *J Orthop Trauma* 2000;14(1):2-9.

5: Lower Extremity

29. Brumback RJ, Virkus WW: Intramedullary nailing of the femur: Reamed versus nonreamed. *J Am Acad Orthop Surg* 2000;8(2):83-90.

30. Mousavi M, David R, Schwendenwein I, et al: Influence of controlled reaming on fat intravasation after femoral osteotomy in sheep. *Clin Orthop Relat Res* 2002;394: 263-270.

31. Canadian Orthopaedic Trauma Society: Nonunion following intramedullary nailing of the femur with and without reaming: Results of a multicenter randomized clinical trial. *J Bone Joint Surg Am* 2003;85(11):2093-2096.

32. Ricci WM, Bolhofner BR, Loftus T, Cox C, Mitchell S, Borrelli J Jr: Indirect reduction and plate fixation, without grafting, for periprosthetic femoral shaft fractures about a stable intramedullary implant. *J Bone Joint Surg Am* 2005;87(10):2240-2245.

   Fifty consecutive patients with a periprosthetic femoral shaft fracture about a stable intramedullary implant were treated with a protocol of open reduction and internal fixation with biologic reduction techniques and a single lateral plate. No bone grafts or bone graft substitutes were used. All fractures healed in satisfactory alignment after the index procedure.

33. Ricci WM, Borrelli J Jr: Operative management of periprosthetic femur fractures in the elderly using biological fracture reduction and fixation techniques. *Injury* 2007;38(Suppl 3):S53-8.

   Fifty-nine patients with a periprosthetic femoral shaft fracture (*n* = 29) or a periprosthetic supracondylar fracture (*n* = 30) were treated with biologic open reduction and internal fixation techniques without bone graft or bone graft substitutes. All but one patient healed after the index procedure and three had progressive malalignment and then healed without further surgery.

34. Ricci WM, Haidukewych GJ: Periprosthetic femoral fractures. *Instr Course Lect* 2009;58:105-115.

   The optimal treatment of periprosthetic fractures should be individualized considering fracture location relative to the arthroplasty component, implant stability, bone quality, and medical and functional status of the patient.

35. Krettek C, Muller M, Miclau T: Evolution of minimally invasive plate osteosynthesis (MIPO) in the femur. *Injury* 2001;32 Suppl 3:SC14-SC23.

36. Kanlic EM, Anglen JO, Smith DG, Morgan SJ, Pesántez RF: Advantages of submuscular bridge plating for complex pediatric femur fractures. *Clin Orthop Relat Res* 2004;426:244-251.

   A review of 51 pediatric patients (average age, 10 years) treated with submuscular plating of femoral shaft fractures is presented. All fractures were followed to union. One case of hardware failure occurred using a 3.5-mm titanium plate that was revised to a 4.5-mm plate. There was one case of plate deformation after a fall at 2 weeks postoperatively and one refracture through a nonossifying fibroma after plate removal. There were no symptomatic malalignments or limb-length discrepancies.

37. Sink EL, Hedequist D, Morgan SJ, Hresko T: Results and technique of unstable pediatric femoral fractures treated with submuscular bridge plating. *J Pediatr Orthop* 2006;26(2):177-181.

   A retrospective review of 27 pediatric patients (average age, 9 years) with femoral shaft fractures treated with submuscular plating is presented. There were no intraoperative or postoperative complications. In one patient, fracture fixation was in 8° of valgus with no other malalignment or shortening. All fractures displayed stable bridging callous on three or four cortices by 12 weeks.

38. Zlowodzki M, Vogt D, Cole PA, Kregor PJ: Plating of femoral shaft fractures: Open reduction and internal fixation versus submuscular fixation. *J Trauma* 2007; 63(5):1061-1065.

   The authors present a retrospective cohort study comparing open plating and submuscular plating of femoral shaft fractures. There were no malreductions in the open plating group (19 patients) and 6 in the submuscular group (21 patients). Infectious complications were equivalent. The authors concluded that submuscular plating of the femur is technically challenging and may not provide a clear advantage over open plating techniques with appropriate soft-tissue management.

39. Copeland CE, Mitchell KA, Brumback RJ, Gens DR, Burgess AR: Mortality in patients with bilateral femoral fractures. *J Orthop Trauma* 1998;12(5):315-319.

40. Nork SE, Agel J, Russell GV, Mills WJ, Holt S, Routt ML Jr: Mortality after reamed intramedullary nailing of bilateral femur fractures. *Clin Orthop Relat Res* 2003; 415:272-278.

41. Lundy DW, Johnson KD: "Floating knee" injuries: Ipsilateral fractures of the femur and tibia. *J Am Acad Orthop Surg* 2001;9(4):238-245.

42. Yokoyama K, Nakamura T, Shindo M, et al: Contributing factors influencing the functional outcome of floating knee injuries. *Am J Orthop* 2000;29(9):721-729.

43. Fraser RD, Hunter GA, Waddell JP: Ipsilateral fracture of the femur and tibia. *J Bone Joint Surg Br* 1978;60(4): 510-515.

44. Yokoyama K, Tsukamoto T, Aoki S, et al: Evaluation of functional outcome of the floating knee injury using multivariate analysis. *Arch Orthop Trauma Surg* 2002; 122(8):432-435.

45. Ostrum RF: Treatment of floating knee injuries through a single percutaneous approach. *Clin Orthop Relat Res* 2000;375:43-50.

46. Al-Arabi YB, Nader M, Nader M, Hamidian-Jahromi AR, Woods DA: The effect of the timing of antibiotics and surgical treatment on infection rates in open long-

bone fractures: A 9-year prospective study from a district general hospital. *Injury* 2007;38(8):900-905.

A prospective study of 248 open long bone fractures is presented. Surgical débridement was performed within 6 hours of injury in 62% of fractures, and after 6 hours in 38%. Infection rates were 7.8% in fractures débrided within 6 hours and 9.6% in fractures débrided after 6 hours, a difference that was not statistically significant ($P = 0.6438$). Additionally, the timing of antibiotic administration did not significantly affect the rate of infection.

47. Noumi T, Yokoyama K, Ohtsuka H, Nakamura K, Itoman M: Intramedullary nailing for open fractures of the femoral shaft: Evaluation of contributing factors on deep infection and nonunion using multivariate analysis. *Injury* 2005;36(9):1085-1093.

A retrospective review of 89 open femoral fractures in 88 patients evaluated contributing factors affecting deep infection and nonunion of open femoral fractures treated with locked intramedullary nailing (IMN). Patients were divided into three groups: group 1, immediate IMN at the time of initial débridement (n = 36); group 2, delayed IMN following nonsurgical treatment such as skeletal traction or splint (n = 44); group 3, delayed IMN following external fixation (n = 9). Patients were also divided into a reamed IMN group (n = 67) and an unreamed group (n = 22). Multivariate analysis showed that only Gustilo type fracture significantly correlated with deep infection ($P < .05$) and that only fracture grade by AO type significantly correlated with occurrence of nonunion ($P < .02$).

48. Ricci WM, Gallagher B, Haidukewych GJ: Intramedullary nailing of femoral shaft fractures: Current concepts. *J Am Acad Orthop Surg* 2009;17(5):296-305.

The authors review the various nailing options for treatment of femoral shaft fractures. The relative advantages and disadvantages of various starting points (piriformis, trochanteric, and retrograde), patient positions (supine or lateral with or without traction), and reaming are discussed.

49. Bartlett CS, Helfet DL, Hausman MR, Strauss E: Ballistics and gunshot wounds: Effects on musculoskeletal tissues. *J Am Acad Orthop Surg* 2000;8(1):21-36.

50. Cannada LK, Jones TR, Guerrero-Bejarano M, et al: Retrograde intramedullary nailing of femoral diaphyseal fractures caused by low-velocity gunshots. *Orthopedics* 2009;32(3):162.

Seventy-three patients with 74 femoral shaft fractures from gunshot wounds were treated with reamed, retrograde, statically locked nails. Three patients had shortening greater than 10 mm and one was malaligned in 13° of recurvatum. One patient had a hypertrophic nonunion that healed after dynamization. There were no cases of septic knee arthritis.

51. McHenry TP, Holcomb JB, Aoki N, Lindsey RW: Fractures with major vascular injuries from gunshot wounds: Implications of surgical sequence. *J Trauma* 2002;53(4):717-721.

52. Jaarsma RL, van Kampen A: Rotational malalignment after fractures of the femur. *J Bone Joint Surg Br* 2004;86(8):1100-1104.

The authors assess rotational malalignment after femoral nailing by various means, including clinical examination and CT. The incidence, causes, methods to avoid, and clinical consequences of rotational malalignment are discussed.

53. Jaarsma RL, Pakvis DF, Verdonschot N, Biert J, van Kampen A: Rotational malalignment after intramedullary nailing of femoral fractures. *J Orthop Trauma* 2004;18(7):403-409.

Rotational alignment was analyzed clinically and with CT in 76 patients after antegrade IM nailing of the femur. Clinical examination was found to be inaccurate in comparison with CT measurements, which revealed at least 15° of malrotation in 28% of patients. Malrotation was found to be independent of fracture level. Patients with rotational deformity had difficulty with running, sports activity, and stair climbing. These difficulties were more pronounced with an external rotation deformity than with internal rotation deformity.

54. Braten M, Tveit K, Junk S, et al: The role of fluoroscopy in avoiding rotational deformity of treated femoral shaft fractures: An anatomical and clinical study. *Injury* 2000;31:311-315.

55. Tornetta P III, Ritz G, Kantor A: Femoral torsion after interlocked nailing of unstable femoral fractures. *J Trauma* 1995;38(2):213-219.

56. Hilgert RE, Ohrendorf K, Schäfer FK, et al: Preventing malrotation during intramedullary nailing of femoral fractures. *Unfallchirurg* 2006;109(10):855-861.

A C-arm based measurement of femoral anteversion is presented. A true lateral view of the distal femur and the femoral neck are obtained. The difference in C-arm angle to obtain these views for the uninjured leg is used as a guide for obtaining proper rotation of the fractured femur using the same method. Intraobserver variation of this method was 5°.

57. Jaarsma RL, Verdonschot N, van der Venne R, van Kampen A: Avoiding rotational malalignment after fractures of the femur by using the profile of the lesser trochanter: An in vitro study. *Arch Orthop Trauma Surg* 2005;125(3):184-187.

A cadaver study to evaluate the accuracy of using the profile of the lesser trochanter to guide rotational alignment is presented. With the distal femur in neutral rotation, the proximal fragment was rotated until the lesser trochanter was also neutral. This method resulted in an average malrotation of only 2.2°.

58. Krettek C, Rudolf J, Schandelmaier P, Guy P, Könemann B, Tscherne H: Unreamed intramedullary nailing of femoral shaft fractures: Operative technique and early clinical experience with the standard locking option. *Injury* 1996;27(4):233-254.

5: Lower Extremity

59. Langer J, Gardner MJ, Ricci WM: The cortical step sign as a tool for assessing and correcting rotational deforify in femoral shaft fractures. *J Orthop Trauma* 2010;24: 82-88.

The authors present a cadaver study demonstrating that the cortical step sign is indicative of rotational malreduction of the femur.

60. Jaarsma RL, Bruggeman AW, Pakvis DF, Verdonschot N, Lemmens JA, van Kampen A: Computed tomography determined femoral torsion is not accurate. *Arch Orthop Trauma Surg* 2004;124(8):552-554.

CT scans used to determine rotational malalignment were found to be associated with an intraobserver difference of 3.9° and an interobserver difference of 4.1°. The inaccuracies were principally due to difficulty defining a line through the femoral neck.

61. Hak DJ, Lee SS, Goulet JA: Success of exchange reamed intramedullary nailing for femoral shaft nonunion or delayed union. *J Orthop Trauma* 2000;14(3):178-182.

62. Weresh MJ, Hakanson R, Stover MD, Sims SH, Kellam JF, Bosse MJ: Failure of exchange reamed intramedullary nails for ununited femoral shaft fractures. *J Orthop Trauma* 2000;14(5):335-338.

63. Brinker MR, O'Connor DP, Monla YT, Earthman TP: Metabolic and endocrine abnormalities in patients with nonunions. *J Orthop Trauma* 2007;21(8):557-570.

Thirty-seven patients with nonunion and an endocrine evaluation were studied. The indications for endocrine evaluation were varied. Eighty-four percent were found to have metabolic or endocrine abnormalities, with 64% having a vitamin deficiency.

64. Bellabarba C, Ricci WM, Bolhofner BR: Results of indirect reduction and plating of femoral shaft nonunions after intramedullary nailing. *J Orthop Trauma* 2001; 15(4):254-263.

65. Thonse R, Conway J: Antibiotic cement-coated interlocking nail for the treatment of infected nonunions and segmental bone defects. *J Orthop Trauma* 2007;21(4): 258-268.

Twenty patients with an infected nonunion were treated with an antibiotic cement-coated interlocking IM nail. Seventeen patients achieved union, one had a persistent nonunion without infection, and two had residual bone defects (one with persistent infection). Cement-nail debonding occurred during nail removal (four patients) and during nail insertion (one patient).

66. Helmy N, Jando VT, Lu T, Chan H, O'Brien PJ: Muscle function and functional outcome following standard antegrade reamed intramedullary nailing of isolated femoral shaft fractures. *J Orthop Trauma* 2008;22(1):10-15.

Twenty-one patients with isolated femoral shaft fractures treated with antegrade nailing through the piriformis fossa were examined at least 1 year after fracture for muscle strength. Ten also underwent gait analysis. Patients demonstrated lower hip abductor and hip extensor strength than on the uninjured side but without important gait changes or significant disability according to Musculoskeletal Function Assessment and Short Form-36 results.

Chapter 34

Fractures of the Distal Femur

Cory A. Collinge, MD   Jeffrey M. Smith, MD

5: Lower Extremity

Introduction

The treatment of distal femoral fractures has evolved over the past few decades with more predictable and improved outcomes, although no single method of management has overcome all of the problems associated with these injuries. Before 1970, most distal femur fractures were treated nonsurgically. However, difficulties with malunion, joint incongruity, loss of knee motion, and delayed mobilization (especially in patients with multiple injuries) were common. During the past few decades, surgical techniques and technology have improved, and currently internal fixation is favored for most displaced distal femur fractures. The surgical goals of treatment are anatomic reduction of the articular surface; restoration of limb alignment, length, and rotation; and stable fixation that allows for early mobilization. Although improved methods of fixation have dramatically improved clinical results, the surgical management of these difficult fractures is not uniformly successful.

The demographic pattern of patients with distal femur fractures demonstrates a bimodal age distribution, including younger patients with high-energy trauma and elderly patients with low-energy trauma. However, an increasing number of higher-energy injuries are being seen in elderly patients, blurring this distinction. Although not without potential complication, simple fractures in good-quality bone often have good results with any one of the many various techniques and implants that are available. In higher energy fractures, there may be considerable fracture displacement, comminution, open wounds, and associated injuries that make stable fixation more difficult to achieve. Similarly, obtaining reliable, stable fixation in elderly patients with osteoporosis can be a significant challenge.

Dr. Collinge or an immediate family member has received royalties from Biomet, Smith & Nephew, and Advanced Orthopedic System; is a member of a speakers' bureau or has made paid presentations on behalf of Smith & Nephew; and serves as a paid consultant to or is an employee of Smith & Nephew. Dr. Smith or an immediate family member serves as a board member, owner, officer, or committee member of Orthopaedic Trauma Association; is a member of a speakers' bureau or has made paid presentations on behalf of AO North America; and serves as a paid consultant to or is an employee of Smith & Nephew and Stryker.

The unique anatomy of the distal femur must be clearly understood to successfully manage these fractures surgically. The distal femur broadens into two curved condyles that, if viewed on end, are trapezoidal in shape (narrower anteriorly than posteriorly) with an angle of inclination of the medial surface of approximately 25° (Figure 1). This anatomy becomes important when placing implants across the condyles. On AP radiographs, implants that appear of appropriate length may be too long and cause painful irritation. Anteriorly, the articular surfaces of the two condyles come together to form a joint for articulation with the patella, and posteriorly they are separated by a deep intercondylar fossa that contains the origins of the cruciate ligaments. The lateral condyle is broader and extends farther proximally. The knee joint normally is oriented parallel to the ankle and ground. The anatomic axis of the femur relative to the knee averages about 8° of valgus, with some variability between individuals (range, 5° to 12°). The contralateral limb can usually be used to radiographically define the limb axis for each person.

Initial Evaluation

Forces that are sufficient to fracture the distal femur may produce additional injuries in the same extremity and to other body parts. These injuries and their sequelae may complicate treatment or delay definitive fracture fixation. Without thoughtful treatment, this delay may increase the technical difficulty of the procedure, contribute to patient morbidity, and compromise the full benefits of internal fixation.

If there are differences in distal pulses between the injured and uninjured sides, or if there is suspicion of an occult vascular injury, ankle-ankle or ankle-brachial indices should be measured. The ankle-brachial indices or Doppler-derived pressure on the injured side should be 90% of the uninjured side; vascular injury is then unlikely. Conventional and CT angiography can also be useful tools for evaluating for vascular injury. A gentle reduction and splinting of the injured limb should be performed early after arrival at the emergency department, if not already done by prehospital caregivers.

Quality AP and lateral radiographs of the knee and distal femur are usually sufficient for diagnosis. Traction radiographs are often helpful if there is significant

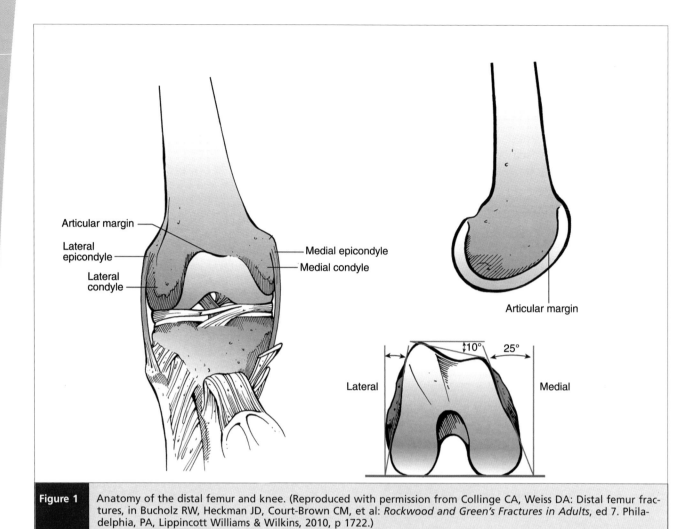

Figure 1   Anatomy of the distal femur and knee. (Reproduced with permission from Collinge CA, Weiss DA: Distal femur fractures, in Bucholz RW, Heckman JD, Court-Brown CM, et al: *Rockwood and Green's Fractures in Adults*, ed 7. Philadelphia, PA, Lippincott Williams & Wilkins, 2010, p 1722.)

shortening and deformity, and they provide a better understanding of the fracture morphology. This radiographic maneuver can be combined with the reduction and splinting process. Radiographs of the entire femur should be obtained to assess for more proximal femur fractures. CT scans with axial, coronal, and sagittal reconstructions are an important adjunct to plain radiographs and are recommended with most displaced fractures. Intra-articular injuries are better delineated, and several potentially important occult fractures may be identified. One study recently showed a 40% rate of coronal plane or Hoffa fracture with intercondylar fractures, many of which are missed with plain radiographs alone.[1] If osteoporosis is evident on plain radiographs, a loss of bone density of 40% or greater has occurred, and these patients should be identified, educated, and considered for treatment to avoid future fragility fractures.

Open fractures occur in 5% to 25% of distal femur fractures. The traumatic wound is usually anterior and is associated with a variable degree of damage to the extensor mechanism. Early antibiotic administration and thorough irrigation and débridement of the frac-

ture and traumatic wounds are critical in preventing infection. Serial débridements, antibiotic beads, and negative pressure wound dressings are useful tools in higher-grade open fractures. Immediate internal fixation is not indicated for all injury patterns, and the risk-benefit ratio for each individual patient must be carefully assessed when contemplating primary internal fixation. In stable patients with type I, II, and IIIA open distal femur fractures, early definitive internal fixation is indicated after débridement of the traumatic wounds if the wounds can be made "clean" and appropriate resources are available. However, most type IIIB and IIIC open distal femur fractures are more safely treated with initial knee-spanning external fixation and delayed internal fixation. Subsequent surgery can be carefully planned with optimal operating room personnel and resources, or patients can be transferred to a tertiary care center if desired.

Distal femoral fractures following total knee replacement are increasing in incidence, with an estimated frequency of 0.5% to 2.5%. These complex injuries are likely to increase as the number of knee replacements continues to rise. Treatment is often difficult, and until recently most published studies report relatively small numbers of patients. Risk factors for fractures include osteopenia, rheumatoid arthritis, prolonged corticosteroid therapy, anterior notching of the femoral cortex, and revision arthroplasty. Results of internal fixation have improved dramatically in the past few years, and the principles for successful treatment of most types of periprosthetic distal femur fractures are now established and thoroughly discussed in chapter 43.

Classification

There is no universally accepted classification for distal femur fractures. Essentially, all classifications distinguish between extra-articular, intra-articular, and isolated condylar lesions. Fractures are further subdivided according to the degree and direction of displacement, the amount of comminution, and the involvement of the joint surfaces. Unfortunately, anatomic fracture classifications fail to address the conditions commonly associated with fractures of the distal femur, which often influence treatment or outcome. These factors play a dynamic role in management and determine the "personality" of a fracture.

The Orthopaedic Trauma Association (OTA) classification system[2] (**Figure 2**) distinguishes between extra-articular (type A), partial articular (type B), and complete intra-articular (type C) injuries, and it accounts for fracture complexity with subclassifications. A basic treatment plan for distal femur fractures can usually be formulated based on this classification system. Because of the large number of fracture patterns seen in clinical practice, however, some fractures do not fit neatly into any classification scheme. This emphasizes the fact that every case must be individually evaluated, and the "personality" of the fracture must be considered in selecting the method of treatment (**Table 1**).

Role of Temporizing External Fixation

The prerequisites for definitive surgical intervention for a distal femur fracture include a well-resuscitated patient without life-threatening injuries, a good understanding of the injury, and adequate surgical resources. If these circumstances are not in place, the use of a temporizing external fixator to stabilize the fracture helps prevent further soft-tissue trauma to the area and allows for patient mobilization and nursing care. Temporizing fracture stabilization for open fractures is particularly useful in patients with multiple injuries, mutilating limb injuries, vascular injuries, and open intra-articular factures. Advantages of immediate internal or external fixation in settings such as these (when definitive internal fixation cannot be safely performed) include stabilization of the fracture and surrounding soft tissues, ease of wound care, pain relief, and mobilization of the patient and the injured limb.

With careful fixator application (for example, avoiding overlap of pin tracts with future plate placement), no increase in complications is expected. A knee-spanning external fixator can be applied with two pins laterally or anteriorly in the midproximal and proximal femur and two pins anteriorly in the middle and mid-proximal tibia[3] (**Figure 3**). Closed reduction to restore axial alignment and length appear to be important factors with frame application.

In a retrospective study, complications and healing rates in 47 patients treated with temporary external fixation and subsequent open reduction and internal fixation for high-energy distal femoral (16 patients) or proximal tibial fractures (36 patients) were evaluated.[4] Of 40 patients with 1-year follow-up, 36 (91%) had healed both radiographically and clinically. There were eight deep infections (16%) that all occurred in open fractures, one hematoma, and one pin site infection. The authors concluded that temporary bridging external fixation was safe and offered the advantage of early soft-tissue and bone stabilization without the potential local risks of immediate open reduction and internal fixation in severely injured soft tissues or the potential systemic risks in a severely traumatized patient.

Indications for Fixation

Most displaced distal femur fractures in adults are best treated with internal fixation, usually with angular stable plating or intramedullary nailing. Regardless of the implant used, the goal is anatomic reduction of the joint surface, restoration of axial alignment, and stable internal fixation to safely start knee range of motion. Because the spectrum of injuries to the distal femur is so great, no single implant will be optimal for every case. Careful assessment of the patient and critical review of the radiographs and the "personality" of the fracture are essential. Some of the factors to be considered in the surgical decision-making process include (1) the ambulatory status, (2) the degree of osteopenia, (3) the degree of comminution, (4) the involvement of the joint surfaces, (5) the condition of the soft tissues, (6) the presence or absence of open wounds, and (7) whether the fracture is an isolated injury or one of multiple injuries.

The role of supplemental grafting with bone or bone substitutes has become less clear with the increased use of indirect reduction techniques and soft-tissue preserving methods. The current role of autogenous bone graft and bone morphogenetic proteins is not yet scientifically clarified. Relative indications for bone grafting include fractures with bone loss or residual major bone defects and severe open fractures treated on a delayed basis to prevent nonunion. In many cases, where a comminuted fracture or one with bone loss has been bridged with a flexible implant, early callus formation will be seen that provides a sentinel for progression to early healing without grafting.

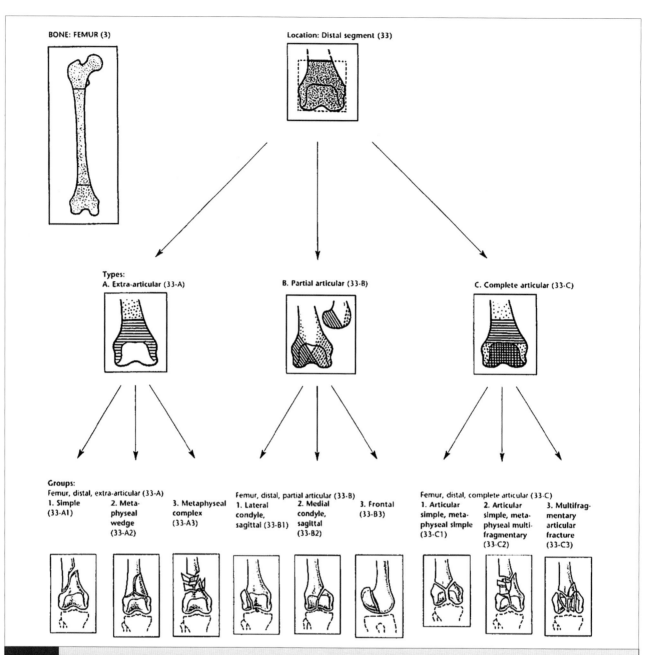

Figure 2 The OTA classification of distal femur fractures (types 33-A through 33-C). (Reproduced with permission from Marsh JL, Slongo TF, Agel J: Fracture and Dislocation Classification Compendium 2007: Orthopaedic Trauma Association Classification, Database and Outcomes Committee. *J Orthop Trauma* 2007;21(suppl 10):S1-S163.)

Using more biologic approaches and improved implants (for example, locked plating and improved retrograde intramedullary nails) has made treatment of distal femur fractures much more predictable and successful. The fixation method should be based on a formal preoperative plan that incorporates fracture pattern, soft-tissue injury, patient factors, surgeon's preference/familiarity, and hospital resources. Executed properly, this surgical tactic shortens operating room time, minimizes the need for intraoperative decision making, and likely improves results. The sequential steps in the surgical management of distal femoral frac-

tures include (1) restoration and fixation of the articular surface, (2) reestablishment of axial alignment (and length in younger active patients), (3) stable internal fixation, (4) consideration for biologic grafting (autogenous bone graft or bone morphogenetic proteins), (5) repair of associated knee injuries, (6) early knee range of motion, and (7) protected weight bearing.

As late as the 1980s, surgically treated distal femoral fractures were most commonly repaired with a relatively anatomically contoured distal femoral plate using conventional screws. Relatively high complication rates were reported that adversely affected clinical results, in-

Table 1

General Surgical Tactics for Bony Reconstruction by OTA Classification

Type A
Open locked plating (or 95° blade plate or DCS) using lateral approach
Minimally invasive locked plating
Locked retrograde nailing

Type B
Buttress plating for lateral or medial condyle fracture (or lag screws alone in rare cases)
Countersunk anterior to posterior screws for coronally oriented (Hoffa) fracture

Type C
Strong consideration for extended lateral parapatellar arthrotomy for open reduction and internal fixation of articular fracture(s) followed by:

    Open locked plating (or 95° blade plate or DCS) using lateral approach
    Minimally invasive locked plating
    Locked retrograde nailing

DCS = dynamic compression plate
(Adapted with permission from Baker BJ, Escobedo EM, Nork SE, Henley MB: Hoffa fracture: A common association with high-energy supracondylar fractures of the distal femur. *Am J Roentgenol* 2002;178:994.)

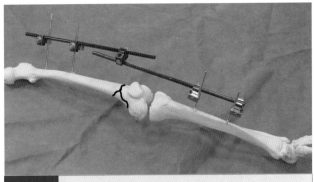

Figure 3   A knee-spanning external fixator is a useful tool in complex open fractures and polytrauma patients. Note that the femur pins are applied proximally so as not to overlap with a plate at the time of reconstruction.

cluding infection, nonunion or delayed union, malunion (especially varus collapse), the need for bone graft, and knee stiffness. Many of these complications may also reflect the wide dissection commonly used for fracture reduction and fixation at that time.

Alternative methods were proposed, including fixed angled plates (for example, the 95° angled blade plate or dynamic compression plate [DCS]), the use of which resulted in improved mechanical stability of the repaired fracture. About this time, indirect fracture reduction with minimal soft-tissue stripping became popular in an effort to maintain the fracture biology. When these two methods of fixed-angle plating and indirect fracture reduction were combined, dramatically improved rates of bone healing with fewer complications were found compared to previous results.[5,6]

More recently, locked plating systems have been developed in which screws are inserted that lock into the plate and form a fixed-angle construct (**Figure 4**). Most of these systems are designed with options for insertion through minimally invasive techniques that theoretically may further decrease complications with fracture healing and infection. Condylar fixation is mechanically improved over earlier fixed-angle implants (for example, blade plate or DCS) by spreading out fixation points among several locking screws.[7-9] Multiple published studies have shown the distal femur Less Invasive Stabilization System (LISS; Synthes, Paoli, PA) to be effective in achieving stable fixation with good short-term and midterm results.[10-14] A learning curve was clearly seen, with emphasis on accurately restoring

alignment intraoperatively and using minimally invasive reduction techniques. A variety of plating systems have since been developed that offer some potential advantages for distal femur fractures, including better anatomic contouring, improved fixation in the condylar segment, and options for conventional screws, bicortical or unicortical solid locking screws, cannulated nonlocking or locking screws, and either conventional open plating or percutaneous fixation.

There was a movement in the late 1980s and 1990s toward using retrograde intramedullary nails for distal femur fractures, although widespread success was hampered by shortcomings of the implants and the technique. Potential advantages of nailing for distal femur fractures include (1) the intramedullary nail is a load-sharing device compared with a plate; (2) it has the potential to stabilize complex or segmental fractures with minimal soft-tissue dissection; and (3) it can often be inserted quickly in a patient with multiple injuries. Like plating techniques, aspects of intramedullary nailing for distal femoral fractures have evolved over the past decade, resulting in improved fracture stabilization capabilities. Modern techniques include the use of long nails inserted to the level of or just above the lesser trochanter to avoid potential problems with injuring local anatomy and to prevent the windshield-wiper effect caused by nail-canal mismatch (improving stability). Most nailing systems now allow for three or four locking screws in the condylar segment that can be placed in multiple planes, and some even lock to the nail to create a fixed-angle device. In patients with ipsilateral hip and distal femur fractures, both fractures can be independently stabilized and the distal fracture securely fixed with a retrograde nail. Antegrade nailing has been advocated for distal femur fractures and may be especially useful in segmental fractures, although retrograde femoral nailing is more effective than antegrade nailing for maintaining alignment of the distal fracture.

The Hoffa fracture, a coronally oriented shear fracture involving the lateral or medial condyle, is common and is usually seen with other bony or ligamentous in-

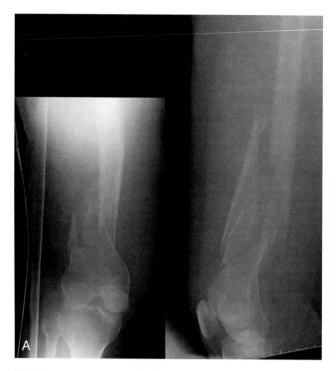

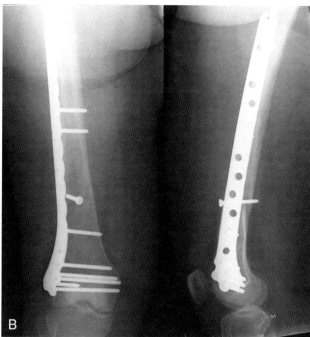

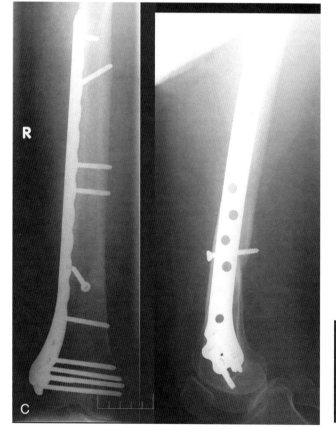

Figure 4 Imaging studies of a patient with a distal femur fracture. **A**, Injury AP (left) and lateral (right) radiographs. **B**, AP (left) and lateral (right) postoperative radiographs after internal fixation with a locked plate. **C**, Final AP (left) and lateral (right) radiographs taken at 5 months show a healed fracture with no change in alignment.

juries around the knee. This fracture pattern is often missed on plain radiographs but is readily seen on CT scans, which should be ordered in most cases.[1] The posterior condyle fragment is mostly covered with articular cartilage, and fixation may be difficult.

Plating

Several approaches to the distal femur have been described, and one is chosen based on a preoperative plan incorporating the fracture and soft-tissue injury pattern, patient factors, implant selection, and surgical ex-

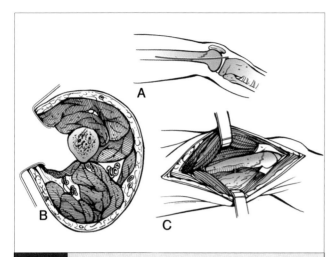

Figure 5 Standard lateral approach to the distal femur provides sufficient exposure for nonarticular (type A) and many simple articular (type C1) fractures. **A**, The skin incision (*solid red line*). **B** and **C**, Deep exposure. (Reproduced with permission from Collinge CA, Weiss DA: Distal femur fractures, in Bucholz RW, Heckman JD, Court-Brown CM, et al: *Rockwood and Green's Fractures in Adults*, ed 7. Philadelphia, PA, Lippincott Williams & Wilkins, 2010, p 1724.)

perience. For extra-articular (OTA type A) fractures, no visualization of the joint is necessary and minimally invasive fixation techniques with a submuscular plate (or open) or retrograde intramedullary nail may be effective. For most intra-articular fractures (OTA types B and C), optimal treatment requires an arthrotomy to visualize, anatomically reduce, and stabilize the articular injury. Standard open or submuscular plating or retrograde intramedullary nailing can then be used to reconstruct the stabilized condylar segment to the femoral shaft.

A direct lateral approach is the most commonly used exposure for open reduction and plating of the distal femur (**Figure 5**). The patient is positioned supine with a bump beneath the ipsilateral hip to internally rotate the leg. The skin incision is longitudinal and centered over the lateral epicondyle. The incision should be long enough to allow gentle soft-tissue retraction. The fascia lata is incised in line with its fibers, exposing the vastus lateralis, which is reflected off the intermuscular septum along the linea aspera in the anterior direction. Perforators are identified and ligated or cauterized. This careful dissection is started distally and carried proximally. Wide soft-tissue stripping is avoided and no soft-tissue dissection should be performed on the medial side of the femur to minimize disruption of the soft tissues. Visualization of the articular surface of the lateral condyle is satisfactory, but exposure of the intercondylar notch and medial condyle are more limited. When more access to the knee joint is needed, the incision can be extended distally and curved medially to allow for greater patellar subluxation. Rarely, a tibial tubercle osteotomy can be performed to allow for

reflection of the extensor mechanism and wide articular exposure. Knee flexion must be restricted for a period of time following tibial tubercle osteotomy; thus, its use has been limited. Alternatively, an anterolateral peripatellar arthrotomy can be used; when combined with medial subluxation of the patella, complete visualization of the articular surface, including the intercondylar notch, is possible. Plates can still be readily applied to the lateral surface of the femoral condyle, and the plates may be passed proximally in a submuscular fashion. A second lateral approach can be made to the femoral shaft for proximal plate fixation.

If a minimally invasive technique is to be used for plating of selected distal femur fractures, a 5- to 6-cm lateral incision limited to the area of the lateral condyle and distal metaphysis is used. The incision is placed more distal to allow for retrograde submuscular plate insertion. Condylar screws are placed through the incision used for plate insertion. Proximal screws are placed using multiple stab incisions or a short open lateral approach and using a radiolucent guide. In this setting, a longer plate may be desirable to increase construct stability and minimize dissection in the zone of injury.

Although adequate exposure with anatomic reduction and rigid fixation is a basic principle of treatment of articular portions of distal femur injury, indirect (or biology-sparing) reduction is recommended for the metaphyseal and metadiaphyseal regions, where tampering with the fracture environment is likely to have negative biologic consequences. Reduction can typically be achieved and assessed without extensive soft-tissue stripping in these areas, and then a plate can be applied using minimally invasive or biology-sparing open tactics. Useful reduction techniques[15] include chemical paralysis by anesthesia, longitudinal traction using a femoral distractor or external fixator, careful application of pointed clamps or the King tongs, a well-placed towel roll (to correct sagittal plane alignment), carefully applied Kirschner wires for provisional fixation or to use as joysticks for fracture fragment manipulation, and use of the plate and standard screws themselves as reduction tools.

Combining standard nonlocking screws to lag the bone to the plate and locked screws to aid in construct stability is a useful tactic and uses benefits of both screw types. If a combination of nonlocking screws and locking screws is used, the nonlocking cortical screws must be inserted first. Plain radiographs or intraoperative fluoroscopy must be carefully scrutinized to assess limb alignment, rotation, and length. Malunion is the most common complication for distal femur fractures repaired with indirect reduction methods. Fluoroscopic AP view of the hip relative to the knee in the well leg can be compared to the reconstructed limb side to assess for rotation and length.

Plate application has become more complex with the evolution of locked implants, but also potentially more effective with multiple options for screws. When using the plate as a reduction tool it is important to align the

5: Lower Extremity

most distal screws parallel to the knee joint to ensure that the 8° or so of valgus built into the plate is achieved. When appropriate, compression should be applied to optimize stability in simple transverse or short oblique fracture patterns (for example, OTA A1 patterns) to allow for earlier weight bearing. When significant comminution is present, the plate is fixed to the proximal and distal fragments, bridging the zone of comminution.

The length of the plate and the number and placement of screws is based on a growing understanding of modern nonlocking, locking, and hybrid fixation principles. In general, a longer plate with spaced screws provides better mechanical stability compared to a shorter plate. The surgeon should be familiar with the specific technique suggested for a given plate to achieve proper coronal plate alignment (varus-valgus). Typically, this involves inserting a specific guide pin parallel to the articular surface of the distal femur. The condylar segment is stabilized with all or nearly all locked screws; the specific number necessary to provide adequate stability in normal versus osteoporotic bone has not been determined. Locked plates must be centered on the diaphysis to minimize the risk of cutout and catastrophic failure. Standard screws through the plate may be used to bring a plate closer to the bone, to assist in reducing the bone to the plate, or to lag a simple oblique fracture fragment but should not be placed within a bone segment after the placement of a locking screw within that segment. A series of standard screws followed by locked screws (hybrid technique) allows the benefits of both screw types to be realized. When addressing a more comminuted metaphyseal segment, it is recommended to select a plate length with several screw holes above the most proximal extent of the fracture to leave a fairly long working length. The number, distribution, and choice of locking versus nonlocking screws is the subject of ongoing research and appears to be an area of surgical judgment that can lead to complications of fixation failure or fracture healing. While fixation is important, reduction and alignment still remain more important determinants of outcome.

Intramedullary Nailing

The concept of preoperative planning is no less important for intramedullary nailing than it is for osteosynthesis with plates and screws. Limitations of nails used for distal femur fractures make planning very important, such as the size of the condylar segment, the insertional depth of the nail, and the number and distances of locking screws from the nail's end. Significant advances have been made in nailing techniques and technology in the past decade. Nonetheless, the goals of surgery remain the same as for plating (**Figure 6**). Two particular problems exist with nailing relative to plating.[16,17] First, for extra-articular fractures, infection after nailing may allow for knee joint sepsis, and second, leaving the nail proud by even 1 mm in the notch or inadvertently reaming the patella places the patellofemoral joint at risk for destruction.

The patient is positioned supine and the affected limb supported on a radiolucent triangle or large bump to a 20° or 30° angle. The C-arm unit should come in from the opposite side of the table, and the underside of the table should allow free navigation of the C-arm distal to the knee and proximal beyond the intertrochanteric region for AP and lateral radiographs. When possible, the fracture should be reduced before nailing. Many of the indirect reduction methods described in femoral plating are useful for nailing.

With most OTA type A and some type C distal femur fractures, a limited medial parapatellar arthrotomy is used for retrograde femoral nailing. The patella and local soft tissues should be protected from reamers and other instrumentation during nailing. Most displaced intra-articular fractures (displaced type C1 and C2, C3) should be exposed, reduced, and stabilized using an open medial or lateral parapatellar arthrotomy based on the fracture pattern. The intramedullary nail can then be inserted through the open incision. Interfragmentary screws used for the fixation of condylar fractures must be placed anteriorly or posteriorly so as not to block nail passage. The portal of entry for the nail is in the intercondylar notch just anterior to the femoral attachment of the posterior cruciate ligament (just anterior to Blumensaat's line). A threaded tipped guide pin and cannulated drill are used to prepare the distal femur before nailing, with the pin inserted in line with the femoral shaft to ensure restoration of alignment on the AP image. This pin is started at the apex of the intercondylar notch and aimed centrally through the supracondylar region.

A beaded tip guidewire is inserted into the intramedullary canal and advanced past the fracture site, into the proximal femur under fluoroscopic control. With the fracture reduced, the position of the guidewire is confirmed to be center-center in the AP and lateral views. Blocking screws are sometimes used to narrow the effective canal diameter of distal femur to improve alignment and prevent deformity. The fracture should be reduced and out to length during reaming and insertion of the nail. The nail must be countersunk several millimeters to prevent cartilage damage to the patellofemoral articulation. Final nail positioning should be checked in both the AP and lateral radiographs to ensure nail depth and proper alignment.

Distal locking bolts are placed through cannulated sleeves using a radiolucent guide. Proximal locking is accomplished typically in the AP plane using a freehand technique. The knee joint is thoroughly lavaged and suctioned to remove reamings or other debris that may cause mechanical problems or heterotopic bone formation. The arthrotomy is anatomically repaired and the skin closed in standard fashion.

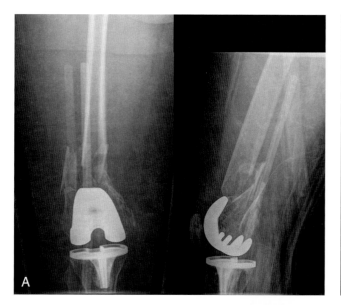
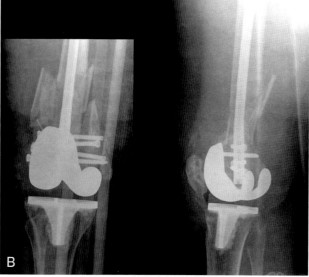
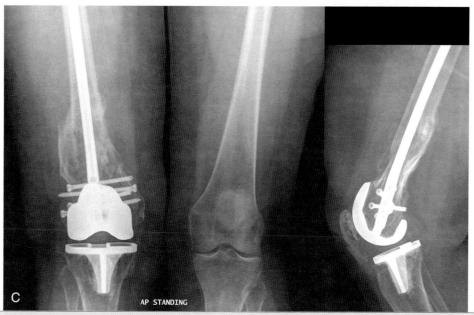

Figure 6 **A**, Injury AP (left) and lateral (right) radiographs of an elderly patient with osteoporosis and a periprosthetic distal femur fracture. **B**, AP (left) and lateral (right) postoperative radiographs after retrograde intramedullary nailing. **C**, Final standing AP (left) and lateral (right) radiographs taken at 6 months show a healed fracture with no change in alignment.

Type C Fractures

For OTA type C injuries, the principles and goals of treatment are precise anatomic reduction and fixation of the articular surface and stabilization of the metadiaphyseal component. With nondisplaced or minimally displaced simple articular splits in type C1 injuries, the condyles can often be anatomically held or reduced with a large clamp, and stabilized through a standard open or minimally invasive lateral approach using long 3.5-, 4.5-, or 6.5-mm lag screws applied outside the footprint of the plate on the lateral femoral condyle or avoiding the path of the nail, depending on the choice of fixation. Some-

times inserting lag screws from the medial side simplifies their placement.

In patients with more complex intra-articular involvement (most C2, C3 fractures), the modified lateral (or medial) parapatellar approach is preferable, to allow access to the joint.[18] After adequate surgical exposure, the femoral condyles are reduced and provisionally fixed with Kirschner wires. Once reduction is confirmed clinically and/or radiographically, the condyles are definitively fixed with long screws anterior and/or posterior in the condyles, allowing sufficient room for the plate. If a posterior coronal or Hoffa fracture is present, fixation can be obtained by placing

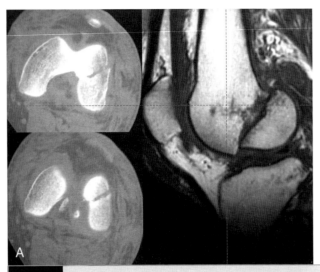
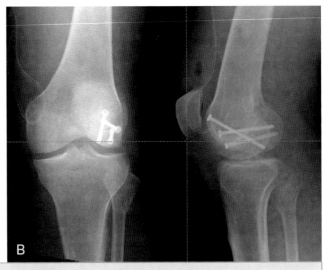

Figure 7 A type B Hoffa fracture. **A,** Injury MRIs. **B,** Postoperative AP (left) and lateral (right) radiographs after internal fixation with a locked plate.

countersunk 2.7- or 3.5-mm cortical or 4.0-mm cancellous screws through the articular surface from anterior to posterior. In these cases small fragment fixation for the condylar injuries in conjunction with distal femur locked plates is preferred.

Type B Fractures

Isolated fractures of the medial or lateral femoral condyle are uncommon. Open reduction and internal fixation is the most reliable method to ensure articular surface restoration. In patients with good bone quality where anatomic reduction is achieved with closed means, the fracture may be stabilized with several percutaneous lag screws. In displaced fractures, an open approach and plate fixation along with lag screws is routinely used. A direct lateral or medial approach may be used for simple B1 fracture patterns where anatomic reduction of the joint can be gained without arthrotomy. In comminuted fractures such as B2 or B3 fractures, a medial or lateral parapatellar approach is preferred, and extended proximally as necessary. Fixation of the articular surface must be anatomic and stable because shearing stresses are common even without weight bearing. With the typical vertical condylar fracture (medial or lateral), the use of an antiglide or buttress plate with supplemental lag screws is recommended. The Hoffa fracture, a coronally-oriented shear fracture involving the lateral or medial condyle, is common with other fracture patterns but also occasionally occurs as an isolated bony fracture with associated ligament injury (**Figure 7**). The posterior condyle fragment is mostly articular and fixation may be problematic. In isolated fractures a limited arthrotomy can be performed and screw fixation applied as previously discussed. Occasionally, a nonarticular fracture spike extends superiorly from the posterior fragment and is useful for assessing reduction and may benefit from application of an antiglide plate.

Postoperative Protocols

Postoperatively, early mobility with gentle active knee motion is initiated in the conscious patient, whereas a continuous passive motion machine may be useful in patients remaining intubated or in the intensive care unit. Instruction in early isometric muscle-strengthening exercises and active-assisted range of motion is encouraged. Early or immediate range of motion has been shown to improve clinical outcome as it pertains to ultimate range of motion and avoidance of the need for manipulation under anesthesia and/or surgical release.

Little clinical evidence is available to guide recommendations for postoperative weight bearing. In patients with intra-articular injuries, most surgeons will recommend either no weight bearing or touchdown weight bearing for 10 to 12 weeks to allow the articular injury to heal. In patients with extra-articular injuries, even more variability exists, but partial weight bearing with progression over 4 to 12 weeks is common. Progressive weight bearing is encouraged once there is radiographic evidence of healing. By 12 weeks, most patients should tolerate substantial weight bearing, although most patients still require an assistive device.

Although the use of biologic approaches and state-of-the-art implants has improved results, their use does not guarantee a favorable outcome. The surgeon must have a thorough understanding of the local anatomy, the mechanics of fracture fixation, and patterns of fracture healing after internal fixation if consistently good results are to be achieved and must be aware of the common problems associated with surgical treatment.

Complications

Malalignment/Malunion

Malalignment resulting in deformity of the distal femur carries an increased risk of subsequent arthrosis, as well as a negative impact on gait, range of motion, and activities of daily living. In early series using traditional plates and screws, problems with fixation failure, varus collapse, and malalignment for unstable injuries were common. Multiple studies using locking plates or retrograde nails have shown improved fixation in the relatively osteopenic distal condylar segment, but newer methods using indirect reduction have resulted in an increased incidence of operative malalignment leading to malunion. For example, one study reported early experience with the LISS implant in 62 patients with 66 OTA 33-A or 33-C fractures.[13] Although healing was reasonably achieved, assessment of valgus/varus alignment showed correct axial alignment (<5°) in only 49 patients (74%) and correct sagittal alignment in 56 patients (85%). Incorporating alignment assessment into the preoperative plan and vigilant attention to detail in the operating room is essential to ensure correct alignment.

Nonunion

Historically, open anatomic reduction and rigid internal fixation with traditional plates of distal femur fractures was associated with delayed union or nonunion in 29% to 38% of fractures, presumably due to wide surgical dissection and less stable implants. Dramatically improved results have been reported in patients with similar injuries when more biologic approaches and improved implants were used for treatment. Union rates of 93% to 100% were reported in distal femur fractures treated with indirect fracture reduction and internal fixation using 95° fixed-angle devices.[5,6] One study described the results of surgical treatment of distal femur fractures from multiple European centers using LISS, and healing was noted in 37 of 40 patients (93%).[19] Another study reported union in 58 of 61 patients (95%) treated with the femoral LISS device, and successful early healing was attributed to maintenance of the fracture biology and strict adherence to the fixation principles of locked plating.[10] Similar methods were used in a selected high-energy cohort of patients with mechanically unstable distal femur fractures; a high union rate without bone grafting was reported, and there were no problems with maintaining alignment in this "at-risk" population.[14]

Nonunions may be difficult to treat because of preexisting or disuse osteopenia, proximity to the knee joint, and prior surgical procedures. Aseptic nonunions in patients with reasonable bone stock should be treated by bone grafting with or without repeat osteosynthesis. Hypertrophic nonunions usually respond to stable internal fixation of the nonunion site. The 95° condylar blade plate remains an excellent tool for treating nonunions (and malunions); compression can be applied to increase stability.

Infection

One of the major drawbacks of surgical fixation of distal femoral fractures is the risk of infection, although with modern treatment principles the risk of infection is 2% or less. If deep infection develops postoperatively, aggressive irrigation and débridement are indicated. A deep infection with abscess formation should be treated with a thorough débridement and irrigation and possible adjunctive treatment with a negative pressure wound dressing or an antibiotic bead pouch. The wound is closed secondarily when it appears "clean" and the signs of infection have resolved. Appropriate antibiotics are typically given intravenously for 3 to 6 weeks. In the presence of infection, implants that provide stability are often best retained. If the implant is clearly loose, it should be removed and the fracture treated temporarily with external fixation.

Knee Stiffness

Stiffness has been a very common complication following distal femur fractures, but newer implants have allowed for earlier mobility, and regaining knee motion has been less problematic. Quadriceps scarring with or without arthrofibrosis of the knee or patellofemoral joint is thought to restrict knee movement, and these effects are greatly magnified by immobilization after fracture or internal fixation. Early stable internal fixation of the fracture with meticulous soft-tissue handling and immediate mobilization of the knee joint maximize the chance for an optimal outcome after a distal femur fracture. Patients who fail to regain knee motion during the first month after surgery are best treated with aggressive range-of-motion exercises under the direction of a physician and physical therapist. Patients with persistent or ongoing loss of motion after injury may be candidates for quadricepsplasty as a late reconstructive procedure.

Hardware Problems

The relatively bulky nature of the implants as well as the anatomy of the distal thigh and knee often leads to local symptoms (for example, iliotibial band tendinitis over a lateral plate). There are no firmly established criteria for hardware removal after distal femur fracture fixation, but the most common indication for metal removal is local discomfort over the implant with activity in a physiologically young patient with a healed fracture. It is recommended that hardware removal be delayed for 18 to 24 months in most patients to avoid refracture.

Posttraumatic Arthritis

The incidence of posttraumatic arthritis after distal femur fractures is unknown because no long-term outcome studies have been published. However, incongruity of the joint surfaces is thought to be a cause of early arthritis and highlights the importance of anatomic reduction and rigid internal fixation of articular fractures (OTA B and C). Unfortunately, many patients with degenerative arthritis of the knee occurring after fracture are young adults and are not ideal candidates for knee arthroplasty. If the arthritis is limited to the medial or lateral compartment, a corrective osteotomy may be appropriate, but in patients with more global and disabling bicompartmental or tricompartmental arthritis, a total knee replacement may be indicated.

Outcomes

A 2006 study reviewed the English-language literature summarizing and comparing the results of different fixation techniques (traditional compression plating, antegrade nailing, retrograde nailing, submuscular locked internal fixation and external fixation) in the surgical management of acute nonperiprosthetic distal femur fractures (AO/OTA type 33-A and 33-C), and no large, prospective, randomized studies (level I evidence) were found.[20] Several comparative studies are available (level II evidence) in the treatment of distal femoral fractures. A prospective cohort study compared 20 patients treated with locked plating using LISS and 19 treated with locked retrograde femoral nailing.[21] No significant differences with nonunion (both 10%), fixation failure (both 0%), infection (locked plating 0% versus nailing 6%), and secondary surgical procedures (both 10%) were found at 1-year follow-up. There were 45 case series (level IV evidence) reporting 1,614 patients treated with compression plating, antegrade nailing, retrograde nailing, and internal (locked) or external fixation. In all treatment options, additional internal screw and/or plate fixation was performed first if the articular surface was fractured. The average follow-up was 2.5 years. The articular surface was fractured in 58% of the cases; severe fracture was present in 22% (OTA type C3). Twenty-seven percent of all fractures were open, and according to the Gustilo-Anderson classification, 10% were type III. Overall, the average nonunion rate was 6.0%, the fixation failure rate was 3.3%, the deep infection rate was 2.7%, and the average secondary surgical procedure rate was 16.8%. The injury/fracture spectrum was different for the four fixation techniques; therefore, a comparison of outcome parameters was limited. A comparison of outcome parameters between compression plating and locked internal fixation revealed no statistically significant differences for any outcome parameter. However, there was a statistically nonsignificant relative risk (RR) reduction of 55% for deep infection when submuscular locked internal fixation was performed as opposed to traditional compression-plating techniques ($P = 0.056$) despite a significantly higher percentage of all open fractures (36% versus 25%, $P < 0.001$) and grade III open fractures (17% versus 7%, $P < 0.001$) in the locked inter-

nal fixation group. On the other hand, there was a nonsignificant RR increase in secondary surgical procedures of 28% ($P = 0.062$) and a nonsignificant RR increase in fixation failure of 89% ($P = 0.062$).

Several case series of distal femur fractures treated with the principles of minimally invasive locked plating have shown promising early and midterm results in several injury patterns. For example, the early clinical results of 103 distal femur fractures (68 closed fractures and 35 open fractures) in 99 patients treated with the LISS device were reported.[11] Ninety-six of 103 fractures (93%) healed without bone grafting, and no varus collapse or screw loosening in the distal femur fragment was observed. Malreduction of the femoral fracture was seen in six fractures (6%). The authors attributed successful early healing to vigilant maintenance of the fracture biology and strict adherence to modern fixation principles, but early in these series, malalignment was recognized as a significant potential problem with these methods. The results of periprosthetic distal femur fractures above a total knee arthroplasty treated with a locked distal femur plate were evaluated in a 2006 study.[22] Patients with 22 consecutive distal femur fractures (OTA type 33-A) above a well-fixed nonstemmed total knee arthroplasty were treated with locked plating. Nineteen of 22 fractures (86%) healed after the index procedure. Three patients with healing complications were obese and had type I diabetes mellitus. Infected nonunions developed in two of these patients and an aseptic nonunion in one patient. Postoperative alignment was within 5° for 20 of 22 fractures. Three patients had loss of fixation and progressive coronal plane deformity requiring further surgery. According to a 2004 study, it was reported that by using minimally invasive plating with LISS, fracture alignment was maintained and early healing occurred in all 27 patients in a cohort of high-energy, mechanically unstable fractures (OTA types 33-A2, 33-A3, 33-C2, and 33-C3).[14]

Published reports over the past decade using retrograde nailing for distal femur fractures have indicated mostly good results with relatively few complications. There are no large randomized studies comparing retrograde nailing to plating for these injuries. Nevertheless, three small series have been published comparing the two implants. A 2006 study reported on 23 distal femoral fractures randomized to a retrograde intramedullary nail fixation (n = 12) or a fixed-angle blade plate fixation (n = 11).[23] Both fixation methods gave generally good outcomes, but three patients treated with a retrograde nail required revision surgery for removal of implants and experienced more pain on Medical Outcomes Study 36-Item Short Form (SF-36) measures. In a 2005 study, the management of distal femur fractures (OTA types A and C) in mostly elderly patients with the use of a DCS or a retrograde nail was assessed.[24] Seventy-two patients were randomized to nailing (n = 35) or plating (n = 37). Mean operating room time and estimated blood loss were lower in the nailing group (P

< 0.001). Healing times were comparable, and clinical results were similar with good-excellent results in 80% or more of the patients. Midterm outcomes of 11 patients with traditional open reduction internal fixation versus 11 others treated with limited open reduction with retrograde intramedullary nailing for C-type distal femoral fractures were evaluated in a 2008 study.[25] The rate of subsequent bone-grafting procedures (67% versus 9%) and malunion (42% versus 0%) were significantly higher with open reduction and internal fixation in comparison with the less invasive retrograde intramedullary nailing treatment. A trend toward increased infection (25% versus 0%) and nonunion (33% versus 9%) in the open plating group was noted. The physical function component of the SF-36 was approximately 2 standard deviations below that of the US population mean, and 50% of patients demonstrated radiographic changes of posttraumatic arthritis for all patients. There was no significant difference in any domain of the SF-36 or Short Musculoskeletal Functional Assessment, or the Iowa Knee Score between the two treatment groups.

The midterm to long-term (5 to 25 years) functional and radiologic results of surgically treated intra-articular fractures of the distal femur were analyzed.[26] Follow-up was 1 year in all 67 patients, and 32 patients were seen for a long-term follow-up visit. After a mean follow-up of 14 years (range, 5 to 25 years), the mean knee range of motion was 118° (range, 10° to 145°), the Neer Score showed good to excellent results in 84% of the patients, and the Hospital for Special Surgery Knee Score showed good to excellent results in 75% of the patients. The Ahlback Score showed a moderate to severe development of secondary osteoarthritis in 36% of all patients, although 72% of these patients still scored a good to excellent functional result.

Summary

Notable advances in the treatment of distal femoral fractures have been achieved over the past decade yielding improved clinical results. Surgical treatment currently is indicated for most patients with a distal femoral fracture. For OTA types 33-A and 33-C injuries, either locked plating or intramedullary nailing appears appropriate for fixation, as long as modern treatment principles such as anatomic reduction of articular injury, restoration of axial alignment, and maintenance of fracture biology are followed.

Annotated References

1. Baker BJ, Escobedo EM, Nork SE, Henley MB: Hoffa fracture: A common association with high-energy supracondylar fractures of the distal femur. *AJR Am J Roentgenol* 2002;178(4):994.

2. Marsh JL: OTA fracture classification. *J Orthop Trauma* 2009;23(8):551.

    The author presents a review of the OTA fracture classification system.

3. Haidukewych GJ: Temporary external fixation for the management of complex intra- and periarticular fractures of the lower extremity. *J Orthop Trauma* 2002; 16(9):678-685.

4. Parekh AA, Smith WR, Silva S, et al: Treatment of distal femur and proximal tibia fractures with external fixation followed by planned conversion to internal fixation. *J Trauma* 2008;64(3):736-739.

    This is a retrospective review of patients with 44 high-energy distal femur and tibial plateau fractures receiving initial treatment of high-energy periarticular knee fractures with bridging external fixation, followed by planned conversion to internal fixation. The authors concluded that this treatment is a safe option in patients who are unsuitable for initial definitive surgery.

5. Bolhofner BR, Carmen B, Clifford P: The results of open reduction and internal fixation of distal femur fractures using a biologic (indirect) reduction technique. *J Orthop Trauma* 1996;10(6):372-377.

6. Ostrum RF, Geel C: Indirect reduction and internal fixation of supracondylar femur fractures without bone graft. *J Orthop Trauma* 1995;9(4):278-284.

7. Bong MR, Egol KA, Koval KJ, et al: Comparison of the LISS and a retrograde-inserted supracondylar intramedullary nail for fixation of a periprosthetic distal femur fracture proximal to a total knee arthroplasty. *J Arthroplasty* 2002;17(7):876-881.

8. Egol KA, Bazzi J, McLaurin TM, Tejwani NC: The effect of knee-spanning external fixation on compartment pressures in the leg. *J Orthop Trauma* 2008;22(10):680-685.

    The authors evaluated 25 patients (mean age 52 years) to determine if the application of external fixation for the temporary stabilization of high-energy proximal tibial fractures and dislocation would have an effect on compartment pressures in the leg. Results showed that transient elevation of intracompartment pressures occurred in some instances but did not appear to lead to compartment syndrome.

9. Higgins TF, Pittman G, Hines J, Bachus KN: Biomechanical analysis of distal femur fracture fixation: Fixed-angle screw-plate construct versus condylar blade plate. *J Orthop Trauma* 2007;21(1):43-46.

    The relative strength of fixation with a locking distal femoral plate was compared with a condylar blade plate in this study using eight matched pairs of fresh-frozen cadaver femurs. In biomechanical testing of a simulated distal femoral fracture, the locking screw-plate construct was found to be stronger than the condylar blade plate in cyclic loading and ultimate strength. The authors concluded that there was some support for using the locking plate rather than the blade plate in comminuted distal femoral fracture fixation.

10. Kregor PJ: Distal femur fractures with complex articular involvement: Management by articular exposure and submuscular fixation. *Orthop Clin North Am* 2002; 33(1):153-175.

11. Kregor PJ, Stannard JA, Zlowodzki M, Cole PA: Treatment of distal femur fractures using the less invasive stabilization system: Surgical experience and early clinical results in 103 fractures. *J Orthop Trauma* 2004;18(8): 509-520.

    This is a retrospective study evaluating early results of patients with 103 distal femur fractures treated with minimally invasive reduction and locking plate-screw fixation using the LISS system. The authors reported high union rates without autogenous bone grafting (93%), a low incidence of infection (3%), and maintenance of distal femoral fixation (100%).

12. Ricci AR, Yue JJ, Taffet R, Catalano JB, DeFalco RA, Wilkens KJ: Less Invasive Stabilization System for treatment of distal femur fractures. *Am J Orthop* 2004; 33(5):250-255.

    In a prospective, nonrandomized study, the authors evaluated LISS plating to determine its value in treating distal femoral fractures. Twenty-five multiply injured patients with 26 unstable distal femoral fractures were treated with LISS plating. Result showed no nonunions, infections, or need for bone grafting. Excellent range of motion and alignment were achieved.

13. Schütz M, Müller M, Regazzoni P, et al: Use of the less invasive stabilization system (LISS) in patients with distal femoral (AO33) fractures: A prospective multicenter study. *Arch Orthop Trauma Surg* 2005;125(2):102-108.

    This is a retrospective study of minimally invasive plating with the LISS device performed at multiple European centers early in the learning curve for these techniques. Reasonably good healing rates were seen (85%), with few bone grafts and infections. However, malunion of 5° or more was seen in 39% of cases, highlighting the significance of intraoperative assessment of limb alignment in these cases.

14. Weight M, Collinge C: Early results of the less invasive stabilization system for mechanically unstable fractures of the distal femur (AO/OTA types A2, A3, C2, and C3). *J Orthop Trauma* 2004;18(8):503-508.

    The authors evaluated 26 patient with 27 high-energy fractures of the distal femur (AO/OTA type A2, A3, C2, and C3) treated with LISS fixation. All the fractures healed at a mean of 13 weeks, with no failed fixations, infections, or implant breakage. It was concluded that LISS allowed early healing and stable fixation in unstable fractures of the distal femur.

15. Collinge CA, Sanders RW: Percutaneous plating in the lower extremity. *J Am Acad Orthop Surg* 2000;8(4): 211-216.

16. Gliatis J, Megas P, Panagiotopoulos E, Lambiris E: Midterm results of treatment with a retrograde nail for supracondylar periprosthetic fractures of the femur following total knee arthroplasty. *J Orthop Trauma* 2005; 19(3):164-170.

    Midterm results of periprosthetic fracture healing and knee function in nine patients (10 fractures) were evaluated after treatment with a supracondylar nail. The authors reported that all the fractures healed within 3 months, with no infections and no loosening of the prosthesis. One patient required revision because the fracture united in extreme valgus. It was concluded that retrograde nailing is the treatment of choice for a periprosthetic fracture with a stable prosthesis.

17. Patel K, Kapoor A, Daveshwar R, Golwala P: Percutaneous intramedullary supracondylar nailing for fractures of distal femur. *Med J Malaysia* 2004;59(suppl B): 206-207.

    In this prospective study, the authors report on 25 patients with supracondylar and intercondylar fractures treated with percutaneous supracondylar nailing. No complications occurred that were related to the fracture treatment. Based on the Hospital for Special Surgery rating scale, 84% of patients had excellent results, 8% had good results, and 8% had fair results. The authors concluded that supracondylar nailing was an excellent method for treating distal femoral fractures.

18. Starr AJ, Jones AL, Reinert CM: The "swashbuckler": A modified anterior approach for fractures of the distal femur. *J Orthop Trauma* 1999;13(2):138-140.

19. Schütz M, Müller M, Krettek C, et al: Minimally invasive fracture stabilization of distal femoral fractures with the LISS: a prospective multicenter study: Results of a clinical study with special emphasis on difficult cases. *Injury* 2001;32(suppl 3):SC48-SC54.

20. Zlowodzki M, Bhandari M, Marek DJ, Cole PA, Kregor PJ: Operative treatment of acute distal femur fractures: Systematic review of 2 comparative studies and 45 case series (1989 to 2005). *J Orthop Trauma* 2006;20(5): 366-371.

    This is a systematic review of the English literature that summarized and compared the results of different fixation techniques in the surgical management of acute nonperiprosthetic distal femur fractures (AO/OTA types 33-A and 33-C) and the characteristics of the fractures for each treatment (articular/nonarticular and open/ closed).

21. Markmiller M, Konrad G, Südkamp N: Femur-LISS and distal femoral nail for fixation of distal femoral fractures: Are there differences in outcome and complications? *Clin Orthop Relat Res* 2004;426:252-257.

    A prospective cohort study compared 20 patients treated with locked plating using LISS and 19 treated with locked retrograde femoral nailing. No significant differences with nonunion (both 10%), fixation failure (both 0%), infection (locked plating 0% versus nailing 6%), and secondary surgical procedures (both 10%) were reported at 1-year follow-up.

22. Ricci WM, Loftus T, Cox C, Borrelli J: Locked plates combined with minimally invasive insertion technique for the treatment of periprosthetic supracondylar femur fractures above a total knee arthroplasty. *J Orthop Trauma* 2006;20(3):190-196.

Patients with 22 consecutive distal femur fractures (OTA type 33-A) above a well-fixed nonstemmed total knee arthroplasty were treated with locked plating. Nineteen of 22 fractures (86%) healed after the index procedure. Three patients with healing complications were obese and had type I diabetes mellitus. Infected nonunions developed in two of these patients and an aseptic nonunion in one patient. Postoperative alignment was within 5° for 20 of 22 fractures. Three patients had loss of fixation and progressive coronal plane deformity requiring further surgery.

23. Hartin NL, Harris I, Hazratwala K: Retrograde nailing versus fixed-angle blade plating for supracondylar femoral fractures: A randomized controlled trial. *ANZ J Surg* 2006;76(5):290-294.

The authors reported on 23 distal femoral fractures randomized to a retrograde intramedullary nail fixation (n = 12) or a fixed-angle blade plate fixation (n = 11). Both fixation methods achieved generally good outcomes; however, three patients treated with a retrograde nail required revision surgery for removal of implants and experienced more pain on SF-36 measures.

24. Christodoulou A, Terzidis I, Ploumis A, Metsovitis S, Koukoulidis A, Toptsis C: Supracondylar femoral fractures in elderly patients treated with the dynamic condylar screw and the retrograde intramedullary nail: A comparative study of the two methods. *Arch Orthop Trauma Surg* 2005;125(2):73-79.

The management of distal femur fractures (OTA types A and C) in mostly elderly patients with the use of a DCS or a retrograde nail was assessed. Seventy-two patients were randomized to nailing (n = 35) or plating (n = 37). The mean operating room time and estimated blood loss were lower in the nailing group (*P* < 0.001). Healing times were comparable, and clinical results were similar with good-excellent results in 80% or more of the patients.

25. Thomson AB, Driver R, Kregor PJ, Obremskey WT: Long-term functional outcomes after intra-articular distal femur fractures: ORIF versus retrograde intramedullary nailing. *Orthopedics* 2008;31(8):748-750.

The authors compared the midterm outcomes of 11 patients with traditional open reduction internal fixation versus 11 others treated with limited open reduction with retrograde intramedullary nailing for C-type distal femoral fractures. The rate of subsequent bone-grafting procedures (67% versus 9%) and malunion (42% versus 0%) were significantly higher with open reduction and internal fixation compared with the less invasive retrograde intramedullary nailing treatment. There was a trend toward increased infection (25% versus 0%) and nonunion (33% versus 9%) in the open plating group. The physical function component of the SF-36 was approximately 2 standard deviations below that of the US population mean, and 50% of patients showed radiographic changes of posttraumatic arthritis for all patients. There was no significant difference in any domain of the SF-36 or Short Musculoskeletal Functional Assessment, or the Iowa Knee Score between the two treatment groups.

26. Rademakers MV, Kerkhoffs GM, Sierevelt IN, Raaymakers EL, Marti RK: Intra-articular fractures of the distal femur: A long-term follow-up study of surgically treated patients. *J Orthop Trauma* 2004;18(4):213-219.

This retrospective study included 32 patients with 5- to 25-year follow-up after surgical treatment of a distal femur fracture. The mean knee range of motion was 118°. The Neer Score showed good to excellent results in 84% of the patients and the Hospital for Special Surgery Knee Score showed good to excellent results in 75% of the patients. There was moderate to severe secondary osteoarthritis in 36% of all patients, although 72% of these patients still had a good to excellent functional result.

Chapter 35

Knee Injuries

Bruce A. Levy, MD   Michael J. Stuart, MD   Stephen A. Kottmeier, MD

Knee Dislocations

Introduction

Optimal treatment strategies for the dislocated knee remain highly debated. Currently, there is a paucity of data to help guide decision making. These limb-threatening injuries have a high rate of neurovascular compromise and the potential for significant functional impairment. Moreover, many knee dislocations present after a spontaneous reduction and are never recognized as true dislocations. It is important to be knowledgeable about all aspects of the multiligament-injured knee including vascular assessment, timing of surgery, technical considerations, rehabilitation, and current evidence-based medicine.

Initial Evaluation

Vascular Assessment

The most effective screening method for assessing possible vascular injury in a dislocated knee remains controversial. The options include physical examination, the ankle-brachial index (ABI), duplex ultrasonography, conventional arteriography, and CT arteriography.

When patients present with obvious physical ("hard") signs of ischemia (a cold, pulseless limb) and the location of the vascular injury is known (the popliteal artery), the vascular surgeon may opt for emergent surgical exploration without obtaining confirmatory studies. However, those patients who present with subtle ("soft") signs of ischemia (for example, asymmetric pulses, warmth, color of limb) require further screening to rule out a vascular injury.

Physical Examination

Many studies in the recent literature validate the use of selective arteriography in patients who demonstrate ab-

Dr. Levy or an immediate family member serves as a paid consultant to or is an employee of Arthrex and Valpo Orthotec; and has received research or institutional support from DePuy. Dr. Stuart or an immediate family member has received royalties from Fios; serves as a paid consultant to or is an employee of Arthrex and Fios; and has received research or institutional support from DePuy, Biomet, Stryker, and Zimmer. Dr. Kottmeier or an immediate family member is a member of a speakers' bureau or has made paid presentations on behalf of Smith & Nephew.

normal findings on physical examination. Prospective studies involving patients with knee dislocation concluded that clinically significant vascular injuries could be discerned by physical examination alone. However, it is important to recognize that collateral blood flow can produce palpable distal pulses, despite a major arterial occlusion.

Ankle-Brachial Index

Utilization of the ABI, combined with physical examination and selective use of arteriography, has been recommended by some authors.[1] The sensitivity, specificity, and positive predictive value of ABI for significant arterial injury has been reported at 100% in patients with an ABI of less than 0.9.[2] Measurement of the ABI is obtained by placing a blood pressure cuff on the supine patient's injured lower extremity proximal to the ankle and determining the systolic pressure at the posterior tibial artery or dorsalis pedis artery with a Doppler probe. A similar reading of the systolic blood pressure is obtained in the ipsilateral uninjured upper extremity. This technique is illustrated in **Figure 1**. The ABI is calculated as follows:

$$ABI = \frac{\text{Doppler systolic arterial pressure in injured limb (ankle)}}{\text{Doppler systolic arterial pressure in uninjured limb (brachial)}}$$

Duplex Ultrasonography, Conventional Angiography, and CT Angiography

Duplex ultrasonography is a noninvasive and fast screening tool with excellent sensitivity (90%) but less specificity (68%) than conventional angiography. Ultrasonography is technician dependent, and not all facilities have a full-time technician available.[1]

Conventional angiography has long been considered the "gold standard" screening tool for vascular injury despite the fact that it is more invasive, expensive, and time consuming than duplex ultrasonography. Risks include allergic reaction, nephrotoxicity, and pseudoaneurysm. False positive rates of 5% to 7% have been reported.[1,3]

The recent advent of CT angiography has offered a new avenue for vascular evaluation in the setting of the multiligament-injured knee. CT angiography is less invasive than the conventional method, uses one quarter

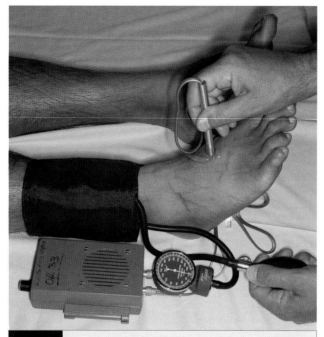

Figure 1 | Technique for the measurement of ABI. (Courtesy of Bruce A. Levy, MD, Rochester, MN.)

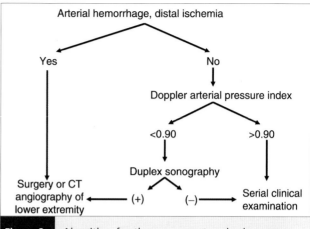

Figure 2 | Algorithm for the assessment and subsequent treatment of a vascular injury. (Adapted with permission from Mills WJ, Barei DP, McNair P: The value of the ankle-brachial index for diagnosing arterial injury after knee dislocation: A prospective study. *J Trauma* 2004;56:1261-1265.)

the radiation, and has excellent sensitivity and specificity. One study of 63 patients who underwent CT angiography demonstrated 100% sensitivity and specificity confirmed by conventional angiography and surgical findings.[4]

Current Recommendations

An algorithm for assessment of vascular injury in the dislocated knee is shown in **Figure 2**.[1] If the patient presents with "hard" signs of ischemia, a vascular surgeon will proceed with immediate surgical exploration (if the location of the lesion is known) or CT angiography. ABI can be determined in all patients with knee dislocation who do not have evidence of a dysvascular limb. If the ABI is greater than 0.9, the patient is carefully monitored by serial physical examinations every 4 hours for 48 hours. If the ABI is less than 0.9, duplex ultrasonography is performed. When the duplex ultrasound yields abnormal results, CT angiography is required to further define the lesion.

Diagnostic Imaging

Plain radiographs are often normal after knee dislocation because of the high rate of spontaneous reduction. Subtle changes in joint space width, tibiofemoral subluxation, or rim and/or avulsion fractures may be indicative of a reduced knee dislocation. MRI is the diagnostic imaging method of choice to identify the injured anatomic structures. If a spanning-joint external fixator is placed before MRI is obtained, it is important to use an MRI-compatible frame. Comparative stress radiographs of both knees using fluoroscopy (under anesthesia when applicable), have proven valuable. Varus-valgus laxity is assessed with AP views at 30° of knee flexion to evaluate the medial collateral ligament (MCL) and fibular collateral ligament (FCL). Posterior tibial translation is assessed with lateral views at 90° of knee flexion to evaluate the posterior cruciate ligament (PCL).

At the time of definitive surgical intervention, diagnostic arthroscopy identifies and confirms all associated intra-articular pathology (meniscus, articular cartilage, loose bodies). The surgeon should ensure adequate outflow to prevent excessive fluid extravasation in the setting of joint capsule disruption

Outcomes

Reports of outcomes after knee dislocation are generally case series (level IV), with few comparative studies. Scientific investigation is also hampered by the heterogeneous nature of multiligament knee injuries in regard to patient demographics, injury patterns, surgical techniques, and rehabilitation protocols.

Treatment Options

Surgical Versus Nonsurgical Management

Absolute indications for immediate surgery include an irreducible dislocation, a dysvascular limb, and an open injury. Associated fractures and/or avulsion-type injuries are also amenable to early surgical treatment.

A meta-analysis of mostly retrospective studies compared surgical and nonsurgical treatment of these injuries.[5] Surgical reconstruction led to improved motion in a collective cohort of 132 knees. Although no significant differences in stability were noted, average Lysholm scores were almost 20 points higher in the surgically treated group. These data have been used to support the rationale for acute surgical treatment. Subsequent studies have reported similar findings after surgical reconstruction.[6] In a recent report on 50 knees comparing surgical and nonsurgical treatment, the surgically treated group had improved functional outcome scores, less pain, and higher activity levels.[7]

Repair Versus Reconstruction
Most authors agree that reconstruction as opposed to repair of the cruciate ligaments yields improved outcomes. Controversy persists, however, with regard to optimal treatment of the medial and lateral structures in the multiligament-injured knee. A prospective, nonrandomized trial of combined cruciate ligament and posterolateral corner (PLC) injuries revealed a 37% failure rate for repair of the posterolateral corner. In contrast, PLC reconstruction resulted in a 9% failure rate with significant improvement in postoperative joint stability ($P < 0.05$).[8]

For the MCL/posteromedial corner (PMC), a recent systematic review of the literature in the setting of the multiligament-injured knee found only eight studies that met the authors' inclusion criteria: five on MCL/PMC repair and three on reconstruction. Satisfactory outcomes were achieved with repair, reconstruction, or some combination thereof.[9] No studies to date have directly compared repair with reconstruction for medial-sided injuries in the dislocated knee.

Early Versus Delayed Surgery
Several authors have noted improved outcomes with early (<3 weeks after surgery) versus delayed ligament reconstruction after knee dislocation.[10,11] These retrospective studies were all limited by a small sample size and a heterogeneous population. One study reported on 31 patients, 19 of which were treated acutely. Those patients demonstrated improved functional outcome scores and stability, although there was a slightly higher rate of arthrofibrosis in this group.[10] In a more recent study, 35 of 45 patients treated acutely demonstrated improved functional outcomes and no difference in their final knee range of motion.[11]

Several potential differences between the acute and chronic groups in these studies may have affected clinical and functional outcomes. Multiligament knee reconstruction for patients with severe soft-tissue trauma or concomitant orthopaedic and/or nonorthopaedic injuries may have been delayed for many weeks before definitive surgical treatment, resulting in worse outcomes. The current recommendation is to proceed with multiligament knee reconstruction when the soft tissues are amenable to surgical intervention and the patient is able to undergo an extensive postoperative rehabilitation protocol.

Current Treatment Strategies
Staged Protocol Approach
As for tibial plateau or pilon fractures, many knee surgeons follow a staged protocol for managing the multiligament-injured knee. Patients are treated initially with expedient joint reduction and splinting or the se-

lective use of knee-spanning external fixation, followed by initiation of deep venous thrombosis prophylaxis. Multiligament knee reconstruction is performed approximately 3 weeks after injury. Initial indications for knee-spanning external fixation include vascular injury, gross instability with failure to maintain reduction in a brace, open knee dislocation, and patient inability to mobilize in a brace or splint. Once surgery is performed, single-stage reconstruction can often be done regardless of the injury combinations. However, in the setting of an open knee dislocation, depending on the specific structures involved, primary repair at the initial or subsequent irrigation/débridement procedures may be performed for some portions of the injury, with delayed reconstruction of the remaining injured ligaments when the soft tissues allow. This staged-protocol approach has been deemed safe with regard to the development of deep venous thrombosis.[12]

Graft Selection
Satisfactory outcomes after multiligament knee reconstruction have been demonstrated with the use of either autograft or allograft tissue.[13,14] There are many advantages to the use of allograft tissue, including lack of donor site morbidity, flexibility with graft sizes, and shorter operating room time.[13-15] A disadvantage of allograft tissue is the potential for disease transmission. In particular, the risk of HIV transmission is estimated at 1 in 1.6 million provided that the graft has been appropriately sterilized and the donor adequately screened. In contrast, autograft tissue carries no risk of disease transmission, and multiple sources are readily available from either the ipsilateral or contralateral knee, including patellar, quadriceps, or hamstring tendons. Donor site morbidity should be an important consideration when choosing autograft tissue.

Technical Advances
Anterior Cruciate Ligament
In the isolated anterior cruciate ligament (ACL)-injured knee, much debate continues surrounding single-bundle versus double-bundle techniques. In the dislocated knee, double-bundle reconstruction would be difficult because of the numerous tunnels required for multiligament knee reconstruction. For example, in an ACL/PCL lateral-side injury, two tunnels are created on the tibial side (one for the ACL, one for the PCL), and several tunnels are created on the femoral side (one for the ACL, one or more for the PCL). Thus, single-bundle ACL reconstructions using standard ACL techniques are appropriate in the setting of knee dislocations.

Posterior Cruciate Ligament
PCL reconstruction can be performed through a transtibial or tibial-inlay technique. Both techniques have demonstrated excellent biomechanical[16] and clinical success.[13,14] Similar to the ACL, double-bundle PCL reconstruction has recently gained popularity. Several biomechanical cadaver studies have shown improved

stability with a double-bundle technique;[17,18] however, this has not been demonstrated clinically. Only two series have compared single- and double-bundle PCL reconstruction in the multiligament-injured knee, and neither demonstrated significant differences in knee stability or functional outcomes.[19,20] Further prospective randomized trials are needed to determine the efficacy and safety of the double-bundle technique.

Many surgeons perform a transtibial single-bundle (anterolateral) reconstruction using Achilles tendon with bone allograft. An important technical consideration when performing PCL reconstruction is the establishment of a posteromedial portal to clearly identify the attachment site of the PCL on the tibia and protect the neurovascular bundle. The tibial tunnel is approached through the anteromedial aspect of the tibia, although recently, some authors have advocated an anterolateral approach in an effort to avoid a steep graft angle ("killer turn") at the back of the knee. On the femoral side, debate continues regarding drilling from outside-in versus inside-out. The proponents for the outside-in technique advocate less "killer turn" on the femoral side. Clinical advantages to these techniques have yet to be elucidated.

Medial Collateral Ligament /Posteromedial Corner

The decision to repair or reconstruct the MCL/PMC is based on the timing of surgery and the quality of the native tissue. In the acute setting, the MCL/PMC are repaired if the quality of tissue is found to be adequate. In the chronic setting, reconstruction is typically recommended, because the remaining tissue is scarred and not readily identifiable.

The MCL is repaired via a standard approach, and the torn ligament (either distal or proximal limbs) is reattached to bone with a spiked ligament washer-screw and suture-post construct. The MCL is reconstructed using autograft or allograft tissue.[14] The Achilles tendon allograft calcaneus bone block is anatomically placed in a femoral socket and fixed with an interference screw. The graft is tunneled subcutaneously and fixed to the tibia using a screw and ligament washer. An alternative technique uses ipsilateral semitendinosus/gracilis autografts. These tendons are left attached distally, looped around the epicondylar axis on the femur, and secured both proximally and distally with spiked ligament washer-screw constructs. Several authors have reported satisfactory outcomes with this technique.[9]

Fibular Collateral Ligament /Posterolateral Corner

Because of the high rates of failure with repair alone of the FCL/PLC structures in the setting of the multiligament-injured knee, reconstruction is favored in most cases. The reconstruction is augmented with repair of the remaining FCL, biceps, or popliteus tendons if they are of adequate quality. An exception is the fibular head avulsion fracture with attached, intact FCL and biceps femoris tendon.

Numerous PLC reconstruction techniques have been reported with varying degrees of success.[19,21] A preferred technique has been use of an Achilles tendon with bone allograft with two sockets created on the femoral side and one through the fibula, reconstructing the tendinous portion of the popliteus, the popliteofibular ligament, and the FCL.[22] In the presence of combined PCL/PLC injuries, the "anatomic" reconstruction technique is usually performed.[23] By drilling a separate tibial tunnel for the popliteus and attaching the graft to the femur, there may be an advantage to this technique in this combined injury pattern. Each tibial tunnel graft (the PCL graft and the popliteus graft) may offload each other. To date, biomechanical and clinical advantages of one technique over another have not been documented.

Rehabilitation

Specific rehabilitation protocols have been developed after multiligament knee reconstruction. Controversy exists with regard to early versus delayed range of motion (ROM). The process of protecting the reconstructed/repaired ligaments while restoring ROM in a timely fashion proves a delicate balancing act.

The rehabilitation protocol described in a 2002 study has demonstrated excellent long-term results.[14] Patients are immobilized in full extension for the first 3 weeks after surgery and then allowed to progress to pain-free prone passive ROM. They refrain from bearing weight for the first 6 weeks after surgery and then begin progressive weight bearing as tolerated. Open kinetic chain exercises are avoided because they are thought to produce undue stress on the grafts. Patients are maintained in a functional brace for up to 1 year after reconstruction and typically return to work or recreational activities by 9 to 12 months postoperatively.

Patella Fractures

Introduction

Fractures of the patella represent 1% of all fractures and 3% of all lower extremity fractures. Injury to the patella may result in compromise of the articular surface of the patellofemoral joint as well as incompetence of the knee extensor apparatus. Treatment goals include accurate restoration of joint congruity and extensor mechanism integrity. The patella is the largest sesamoid bone of the body and possesses the thickest chondral surface of any articulation. It has vertically oriented facets defined by major and lesser vertical ridges as well as two transverse ones. The inferior third of the patella is nonarticular and devoid of chondral surface. The quadriceps tendon, patella, and patellar ligament make up the extensor mechanism of the knee. The four muscle groups of the quadriceps mechanism envelope the patella, offering distal continuity to the proximal tibia in the form of aponeurotic retinacula. The extensor retinaculum serves as a secondary knee extensor, potentially affording active knee extension in the presence of a patella fracture.

The blood supply to the patella is composed of an extraosseous arterial anastomotic ring supplied by the genicular arteries. The patella is an integral part of the extensor mechanism and serves to increase the moment arm of the extensor mechanism by displacing it from the center of knee rotation. Its contribution is most evident in the terminal 15° of active knee extension, during which increasing torque is required to elevate the leg.

No generally accepted classification of patella fractures currently exists. Fractures, in most schemes, are assigned based on the mechanism of injury, fracture pattern, or combinations of both. Common descriptive terms include transverse, vertical, and comminuted (stellate). Transverse factures are the result of forceful tensile forces (quadriceps contraction) in the presence of knee hyperflexion. Because transverse fractures are primarily the result of tensile rather than compressive loads, neither femoral trochlear nor retropatellar chondral surfaces may have significant compromise.

Mechanism of Injury

Forces directly applied to the anterior aspect of the knee (in a fall or vehicular injury) may result in comminuted fracture patterns. In the absence of displacement, retinacular tissues and the extensor mechanism may remain intact with active knee extension maintained. Direct impaction forces may injure the chondral surfaces regardless of the displacement of the fracture.

Fractures of the patellar pole are often the result of combined indirect and direct forces. Inferior pole variants may have limited articular involvement. They can present with discontinuity of the extensor mechanism and, because of associated comminution, pose unique reconstructive challenges. Vertical fractures are typically minimally displaced and not associated with retinacular injury and extensor insufficiency. Therefore, most vertical fractures do not require surgical treatment.

Preoperative Assessment

The integrity of the extensor mechanism must be established. Fractures with interfragmentary displacement suggest absence of extensor mechanism continuity and rupture of the medial and lateral retinacula. In contrast, comminuted fractures without significant displacement likely have intact retinacular and surrounding soft tissues, rendering the extensor apparatus functionally intact. Absence of active knee extension and the presence of a palpable defect imply discontinuity of the extensor mechanism.

Radiographic imaging of patella fractures begins with conventional radiographs in AP, lateral, and axial projections. Subtle fractures may be difficult to identify on the standard AP view because of superimposition of the femur. The lateral view may more adequately reveal the extent of both displacement and comminution of the patella. Vertically oriented fractures and those with chondral defects are appreciated most on the axial view. Conventional radiography offers sufficient detail pertaining to fracture pattern and comminution to adequately determine treatment. Additional imaging modalities serve primarily to identify associated chondral and soft-tissue (ligamentous and meniscal) concerns.

Treatment

Rigid criteria for intervention, from the standpoints of acceptable amounts of fracture displacement, comminution, and morphology, are lacking. Nonsurgical treatment is appropriate for nondisplaced or minimally displaced fractures, particularly if the retinacular tissues and the extensor mechanism remain intact. Some stellate and most vertical fractures present in this fashion. Patients with low physical demands, particularly those with considerable medical comorbidities, may be preferentially managed with nonsurgical treatment.

Those lesions with joint incongruity and significant displacement are most predictably managed with extensor mechanism and articular surface reconstitution. The clinical goal is preservation of motion and restoration of the competence of the knee extensor apparatus, as well as prevention of posttraumatic arthrosis. The surgical goals must be anatomic articular restoration, rigid fixation, and the early introduction of knee joint mobilization. Displaced transverse fractures result in structural failure of the extensor mechanism and require repair. Displaced inferior pole fractures, although relatively nonarticular, present with discontinuity of the extensor mechanism, mandating surgical treatment.

As the severity of the injury increases and articular reconstruction becomes less plausible, the indication for complete or partial patellectomy increases. Complete patellectomy is regarded as a salvage effort because it contributes to both functional and cosmetic concerns. It may result in functional lengthening of the knee extensor mechanism and a reduction of its fulcrum, resulting in loss of mechanical strength. From the patient's perspective, the knee remains in a flexed and loaded position at terminal extension, offering the perception of instability. Because total patellectomy reduces extensor mechanism efficiency by 30%, it should be reserved for those cases in which severe comminution precludes adequate fixation. When possible, retention of portions of the patella may be sufficient to maintain the biomechanical advantage of the extensor mechanism. Partial patellectomy, in such cases, may offer satisfactory results.

There are three general methods of surgical treatment of patella fractures: surgical fixation, partial patellectomy, and complete patellectomy. A variety of fixation techniques have been adopted, including interfragmentary fixation with screws, wires, cerclage, and combinations of each. Simple transverse patterns are amenable to modified tension band fixation with or without the addition of cerclage fixation. Screw fixation alone for these patterns is often biomechanically insufficient and overcome by the strong tensile forces

5: Lower Extremity

generated by the extensor mechanism. Partial patellectomy, with tendinous reattachment, is reserved for fractures of either patellar pole.

Surgical exposure of the patella begins with a midline vertical incision that is extensile and allows for a thorough assessment of the extent of extensor mechanism injury. Surgical dissection should include skin, subcutaneous tissues, and superficial fascia in a single layer to maintain perfusion to overlying soft tissue. Fracture margins are identified and cleaned without surgical devitalization of individual fragments. The status of the extensor retinaculum is established and the fragments reduced to one another. Reduction can be maintained by large, pointed reduction clamps or Kirschner wires. An assessment of the quality of reduction based on the anterior surface topography of the patella may prove misleading. The adequacy of articular reconstruction and extra-articular implant position is best confirmed by palpation or direct visualization of the chondral surface using an existing retinacular tear or a limited arthrotomy.

Various forms of fixation of simple transverse fractures have been studied, including tension band fixation with simpler wire constructs and screw fixation. Tension band fixation has superior biomechanical attributes. The application of tension band fixation is ideally suited for tranverse patterns that can accept interfragmentary compression. In theory, this construct neutralizes anterior surface tensile forces, transforming them instead into compressive forces. Accordingly, tension band constructs have limited application when managing comminuted fractures.

Recently, the traditional tension band fixation has been modified in technique and materials. A modified technique using vertically oriented transosseous wires has been shown to diminish fracture fragment separation. Both circular and figure-of-8 configurations with single or dual twists have been described.[24] More uniform compression can be expected from a circular band with dual twists. Historically, most described techniques have advocated the use of simple stainless steel wire. Braided cable and braided polyester outperform monofilament wire in biomechanical tests.[25] Some authors support the use of biodegradable materials to lessen both implant-related discomfort and the need for later removal.[26]

Tension band fixation may exhibit fracture site displacement with early knee motion. Another recent modification of the tension band technique is to use cannulated screws for primary interfragmentary compression and fixation, with the wires of the tension band placed through the screws. Reduction in implant-related discomfort and improved construct rigidity have been observed. This is primarily evident in the terminal phases of knee extension. Newer trends in patella fracture fixation techniques include the adoption of minimally invasive methods.[27] These methods may involve, but do not demand, the inclusion of arthroscopically assisted reduction. Proponents suggest these methods may offer less threat to parapatellar soft tissues.[28,29] These minimally invasive methods may result in preservation of the osseous blood supply and diminished adhesion formation. It is further maintained that operating room times, complications, and required analgesics are diminished while patient satisfaction and functional scores are improved. Only fractures within the midcentral portion of the patella and with limited or no comminution should be considered; thus, these methods are limited to simple transverse fracture patterns with intact retinacular tissues that are amenable to screw fixation.

Fractures of the proximal or distal poles of the patella pose unique therapeutic challenges. Those involving the inferior pole are most common. Typically the extensor mechanism is disrupted, and the inferior pole itself is comminuted. These injuries may be treated by surgical fixation of the fracture or excision of the inferior pole fragments with reattachment of the patellar tendon to the proximal part of the patella. Although encouraging results have been described with partial patellectomy, studies have raised concerns regarding sustained quadriceps atrophy, elevated residual patellofemoral contact area, and subsequent osteoarthritis.[30] The negative effects of residual patella baja and protocols limiting postoperative ROM may contribute to these findings. Recent trends suggest that restoration of patella height and reconstitution of as much articular surface as possible may optimize results.

Partial patellectomy should be reserved for nonreconstructable fractures that have limited or no articular involvement. Excision of the inferior pole is followed by reattachment of the patellar tendon via vertical transosseous sutures. The tendon should be secured close to the articular (posterior) surface. Anterior attachment of the patellar tendon may result in posterior rotation of the distal pole, precipitating altered kinematics and resulting in degenerative changes to the articular surface.[30] The completed construct may be neutralized, and ROM initiated, by the inclusion of a load-sharing device similar to a cerclage from the superior patella pole to the tibial tubercle. Avoidance of patella baja is of paramount importance because its adverse impact on outcome is considerable.

More recently, preservation of the inferior patellar pole, and accordingly patellar height, has been proposed to offer better biomechanical and clinical results than excision.[31,32] In a study comparing preservation with excision of the inferior pole of the patella, increased range of motion, better functional activity, and diminished pain were observed in the former group.[33] The authors' protocol encouraged immediate weight bearing and range of motion. They contend that restoration of patella height, contact area, and mobility contributed to observed favorable results. To satisfy the requirements of sufficient fixation, a basket plate was designed to collect the inferior pole fragments.

Extensively comminuted fractures of the patella offer a challenging therapeutic dilemma. Major fragments should be meticulously defined and anatomically reduced. Smaller fragments are indirectly reduced with preservation of surrounding soft tissues to limit devitalization and destabilization. Fractures with lesser degrees of comminution may be converted to a two-part pattern with introduction of smooth wires and screws. The inclusion of a tension band may be pursued in combination with such constructs. However, the biomechanical efficacy of the tension band is questionable when interfragmentary compression cannot be achieved. Cerclage techniques, supplemented with independent interfragmentary screws and wires, are reserved for those fractures that are too comminuted to adhere to the principles of tension band fixation.

An assessment of reduction based on anterior surface inspection, particularly with comminuted fracture variants, may prove misleading. In addition to performing a limited arthrotomy to assess articular reduction, some authors have encouraged more extensile exposures. These include inversion of the patella[34] as well as osteotomy of the tibial tubercle.

Occasionally, the degree of comminution exceeds the limitations of internal fixation. In such instances, either partial or complete patellectomy may be the only option possible. When compared with patellectomy, preservation of a portion of the patella may offer enhanced satisfaction with activities of daily living, enhanced perception of stability, and diminished discomfort.[33] Conflicting reports exist regarding the optimum size of retained fragments and a threshold for complete excision of the patella. Some authors contend that a poorly reconstituted articular surface of limited size may precipitate arthrosis and pain. Complete patellectomy should be reserved for extensively comminuted fractures, many of which are associated with considerable soft-tissue compromise. Surgical patellectomy demands proper integration of retinacular tissues to maintain the integrity and suitable length of the extensor apparatus.

Extensor Mechanism Disruption

Introduction
Extensor mechanism disruption occurs infrequently but is most common in men, African-Americans, and individuals older than 40 years.[35,36] Knowledge of pertinent anatomy, physical examination findings, and diagnostic imaging helps in the implementation of specific management strategies for acute and chronic rupture of both the patellar and quadriceps tendons.

Anatomy
The four muscles comprising the quadriceps femoris converge to form a single tendinous insertion—the quadriceps tendon—on the proximal pole of the patella. The patellar tendon originates on the distal pole of the patella and inserts on the anterior tibial tubercle. The central quadriceps tendon is twice as thick as the patellar tendon. The patella is a sesamoid bone that in-

creases the moment arms of both the quadriceps and patellar tendons, providing an efficient fulcrum for knee extension.

Physical Examination
Extensor mechanism disruption results in knee swelling, giving way in flexion, limp, or a hyperextension gait pattern. Point tenderness and a palpable gap may be appreciated at the site of the tendon injury. Passive knee range of motion is normal, but active knee extension is limited (a seated active-extension lag). The patient may be able to perform a straight-leg raise if the patellar retinaculum is intact.

Diagnostic Imaging
AP and lateral radiographs may reveal normal patellar height, patella alta (patellar tendon rupture), patella infera (quadriceps tendon rupture), and an inferior patellar fat pad sign.[37] The identification of a proximal patellar enthesophyte may increase suspicion for a quadriceps tendon rupture, because chronic tendinopathy has been demonstrated to be a risk factor.[38]

Ultrasound is an inexpensive diagnostic tool that is performed in real time and does not use ionizing radiation.[39-41] Patellar and quadriceps tendon ruptures are easily identified, but the technique is operator dependent.

MRI depicts the soft-tissue structures in great detail, which allows for diagnosis and preoperative planning. In addition, MRI provides information on the underlying bone and intra-articular knee structures.

Patellar Tendon Rupture
Rupture of the patellar tendon typically occurs in young male athletes as a result of repetitive microtrauma (end-stage jumper's knee). Acute patellar tendon rupture is best treated with early surgical repair and rehabilitation.[42] Tendon repair is performed with nonabsorbable locking whipstitch sutures passed through longitudinal, transosseous patellar tunnels combined with reapproximation of the retinaculum.[43] The addition of suture anchors placed in the distal pole of the patella may add to the strength of the repair and better replicate the natural tendon footprint.[43] Some authors recommend protection of the repair with a cerclage wire or relaxing suture.[44,45]

These injuries can also be iatrogenic as a result of steroid injection, ACL reconstruction autograft harvest, or total knee arthroplasty.[46-48] Patellar tendon rupture in adult patients is often associated with chronic renal failure, secondary hyperparathyroidism, rheumatoid arthritis, systemic lupus erythematosus, obesity, diabetes mellitus, and chronic steroid use.[46,49-52] In these settings, augmentation of the repair with semitendinosus and/or gracilis tendon autograft or a medial gastrocnemius flap can provide a stronger construct and facilitate postoperative rehabilitation.[53,54]

In the chronic setting, poor tissue quality and delayed diagnosis and treatment may result in quadriceps

5: Lower Extremity

weakness, tendon contracture, and poor knee flexion.[55] Patellar tendon reconstruction with a contralateral knee bone-patellar tendon-bone autograft with subsequent double-wire loop reinforcement and early postoperative mobilization has demonstrated excellent isokinetic strength and functional outcomes.[56] Achilles tendon allograft reconstruction has also been touted as a successful technique, especially after a failed tendon repair.[55] Reconstruction in the chronic setting results in less favorable outcomes than an acute repair, but extensor mechanism function can typically be restored.[57]

Quadriceps Tendon Rupture

Vascular insufficiency, tendinopathy, and repetitive trauma contribute to quadriceps tendon rupture.[58] Early suture repair using the transosseous tunnel technique with or without graft augmentation has demonstrated satisfactory outcomes.[59-61] As in patellar tendon repair, the use of suture anchors may strengthen the construct and allow for early postoperative range of motion.[62]

Quadriceps tendon rupture in the chronic setting can also be attributed to systemic disease, age-related tendon degeneration, or the use of fluoroquinolone antibiotics (ciprofloxacin).[63] Because tissue quality is usually suboptimal, reconstruction techniques using autograft or allograft are commonly employed to ensure successful long-term results.

Postoperative Rehabilitation

In the past, the knee was immobilized for 6 weeks in a cylinder cast after patellar and quadriceps tendon repair. Modern practice encourages early mobilization to promote muscle tone, joint mobility, and tendon healing.[42] A rehabilitation brace with an extension lock and flexion stops allows for gradual progression of an active flexion–passive extension ROM program and partial weight bearing in full extension. Early surgical treatment and aggressive rehabilitation after acute rupture of the patellar tendon can be expected to produce an excellent outcome.

Summary

Ideal management of the dislocated knee remains controversial. Based on the best available evidence, the following are currently recommended: vascular assessment including serial physical examination and ABI measurement with the selective use of arteriography, acute surgical management of all damaged ligamentous structures, selective use of preoperative joint-spanning external fixation when indicated, the use of allograft or autograft tissue (accounting for donor site morbidity), reconstruction as opposed to repair of the ACL, PCL, and FCL/PLC, and primary open repair or reconstruction of the MCL/PMC.

Fractures of the patella present with a spectrum of injury. Reconstitution of the extensor mechanism is required when managing displaced fractures. This can be achieved in the form of fracture osteosynthesis, or partial or complete patellectomy. Contemporary standards of care encourage patella preservation and articular restoration when feasible.

Disruption of the extensor mechanism is a severe, debilitating injury. Acute tendon rupture can usually be attributed to repetitive trauma, whereas chronic injuries are more likely a result of systemic illness or degenerative processes. Early surgical repair and aggressive postoperative rehabilitation are recommended for the most successful outcomes. Techniques for repair and reconstruction have shown similar efficacy and are chosen based on surgeon preference in response to the quality of tissue and pattern of injury.

Annotated References

1. Redmond JM, Levy BA, Dajani KA, Cass JR, Cole PA: Detecting vascular injury in lower-extremity orthopedic trauma: The role of CT angiography. *Orthopedics* 2008;31(8):761-767.

    CT angiography demonstrates excellent sensitivity and specificity as a screening tool for vascular injury in the setting of trauma to the lower extremity and has several advantages compared to conventional arteriography.

2. Mills WJ, Barei DP, McNair P: The value of the ankle-brachial index for diagnosing arterial injury after knee dislocation: A prospective study. *J Trauma* 2004;56(6): 1261-1265.

    This prospective study of 38 patients with knee dislocation evaluated the diagnostic effectiveness of ABIs below 0.90 for vascular injury in this setting. Sensitivity, specificity, and positive predictive value of an ABI less than 0.90 were 100%.

3. Stannard JP, Sheils TM, Lopez-Ben RR, McGwin G Jr, Robinson JT, Volgas DA: Vascular injuries in knee dislocations: The role of physical examination in determining the need for arteriography. *J Bone Joint Surg Am* 2004;86(5):910-915.

    This prospective study of 134 knees with mean 19-month follow-up concluded that selective arteriography based on serial physical examinations is a safe and prudent practice, especially for KD-IV (Schenck class 4) dislocations, for which serial examinations are mandated for at least 48 hours.

4. Inaba K, Potzman J, Munera F, et al: Multi-slice CT angiography for arterial evaluation in the injured lower extremity. *J Trauma* 2006;60(3):502-506.

    This retrospective study evaluated the diagnostic accuracy of multislice helical CT angiography for arterial injury in the traumatized lower extremity in 59 patients. This scan was 100% sensitive and specific for clinically significant arterial injury.

5. Dedmond BT, Almekinders LC: Operative versus non-operative treatment of knee dislocations: A meta-analysis. *Am J Knee Surg* 2001;14(1):33-38.

6. Levy BA, Dajani KA, Whelan DB, et al: Decision making in the multiligament-injured knee: An evidence-based systematic review. *Arthroscopy* 2009;25(4):430-438.

   This systematic review suggested that early surgical treatment of the multiligament-injured knee produces improved functional and clinical outcomes compared with nonsurgical management or delayed surgery and that repair of the PLC yields higher revision rates compared with reconstruction.

7. Plancher KD, Siliski J: Long-term functional results and complications in patients with knee dislocations. *J Knee Surg* 2008;21(4):261-268.

   Fifty knees in 48 patients were evaluated retrospectively for outcomes after surgical versus nonsurgical treatment with mean 8.3-year follow-up. Significantly better Hospital for Special Surgery and Lysholm scores were observed in the surgery cohort, suggesting that this treatment yields better functional results.

8. Stannard JP, Brown SL, Farris RC, McGwin G Jr, Volgas DA: The posterolateral corner of the knee: Repair versus reconstruction. *Am J Sports Med* 2005;33(6):881-888.

   Outcomes of repair versus reconstruction of the PLC were evaluated prospectively in 64 knees with minimum 2-year follow-up. Failure rates of 37% and 9% were observed for repair and reconstruction respectively, suggesting reconstruction is more effective for PLC tears.

9. Kovachevich R, Shah JP, Arens AM, Stuart MJ, Dahm DL, Levy BA: Operative management of the medial collateral ligament in the multi-ligament injured knee: An evidence-based systematic review. *Knee Surg Sports Traumatol Arthrosc* 2009;17(7):823-829.

   This systematic review examined evidence in the literature comparing outcomes of repair versus reconstruction of the MCL in multiligament knee injuries. Satisfactory results were observed with both techniques. Treatment decisions should be made on a case-by-case basis.

10. Harner CD, Waltrip RL, Bennett CH, Francis KA, Cole B, Irrgang JJ: Surgical management of knee dislocations. *J Bone Joint Surg Am* 2004;86(2):262-273.

    Outcomes after early versus delayed multiligament knee reconstruction were evaluated in 31 patients with knee dislocations at a minimum 2-year follow-up. Patients treated acutely demonstrated better clinical and functional outcomes than those treated more than 3 weeks postinjury.

11. Tzurbakis M, Diamantopoulos A, Xenakis T, Georgoulis A: Surgical treatment of multiple knee ligament injuries in 44 patients: 2-8 years follow-up results. *Knee Surg Sports Traumatol Arthrosc* 2006;14(8):739-749.

    Forty-eight patients with multiligament knee injuries were treated with acute or chronic surgical intervention and followed for a mean of 51.3 months. Analysis of functional outcome scores showed no statistically significant difference in surgical timing, although acute treatment generally led to higher scores.

12. Sems SA, Levy BA, Dajani K, Herrera DA, Templeman DC: Incidence of deep venous thrombosis after temporary joint spanning external fixation for complex lower extremity injuries. *J Trauma* 2009;66(4):1164-1166.

    This prospective study evaluated the incidence of deep venous thrombosis in 136 consecutive patients treated with early spanning external fixation and low–molecular weight heparin after high-energy lower extremity trauma, reporting a value of 2.1%, consistent with historical controls.

13. Cooper DE, Stewart D: Posterior cruciate ligament reconstruction using single-bundle patella tendon graft with tibial inlay fixation: 2- to 10-year follow-up. *Am J Sports Med* 2004;32(2):346-360.

    This study prospectively followed 41 patients with PCL reconstruction using a single-bundle bone-patellar tendon-bone graft tibial inlay fixation technique for 2 to 10 years, with excellent functional outcomes. This technique is recommended for PCL reconstruction.

14. Fanelli GC, Edson CJ: Arthroscopically assisted combined anterior and posterior cruciate ligament reconstruction in the multiple ligament injured knee: 2- to 10-year follow-up. *Arthroscopy* 2002;18(7):703-714.

15. Wascher DC, Becker JR, Dexter JG, Blevins FT: Reconstruction of the anterior and posterior cruciate ligaments after knee dislocation: Results using fresh-frozen nonirradiated allografts. *Am J Sports Med* 1999;27(2):189-196.

16. McAllister DR, Markolf KL, Oakes DA, Young CR, McWilliams J: A biomechanical comparison of tibial inlay and tibial tunnel posterior cruciate ligament reconstruction techniques: Graft pretension and knee laxity. *Am J Sports Med* 2002;30(3):312-317.

17. Markolf KL, Feeley BT, Jackson SR, McAllister DR: Biomechanical studies of double-bundle posterior cruciate ligament reconstructions. *J Bone Joint Surg Am* 2006;88(8):1788-1794.

    Biomechanical testing of double-bundle PCL reconstruction demonstrated that a single anterolateral graft best reproduced normal PCL force profiles but increased laxity at 0° to 30° of flexion. Adding a posteromedial graft reduced laxity but increased forces in the graft.

18. Whiddon DR, Zehms CT, Miller MD, Quinby JS, Montgomery SL, Sekiya JK: Double compared with single-bundle open inlay posterior cruciate ligament reconstruction in a cadaver model. *J Bone Joint Surg Am* 2008;90(9):1820-1829.

    Posterior tibial translation and external rotation after single- and double-bundle PCL tibial-inlay reconstruction were compared in nine cadaver knees with a deficient and repaired posterolateral corner. The double-bundle technique resulted in significantly greater rotational and anterior-posterior stability.

5: Lower Extremity

19. Fanelli G, Edson C, Reinheimer K, Beck J: Arthroscopic single-bundle versus double-bundle posterior cruciate ligament reconstruction (SS-46). *Arthroscopy* 2008;24: e26-e26.

This prospective study examined postoperative outcome scores after single- versus double-bundle PCL reconstruction in 90 consecutive patients followed for 15 to 72 months. Both techniques achieved excellent functional outcomes, with neither procedure demonstrating clear superiority over the other.

20. Wang CJ, Weng LH, Hsu CC, Chan YS: Arthroscopic single- versus double-bundle posterior cruciate ligament reconstructions using hamstring autograft. *Injury* 2004; 35(12):1293-1299.

This study compared outcomes after single- and double-bundle PCL reconstruction with hamstring autograft in 35 patients with minimum 2-year follow-up. No significant difference in clinical or functional outcomes was observed during this medium-term follow-up period.

21. Fanelli GC, Edson CJ: Combined posterior cruciate ligament-posterolateral reconstruction with Achilles tendon allograft and biceps femoris tendon tenodesis: 2 to 10 year follow up. *Arthroscopy* 2004;20:339-345.

The authors determined that chronic combined PCL injuries can be treated with arthroscopic PCL reconstruction using fresh-frozen Achilles tendon allograft with PCL reconstruction. Successful results and statistically significant improvement (*P* = .001) were noted. Level of evidence: IV.

22. Schechinger SJ, Levy BA, Dajani KA, Shah JP, Herrera DA, Marx RG: Achilles tendon allograft reconstruction of the fibular collateral ligament and posterolateral corner. *Arthroscopy* 2009;25(3):232-242.

FCL and PLC reconstruction via a single Achilles tendon allograft construct was evaluated in 16 knees (minimum 2-year follow-up). No significant difference in clinical or functional outcomes was observed between two-ligament and multiligament PLC-based reconstructions.

23. LaPrade RF, Ly TV, Wentorf FA, Engebretsen L: The posterolateral attachments of the knee: A qualitative and quantitative morphologic analysis of the fibular collateral ligament, popliteus tendon, popliteofibular ligament, and lateral gastrocnemius tendon. *Am J Sports Med* 2003;31(6):854-860.

The purpose of this study was to qualitatively and quantitatively determine the anatomic attachment sites of the main posterolateral knee structures and their relationships to pertinent bony landmarks. A cadaver study in which dissections were performed and measurements taken on 10 nonpaired fresh-frozen cadaver knees revealed that these structures had a consistent attachment pattern. This information will prove useful in the study of anatomic repair and reconstruction of the posterolateral structures of the knee.

24. John J, Wagner WW, Kuiper JH: Tension-band wiring of transverse fractures of patella: The effect of site of wire twists and orientation of stainless steel wire loop. A biomechanical investigation. *Int Orthop* 2007;31(5): 703-707.

The authors designed a biomechanical model to compare figure-of-8 tension band constructs. Figure-of-8 constructs positioned horizontally rather than vertically, had lower failure rates with cyclic loading. Location of wire twists influenced construct stability as well.

25. Hughes SC, Stott PM, Hearnden AJ, Ripley LG: A new and effective tension-band braided polyester suture technique for transverse patellar fracture fixation. *Injury* 2007;38(2):212-222.

The authors designed a model and rig to monitor fracture gap and compression with strain gauge assessment. Tension band constructs employing suture and wire were compared. Braided polyester constructs, although less rigid, offered favorable biomechanical characteristics, warranting their consideration for clinical use.

26. Sturdee SW, Templeton PA, Oxborrow NJ: Internal fixation of a patella fracture using an absorbable suture. *J Orthop Trauma* 2002;16(4):272-273.

27. Luna-Pizarro D, Amato D, Arellano F, Hernández A, López-Rojas P: Comparison of a technique using a new percutaneous osteosynthesis device with conventional open surgery for displaced patella fractures in a randomized controlled trial. *J Orthop Trauma* 2006;20(8): 529-535.

A randomized controlled study comparing percutaneous and open osteosynthesis of displaced noncomminuted patella fractures was performed. Percutaneous methods offered fewer complications, less pain, and higher functional scores up to 2 years.

28. El-Sayed AM, Ragab RK: Arthroscopic-assisted reduction and stabilization of transverse fractures of the patella. *Knee* 2009;16(1):54-57.

The results of 14 cases treated with arthroscopic assisted reduction and percutaneous screw stabilization of transverse patella fractures were assessed. The authors deemed this technique appropriate for lesions without significant separation or comminution. Good functional outcomes were achieved with only minimal complications.

29. Tandogan RN, Demirors H, Tuncay CI, Cesur N, Hersekli M: Arthroscopic-assisted percutaneous screw fixation of select patellar fractures. *Arthroscopy* 2002; 18(2):156-162.

30. Marder RA, Swanson TV, Sharkey NA, Duwelius PJ: Effects of partial patellectomy and reattachment of the patellar tendon on patellofemoral contact areas and pressures. *J Bone Joint Surg Am* 1993;75:35-45.

31. Matejcić A, Smiljanić B, Bekavac-Beslin M, Ledinsky M, Puljiz Z: The basket plate in the osteosynthesis of comminuted fractures of distal pole of the patella. *Injury* 2006;37(6):525-530.

An inferior pole basket plate was used to collect and incorporate comminuted fragments in a fixation construct. Fifty of more than 100 procedures were available for review, and a knee scoring system was applied. Excellent and good results were achieved in 46 cases. A protocol permitting full weight bearing and immediate range of motion was instituted.

32. Matejčić A, Puljiz Z, Elabjer E, Bekavac-Beslin M, Ledinsky M: Multifragment fracture of the patellar apex: Basket plate osteosynthesis compared with partial patellectomy. *Arch Orthop Trauma Surg* 2008;128(4):403-408.

A retrospective assessment of long-term results comparing inferior pole preservation and partial patellectomy was performed. The postoperative protocol in the former group, permitting immediate motion and weight bearing, was suggested to offer superior knee-scoring results.

33. Kastelec M, Veselko M: Inferior patellar pole avulsion fractures: Osteosynthesis compared with pole resection. *J Bone Joint Surg Am* 2004;86(4):696-701.

Long-term results were reviewed comparing two methods toward managing inferior pole patella fractures. Fourteen cases were assigned to each category, most of which were followed for almost 5 years. Osteosynthesis with patella pole preservation permitted restoration of patella height. This variable appeared to correlate favorably with functional outcome.

34. Gardner MJ, Griffith MH, Lawrence BD, Lorich DG: Complete exposure of the articular surface for fixation of patellar fractures. *J Orthop Trauma* 2005;19(2):118-123.

The authors offer a technical solution toward improved fixation and assessment of quality of reduction when managing complex comminuted fractures of the patella. An extended lateral parapatellar arthrotomy is performed and the patella internally rotated 90°. The retropatellar chondral surface is exposed and accessed in its entirety.

35. Clayton RA, Court-Brown CM: The epidemiology of musculoskeletal tendinous and ligamentous injuries. *Injury* 2008;39(12):1338-1344.

This is a study describing the epidemiology of adult musculoskeletal soft-tissue injuries. Demographic details over 5 years were recorded prospectively. Eighteen injury types were studied. A total of 2,794 patients presented with ligamentous or tendinous injuries over 5 years. Meniscal injury of the knee was the most common injury. All injuries were more common in males.

36. White DW, Wenke JC, Mosely DS, Mountcastle SB, Basamania CJ: Incidence of major tendon ruptures and anterior cruciate ligament tears in US Army soldiers. *Am J Sports Med* 2007;35:1308-1314.

Race is a risk factor for major tendon ruptures. All patients with surgical management for tendon rupture were evaluated for risk factors. There were 52 major tendon ruptures: 29 Achilles, 12 patellar, 7 pectoralis major, and 4 quadriceps tendon ruptures. The rate of major tendon rupture was 13 times greater for black men when compared with white men. Level of evidence: II.

37. Chin KR, Sodl JF: Infrapatellar fat pad disruption: A radiographic sign of patellar tendon rupture. *Clin Orthop Relat Res* 2005;440:222-225.

Disruption of the infrapatellar fat pad contour on radiographs is a sign of tendon rupture. Two blinded reviewers independently analyzed randomly selected lateral radiographs of the knees of 14 patients with knee injuries. Disruption in the contour was a reasonably reliable sign of patellar tendon rupture when used with the patient's history, physical examination, and other radiographic signs.

38. Hardy JR, Chimutengwende-Gordon M, Bakar I: Rupture of the quadriceps tendon: An association with a patellar spur. *J Bone Joint Surg Br* 2005;87(10):1361-1363.

This retrospective study evaluated the incidence of patellar osteophytes in 107 cases of extensor mechanism disruption. This concomitant pathology was found in 79% of patients with quadriceps tendon rupture and 27% of patients with patellar tendon rupture.

39. LaRocco BG, Zlupko G, Sierzenski P: Ultrasound diagnosis of quadriceps tendon rupture. *J Emerg Med* 2008;35(3):293-295.

A case report of bilateral quadriceps tendon rupture is presented, demonstrating the utility and ease of bedside ultrasound to rapidly confirm the diagnosis.

40. Goelitz BW, Lomasney LM, Demos TC: Radiologic case study: Quadriceps tendon rupture. *Orthopedics* 2004; 27(8):872-875.

Quadriceps tendon ruptures usually occur in people age 40 years or older who have underlying medical conditions. The injury is disabling and outcome is optimized with early management. The classic clinical symptoms may not be present, in which case radiographs, ultrasound, and MRI often are essential for early diagnosis.

41. Heyde CE, Mahlfeld K, Stahel PF, Kayser R: Ultrasonography as a reliable diagnostic tool in old quadriceps tendon ruptures: A prospective multicentre study. *Knee Surg Sports Traumatol Arthrosc* 2005;13(7):564-568.

This prospective study evaluated the use of ultrasonography in diagnosis of chronic quadriceps tendon rupture over 6 years in seven knees. Ultrasound is recommended as part of the diagnostic work-up with suspicion for knee tendon injuries.

42. Greis PE, Holmstrom MC, Lahav A: Surgical treatment options for patella tendon rupture: Part I. Acute. *Orthopedics* 2005;28(7):672-679.

In patients with a ruptured patella tendon that is promptly diagnosed, securely repaired, and followed closely throughout rehabilitation, good results can be expected. In acute injuries with inadequate tissue, augmentation with hamstring tendon or allograft generally is necessary.

43. Lighthart WA, Cohen DA, Levine RG, Parks BG, Boucher HR: Suture anchor versus suture through tunnel fixation for quadriceps tendon rupture: A biomechanical study. *Orthopedics* 2008;31(5):441.

This study compares biomechanical characteristics of transosseous suture and suture anchor techniques for quadriceps tendon repair. No significant difference was observed, and the use of suture anchor technique is justified.

44. Bhargava SP, Hynes MC, Dowell JK: Traumatic patella tendon rupture: Early mobilisation following surgical repair. *Injury* 2004;35(1):76-79.

Postoperative immobilization in a cast is unnecessary following suture repair of the patella tendon and retinacula protected by a cerclage wire. The differences between the operated and control knee at the time of assessment were a mean loss of power of 6% (range, 2% to 11%) when measuring concentric extension and a mean loss of power of 7% (range, 13% to an increase of 12%) in concentric flexion.

45. West JL, Keene JS, Kaplan LD: Early motion after quadriceps and patellar tendon repairs: Outcomes with single-suture augmentation. *Am J Sports Med* 2008; 36(2):316-323.

This case series retrospectively evaluated early mobilization after primary repair of extensor mechanism disruption augmented with a single no. 5 Ethibond suture. Satisfactory outcomes were observed in all 50 patients.

46. Chen SK, Lu CC, Chou PH, Guo LY, Wu WL: Patellar tendon ruptures in weight lifters after local steroid injections. *Arch Orthop Trauma Surg* 2009;129(3):369-372.

The purpose of this report is to describe incidence of rupture of the patellar tendon after multiple local steroid injections in weight lifters. Seven weightlifters with a history of multiple local steroid injections into the patellar tendon presented with ruptured patellar tendon. All seven athletes returned to full competition 18 months after surgery.

47. Busfield BT, Safran MR, Cannon WD: Extensor mechanism disruption after contralateral middle third patellar tendon harvest for anterior cruciate ligament revision reconstruction. *Arthroscopy* 2005;21(10):1268.

Although contralateral middle third patellar tendon autograft for primary and revision ACL reconstruction is established in the literature, extensor mechanism complications can occur. Technical considerations are important to avoid weakening the remaining patellar tendon insertion. Postoperative nerve blocks or local anesthetics may alter pain feedback for regulation of weight bearing and contribute to overload of the donor knee.

48. Rust PA, Tanna N, Spicer DD: Repair of ruptured quadriceps tendon with Leeds-Keio ligament following revision knee surgery. *Knee Surg Sports Traumatol Arthrosc* 2008;16(4):370-372.

The use of the Leeds-Keio ligament to reconstruct a neglected quadriceps tendon rupture following revision knee arthroplasty is described. The Leeds-Keio ligament has been used in the treatment of patellar tendon ruptures complicating primary knee arthroplasty with good results, but may, as this report shows, also be successfully applied to address deficiencies of the quadriceps tendon in the revision setting, with continued good function for 2 years.

49. Muratli HH, Celebi L, Hapa O, Biçimoğlu A: Simultaneous rupture of the quadriceps tendon and contralateral patellar tendon in a patient with chronic renal failure. *J Orthop Sci* 2005;10(2):227-232.

Simultaneous quadriceps and patellar tendon rupture is rare. Mechanical factors and coexisting systemic and local factors are taken into consideration in the pathogenesis of these ruptures. In patients with some chronic systemic diseases, simultaneous rupture can occur spontaneously or with minor traumas. The authors present a case of simultaneous quadriceps and patellar tendon rupture in a 21-year-old man with chronic renal failure. He was treated surgically with osseotendinous repair with suture anchors and supplemental cerclage wire fixation on both sides. He regained normal knee joint function 18 months after the operation.

50. Chen CM, Chu P, Huang GS, Wang SJ, Wu SS: Spontaneous rupture of the patellar and contralateral quadriceps tendons associated with secondary hyperparathyroidism in a patient receiving long-term dialysis. *J Formos Med Assoc* 2006;105(11):941-945.

Although spontaneous rupture of the extensor tendon of the knee is more likely to occur in uremic patients with secondary hyperparathyroidism, simultaneous ruptures of bilateral knee extensor tendons is rarely reported. The authors describe a 30-year-old man who sustained spontaneous simultaneous ruptures of the right patellar tendon and left quadriceps tendon 2 weeks after he underwent subtotal parathyroidectomy. The tendon ruptures were surgically repaired. The mechanism of spontaneous tendon rupture in uremic patients with secondary hyperparathyroidism seems to be related to high parathyroid hormone level, which results in osteolytic bone resorption at the tendon insertion site.

51. Cree C, Pillai A, Jones B, Blyth M: Bilateral patellar tendon ruptures: A missed diagnosis. Case report and literature review. *Knee Surg Sports Traumatol Arthrosc* 2007;15(11):1350-1354.

Disruption of the patellar tendon is often associated with systemic diseases such as rheumatoid arthritis and systemic lupus erythematosus. Surgical management is required to repair the patellar tendon after clinical assessment and diagnosis. The authors present the case of a 75-year-old man without any known predisposing systemic disease presenting on several occasions before accurate diagnosis and treatment.

52. Alpantaki K, Papadokostakis G, Katonis P, Hadjpavlou A: Spontaneous and simultaneous bilateral rupture of the quadriceps tendon: A case report. *Acta Orthop Belg* 2004;70(1):76-79.

Simultaneous bilateral rupture of the quadriceps tendon generally occurs in association with chronic metabolic disorders, such as chronic renal failure, obesity, diabetes mellitus, and secondary hyperparathyroidism. The case presented here is that of an 85-year-old man with no known risk factors who sustained simultaneous and spontaneous rupture of both quadriceps tendons. These findings suggest that quadriceps weakness as a result of spinal stenosis may have played a significant role in the pathogenesis of this injury.

53. Gokce A, Ekici H, Erdogan F: Arthroscopic reconstruction of a ruptured patellar tendon: A technical note. *Knee Surg Sports Traumatol Arthrosc* 2008;16(6):581-584.

A traumatic patellar tendon rupture of a 35-year-old patient was reconstructed with semi-tendinosis and gracilis tendons. It was demonstrated that arthroscopic reconstruction of a ruptured patellar tendon may be the optimal surgical choice to minimize trauma and begin early rehabilitation.

54. Park JW, Lee YS, Oh JK, Park JH, Lee JW, Park JS: Knee extensor mechanism reconstruction with an extended gastrocnemius flap and a saphenous neurocutaneous flap. *J Orthop Trauma* 2009;23(4):309-312.

An open comminuted patellar fracture was initially managed with a tension band and cerclage wiring and primary closure of the wound. Unfortunately, the fractured patella and overlying soft tissue became totally infected and a wide necrosis occurred. At 12 months after surgery, the patient showed complete extension, 135 degrees of flexion, and grade IV knee extensor power and was able to ambulate without a walking aid.

55. Lewis PB, Rue JP, Bach BR Jr: Chronic patellar tendon rupture: Surgical reconstruction technique using 2 Achilles tendon allografts. *J Knee Surg* 2008;21(2):130-135.

Delayed reconstruction of chronic patellar tendon ruptures classically has yielded suboptimal results. Quadriceps contracture, distal patella mobilization, quadriceps lengthening (for example, V-Y lengthening), prolonged postoperative immobilization, residual quadriceps weakness, surgical macrofailure, and loss of knee flexion are some of the complications associated with treatment for chronic patellar tendon rupture. Reinforcement hardware (cerclage wire) may necessitate subsequent removal and the possibility of breaking, with migration through the body. This article details use and short-term success of a surgical technique using two Achilles tendon allografts for reconstruction of a chronic patellar tendon rupture.

56. Milankov MZ, Miljkovic N, Stankovic M: Reconstruction of chronic patellar tendon rupture with contralateral BTB autograft: A case report. *Knee Surg Sports Traumatol Arthrosc* 2007;15(12):1445-1448.

Chronic patellar tendon rupture is a rare, disabling injury that is technically difficult to repair. Many different surgical methods have been reported for the reconstruction of chronic patellar tendon ruptures. This article reports on the use of contralateral bone-tendon-bone autograft for chronic patellar tendon rupture reconstruction followed by double-wire loop reinforcement without postoperative immobilization. The patient returned to playing basketball in his spare time, without having any limitation.

57. Greis PE, Lahav A, Holmstrom MC: Surgical treatment options for patella tendon rupture, part II: chronic. *Orthopedics* 2005;28(8):765-769.

Patella tendon rupture is a debilitating injury that often occurs in the setting of preexisting tendon degeneration. Prompt diagnosis and treatment is essential to prevent retraction of the patella with subsequent adhesions and quadriceps contractures. In the setting of a chronic rupture, augmentation with hamstring tendons or allograft reconstruction generally is necessary. Patients who undergo delayed repair are at risk for a compromised result secondary to loss of full knee flexion and decreased quadriceps strength, although a functional extensor mechanism is likely to be reestablished. The overall results of chronic repair are less satisfactory than the acute repair, but still provide an extensor mechanism for the patient and thus provide function.

58. Yepes H, Tang M, Morris SF, Stanish WD: Relationship between hypovascular zones and patterns of ruptures of the quadriceps tendon. *J Bone Joint Surg Am* 2008;90(10):2135-2141.

This study evaluates the vascularity of 33 cadaver quadriceps tendons via angiographic techniques after arterial perfusion with a preservative mixture. A hypovascular zone was consistently identified, warranting awareness of this zone's healing properties for decision-making regarding the need for surgical management.

59. Puranik GS, Faraj A: Outcome of quadriceps tendon repair. *Acta Orthop Belg* 2006;72(2):176-178.

This study is a retrospective analysis of patients who had surgical repair of their quadriceps tendon over a 13-year period, totaling 21 patients. Most of the patients returned to their preinjury level of activity. Patients who had direct repair of the tendon using the Bunnell technique had lower Rougraff scores than the rest.

60. Ramseier LE, Werner CM, Heinzelmann M: Quadriceps and patellar tendon rupture. *Injury* 2006;37(6):516-519.

This prospective study of 33 extensor mechanism disruptions evaluated risk factors and functional and isokinetic outcomes at minimum 2-year follow-up. Patients with multiple injuries demonstrated a significant reduction in muscle strength and circumference.

61. Wenzl ME, Kirchner R, Seide K, Strametz S, Jürgens C: Quadriceps tendon ruptures: Is there a complete functional restitution? *Injury* 2004;35(9):922-926.

In 35 patients with 36 traumatic ruptures of the quadriceps tendon, all without medical risk factors were treated surgically. The type of repair (direct or transosseous suture with or without augmentation), the kind of postoperative physiotherapy, age, and body mass index had no influence on the final outcome.

62. Bushnell BD, Whitener GB, Rubright JH, Creighton RA, Logel KJ, Wood ML: The use of suture anchors to repair the ruptured quadriceps tendon. *J Orthop Trauma* 2007;21(6):407-413.

Quadriceps tendon rupture is an incapacitating injury that usually requires surgical repair. Traditional repair methods involve transpatellar suture tunnels, but recent reports have introduced the idea of using suture anchors to repair the ruptured tendon. The authors discuss five cases in which suture anchors were used to repair the ruptured quadriceps tendon.

5: Lower Extremity

63. Karistinos A, Paulos LE: "Ciprofloxacin-induced" bilateral rectus femoris tendon rupture. *Clin J Sport Med* 2007;17(5):406-407.

This case report describes bilateral quadriceps tendon rupture attributed to the use of ciprofloxacin.

Chapter 36

Tibial Plateau Fractures

Thomas F. Higgins, MD   Erik P. Severson, MD

Introduction

Fractures of the tibial plateau comprise a wide range of periarticular injuries of varying severity. In addition to the osseous injury immediately apparent on radiographs, plateau fractures may be accompanied by soft-tissue injury to the ligaments and menisci as well as the surrounding muscle, capsular tissue, and skin. The past four decades have seen a marked shift toward surgical management of these injuries, which was led by early encouraging results of surgical treatment.[1]

The current surgical treatment of these injuries focuses on three goals: (1) restoring articular congruity, (2) restoring axial alignment and joint stability, and (3) treating associated soft-tissue injuries to minimize complications and maximize functional restoration. As additional data regarding patient outcomes become available, the long-term impact of these articular injuries on patients' lives and long-term function is gaining new respect.[2-4]

Incidence and Epidemiology

In the adult population, tibial plateau fractures can be separated into two broad categories. One category comprises high-energy injuries that usually occur in a younger population, and more often in males than females. The second group is composed of low-energy injuries, which often occur in an older population (usually female), and may be categorized as insufficiency fractures. The high-energy fracture patterns show a greater degree of comminution and carry a higher likelihood of associated soft-tissue damage and subsequent complications.

Classification

Two systems, the Orthopaedic Trauma Association (OTA)/AO classification system (**Figure 1**) and the

Dr. Higgins receives a teaching stipend from Smith-Nephew and AO North America for teaching of resident courses. Neither Dr. Severson nor any immediate family member has received anything of value from or owns stock in a commercial company or institution related directly or indirectly to the subject of this chapter.

Schatzker system (**Figure 2**) are predominantly used for classifying tibial plateau fractures, although neither system accounts for knee fracture–dislocations. Prior data have shown that the OTA/AO system has higher interobserver reliability, whereas the two systems have approximately equal intraobserver reliability.[5] Despite this, the Schatzker classification system has maintained widespread use. Types I through IV are unicondylar fractures and types V and VI are bicondylar. The bicondylar injuries are the most difficult to classify because they may include a variety of distinct fracture patterns, and many bicondylar injuries represent fracture–dislocations, which are fundamentally different from fractures without knee dislocation. A true Schatzker type V injury is rare and may be differentiated from a type VI fracture based on the presence of metaphyseal-diaphyseal dissociation in type VI injuries. A Schatzker type IV fracture is unicondylar on the medial side but may be accompanied by articular impaction in the central portion of the lateral condyle without violation of the lateral cortex. Displaced Schatzker type IV fractures, which should be considered the equivalent of a knee fracture–dislocation, have a higher rate of vascular and nerve injuries.[1,6,7] A study that used MRI to evaluate proximal tibial fractures questioned whether a Schatzker type III (isolated lateral compartment depression) fracture actually exists, noting that there appears to be an extension from the lateral depressions into the metaphyseal cortex visible on MRI in virtually all lateral tibial plateau fractures.[8]

A reliable method of grading soft-tissue swelling would be helpful in classifying tibial plateau fractures. The Tscherne classification system has been proposed to grade soft-tissue injury, but it is neither widely used nor highly reliable.

Physical Examination

In a patient with a tibial plateau fracture, an accurate physical examination of the injured limb is critical to planning and timing treatment. The initial examination should include circumferential inspection of the extremity to evaluate skin integrity and soft-tissue swelling and to rule out an open fracture. In addition to assessing the condition of the soft tissues, the examiner should determine if the injured limb is grossly shortened compared with the contralateral uninjured limb because this factor

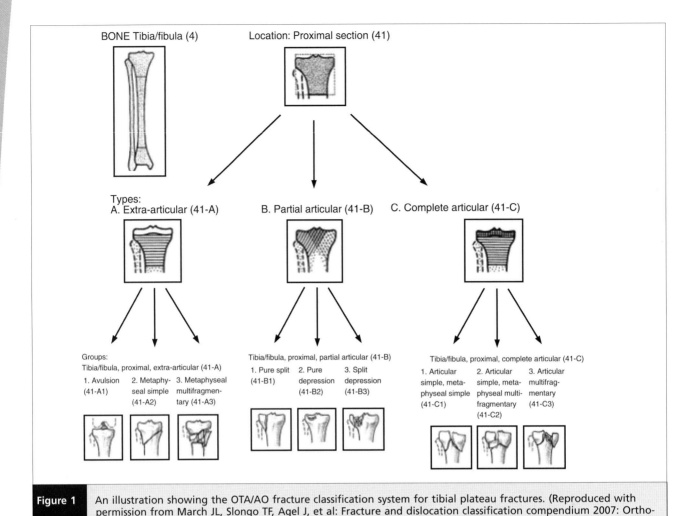

Figure 1 An illustration showing the OTA/AO fracture classification system for tibial plateau fractures. (Reproduced with permission from March JL, Slongo TF, Agel J, et al: Fracture and dislocation classification compendium 2007: Orthopaedic Trauma Association Classification, Database and Outcomes Committee. *J Orthop Trauma* 2007;21(suppl 10): S1-S163.)

may influence the decision for temporary spanning external fixation. Dorsalis pedis and tibial pulses can be assessed manually. Assuming an intact contralateral limb, pulses may be compared side to side. When pulses are asymmetric, the ankle brachial index may be assessed on each lower limb. An ankle-brachial index less than 0.8 or 0.9 is often an indication for further diagnostic vascular evaluation.[9] Complete motor and sensory examinations should be conducted, particularly to evaluate the possibility for compartment syndrome.

In the emergency department, if the diagnosis has been established with plain radiographs, a well-padded dressing and a splint or brace is generally placed across the knee to stabilize the limb before further imaging is attempted.

Imaging Studies

Routine AP and lateral radiographs are usually adequate to diagnose a tibial plateau fracture. For further assessment of the articular surface, a 10° caudal radiograph may be obtained in the AP plane. This view accounts for the posterior slope of the proximal tibial articular surface. Traction radiographs may be helpful in surgical planning in patients with highly comminuted or bicondylar tibial plateau injuries. These radiographs may be obtained with manual traction or after applying knee-spanning external fixation. Plain radiographs of lateral plateau fractures may be useful in predicting lateral meniscal injury.[10] A finding of greater than 5 mm of articular depression and 6 mm of widening is predictive of lateral meniscal pathology.

Axial CT scans, with or without two- or three-dimensional reconstruction, can provide excellent detail of the bony anatomy and have become a standard part of the diagnostic algorithm at most centers. CT may be most helpful in identifying an intra-articular depression that may be obscured by overlying fracture lines. CT also aids in assessing the size, location, plane, and displacement of the posteromedial fragment in bicondylar injuries.

During the past 7 years, there has been a growing interest in the use of MRI for evaluating tibial plateau fractures. Studies have shown the value of MRI in identifying meniscal and cruciate pathology as well as in further delineating subtle nondisplaced fracture lines.[8,11]

Associated Soft-Tissue Injuries

The importance of identifying compartment syndrome in a patient with a tibial plateau fracture cannot be overemphasized. When a fasciotomy is indicated, the surgeon must consider placement of incisions to permit subsequent definitive internal fixation. The incidence of compartment syndrome in tibial plateau fractures ranges from 14% to 22%.[6,12-14] Determining the incidence of open tibial plateau fractures is difficult because of the heterogeneous nature of the studies in the literature. In studies of higher-energy tibial plateau fractures, the open fracture rate has been reported to range from 4% to 13%.[12,14]

The incidence of meniscal and cruciate pathology in patients with tibial plateau fractures is likely much higher than once believed. A retrospective review of the arthroscopic assessment of 98 tibial plateau fractures showed a soft-tissue injury in 71% of all knees, with a meniscal injury in 57% and an anterior cruciate injury in 25%.[15] CT has been shown to predict torn ligaments with 80% sensitivity and 98% specificity; however MRI is needed to reliably detect meniscal pathology.[16]

An MRI study of all types of tibial plateau fractures showed a complete tear or avulsion of one or more of the cruciate or collateral ligaments in 77%, evidence of lateral meniscal pathology in 91%, and medial meniscal tears in 44%.[8] Tears of one or more of the posterolateral corner structures of the knee occurred in 68% of tibial plateau fractures. However, 60% of the fractures in this study were Schatzker type II, representing only a small cross section of the tibial plateau fracture population. A small study of tibial plateau fractures treated nonsurgically showed 80% with meniscal tears and 40% with complete ligament disruptions.[17]

The significance of these findings and their impact on the eventual management of tibial plateau fractures is unclear. Debate exists regarding whether a cruciate ligament injury with a tibial plateau fracture should be treated acutely at the time of osteosynthesis or if expectant management is best. This question remains unanswered.

Staged Treatment

Immediate open reduction and internal fixation (ORIF) of very swollen tibial plateau fractures has led to soft-tissue complications.[12,18-20] In bicondylar plateau fractures with a high degree of swelling, a staged treatment protocol has been adopted by many centers.[12,18] The protocol entails bridging external fixation (with or without fasciotomies, as indicated) in the first 24 hours

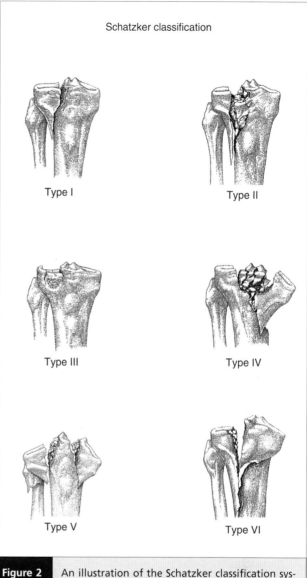

Schatzker classification

Type I

Type II

Type III

Type IV

Type V

Type VI

| Figure 2 | An illustration of the Schatzker classification system for tibial plateau fractures. Type I, lateral plateau split; type II, lateral split-depression; type III, lateral depression; type IV, medial plateau fracture; type V, bicondylar injury; and type VI, tibial plateau fracture with metaphyseal-diaphyseal dissociation. (Reproduced from Beaty JH, ed: *Orthopaedic Knowledge Update 6.* Rosemont, IL, American Academy of Orthopaedic Surgeons, 1999, 521-532.) |

after admission, followed by close monitoring of the soft tissues until the treating surgeon deems the tissue envelope safe for surgical treatment. The decision for immediate surgery versus delayed surgery may be based on the presence or absence of wrinkles in the skin about the knee and on the surgeon's experience in judging the condition of the soft tissues. Even with a staged protocol and treatment by an experienced surgeon, high rates of complications and deep infection (ranging from 5.9% to 27%) occur in patients with severe injuries.[12,13,19]

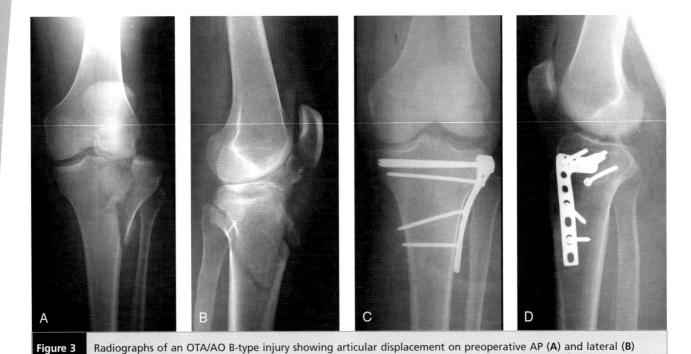

Figure 3 Radiographs of an OTA/AO B-type injury showing articular displacement on preoperative AP (**A**) and lateral (**B**) views. AP (**C**) and lateral (**D**) views after treatment of this B-type injury with nonlocking buttress fixation.

Nonsurgical Treatment

A compelling argument for nonsurgical treatment was based on a study of 131 tibial plateau fractures. Valgus alignment of up to 5°, articular step-off up to 3 mm, and condylar widening up to 5 mm resulted in minimal long-term ill effects.[21] In this study, any varus malalignment or medial unicondylar fractures with instability were indications for surgical treatment. A subsequent outcome study suggested that axial alignment may potentially be an equally important prognostic outcome factor as articular congruity.[3] Currently, the nonsurgical management of tibial plateau fractures is more frequently elected for elderly patients.

Most of the indications for surgical treatment are predicated on restoring articular congruity and axial alignment. Cartilage defects in the proximal tibia produce changes in trabecular bone strain that are postulated to be associated with the subsequent development of posttraumatic arthritis.[22] It has been shown that increasing articular step-off in the lateral compartment leads to significant increases in average and peak contact pressures as well as increasing valgus malalignment.[23] Articular step-off that is less than the thickness of the cartilage may be tolerated and compensated for, at least in an animal model.[24]

Internal Fixation

Biomechanics

Tibial plateau fractures may be caused by a combination of axial loading, three-point bending, and shear forces. Ideally, the selected internal or external fixation repair construct should resist the forces likely to reproduce fracture displacement. Maintaining articular reduction and the stability of metaphyseal alignment are primary goals when selecting a method of fixation.

The advent of locking plates has led to widespread use of these devices around the metaphysis for the stabilization of articular and metaphyseal injuries. In the tibial plateau, particularly, there has been active debate regarding the isolated use of locking implants on the lateral aspect of the proximal tibia. Many investigators have performed biomechanical studies to determine whether a single lateral locked plate provides an adequately secure construct to prevent varus displacement of the medial metaphysis in a bicondylar injury and if it can maintain reduction of posteromedial fracture fragments when they are present.[25-27] A definitive answer to this debate has not been achieved. Some authors have shown that lateral locked fixation alone is adequate to maintain alignment of the medial articular surface,[13,28] whereas others have advocated the need for a separate incision and buttress plating to treat the posteromedial side.[26,29-31] The clinical application of isolated lateral locked plating for bicondylar injuries has led to malreduction rates ranging from 13% to 26%.[13,28] Unicondylar injuries in healthy bone should usually be treated with nonlocking buttress fixation (**Figure 3**). In a few patients with severe osteopenia, unicondylar injuries may benefit from fixation with locking periarticular implants.

"Rafting" of the articular surface is most often used to maintain articular reduction. This technique entails spreading screws across the subchondral region of the bone immediately under the articular surface in an effort to maintain articular reduction and support the articular surface against further subsidence (**Figure 4**).

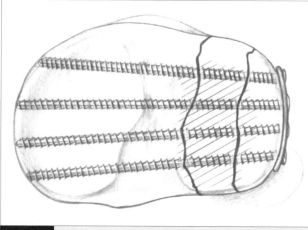

Figure 4 Illustration of the tibial plateau surface, as viewed from above, with rafting screws splayed out across the subchondral region of the bone immediately under the articular surface to maximize support of the articular surface and maintain articular reduction.

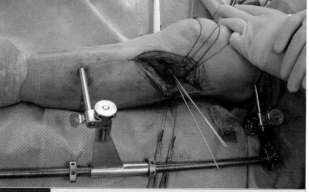

Figure 5 Intraoperative photograph showing placement of a femoral distractor to assist in reducing alignment and visualizing the joint surface.

Bone graft substitutes have gained popularity for use in supporting the disimpacted plateau articular surface.[32-34] A prospective randomized trial showed greater resistance to articular subsidence when a bone void was filled with calcium phosphate cement compared with bone graft,[33] corroborating the findings of a 2005 cadaver study.[34]

Surgical Approaches and Indications

Lateral Approach

A lateral approach to the proximal tibia may be used with a so-called hockey stick or inverted L incision immediately lateral to the tubercle, elevating the proximal aspect of the anterior compartment from the metaphyseal proximal tibia. More often, a lazy S approach is used, with a gentler curve extending up to the lateral aspect of the distal thigh, allowing wider exposure at the level of the knee. A straight midline incision has been advocated by some, but does not offer the same visualization of the posterior portion of the lateral plateau. Dissection is taken down to the level of the iliotibial band, which may be divided in line with fibers or in line with the skin incision. The soft tissues of the anterior compartment are elevated off the proximal tibial metaphysis and the capsule is incised. The lateral meniscus is identified and should be inspected for tears and tagged for subsequent repair. The meniscus is generally elevated off the lateral plateau for better visualization.

A large femoral distractor may be applied between the femur and the tibia. Pin placement should allow adequate visualization of the joint both directly and radiographically (**Figure 5**). This approach is most frequently used in isolation for lateral unicondylar injuries or may be used in conjunction with a secondary approach for bicondylar injuries.

Posteromedial Approach

The need to identify the posteromedial articular fragment of the tibial plateau has gained attention in recent years.[23,31] This fragment is found in more than 50% of bicondylar injuries and comprises approximately 25% of the joint surface. Failure to identify and reduce this fragment may lead to poor results (**Figure 6**). To achieve reduction and apply buttress fixation directly, a posteromedial approach, which entails a medially based incision just posterior to the posteromedial border of the tibia and extending proximally over the medial hamstrings, is most commonly used. The tendons of the pes anserinus are identified and the medial aspect of the gastrocnemius muscle is elevated off the posteromedial metaphysis. The popliteus is elevated directly off the bone. This dissection may be extended proximally or distally. Arthrotomy and articular visualization may also be achieved. A femoral distractor can be used on the medial side. Lateral and posteromedial approaches may often be used in concert for bicondylar injuries.

Direct Posterior Approach

The Lobenhoffer approach has been advocated for the direct approach to posterior shear fractures.[35] This prone approach facilitates adequate visualization and stabilization of posterior fragments but may complicate the ability to treat the anterolateral surface of the joint, if necessary. This approach uses an incision along the direct posterior aspect toward the medial side. The gastrocnemius muscle is elevated and the medial head of the gastrocnemius muscle may be released. The popliteus is elevated and the exposure may be taken from the posteromedial border of the tibia to the fibula. Visualization of the meniscus as well as direct repair of the posterior cruciate ligament can be achieved with this approach.

Approaches to Treat Isolated Medial Fractures

For isolated medial fractures, a posteromedial approach, a direct medial approach, or a midline parapa-

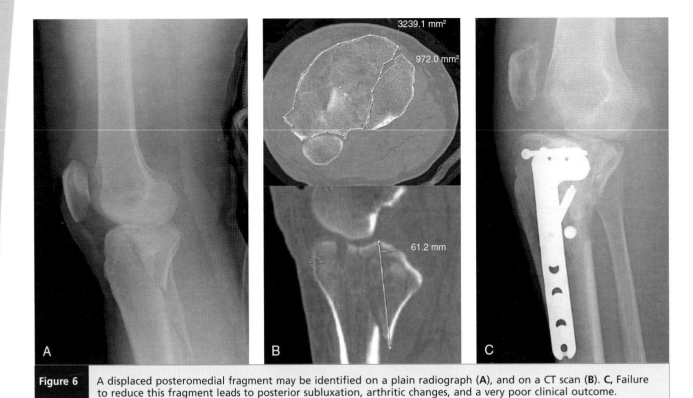

Figure 6 A displaced posteromedial fragment may be identified on a plain radiograph (**A**), and on a CT scan (**B**). **C**, Failure to reduce this fragment leads to posterior subluxation, arthritic changes, and a very poor clinical outcome.

tellar anterior approach raising a full-thickness medial flap have been advocated.[36]

Fixation Techniques

Internal Fixation

Prior to attempting ORIF, the readiness of the soft-tissue envelope should be evaluated. This may best be determined through serial examinations, the absence of blisters, and the surgeon's judgment. The timing of internal fixation in the setting of fasciotomies remains somewhat controversial. Recent data suggest that proceeding with internal fixation in the presence of open fasciotomies results in a soft-tissue or bone infection complication rate similar to that achieved by waiting for the fasciotomies to be closed and sealed. [37]

The patient is generally placed supine on a radiolucent table. A bump may be placed under the ipsilateral hip to maximize the exposure of the lateral side or under the contralateral hip to maximize exposure of the posteromedial side while in the supine position. Regional anesthetic should not be used because it may disguise the development of postoperative compartment syndrome. A tourniquet may be placed, and the lower extremity should be prepped and draped free. Prepping the external fixation frame, if present, is done at the surgeon's discretion. The frame may be used intraoperatively as a means of distraction to aid reduction. If two incisions are planned, both should be drawn on the skin (before any incision is made) to assess the skin

bridge before retracting the tissues.

If a second incision is planned, both incisions may be opened simultaneously. Some surgeons treat the posteromedial corner first, whereas others treat the lateral side first.[30] Articular reduction is obtained and metaphyseal/diaphyseal alignment is reestablished (**Figure 7**).

For unicondylar injuries, nonlocking buttress fixation should be adequate except in severe osteopenic bone. Rafting of the joint may be done primarily or after reestablishment of the metaphyseal-diaphyseal relationship. If lateral locked fixation is used in a bicondylar injury, nonlocked buttress fixation is usually adequate to buttress the medial side.

Fluoroscopy should be used to obtain AP, lateral, and possibly 10° caudad AP views to correctly assess the articular congruity. Other landmarks that should be fluoroscopically assessed include flexion or extension of one condyle relative to the other, restoration of condylar width, and anterior to posterior widening on the medial side. The relationship between the joint surface and the diaphysis may be difficult to interpret fluoroscopically and may require intraoperative plain radiography before definitive fixation is completed.

At the conclusion of internal fixation, closure is completed based on the surgeon's preference. Some surgeons leave the anterior compartment fascia open if the incision has already been extended well into the diaphysis. The swelling and vascular status of the leg should be assessed at this point. The leg is generally placed in a soft dressing and a removable brace. Ideally, passive range of motion begins immediately postoperatively.[38]

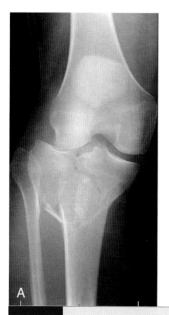
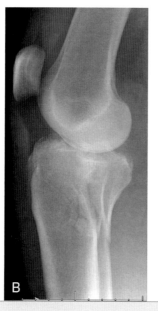
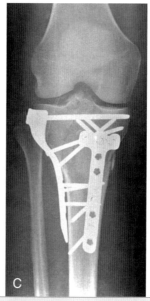
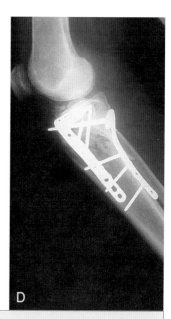

Figure 7   AP (**A**) and lateral (**B**) radiographs of a displaced bicondylar fracture. AP (**C**) and lateral (**D**) radiographs after ORIF. Good functional and radiographic results were achieved.

The long-term benefit of therapy with a continuous passive motion machine after a tibial plateau fracture has not been established.

Complications of internal fixation are well established.[12,13,19,30] The deep infection rate for high-energy bicondylar tibial plateau fractures ranges from 8% to 22%.

Thin Wire Fixation

For many surgeons, thin wire fixation is the preferred method of treating bicondylar injuries with significant diaphyseal extension, and this technique may be most advantageous when a swollen or tenuous soft-tissue envelope is present.[39-43] Conversely, this technique is contraindicated in B-type (partial articular) fractures. The principles of thin wire fixation are the same as for standard internal fixation. Small incisions may be made about the joint to obtain articular reduction. With this technique, internal fixation may be placed percutaneously to maintain the reduction. Thin wires about the joint are then placed and tensioned to a circular frame. Alignment to the diaphysis is then definitively established.

In a multicenter, prospective, randomized trial, percutaneous reduction and application of a circular fixator resulted in a shorter hospital stay, a marginally faster return of function, and similar clinical outcomes compared with patients treated with standard ORIF with medial and lateral plates.[44] The number and severity of complications was much higher in the group treated with standard ORIF compared with the group treated with thin wire fixation.

Outcomes

Overall

A study of 131 tibial plateau fractures followed over a 9-year period (average follow-up, 7.6 years) attempted to identify factors associated with the development of posttraumatic arthritis.[3] Seventy-six of the fractures were treated surgically and 55 were treated nonsurgically. Moderate and severe forms of osteoarthritis occurred more frequently in the surgical group, perhaps as the result of selection bias because more severe injuries are indicated for surgical treatment. Four primary risk factors for progression of osteoarthritis were identified: meniscectomy during surgery, axial malalignment, intra-articular infection, and joint instability.

In a retrospective review, the long-term functional results of the surgical treatment of tibial plateau fractures using ORIF were assessed. Forty-seven fractures in 46 patients (average age, 40 years) with an average follow-up of 8.3 years were reviewed. Although a high rate of secondary procedures was required, a high rate (92%) of good functional outcomes was reported in patients younger than 40 years at the time of injury, which were similar to age-matched control subjects. Using 36-Item Short Form scores, approximately 43% of the patients older than 40 years at the time of injury scored worse than age-matched control subjects. Despite the report of comparable 36-Item Short Form scores in the patients younger than 40 years with age-matched control subjects, it should be noted that in this group only 17 of 25 patients (68%) were able to return to full-time employment.[14]

Open Reduction and Internal Fixation

A 2006 study highlighted both the importance of articular reduction and the significant residual dysfunction that occur in patients with high-energy bicondylar plateau fractures.[2] This study calls into question previous studies that suggest that residual articular incongruity of the tibial plateau does not compromise long-term functional outcomes. The authors reported that 17 of 31 patients (55%) had a satisfactory articular reduction of 2 mm or less of step-off or gap, but 28 of 31 (90%) obtained satisfactory coronal plane alignment. A correlation between a lower functional outcome score and an inaccurate articular reduction was identified. Increasing patient age and the presence of polytrauma contributed to worse musculoskeletal functional assessment scores. It was concluded that the severity of an injury to the tibial plateau is associated with the functional outcome and that a satisfactory reduction positively affects patient outcome.

The complication rates for dual-plating internal fixation of high-energy tibial plateau fractures showed an 8.4% deep infection rate, a 3.6% rate of pyarthrosis, and a 19.3% rate of deep venous thrombosis.[12] A 14% deep infection rate in 29 bicondylar fractures was reported in a 2007 study.[19] In a retrospective review of 42 surgically repaired tibial plateau fractures, a 31% failure rate for internal fixation was reported, with the highest failure rates in elderly patients.[45]

Thin Wire Fixation

Authors of a randomized trial comparing ORIF and circular frame thin wire fixation of bicondylar tibial plateau fractures reported no significant differences at 2-year follow-up in Hospital for Special Surgery knee scores, Western Ontario and McMaster Universities Osteoarthritis Index scores, and arc of motion.[44] The quality of reduction was deemed similar in both groups. The deep infection rate (18%) and the number of unplanned secondary procedures were higher in the group treated with standard ORIF.

A retrospective study reviewed the results of combined thin wire circular frame fixation with limited internal fixation performed over an 11-year period in 129 fractures in 127 patients.[41] At 5-year follow-up, 38 of 129 fractures (29%) had excellent results, 63 of 129 (49%) had good results, 18 of 129 (14%) had fair results, and 10 of 129 (8%) had poor results based on patient questionnaire responses. A statistically significant correlation was recorded between the magnitude of the articular step-off and the radiologic result. An interesting finding in this study was the worsening of the radiologic results between the 3- and 5-year follow-up. This change also correlated with loss of knee motion.

Minimally Invasive Surgery

Percutaneous plating of tibial plateau factures in the United States was largely introduced using the Less Invasive Stabilization System (LISS; Synthes USA, Paoli, PA). Most reports to date specifically detail experience with this device. Short-term clinical results from a prospective study using the LISS plate and a minimally invasive technique were reported in a 2004 study.[46] All fractures were Schatzker types V or VI, and 34 fractures were followed for a minimum of 1 year. All fractures united at a mean of 15.6 weeks with a mean knee range of motion from 1° extension (range, 0° to 10°) to 127° flexion (range, 90° to 145°). The overall incidence of infection was 5.9%. LISS plate removal was needed in 10 of 34 patients (29%).

In a study of complication rates of LISS plate fixation in complex proximal tibia injuries, 37 patients were followed until fracture union was achieved and wound healing was completed.[13] Complications were reported in 25 of 37 patients (68%), including 22% with deep infection and 8% with loss of alignment.

Elderly Patients

Multiple reports have shown that older age at the time of sustaining a tibial plateau fracture is associated with a poorer outcome.[14,45] However, a 2004 study showed that the surgical treatment of 39 fractures in patients older than 55 years achieved acceptable clinical and radiographic results in 80% of the patients, and that preexisting arthritis did not correlate with outcomes.[47] Of note, insufficiency fractures of the tibial plateau in elderly patients may go undiagnosed based on plain radiography.

Total knee arthroplasty (TKA) may eventually be needed to treat some tibial plateau fractures. TKA may be more technically demanding when performed in a patient with a prior tibial plateau fracture, and TKA outcomes have a markedly diminished success rate in this patient population.[48,49] In a study of 62 TKAs in patients with prior tibial plateau fractures (61% had been surgically repaired), a significant improvement in knee scores for both pain and function were reported; however, there was a 26% postoperative complication rate and a 21% reoperation rate.[49] With a minimum 5-year follow-up of 15 TKAs after ORIF of a tibial plateau fracture, 4 of 15 patients (27%) had poor wound healing, 2 of 15 (13%) required prosthesis removal and subsequent arthrodesis, 2 of 15 (13%) had patella tendon rupture within the first month of TKA, and 3 of 15 (20%) required manipulation for poor motion.[48] In TKAs done in patients with tibial plateau fractures and prior infections, previously infected knees were 4.1 times more likely to require a secondary procedure compared with knees with no prior infection.[50]

Arthroscopically-Assisted ORIF

Arthroscopically assisted ORIF has produced satisfactory results based on clinical and radiographic studies. This technique had primarily been used to treat Schatzker types I through III fractures, but the recent literature has shown similar results in bicondylar injuries.[51,52] Proposed advantages of arthroscopically assisted ORIF include the benefit of intra-articular lavage, easier retrieval of intra-articular loose bodies, and the capability to perform a complete diagnostic ligamentous examination and to directly visualize the intra-articular reduction. Concerns with the technique include the development of compartment syndrome, prolonged surgical time, and a steep learning curve for the surgeon.[53,54]

Summary

The evaluation and treatment of tibial plateau fractures must include an understanding of the injury mechanism (high- or low-energy), associated soft-tissue injuries, the patient's age and physical demands, and radiographic and clinical goals.

If surgical treatment is indicated, the focus should be on restoring articular congruity and axial alignment, treating the soft-tissue envelope, and minimizing further complications. Careful treatment may yield satisfactory results for patients, but more comprehensive data are needed on the overall functional outcomes of patients with these fractures.

Annotated References

1. Schatzker J, McBroom R, Bruce D: The tibial plateau fracture: The Toronto experience 1968–1975. *Clin Orthop Relat Res* 1979;138:94-104.

2. Barei DP, Nork SE, Mills WJ, Coles CP, Henley MB, Benirschke SK: Functional outcomes of severe bicondylar tibial plateau fractures treated with dual incisions and medial and lateral plates. *J Bone Joint Surg Am* 2006;88(8):1713-1721.

   This comprehensive review of ORIF for 83 bicondylar plateau fractures showed that age, polytrauma, and articular reduction correlated with patient outcomes. Patients showed significant residual dysfunction compared with normative data.

3. Honkonen SE: Degenerative arthritis after tibial plateau fractures. *J Orthop Trauma* 1995;9(4):273-277.

4. Weigel DP, Marsh JL: High-energy fractures of the tibial plateau: Knee function after longer follow-up. *J Bone Joint Surg Am* 2002;84(9):1541-1551.

5. Walton NP, Harish S, Roberts C, Blundell C: AO or Schatzker? How reliable is classification of tibial plateau fractures? *Arch Orthop Trauma Surg* 2003;123(8): 396-398.

6. Stark E, Stucken C, Trainer G, Tornetta P III: Compartment syndrome in Schatzker type VI plateau fractures and medial condylar fracture-dislocations treated with temporary external fixation. *J Orthop Trauma* 2009; 23(7):502-506.

   This retrospective review of 67 patients reported an 18% rate of compartment syndrome for Schatzker type VI fractures and a more than 50% rate for medial fracture-dislocations.

7. Wahlquist M, Iaguilli N, Ebraheim N, Levine J: Medial tibial plateau fractures: A new classification system. *J Trauma* 2007;63(6):1418-1421.

   Although the new classification system described in this article may be of limited value, the study confirms the increased rate of soft-tissue compromise and compartment syndrome in medial plateau fractures.

8. Gardner MJ, Yacoubian S, Geller D, et al: The incidence of soft tissue injury in operative tibial plateau fractures: A magnetic resonance imaging analysis of 103 patients. *J Orthop Trauma* 2005;19(2):79-84.

   A high rate of meniscal and cruciate pathology was documented in this study, which predominantly reviewed lateral plateau fractures.

9. Johansen K, Lynch K, Paun M, Copass M: Non-invasive vascular tests reliably exclude occult arterial trauma in injured extremities. *J Trauma* 1991;31(4):515-519.

10. Gardner MJ, Yacoubian S, Geller D, et al: Prediction of soft-tissue injuries in Schatzker II tibial plateau fractures based on measurements of plain radiographs. *J Trauma* 2006;60(2):319-323.

    The authors correlate plain radiographic findings with MRI results for meniscal pathology in lateral plateau fractures.

11. Mustonen AO, Koivikko MP, Lindahl J, Koskinen SK: MRI of acute meniscal injury associated with tibial plateau fractures: Prevalence, type, and location. *AJR Am J Roentgenol* 2008;191(4):1002-1009.

    An incidence study on meniscal injury from the radiology literature is presented.

12. Barei DP, Nork SE, Mills WJ, Henley MB, Benirschke SK: Complications associated with internal fixation of high-energy bicondylar tibial plateau fractures utilizing a two-incision technique. *J Orthop Trauma* 2004; 18(10):649-657.

    This review of 83 patients with OTA/AO type 41-C3 fractures treated with dual incisions and plating showed an 8.4% rate of deep infection and a 19.3% rate of DVT. Dysvascular limbs requiring repair were significantly associated with infection. This paper showed that staged management, two approaches, and proper soft-tissue handling may lead to lower complication rates than previously reported for bicondylar injuries.

13. Phisitkul P, McKinley TO, Nepola JV, Marsh JL: Complications of locking plate fixation in complex proximal tibia injuries. *J Orthop Trauma* 2007;21(2):83-91.

    A retrospective review of the LISS plate when used in high-energy proximal tibial fractures showed a high complication rate (68%), including malalignment (8%) and infection (22%).

14. Stevens DG, Beharry R, McKee MD, Waddell JP, Schemitsch EH: The long-term functional outcome of operatively treated tibial plateau fractures. *J Orthop Trauma* 2001;15(5):312-320.

5: Lower Extremity

15. Abdel-Hamid MZ, Chang CH, Chan YS, et al: Arthroscopic evaluation of soft tissue injuries in tibial plateau fractures: Retrospective analysis of 98 cases. *Arthroscopy* 2006;22(6):669-675.

    A review of the surgical records documenting the rate of cruciate and meniscal injury in tibial plateau fractures is presented.

16. Mui LW, Engelsohn E, Umans H: Comparison of CT and MRI in patients with tibial plateau fracture: Can CT findings predict ligament tear or meniscal injury? *Skeletal Radiol* 2007;36(2):145-151.

    The authors of this study report that CT may be reasonably sensitive for cruciate pathology but inadequate for meniscal imaging.

17. Shepherd L, Abdollahi K, Lee J, Vangsness CT Jr: The prevalence of soft tissue injuries in nonoperative tibial plateau fractures as determined by magnetic resonance imaging. *J Orthop Trauma* 2002;16(9):628-631.

18. Egol KA, Tejwani NC, Capla EL, Wolinsky PL, Koval KJ: Staged management of high-energy proximal tibia fractures (OTA types 41): The results of a prospective, standardized protocol. *J Orthop Trauma* 2005;19(7):448-455.

    A staged technique of external fixation and delayed ORIF used at two centers to treat 57 patients with high-energy proximal tibial fractures showed a low rate of wound complications but residual knee stiffness.

19. Shah SN, Karunakar MA: Early wound complications after operative treatment of high energy tibial plateau fractures through two incisions. *Bull NYU Hosp Jt Dis* 2007;65(2):115-119.

    The authors present a retrospective review of 29 patients with high-energy tibial plateau fractures who were treated with a two-incision technique. A 14% infection rate was reported.

20. Young MJ, Barrack RL: Complications of internal fixation of tibial plateau fractures. *Orthop Rev* 1994;23(2):149-154.

21. Honkonen SE: Indications for surgical treatment of tibial condyle fractures. *Clin Orthop Relat Res* 1994;302:199-205.

22. McKinley TO, Bay BK: Trabecular bone strain changes associated with cartilage defects in the proximal and distal tibia. *J Orthop Res* 2001;19(5):906-913.

23. Bai B, Kummer FJ, Sala DA, Koval KJ, Wolinsky PR: Effect of articular step-off and meniscectomy on joint alignment and contact pressures for fractures of the lateral tibial plateau. *J Orthop Trauma* 2001;15(2):101-106.

24. Trumble T, Allan CH, Miyano J, et al: A preliminary study of joint surface changes after an intraarticular fracture: A sheep model of a tibia fracture with weight bearing after internal fixation. *J Orthop Trauma* 2001;15(5):326-332.

25. Gösling T, Schandelmaier P, Marti A, Hufner T, Partenheimer A, Krettek C: Less invasive stabilization of complex tibial plateau fractures: A biomechanical evaluation of a unilateral locked screw plate and double plating. *J Orthop Trauma* 2004;18(8):546-551.

    This cadaveric study was not able to show any difference between these two constructs for vertical subsidence.

26. Higgins TF, Klatt J, Bachus KN: Biomechanical analysis of bicondylar tibial plateau fixation: How does lateral locking plate fixation compare to dual plate fixation? *J Orthop Trauma* 2007;21(5):301-306.

    This biomechanical study reported less articular subsidence with medial and lateral nonlocked plating than with lateral locked plating in a bicondylar plateau fracture model.

27. Mueller KL, Karunakar MA, Frankenburg EP, Scott DS: Bicondylar tibial plateau fractures: A biomechanical study. *Clin Orthop Relat Res* 2003;412:189-195.

28. Gosling T, Schandelmaier P, Muller M, Hankemeier S, Wagner M, Krettek C: Single lateral locked screw plating of bicondylar tibial plateau fractures. *Clin Orthop Relat Res* 2005;439:207-214.

    The authors of a multicenter review of 69 bicondylar fractures fixed with lateral locked plating showed 9% postoperative varus and an 11% subsequent varus loss of reduction.

29. Barei DP, O'Mara TJ, Taitsman LA, Dunbar RP, Nork SE: Frequency and fracture morphology of the posteromedial fragment in bicondylar tibial plateau fracture patterns. *J Orthop Trauma* 2008;22(3):176-182.

    A review of 57 bicondylar plateau fractures with medial involvement showed 74% had a posteromedial fragment, accounting for 23% of the joint surface; the fracture line was usually vertically oriented.

30. Eggli S, Hartel MJ, Kohl S, Haupt U, Exadaktylos AK, Röder C: Unstable bicondylar tibial plateau fractures: A clinical investigation. *J Orthop Trauma* 2008;22(10):673-679.

    The authors present the result of a small study of ORIF via a two-incision technique, specifically starting with medial buttress plating.

31. Higgins TF, Kemper D, Klatt J: Incidence and morphology of the posteromedial fragment in bicondylar tibial plateau fractures. *J Orthop Trauma* 2009;23(1):45-51.

    A review of 111 bicondylar plateau fractures confirmed the frequency (65%) and vertical morphology of the posteromedial fragment.

32. Lobenhoffer P, Gerich T, Witte F, Tscherne H: Use of an injectable calcium phosphate bone cement in the treatment of tibial plateau fractures: A prospective study of twenty-six cases with twenty-month mean follow-up. *J Orthop Trauma* 2002;16(3):143-149.

33. Russell TA, Leighton RK, Alpha-BSM Tibial Plateau

Fracture Study Group: Comparison of autogenous bone graft and endothermic calcium phosphate cement for defect augmentation in tibial plateau fractures: A multicenter, prospective, randomized study. *J Bone Joint Surg Am* 2008;90(10):2057-2061.

This prospective randomized trial showed that less articular subsidence occurs with cement than with bone graft.

34. Trenholm A, Landry S, McLaughlin K, et al: Comparative fixation of tibial plateau fractures using alpha-BSM, a calcium phosphate cement, versus cancellous bone graft. *J Orthop Trauma* 2005;19(10):698-702.

This cadaver study showed less articular subsidence with the use of calcium phosphate cement than with cancellous bone graft.

35. Fakler JK, Ryzewicz M, Hartshorn C, Morgan SJ, Stahel PF, Smith WR: Optimizing the management of Moore type I postero-medial split fracture dislocations of the tibial head: Description of the Lobenhoffer approach. *J Orthop Trauma* 2007;21(5):330-336.

Description and case examples of the direct posterior approach for posterior shear fractures are presented.

36. Espinoza-Ervin CZ, Starr AJ, Reinert CM, Nakatani TQ, Jones AL: Use of a midline anterior incision for isolated medial tibial plateau fractures. *J Orthop Trauma* 2009;23(2):148-153.

An alternative approach is described for ORIF of isolated medial plateau fractures.

37. Zura RD, Adams SB Jr, Jeray KJ, Obremskey WT, Stinnett SS, Olson SA; for the Southeastern Fracture Consortium Foundation: Timing of definitive fixation of severe tibial plateau fractures with compartment syndrome does not have an effect on the rate of infection. *J Trauma* 2010 May 20 [Epub ahead of print].

This retrospective review of 81 patients with tibial plateau fractures and four compartment fasciotomies could not establish a difference in infection rate among those who underwent osteosynthesis before, during, or after definitive fasciotomy closure.

38. Gausewitz S, Hohl M: The significance of early motion in the treatment of tibial plateau fractures. *Clin Orthop Relat Res* 1986;202:135-138.

39. Gaudinez RF, Mallik AR, Szporn M: Hybrid external fixation of comminuted tibial plateau fractures. *Clin Orthop Relat Res* 1996;328:203-210.

40. Hall JA, Beuerlein MJ, McKee MD; Canadian Orthopaedic Trauma Society: Open reduction and internal fixation compared with circular fixator application for bicondylar tibial plateau fractures: Surgical technique. *J Bone Joint Surg Am* 2009;91(suppl 2 pt 1):74-88.

The surgical technique of skinny wire fixation versus ORIF for bicondylar tibial plateau fractures is described.

41. Katsenis D, Dendrinos G, Kouris A, Savas N, Schoino-choritis N, Pogiatzis K: Combination of fine wire fixation and limited internal fixation for high-energy tibial plateau fractures: Functional results at minimum 5-year follow-up. *J Orthop Trauma* 2009;23(7):493-501.

Review of 129 fractures treated with skinny wire frames showed a high incidence of posttraumatic arthrosis but satisfactory functional results.

42. Marsh JL, Smith ST, Do TT: External fixation and limited internal fixation for complex fractures of the tibial plateau. *J Bone Joint Surg Am* 1995;77(5):661-673.

43. Watson JT, Ripple S, Hoshaw SJ, Fhyrie D: Hybrid external fixation for tibial plateau fractures: Clinical and biomechanical correlation. *Orthop Clin North Am* 2002;33(1):199-209.

44. Canadian Orthopaedic Trauma Society: Open reduction and internal fixation compared with circular fixator application for bicondylar tibial plateau fractures: Results of a multicenter, prospective, randomized clinical trial. *J Bone Joint Surg Am* 2006;88(12):2613-2623.

A nationwide prospective randomized trial of fixation with a circular fixator compared with ORIF show similar results for both techniques. The group treated with ORIF had a higher complication rate.

45. Ali AM, El-Shafie M, Willett KM: Failure of fixation of tibial plateau fractures. *J Orthop Trauma* 2002;16(5):323-329.

46. Stannard JP, Wilson TC, Volgas DA, Alonso JE: The less invasive stabilization system in the treatment of complex fractures of the tibial plateau: Short-term results. *J Orthop Trauma* 2004;18(8):552-558.

All fractures were Schatzker types V or VI, and 34 fractures were followed for a minimum of 1 year. All fractures united at a mean of 15.6 weeks with a mean knee range of motion from 1° extension (range, 0° to 10°) to 127° flexion (range, 90° to 145°). The overall incidence of infection was 5.9%. LISS plate removal was needed in 10 of 34 patients (29%).

47. Su EP, Westrich GH, Rana AJ, Kapoor K, Helfet DL: Operative treatment of tibial plateau fractures in patients older than 55 years. *Clin Orthop Relat Res* 2004;421:240-248.

This retrospective review of 39 older patients with tibial plateau fractures with mean follow-up of 2.5 years showed increasing age was associated with poorer clinical and self-assessment scores, but pre-existing degenerative joint disease was not.

48. Saleh KJ, Sherman P, Katkin P, et al: Total knee arthroplasty after open reduction and internal fixation of fractures of the tibial plateau: A minimum five-year follow-up study. *J Bone Joint Surg Am* 2001;83-A(8):1144-1148.

49. Weiss NG, Parvizi J, Trousdale RT, Bryce RD, Lewallen DG: Total knee arthroplasty in patients with a prior fracture of the tibial plateau. *J Bone Joint Surg Am* 2003;85-A(2):218-221.

5: Lower Extremity

50. Larson AN, Hanssen AD, Cass JR: Does prior infection alter the outcome of TKA after tibial plateau fracture? *Clin Orthop Relat Res* 2009;467(7):1793-1799.

    TKA after a tibial plateau fracture with a history of infection results in a fourfold increase in the risk for a secondary procedure.

51. Chan YS, Chiu CH, Lo YP, et al: Arthroscopy-assisted surgery for tibial plateau fractures: 2- to 10-year follow-up results. *Arthroscopy* 2008;24(7):760-768.

    The authors present their findings of a retrospective review of clinical and radiographic outcomes in 54 patients, including those with bicondylar injuries.

52. Rossi R, Bonasia DE, Blonna D, Assom M, Castoldi F: Prospective follow-up of a simple arthroscopic-assisted technique for lateral tibial plateau fractures: Results at 5 years. *Knee* 2008;15(5):378-383.

    A follow-up study of lateral plateau fractures repaired with arthroscopic assistance showed satisfactory clinical and radiographic results.

53. Belanger M, Fadale P: Compartment syndrome of the leg after arthroscopic examination of a tibial plateau fracture: Case report and review of the literature. *Arthroscopy* 1997;13(5):646-651.

54. Lubowitz JH, Elson WS, Guttmann D: Part I: Arthroscopic management of tibial plateau fractures. *Arthroscopy* 2004;20(10):1063-1070.

    This review article includes a detailed technique description for arthroscopically-aided repair of tibial plateau fractures.

Chapter 37

Fractures of the Tibial Shaft

Michael J. Prayson, MD   David Dalstrom, MD   Michael Sirkin, MD

Introduction

Tibial shaft fractures are the most common type of large long-bone fractures. Successful treatment involves evaluating multiple factors, including bony and soft-tissue injuries, along with early recognition of complications to avoid adverse outcomes. As indications for surgical management evolve, a thorough understanding of the varying injury patterns as well as functional expectations for different treatments will help optimize clinical outcomes.

Evaluation and Classification

The well-established Advanced Trauma Life Support guidelines should be used to initially assess a patient with a tibial shaft fracture. Early evaluation begins with a detailed neurovascular examination of the injured limb and a careful assessment of associated soft-tissue injuries. Radiographs of the extremity, including the knee and ankle, are paramount in detailing the extent of bony injury and assisting in the initial treatment decisions.

The potential for the development of a compartment syndrome should be considered early in the evaluation process.[1,2] Clinical assessment and vigilance remain the cornerstones to early recognition of compartment syndrome. Intracompartmental pressure measurements serve as an adjunct to clinical assessment in equivocal cases and aid in the diagnosis of compartment syndrome in the obtunded or uncooperative patient. Fasciotomies serve as definitive treatment and are generally considered when the pressure difference (Δ-P) between the diastolic pressure and intracompartmental

Dr. Prayson or an immediate family member serves as a board member of Wright State Physicians; is a member of a speakers' bureau or has made paid presentations on behalf of Smith & Nephew and Synthes; serves as a paid consultant to Smith & Nephew; and has received research or institutional support from Synthes, Smith & Nephew, I-Flow, Aquacel, the Orthopaedic Trauma Association, and DAGMEC. Dr. Dalstrom or an immediate family member has stock or stock options held in Roche. Dr. Sirkin or an immediate family member has received royalties from Biomet; serves as a paid consultant to or is an employee of Biomet; and has received research or institutional support from Biomet, Synthes, Smith & Nephew, Wright Medical Technology, and the Musculoskeletal Transplant Foundation.

pressure falls below 30 mm Hg. Other noninvasive methods for early detection of compartment syndrome have been investigated with varying results and may hold promise for the future.[3,4]

Bony injury is initially described by the location of the fracture (proximal, middle, or distal) and the fracture pattern (transverse, spiral, segmental, or comminuted). The Orthopaedic Trauma Association classification system ensures consistent communication of fracture location and pattern and is currently favored by surgeons and investigators.[5] The tibial diaphysis is designated as "42," and the fracture is assigned an associated letter (A through C) representing increasing amounts of fracture comminution and complexity (Figure 1). Additional subcategories indicate the presence and level of any associated fibular fracture.

Soft-tissue injury in closed tibial shaft fractures is typically described according to the classification system of Oestern and Tscherne[6] (Table 1). The management of soft-tissue injuries should occur concomitantly with fracture management. Versatility with bone stabilization methods combined with modern soft-tissue and wound care approaches can optimize limb salvage and functional outcomes. In certain instances, the soft-tissue injury warrants a multiple-stage treatment approach (Figure 2). Such staged surgical management is less common in midtibial fractures in comparison with those of the proximal and distal ends of the bone.

Open tibial shaft fractures are most commonly classified according to the system of Gustilo and Anderson, developed in 1976 and later modified in 1984[7,8] (Table 2). This classification scheme is widely used for all open fractures and serves as a basis for treatment decisions as well as comparison of published treatment results. The interobserver reliability, however, has been shown in several studies to be moderate at best.[9,10] Therefore, caution is warranted for management recommendations and studies based on its use. Current principles for open tibial fracture care are detailed in the literature. The traditional 6-hour window for surgical débridement of open fractures has been challenged in the recent literature. Although several studies have reported no increase in the infection rate if surgical débridement of an open fracture is performed after 6 to 8 hours,[11,12] there have been no strong recommendations for delaying treatment of an open fracture. There does not, however, appear to be a statistically significant increase in infection rates if débridement is delayed be-

5: Lower Extremity

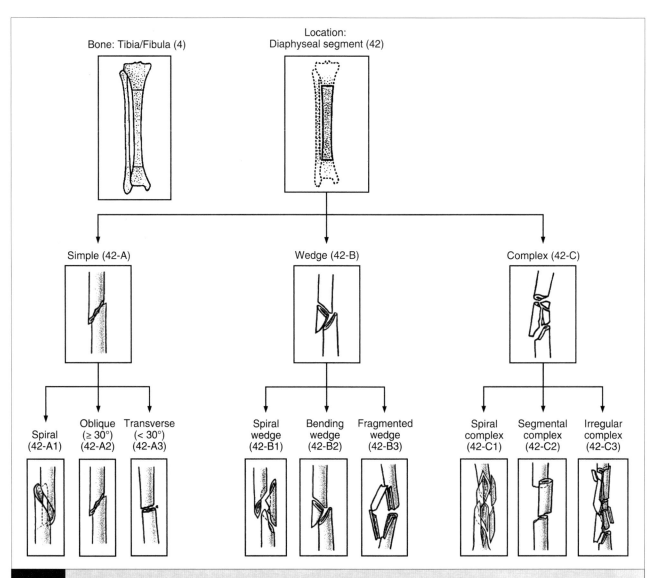

Figure 1 Illustration showing the Orthopaedic Trauma Association classification of tibial diaphyseal fractures. (Reproduced with permission from Marsh JL, Slongo TF, Agel J, et al: Fracture and Dislocation Classification Compendium 2007: Orthopaedic Trauma Association Classification, Database and Outcomes Committee. *J Orthop Trauma* 2007;21[suppl 10]:S1-S163.)

Table 1

Oestern and Tscherne Classification of Closed-Fracture Soft-Tissue Injury

Grade	Description
0	Injuries from indirect forces with negligible soft-tissue damage
I	Superficial contusion/abrasion, simple fractures
II	Deep abrasions, muscle/skin contusion; direct trauma, impending compartment syndrome
III	Excessive skin contusion; crushed skin or destruction of muscle, subcutaneous degloving, acute compartment syndrome, and rupture of major blood vessel or nerve

Reproduced with permission from Oestern HJ, Tscherne H: Pathophysiology and classification of soft tissue injuries with fractures, in Tscherne H, Gotzen L (eds): *Fractures With Soft Tissue Injuries*. Berlin, Germany: Springer-Verlag, 1984, pp 1-9.

yond 6 hours. Certain conditions (for example, gross contamination, substantial muscle damage, neurovascular compromise, or evolving compartment syndrome) demand emergent surgical intervention. Early prophylactic antibiotics remain a critical aspect of initial care. Placing antibiotic beads has been shown to reduce the incidence of infection, especially in more severe types of open fractures. More information on soft-tissue injuries is available in chapter 6.

Choosing a treatment method for a tibial shaft fracture requires consideration of fracture stability, the need for observation and management of associated soft-tissue injuries, and the need for restoration of limb length, alignment, and rotation. Early joint range of motion and patient mobility also should be considered, particularly in a polytraumatized patient.

Treatment Choices

Nonsurgical Treatment

Traditionally, nonsurgical treatment has been recommended for the more stable fracture patterns characterized by more than 50% cortical overlap, minimal initial shortening, and only minor comminution. Acceptable fracture reduction for continued nonsurgical treatment includes less than 1 to 1.2 cm of shortening, less than 5° to 8° of coronal plane angulation, less than 10° of sagittal plane angulation, and less than 5° of malrotation.[13,14] Relative contraindications to nonsurgical care include the inability to tolerate prolonged cast or brace treatment, the presence of an intact fibula (Figure 3), unstable fracture patterns, open fractures, concomitant compartment syndrome, a floating knee, and fractures with neurovascular injury.

The incidence of malunion is consistently higher in patients with closed tibial shaft fracture who are treated with casting compared with those treated surgically. The incidence of problematic malunion is unknown and likely varies among individuals. Patients treated with intramedullary nail fracture stabilization had better results for time to union, function, and Medical Outcomes Study Short Form-36 Health Survey (SF-36) scores compared with those treated with casting.[15] With nonsurgical treatment, an intact fibula will serve as a lateral-sided strut and commonly lead to varus malunion or nonunion.[16]

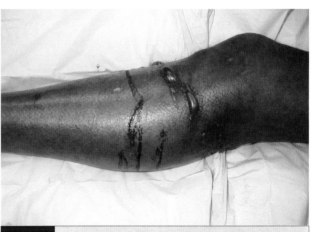

Figure 2 A clinical photograph of a high-energy tibial shaft fracture with significant soft-tissue swelling and blistering. Intracompartmental pressure measurements were taken to confirm the clinical suspicion of lower leg compartment syndrome.

Table 2

Classification of Open Fractures

Type	Wound	Level of Contamination	Soft Tissue Injury	Bone Injury
I	< 1 cm long	Clean	Minimal	Simple, minimal comminution
II	> 1 cm long	Moderate	Moderate, some muscle damage	Moderate comminution
III[a]				
A	Usually >10 cm long	High	Severe with crushing	Usually comminuted: soft tissue coverage of bone possible
B	Usually >10 cm long	High	Very severe loss of coverage; usually requires soft tissue reconstructive surgery	Bone coverage poor; variable, may be moderate to severe comminution
C	Usually >10 cm long	High	Very severe loss of coverage plus vascular injury requiring repair; may require soft-tissue reconstructive surgery	Bone coverage poor; variable, may be moderate to severe comminution

[a] Segmental fractures, farmyard injuries, fractures occurring in a highly contaminated environment, shotgun wounds, or high-velocity gunshot wounds automatically result in classification as type III open fracture.
Reproduced with permission from Chapman MW: The role of intramedullary fixation in open fractures. *Clin Orthop* 1986;212:27.

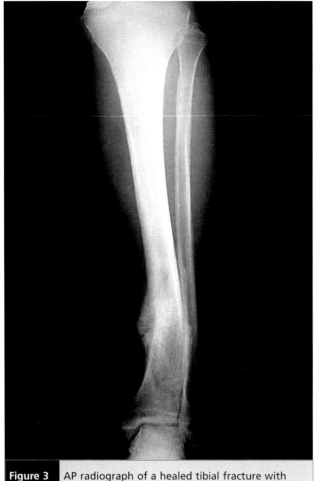

Figure 3 AP radiograph of a healed tibial fracture with varus angulation in the presence of an intact fibula.

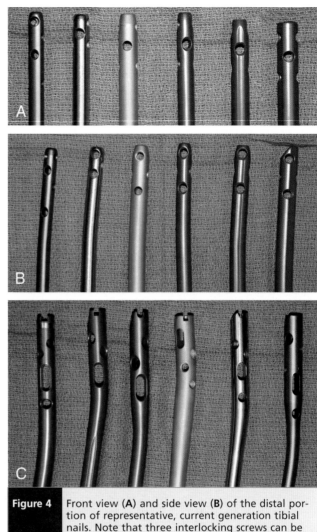

Figure 4 Front view (**A**) and side view (**B**) of the distal portion of representative, current generation tibial nails. Note that three interlocking screws can be placed within 3 cm from the distal tip of the nails. Side view (**C**) of the proximal portion of the same nails shows a similar ability to achieve multiplanar interlocking for proximally located fractures.

Surgical Treatment

Consideration for the surgical treatment of a tibial shaft fracture should begin with a discussion of the potential surgical risks, including infection, malunion, nonunion, the possible need for future surgeries, anterior knee pain, hardware irritation, and the potential for limb loss.[17-20] Definite indications for surgical treatment include an open fracture, the inability to maintain acceptable alignment with closed treatment, concomitant compartment syndrome, ipsilateral femoral fracture, and a severe soft-tissue injury requiring graft or flap coverage.

Many methods have been developed for the definitive surgical management of tibial shaft fractures. Most surgeons prefer to implant an intramedullary nail to stabilize both closed and open tibial diaphyseal fractures. Other methods, such as external fixation and plating, are considered based on various factors such as surgeon experience, fracture location and severity, and the degree of soft-tissue injury. With modern nail designs, more proximal and distal fractures can be successfully treated with intramedullary implants[21-23] (Fig-

ure 4). Recently, high rates of associated ankle injury have been reported and should prompt closer inspection of the ankle joint (**Figure 5**). Pronation-eversion patterns, spiral fracture patterns, proximal fibular fractures, and an intact fibula may be associated risk factors for unrecognized ankle joint injury.[24]

After intramedullary nailing, long-term outcomes have generally been good. SF-36 and Short Musculoskeletal Functional Assessment (SMFA) scores are similar to reference population norms. Knee pain, ankle stiffness, and quadriceps atrophy are cited as common residual sequelae.[25]

Definitive treatment of tibial shaft fractures through external fixation has traditionally been reserved for patients with medullary canal diameters of less than 8 mm, open physes, severe open fractures, or complex periarticular injuries. More commonly, external fixa-

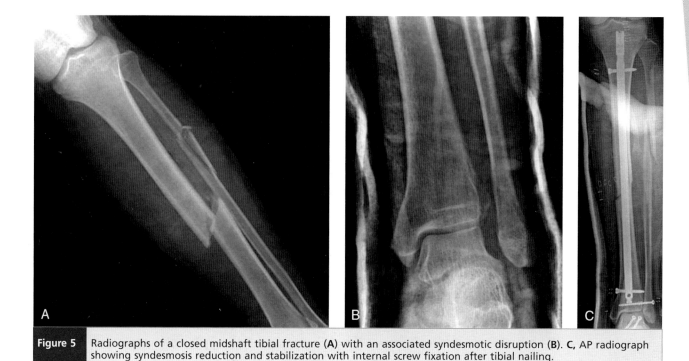

Figure 5 Radiographs of a closed midshaft tibial fracture (**A**) with an associated syndesmotic disruption (**B**). **C,** AP radiograph showing syndesmosis reduction and stabilization with internal screw fixation after tibial nailing.

tion is used as provisional stabilization for fractures in unstable trauma victims or for fractures with significant contamination and soft-tissue injury. Recently, the safety and timing of conversion to definitive fixation with intramedullary nails have been studied. In an evidence-based analysis of the literature, sequential tibial nailing following external fixation results in an infection rate average of 9% and a union rate average of 90%. A length of external fixation with 28 days reduces the risk of infection by 83% in the tibia.[26] Other relative indications for external fixation include significant intramedullary contamination that cannot be thoroughly cleaned or the need for a second surgical evaluation of the intramedullary canal. Reevaluation of muscle damage behind the fracture is also an indication for temporizing external fixation. The fixator can be loosened, the fracture displaced, and the muscle or intramedullary canal examined as needed.

External fixation has achieved promising results in managing severe limb-threatening injuries from blast or high-velocity gunshot wounds with deep contamination and segmental bone loss.[27] For the treatment of severe combined bony and soft-tissue injuries, the Taylor Spatial Frame (Smith & Nephew, Memphis, TN) allows the combination of acute shortening and/or angulation (to facilitate wound closure), and subsequent gradual alignment restoration.[28] Although early results are encouraging, such indications for external fixation remain controversial. Successful treatment of the tibia using external fixation remains technically challenging.

Open reduction and internal fixation of diaphyseal tibial fractures with plates and screws has notably declined since the popularization of intramedullary nail fixation.[29] Plate utilization in this area has diminished because of several concerns, including soft-tissue stripping, bony fragment devitalization, periosteal blood supply disruption, and complications such as infection.[30] Plate fixation continues to be a viable option in two circumstances: (1) the treatment of proximal and distal metadiaphyseal tibial fractures, especially those with an articular extension, and (2) when intramedullary nailing is difficult or contraindicated, such as below a total knee prosthesis or if previous deformity precludes the use of intramedullary fixation.

The use of plating versus nailing in extra-articular distal tibial fractures between 4 and 11 cm proximal to the tibial plafond has been retrospectively studied.[31] Lower rates of delayed union, malunion, and secondary procedures have been reported with plating of these injuries. In a study of minimally invasive plate osteosynthesis in high-energy distal tibial fractures with little to no articular involvement, a high rate of reoperation (35%) and a prolonged time to union (22%) was reported in this patient population.[32] Risk factors identified for poor healing include open fractures, highly comminuted fractures, and bone loss. Early intervention (bone grafting) was recommended within 8 to 10 weeks after the injury if little callus formation was seen along the lateral or posterolateral cortex. Plating also has been used in combination with intramedullary fixation. A 2008 study detailed the treatment of unicondylar tibial plateau fractures combined with noncontiguous shaft fractures.[33] Excellent results were reported using minimally invasive plating techniques in concert with intramedullary nail stabilization.

5: Lower Extremity

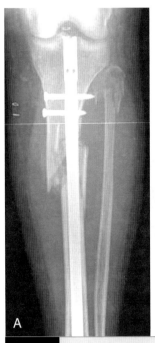
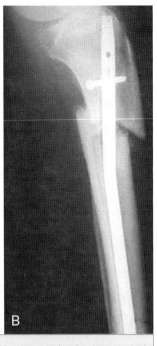

Figure 6 AP (**A**) and lateral (**B**) radiographs showing typical deformities seen with intramedullary nailing of a proximal tibia fracture. The deformities include valgus, procurvatum (apex anterior angulation), and posterior translation.

Reduction Techniques

Proper intramedullary nail insertion begins with precisely locating the proximal entry site. Three starting points, the medial parapatellar, the transpatellar, and the suprapatellar, have been used for placing a tibial nail. The medial parapatellar and transpatellar portals are most commonly used for routine diaphyseal fractures. Entry into the bone is slightly medial to the lateral tibial spine on the AP radiographic view, colinear with the anatomic axis of the medullary canal. On the lateral view, the proper entry portal begins directly adjacent to the anterior articular margin. Prior to intramedullary reaming and nail placement, achieving adequate reduction of the fracture is mandatory, especially for metaphyseal fractures. The implant should not be relied on to reduce the fracture. Most often, reduction is obtained using a combination of traction and local manipulation with the aid of intraoperative fluoroscopy. Traction can be provided manually or with an external fixator or universal distractor. Additional techniques (for example, blocking [Poller] screws, unicortical plates, joy sticks, and percutaneously placed clamps) have been used to obtain and maintain reduction in complicated or problematic fracture patterns.

Metadiaphyseal fractures are particularly prone to malalignment because of the mismatch between the canal and implant diameters. Proper entry portal place-ment is paramount for minimizing iatrogenic malalignment from the implant insertion, and is critical when nailing a fracture in the proximal third of the tibia. The lateral parapatellar approach can be used to keep the nail directed laterally and to avoid valgus malalignment. The suprapatellar portal, coupled with maintaining the knee in a semiextended position, has recently gained acceptance for this indication.[22] This approach minimizes the procurvatum deformity created by the nail and the extensor mechanism. Care must be taken to avoid intra-articular cartilaginous injury when using the suprapatellar portal. Reduced knee pain also has been cited as a potential advantage of this approach, although comparative studies of outcomes of these various approaches, including knee pain, have not been performed in a prospective fashion. Poller screws, which artificially constrain the implant within the medullary cavity and work to counter the forces causing malreduction, can also reduce the potential for malalignment.[34] Such screws serve as new boundaries or cortices (cortical substitution) for the nail. Poller screws are especially helpful in treating proximal third tibial fractures.[35] These fractures are prone to valgus malalignment, apex anterior (procurvatum) deformity, and posterior translation secondary to deforming forces on the proximal tibial segment (**Figure 6**). Strategies to treat this problematic fracture include a more lateral and vertical starting point, placing poller screws lateral and posterior to the intended intramedullary nail path, and placing the proximal interlocking screws with the knee in relative extension.[22]

Provisional unicortical plates have been used for reducing and stabilizing open fractures before intramedullary nail placement.[36] The plate is placed prior to insertion of the intramedullary nail, often through minimal incision(s).[37] Unicortical plates may be retained or removed after nail stabilization, depending on the fracture. No increased risk of infection has been reported using limited open reduction techniques for closed tibial shaft fractures.[38]

The use of percutaneously placed reduction clamps to obtain acceptable reduction before reaming and placing intramedullary nails in the tibia has been described. Placing such clamps may result in improved reduction and minimal disruption to the soft-tissue envelope surrounding the tibia (**Figure 7**). Good results have been reported using these techniques without a concomitant increase in morbidity.

Adjuncts to Nailing and Healing

A notable amount of recent research has focused on treatment strategies designed to improve the rate of union of tibial shaft fractures, both by altering techniques and through the use of adjunctive measures.

There is an ongoing debate regarding the use of reaming in the preparation of the tibial canal before intramedullary nail insertion. The Study to Prospectively

Evaluate Reamed Intramedullary Nails in Tibial Fractures found no significant difference between the results achieved with either reamed or unreamed intramedullary nailing of open tibial shaft fractures.[39] This multicenter randomized trial included more than 1,300 patients treated at 29 clinical sites by more than 200 surgeons. The primary outcome measure was reoperation after 6 months. Closed tibial fractures treated with reamed intramedullary nails had an 11% reoperation rate, whereas those treated with unreamed techniques required additional procedures 17% of the time. It was believed that reaming had a possible effect on closed fracture union. Surgeons were not permitted to reoperate during the 6-month period following the initial procedure to allow time for adequate healing. A higher rate of nonunion was reported in patients who both smoked and were treated with reamed intramedullary nailing for an open fracture. Patients with closed fractures had better 1-year SF-36 and SMFA scores than those with open fractures; patients with isolated tibial shaft fractures had superior outcomes compared with polytraumatized patients.[39]

The treatment of an associated fibular fracture also has been investigated. It has been shown in a cadaver study that fibular fixation (using plate fixation or Enders nails) did not substantially reduce tibial defect motion in cadaveric specimens stabilized with locked intramedullary nails in the tibia.[40] A positive impact of concomitant fibular fixation does appear to exist as the fracture level approaches the ankle. Fewer losses of tibial reductions (4% versus 13%) were reported when fibular fractures were stabilized in conjunction with distal tibial intramedullary nailing.[41]

There has been increasing use of bone morphogenetic protein (BMP) to augment the healing of problematic tibial shaft fractures.[42-45] BMP-2 is currently approved for use in open tibial shaft fractures treated with intramedullary nailing within 14 days of injury. Contraindications for BMP use include pregnancy, skeletal immaturity, active infection, current or previous history of cancer, and known allergy to the product. Treatment with recombinant BMP-2 has shown promising results with a 44% decrease in delayed union, faster overall rates of union, fewer hardware failures, and a significant reduction in infections for type III open tibial shaft fractures (24% with versus 44% without).[45]

Bone stimulation can be used as an adjunct for accelerating bone healing or union. In a randomized, double-blinded trial of tibial fractures treated nonsurgically, in which 67 patients were assigned to receive ultrasound bone stimulation or treatment with a placebo control device, the authors reported accelerated clinical (86 days versus 114 days) and radiographic (96 days versus 154 days) healing. Other studies have reported some success with the use of an electrical version of external bone stimulation.[46]

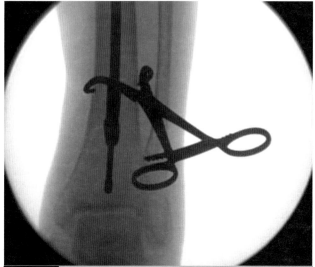

| **Figure 7** | Intraoperative fluoroscopic image of a distal tibial fracture shows anatomic reduction secured with a percutaneous clamp. When used, the clamp should be maintained through placement of the guidewire, reaming, insertion of the nail, and nail interlocking. Strategic placement is warranted so as not to crush adjacent soft tissues with the clamp itself. |

Deterrents to Healing

Nonsteroidal anti-inflammatory medication has been shown to inhibit fracture healing.[47] Recent evidence shows that cyclooxygenase-2 (COX-2)-specific agents deter healing more than their nonspecific counterparts in an animal model.[48] If given within the first 2 weeks of fracture occurrence, fracture healing is impaired. If COX-2 agents are given after 2 weeks or before the fracture occurred, there appears to be no detrimental effects on fracture healing.[49]

Smoking has been shown to impair fracture healing. Smokers with limb-threatening open tibial fractures have an increased time to union and a greater infection rate.[50] Injured patients with a previous history of smoking are at higher risk for nonunion, osteomyelitis, and other complications.[51] Compared with nonsmokers, smokers with closed tibia fractures treated with an intramedullary nail or external fixation showed a statistically significant reduction in healing.[52] Tibial fracture healing in smokers treated with casts took 62% longer compared with healing in nonsmokers; however, the delay was not statistically significant.

Summary

The treatment of tibial shaft fractures continues to evolve. Early evaluation includes adequate bony and soft-tissue assessment. Initial reduction and splinting are performed while the preoperative plan is developed.

Prophylactic antibiotics are administered expeditiously in patients with an open fracture. The fracture is initially assessed for nonsurgical treatment. Most surgically treated tibial fractures are stabilized with intramedullary nails. Various reduction techniques are used as necessary to maintain satisfactory alignment. External fixation or plating is used in circumstances in which nailing is undesirable or if there is risk to the patient. Adjuncts are available to improve fracture healing outcomes, especially in patients with high-energy or open fractures. Satisfactory functional return is common, except with the most severe injuries. Common extraneous factors such as nonsteroidal anti-inflammatory medication and smoking should be avoided to minimize delays in fracture healing.

Annotated References

1. Shadgan B, Menon M, O'Brien PJ, Reid WD: Diagnostic techniques in acute compartment syndrome of the leg. *J Orthop Trauma* 2008;22(8):581-587.

   Diagnostic techniques for compartment syndrome are reviewed in this meta-analysis of the literature extending from 1950 through May 2007. Early diagnosis is important. Clinical assessment remains the cornerstone for diagnosing acute compartment syndrome. Intracompartmental pressure measurements can confirm the diagnosis and are useful in patients in whom a clinical examination is not possible.

2. Tiwari A, Haq AI, Myint F, Hamilton G: Acute compartment syndromes. *Br J Surg* 2002;89(4):397-412.

3. Dickson KF, Sullivan MJ, Steinberg B, Myers L, Anderson ER III, Harris M: Noninvasive measurement of compartment syndrome. *Orthopedics* 2003;26(12):1215-1218.

4. Wiemann JM, Ueno T, Leek BT, Yost WT, Schwartz AK, Hargens AR: Noninvasive measurements of intramuscular pressure using pulsed phase-locked loop ultrasound for detecting compartment syndromes: A preliminary report. *J Orthop Trauma* 2006;20(7):458-463.

   Pulsed, phase-locked, loop fascial displacement waveform analysis showed potential as a method for noninvasively measuring intramuscular pressure and diagnosing compartment syndrome. A linear correlation was found between pulsed, phase-locked loop measurements and invasive intramuscular pressures.

5. Marsh JL, Slongo TF, Agel J, et al: Fracture and dislocation classification compendium, 2007: Orthopaedic Trauma Association classification, database and outcomes committee. *J Orthop Trauma* 2007;21(suppl 10) S1-S133.

   The revised and most recent version of the Orthopaedic Trauma Association's classification of fractures and dislocations is presented.

6. Oestern HJ, Tscherne H: Pathophysiology and classification of soft tissue injuries associated with fractures, in Tscherne H, Gotzen L (eds): *Fractures with soft tissue injuries*. Berlin, Germany, Springer-Verlag, 1984, pp 1-9.

7. Gustilo RB, Anderson JT: Prevention of infection in the treatment of one thousand and twenty-five open fractures of long bones: Retrospective and prospective analyses. *J Bone Joint Surg Am* 1976;58(4):453-458.

8. Gustilo RB, Mendoza RM, Williams DN: Problems in the management of type III (severe) open fractures: A new classification of type III open fractures. *J Trauma* 1984;24(8):742-746.

9. Brumback RJ, Jones AL: Interobserver agreement in the classification of open fractures of the tibia. The results of a survey of two hundred and forty-five orthopaedic surgeons. *J Bone Joint Surg Am* 1994;76(8):1162-1166.

10. Horn BD, Rettig ME: Interobserver reliability in the Gustilo and Anderson classification of open fractures. *J Orthop Trauma* 1993;7(4):357-360.

11. Khatod M, Botte MJ, Hoyt DB, Meyer RS, Smith JM, Akeson WH: Outcomes in open tibia fractures: Relationship between delay in treatment and infection. *J Trauma* 2003;55(5):949-954.

12. Charalambous CP, Siddique I, Zenios M, et al: Early versus delayed surgical treatment of open tibial fractures: Effect on the rates of infection and need of secondary surgical procedures to promote bone union. *Injury* 2005;36(5):656-661.

    The authors report on 383 open tibial fractures in which early surgical treatment (≤ 6 hours from hospital arrival) was instituted in 184 of the fractures and late treatment (> 6 hours after hospital arrival) was instituted in 199 fractures. There were no differences between early and late groups with regard to infection and the rate of secondary procedures needed to achieve fracture union.

13. Sarmiento A, Latta LL: Functional fracture bracing. *J Am Acad Orthop Surg* 1999;7(1):66-75.

14. Lindsey RW, Blair SR: Closed tibial-shaft fractures: Which ones benefit from surgical treatment? *J Am Acad Orthop Surg* 1996;4(1):35-43.

15. Bone LB, Sucato D, Stegemann PM, Rohrbacher BJ: Displaced isolated fractures of the tibial shaft treated with either a cast or intramedullary nailing. An outcome analysis of matched pairs of patients. *J Bone Joint Surg Am* 1997;79(9):1336-1341.

16. Teitz CC, Carter DR, Frankel VH: Problems associated with tibial fractures with intact fibulae. *J Bone Joint Surg Am* 1980;62(5):770-776.

17. Keating JF, Orfaly R, O'Brien PJ: Knee pain after tibial nailing. *J Orthop Trauma* 1997;11(1):10-13.

18. Court-Brown CM, Gustilo T, Shaw AD: Knee pain after intramedullary tibial nailing: Its incidence, etiology, and outcome. *J Orthop Trauma* 1997;11(2):103-105.

19. Väistö O, Toivanen J, Kannus P, Järvinen M: Anterior knee pain and thigh muscle strength after intramedullary nailing of a tibial shaft fracture: An 8-year follow-up of 28 consecutive cases. *J Orthop Trauma* 2007;21(3):165-171.

In this prospective study of 40 patients with an average follow-up of 8.1 years, 7 patients had no initial anterior knee pain, 13 had initial anterior knee pain that resolved, and 8 had anterior knee pain initially and at final follow-up. Quadriceps weakness and lower functional knee scores were associated with persistent anterior knee pain at 8-year follow-up.

20. Cartwright-Terry M, Snow M, Nalwad H: The severity and prediction of anterior knee pain post tibial nail insertion. *J Orthop Trauma* 2007;21(6):381-385.

The authors reported a significant preinjury prevalence of anterior knee pain. The severity of anterior knee pain after nailing significantly correlated with that of the uninjured limb. The relative risk of anterior knee pain after tibial nailing was twice that of a comparative population.

21. Nork SE, Barei DP, Schildhauer TA, et al: Intramedullary nailing of proximal quarter tibial fractures. *J Orthop Trauma* 2006;20(8):523-528.

The authors of this retrospective study analyzed 37 fractures of the proximal quarter of the tibia that were stabilized with an intramedullary nail. Acceptable alignment was achieved in 91.9% of fractures. Four patients were lost to follow-up. In the remaining 33 fractures, 31 united without additional procedures. The authors emphasized adjunctive techniques (the choice of a proper starting point, the use of unicortical plates, and the use of a femoral distractor) to successfully manage these injuries with intramedullary nails.

22. Tornetta P III, Collins E: Semiextended position of intramedullary nailing of the proximal tibia. *Clin Orthop Relat Res* 1996;328(328):185-189.

23. Nork SE, Schwartz AK, Agel J, Holt SK, Schrick JL, Winquist RA: Intramedullary nailing of distal metaphyseal tibial fractures. *J Bone Joint Surg Am* 2005; 87(6):1213-1221.

The authors reported on 36 tibial fractures within 5 cm of the plafond treated with intramedullary nailing. Ten of the fractures had a simple articular extension, which was stabilized with supplemental screw fixation before the nailing. Of the 30 patients followed, union was achieved at an average of 23.5 weeks. Acceptable alignment was achieved in 92% of all patients. Functional outcomes improved over time.

24. Stuermer EK, Stuermer KM: Tibial shaft fracture and ankle joint injury. *J Orthop Trauma* 2008;22(2):107-112.

This prospective study detected 43 associated ankle joint injuries in 214 tibial fractures (20.1%). Risk factors for ankle injury included pronation-eversion mechanisms, spiral fractures of the tibia, proximal fibular fractures, and fractures with an intact fibula.

25. Lefaivre KA, Guy P, Chan H, Blachut PA: Long-term follow-up of tibial shaft fractures treated with intramedullary nailing. *J Orthop Trauma* 2008;22(8):525-529.

The authors evaluated 56 of 250 eligible patients with isolated tibial fractures treated with an intramedullary nail. At median-term follow-up of 14 years, the patients' function was comparable to population norms, but objective and subjective evaluation showed persistent sequelae. Of note, 73.2% of patients had at least moderate knee pain, 33.9% had asymmetric swelling, 27.3% had persistent quadriceps atrophy, and 35.4% had evidence of arthritis.

26. Bhandari M, Zlowodzki M, Tornetta P III, Schmidt A, Templeman DC: Intramedullary nailing following external fixation in femoral and tibial shaft fractures. *J Orthop Trauma* 2005;19(2):140-144.

The authors present an evidence-based summary of intramedullary nailing after external fixation in femoral and tibial shaft fractures. For tibial fractures, the infection rate for intramedullary nailing following external fixation was 9% and the union rate was 90%. External fixation applied at 28 days or fewer from the time of injury reduced the risk of infection by 83%.

27. Pollak AN, Ficke JR; Extremity War Injuries III Session Moderators: Extremity war injuries: Challenges in definitive reconstruction. *J Am Acad Orthop Surg* 2008; 16(11):628-634.

The authors summarize the findings and recommendations from the third annual Extremity War Injuries Symposium held in January 2008.

28. Nho SJ, Helfet DL, Rozbruch SR: Temporary intentional leg shortening and deformation to facilitate wound closure using the Ilizarov/Taylor spatial frame. *J Orthop Trauma* 2006;20(6):419-424.

A technique combining acute shortening with temporary bony deformation using an Ilizarov apparatus to facilitate wound closure without soft-tissue reconstructive procedures is detailed. After soft-tissue healing occurs, the bone deformity and shortening are subsequently corrected through distraction osteogenesis.

29. Court-Brown CM: Reamed intramedullary tibial nailing: An overview and analysis of 1106 cases. *J Orthop Trauma* 2004;18(2):96-101.

The author provides an overview on reamed tibial nailing as well as an analysis of 1,106 cases. The average time to union for closed fractures was 18.5 weeks and for open fractures was 30 weeks. The infection rate was 1.9% in closed fractures and 7.7% in open fractures.

30. Jensen JS, Hansen FW, Johansen J: Tibial shaft fractures: A comparison of conservative treatment and internal fixation with conventional plates or AO compression plates. *Acta Orthop Scand* 1977;48(2):204-212.

31. Vallier HA, Le TT, Bedi A: Radiographic and clinical comparisons of distal tibia shaft fractures (4 to 11 cm proximal to the plafond): Plating versus intramedullary nailing. *J Orthop Trauma* 2008;22(5):307-311.

The authors retrospectively reviewed 113 extra-articular

5: Lower Extremity

distal tibial fractures from two level I trauma centers. Seventy-six fractures were treated with an intramedullary nail and 37 with a medial plate. Reasonable success was achieved with both methods; however, delayed union, malunion, and secondary procedures were needed more often after intramedullary nailing.

32. Collinge C, Kuper M, Larson K, Protzman R: Minimally invasive plating of high-energy metaphyseal distal tibia fractures. *J Orthop Trauma* 2007;21(6):355-361.

The authors present a retrospective analysis of 26 patients with high-energy injuries of the metaphyseal distal tibia with minimal or no articular involvement treated by minimally invasive plating techniques. Mean fracture healing time was 35 weeks. Secondary surgeries to achieve union were performed in nine patients (35%). Risk factors for healing complications included bone loss, high-grade comminution, and high-grade open fractures.

33. Kubiak EN, Camuso MR, Barei DP, Nork SE: Operative treatment of ipsilateral noncontiguous unicondylar tibial plateau and shaft fractures: Combining plates and nails. *J Orthop Trauma* 2008;22(8):560-565.

The use of combined plates and intramedullary nails for fixing noncontiguous ipsilateral unicondylar tibial plateau and shaft fractures are reviewed.

34. Krettek C, Miclau T, Schandelmaier P, Stephan C, Möhlmann U, Tscherne H: The mechanical effect of blocking screws ("Poller screws") in stabilizing tibia fractures with short proximal or distal fragments after insertion of small-diameter intramedullary nails. *J Orthop Trauma* 1999;13(8):550-553.

35. Ricci WM, O'Boyle M, Borrelli J, Bellabarba C, Sanders R: Fractures of the proximal third of the tibial shaft treated with intramedullary nails and blocking screws. *J Orthop Trauma* 2001;15(4):264-270.

36. Matthews DE, McGuire R, Freeland AE: Anterior unicortical buttress plating in conjunction with an unreamed interlocking intramedullary nail for treatment of very proximal tibial diaphyseal fractures. *Orthopedics* 1997;20(7):647-648.

37. Archdeacon MT, Wyrick JD: Reduction plating for provisional fracture fixation. *J Orthop Trauma* 2006;20(3): 206-211.

The authors review the use of provisional unicortical plates to maintain fracture reduction until definitive internal fixation is applied.

38. Tang P, Gates C, Hawes J, Vogt M, Prayson MJ: Does open reduction increase the chance of infection during intramedullary nailing of closed tibial shaft fractures? *J Orthop Trauma* 2006;20(5):317-322.

The authors of this retrospective analysis of 119 fractures evaluated whether open reduction increased the risk of infection during intramedullary nailing of a closed tibial shaft fracture. There were no infections in the 79 fractures nailed in a closed fashion, and two infections (5%) in the 40 fractures treated with some type

of open reduction (formal incisions > 1 cm, percutaneous incisions < 1 cm, or through fasciotomy incisions). The difference was not statistically significant.

39. SPRINT Investigators: Randomized trial of reamed and unreamed intramedullary nailing of tibial shaft fractures. *J Bone Joint Surg* 2008:90A(12):2567-2578.

This multicenter, randomized trial of 1,319 patients compared reamed and unreamed intramedullary nailing of the tibia. Reaming had a possible benefit in closed fractures (11% reoperation rate by 1 year versus 17% for unreamed nails). No differences were seen in open fractures. Delaying surgery for a delayed union or nonunion for at least 6 months decreased the need for reoperation.

40. Weber TG, Harrington RM, Henley MB, Tencer AF: The role of fibular fixation in combined fractures of the tibia and fibula: A biomechanical investigation. *J Orthop Trauma* 1997;11(3):206-211.

41. Egol KA, Weisz R, Hiebert R, Tejwani NC, Koval KJ, Sanders RW: Does fibular plating improve alignment after intramedullary nailing of distal metaphyseal tibia fractures? *J Orthop Trauma* 2006;20(2):94-103.

This retrospective review from three level I trauma centers examined 72 distal tibial metaphyseal fractures treated with fibular plating after intramedullary nailing. Those fractures in which the associated fibular fracture was stabilized (*n* = 25) achieved and maintained better alignment at 12 weeks or later after tibial nailing compared with the nonsurgically treated fibular fractures.

42. Jones CB, Mayo KA: Nonunion treatment: Iliac crest bone graft techniques. *J Orthop Trauma* 2005;19 (suppl 10):S11-S13.

This review article details the classification of nonunions and indications for autogenous iliac crest bone grafting.

43. McKee MD: Recombinant human bone morphogenic protein-7: Applications for clinical trauma. *J Orthop Trauma* 2005;19(suppl 10):S26-S28.

The authors of this review article summarize the results of three clinical trials showing promise for recombinant human BMP-7 for treating tibial nonunion, long-bone nonunion, and open tibial fractures.

44. Swiontkowski MF, Aro HT, Donell S, et al: Recombinant human bone morphogenetic protein-2 in open tibial fractures: A subgroup analysis of data combined from two prospective randomized studies. *J Bone Joint Surg Am* 2006;88(6):1258-1265.

The authors present the result of an analysis of 510 patients from two randomized trials investigating the effect of recombinant human BMP-2 on open tibial fractures. Recombinant human BMP-2 delivered on absorbable collagen sponges reduced the frequency of bone graft procedures and other secondary interventions in severe open tibial fractures.

45. Govender S, Csimma C, Genant HK, et al: Recombinant human bone morphogenic protein-2 for treatment

of open tibial fractures: A prospective, controlled, randomized study of four hundred and fifty patients. *J Bone Joint Surg Am* 2002;84(12):1223-1234.

46. Heckman JD, Ryaby JP, McCabe J, Frey JJ, Kilcoyne RF: Acceleration of tibial fracture-healing by non-invasive, low-intensity pulsed ultrasound. *J Bone Joint Surg Am* 1994;76(1):26-34.

47. Harder AT, An YH: The mechanisms of the inhibitory effects of nonsteroidal anti-inflammatory drugs on bone healing: A concise review. *J Clin Pharmacol* 2003;43(8): 807-815.

48. Simon AM, O'Connor JP: Dose and time-dependent effects of cyclooxygenase-2 inhibition on fracture-healing. *J Bone Joint Surg Am* 2007;89(3):500-511.

COX-2 nonsteroidal anti-inflammatory drugs given at the early stages of fracture healing reduced the mechanical properties of callus at later stages of healing. The nonunion rate was also higher in rats exposed to COX-2 medications.

49. Gerstenfeld LC, Al-Ghawas M, Alkhiary YM, et al: Selective and nonselective cyclooxygenase-2 inhibitors and experimental fracture healing. Reversibility of effects after short-term treatment. *J Bone Joint Surg Am* 2007; 89(1):114-125.

COX-2 specific drugs inhibited fracture healing in this rat model more than nonspecific nonsteroidal anti-inflammatory drugs. The magnitude of the effect was related to the duration of treatment. The negative effects on bone healing gradually disappeared when the medication was discontinued.

50. Castillo RC, Bosse MJ, MacKenzie EJ, Patterson BM; LEAP Study Group: Impact of smoking on fracture healing and risk of complications in limb-threatening open tibia fractures. *J Orthop Trauma* 2005;19(3):151-157.

This evaluation of 268 patients with open tibial fractures from eight level I trauma centers showed that patients who currently smoke (n = 105) and previously smoked (n = 82) were 37% and 32% less likely, respectively, to achieve union compared with nonsmokers. Osteomyelitis was also more likely to develop in current and previous smokers.

51. Harvey EJ, Agel J, Selznick HS, Chapman JR, Henley MB: Deleterious effect of smoking on healing of open tibia-shaft fractures. *Am J Orthop (Belle Mead NJ)* 2002;31(9):518-521.

52. Schmitz MA, Finnegan M, Natarajan R, Champine J: Effect of smoking on tibial shaft fracture healing. *Clin Orthop Relat Res* 1999;365(365):184-200.

5: Lower Extremity

Chapter 38

Fractures of the Ankle and Distal Tibial Pilon

David P. Barei, MD   Brett D. Crist, MD, FACS

Fractures of the Ankle

Introduction

Ankle fractures remain one of the most common injuries treated by the orthopaedic surgeon. Despite their commonality, their mechanisms and injury severity can be quite disparate. Optimal treatment requires an understanding of the injury mechanism, fracture pattern, and associated ligamentous and soft-tissue injuries. Associated patient factors such as the presence of diabetes, chronologic age, and bone quality are variables outside of the surgeon's control but may have significant influence on the final outcome. Successful treatment requires the restoration of normal anatomy, early functional rehabilitation, and avoidance of complications.

Ankle instability results from the loss of osseous and/or ligamentous supports that constrain the talus in the mortise. Subsequent abnormal talar translation relative to the tibia results in ankle arthritis and a poor functional result. One recent study noted that most ankle osteoarthritis is attributable to a posttraumatic etiology and that primary osteoarthritis of the ankle is a relatively rare event.[1] The authors found that most of the posttraumatic osteoarthritis cohort had a history of a malleolar fracture, followed by those with chronic ligamentous instability, and finally, tibial pilon fractures.

Ankle fractures can be classified according to their mechanism of injury, their radiographic appearance, or from combinations of these. The well-known Lauge-Hansen classification describes four categories of injuries based on foot position and the direction of the subsequently applied force. Each category produces stereotyped injury patterns that are further divided into stages based on a theorized sequence of disruption of osseous and ligamentous ankle joint supporting structures. Although the Lauge-Hansen system is useful as an attempt to categorize and predict injury patterns, its accuracy is questionable. In one study, MRI was used to analyze the associated soft-tissue injuries in a series of surgically treated ankle fractures and failed to predict the observed ligamentous injury in more than half the cases.[2] It was recommended that, although the Lauge-Hansen classification should still be used as the first step in understanding the entire picture of an ankle fracture, supplemental tests such as stress views, CT, and MRI may be useful adjuncts to completely elucidate the injury. A decision tree for ankle fracture management emphasizing stability criteria has recently been introduced and may be complementary to the Lauge-Hansen and Weber systems.[3] This system can aid in determining which ankle fractures should be considered for surgical repair, but it is not detailed enough to adequately describe the fracture patterns clinically. This latter parameter, which is useful for guiding the application of internal fixation in those fractures deemed unstable and thus requiring surgery, can continue to be served by the currently used Lauge-Hansen or Weber systems.

Ankle Syndesmosis Injuries

Three ligaments ensure the stability of the tibiofibular mortise: the interosseous tibiofibular ligament (a distal continuation of the interosseous membrane), the anterior tibiofibular ligament, and the posterior tibiofibular ligament. Though commonly cited as a separate supporting fourth ligament, the so-called inferior transverse tibiofibular ligament is likely a strong horizontal expansion of the posterior tibiofibular ligament, rather than a separate ligamentous structure.[4] Clinically, external rotation forces applied to the foot are thought to be the main mechanism of injury to the ankle syndesmosis, and are invariably accompanied by a medial ankle disruption, such as a medial malleolar fracture or deltoid ligament disruption.

Injuries to the distal tibiofibular syndesmosis are incompletely understood and demonstrate a wide variation in presentation. Although certain associated frac-

Dr. Barei or an immediate family member serves as a board member, owner, officer, or committee member of Orthopaedic Trauma Association; is a member of a speakers' bureau or has made paid presentations on behalf of AO, Smith & Nephew, Synthes, and Zimmer; serves as a paid consultant to or is an employee of Zimmer; and has received research or institutional support from Synthes and Zimmer. Dr. Crist or an immediate family member has received research or institutional support from Synthes, KCI, Medtronic, and Pfizer.

ture patterns are commonly observed, injury to the syndesmosis should be suspected and specifically evaluated in virtually all ankle fractures. Although more commonly used to diagnose syndesmosis injuries without lateral malleolus fractures, the squeeze test, external rotation stress test, and direct palpation of the syndesmosis all have been recommended to clinically evaluate injuries to the distal tibiofibular ankle syndesmosis. Because of poor interobserver variability and the imperfect sensitivity of these physical examination tests, adjunctive diagnostic methods are frequently required. Radiographic parameters commonly used to suggest injury to the syndesmosis include the level of the fibular fracture relative to the tibial plafond and loss of the normal relationship between the fibula and the tibia, such as the tibiofibular clear space and overlap. Fibular fractures above the level of the ankle joint (especially ≥ 4.5 cm above the joint) are more commonly associated with syndesmotic instability, particularly when associated with a deltoid ligament disruption. However, the reverse is not necessarily true. Recent investigations have challenged the long-standing cadaver data that suggest that fibula fractures within 3.5 to 4 cm of the tibiotalar articulation should not be associated with pathologic instability. After lateral malleolar fixation, one study identified 39% of Weber B ankle fractures to have syndesmotic instability identified intraoperatively under direct vision and fluoroscopy after applying an external rotation stress test.[5] Given these findings, the authors strongly recommended intraoperative evaluation of the syndesmosis in unstable Weber B supination-external rotation injuries after lateral malleolar fixation. Other authors have also corroborated this unexpectedly high incidence of syndesmotic injuries associated with Weber B supination-external rotation injury patterns.[6] Although gross disruptions of the normal tibiofibular clear space and overlap are indicative of syndesmotic disruption, subtle injuries can be easily missed and limit the utility of these radiographic measurements. CT, particularly when compared with imaging studies of the normal contralateral ankle, has demonstrated improved ability to identify subtle alterations in syndesmotic widening, anterior or posterior displacement, and retained osteochondral fragments within the syndesmosis. MRI has become increasingly important in directly diagnosing injury of the ligamentous supports responsible for syndesmotic stability, rather than inferring injury based on the relationship of the tibia and fibula at the level of the syndesmosis. In a recent prospective and blinded study, in 70 patients with closed ankle fracture, plain radiographs and MRI were obtained. The authors found that a medial clear space of greater than 4 mm correlated with disruption of the deltoid and tibiofibular ligaments, but there was no correlation between syndesmotic injury and either tibiofibular clear space or overlap measurements.[7] Additionally, in a clinical prelude to a biomechanical cadaver study, 15 patients with pronation-external rotation fracture patterns associated

with a posterior malleolar fracture were evaluated with radiographs and MRI. No cases of posterior-inferior tibiofibular ligament injury were observed despite findings of syndesmotic injury.[8] Finally, other authors have confirmed the usefulness of intraoperative dynamic fluoroscopic stress testing to evaluate the syndesmosis.[5,9] In these studies, a standardized and reproducible external rotation force was applied to the foot that identified unpredicted syndesmotic instability in almost 40% of the ankles tested. Currently, most stress examinations rely on alterations of the tibiofibular clear space (or overlap) using an external rotation force applied through the foot, or by pulling on the fibula with a bone hook in the coronal plane (hook test). A recent cadaver ligamentous sectioning study applied the hook test in both the coronal and sagittal planes, identifying substantially greater sagittal rather than coronal plane motion for a given combination of sectioned ligamentous supports.[10] This suggests that dynamic sagittal plane testing of the syndesmosis may be even more sensitive at diagnosing syndesmotic injury than dynamic coronal plane testing.

In short, the sensitivity of physical examination signs in identifying syndesmotic injuries of the ankle is limited. Static plain radiographic parameters and classification systems, though an improvement in increasing the diagnostic sensitivity, still fail to consistently diagnose or predict syndesmotic injuries. Previous cadaver biomechanical data also appear to potentially underestimate the clinical incidence of syndesmotic injury. Because missed or untreated syndesmotic injuries are associated with extremely poor results, the surgeon should be vigilant in assessing for their presence, even in injury patterns thought previously to be unassociated with syndesmotic disruption. Ankle stress tests, MRI, and CT have clearly demonstrated an improved ability at diagnosing these injuries and should be considered when the physical examination and static plain radiographic investigations remain equivocal.

Treatment of static syndesmotic instability and/or pronounced dynamic instability includes an accurate surgical reduction of the distal tibiofibular joint and syndesmotic stabilization. In the setting of a fibula fracture, anatomic restoration of fibular length, alignment, and rotation must be achieved. Furthermore, accurate reduction of the fibular relationship with the tibial incisura is critical to completing a satisfactory syndesmotic reduction. While seemingly simple, accurate and consistent reduction of the distal tibiofibular syndesmosis has been noted by several authors to be surprisingly elusive. Using postoperative CT, two separate but related publications noted an approximate 50% malreduction rate in distal tibiofibular syndesmotic reductions when indirect reduction and intraoperative fluoroscopic control were used.[11,12] In these studies, 25 patients underwent surgical reduction and fixation of their unstable ankle fractures with associated syndesmotic instability. The authors noted that although the syndesmotic malreductions could be easily identified on

CT scanning, plain radiographic measurements failed to accurately reflect the status of the distal tibiofibular joint. Additionally, a common malreduction was excessive internal rotation of the fibula or anterior fibular translation within the incisura, which is likely caused by percutaneous clamps that are commonly applied for the provisional reduction and stabilization of the syndesmosis.[11] In a related publication, 149 consecutive patients with syndesmotic disruptions were treated prospectively with open reduction and direct visualization, followed by stabilization. Postoperative CT confirmed a substantial decrease in the rate of syndesmotic malreductions, but malreduction still occurred in 16% despite the open visualization.[12] One of the main strategies that the authors identified as being responsible for decreasing the malreduction rate was the liberal use of open reduction and internal fixation (ORIF) of any posterior malleolar fracture fragments. Because the posterior tibiofibular ligament is rarely disrupted in the setting of a posterior malleolar fracture, accurate reduction of the posterior malleolus, therefore, restores the osseous anatomy of the incisura, creates a posterior buttress to help prevent the fibula from rotating out of the incisura posteriorly, and directly reduces the fibula to an accurate position relative to the tibia by virtue of the intact posterior tibiofibular ligament. In addition to potentially improving the accuracy of syndesmotic reduction, ORIF of the posterior malleolus may also substantially improve the syndesmotic stability. In a recent cadaver biomechanical study, a syndesmotic injury was created by sectioning the deep and superficial deltoid and the anterior tibiofibular ligament, and by dividing the interosseous membrane 6 cm above the plafond. After creating a simulated posterior malleolar fracture without injuring the posterior inferior tibiofibular ligament, the specimens were randomized into ORIF of the posterior malleolus or syndesmotic fixation. ORIF of the posterior malleolus using a single bicortical 3.5-mm screw restored the distal tibiofibular syndesmosis to 70% of the intact stiffness versus 40% when compared to a single 3.5-mm tricortical syndesmosis screw.[8] These studies have illustrated the potential importance of posterior malleolar reduction and fixation in achieving and strethening syndesmotic reduction.

In many circumstances, however, a posterior malleolar fracture fragment does not occur, and syndesmotic fixation is required. The ideal syndesmosis fixation remains debatable. Current options for fixation include metallic screw fixation, bioabsorbable screw fixation, and suture techniques. Controversy exists regarding the implant material (stainless steel, titanium, bioabsorbable, suture), screw size (3.5-mm versus 4.5-mm screws), the number of cortices engaged by the implant (three versus four cortices), screw location relative to the tibial plafond, and the number of screws used (one versus two).[13] Currently accepted techniques include the placement of screws angled 20° to 30° from posterior to anterior, and ideally located 2 to 4 cm above the tibial plafond. Interestingly, one small study evaluated

syndesmosis screws that were placed in a transsyndesmotic location (plafond to 2 cm above) or suprasyndesmotic (2 to 5 cm above the plafond) location. The authors demonstrated no difference in several radiographic and clinical parameters, including ankle range of motion, pain, osteoarthrosis, patient satisfaction, and the presence of distal tibiofibular synostosis, but given the small sample size, the study is likely underpowered and subject to a beta error.[14] Biomechanical studies have demonstrated no difference between stainless and titanium implants, stainless and bioabsorbable implants, and the number of cortices engaged.[15,16] Recent cadaver biomechanical evidence has also indicated that syndesmotic fixation using a single 3.5-mm syndesmosis screw, either in a tricortical or quadricortical fashion, is inadequate to support weight bearing loads, suggesting that activity modifications are indicated until presumed ligamentous healing has occurred.[15] Interest in the evaluation and utilization of bioabsorbable and suture syndesmotic implants is substantial. In a prospective and randomized study comparing metallic and bioabsorbable screws, the polylevolactic screws were associated with a better return to activities and less swelling, with no loss to joint motion and syndesmotic reduction in comparison with metallic implants.[17] A more recent study evaluated a polylactic bioabsorbable screw used in 75 patients. Seventy patients were available with a minimum 12-month follow-up period, and a mean follow-up period of almost 3 years. The authors demonstrated no radiographic loss of syndesmotic stability, mortise congruency, or osteoarthrosis changes at the syndesmosis. No patient required a revision, and excellent outcomes were noted when evaluated with a standardized outcome test.[18] Although further study is necessary to unequivocally recommend bioabsorbable implants, there is continuing evidence to support their use. Syndesmotic fixation using suture constructs is an area of continuing interest. A recent clinical series has demonstrated successful results in a small number of patients.[19] Cadaver mechanical evidence, however, suggests that metal screw fixation has a significantly greater ability to maintain reduction of the syndesmosis than the suture/implant technique during all external loading conditions.[20] While touted as an alternate method for avoiding the irritation from metallic screws and the need for subsequent screw removal, one study identified two cases of soft-tissue irritation and granuloma formation with the suture technique for syndesmotic fixation.[21]

The need for fibular fixation in high fibular fractures associated with syndesmotic disruption remains controversial. One strategy is to omit fibular fracture reduction and fixation, and to rely solely on the fixation of the fibula to the tibia using syndesmotic screw fixation. However, restoration of accurate fibular length and rotation may be difficult to accomplish and assess at the ankle joint. Because of the increasing evidence that demonstrates the inaccuracy with closed, percutaneous, and even open reduction of the syndesmosis, another strategy is to accurately fix the fibular fracture to restore the accurate anatomic fibular length and rotation. Although subsequent open reduction and fixation of the distal syndesmosis is more likely to be accurate, malreduction may still occur. Regardless of the surgical tactic used, an accurate syndesmotic reduction is of prime importance (**Figure 1**).

Numerous variables are responsible for the outcome after an injury to the distal tibiofibular syndesmosis. One retrospective review of ankle fractures with transsyndesmotic screw fixation, however, found that the most important factor influencing clinically important differences in functional outcome was an accurate reduction of the syndesmosis.[6] A prospective, randomized, clinical study comparing tricortical and quadricortical syndesmotic fixation consisting of either a 4.5-m screw placed through four cortices or two 3.5-mm screws placed through three cortices noted better function at 3 months in the tricortical screw group, but no difference in ankle dorsiflexion, loss of fixation, or function at 1 year was observed.[22] A more recent follow-up study of 48 of the original 64 patients at an average of 8.4 years demonstrated no statistical differences in the tricortical versus quadricortical syndesmosis fixation groups regarding a functional ankle outcome score or osteoarthritis. The authors found that the outcome score was negatively influenced by an increased syndesmotic width of 1.5 mm or greater when compared to the nonoperated ankle, syndesmosis synostosis, the presence of a posterior fracture fragment, and obesity.[23] The timing, potential benefits and drawbacks, and ultimate need for screw removal after surgical stabilization of syndesmotic injuries remains controversial. One recent study assessed functional outcomes and range of motion of ankles after syndesmotic screw and fibular plate removal. The authors identified a significant and nearly immediate improvement in ankle range of motion and outcome scores that persisted at longer follow-up.[24] Implants were removed 4 months after implantation, and no loss of syndesmotic reduction, adverse events, or complications associated with implant removal were noted. Other authors have corroborated these results, noting that an intact syndesmosis screw was associated with a worse functional outcome compared with loose, fractured, or removed screws. Interestingly, there were no differences in functional outcomes comparing loose or fractured screws with removed screws, indicating that broken screw removal is unlikely to benefit patients but that removal of intact syndesmosis screws may have a beneficial effect.[25] An additional study, however, found no statistical difference in clinical outcome of patients with Weber B or C injuries who underwent syndesmosis screw removal and those who did not.[26] Additional results from this study, however, did support the findings of others that broken screw removal is unlikely to improve clinical outcomes. Taken together, these recent studies suggest several key management points: an anatomic reduction of the syndesmosis is critical to maximizing functional outcomes; provided that stability is maintained until soft-tissue healing, numerous techniques are available to adequately stabilize the syndesmosis, without any obviously significant advantages of one technique compared to others; and a rigidly stabilized distal tibiofibular syndesmosis, either secondary to retained intact transsyndesmotic screw fixation or distal tibiofibular synostosis, may be associated with lower functional outcomes than in those with presumed mobile syndesmoses. Patients should be counseled regarding the potential beneficial effects of transsyndesmotic screw removal after syndesmotic ligamentous healing has occurred. They should similarly be counseled that broken syndesmotic screw removal is unlikely to provide significant improvement in clinical function.

Malleolar Ankle Fractures

Malleolar ankle fractures, with a few notable exceptions, occur as a result of rotational mechanisms. Commonly used classification systems include the mechanistic Lauge-Hansen system and the descriptive Weber system that is based on the location of the fibula/lateral malleolus fracture relative to the distal tibiofibular syndesmosis. Significant fracture displacement, talar shift, and the presence of multiple malleoli fractures are features associated with ankle instability and therefore are indications for surgical care.

Fractures of the Lateral Malleolus

Weber A lateral malleolar fractures are those that occur below the level of the tibiofibular syndesmosis. They typically do not result in ankle instability, and surgical stabilization of the fibula is not usually indicated. According to the Lauge-Hansen system, lateral malleolar ankle fractures are often the result of a supination and adduction mechanism, with tension failure of the lateral malleolus in an infrasyndesmotic location. Surgical indication of this injury pattern is frequently dictated by the presence of any medial malleolar fracture. When present, the medial malleolar fracture typically demonstrates a vertical fracture plane, and is commonly associated with chondral impaction of the medial tibial plafond immediately lateral to the vertical fracture plane. This injury pattern requires surgical stabilization of the medial malleolus fracture with reduction, stabilization, and bone grafting of any chondral impaction.[27] A recent biomechanical study has confirmed that fixation of vertical shear fractures of the medial malleolus with a properly applied neutralization plate (one third tubular with 3.5-mm screws) offers significant mechanical advantages over screw-only constructs.[28]

Weber B lateral malleolar fractures occur at the level of the ankle syndesmosis and are the most common malleolar ankle fracture. The injury occurs from a supination-external rotation mechanism, and the fracture typically begins distally and anteromedially at the level of the distal tibiofibular syndesmosis, traveling

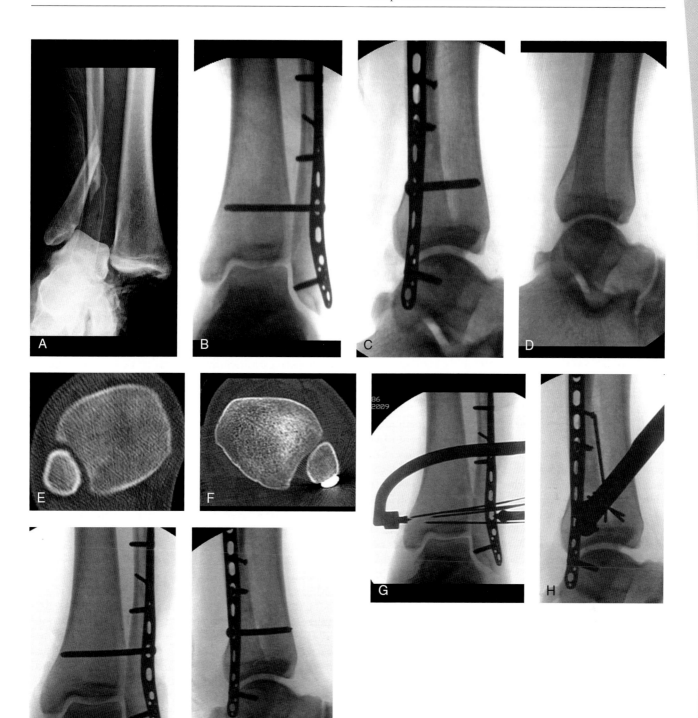

Figure 1 A 21-year-old man involved in a low-velocity motorcycle collision sustained an isolated open injury to the left lower extremity. The injury AP ankle radiograph (**A**) demonstrates a Weber C fibula fracture with obvious tibiotalar dislocation and gross distal tibiofibular syndesmotic disruption. Final mortise (**B**) and lateral (**C**) fluoroscopic images after débridement and ORIF demonstrate an apparent satisfactory reduction of all components of the injury. An open reduction of the distal tibiofibular syndesmosis had been performed. The lateral view, however, suggests slight anterior fibular translation, particularly when compared to the lateral fluoroscopic image of the contralateral, uninjured ankle (**D**). Postoperative CT of the uninjured ankle (**E**) and the surgically treated ankle (**F**) confirms a significant distal syndesmosis malreduction. Syndesmotic revision consisted of syndesmotic screw removal and posterior translation of the fibula approximately 5 mm. Mortise (**G**) and lateral (**H**) intraoperative fluoroscopic images demonstrate the revised syndesmotic reduction with provisional clamp and wire stabilization. A new quadricortical syndesmosis screw was inserted through a new tibial drill path. Final AP and lateral intraoperative fluoroscopic images are shown (**I** and **J**). Note the subtle but discernible posterior translation of the fibula compared with the initial reduction.

proximally and posterolaterally. Because classic biomechanical studies have demonstrated that even a small amount of lateral shift of the talus (1 mm) is associated with altered ankle joint mechanics and a marked increase in tibiotalar contact forces,[29] any shift of the talus within the ankle mortise is an indication for surgical reduction and fixation. The goals of treatment therefore are the anatomic reduction of the talus within the ankle mortise, best accomplished with anatomic reduction of the lateral malleolar fracture. Closed management of lateral malleolar fractures with talar shift is usually contraindicated secondary to the relative high frequency of loss of reduction.

Treatment of isolated Weber B lateral malleolar ankle fractures without obvious talar shift remains relatively controversial and depends on the identification of associated periarticular injury that results in ankle instability, such as a ruptured deltoid ligament or ligamentous syndesmotic disruption. Interestingly, displacement of the lateral malleolus fracture itself may not necessarily indicate a concomitant lateral shift of the talus. The authors of a recent study retrospectively reviewed the injury and postoperative radiographs of 55 adult patients with displaced lateral malleolar fractures.[30] These patients demonstrated fracture displacement of at least 2 mm but with a normal medial clear space on the mortise radiograph and no clinical indication of a medial sided deltoid ligament injury. Compared with the preoperative radiographs, the authors found that reduction of the lateral malleolar fracture simply resulted in a greater distance between the distal end of the proximal fibular fragment relative to the tibia with virtually no change in the distance of the distal lateral malleolar fragment relative to the tibia. These findings suggest that the lateral malleolus remained reduced relative to the talus and that the talus was congruent within the ankle mortise. The fracture displacement appeared to be secondary to an internal rotation deformity of the proximal fibular fragment, corroborating previous studies. Although the results of the preceding study are provocative, incompetence of the deltoid ligament should be actively sought out to aid in the determination of ankle instability.

Determining ankle instability in isolated Weber B lateral malleolus fracture without radiographic evidence of lateral talar shift on the injury radiographs has evolved. If the deltoid ligament is competent, the ankle mortise remains stable, and late talar displacement is unlikely to occur, even with early functional treatment. However, if the deltoid ligament is ruptured, a significant risk of talar displacement is present, and treatment is then directed at obtaining ankle stability, typically with open anatomic lateral malleolar reduction and fixation. Clinical evaluation that elicits medial ankle tenderness and swelling for diagnosing deltoid ligament disruption has been demonstrated to be unreliable.[31-33] Manual stress testing has been demonstrated to be a substantial improvement over clinical examination in the determination of deep deltoid ligament disrup-

tion.[32,33] A recent study compared manual and gravity stress radiographs for the evaluation of supination-external rotation fibular fractures, finding that the gravity stress radiograph was equivalent to the manual stress radiograph for determining deltoid ligament injury.[34] Similar findings were noted by other authors who also demonstrated an increase in patient comfort with the gravity stress view when compared with manual stress testing.[35] The importance of these studies is that, with proper radiology technician training, the gravity stress radiograph may be incorporated into a routine part of the ankle trauma radiograph series, minimizing physician radiation exposure and time, and minimizing patient discomfort. The gravity stress test, however, is indicated only for those isolated lateral malleolar ankle fractures that do not demonstrate other indicators of ankle instability on static plain radiographs, such as evident medial clear space widening, or associated fractures of either the medial or posterior malleolus. Another study has recently demonstrated the limitations of the gravity stress view.[36] Twenty-one patients with a positive ankle stress test (≥ 5 mm of medial clear space widening) underwent MRI scanning. Of these, only two patients demonstrated complete deep deltoid ligament disruptions, with the remaining 19 having only partial deep deltoid ligament disruption. These 19 patients were treated nonsurgically. Fifteen were evaluated at a minimum of 1-year follow-up and demonstrated united fractures without evidence of residual medial clear space widening or posttraumatic joint space narrowing. Overall, excellent functional outcome scores were similarly noted. These results are in contrast with earlier cadaver studies that identified an absolute medial clear space of 5 mm or more on radiographs obtained in dorsiflexion with an external rotation stress as being the most reliable criteria for predicting deep deltoid ligament transection after distal fibular fracture.[37] The dissimilarity between these two studies may be related to sample size differences and the effect of dynamic and static ankle stabilizers between clinical and cadaver biomechanical studies. These studies highlight the importance of understanding that clinical examination, dynamic plain radiographic stress testing, and medial clear space widening are surrogate indicators of deep deltoid ligament disruption and are imperfect diagnostic tests. Despite these controversies, a gravity stress test remains the gold standard in evaluating the integrity of the deep deltoid ligament in minimally displaced isolated lateral malleolar fractures without medial clear space widening on the injury mortise radiograph (**Figure 2**). The literature varies somewhat regarding the absolute definition of a widened medial clear space, with values ranging from 4 mm or greater (with that value being at least 1 mm greater than the superior tibiotalar space), to 5 mm or greater, to an increase in medial clear space of 2 mm from its baseline value. Despite a cadaver study identifying that a medial clear space of 5 mm or greater on radiographs taken with a dorsiflexion-

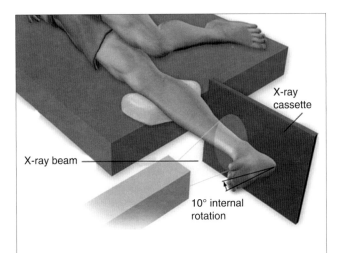

Figure 2 Diagrammatic representation of the patient position used for the gravity stress radiograph. (Reproduced with permission from Schock HJ, Pinzur M, Manion L, Stover M: The use of gravity or manual-stress radiographs in the assessment of supination-external rotation fractures of the ankle. *J Bone Joint Surg Br* 2007;89(8): 1055-1059.)

external rotation stress to be most predictive of deep deltoid ligament disruption after distal fibular fracture,[37] these ankle positions are unlikely to be consistently present during gravity stress examination in the clinical setting, and therefore strict adherence to any absolute value should be done with caution. A recent study presented the results of ultrasound evaluations of the deltoid ligament in the setting of isolated lateral malleolar fractures.[38] Patients who demonstrated complete rupture on ultrasound underwent surgical fibular stabilization, and concomitant exploration of the deltoid ligament corroborated the complete rupture. Those without complete rupture on ultrasound evaluation were treated nonsurgically and all healed uneventfully. Limitations of this study include the small sample size and the lack of a corroborating test, such as MRI, to validate the ultrasound findings in those patients determined to have incomplete deltoid disruption. Nevertheless, ultrasound may hold promise as a simple diagnostic tool for evaluating the status of the deltoid ligament, provided that it can be determined to be an accurate imaging modality for this purpose. Although MRI is presumed to be the most accurate noninvasive imaging modality for soft-tissue injury, its accuracy in evaluating complete or partial deep deltoid disruption has not been fully elucidated. Furthermore, the clinical utility of MRI for evaluating the deltoid ligament in isolated minimally displaced Weber B lateral malleolar fractures is limited secondary to cost and availability concerns, but may be useful in selected individuals.

When surgical intervention is indicated for patients with unstable Weber B lateral malleolar ankle fractures, ORIF typically consists of plate and screw fixation. Fibular reduction should be anatomic, and stabilization

can be accomplished with either a posterior antiglide plate, a lateral neutralization plate combined with a lag screw, or lag screws alone. Lag screw fixation in isolation should be limited to noncomminuted oblique or spiral fracture patterns that allow multiple screw placements at least 1 cm apart.[39] Studies have indicated excellent functional outcomes without loss of reduction and minimal soft-tissue irritation. Posterior plate placement has been shown to have biomechanical advantages compared with lateral plate placement, but surgical outcomes appear to be similar with both techniques.[40] However, to avoid peroneal irritation, extremely distal plate applications and prominent distal screws should be avoided.[41] Medial-sided injury can be purely ligamentous (deltoid disruption), osseous (supracollicular medial malleolar fracture), or a combination thereof. In the latter situation, a fracture of the anterior colliculus of the medial malleolus may occur with disruption of the deep deltoid ligament. The deep deltoid ligament, originating from the posterior colliculus, is the main medial ligamentous stabilizer of the talus within the mortise in the setting of a supination-external rotation injury with a lateral malleolus fracture. In contradistinction to a supracollicular medial malleolus fracture, surgical stabilization of an anterior colliculus fracture may not restore medial stability. Because the incidence of syndesmotic instability present in Weber B lateral malleolar fractures has been estimated at approximately 40%, a stress examination of the syndesmosis should be performed at the conclusion of lateral malleolar fixation and transsyndesmotic stabilization performed if indicated.

Weber C ankle fractures are defined as those fibula fractures that occur in a suprasyndesmotic location. They commonly occur as a result of external rotation mechanisms, but may also occur with abduction mechanisms where the displacing force is translational rather than rotational. These injury patterns are associated with ankle instability and disruption of the distal tibiofibular syndesmosis, and therefore typically require surgical stabilization. Although biomechanical data have been established as a guide to recognizing the potential instability of the distal tibiofibular syndesmosis, these data should be interpreted with caution because several syndesmotic injuries may be underappreciated. In uncertain or equivocal situations, stress examination is indicated and the syndesmosis stabilized accordingly. A recent study evaluated the treatment of pronation-abduction Weber C ankle fractures treated with extraperiosteal plating. The authors noted that their technique was an effective method of stabilization that led to predictable union with satisfactory functional outcome scores.[42]

Fractures of the Posterior Malleolus

Fractures of posterior malleolus may occur as isolated injuries, but are more commonly associated with bimalleolar and trimalleolar fracture patterns. In addition to providing a substantial contribution to the weight-bearing articular surface of the tibial plafond, the posterior malleolus serves as the tibial attachment site of the posterior talofibular ligament, and the posterolateral tibial portion of the distal tibiofibular syndesmosis articulation. Its anatomic location, therefore, is important for maintaining the stability and reduction of the ankle joint. The decision to treat a fracture of the posterior malleolus has traditionally been dictated by the size of the fragment, and with fractures involving less than 25% of the tibial plafond, recommendations have typically been nonsurgical treatment. This recommendation has been based on the lateral plain radiographic view, which is inaccurate for estimating the size of the posterior malleolar fragment. Recently, the pathoanatomy of posterior malleolar fractures has been delineated using CT, identifying the posterolateral oblique fracture as the most common pattern (67%), with extension to the posterior aspect of the medial malleolus (19%) and small-shell fractures (14%) comprising the remaining patterns.[43] This study demonstrates the high variability of posterior malleolar fracture patterns. Given the findings of this study, and combined with the knowledge that the lateral radiographic is inaccurate for estimating the size of the posterior malleolus, CT is indicated for many posterior malleolar fractures.

As noted previously, increasing evidence suggests that surgical reduction and stabilization of posterior malleolar fracture fragments has a positive influence on obtaining and maintaining reduction of the distal tibiofibular syndesmosis.

A recent study evaluated functional outcome and the local morbidity of the posterolateral approach for the displaced posterior malleolus.[44] In a consecutive series of 45 patients with a mean follow-up of 25 months, the authors demonstrated excellent functional outcomes without secondary displacement or significant local soft-tissue complications. Indications for surgical treatment of posterior malleolar fractures in that study were as follows: involvement of more that 25% of the articular surface in patients older than 50 years, greater than 10% articular involvement in patients younger than 50 years, or a greater than 10% articular involvement in any patient with tibiotalar subluxation. Previous investigations have indicated that small posterior malleolar fractures can be treated without surgery (assuming stable fixation of the other components of the ankle injury), with good long-term outcomes documented.[45] Unfortunately, the exact fragment size and configuration that requires surgical intervention remains unknown. As the fragment size increases, however, an accurate restoration of the anatomy is necessary to maintain the stability and congruency of the ankle. Although biomechanical testing has demonstrated a shift in the contact stresses anteriorly and medially in a fracture model with a large posterior malleolar fragment, talar subluxation was not identified.[46] Further investigation is required to determine precise indications for surgical stabilization of posterior malleolar fractures.

Fractures of the Medial Malleolus

Medial malleolar fractures are very commonly associated with lateral and posterior malleolar ankle fractures, but can occur in isolation. Medial malleolar fractures occur either as tension failure by a distracting force applied through the deltoid ligament during displacement of the talus, or in compression secondary to medial displacement of the talus. Tension failure is usually noted by the lateral displacement of the medial malleolar fragment and a relatively horizontal fracture orientation. When associated with lateral and/or posterior malleolar fractures, surgical treatment is indicated to restore tibiotalar congruency and stability. After anatomic reduction, fixation is typically achieved with lag screw fixation. A recent anatomic study has highlighted the potential risk to the posterior tibial tendon with screws placed into the posterior colliculus, and recommends direct visualization of the posterior tibial tendon when screws are inserted in this location.[47] Compression failures typically demonstrate a vertical medial malleolar fracture orientation, medial displacement of the medial malleolus, and a varus angulation of the talus relative to the tibial plafond. Associated chondral impaction may be identified. In these fractures, plate stabilization is preferred.[28]

Occasionally medial malleolar fractures occur in isolation. Careful radiographic examination must be performed to exclude instability patterns, such as the presence of a proximal fibular fracture, syndesmotic disruption, or chondral impaction of the medial aspect of the tibial plafond. A recent retrospective study evaluated 57 patients with closed isolated medial malleolar fractures treated nonsurgically with cast immobilization in slight inversion for 6 weeks.[48] All fractures were treated closed regardless of fracture gap or displacement. The authors noted a 96% union rate, excellent range of motion, and good functional results. The lack of a concurrent control group and the relatively short follow-up time were noted limitations to the study. The authors recommend that surgical stabilization of medial malleolar fractures should be reserved for bimalleolar or trimalleolar fractures, open fractures, injuries that compromise the skin, those involving the plafond, or for those patients who develop a painful nonunion.

Outcomes

Several recent prospective studies have provided outcomes data after fixation of ankle fractures. One study evaluated functional outcomes 1 year after surgical stabilization of unstable ankle fractures and fracture-dislocations. The authors noted that, at 1 year, patients were doing generally well with most experiencing little or mild pain and few restrictions in functional activities. A significant functional improvement was noted between the 6- and 12-month points. Older age, an American Society of Anesthesiologists classification of 3 or 4 (indicative of a generally sicker baseline), the presence of diabetes mellitus, and the female sex were factors significantly associated with a delay in functional recovery at 1 year.[49] Another prospective observational study of patients with unstable Weber B ankle fractures treated surgically found significant limitations even 2 years after treatment. Worse outcomes were associated primarily with social factors (smoking, less education, alcohol use, increasing age) and the presence of a medial malleolar fracture.[50] Poorer functional outcomes were similarly noted in patients sustaining a bimalleolar ankle fracture compared with those who had a medial ligamentous injury only.[51] Although it was hypothesized that the dissimilar results between the ruptured deltoid group and the medial malleolar fracture group may even out over time, a study examining surgically managed stage 4 supination-external rotation injuries at a mean of 13 years found that patients with partial or complete rupture of the medial deltoid ligament still tended to have a better functional result than those with a medial malleolar fracture, although pain and alignment showed no differences.[52] A true estimate of the end result of an ankle fracture, however, appears to require prolonged follow-up. One study found a latency time of almost 21 years between ankle related fractures and the occurrence of end-stage osteoarthritis.[53] Although some ankle injuries, such as pilon fractures or those that develop a complication during the healing process, appear to have an accelerated time course toward end-stage arthritis, most instances of end-stage osteoarthritis of the ankle are secondary to malleolar ankle fractures. This is almost certainly due to the frequency of malleolar fractures, as the true incidence of end-stage osteoarthritis of the ankle after a malleolar fracture is currently unknown.

Although a long-held tenet of fracture surgery is the importance of early active range-of-motion activities, little evidence exists to support this concept following ankle surgery. One recent systematic review of early mobilization of ankle fracture ORIF examined several randomized, controlled trials that compared early motion of the ankle joint to immobilization in a cast for 6 weeks.[54] The evidence suggested that, with early mobilization, there was an earlier return to work and improved range of motion at 12 weeks. Despite these positive findings, there was no difference in functional outcome scores or range of motion at 1 year, and the early range of motion group appeared to have a significantly increased risk of wound infection. Early functional rehabilitation, therefore, should be approached cautiously with achievement of adequate wound healing being the early postoperative focus.

Ankle Fractures in Patients With Diabetes

Impaired wound healing, delayed bone healing, pain insensitivity and altered proprioception, and the potential for Charcot changes make the management of ankle fractures in patients with diabetes extremely challenging. A recent review article succinctly describes the pitfalls and a treatment algorithm in this patient population.[55] The authors recommend a multidisciplinary approach with the initial management focused on blood glucose control and management of the soft-tissue envelope. In patients with unstable injuries identified by the presence of a dislocation or persistent subluxation, staged ORIF should be considered, using an external fixator to maintain alignment while awaiting soft-tissue recovery. In fractures that are reducible and stable, surgical management can proceed once the soft-tissue envelope is satisfactory. The injured limb should be supported with a well-padded and secure splint to maintain fracture and joint stability until ORIF can proceed. Nondisplaced fractures should be aggressively managed with serial short leg casting and close follow-up. The principles of surgical management are the meticulous handling of the soft-tissue envelope, achieving anatomic and rigid internal fixation with whatever means are necessary, and joint immobilization with casting or even external fixation to ensure adequate healing. Whether surgical or nonsurgical treatment was used, patients should be instructed to refrain from bearing weight for a minimum of 8 weeks; delayed weight bearing for up to 12 weeks should be considered in patients with additional risk factors for delayed bone healing, such as wide initial displacements, dislocations, or comminution. Once weight bearing begins, a total contact casting protocol may be considered for 3 to 6 additional months depending on the individual situation. Ankle fractures for which diagnosis is delayed or those displaced ankle fractures that are treated nonsurgically appear to have a higher risk of developing Charcot arthropathy.

Ankle Fractures in the Elderly

The management of ankle fractures in the elderly remains relatively controversial. Although associated osteoporosis may be a causative factor, it appears that increased weight, polypharmacy, and an increased propensity for falls also play important roles. A recent study noted that earlier investigations cited high complication rates and relatively poor outcomes following operative management; however, more recent investigations have demonstrated successful functional outcomes.[56] Another study reviewed the outcomes of surgical management of unstable ankle fractures in patients older than 80 years.[57] The authors noted that their complications of fixation failure and infection occurred exclusively in patients who were noncompliant. Current evidence, therefore, suggests that surgical treatment of unstable ankle fractures in the elderly can provide satisfactory outcomes with low complication rates, but patient selection is critical. Patients who are likely to be noncompliant with weight-bearing restrictions are at higher risk for fixation failure and wound infections. The surgeon should be prepared to encounter poor quality bone and have techniques available to maintain fracture stability, such as small and minifragment locking plates, medullary Kirschner wires, tibia-pro-fibula screws, and transarticular external fixation.

Distal Tibial Pilon Fractures

Introduction

In contrast to the rotational mechanisms that result in malleolar fractures and fracture-dislocations of the ankle, distal tibial pilon fractures typically result from high-energy axial-loading mechanisms. This mechanistic difference is the key characteristic that distinguishes "ankle" fractures and fracture-dislocations from distal tibial pilon fractures. The clinical manifestation of this mechanistic difference is the generation of osteochondral fracturing, comminution, and displacement of the weight-bearing articular portion of the tibial plafond and distal tibial metaphysis, as well as the development of marked swelling, blistering, and devitalization of the surrounding soft-tissue envelope typically identified in tibial pilon fractures. Although marginal areas of impaction, particularly along the posterior malleolar and medial malleolar fracture lines, can be identified in ankle fractures and fracture-dislocations, most fragment displacement is secondary to translational and rotational forces rather than compressive forces.

The initial management includes a careful and thorough evaluation of the soft-tissue envelope, provisional realignment of the limb, and radiographic assessment. Plain radiographs include standard ankle views and orthogonal full-length tibia and fibula images. To aid in fracture comprehension, CT is indicated in virtually all fractures of the tibial plafond, but is typically deferred until a provisional reduction is performed to maximize the information obtained. The simplistic Rüedi and Allgöwer classification system, and the comprehensive AO/Orthopaedic Trauma Association (OTA) classification system have not demonstrated optimal observer variability and have limited clinical utility in terms of guiding treatment or prognostication. Data suggest that the tibiotalar joint is intolerant of articular incongruity and subluxation,[53] but the degree to which residual incongruity affects long-term functional outcomes, posttraumatic arthrosis, and subsequent surgical intervention, remains controversial. Although strict guidelines are lacking, a visible incongruity at the tibial plafond identified on plain radiographs should be considered an indication for operative reduction and fixation in properly selected patients. Associated angular malalignment and/or talar subluxation are also strong indications for surgical treatment. Nonsurgical treatment is typically reserved for those rare instances where the fracture is nondisplaced and axially stable, or if the patient is nonambulatory or a poor candidate for surgery without impending skin breakdown.

Surgical Treatment

ORIF of pilon fractures has evolved over the past 40 years. Initially, Rüedi and Allgöwer reported 74% good and excellent results with primary ORIF following four classic principles: (1) restoring length with ORIF of the associated fibula fracture, (2) anatomic reduction of the tibial articular surface, (3) bone grafting metaphyseal defects, and (4) using a medial tibial buttress plate to prevent varus collapse and neutralize rotational forces to allow for early ankle motion.[58] However, these injuries were typically the result of rotational mechanisms in skiers, and the experiences of those treating higher-energy injuries were vastly different. Clinical series from the 1980s and 1990s using primary ORIF had complication rates of greater than 50%, most related to soft-tissue complications and infection, including amputation rates as high as 17%.[59,60] Disastrous results tempered enthusiasm for ORIF, and led to the evolution of using external fixation with limited articular internal fixation in an effort to decrease septic and soft-tissue complications. Subsequent studies, however, indicated increased rates of malunion, nonunion, and lower clinical scores with external fixation when compared with ORIF. With improved understanding of the importance of the associated soft-tissue injury, open treatment was reconsidered, but after a period of soft-tissue recovery. Definitive fixation of pilon fractures should be done when the soft-tissue envelope can withstand the added surgical insult. Surgical timing appeared to be a major contributing factor to the high complication rates seen in high-energy pilon fractures that underwent early definitive fixation. To minimize these unacceptable complication rates of early ORIF, a two-stage approach led to complication rates of less than 10%.[61,62]

Staged ORIF

Staged ORIF of tibial pilon fractures is a surgical tactic developed in response to the historically high soft-tissue complication rate encountered with early definitive open reduction and internal fixation of high-energy tibial pilon fractures. The initial stage is performed acutely to generally realign the limb and restore tibial and fibular length, provide provisional stability, and facilitate soft-tissue recovery. The second stage is performed when the soft-tissue swelling has abated, allowing definitive stabilization of the tibial component to proceed with a lessened risk of wound dehiscence and sepsis.

The key features of the initial stage are fibular reduction and fixation and ankle-spanning external fixation of the tibial pilon component. These procedures are performed acutely when the patient's general condition permits. Anatomic ORIF of the fibula accurately regains leg length, realigns the tibia, indirectly reduces the anterolateral and posterolateral articular tibial segments, and centers the talus beneath the tibia. On the other hand, malreduction of the fibula will limit the ability to reduce the tibia during the second stage.[63] If anatomic reduction cannot be achieved, fibular fixation should be delayed. Several options exist for surgical approaches to the distal tibia; most of these approaches comprise anterior exposures. A posterolateral surgical approach to the fibula maximizes the skin bridge available for these subsequent tibial approaches. ORIF of the associated fibula fracture with a plate and screws

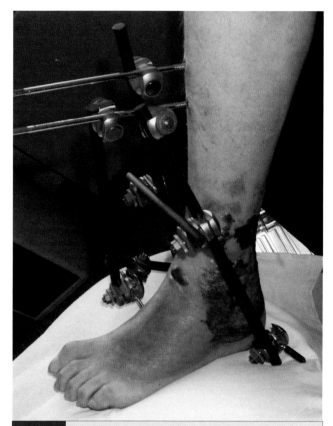

Figure 3 Clinical photograph showing a delta ankle-spanning external fixator frame and an ankle with hemorrhagic blisters.

has been shown to have a better clinical outcome with decreased tibial malunion and posttraumatic arthrosis.[64]

Ankle-spanning temporary external fixation is used to restore general limb alignment and displaced articular fragments through distraction and ligamentotaxis. By maintaining length and alignment, the limb is more effectively stabilized than with splinting, aiding in resolution of the soft-tissue injury and allowing for easier monitoring of the soft tissues. CT is most beneficial when performed after the external fixator is applied. The indirect reduction of displaced osseous fragments by ligamentotaxis is maintained by the external fixator, allowing for easier delineation of articular fracture patterns, and in turn more effectively helps plan the surgical approach and reduction and fixation strategy.[65] Although numerous external fixation devices and constructs are available, simple external fixator frames are favored for the initial stage of treatment. A simple external fixator frame can be used to minimize expense and can range from a simple transtibial and transcalcaneal pin ("traveling traction") to a delta-type frame (**Figure 3**). Either a posterior splint or forefoot pins should be added to maintain the foot and ankle in a plantigrade position, avoiding an acquired ankle or midfoot equinus contracture. Forefoot pins can be

placed across the cuneiforms or into the bases of the first and fifth metatarsals. It is important to avoid a metatarsal base pin that crosses the first intermetatarsal space because of the risk of vascular injury.[66] The critical aspects of using the external fixator are to restore length and ensure that the talus is beneath the tibia on both the anteroposterior and lateral radiographic views. Trying to restore each of these in a delayed fashion is much more difficult and dramatically lengthens the time of definitive surgery, which in turn increases the risk of complications. Additionally, any direct pressure on the skin or soft tissues by osseous fragments must be corrected to avoid skin compromise. The second stage, definitive ORIF of the tibial pilon component, is undertaken when the soft-tissue injury has resolved. This typically occurs between 10 and 24 days after injury.[61,62] Percutaneous methods and limited open surgical approaches have been successfully used with early definitive external fixation, but the condition of the soft-tissue envelope should determine whether this can be performed acutely. Reepithelialization of fracture blisters, healing of open fracture wounds, resolution of ecchymosis, and wrinkling of the affected skin are clinical objective parameters that indicate recovery of the soft-tissue injury and that definitive surgery may occur.

Multiple surgical approaches have been described for ORIF of pilon fractures. The surgical approach should be determined by the soft-tissue injury (for example, presence of open wounds) and fracture pattern. The classic approach is the anteromedial exposure with the incision beginning proximally lateral to the tibial crest and continuing distally parallel to the tibialis anterior tendon. With development of precontoured anterolateral plates and soft-tissue complications associated with medial distal tibial plating, the anterolateral approach has become more popular for complex articular fracture patterns, allowing adequate ability to visualize the articular surface, direct access to the Chaput fragment, and improved soft-tissue coverage for implants. Several surgical exposures to the distal tibia have recently been described, including an extensile modified anteromedial, a posterolateral, and an extensile lateral approach. The latter exposure allows for fixation of the fibula and tibia through a single incision.[63,67,68] Recent reports have also focused on the use of multiple surgical approaches to address complex articular fractures. These studies have shown that with appropriate surgical technique, complications related to multiple incisions are less than 10%, and they have challenged the need for a 7-cm skin bridge between incisions[69,70] (**Figure 4**).

Minimally invasive plating and "biologically friendly" surgical techniques have been used in an attempt to decrease complication rates. The general principles of these techniques include: a formal surgical approach to the articular surface alone for direct reduction and absolute stability; indirect reduction techniques for the metaphyseal and diaphyseal components; and percutaneous techniques for fixation proxi-

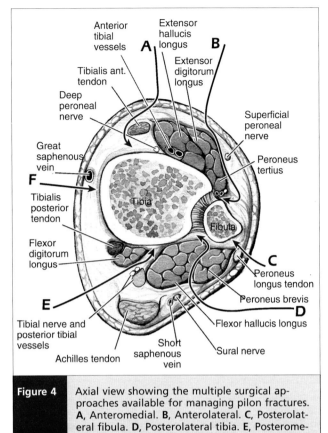

Figure 4 Axial view showing the multiple surgical approaches available for managing pilon fractures. **A**, Anteromedial. **B**, Anterolateral. **C**, Posterolateral fibula. **D**, Posterolateral tibia. **E**, Posteromedial. **F**, Medial. (Reproduced with permission from Howard JL, Agel J, Barei DP, Benirschke SK, Nork SE: A prospective study evaluating incision placement and wound healing for tibial plafond fractures. *J Orthop Trauma* 2008:22:299-305.)

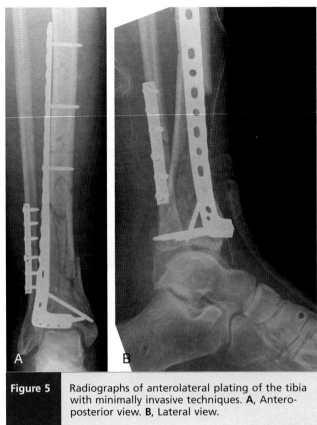

Figure 5 Radiographs of anterolateral plating of the tibia with minimally invasive techniques. **A**, Anteroposterior view. **B**, Lateral view.

mal to the articular surface.[71-75] Low profile, precontoured, and locking plates with percutaneous insertion techniques have been used to potentially improve fixation and decrease soft-tissue complications (**Figure 5**). Minimally invasive plating techniques have led to early attempts at definitive fixation, including the use of arthroscopically assisted articular reduction, and have had mixed results.[76,77]

Definitive Management With External Fixation

The high rate of soft-tissue complications associated with primary ORIF of pilon fractures led to the use of external fixation, with limited internal fixation as an alternative technique for definitive management. Ankle-spanning with or without articulation, Ilizarov, and hybrid external fixation have been used. All methods may be supplemented with percutaneous or limited surgical approaches for articular reduction and fixation with lag screws when the soft tissues permit. The external fixator acts as a neutralization device to maintain length, alignment, and rotation. Fibular fixation has been performed in some series and led to fewer malunions but a higher risk of fibular complications and no significant outcome difference.

Through ligamentotaxis, the ankle-spanning external fixator helps reduce the articular surface. A concern over prolonged ankle-spanning external fixation relates to the effect on ankle range of motion. In a small, prospective, multicenter, randomized trial comparing early motion with no motion with an articulated ankle-spanning external fixator, there was no range-of-motion or validated outcome score differences at 2 years.[78] Ankle-spanning and ankle-sparing Ilizarov fixation has also been successfully used in small series involving high-energy pilon fractures with pin tract infections being the most common complication.[79-81] Hybrid external fixation has been used to allow early ankle motion and provide more control of the articular segment than ankle-spanning external fixation. It is typically used for fractures with large articular fragments, metaphyseal comminution, complicated open fracture wounds, or in patients with comorbidities that significantly increase the risk of complications, such as diabetic neuropathy (**Figure 6**). Hybrid external fixation has been shown to have a significantly lower rate of malunion than ankle-spanning external fixation.[82]

Comparing Treatment Methods

With the increased success of staged ORIF of pilon fractures with plates, few recent studies have directly compared delayed definitive plating with definitive external fixation. Most of the available studies are retro-

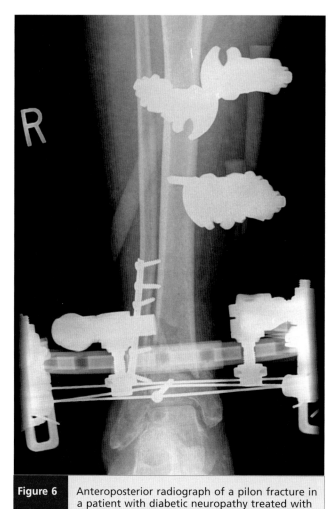

Figure 6 Anteroposterior radiograph of a pilon fracture in a patient with diabetic neuropathy treated with hybrid external fixation and limited internal fixation.

ited internal fixation or two-stage ORIF with plating.[79] Although no significant differences were found, twice as many patients were in the staged plating group and there was a trend toward lower rate of nonunion, malunion, and infection.

Although conflicting and insufficient data exist comparing treatment methods, the literature shows that, for pilon fractures, the condition of the soft tissue may be the most important determining factor as to when and what type of treatment should be undertaken. Surgeons ultimately must choose the treatment strategy based on the fracture pattern, soft-tissue condition, patient comorbidities, and surgeon experience.

Soft-Tissue Management Strategies

Soft-tissue management in high-energy pilon fractures can be challenging. Although appropriate surgical timing, approaches, and techniques are critical, negative pressure wound therapy has been investigated to determine its role in managing these injuries. In addition to its use in open wound management, negative pressure wound therapy has been beneficial when applied over primarily closed incisions for removal of postoperative hematoma, and it decreased postoperative drainage and edema in high-risk injuries and patients.[84,85]

Summary

The commonality of ankle fractures requires that the treating orthopaedist have a thorough understanding of the determinants of tibiotalar stability. Increasing use of CT to delineate fracture morphology, particularly of the syndesmosis and posterior malleolus, as well as the use of preoperative and intraoperative dynamic plain radiography, facilitate the identification of unstable injuries and allow a surgical tactic for successful treatment. The importance of recognizing distal tibiofibular syndesmotic injury has become increasingly apparent. Although specific details regarding the technique of stabilization are debatable, the importance of obtaining an accurate syndesmotic reduction is critical for maximizing the chances of obtaining a satisfactory outcome. The axial-loading tibial pilon fractures remain a therapeutic challenge. Staged approaches that allow for the resolution of the associated soft-tissue injury prior to definitive ORIF have demonstrated durable success in decreasing the previously high wound and deep septic complication rates. Fracture pattern-specific approaches, determined with the use of CT, combined with improved plate-screw designs, are also important variables responsible for decreasing wound complication rates. Despite these advances, the outcome of tibial pilon fractures remains problematic, with a substantial number of patients reporting problems with stiffness, swelling, and pain. Although accurate surgical reconstruction with minimization of soft-tissue complications should remain the goal, factors outside of the surgeon's control may have substantial influence on the final outcome.

spective comparative studies that have evaluated implemented protocols. Most series from the past 10 years that compared hybrid or circular external fixation to delayed plating showed that fractures treated with external fixation had typically more complex fracture patterns accompanied by worse soft-tissue injuries, which induces selection bias and makes direct comparison difficult.[83] Despite this potential selection bias, conflicting data exist regarding which method has a higher rate of complications. Only one series had a higher rate of complications in the delayed plating group, which was composed of all closed fractures with Tscherne grade 0 and 1 soft-tissue injuries.[83] This finding may have resulted in part from definitive plating being performed an average of only 5 days after injury. A previous direct comparison of primary ORIF on day 3 to 5 with hybrid external fixation showed significantly higher rates of complications in the ORIF group.[60] Recently, a retrospective comparative series was done for AO/OTA type C fractures treated either by ankle-spanning Ilizarov external fixation with lim-

5: Lower Extremity

Annotated References

1. Valderrabano V, Horisberger M, Russell I, Dougall H, Hintermann B: Etiology of ankle osteoarthritis. *Clin Orthop Relat Res* 2009;467(7):1800-1806.

   This study evaluated the etiologies leading to ankle arthritis. Posttraumatic ankle OA was seen in 78% of the cases, secondary arthritis in 13%, and primary OA in 9%. Currently, trauma is the main cause of ankle OA, and primary OA is rare. Level of evidence: IV.

2. Gardner MJ, Demetrakopoulos D, Briggs SM, Helfet DL, Lorich DG: The ability of the Lauge-Hansen classification to predict ligament injury and mechanism in ankle fractures: An MRI study. *J Orthop Trauma* 2006; 20(4):267-272.

   This retrospective study evaluated the accuracy of predicted injury sequences using MRI in a series of patients with ankle fractures. A standard ankle radiographic series was assigned to a Lauge-Hansen category, then MRIs evaluated the integrity of the ankle ligaments. The results demonstrated that the Lauge-Hansen classification system might have some limitations as a predictor of the mechanism of injury and the presence of soft-tissue damage associated with ankle fractures.

3. Michelson JD, Magid D, McHale K: Clinical utility of a stability-based ankle fracture classification system. *J Orthop Trauma* 2007;21(5):307-315.

   The results of this study suggest that a stability-based ankle fracture classification system can be prognostic. For unstable ankle fractures, the radiographic outcomes were better after surgery when the decision for surgery was made on the basis of stability. Overall, nonsurgical treatment results were also better with stability-based treatment.

4. Bartonícek J: Anatomy of the tibiofibular syndesmosis and its clinical relevance. *Surg Radiol Anat* 2003;25(5-6):379-386.

5. Stark E, Tornetta P III, Creevy WR: Syndesmotic instability in Weber B ankle fractures: A clinical evaluation. *J Orthop Trauma* 2007;21(9):643-646.

   This retrospective cohort, consecutive series found syndesmotic instability to be common after anatomic ORIF in unstable Weber B SE pattern lateral malleolar fractures. Previous cadaver study criteria for syndesmotic instability are not clinically representative. Syndesmotic instability in these fractures can and should be identified intraoperatively with a stress examination.

6. Weening B, Bhandari M: Predictors of functional outcome following transsyndesmotic screw fixation of ankle fractures. *J Orthop Trauma* 2005;19(2):102-108.

   This retrospective observational study found: (1) technical aspects of syndesmotic screw fixation vary between surgeons; (2) 16% of syndesmotic screws may have been unnecessary; and (3) despite variability in technique and indications, anatomic reduction of syndesmosis was significantly associated with improved functional outcome. Level of evidence: IV.

7. Nielson JH, Gardner MJ, Peterson MG, et al: Radiographic measurements do not predict syndesmotic injury in ankle fractures: An MRI study. *Clin Orthop Relat Res* 2005;436:216-221.

   Prospectively, 70 ankle fractures had plain radiographic evaluations and MRI. Several radiographic measurements and MRI findings were analyzed. A medial clear space measurement > 4 mm correlated with deltoid and tibiofibular ligament disruption. There was no association between the tibiofibular clear space and overlap measurements on radiographs with syndesmotic injury on MRI. Level of evidence: II-1.

8. Gardner MJ, Brodsky A, Briggs SM, Nielson JH, Lorich DG: Fixation of posterior malleolar fractures provides greater syndesmotic stability. *Clin Orthop Relat Res* 2006;447:165-171.

   A pronation-external rotation fracture pattern with a posterior malleolar fragment was created in 10 cadavers randomly assigned to posterior malleolus or syndesmotic fixation. Compared with the intact specimens, stiffness was restored to 70% after fixation of the posterior malleolus, and to 40% after syndesmosis stabilization.

9. Jenkinson RJ, Sanders DW, Macleod MD, Domonkos A, Lydestadt J: Intraoperative diagnosis of syndesmosis injuries in external rotation ankle fractures. *J Orthop Trauma* 2005;19(9):604-609.

   In a prospective, consecutive series, intraoperative fluoroscopy detected unpredicted syndesmotic instability in 37% of ankles. Specifically, unpredicted syndesmosis instability was found in 33% of supination-external rotation injuries, and 57% of pronation-external rotation injuries. Intraoperative stress fluoroscopy is valuable for detecting unstable syndesmotic injuries.

10. Candal-Couto JJ, Burrow D, Bromage S, Briggs PJ: Instability of the tibio-fibular syndesmosis: Have we been pulling in the wrong direction? *Injury* 2004;35(8):814-818.

    Using a ligament-sectioning cadaver model, the authors demonstrated substantially greater sagittal plane displacements of the fibular relative to the tibia compared with the coronal plane, for a given set of ligamentous disruptions.

11. Gardner MJ, Demetrakopoulos D, Briggs SM, Helfet DL, Lorich DG: Malreduction of the tibiofibular syndesmosis in ankle fractures. *Foot Ankle Int* 2006; 27(10):788-792.

    Twenty-five patients with ankle fractures and syndesmotic instability who had open reduction and syndesmotic fixation were evaluated. Postoperatively, all had a standard radiographic series and CT. Many syndesmoses were malreduced on CT scan but went undetected by plain radiographs; postreduction radiographic measurements were inaccurate for assessing reduction quality.

12. Miller AN, Carroll EA, Parker RJ, Boraiah S, Helfet DL, Lorich DG: Direct visualization for syndesmotic stabilization of ankle fractures. *Foot Ankle Int* 2009; 30(5):419-426.

In this study, direct visualization and reduction of the syndesmosis demonstrated a 16% incongruity incidence, compared with 52% of controls. Although malreductions were significantly decreased in the direct visualization group, they were not eliminated. Posterior malleolar reconstruction was more accurate than syndesmotic screw fixation.

13. Thordarson DB, Samuelson M, Shepherd LE, Merkle PF, Lee J: Bioabsorbable versus stainless steel screw fixation of the syndesmosis in pronation-lateral rotation ankle fractures: A prospective randomized trial. *Foot Ankle Int* 2001;22(4):335-338.

14. Kukreti S, Faraj A, Miles JN: Does position of syndesmotic screw affect functional and radiological outcome in ankle fractures? *Injury* 2005;36(9):1121-1124.

    This small, retrospective cohort study demonstrated no difference in radiologic or clinical outcomes in patients with distal tibiofibular syndesmotic injuries treated using transsyndesmotic screw fixation or suprasyndesmotic screw fixation.

15. Beumer A, Campo MM, Niesing R, Day J, Kleinrensink GJ, Swierstra BA: Screw fixation of the syndesmosis: A cadaver model comparing stainless steel and titanium screws and three and four cortical fixation. *Injury* 2005; 36(1):60-64.

    Syndesmotic set screw strength and fixation capacity during cyclical testing in a cadaver model simulating protected weight bearing was assessed. The authors concluded that the syndesmotic set screw cannot prevent excessive syndesmotic widening when loaded with a load comparable with body weight.

16. Cox S, Mukherjee DP, Ogden AL, et al: Distal tibiofibular syndesmosis fixation: A cadaveric, simulated fracture stabilization study comparing bioabsorbable and metallic single screw fixation. *J Foot Ankle Surg* 2005; 44(2):144-151.

    This cadaver biomechanical study demonstrated equivalent distal tibiofibular syndesmotic stability when comparing a 5.0-mm bioabsorbable screw with a 5.0-mm stainless steel screw.

17. Kaukonen JP, Lamberg T, Korkala O, Pajarinen J: Fixation of syndesmotic ruptures in 38 patients with a malleolar fracture: A randomized study comparing a metallic and a bioabsorbable screw. *J Orthop Trauma* 2005; 19(6):392-395.

    In a clinical randomized controlled trial, the performance of a metallic and a biodegradable screw in the fixation of tibia-fibula syndesmotic ruptures in 38 patients was evaluated. More patients with a polylevolactic acid screw returned to their previous activity level, and there was less swelling in the ankles of these patients, but joint motion was similar between the groups.

18. Ahmad J, Raikin SM, Pour AE, Haytmanek C: Bioabsorbable screw fixation of the syndesmosis in unstable ankle injuries. *Foot Ankle Int* 2009;30(2):99-105.

    This study retrospectively evaluated the clinical and radiographic outcomes of medium and long-term results of bioabsorbable screw fixation of unstable ankle syndesmosis injuries in 75 patients. This study demonstrated that bioabsorbable syndesmotic screw fixation is associated with satisfactory restoration of ankle function and syndesmotic stability.

19. Cottom JM, Hyer CF, Philbin TM, Berlet GC: Treatment of syndesmotic disruptions with the Arthrex Tightrope: A report of 25 cases. *Foot Ankle Int* 2008; 29(8):773-780.

    Twenty-five patients with distal tibiofibular joint disruption underwent stabilization with a suture technique. Mean time to full weight bearing was 5.5 weeks and good results ensued. Benefits included quick and minimally invasive intraoperative placement obviating later hardware removal. In this series, excellent syndesmotic reduction was maintained.

20. Forsythe K, Freedman KB, Stover MD, Patwardhan AG: Comparison of a novel FiberWire-button construct versus metallic screw fixation in a syndesmotic injury model. *Foot Ankle Int* 2008;29(1):49-54.

    This cadaver biomechanical study evaluated the ability of a suture implant to maintain syndesmotic reduction when compared with a metallic screw. The suture implant was unable to maintain syndesmotic reduction at any of the forces applied, with significantly greater syndesmotic widening compared to screw fixation, at all loads.

21. Willmott HJ, Singh B, David LA: Outcome and complications of treatment of ankle diastasis with tightrope fixation. *Injury* 2009;40(11):1204-1206.

    This series showed a significant incidence of soft-tissue complications with the use of suture fixation technique and subsequent need for removal.

22. Høiness P, Strømsøe K: Tricortical versus quadricortical syndesmosis fixation in ankle fractures: A prospective, randomized study comparing two methods of syndesmosis fixation. *J Orthop Trauma* 2004;18(6):331-337.

    This randomized clinical study concluded that syndesmosis fixation with two tricortical screws provided adequate stability and improved function at 3 months compared with quadricortical screw fixation. After 1 year, however, there were no significant differences between the two groups in functional score, pain, and dorsiflexion. Unfortunately, because of other uncontrolled variables (differences in screw diameter and implant removal), robust conclusions could not be made.

23. Wikerøy AK, Høiness PR, Andreassen GS, Hellund JC, Madsen JE: No difference in functional and radiographic results 8.4 years after quadricortical compared with tricortical syndesmosis fixation in ankle fractures. *J Orthop Trauma* 2010;24(1):17-23.

    Follow-up 8.4 years after surgery of ankle fractures with syndesmotic injury showed satisfactory functional results with only minor differences between the tricortical and quadricortical fixation groups. Synostosis, a posterior fracture fragment, obesity, and syndesmotic width ≥ 1.5 mm more than the contralateral normal ankle predicted impaired ankle function.

5: Lower Extremity

24. Miller AN, Paul O, Boraiah S, Parker RJ, Helfet DL, Lorich DG: Functional outcomes after syndesmotic screw fixation and removal. *J Orthop Trauma* 2010; 24(1):12-16.

    This study examined the effects of syndesmotic and fibular implant removal after ankle fracture. Significant improvement in range of motion and functional scores at the immediate postoperative visit was noted. This did not significantly change with longer follow-up. There was no loss of syndesmotic reduction after screw removal.

25. Manjoo A, Sanders DW, Tieszer C, MacLeod MD: Functional and radiographic results of patients with syndesmotic screw fixation: Implications for screw removal. *J Orthop Trauma* 2010;24(1):2-6.

    This study sought to determine whether functional outcomes and radiographic results after ankle fracture were affected by the status of the syndesmosis screw. An intact syndesmosis screw was associated with a worse functional outcome compared with loose, fractured, or removed screws. There were no differences in functional outcomes comparing loose or fractured screws with removed screws.

26. Hamid N, Loeffler BJ, Braddy W, Kellam JF, Cohen BE, Bosse MJ: Outcome after fixation of ankle fractures with an injury to the syndesmosis: The effect of the syndesmosis screw. *J Bone Joint Surg Br* 2009;91(8):1069-1073.

    Patient outcomes were compared after ankle fractures relative to the syndesmosis screw status. There was no difference in outcome with intact or removed syndesmotic screws. Patients with a broken syndesmosis screw had the best outcome. These data do not support the removal of intact or broken syndesmosis screws.

27. McConnell T, Tornetta P III: Marginal plafond impaction in association with supination-adduction ankle fractures: A report of eight cases. *J Orthop Trauma* 2001;15(6):447-449.

28. Dumigan RM, Bronson DG, Early JS: Analysis of fixation methods for vertical shear fractures of the medial malleolus. *J Orthop Trauma* 2006;20(10):687-691.

    Fixation of vertical shear fractures of the medial malleolus with a properly applied neutralization plate offers a significant mechanical advantage over screw-only constructs.

29. Ramsey PL, Hamilton W: Changes in tibiotalar area of contact caused by lateral talar shift. *J Bone Joint Surg Am* 1976;58(3):356-357.

30. van den Bekerom MP, van Dijk CN: Is fibular fracture displacement consistent with tibiotalar displacement? *Clin Orthop Relat Res* 2010;468(4):969-974.

    The authors concluded that tibiotalar displacement cannot be reliably assessed at the level of the fracture. Based on this and other studies, the authors believe there is little evidence to support performing open reduction and internal fixation of supination-external rotation II ankle fractures. Level of evidence: IV.

31. DeAngelis NA, Eskander MS, French BG: Does medial tenderness predict deep deltoid ligament incompetence in supination-external rotation type ankle fractures? *J Orthop Trauma* 2007;21(4):244-247.

    In this study, there was no statistical significance between medial ankle tenderness and deep deltoid ligament incompetence. Medial tenderness in a Weber B ankle fracture with a normal clear space on plain radiographs does not ensure the presence of a positive external rotation stress test.

32. Egol KA, Amirtharajah M, Amirtharage M, Tejwani NC, Capla EL, Koval KJ: Ankle stress test for predicting the need for surgical fixation of isolated fibular fractures. *J Bone Joint Surg Am* 2004;86(11):2393-2398.

    This study confirmed a high rate of positive stress radiographs for patients who present with an isolated fibular fracture and an intact ankle mortise on the initial plain radiographs. However, the presence of medial symptoms was not sensitive with regard to medial clear space stress widening. Additionally, a number of patients with radiographic widening but no clinical symptoms were treated successfully without surgery.

33. McConnell T, Creevy W, Tornetta P III: Stress examination of supination external rotation-type fibular fractures. *J Bone Joint Surg Am* 2004;86(10):2171-2178.

    The authors concluded that stress radiographs allow for the accurate diagnosis of deltoid incompetence in patients with isolated Weber B-type supination-external rotations fibular fractures. In this clinical study, medial soft tissue indicators (bruising tenderness, swelling) were not accurate predictors of instability.

34. Gill JB, Risko T, Raducan V, Grimes JS, Schutt RC Jr: Comparison of manual and gravity stress radiographs for the evaluation of supination-external rotation fibular fractures. *J Bone Joint Surg Am* 2007;89(5):994-999.

    The gravity stress radiograph is equivalent to the manual stress radiograph for determining deltoid ligament injury in association with an isolated distal fibular fracture, and thus it can be used to determine ankle stability in patients who present with an isolated distal fibular fracture.

35. Schock HJ, Pinzur M, Manion L, Stover M: The use of gravity or manual-stress radiographs in the assessment of supination-external rotation fractures of the ankle. *J Bone Joint Surg Br* 2007;89(8):1055-1059.

    Supination-external rotation ankle fractures may present with a medial ligamentous injury that is not radiographically apparent. This study demonstrated that gravity-stress is as reliable and perceived as more comfortable than that of manual stress for the detection of occult medial ligamentous injuries in supination-external rotation fractures of the ankle.

36. Koval KJ, Egol KA, Cheung Y, Goodwin DW, Spratt KF: Does a positive ankle stress test indicate the need for operative treatment after lateral malleolus fracture? A preliminary report. *J Orthop Trauma* 2007;21:449-455.

This study evaluated patients with isolated Weber B lateral malleolus fracture and a positive ankle stress test (≥ 5 mm clear space widening) with MRI to determine the status of the deep deltoid ligament. Ninety percent had evidence of partially torn deep deltoid ligament on MRI and were treated nonsurgically. Excellent functional scores at 1 year were noted without evidence of residual medial clear space widening or posttraumatic joint space narrowing. This protocol was able to identify and provide effective nonsurgical care to 19 patients who otherwise might have undergone surgical treatment after an isolated lateral malleolus fracture.

37. Park SS, Kubiak EN, Egol KA, Kummer F, Koval KJ: Stress radiographs after ankle fracture: The effect of ankle position and deltoid ligament status on medial clear space measurements. *J Orthop Trauma* 2006;20(1):11-18.

In a cadaver fracture model, ankle stress radiographs taken in dorsiflexion-external rotation were most predictive of deep deltoid ligament disruption after distal fibular fracture. Under this stress condition, a medial clear space of ≥ 5 mm was the most reliable predictor of deep deltoid ligament status.

38. Chen PY, Wang TG, Wang CL: Ultrasonographic examination of the deltoid ligament in bimalleolar equivalent fractures. *Foot Ankle Int* 2008;29(9):883-886.

Ultrasonography showed complete rupture of the deltoid ligament in a small number of patients. Subsequent exploration confirmed the sonographic findings in all. In nine patients, the deltoid ligament was not completely ruptured on ultrasound; conservative treatment yielded uneventful healing.

39. McKenna PB, O'Shea K, Burke T: Less is more: Lag screw only fixation of lateral malleolar fractures. *Int Orthop* 2007;31(4):497-502.

This clinical study demonstrated the effectiveness of lag screw-only fixation of selected lateral malleolus fractures.

40. Lamontagne J, Blachut PA, Broekhuyse HM, O'Brien PJ, Meek RN: Surgical treatment of a displaced lateral malleolus fracture: The antiglide technique versus lateral plate fixation. *J Orthop Trauma* 2002;16(7):498-502.

41. Weber M, Krause F: Peroneal tendon lesions caused by antiglide plates used for fixation of lateral malleolar fractures: The effect of plate and screw position. *Foot Ankle Int* 2005;26(4):281-285.

The authors of this clinical study identified a high rate of later implant removal required to treat peroneal tendon irritation. Very distal plate placement and protruding distal screw heads correlated with peroneal tendon lesions and symptoms.

42. Siegel J, Tornetta P III: Extraperiosteal plating of pronation-abduction ankle fractures. *J Bone Joint Surg Am* 2007;89(2):276-281.

Extraperiosteal plating of pronation-abduction ankle fractures proved to be an effective method leading to predictable fibular union. The results were considered to be at least as good as those of other techniques of open reduction and internal fixation of the ankle.

43. Haraguchi N, Haruyama H, Toga H, Kato F: Pathoanatomy of posterior malleolar fractures of the ankle. *J Bone Joint Surg Am* 2006;88(5):1085-1092.

This CT study identified that the fracture lines associated with posterior malleolar fractures appear to be highly variable, with 20% of the posterior malleolar fractures in this study extending to the medial malleolus. Because of the great variation in fracture configurations, preoperative use of CT may be justified.

44. Forberger J, Sabandal PV, Dietrich M, Gralla J, Lattmann T, Platz A: Posterolateral approach to the displaced posterior malleolus: Functional outcome and local morbidity. *Foot Ankle Int* 2009;30(4):309-314.

In this study, the posterolateral approach allowed good exposure and stable fixation of a displaced posterior malleolar fragment with few local complications. The anatomic repositioning and stable fixation led to good functional and subjective outcome.

45. De Vries JS, Wijgman AJ, Sierevelt IN, Schaap GR: Long-term results of ankle fractures with a posterior malleolar fragment. *J Foot Ankle Surg* 2005;44(3):211-217.

This long-term clinical study evaluated the results of ankle fractures with a posterior malleolar fragment. The authors concluded that patients showed good results after 13-year follow-up, and there was no evidence for the need of fixation of fragments smaller than 25% of the width of the plafond.

46. Fitzpatrick DC, Otto JK, McKinley TO, Marsh JL, Brown TD: Kinematic and contact stress analysis of posterior malleolus fractures of the ankle. *J Orthop Trauma* 2004;18(5):271-278.

Using a cadaver fracture model, the authors simulated a variety of posterior malleolar fracture situations, including step and gap malreductions, an unsecured fragment, and an anatomically reduced fragment. The authors found no talar subluxation and no increase in contact stresses near the articular incongruity, making it unlikely that these factors explain the increased incidence of arthrosis after trimalleolar ankle fractures.

47. Femino JE, Gruber BF, Karunakar MA: Safe zone for the placement of medial malleolar screws. *J Bone Joint Surg Am* 2007;89(1):133-138.

Screws inserted posterior to the anterior colliculus place the posterior tibial tendon at significant risk for injury or abutment.

48. Herscovici D Jr, Scaduto JM, Infante A: Conservative treatment of isolated fractures of the medial malleolus. *J Bone Joint Surg Br* 2007;89(1):89-93.

Fifty-seven isolated fractures of the medial malleolus were treated by cast immobilization. Fifty-five healed without further treatment. There was no evidence of medial instability, mortise malalignment, or posttraumatic arthritis. Isolated medial malleolus fractures can obtain high rates of union and good functional results with conservative treatment.

49. Egol KA, Tejwani NC, Walsh MG, Capla EL, Koval KJ: Predictors of short-term functional outcome following ankle fracture surgery. *J Bone Joint Surg Am* 2006; 88(5):974-979.

One year after ankle fracture surgery, patients are generally well, with most experiencing little or mild pain and few restrictions in functional activities. Younger age, male sex, absence of diabetes, and a lower ASA class were predictive of functional recovery at 1 year.

50. Bhandari M, Sprague S, Hanson B, et al: Health-related quality of life following operative treatment of unstable ankle fractures: A prospective observational study. *J Orthop Trauma* 2004;18(6):338-345.

As is the case in many other areas, social factors may be important determinants of outcome in patients with traumatic fractures. Optimal orthopaedic care may involve attention to modifiable risk factors, including smoking and alcohol consumption.

51. Tejwani NC, McLaurin TM, Walsh M, Bhadsavle S, Koval KJ, Egol KA: Are outcomes of bimalleolar fractures poorer than those of lateral malleolar fractures with medial ligamentous injury? *J Bone Joint Surg Am* 2007;89(7):1438-1441.

At 1 year after surgical stabilization of an unstable ankle fracture, most patients experience little or mild pain and have few restrictions in functional activities. However, the functional outcome for those with a bimalleolar fracture is worse than that for those with a lateral malleolar fracture and disruption of the deltoid ligament, possibly because of the injury pattern and the energy expended.

52. Stufkens SA, Knupp M, Lampert C, van Dijk CN, Hintermann B: Long-term outcome after supination-external rotation type-4 fractures of the ankle. *J Bone Joint Surg Br* 2009;91(12):1607-1611.

At a mean follow-up of 13 years after surgical treatment of a supination-external rotation type 4 ankle fracture, patients with partial or complete rupture of the medial deltoid ligament tended to have a better result than those with a medial malleolar fracture.

53. Horisberger M, Valderrabano V, Hintermann B: Post-traumatic ankle osteoarthritis after ankle-related fractures. *J Orthop Trauma* 2009;23(1):60-67.

The latency time between injury and end-stage ankle osteoarthritis was approximately 21 years. Malleolar fracture was the most common fracture (53.2%). A negative correlation of the osteoarthritis latency time with the fracture severity was observed for pilon fractures and patients with complications during the healing process.

54. Thomas G, Whalley H, Modi C: Early mobilization of operatively fixed ankle fractures: A systematic review. *Foot Ankle Int* 2009;30(7):666-674.

Nine randomized, controlled trials were identified that compared early ankle joint motion to immobilization in a cast for 6 weeks after ankle ORIF. The evidence suggested that earlier range of motion provides an earlier return to work but has a significant risk of wound complications. Outcomes at 1 year were similar between the groups.

55. Chaudhary SB, Liporace FA, Gandhi A, Donley BG, Pinzur MS, Lin SS: Complications of ankle fracture in patients with diabetes. *J Am Acad Orthop Surg* 2008; 16(3):159-170.

Ankle fractures in patients with diabetes mellitus have long been recognized as a challenge to practicing clinicians. Adherence to the basic principles of preoperative planning, meticulous soft-tissue management, and attention to stable, rigid fixation with prolonged, protected immobilization are paramount in minimizing problems and yielding good functional outcomes.

56. Strauss EJ, Egol KA: The management of ankle fractures in the elderly. *Injury* 2007;38(suppl 3):S2-S9.

This review article suggests that based on the current evidence, the literature appears to support surgical fixation of displaced ankle fractures in the elderly patient population.

57. Fong W, Acevedo JI, Stone RG, Mizel MS: The treatment of unstable ankle fractures in patients over eighty years of age. *Foot Ankle Int* 2007;28(12):1256-1259.

The study examined the outcomes of ankle fractures ORIF in patients 80 years or older. When noncompliant patients who developed complications were removed from analysis, fixation failure and deep infection rates were eliminated. Patient compliance and non–weight-bearing status are important in the treatment of ankle fractures in octogenarians.

58. Rüedi T, Allgöwer M: Fractures of the lower end of the tibia into the ankle-joint. *Injury* 1969;1:92-99.

59. McFerran MA, Smith SW, Boulas HJ, Schwartz HS: Complications encountered in the treatment of pilon fractures. *J Orthop Trauma* 1992;6(2):195-200.

60. Wyrsch B, McFerran MA, McAndrew M, et al: Operative treatment of fractures of the tibial plafond: A randomized, prospective study. *J Bone Joint Surg Am* 1996; 78(11):1646-1657.

61. Patterson MJ, Cole JD: Two-staged delayed open reduction and internal fixation of severe pilon fractures. *J Orthop Trauma* 1999;13(2):85-91.

62. Sirkin M, Sanders R, DiPasquale T, Herscovici D Jr: A staged protocol for soft tissue management in the treatment of complex pilon fractures. *J Orthop Trauma* 1999;13(2):78-84.

63. Assal M, Ray A, Stern R: The extensile approach for the operative treatment of high-energy pilon fractures: Surgical technique and soft-tissue healing. *J Orthop Trauma* 2007;21(3):198-206.

This article illustrates an extensile approach and its effect on soft-tissue healing. Complete access to the ankle joint to achieve reduction and fixation of the articular surface, as far medially or laterally as is necessary is demonstrated. Proximally, plates can be placed subcutaneously from distal to proximal through the open incision.

64. Lee YS, Chen SW, Chen SH, Chen WC, Lau MJ, Hsu TL: Stabilisation of the fractured fibula plays an important role in the treatment of pilon fractures: A retrospective comparison of fibular fixation methods. *Int Orthop* 2009;33(3):695-699.

Ninety-eight pilon fractures associated with ipsilateral distal fibular fracture were included in this study. For pilon fractures associated with ipsilateral fibular fractures, stabilization of the fractured fibula played an important role in the decrease of distal tibial malunion and posttraumatic ankle arthrosis as well as improvement of clinical outcomes.

65. Topliss CJ, Jackson M, Atkins RM: Anatomy of pilon fractures of the distal tibia. *J Bone Joint Surg Br* 2005;87(5):692-697.

In a series of 126 consecutive pilon fractures, anatomically explicable fragments are identified. Fracture lines describing these fragments revealed 10 types of pilon fracture belonging to 2 families, sagittal and coronal. Fracture type was dictated by the energy of injury, direction of the injurious force, and patient age.

66. Barrett MO, Wade AM, Della Rocca GJ, Crist BD, Anglen JO: The safety of forefoot metatarsal pins in external fixation of the lower extremity. *J Bone Joint Surg Am* 2008;90(3):560-564.

This anatomic study evaluated the safety of external fixation pins placed across the bases of the first and second metatarsals, spanning the first intermetarsal space. Placement of pins through the proximal bases of the first and second metatarsals, within 2 cm of the first tarsometatarsal joint, consistently places the deep plantar branch of the dorsalis pedis artery at risk.

67. Bhattacharyya T, Crichlow R, Gobezie R, Kim E, Vrahas MS: Complications associated with the posterolateral approach for pilon fractures. *J Orthop Trauma* 2006;20(2):104-107.

A review of complication rates of ORIF of tibial pilon fractures using the posterolateral approach is presented. This approach did not eliminate the complications common to other approaches, but does offer an alternative when soft-tissue concerns prevent other approaches.

68. Grose A, Gardner MJ, Hettrich C, et al: Open reduction and internal fixation of tibial pilon fractures using a lateral approach. *J Orthop Trauma* 2007;21(8):530-537.

An extensile lateral approach to the distal tibia is described. When applied in a staged fashion, this approach for pilon fractures provided excellent protection of the soft-tissue envelopes by creating thick flaps while allowing excellent visualization for reconstruction of the anterior and lateral distal tibia.

69. Chen L, O'Shea K, Early JS: The use of medial and lateral surgical approaches for the treatment of tibial plafond fractures. *J Orthop Trauma* 2007;21(3):207-211.

This study describes a two-incision approach using medial and lateral incisions for ORIF of tibial pilon fractures. It was found to allow improved visualization of the tibial articular surface and talus, ease of plate application, and a low soft-tissue complication rate.

70. Howard JL, Agel J, Barei DP, Benirschke SK, Nork SE: A prospective study evaluating incision placement and wound healing for tibial plafond fractures. *J Orthop Trauma* 2008;22(5):299-305.

This prospective study noted that, despite a skin bridge of less than 7 cm in 83% of instances, the soft-tissue complication rate was low in this group of tibial plafond fractures. With attention to soft-tissue management and timing, incisions for tibial plafond fractures may be placed less than 7 cm apart.

71. Bahari S, Lenehan B, Khan H, McElwain JP: Minimally invasive percutaneous plate fixation of distal tibia fractures. *Acta Orthop Belg* 2007;73(5):635-640.

This study reports satisfactory outcomes with the use of the AO distal tibia locking plate in treatment of unstable distal tibial fractures. Eighty-nine percent of the patients thought that they were able to go back to their preinjury status and 95% back to their previous employment.

72. Borens O, Kloen P, Richmond J, Roederer G, Levine DS, Helfet DL: Minimally invasive treatment of pilon fractures with a low profile plate: Preliminary results in 17 cases. *Arch Orthop Trauma Surg* 2009;129(5):649-659.

Based on these initial results of this study, it appears that a minimally invasive surgical technique for tibial plafond fracture ORIF, including a new low profile plate, can decrease soft-tissue problems while leading to fracture healing and obtaining results comparable with other more recent series.

73. Hasenboehler E, Rikli D, Babst R: Locking compression plate with minimally invasive plate osteosynthesis in diaphyseal and distal tibial fracture: A retrospective study of 32 patients. *Injury* 2007;38(3):365-370.

This clinical study retrospectively evaluated the healing pattern of diaphyseal and distal tibial shaft fractures treated with minimally invasive locked plating. Despite the potential soft-tissue and osseous biologic advantages, careful technique is required as the authors noted prolonged healing in simple fracture patterns treated with bridge plating.

74. Hazarika S, Chakravarthy J, Cooper J: Minimally invasive locking plate osteosynthesis for fractures of the distal tibia—results in 20 patients. *Injury* 2006;37(9):877-887.

Minimally invasive locking plate osteosynthesis was used for definitive fixation of high-energy, open and closed, periarticular distal tibia fractures. This approach aims to preserve bone biology and minimize surgical soft-tissue trauma. This surgical approach appears successful in treating a challenging group of fractures but requires further research.

75. Lee T, Blitz NM, Rush SM: Percutaneous contoured

locking plate fixation of the pilon fracture: Surgical technique. *J Foot Ankle Surg* 2008;47(6):598-602.

The authors describe their technique of minimally invasive percutaneous locked plating of distal tibial pilon fractures.

76. Lau TW, Leung F, Chan CF, Chow SP: Wound complication of minimally invasive plate osteosynthesis in distal tibia fractures. *Int Orthop* 2008;32(5):697-703.

This study evaluated the clinical outcome of minimally invasive plate osteosynthesis of distal tibia fractures. Minimally invasive plate osteosynthesis fixation using a metaphyseal locking plate appeared to be safe and efficient. However, complications such as late wound infection and impingement were relatively common.

77. Leonard M, Magill P, Khayyat G: Minimally-invasive treatment of high velocity intra-articular fractures of the distal tibia. *Int Orthop* 2009;33(4):1149-1153.

The purpose of this prospective study was to evaluate the outcome of minimally invasive techniques in management of these tibial pilon fractures. An excellent American Orthopaedic Foot and Ankle Surgeons result was obtained in 83% of patients at a minimum of 2 years' follow-up.

78. Marsh JL, Muehling V, Dirschl D, Hurwitz S, Brown TD, Nepola J: Tibial plafond fractures treated by articulated external fixation: A randomized trial of postoperative motion versus nonmotion. *J Orthop Trauma* 2006;20(8):536-541.

The results indicate that long periods of cross-joint ankle-immobilizing external fixation for definitive treatment of pilon fractures result in similar patient outcomes compared to otherwise identical treatment protocols that incorporate and use an articulated hinge for ankle motion.

79. Bacon S, Smith WR, Morgan SJ, et al: A retrospective analysis of comminuted intra-articular fractures of the tibial plafond: Open reduction and internal fixation versus external Ilizarov fixation. *Injury* 2008;39(2):196-202.

The authors compared a subset of AO/OTA-type-C pilon fractures treated by a staged ORIF versus definitive Ilizarov fixation. There were no statistically significant differences in nonunion, malunion, or infection rates between the groups. Based on these results, no recommendation could be made regarding optimal treatment.

80. Leung F, Kwok HY, Pun TS, Chow SP: Limited open reduction and Ilizarov external fixation in the treatment of distal tibial fractures. *Injury* 2004;35(3):278-283.

Thirty-one distal tibial fractures were treated with Ilizarov external fixation. Results were comparable to previous studies using ORIF. Twenty-nine percent of the patients had pin tract infection, which remained the most important complication of this method.

81. Vidyadhara S, Rao SK: Ilizarov treatment of complex tibial pilon fractures. *Int Orthop* 2006;30(2):113-117.

Twenty-one consecutive patients with tibial pilon fractures were treated using percutaneous reduction and fixation with the small diameter Ilizarov apparatus. All fractures united. The average American Orthopaedic Foot and Ankle Surgeons score was excellent in 11 patients, good in five, fair in four, and poor in one.

82. Papadokostakis G, Kontakis G, Giannoudis P, Hadjipavlou A: External fixation devices in the treatment of fractures of the tibial plafond: A systematic review of the literature. *J Bone Joint Surg Br* 2008;90(1):1-6.

The outcomes of external fixation devices for spanning or sparing the ankle joint in tibial plafond fracture treatment were compared. There were no statistically significant differences regarding infection rates, nonunion, and time to union between groups. Patients treated with spanning frames had significantly greater incidence of malunion compared with patients treated with sparing frames.

83. Watson JT, Moed BR, Karges DE, Cramer KE: Pilon fractures: Treatment protocol based on severity of soft tissue injury. *Clin Orthop Relat Res* 2000;375:78-90.

84. Gomoll AH, Lin A, Harris MB: Incisional vacuum-assisted closure therapy. *J Orthop Trauma* 2006;20(10):705-709.

Postoperative swelling and prolonged drainage from surgical incisions result in practical and medical burdens, and potentially higher rates of wound infection. This article presents a technique to apply a vacuum-assisted closure therapy sponge as a postoperative dressing to provide a clean, dry wound environment in the immediate postoperative period.

85. Stannard JP, Robinson JT, Anderson ER, McGwin G Jr, Volgas DA, Alonso JE: Negative pressure wound therapy to treat hematomas and surgical incisions following high-energy trauma. *J Trauma* 2006;60(6):1301-1306.

Negative pressure wound therapy may augment healing of surgical incisions and hematomas after high-energy trauma. Potential mechanisms of action include angiogenesis, increased blood flow, and decreased interstitial fluid. This ongoing randomized study demonstrated decreased drainage and improved wound healing following both hematomas and severe fractures.

Foot Injuries

Nirmal C. Tejwani, MD   Kevin J. Pugh, MD

Talus Fractures

Fractures of the talus are uncommon and can lead to a poor outcome if not treated appropriately. The incidence of talus fractures is reported to be 3% of all foot fractures; these are usually high-energy injuries with 50% of them being fractures of the talar neck.[1] Other fracture patterns including those of the talar dome and of the lateral process (snowboarder's fracture) have been reported.[2,3] Combined fractures of the talus and calcaneus are very rare, but have been reported to have significant associated morbidity.[4,5]

The diagnosis of talus fractures is based on the standard three radiographs of the ankle. The Canale view allows visualization of the talar neck and the subtalar joint. A CT scan is useful in delineating the fracture pattern, especially those involving the talar body and the lateral process. MRI may be needed for later detection of osteonecrosis, but provides little additional information in acute fractures.

Talar neck fractures are classified based on displacement of the fracture and associated disruption of the surrounding joints. Hawkins classified talar neck fractures into three types, with a fourth type later described by Canale et al. Type 1 is a nondisplaced fracture of the talus neck; type 2 is a displaced talar neck fracture with dislocation or subluxation of the subtalar joint; type 3 is displaced fracture with dislocation of both the subtalar and ankle joints; type 4 is associated talonavicular dislocation in addition to the above-mentioned injuries.[6,7] Because the blood supply of the talus courses from distal to proximal, any disruption of the talar neck can result in osteonecrosis of the body of the talus. This risk increases with the degree of displacement, with rates of osteonecrosis ranging from 10% for type 1 and up to 70% for type 4 injuries.

Dr. Tejwani or an immediate family member has received royalties from Biomet; is a member of a speakers' bureau or has made paid presentations on behalf of Stryker and Zimmer; and has received research or institutional support from Biomet. Dr. Pugh or an immediate family member is a member of a speakers' bureau or has made paid presentations on behalf of Medtronic and Smith & Nephew and serves as a paid consultant to or is an employee of Medtronic and Smith & Nephew

Treatment

Closed reduction and casting may be attempted for nondisplaced (type 1) fractures, with the cast in place for a minimum of 6 weeks, followed by a protective boot and no weight bearing for another 6 weeks. Alternatively, percutaneous screw fixation may be undertaken,[8] followed by cast treatment and no weight bearing.

Open reduction using two approaches is recommended for achieving anatomic reduction and optimal fixation using a combination of screws and plates. Small and mini fragment plates are useful in fixing these fractures, and good results have been reported.[9,10] Medial plate fixation can prevent varus deformity that may occur if a screw alone is used for fixation, especially in the presence of comminution. Lateral talar neck plates can also be safely used, and avoid the potential damage to the vascular supply of the talus that can result from medial plating.

Timing of Surgery

Traditionally, talar neck fractures have been considered orthopaedic emergencies requiring urgent reduction and fixation, preferably within the first 6 hours. However, a recent study found no correlation between surgical delay in fixation of the fracture and the development of osteonecrosis as long as the associated dislocation was reduced urgently. Instead, osteonecrosis was associated with comminution of the talar neck ($P < 0.03$) and open fractures ($P < 0.05$).[10]

Complications

Osteonecrosis and posttraumatic arthritis have been reported as the most common complications of these fractures, with incidences varying from 10% to 100%.[9] The incidence increases with higher fracture grade and also with higher energy injuries, as may be seen in open fractures or those with increased comminution. In a series of 26 fractures, osteonecrosis reportedly was seen after 13 of the 26 fractures overall and after 6 of the 7 open fractures.[11]

The presence of a Hawkins' sign, a subchondral lucency best seen on mortise view radiographs taken 6 weeks or more after injury or fixation, indicates the presence of vascularity. However, its absence does not necessarily indicate lack of vascularity. The treatment of osteonecrosis is based on fracture healing and presence of collapse, if any. There is also no reported benefit to keeping patients from bearing weight for a prolonged period to prevent collapse or subtalar arthritis.

Subtalar arthritis is the most common complication, with an incidence of about 50%. This condition may require arthrodesis if symptoms persist in spite of orthotics and shoe modification for pain relief. Malunion of talar neck fractures classically occurs in varus and leads to stiffening of the midfoot and hindfoot joints secondary to lack of eversion at the subtalar joints. Treatment ranges from corrective osteotomy to midfoot fusion or triple arthrodesis, depending on the status of the pantalar articulations.

Outcomes

Outcomes of talar neck fractures vary with the severity of injury including Hawkins type, open fracture, and presence of associated foot injuries. The authors of a 2004 study reported that 21 of 39 patients (54%) developed posttraumatic arthritis, which was more common after comminuted fractures ($P < 0.07$) and open fractures ($P = 0.09$).[10] Patients with comminuted fractures also had worse functional outcome scores. Another study found that posttraumatic arthritis of the subtalar joint was a ubiquitous complication in 26 patients, 16 of whom had involvement of more than one joint, whereas those patients with open fractures posed a more pronounced risk for poor outcome.[11]

Talar Process and Body Fractures

Also known as snowboarder's fractures, lateral process injuries are commonly missed on plain radiographs, and CT may be required for diagnosis and treatment planning. The most common mechanism is axial impaction with dorsiflexion of the ankle. Small, nondisplaced fractures may be treated nonsurgically. However, larger fragments require fixation using a lag screw or a small plate. Primary surgical treatment leads to better outcomes, reducing the risk of subtalar arthritis, and allowing patients to resume the same level of sports activity as before their injury.[2]

Excision of small, comminuted, displaced fractures may be done when painful (usually delayed) or when intra-articular fragments are present. Medial process fractures are commonly caused by inversion and axial load of the ankle and may also be missed on plain radiographs. Both management and outcomes are similar to those of lateral process fractures, and subtalar arthritis and varus deformity may occur secondary to large untreated fragments.

Talar body fractures are more common than talar neck fractures and may result from axial load and shear forces. Displaced fractures usually require surgical treatment and in severe injuries may be associated with neck fractures. Treatment of severe talar dome fractures may require an osteotomy of the medial malleolus for visualization, reduction, and fixation. The medial malleolus osteotomy allows preservation of the deltoid ligament and the associated vascularity to the talus body.

In a series of 56 patients with talar body fractures, it was reported that 23 patients (50%) had associated talar neck fractures. Most patients had radiographic evidence of osteonecrosis and/or posttraumatic arthritis. Associated talar neck fractures and open fractures more commonly resulted in osteonecrosis or advanced arthritis.[12] Fractures of the body of the talus were associated with the highest incidence of degenerative joint disease of both the subtalar and ankle joints.[9]

Associated Injuries

Ipsilateral fractures of the calcaneus and talus are rare, have been reported sporadically, and have poor results. The authors of a 2009 study reported on 45 patients with this combined injury. Five patients required an early below-knee amputation (BKA). Five patients were treated with a primary subtalar arthrodesis. Twenty-eight of the 35 patients who did not undergo early BKA or primary subtalar arthrodesis developed subtalar arthritis. Five patients had deep wound complications. Four patients had talar body collapse from osteonecrosis. There were 13 open fractures, 8 of which resulted in eventual BKA.[4]

Subtalar Dislocations

Subtalar dislocations are uncommon injuries and may be either medial (65% to 70%) or lateral, based on the position of the calcaneus with respect to the talus. They may be associated with fractures of the articular surface and on presentation have significant skin tenting and obvious deformity. Most of the dislocations can be treated with closed reduction (done with knee flexion, ankle plantar flexion, and distraction) after diagnostic standard radiographs. A postreduction CT scan is recommended to identify any intra-articular loose bodies, because their presence necessitates surgical removal.

Occasionally, subtalar dislocations may be irreducible because of soft-tissue interposition. In lateral dislocations this is due to the posterior tibialis tendon or the flexor hallucis longus; in medial dislocation, the talar head may buttonhole through the inferior retinaculum, the joint capsule, or the extensor digitorum brevis.

Immobilization and no weight bearing for 6 weeks is recommended as definitive treatment. Subtalar and midtarsal arthritis occur frequently, but few require surgical treatment of this. A 10% subtalar fusion rate was noted during midterm follow-up of these injuries treated nonsurgically initially, with 70% good to excellent results.[13]

Calcaneus Fractures

Pathoanatomy

The calcaneus has a complex shape; its multiple articulations with the talus form the three facets of the subtalar joint, in addition to the calcaneocuboid joint. Calcaneal morphology is essential to hindfoot and ankle function. A normally aligned and congruent subtalar joint allows the foot to accommodate to uneven ground, and normal calcaneal height provides for a normal tibiotalar relationship and normal ankle dorsiflexion. The tuber of the calcaneus is located lateral to the mechanical axis of the body in neutral stance, and this valgus alignment of the bone allows unlocking of the midfoot and thus foot flexibility during the gait cycle.

The calcaneus is the most frequently fractured tarsal bone. Most of these injuries are associated with a high energy mechanism and are the result of axial loading during falls from a height or motor vehicle crashes. Because the point of contact of the calcaneus with the ground is lateral to the mechanical axis of the body, during axial loading the talus acts as a wedge to create a shearing force, and an oblique primary fracture line divides the sustentaculum from the tuber across the posterior facet. The sustentacular fragment remains connected to the talus, and becomes a "constant fragment" that serves as a useful cornerstone for surgical reconstruction. Further energy is dissipated creating secondary fracture lines that divide the calcaneus into anterior and posterior fragments, as well as causing comminution of the posterior facet and blowout of the lateral wall. The resulting four characteristic deformities of the fractured calcaneus are therefore loss of calcaneal height, widening, hindfoot varus, and disruption of the subtalar joint. Open calcaneus fractures usually have a medial wound caused by the sustentaculum being driven through the skin on the medial side. Surgical débridement often includes removing medial sided tendons and neurovascular structures from the fracture site.

Evaluation

A thorough history and physical examination are required to understand the personality of the injury. Patients who have fallen often have associated injuries to cancellous bone in the lower extremities and spine. The hindfoot should be placed in a well-padded splint in neutral position to prevent equinus deformity. Swelling can be severe and patients should elevate the extremity as much as possible. Fracture blisters are common and reflect the extent of the soft-tissue injury that can occur. Surgical treatment must be delayed until the resolution of swelling and reepithelialization of any fracture blisters (**Figure 1**). It is generally safe to proceed when wrinkles reappear on the foot with dorsiflexion and eversion of the hindfoot. Patients with a tongue-type or avulsion fracture of the Achilles tendon may require urgent reduction to avoid skin necrosis at the posterior aspect of the heel.

All patients with a suspected calcaneus fracture should have standard radiographs including a true lateral of the foot and ankle, an oblique view of the foot, a mortise view of the ankle, and an axial view of the calcaneus. The lateral view confirms the diagnosis and allows assessment of radiographic landmarks. The

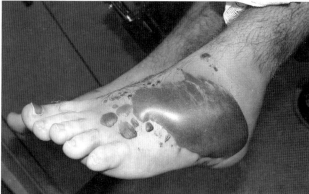

Figure 1 Photograph showing severe blistering of a foot after a motorcycle accident. (Reproduced from Schwartz AK, Brage ME, Laughlin RT, Stephen D: Foot injuries, in Baumgaertner MR, Tornetta P III [eds]: *Orthopaedic Knowledge Update: Trauma 3.* Rosemont, IL, American Academy of Orthopaedic Surgeons, 2005, pp 453-468.)

Bohler angle, which serves as an indicator of prognosis, is formed by a line from the posterior tuber to the back of the posterior facet and another from the posterior facet to the anterior process and is normally 20° to 40°. Angles smaller than this are the result of joint depression. A line along the posterior facet and a line from the most distal point of the posterior facet to the tip of the anterior process form the crucial angle of Gissane. This angle represents the junction of the anterior calcaneus with the posterior facet and is crucial to the restoration of the anatomy during surgical reconstruction. A joint depression fracture has a posterior facet that is dissociated from the tuber and is located in the relatively osteopenic midportion of the bone. A tongue-type fracture has continuity of the posterior facet and the tuberosity and often threatens the skin at the back of the heel.

The oblique view of the foot allows visualization of the calcaneocuboid joint and demonstrates any subluxation of the talonavicular joint. The mortise view of the ankle provides a good view of the subtalar joint to assess fracture or subluxation, and also may reveal ligamentous injuries about the ankle joint. The axial view, or Harris heel view, shows the tuberosity, the sustentaculum, the posterior facet, and the extra-articular deformities associated with fracture.

CT has become a routine aspect of the preoperative evaluation of this injury. Axial and coronal scanning both add to the surgeons' three-dimensional understanding of this fracture. The axial view shows comminution of the joint, widening of the lateral wall and the injury to the calcaneocuboid joint. Coronal views allow identification of the number of joint fragments within the posterior facet, as well as displacement, the size of the sustentaculum, widening of the calcaneous, hindfoot alignment, and impingement of the peroneal tendons.

The most commonly used classification system is the Sanders classification,[14] based on the coronal CT scan at the widest point of the posterior facet. The posterior facet is divided by three lines (A, B, C) into four fragments: lateral, central, medial, and sustentacular. A Sanders I is a nondisplaced fracture, no matter the number of fracture lines. A Sanders II is a two-part fracture and is subclassified based on the location of the fracture line (IIA, IIB, IIC). Type III fractures are three-part fractures, and are divided into IIIAB, IIIAC, and IIIBC. Type IV fractures have four or more articular pieces. This system has been found to be predictive of outcome after surgical treatment.

Treatment Options

Historically, calcaneus fractures were treated nonsurgically because of extremely poor outcomes with surgical treatment. Although outcomes with surgical management have improved dramatically, the decision to operate on a calcaneus fracture should not be made lightly. The patient may have poor soft tissues, be a poor physiologic host, or have the potential for noncompliance with postoperative instructions.

Patients with gross swelling, blistering, or open wounds are poor candidates for definitive surgical treatment. A long history of smoking or diabetes with associated vascular disease, as well as a history of venous stasis, increases risk of wound complications. Patients with immunocompromise, malnutrition, very low physical demands, and chronic disease such as renal failure should be strongly considered for nonsurgical treatment. In addition, those with drug or alcohol issues and those with organic brain disease such as dementia may have issues with postoperative compliance and do better with closed management. Nondisplaced fractures should be treated nonsurgically.

In general, younger active patients with displaced but reconstructable articular fractures (Sanders II, III), those with discontinuity of the Achilles tendon, and those with gross extra-articular displacement should be considered for surgical intervention. It is clear that displaced fractures can have safe and effective surgical treatment, but fractures with high-energy injury mechanisms that are more comminuted have less desirable results. Anatomic restoration of the calcaneus has been shown to be necessary for a good functional outcome, but does not guarantee one.[15,16]

Surgical treatment is delayed until the soft-tissue swelling has subsided and the "wrinkle sign" has appeared, usually by 3 weeks after injury. Fracture reduction becomes more difficult with time, however, and there is contraction of the flap used in the preferred lateral exposure, leading to more difficulty in tension-free wound closure. Surgical management of calcaneus fractures can be challenging and has a well-documented learning curve. In a meta-analysis of 236 studies dealing with calcaneal fractures, the authors found a relationship between deep infection, subtalar arthritis, and the fracture volume of the institution treating the patient, suggesting that treatment by experienced providers leads to better outcomes.[17]

Surgical Approach

The extensile lateral approach is most commonly used for surgical treatment. This approach allows for direct reduction and visualization of the posterior facet, the calcaneocuboid joint, and the extra-articular anatomy of the calcaneus. The medial side can be reduced indirectly through this approach. The patient is placed in the lateral or prone position, and image intensification is used to obtain lateral and axial images, confirming reduction and hardware placement. After fracture reduction, a void is created once the depressed joint segment has been reduced. Autogenous bone grafting has not been shown to improve outcomes. Bone void fillers such as allograft and cements are often used as a scaffold to promote healing, but do not yet have a proven role.[18-20]

The implants typically used for fracture fixation now include low-profile, calcaneal-specific plates. Locking technology has been introduced, and biomechanical studies show that these plates may provide an advantage in cyclic loading of the fracture. However, no clinical data are available on the efficacy of locked calcaneal plating, and further work is required to determine its usefulness.[21-24]

Medial approaches allow for direct visualization of the sustentaculum and are often used for isolated fractures of this structure. Through this approach, which avoids the tenuous skin of the lateral side, the medial wall and tuberosity can be reduced directly, but the joint is not well visualized and must be reduced indirectly. In addition, the calcaneocuboid joint is not visualized, and the lateral wall cannot be assessed through this approach. Medial approaches require a careful dissection around the neurovascular structures and have a high incidence of injury to the medial calcaneal sensory branch.

Minimally invasive techniques are useful when the risk of surgical treatment is too great to consider an extensile approach, yet the fracture position is unacceptable for the patient. Originally described as the Essex-Lopresti approach for reducing and stabilizing tongue-type fractures, these methods have been expanded to treat patients with selected joint depression fractures. Treatment using a percutaneous technique must be undertaken early, before the fracture hematoma organizes. These techniques have the potential to improve fracture position while reducing wound complications in high-risk patients. External fixation is used infrequently, but may be helpful in severe injuries or those with open or poor-quality soft tissues.[25-31]

Primary arthrodesis of the subtalar joint combined with open reduction and internal fixation of the extra-articular calcaneal anatomy has been advocated for fractures with highly comminuted articular surfaces. Support exists for primary arthrodesis in Sanders IV fractures. Intraoperatively, the extra-articular fractures

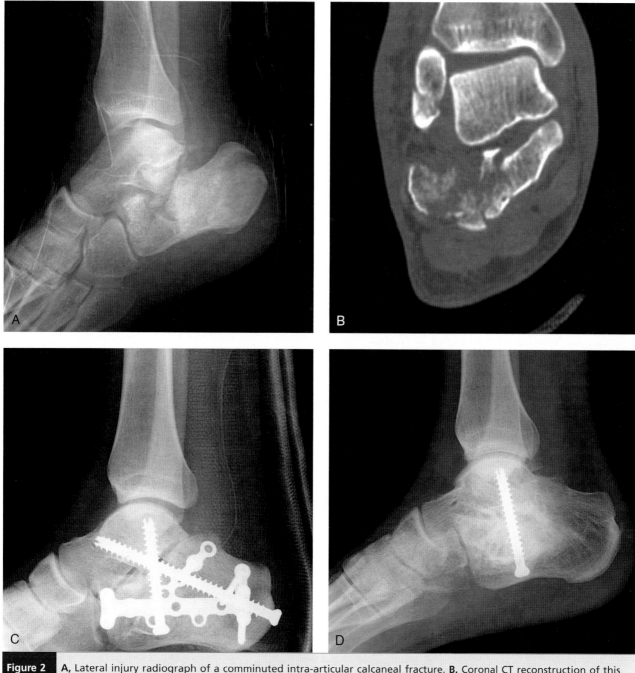

Figure 2 **A,** Lateral injury radiograph of a comminuted intra-articular calcaneal fracture. **B,** Coronal CT reconstruction of this Sanders IV fracture at the level of the posterior facet. The lateral wall is blown out; the calcaneofibular ligaments are incompetent, leading to a subluxated ankle joint; there is an associated fibular fracture due to shortening at the time of injury. **C,** Postoperative lateral radiograph showing restoration of calcaneal anatomy with primary subtalar arthrodesis. **D,** Lateral radiograph at union after removal of painful screws.

are reduced and stabilized with screws and the lateral wall buttressed with a plate. Instead of reducing the joint, the remaining cartilage is removed from both sides of the subtalar joint, and the joint is stabilized with cannulated screws[32] (**Figure 2**).

Complications

Compartment syndrome occurs in 10% of patients with calcaneus fractures. Long-term sequelae of a foot compartment syndrome include claw toes, stiffness, pain, and dysesthesia. Compartment syndromes can be treated by prompt fasciotomies, but creating large wounds on the foot can be problematic in the face of tenuous soft tissues and gross swelling. Some have argued that in selected cases, the morbidity of treating toe deformities resulting from compartment syndromes is less than that caused by acute fasciotomy. Long-term results of this approach are not yet available.

Although the lateral approach provides surgical access for direct reduction of the subtalar joint, the calcaneocuboid joint, the lateral wall, and the body of the calcaneus, the bone is subcutaneous in this area. This lateral flap is perfused by the lateral calcaneal artery, and poor quality soft tissues, poorly placed incisions, and poor soft-tissue technique can lead to wound healing problems. The tip of the flap is most susceptible to breakdown. Wound issues should be taken seriously and treated with appropriate dressing changes, antibiotics, and surgical débridement if warranted. Risk factors for wound complication include single layer closure, high body mass index, and history of diabetes and smoking. An infected calcaneal fracture is a devastating complication. Deeply infected fractures may require hardware removal, flap coverage, and even amputation.[33-38]

Symptomatic nonunion and malunion are difficult issues for the treating physician and the patient. Symptomatic nonunion can be treated safely, whereas malunion may benefit from restoration of the normal extra-articular anatomy. Symptomatic subtalar joints can be arthroscopically released if restricted by fibrous tissue, or fused to provide pain relief. Lateral wall blowout followed by peroneal-fibular-calcaneal impingement may benefit from lateral wall decompression.[39-44]

Outcomes

Fractures of the calcaneus have been successfully treated by both surgical and nonsurgical methods. With the potential for complications being high, it is incumbent upon the surgeon to select the patient for whom surgical treatment will be optimal. In a study of intra-articular fractures followed sequentially for two decades, the authors found that outcomes correlate with the presence of arthrosis on CT scanning. Patients with arthrosis reported increased pain and decreasing function in the second decade. Patients without signs of arthritis remained stable.[45] In a study assessing patient satisfaction with gait at long-term follow-up, there was no difference in outcome scoring between those treated operatively or nonsurgically. However, patients had better scores if their age was less than 30 years, they were not receiving workers' compensation, they had moderate workloads, and the Bohler angle was restored above 5°. Subtalar motion at 12 weeks has been correlated with improved outcome at 2 years. Women had statistically significant better results than men when treated surgically.[46] In a study of 312 patients with displaced intra-articular fractures who were followed long term, Short Form-36 scores were altered from population norms, and were worse than for other orthopaedic conditions as well as for those patients with organ transplantation or myocardial infarction.[47]

In a study of patients in whom surgical or nonsurgical treatment failed and who required late subtalar arthrodesis, the authors found several prognostic factors. Patients with higher degree of initial injury, Sanders type IV fracture, the presence of a workers' compensa-

tion claim, and those with nonsurgical care were more likely to need a fusion.[32] In an economic analysis of calcaneal fracture patients, those who underwent surgical treatment had less time off work and a lower rate of late fusion. When indirect costs are considered, those patients treated surgically were $19,000 (Canadian dollars) less expensive to manage per patient.[48-51]

Midfoot Injuries

Fractures of the midfoot are uncommon and include those of the cuboid, navicular, and cuneiforms. Usually they are associated with either Lisfranc or Chopart joint subluxations or dislocations. There is very little motion at the midfoot joints, and fixation of these injuries may be performed using implants that cross the joints without sacrificing foot flexibility. Strong interosseous ligaments, particularly the plantar Lisfranc ligament that runs from the medial cuneiform to the base of the second metatarsal, provide the primary stability to the midfoot. Midfoot injury is often accompanied by other hindfoot or forefoot injury.

Navicular Fractures

Navicular body fractures have been classified into three types: type 1, coronal plane fracture; type 2, dorsal-lateral to plantar-medial fracture plane; and type 3, comminuted sagittal plane fracture with the forefoot laterally displaced. Accuracy of reduction and fracture severity determine the final outcome.[52]

Avulsion fractures of the navicular tuberosity may result from posterior tibial tendon forces and may require excision with tendon advancement if symptomatic. Rarely dorsal lip fractures may be seen with forced plantar flexion and inversion injuries and are usually treated nonsurgically.

Cuboid Fractures

Compression fracture of the cuboid, the so-called "nutcracker fracture," is usually associated with a medial column injury. Comminuted fractures may result in shortening of the lateral column or disruption of the fifth tarsometatarsal joint. Depressed articular pieces or shortening require either open reduction and internal fixation with bone grafting or the application of an external fixator to restore length and alignment of the midfoot. More commonly, small avulsion fractures of the cuboid are seen at the calcaneocuboid joint and are diagnosed on oblique foot radiographs. These injuries can be treated nonsurgically with satisfactory results.

Lisfranc Fracture-Dislocation

These high-energy injuries result from disruption of the Lisfranc ligament usually secondary to axial load on a plantar-flexed foot. There is disruption of the second metatarsal articulation (the keystone) with the middle cuneiform, resulting in loss of midfoot stability. Disruption of the Lisfranc ligament results in loss of the mid-tarsal articulation stability. Isolated ligamentous injury may result in widening between the first and second metatarsal bases and may be missed on initial radiographs. A fleck sign may indicate avulsion of the Lisfranc ligament and is seen on oblique radiographs.

These injuries are classified based on the direction of dislocation and the extent of injury to the ligamentous structures. Associated fractures of the bases of the metatarsals, usually second through fourth, and the cuboid, may commonly be present. The diagnosis is based on the clinical finding of significant tenderness and the presence of plantar ecchymosis. On AP and lateral radiographs, alignment of the second metatarsal with the middle cuneiform and the third metatarsal with the lateral cuneiform, respectively, is noted. A lateral radiograph shows the presence of dorsal displacement of the first metatarsal, indicating medial column displacement, or a dorsal displacement of the second metatarsal base may be observed. Use of weight-bearing or stress radiographs is helpful in the diagnosis of subtle injuries; however, pain control medications may be required for acute injuries. CT is useful for identification of the fracture pattern and deciding the treatment. MRI aids in diagnosing isolated Lisfranc ligament injury and is particularly useful in cases of missed injuries.

Open reduction and internal fixation with anatomic reduction is advocated for these injuries. Because of the associated soft-tissue swelling, compartment syndrome must be considered. A spanning external fixator may be applied to restore length while waiting for soft tissues to recover and swelling to abate for open surgery. Two incisions are usually required when all tarsometatarsal joints are disrupted. Fixation of the medial three tarsometatarsal joints may be accomplished using screw fixation across the joint, while the lateral two joints are typically fixed with Kirschner wires that are removed before weight bearing to allow for restoration of motion.

Outcomes

The outcome is correlated with the quality of reduction and stable fixation. In a study of 48 patients, the major determinant of a good result was anatomic reduction ($P = 0.05$). The subgroup of patients with purely ligamentous injury showed a trend toward poorer outcomes despite anatomic reduction and screw fixation.[53] Early fixation of these injuries usually provides the patient with a better outcome than delayed fusion and corrective surgery.[54] However, a randomized trial showed that early primary arthrodesis of the medial two or three rays had better 2-year outcome than open reduction and internal fixation with improved American Orthopaedic Foot and Ankle Society scores.[55] Associated injuries to the ipsilateral foot, including Chopart joint or the limb, results in poorer outcomes.[56]

Complications

The most common problem is midtarsal arthritis and planovalgus deformity secondary to collapse of the longitudinal arch. Secondary fusion may be required for pain relief as well as for missed injuries with persistent symptoms.

Forefoot Injuries

Fractures of the forefoot encompass those of the metatarsals and the phalanges of the toes. These are the most commonly missed injuries in patients with polytrauma and multiple life- or limb-threatening injuries. Yet at long-term follow-up these injuries may be responsible for significant residual problems.

In an epidemiologic study, the most common fracture was of the fifth metatarsal, and most multiple metatarsal fractures, if present, were found in contiguous bones.[57] Most of these fractures can be treated nonsurgically, with some exceptions as described in each of the following sections.

First Metatarsal

The first metatarsal bears approximately 40% (half on each of two sesamoids) of the weight through the foot, with the remainder equally distributed across the lesser metatarsals. Displaced fractures require open or closed reduction and fixation, either with Kirschner wires or plate and screws. Intra-articular fractures at either end require open reduction and internal fixation, especially with articular incongruity of more than 2 mm.

Proximal fractures associated with Lisfranc injuries require stabilization of the medial column. Fusion of the first tarsometatarsal joint is recommended by some for comminuted fractures or those diagnosed late.[58] The most problematic late complication is malunion in plantar flexion and shortening that leads to transfer metatarsalgia and stress fracture of the second metatarsal.

Fractures of the sesamoid bones are commonly missed and may be responsible for significant pain and disability. These injuries, when diagnosed early, may benefit from fixation with minifragment screws if displaced.[59] Nonunion may be treated by repair or excision of the smaller fragment. All attempts must be made to preserve the two sesamoids as well as the intersesamoid ligament.

Fifth Metatarsal

Fractures of the base of the fifth metatarsal can be divided into two main categories: proximal "avulsion" fractures, the so-called pseudo-Jones fracture, and more distal metaphyseal fractures that enter the articulation between the fourth and fifth metatarsals. The proximal fractures are usually treated nonsurgically with weight bearing and pain control. The more distal or Jones fracture requires short leg splint with no weight bearing for 4 to 6 weeks. Young athletes may be treated surgi-

5: Lower Extremity

cally with an intramedullary screw to allow early weight bearing and rehabilitation for faster return to sports.[60]

Fractures of the shaft are usually twisting injuries, classically the "dancers fracture." These injuries are also treated with no weight bearing for 4 to 6 weeks with a short leg splint. Fractures that are angulated plantar of more than 20° to 30° may benefit from open reduction and internal fixation. If the plantar flexion is left uncorrected, the patients develop metatarsalgia with excessive weight bearing on the offending metatarsal head.

Second and Fourth Metatarsals

These injuries usually involve contiguous metatarsals and may require fixation if displaced in the plantar direction similar to injuries to the first and fifth metatarsals. Fixation may be performed using Kirschner wires or miniplates and screws. Multiple displaced fractures with shortening of more than 3 to 4 mm may lead to loss of the normal cascade of the metatarsal heads and result in pain with weight bearing. These fractures may require fixation to restore length and alignment.

Stress fractures of the neck of second metatarsal are commonly seen in athletes or military recruits and are treated nonsurgically with elevation and activity modification.[61] Proximal metatarsal stress fractures are usually seen in dancers. These are diagnosed early using MRI, as radiographs are typically negative for the first 2 to 3 weeks.[62]

Summary

Although fractures of the talus and midfoot are rare, the timing of treatment is important to avoid complications. Forefoot injuries, if missed, may lead to significant residual complications. Displaced intra-articular fractures of the calcaneus are serious injuries leading to long-term physical and social problems. By carefully selecting patients for surgical treatment based on risk factors and outcomes data, results can be improved. In general, young patients with displaced fractures do better with surgical management.

Annotated References

1. Juliano PJ, Dabbah M, Harris TG: Talar neck fractures. *Foot Ankle Clin* 2004;9(4):723-736.

   This review article discusses talar neck fractures.

2. Valderrabano V, Perren T, Ryf C, Rillmann P, Hintermann B: Snowboarder's talus fracture: treatment outcome of 20 cases after 3.5 years. *Am J Sports Med* 2005;33(6):871-880.

   This article is a comparison of surgical versus nonsurgical treatment of lateral process fractures. The surgically treated group did significantly better using the AOFAS

scores; 20% of nonsurgically treated patients did not reach the preinjury level of sport activity compared to none in the surgically treated group.

3. von Knoch F, Reckord U, von Knoch M, Sommer C: Fracture of the lateral process of the talus in snowboarders. *J Bone Joint Surg Br* 2007;89(6):772-777.

   In a series of 23 cases, the outcome was dependent on the fracture pattern and adequate treatment, with minimally displaced fractures having much better outcome with nonsurgical treatment.

4. Aminian A, Howe CR, Sangeorzan BJ, Benirschke SK, Nork SE, Barei DP: Ipsilateral talar and calcaneal fractures: a retrospective review of complications and sequelae. *Injury* 2009;40(2):139-145.

   This is a retrospective review of 45 cases, and five had early below-knee amputations, five had primary subtalar arthrodesis, and 28 developed subtalar arthritis.

5. Seybold D, Schildhauer TA, Muhr G: Combined ipsilateral fractures of talus and calcaneus. *Foot Ankle Int* 2008;29(3):318-324.

   In this series of 11 cases, there was a preponderance of extra-articular calcaneus fractures with no preference for either talar neck or body fractures. All underwent open reduction and internal fixation. At an average of 4.5 years, three patients had ankle arthritis and five had subtalar arthritis, but none required fusion.

6. Canale ST, Kelly FB Jr: Fractures of the neck of the talus. Long-term evaluation of seventy-one cases. *J Bone Joint Surg Am* 1978;60(2):143-156.

7. Hawkins LG: Fractures of the neck of the talus. *J Bone Joint Surg Am* 1970;52(5):991-1002.

8. Attiah M, Sanders DW, Valdivia G, et al: Comminuted talar neck fractures: a mechanical comparison of fixation techniques. *J Orthop Trauma* 2007;21(1):47-51.

   Thirty cadaver specimens were randomized to one of three fixation groups. The first group was fixed with three anterior-to-posterior screws. The second group was fixed with two cannulated screws inserted from posterior to anterior. The third group was fixed with one screw from anterior to posterior and a medially applied blade plate. Biomechanical testing showed no significant differences between the groups.

9. Elgafy H, Ebraheim NA, Tile M, Stephen D, Kase J: Fractures of the talus: experience of two level 1 trauma centers. *Foot Ankle Int* 2000;21(12):1023-1029.

10. Vallier HA, Nork SE, Barei DP, Benirschke SK, Sangeorzan BJ: Talar neck fractures: Results and outcomes. *J Bone Joint Surg Am* 2004;86(8):1616-1624.

    A retrospective review of 60 cases (61 patients) with an average follow-up of 36 months showed osteonecrosis in 31% of cases. Mean time to fixation was 3.4 days for those who developed osteonecrosis and 5 days for those who did not. Development of osteonecrosis was associated with comminution of the neck and open fracture, and 54% demonstrated subtalar arthritis.

11. Lindvall E, Haidukewych G, DiPasquale T, Herscovici D Jr, Sanders R: Open reduction and stable fixation of isolated, displaced talar neck and body fractures. *J Bone Joint Surg Am* 2004;86(10):2229-2234.

This is a retrospective review of 26 fractures, with an 88% union rate and 74 months average follow-up. Osteonecrosis was seen in 50% and subtalar arthritis in 100% of cases. They found no effect of surgical timing on development of osteonecrosis.

12. Vallier HA, Nork SE, Benirschke SK, Sangeorzan BJ: Surgical treatment of talar body fractures. *J Bone Joint Surg Am* 2004;86(Pt 2, suppl 1):180-192.

Fifty-six patients with talar body fractures had concomitant neck fractures in 23, and 11 were open fractures. Of the 26 patients with radiographic follow-up, 10 had osteonecrosis, and 17 had subtalar arthritis.

13. DePalma L, Santucci A, Marinelli M, et al: Clinical outcome of closed subtalar isolated dislocations. *Arch Orthop Trauma Surg* 2008;128(6):593-598.

Thirty patients with isolated closed subtalar dislocations (20 medial and 10 lateral) were followed up for 5 to 12 years. Ten percent of the patients had poor results and underwent subtalar arthrodesis. There was no significant difference in outcome between medial or lateral dislocations.

14. Lauder AJ, Inda DJ, Bott AM, Clare MP, Fitzgibbons TC, Mormino MA: Interobserver and intraobserver reliability of two classification systems for intra-articular calcaneal fractures. *Foot Ankle Int* 2006;27(4):251-255.

The authors compared the interobserver and intraobserver reliability of the Crosby-Fitzgibbons and Sanders classifications of calcaneal fractures. The authors were not able to demonstrate excellent reliability with either scheme.

15. Buckley R, Tough S, McCormack R, et al: Operative compared with nonoperative treatment of displaced intra-articular calcaneal fractures: A prospective, randomized, controlled multicenter trial. *J Bone Joint Surg Am* 2002;84(10):1733-1744.

16. Herscovici D Jr, Widmaier J, Scaduto JM, Sanders RW, Walling A: Operative treatment of calcaneal fractures in elderly patients. *J Bone Joint Surg Am* 2005;87(6):1260-1264.

The authors report on 44 fractures treated surgically in patients aged 65 or older. They found that open reduction and internal fixation was an acceptable method of treatment in the elderly, but caution that those with osteopenia, house ambulators or nonambulatory patients, or those with significant comorbidities undergo nonsurgical care.

17. Poeze M, Verbruggen JP, Brink PR: The relationship between the outcome of operatively treated calcaneal fractures and institutional fracture load. A systematic review of the literature. *J Bone Joint Surg Am* 2008;90(5):1013-1021.

A meta-analysis of 236 studies of surgical treatment of calcaneus fractures from 2000-2006 is presented. A sig-nificant inverse correlation was found between fracture volume and subtalar arthrodesis rate. Fracture volume was found to be an independent predictor of infection rate.

18. Longino D, Buckley RE: Bone graft in the operative treatment of displaced intraarticular calcaneal fractures: Is it helpful? *J Orthop Trauma* 2001;15(4):280-286.

19. Thordarson DB, Bollinger M: SRS cancellous bone cement augmentation of calcaneal fracture fixation. *Foot Ankle Int* 2005;26(5):347-352.

Fifteen patients with fracture underwent open reduction and internal fixation. The defect under the posterior facet was filled with SRS bone cement. Preoperative plain films and radiographs were compared with postoperative studies. Patients were allowed to bear weight either 3 or 6 weeks postoperatively. There was no soft-tissue reaction or loss of reduction.

20. Johal HS, Buckley RE, Le IL, Leighton RK: A prospective randomized controlled trial of a bioresorbable calcium phosphate paste (alpha-BSM) in treatment of displaced intra-articular calcaneal fractures. *J Trauma* 2009;67(4):875-882.

A prospective study of 52 displaced intra-articular calcaneus fractures randomized to either open reduction and internal fixation (ORIF) alone with no grafting of bone voids or ORIF with alpha-bioresorbable calcium phosphate paste used as a void filler. Fractures treated with ORIF and bone void filler were radiographically no different at 6 weeks and 3 months, but at 6 months and 1 year had statistically less collapse of the Bohler angle when compared with ORIF groups alone. There were no differences in clinical outcome between the groups.

21. Redfern DJ, Oliveira ML, Campbell JT, Belkoff SM: A biomechanical comparison of locking and nonlocking plates for the fixation of calcaneal fractures. *Foot Ankle Int* 2006;27(3):196-201.

A cadaver biomechanical study of locked or nonlocked fixation in standardized Sanders II fractures is presented. In this model, locked plating provided no advantages over nonlocked plating in terms of the number of cycles until failure.

22. Richter M, Gosling T, Zech S, et al: A comparison of plates with and without locking screws in a calcaneal fracture model. *Foot Ankle Int* 2005;26(4):309-319.

A sawbones biomechanical study of nonlocked plating against three types of locked constructs is presented. Locked constructs performed significantly better with cyclic loading, but did not have a higher load to failure.

23. Richter M, Droste P, Goesling T, Zech S, Krettek C: Polyaxially-locked plate screws increase stability of fracture fixation in an experimental model of calcaneal fracture. *J Bone Joint Surg Br* 2006;88(9):1257-1263.

Four locking plate constructs were tested in a calcaneal fracture model. Three uniaxial constructs and one polyaxial construct were tested. The polyaxial plating constructs demonstrated increased stability during cyclic loading compared with uniaxial constructs.

5: Lower Extremity

24. Stoffel K, Booth G, Rohrl SM, Kuster M: A comparison of conventional versus locking plates in intraarticular calcaneus fractures: A biomechanical study in human cadavers. *Clin Biomech* 2007;22(1):100-105.

A standard intra-articular fracture was created in seven pairs of cadaver calcanei, and each pair was stabilized with a conventional and a locked plate. During mechanical testing, the locked constructs showed a higher load to failure and a lower irreversible deformation during cyclic loading. The authors conclude that this finding supports the use of locked constructs for fixation of calcaneal fractures in osteopenic patients.

25. McGarvey WC, Burris MW, Clanton TO, Melissinos EG: Calcaneal fractures: Indirect reduction and external fixation. *Foot Ankle Int* 2006;27(7):494-499.

Thirty-three fractures in 31 patients were treated with indirect reduction using an Ilizarov external fixator with percutaneous reduction of the articular surface. The authors report very favorable results in open fractures, and describe a shorter time to surgery, immediate weight bearing, few wound issues, and no retained hardware.

26. Magnan B, Bortolazzi R, Marangon A, Marino M, Dall'Oca C, Bartolozzi P: External fixation for displaced intra-articular fractures of the calcaneum. *J Bone Joint Surg Br* 2006;88(11):1474-1479.

The authors report on 54 consecutive closed calcaneus fractures treated with external fixation. The patients were followed for an average of 49 months, and assessed with radiographs, CT, and clinical scoring. The authors recommend the technique based on results similar to published series of internally fixed fractures with a less invasive approach.

27. Weber M, Lehmann O, Sägesser D, Krause F: Limited open reduction and internal fixation of displaced intra-articular fractures of the calcaneum. *J Bone Joint Surg Br* 2008;90(12):1608-1616.

The authors compared 24 patients using an open reduction of the anterior process and posterior facet with percutaneous reduction/fixation of the tuberosity to 26 patients treated with an extensile exposure and traditional plating. The surgical time was less in the percutaneous group, but more secondary procedures and hardware removal were required. The accuracy and maintenance of reduction was similar, with fewer complications in the percutaneous group.

28. Stulik J, Stehlik J, Rysavy M, Wozniak A: Minimally-invasive treatment of intra-articular fractures of the calcaneum. *J Bone Joint Surg Br* 2006;88(12):1634-1641.

The authors report on 287 intra-articular calcaneus fractures treated with minimally invasive reduction and Kirschner wire fixation. The reduction was near-anatomic in 73.9%. Of 176 fractures followed for an average of 43 months, there were 16.5% excellent results, 55.7% good, 14.8% fair, and 13% poor results. Seventy-four percent of patients returned to their preinjury occupation at an average of 5.6 months after injury.

29. Carr JB: Surgical treatment of intra-articular calcaneal fractures: A review of small incision approaches. *J Orthop Trauma* 2005;19(2):109-117.

This review article discusses the use of small incision open reduction and internal fixation of intra-articular calcaneus fractures.

30. Rammelt S, Amlang M, Barthel S, Zwipp H: Minimally-invasive treatment of calcaneal fractures. *Injury* 2004; 35(suppl 2):SB55-SB63.

This review article discusses percutaneous management of calcaneus fractures with local or systemic contraindications to open techniques. Several methods and principles are discussed.

31. Smerek JP, Kadakia A, Belkoff SM, Knight TA, Myerson MS, Jeng CL: Percutaneous screw configuration versus perimeter plating of calcaneus fractures: A cadaver study. *Foot Ankle Int* 2008;29(9):931-935.

A study of 10 paired cadaver feet with Sanders type 2B fractures is presented. One of the pair underwent open reduction and internal fixation with standard perimeter plating. The other was stabilized with a percutaneous screw pattern. Both pairs of feet were then compressed, and there was no significant difference in axial stiffness between the two groups.

32. Csizy M, Buckley R, Tough S, et al: Displaced intra-articular calcaneal fractures: Variables predicting late subtalar fusion. *J Orthop Trauma* 2003;17(2):106-112.

33. Gardner MJ, Nork SE, Barei DP, Kramer PA, Sangeorzan BJ, Benirschke SK: Secondary soft tissue compromise in tongue-type calcaneus fractures. *J Orthop Trauma* 2008;22(7):439-445.

The authors report retrospectively on 139 tongue-type fractures. Twenty-one percent had some degree of posterior soft-tissue compromise at presentation, more common with a nonfall mechanism of injury, smoking, displacement, and delay in presentation. They found that those who underwent emergent reduction and percutaneous stabilization did not progress to skin compromise.

34. Benirschke SK, Kramer PA: Wound healing complications in closed and open calcaneal fractures. *J Orthop Trauma* 2004;18(1):1-6.

A retrospective study of the infection rate in closed and open fractures treated with open reduction and internal fixation through an extensile approach is presented. The authors report serious infection requiring more than oral antibiotics. The rate of infection in closed fractures was 1.8% and 7.7% in the open fracture group. These results compared favorably with the rates reported in the literature. The authors concluded that open reduction and internal fixation with an extensile approach has the advantage of better reduction without an increase in infection.

35. Koski A, Kuokkanen H, Tukiainen E: Postoperative wound complications after internal fixation of closed calcaneal fractures: A retrospective analysis of 126 consecutive patients with 148 fractures. *Scand J Surg* 2005; 94(3):243-245.

This retrospective analysis reports problematic wound healing in 24%, infection in 16%, and wound edge necrosis in 8% of the 126 patients. Fourteen percent of soft-tissue complications required surgical treatment. Stratification of the group identified that a delay in surgery and longer surgical times were risk factors for wound complications.

36. Cavadas PC, Landin L: Management of soft-tissue complications of the lateral approach for calcaneal fractures. *Plast Reconstr Surg* 2007;120(2):459-466.

The authors present their algorithm for treatment of wound edge necrosis in 24 patients. For minor necrosis, a local flap was successful. For moderate wounds, a sural flap was used. In infected wounds with a good bone reconstruction, a free flap was used. For fractures with infection and a poor reconstruction, hardware removal and flap coverage were performed.

37. Loutzenhiser L, Lawrence SJ, Donegan RP: Treatment of select open calcaneus fractures with reduction and internal fixation: An intermediate-term review. *Foot Ankle Int* 2008;29(8):825-830.

The authors present a series of seven patients with stable soft-tissue wounds after open calcaneus fracture, and a bony injury deemed reconstructable. The authors concluded that aggressive treatment of select open calcaneus fractures with an extensile approach can produce satisfactory function.

38. Thornton SJ, Cheleuitte D, Ptaszek AJ, Early JS: Treatment of open intra-articular calcaneal fractures: Evaluation of a treatment protocol based on wound location and size. *Foot Ankle Int* 2006;27(5):317-323.

The authors present a retrospective series of 31 patients with open calcaneus fractures treated at a level I trauma center. Wounds were initially debrided and fractures stabilized with either extensile or percutaneous approaches. Overall, there was a 29% soft-tissue complication rate. The authors concluded that the location and size of the wound dictated treatment. Medial wounds smaller than 4 cm that are stable from antibiotics can be treated with open reduction and internal fixation. Medial wounds larger than 4 cm or unstable wounds should be treated with percutaneous techniques.

39. Molloy AP, Myerson MS, Yoon P: Symptomatic nonunion after fracture of the calcaneum. Demographics and treatment. *J Bone Joint Surg Br* 2007;89(9):1218-1224.

The authors present a series of 15 fractures in 14 patients with nonunion of an intra-articular fracture of the calcaneus. Ninety-three percent went on to union after an average of two procedures. The eventual outcome was subtalar arthrodesis in 67%, triple arthrodesis in 27%, and nonunion in 6%. The authors concluded that despite a high rate of complications, there is a high union rate and good functional outcome.

40. Lee KB, Chung JY, Song EK, Seon JK, Bai LB: Arthroscopic release for painful subtalar stiffness after intra-articular fractures of the calcaneum. *J Bone Joint Surg Br* 2008;90(11):1457-1461.

The authors describe the surgical technique and results of arthroscopic release of 17 stiff and painful subtalar joints after Sanders II or III fractures. Improved motion

was reported in all patients, with most having increased function.

41. Pollard JD, Schuberth JM: Posterior bone block distraction arthrodesis of the subtalar joint: A review of 22 cases. *J Foot Ankle Surg* 2008;47(3):191-198.

The authors present a retrospective series of patients who underwent posterior bone block arthrodesis for loss of heel height, subtalar arthrosis, decreased talar declination, insufficient Achilles function, malalignment, and pain. Successful restoration of anatomy, with a 95.5% union rate, was reported.

42. Savva N, Saxby TS: In situ arthrodesis with lateral-wall ostectomy for the sequelae of fracture of the os calcis. *J Bone Joint Surg Br* 2007;89(7):919-924.

This is a retrospective series of 17 patients who underwent in situ subtalar arthrodesis after fracture with significant loss of talocalcaneal height. The authors found that after fusion, the American Orthopaedic Foot and Ankle Society hindfoot score improved, and despite a decrease in talcalcaneal height and talar declination angle, and the loss of 21% of ankle dorsiflexion compared to the normal side, no patient had anterior impingement.

43. Rammelt S, Grass R, Zawadski T, Biewener A, Zwipp H: Foot function after subtalar distraction bone-block arthrodesis. A prospective study. *J Bone Joint Surg Br* 2004;86(5):659-668.

The authors present a retrospective study of bone block arthrodesis in 31 patients. These patients had no nonunions and an improved American Orthopaedic Foot and Ankle Society hindfoot score with improvement of anatomic relationships. Dynamic pedobarography revealed a return to normal pressure distribution and a more energetic gait.

44. Clare MP, Lee WE III, Sanders RW: Intermediate to long-term results of a treatment protocol for calcaneal fracture malunions. *J Bone Joint Surg Am* 2005;87(5):963-973.

The authors report on 74 calcaneal malunions after nonsurgical treatment. Their protocol is lateral wall ostectomy with peroneal tenolysis for type 1 malunions, ostectomy/tenolysis and subtalar bone block arthrodesis for type 2 malunions, and ostectomy/tenolysis/fusion and calcaneal osteotomy for type 3 malunions. The authors report effective pain relief, plantigrade feet, and improving functional scores. Because of the difficulty of salvaging these feet, they recommend initial surgical treatment to restore the anatomy.

45. Allmacher DH, Galles KS, Marsh JL: Intra-articular calcaneal fractures treated nonoperatively and followed sequentially for 2 decades. *J Orthop Trauma* 2006;20(7):464-469.

A retrospective study of a cohort of nonsurgically treated fractures at two time points is presented. The data suggest that after nonsurgical treatment, clinical results correlate with the presence of subtalar arthrodesis on CT scan. Patients with arthrosis have increased pain and deterioration of function compared with those with no arthrosis or spontaneous fusion of the subtalar joint. Patients without arthrosis have good outcomes that are stable over two decades.

5: Lower Extremity

46. O'Brien J, Buckley R, McCormack R, et al: Personal gait satisfaction after displaced intraarticular calcaneal fractures: A 2-8 year followup. *Foot Ankle Int* 2004; 25(9):657-665.

The authors report data from a randomized prospective study of 351 displaced intra-articular calcaneus fractures. Personal gait satisfaction scores were not different between those treated surgically or nonsurgically, although patients who were younger than 30 years who were not receiving workers compensation, had jobs requiring a moderate work load before injury, and had a Bohler angle restored to greater than 0 degrees had greater satisfaction after surgical treatment.

47. van Tetering EA, Buckley RE: Functional outcome (SF-36) of patients with displaced calcaneal fractures compared to SF-36 normative data. *Foot Ankle Int* 2004; 25(10):733-738.

Data were collected as part of a large, randomized, prospective study of surgical or nonsurgical care. SF-36 scores were not as good across most categories as in other orthopaedic conditions. Outcomes were also worse across most categories than in patients with organ transplants or myocardial infarction. The authors conclude that displaced intra-articular calcaneus fractures are life-changing events.

48. Brauer CA, Manns BJ, Ko M, Donaldson C, Buckley R: An economic evaluation of operative compared with nonoperative management of displaced intra-articular calcaneal fractures. *J Bone Joint Surg Am* 2005;87(12): 2741-2749.

An economic evaluation of surgical versus nonsurgical management of calcaneus fractures is presented. The authors report a lower rate of subtalar fusion and time off work with surgical care. When indirect costs were included, surgical management was less costly overall.

49. Bajammal S, Tornetta P III, Sanders D, Bhandari M: Displaced intra-articular calcaneal fractures. *J Orthop Trauma* 2005;19(5):360-364.

The authors report a meta-analysis of randomized trials comparing surgical and nonsurgical treatment of calcaneus fractures. They concluded that there is not enough evidence to determine with certainty that surgical treatment is superior to nonsurgical treatment.

50. Barla J, Buckley R, McCormack R, et al; Canadian Orthopaedic Trauma Society: Displaced intraarticular calcaneal fractures: Long-term outcome in women. *Foot Ankle Int* 2004;25(12):853-856.

As part of a randomized prospective study, 41 women with 43 intra-articular fractures were studied. Women were 3.18 times more likely to report high SF-36 scores after surgical treatment than nonsurgical treatment, and these scores were better than those reported in men. Women's fractures generally were caused by a lower energy mechanism and produced less severe injuries. Women were more likely to do light to moderate work and not have work-related injuries.

51. Kingwell S, Buckley R, Willis N: The association between subtalar joint motion and outcome satisfaction in patients with displaced intraarticular calcaneal fractures. *Foot Ankle Int* 2004;25(9):666-673.

Data were collected as part of a large randomized prospective study of surgical or nonsurgical care. The amount of subtalar motion at least 12 weeks after fracture is correlated with patient satisfaction at 2-year follow-up regardless of treatment method.

52. Sangeorzan BJ, Benirschke SK, Mosca V, Mayo KA, Hansen ST Jr: Displaced intra-articular fractures of the tarsal navicular. *J Bone Joint Surg Am* 1989;71(10): 1504-1510.

53. Kuo RS, Tejwani NC, Digiovanni CW, et al: Outcome after open reduction and internal fixation of Lisfranc joint injuries. *J Bone Joint Surg Am* 2000;82(11):1609-1618.

54. Rammelt S, Schneiders W, Schikore H, Holch M, Heineck J, Zwipp H: Primary open reduction and fixation compared with delayed corrective arthrodesis in the treatment of tarsometatarsal (Lisfranc) fracture dislocation. *J Bone Joint Surg Br* 2008;90(11):1499-1506.

It was concluded that primary open reduction and internal fixation resulted in significantly better outcomes than corrective arthrodesis for painful malunion. Early open reduction and internal fixation also improved patient satisfaction and allowed early return to work.

55. Ly TV, Coetzee JC: Treatment of primarily ligamentous Lisfranc joint injuries: Primary arthrodesis compared with open reduction and internal fixation. A prospective, randomized study. *J Bone Joint Surg Am* 2006; 88(3):514-520.

A prospective randomized trial comparing fixation to primary arthrodesis with 42.5-month average follow-up found significantly better outcomes with arthrodesis using the American Orthopaedic Foot and Ankle Society midfoot scores and more of the fusion patients returning to preinjury level of activities.

56. Richter M, Thermann H, Huefner T, Schmidt U, Goesling T, Krettek C: Chopart joint fracture-dislocation: Initial open reduction provides better outcome than closed reduction. *Foot Ankle Int* 2004;25(5):340-348.

There were no differences in outcome in bony or ligamentous Chopart injuries; however, the presence of associated Lisfranc joint injury significantly lowered the scores. Anatomic reduction and fixation was essential for good results.

57. Petrisor BA, Ekrol I, Court-Brown C: The epidemiology of metatarsal fractures. *Foot Ankle Int* 2006;27(3):172-174.

This is a demographic study of 411 metatarsal fractures in 355 patients. Multiple metatarsal fractures occurred in contiguous metatarsals, and 63% of third metatarsal fractures were associated with a fracture of either the second or fourth metatarsal. The fifth metatarsal is the bone most commonly injured.

58. Coetzee JC, Ly TV: Treatment of primarily ligamentous Lisfranc joint injuries: Primary arthrodesis compared

Chapter 39: Foot Injuries

with open reduction and internal fixation. Surgical technique. *J Bone Joint Surg Am* 2007;89(suppl 2, Pt.1): 122-127.

The authors present a prospective randomized comparison of 20 pateints with ORIF compared to 21 with primary arthrodesis. At 2 years postoperatively, the mean AOFAS midfoot score was 68.6 points in the open reduction group and 88 points in the arthrodesis group (P < 0.005). The authors state that primary arthodesis of the medial two or three rays was associated with better outcomes.

59. Blundell CM, Nicholson P, Blackney MW: Percutaneous screw fixation for fractures of the sesamoid bones of the hallux. *J Bone Joint Surg Br* 2002;84(8):1138-1141.

60. Leumann A, Pagenstert G, Fuhr P, Hintermann B, Valderrabano V: Intramedullary screw fixation in proximal fifth-metatarsal fractures in sports: Clinical and biomechanical analysis. *Arch Orthop Trauma Surg* 2008;128(12):1425-1430.

Of 14 patients treated with intramedullary fixation at 42-month follow-up, 13 were able to return to sports with fracture healing between 6 and 12 weeks. American Orthopaedic Foot and Ankle Society score was 100 in 13 of 14 patients. The dynamic pedobarography showed complete functional rehabilitation, and the authors recommend this as a safe and effective procedure.

61. Chuckpaiwong B, Cook C, Pietrobon R, Nunley JA: Second metatarsal stress fracture in sport: Comparative risk factors between proximal and non-proximal locations. *Br J Sports Med* 2007;41(8):510-514.

The authors compared two groups of patients with stress fractures of the second metatarsal and found that patients with proximal stress fractures were more likely to be chronically affected, usually exhibited an Achilles contracture, showed differences in length of first compared with second metatarsal, were more likely to experience multiple stress fractures, and exhibited low bone mass. In addition, a high degree of training slightly increased the risk of a nonproximal fracture, whereas low training volume was associated with a proximal stress fracture.

62. Fulkerson E, Razi A, Tejwani N: Review: Acute compartment syndrome of the foot. *Foot Ankle Int* 2003; 24(2):180-187.

5: Lower Extremity

Geriatric and Pediatric Trauma

SECTION EDITOR:
JOHN T. GORCZYCA, MD

Chapter 40

Perioperative and Postoperative Considerations in the Geriatric Patient

Julie A. Switzer, MD   Matthew D. Layman, MD   Earl R. Bogoch, MD, FRCSC

Indications for Surgery

In the past, fractures in geriatric patients were managed nonsurgically more often than similar injuries in younger patients. However, as the management of patient comorbidities is better understood and improved surgical techniques are developed, surgical intervention has become nearly as common in the older orthopaedic trauma patient as it is in younger patients.

The indications that are generally accepted for surgical repair of fractures in the general population are usually equally applicable to geriatric patients. Therefore, the existence of an open fracture, consider articular disruption, significant loss of length, alignment or rotation, or multiple fractures all dictate surgical intervention.

The management of hip fractures, which are common in geriatric patients and associated with substantial morbidity and mortality, has served as the template for the surgical care of the geriatric orthopaedic trauma patient in general. Surgical intervention in the geriatric orthopaedic trauma patient has reduced morbidity and mortality and has proved palliative, even in the most debilitated patients.[1] Only when a hip fracture patient is nonambulatory and can be comfortably mobilized without surgery should nonsurgical management be considered. All other individuals with hip fractures should be treated surgically, either with internal fixation or arthroplasty.

Dr. Switzer or an immediate family member has received research or institutional support from Biomet, Smith & Nephew, Stryker, Synthes, and Zimmer. Dr. Bogoch or an immediate family member serves as a board member, owner, officer, or committee member of International Osteoporosis Foundation, Osteoporosis Canada, Osteoporosis Fracture Line, and St. Michael's Hospital; and serves as an unpaid consultant to Alliance for Better Bone Health (Procter & Gamble Pharmaceuticals Canada). Neither Dr. Layman nor an immediate family member has received anything of value from or owns stock in a commercial company or institution related directly or indirectly to the subject of this chapter.

Two reviews of the surgical treatment of specific upper and lower extremity fractures in geriatric patients have been published; they document higher historic complication rates in those who have undergone surgical fixation. These reviews also point out that more recent literature describes improved outcomes and fewer complications in this patient population.[2,3]

In geriatric patients who have sustained lower extremity fractures other than a hip fracture, the achievement of fracture stability and the reasonable restoration of involved joint surfaces to facilitate early mobilization remain the surgical goals. Therefore, nearly all femur fractures are treated surgically, as are many tibia fractures. Ankle fractures are treated surgically if surgery minimizes the risk of the loss of fracture reduction, allows for early mobilization, and lessens the risk of sustaining complications such as pressure sores from a cast or brace.

Upper extremity fractures in the geriatric population are also often treated surgically.[3] The best indications for surgical treatment of many of these fractures have not been well established by level I evidence. It is known, however, that although approximately 80% of patients with proximal humerus fractures can be treated nonsurgically, approximately 20% will likely have superior outcomes with surgical intervention. Fractures about the elbow and forearm in geriatric patients are often best treated with surgical intervention. Differences in opinion and practice are especially widespread regarding distal radius fractures, which may be treated surgically or nonsurgically. Several randomized controlled trials are currently under way to try to clarify appropriate indications for closed reduction and casting compared with surgery in these patients.

Team Approach

Multiple studies have shown that in hip fracture patients under the care of orthopaedic surgeons working in concert with hospitalists or geriatricians throughout the perioperative period, postoperative complications are decreased and mortality rates are reduced.[4-7] In this scenario, a formal, dedicated orthogeriatric team or a less integrated but nonetheless connected set of teams of orthopaedic surgeons and primary care providers can be used. The multidisciplinary focus provided by these teams includes expeditious medical optimization and clearance; timely surgery; early postoperative mobilization and rehabilitation; implementation of standardized thromboembolism prevention, pressure sore prevention, and delirium prevention programs; good pain management; and the attainment of adequate hemoglobin and oxygen saturation levels. Also recognized and promoted by these programs is a high level of communication among the services caring for the patients in the hospital, and also with the care providers who will assume care of the patients upon discharge.

In a retrospective chart review of 535 hip fracture patients, there was a reduction in postoperative complications from 33% to 20% when a comprehensive multidisciplinary approach to these patients was adopted. This approach included the use of local femoral nerve catheter blocks to replace opioid analgesics, early assessment by the anesthesia team, and detailed attention to nutrition and fluid management. Length of stay was reduced from 15.8 days in the control group to 9.7 days in the intervention group, and 1-year mortality was decreased from 29% to 23%.[5]

In another study, 204 hip fracture patients were admitted to a standard orthopaedic unit, and 116 patients were admitted to a dedicated orthogeriatric unit. The patients managed in the orthogeriatric unit achieved a successful rehabilitation twice as often and stayed 5 fewer days in rehabilitation beds.[8] A 2006 study described the adoption of a perioperative clinical pathway for hip fracture patients that resulted in reduced morbidity postoperatively. Two sequential hip fracture cohorts were evaluated. One cohort (n = 678), the control group, was not enrolled in the pathway that provided multidisciplinary focused care, whereas the other cohort (n = 663) was enrolled after this pathway was adopted. More patients in the control group developed complications (5% congestive heart failure, 5% postoperative arrhythmia, and 51% delirium) than those in the group treated according to the clinical pathway (1% congestive heart failure, 1% postoperative arrhythmia, and 22% delirium).[4]

The use of standardized admission and discharge order forms for the geriatric orthopaedic trauma patient can result in a decrease in complications and an improvement in outcomes in this vulnerable patient population. Some of the benefits of standardization include improved processes of patient transfer to reduce medication administration errors that occur with increased frequency when patients move from one level or state of care, such as from acute care to a transitional care or rehabilitation unit. Other benefits that may be realized are diminished polypharmacy and improved communication between patients, families, and care providers.[7]

Assessment of Risk

Risk assessment is an important principle for guiding interventions in the geriatric orthopaedic trauma patient, so that individual treatment can be tailored to balance anticipated outcome with potential complications and, just as important, for counseling patients and their families regarding the risks and prognosis of a recommended procedure. The number and type of comorbidities, in particular, increase a patient's risk of complications and mortality (which can be as high as 30% 1 year after surgery).[1,9,10] Especially important considerations in the preoperative workup in this population include renal function, cardiac function, pulmonary function, nutritional status, and cognitive status. Also salient in the preoperative evaluation of these patients is preoperative functional status. Levels of electrolytes, hemoglobin, and blood glucose, along with urinalysis, electrocardiogram, and chest radiographs, should be obtained. Depending on a patient's cardiac history and current symptoms, an echocardiogram should be considered. In this population, the utility of an echocardiogram is mainly to provide information to the anesthesia team regarding cardiac function and structure, as opposed to guiding preoperative cardiac intervention.

In a study that used multiple regression analysis to evaluate a cohort of individuals after hip fracture, the diagnoses of dementia, chronic obstructive pulmonary disease, congestive heart failure, and cancer were associated with greater 6-month mortality. Of special note in this review was the finding that men and nonwhite individuals had poorer outcomes, in terms of mobility and mortality.[9] In another study of hip fracture patients, a hip fracture–specific risk assessment tool was developed to predict postoperative mortality. Older age, male sex, and prefracture morbidities such as renal failure, previous myocardial infarction, malignancy, pneumonia, and malnutrition predicted increased in-hospital and 1-year mortality.[11]

In a 2009 study, 193 hip fracture patients age 60 to 90 years were assessed over a 5-year period. There was a 71% prevalence of sarcopenia, 58% prevalence of undernourishment, and 55% prevalence of vitamin D deficiency.[12] Although impaired nutritional status and strength do not necessarily result in in-hospital complications, they do influence recovery potential.

The American Society of Anesthesiologists (ASA) physical status classification provides a rudimentary assessment of the "sickness" of a patient, which may help in anesthetic selection. Although not designed to assess surgical risk, it is often used for this purpose. For example, in one study in which 836 hip fracture patients were studied, excess mortality occurred in patients whose ASA score was 3 or 4.[1] In another study that specifically focused on patients treated in the Veterans Health Administration system between 1998 and 2003, 5,683 community-dwelling individuals 65 years of age or older who sustained a hip fracture were studied.

Table 1

Clinical Predictors of Increased Perioperative Cardiovascular Risk

Major

Unstable coronary syndromes

Acute or recent myocardial infarction (MI) with evidence of important ischemic risk by clinical symptoms or noninvasive study

Unstable or severe† angina (Canadian class III or IV)‡

Decompensated heart failure

Significant arrhythmias

High-grade atrioventricular block

Symptomatic ventricular arrhythmias in the presence of underlying heart disease

Supraventricular arrhythmias with uncontrolled ventricular rate

Severe valvular disease

Intermediate

Mild angina pectoris (Canadian class I or II)

Previous MI by history or pathologic Q waves

Compensated or prior heart failure

Diabetes mellitus (particularly type I)

Renal insufficiency

Minor

Advanced age

Abnormal electrocardiogram (left ventricular hypertrophy, left bundle-branch block, ST-T abnormalities)

Rhythm other than sinus (eg, atrial fibrillation)

Low functional capacity (eg, inability to climb one flight of stairs with a bag of groceries)

History of stroke

Uncontrolled systemic hypertension

*The American College of Cardiology National Database Library defines recent MI as greater than 7 days but less than or equal to 1 month (30 days); acute MI is within 7 days.

† May include "stable" angina in patients who are unusually sedentary.

‡ Campeau L: Grading of angina pectoris. *Circulation* 1976;54:522-523.

Higher ASA category was associated with worse 30-day outcomes.[13]

The American College of Cardiology and the American Heart Association provide guidelines on the preoperative cardiac workup of these patients. Based on the findings obtained with a clinical history, physical examination, and laboratory tests (such as described previously), a geriatric orthopaedic trauma patient can be predicted to have a perioperative risk of a cardiac event such as myocardial infarction, congestive heart failure, or death that is determined by the existence of an individual's major, intermediate, or minor clinical predictors. Major predictors, such as recent myocardial infarction or decompensated congestive heart failure,

require intensive preoperative management to optimize the patient's condition and can represent factors that delay surgery. Intermediate predictors, such as renal insufficiency or mild angina, and minor predictors, such as age or a history of stroke, should not delay surgery but should be noted and optimized, if possible, by the hospitalist and anesthesia services (**Table 1**).

In the hip fracture patient, surgery is an urgent undertaking. Therefore, assessing risk and addressing immediately responsive physiologic parameters should be accomplished as expeditiously as possible. In geriatric patients who have sustained a lower extremity fracture in an area other than the hip, or an upper extremity fracture, surgery is an urgent but elective undertaking. In this setting, more time is available for optimizing a patient's physiology. Addressing modifiable risk factors in a timely fashion, within 1 week if possible, is paramount. Whenever possible during the preoperative evaluation period, patients with nonhip fractures should be mobilized.

Optimization of Patient Physiology Parameters

Optimizing a patient's physiologic state is crucial for obtaining the best surgical outcome. In the geriatric orthopaedic trauma population, optimization includes being certain that a patient is properly resuscitated in terms of oxygenation, volume status, hemoglobin, electrolyte balance, blood glucose control, and reversal/correction of anticoagulation. Inadequate preoperative resuscitation is common. In a review of 571 hip fracture patients, the presence of one major physiologic abnormality not corrected preoperatively was associated with the development of postoperative complications. Normalization of minor physiologic parameters is also warranted, but is not imperative for minimizing surgical risk.[14] Minor and major physiologic abnormalities are presented in **Table 2**.

The results of a prospective randomized study of interventions to reduce the incidence of delirium following hip fracture were published in 2001. These recommendations provide benchmarks for the optimization of all geriatric orthopaedic trauma patients and include adequate oxygenation, appropriate fluid/electrolyte balance with the avoidance of dehydration, treatment of severe pain, elimination of unnecessary medications, regulation of bowel and bladder function, adequate nutritional intake, early mobilization and rehabilitation, prevention of major postoperative complications, provision of appropriate environmental stimuli, and treatment of delirium.[15]

After hip fracture, it is rare that surgery can be safely deferred for more than the few days required to achieve patient optimization. For individuals who have sustained a lower extremity fracture in an area other than the hip, or an upper extremity fracture, the workup can take up to 1 to 2 weeks for completion before the delay significantly alters outcomes. The preoperative reasons

6: Geriatric and Pediatric Trauma

Table 2

Minor and Major Clinical Abnormalities in Hip Fracture Patients Awaiting Surgery

	Minor Abnormalities*	Major Abnormalities†
Blood pressure (BP)	Systolic BP ≥ 181; diastolic BP ≥ 111	Systolic BP ≤ 90
Rate and rhythm	Atrial fibrillation (AF) or supraventricular tachycardia (SVT) 101-120; sinus tachycardia ≥ 121; or heart rate (hr) 46-50 bpm	AF or SVT ≥ 121 bpm; ventricular tachycardia; 3rd degree heart block or hr ≤ 45 bpm
Infection/pneumonia	Temperature (T) ≥ 38.5 C; clinical diagnosis of pneumonia; or infiltrate on chest x-ray (CXR)	T ≤ 35° C; T ≥ 38.5° C with clinical diagnosis of pneumonia or infiltrate on CXR
Chest pain	Chest pain but normal electrocardiogram (EKG)	Any new myocardial infarction on EKG; or chest pain with abnormal EKG‡
Congestive heart failure (CHF)	Dyspnea or pulmonary rales or S3 but a normal CXR; or CHF on CXR with a normal exam and no dyspnea	Pulmonary edema on CXR; or CHF on CXR with dyspnea and/or abnormal exam
Respiratory failure	46 mm Hg < pCO_2 < 55 mm Hg	Pulse oximetry ≤ 90%; pO_2 ≤ 60 mm Hg; or pCO_2 ≥ 55 mm Hg
International normalized ration (INR)	1.4-1.6	> 1.6
Electrolytes	Sodium (Na) = 126-128 or 151-155 mEq/L; Potassium (K) – 2.5-2.9 or 5.6-6.0 mEq/L; or bicarbonate (HCO_3) = 18-19 or 35-36 mEqL	Na ≤ 125 or > 155 mEq/L; K < 2.5 or > 6.1 mEq/L; or HCO_3 < 18 or > 36 mEq/L
Glucose	451-600 mg/dL	> 600 mg/dL
BUN/creatinine	BUN 41-50 mg/dL; or creatinine 2.1-2.5 mg/DL without history of end-stage renal disease	BUN > 50 mg/dL; or creatinine ≥ 2.6 mg/dL without history of end-stage renal disease
Anemia	Hemoglobin (Hgb) 7.6-8 g/dL	Hgb ≤ 7.5 g/dL

* Minor = mildly abnormal but less likely to require correction before surgery
† Major = markedly abnormal and more likely to require correction before surgery
‡ Abnormal EKG = ST depressions or elevations

that a long delay in patients with nonhip fractures can be tolerated probably is a greater capacity for preoperative mobilization in nonhip fracture patients, which leads to fewer perioperative complications such as pneumonia, urinary tract infections, and pressure ulcers. In all geriatric fracture patients, then, patient optimization should occur as expeditiously as is reasonably possible.

Timing of Surgery

Multiple studies have demonstrated that outcomes are best when surgery for hip fracture is undertaken as expeditiously as is safely possible. In a study reporting on the 1-year mortality of 367 hip fracture patients, a surgical delay that exceeded 2 calendar days led to an increase in 1-year mortality.[16] These results were echoed by a prospective study in 2008 of 850 patients admitted in Sweden during the course of 1 year, which showed that surgical repair of a hip fracture more than 48 hours after admission resulted in a decrease in inde-

pendent living, an increase in the development of pressure sores, and a longer hospital stay.[17]

Although the authors of the 2008 study did not find that mortality increased or that function was worse when surgical repair of hip fracture occurred more than 24 hours following admission, authors of a 2004 study reported that in this population of patients who were deemed healthy enough to undergo early surgery, length of stay was decreased and pain was reduced.[18] In the Veterans Health Administration study of community-dwelling hip fracture patients, a delay of more than 4 days resulted in an increase in 1-month mortality. The tendency to delay surgery (to the detriment of the patient) when the patient was admitted on a weekend or holiday was also noted.[13] In each of these studies, the effect of patients' comorbidities was taken into account and the difference in outcomes following surgical delay remained.

Although the data are most compelling in the hip fracture patient, lower extremity trauma other than in the hip in geriatric patients should be managed without unnecessary delay. For example, a distal humerus fracture should be treated within a few days of the injury (to allow elbow mobilization to begin as soon as possible), but a complex ankle fracture in which significant swelling occurs should be treated only when the swelling is subsiding (usually after 5 days).

Thromboembolism Prophylaxis

Although there is no consensus on specific venous thromboembolism (VTE) or deep venous thrombosis (DVT) prophylaxis, there is general agreement that VTE prophylaxis is necessary for the hip fracture patient. Multiple studies, including randomized controlled trials published in the 1970s and 1980s that used venography rather than clinical evidence of DVT, have shown that the rate of DVT in hip fracture patients not treated with prophylaxis ranges from 46% to 75% and the rate of pulmonary embolism (PE) is 4%.[13,19-21] Clinically apparent DVT and PE are much less common.

Methods of VTE prevention include mechanical devices such as sequential compression devices, and pharmacologic intervention, such as low-dose unfractionated heparin, warfarin, and fondaparinux. Although many have advocated the use of aspirin for DVT prevention, this treatment is not currently supported by level I evidence and is specifically recommended against in the American College of Chest Physicians (ACCP) Chest Guidelines for the Prevention of Venous Thromboembolism.[22] ACCP chest guidelines recommend the use of low-molecular-weight heparin, fondaparinux, warfarin, or low dose unfractionated heparin. Pharmacologic therapy is advised for 10 to 35 days after surgery. A common criticism of the literature on VTE is that level I studies are typically industry funded, and most of them do not include aspirin as a treatment option. Interestingly, a recent pooled analysis of 14 studies cited by the AACP guidelines found that the documented VTE rates with aspirin treatment were not significantly different than the rates found in these studies for warfarin, low-molecular-weight heparin, and pentasaccharide, whereas the relative risk of bleeding complications with these agents was more than four times higher than that of aspirin.[23] At least one study has demonstrated some decrease in clinically relevant DVT or PE with aspirin, and other studies to better determine the efficacy of aspirin in DVT prevention in orthopaedic patients are ongoing.[19]

Much of the evidence cited in support of specific VTE prophylaxis is in arthroplasty patients and is extrapolated to hip fracture patients. A few studies have been completed in hip fracture patients, however, and support the use of one of the previously mentioned pharmacologic agents. No standard duration of treatment has been determined. Varying practices, from the administration of VTE prophylaxis only during the in-hospital period to at least 28 days after surgery, have been described as beneficial in reducing DVT and PE.[19,22,24,25]

Patients should receive short-acting VTE prophylaxis when they are admitted to the hospital because surgery is often delayed for preoperative investigation and optimization, and DVT formation has been demonstrated to begin preoperatively in untreated patients. Patients with risk factors for VTE in addition to hip fracture, such as malignancy, obesity, immobility, and thrombophilia, may benefit from longer VTE prophylaxis treatment regimens.

VTE prophylaxis is often used in the setting of lower extremity fractures in areas other than the hip but rarely used in the setting of upper extremity fracture in geriatric patients. Nevertheless, there is evidence that VTE does occur in these other settings. Two recent articles document DVT formation in lower extremity injury and following (nonfracture related) upper extremity surgery. In a study undertaken in the United Kingdom, 100 patients treated with casting for ankle fracture were evaluated for DVT. No clinical DVTs were detected, but five subclinical DVTs were identified by duplex Doppler ultrasound.[26] In a study of shoulder arthroplasty patients, a PE prevalence of 2%, including one fatal PE, and a DVT prevalence of 13% were reported. Although some of these thromboses occurred in the lower extremities, most occurred in the upper extremities. Upper extremity fracture surgery was not described as a predisposing factor for upper extremity DVT; rather, cancer history, thrombophilia, and recent central venous catheter were described as such.[27]

Anesthetic Considerations

As mentioned previously, early consultation with the anesthesia team promotes safe and efficient anesthesia in the geriatric orthopaedic trauma patient. Identification of comorbidities and prompt, well-documented preoperative evaluation allow the anesthesiologist time to consider anesthetic options and the need for invasive monitoring.

Two issues, in particular, often arise and cause confusion for practitioners: the need for an echocardiogram and the need for transfusion. A preoperative echocardiogram, when indicated by past history or current function, gives the anesthesiologist useful information regarding the patient's cardiac structure (critical aortic stenosis, mitral regurgitation, and so on) and cardiac function (diastolic dysfunction, ventricular dilation, wall motion abnormality, and so on) in these geriatric patients, who often have compromised cardiac function. Transfusion also may be necessary in these patients. Therefore, blood type and cross studies are essential, because geriatric patients may have antibodies (either acquired or congenital) that may result in the need for additional time to find matched blood. Additionally, the patients often arrive with borderline hemoglobin levels, they may be hypovolemic at arrival, they will lose blood during surgery, and postoperative anemia will delay physical therapy and increase cardiac risk.

One study has shown that preoperative comorbidities have a greater effect on postoperative complications than does anesthetic technique (regional compared with general).[28] A recent meta-analysis, however, suggests that there could be an improvement in the incidence of postoperative confusion following hip fracture care if regional anesthetic is used.[29]

Invasive hemodynamic monitoring in the operating room has not been shown to provide better outcome in geriatric patients. However, improved outcomes with invasive monitoring were demonstrated in geriatric polytrauma patients who required treatment in the intensive care unit.[30,31] Beta blockade has been shown to improve outcomes in geriatric patients undergoing surgery, but dosing should be individualized. Maintaining normothermia and relative normoglycemia are also important intraoperative goals.[32]

Postoperative cognitive dysfunction, delirium, and confusion are associated with increased mortality. Anesthetic technique has not been shown to increase the risk of these disorders.[33] Inadequate pain control, especially in geriatric patients with dementia, has been shown to increase postoperative delirium.[34] The anesthesia team can help provide a multimodal approach to pain control in the geriatric orthopaedic trauma patient in the form of regional blocks or in the establishment of patient-controlled analgesia.

Treatment of Anemia

Blood loss and anemia in the geriatric fracture population are of concern before, during, and after surgery. It has been reported that preoperative anemia is associated with increased length of stay and increased 1-year mortality.[35]

Estimation of intraoperative blood loss is a notoriously poor indicator of actual blood loss. In a prospective evaluation of 546 hip fracture patients, intraoperative blood loss was measured using blood obtained by suction and in sponges. Total blood loss was calculated based on the hemoglobin level and estimated blood volume. The potential for dehydration to confound the results was taken into account. Blood loss not accounted for in surgery was significantly greater in individuals who underwent arthroplasty rather than treatment with reduction and internal fixation (1,473 mL and 547 mL, respectively). Independent predictors of blood loss were pretreatment with aspirin, intraoperative hypotension, and gastrointestinal bleeding or ulceration.[36]

In a 2004 prospective observational cohort study, 550 hip fracture patients who underwent surgical repair of their hip fractures were evaluated for perioperative anemia, defined as a hemoglobin level of < 12.0 g/dL. Higher preoperative and discharge hemoglobin levels were associated with shorter length of stay and with lower readmission rates.[37]

There is no consensus regarding the optimal hemoglobin level, although a lower limit of 10 g/dL is widely used as a level below which transfusion is considered. In a recently published study, hip fracture patients were randomized to be transfused at a threshold of 8 g/dL hemoglobin or 10 g/dL hemoglobin. Cardiovascular complications and mortality were decreased in the cohort who underwent transfusion at 10 g/dL.[38]

Pain Control

Pain control, both before and after surgery, is important for achieving the best outcome. Overmedication is of concern, but undermedication in this population of patients is a commonly unrecognized cause of clinical problems. Although analgesic overdosage can result in lethargy, bowel and bladder dysfunction, and increased fall risk, poorly controlled pain through undermedication can result in the development or worsening of delirium in the susceptible geriatric trauma patient. Undermedication can also lead to impaired mobility, thereby increasing the risk of pressure sores, pneumonia, and urinary retention. Less than optimal rehabilitation of a surgically treated extremity is also a predictable outcome in the patient whose pain is poorly controlled.

Achieving adequate pain control is particularly difficult in the large population of fracture patients who have dementia. It is well established that these individuals are undermedicated for pain, despite the fact that appropriate pain management in these individuals decreases the likelihood of the development of delirium.[34] Perhaps because the usual cues used to assess pain level can be absent in these patients, it is especially important that physiologic parameters such as tachycardia and behavioral parameters such as moaning, are given special attention in the assessment of pain.

A reasonable approach to pain control in geriatric patients is continuous acetaminophen with supplementary low-dose opioids as needed. Longer-acting opioids can be of benefit in addition to these medications if adequate pain relief is not achieved.

It is equally important to frequently reassess pain levels and attend to physiologic and behavioral cues in the demented or delirious patient.[15] Appropriate dosing to take into account impaired renal clearance and absorption is also important.

Postoperative Mobilization

Immediate postoperative mobilization is important for achieving the best possible outcome following fracture in the geriatric population. Weight bearing, as tolerated in patients with hip fracture, has been demonstrated to result in no increased risk for complications; rather, immediate postoperative weight bearing has been shown to decrease the risk for poor outcomes.[39,40] Pressure sores, muscle atrophy, pneumonia, and urinary retention can also be decreased if early mobilization is encouraged. It is important to note that, when fracture fixation is unstable, fractures may displace secondarily with or without weight bearing. Substantial loads are seen across the hip joint simply with turning in bed. Resting the leg on the ground may expose the hip to less load than when weight bearing is not attempted. Therefore, postoperative mobilization with touchdown (approximately 20%) weight bearing is recommended.

Early joint mobilization is encouraged in older patients who have sustained extremity fractures in areas other than the hip. With the exception of the patient with diabetes who has a lower extremity fracture and in whom early weight bearing could predispose to loss of reduction, early weight bearing is encouraged when fixation is stable. Otherwise, the focus remains on early joint mobilization; weight bearing is delayed until healing is evident on radiographs and pain with weight bearing is minimal.

Rehabilitation

One-year mortality rates after hip fracture are approximately 20% in women and about 25% to 30% in men. Of those patients who survive hip fracture, approximately 50% sustain a substantial loss of independence and require a change in their living environment. Almost all patients experience diminished mobility and function in comparison to their status before hip fracture.[1,41]

Individuals who most benefit from postoperative rehabilitation are cognitively sound and had good prefracture mobility. Just as perioperative care of the geriatric fracture patient is best provided by a multidisciplinary team, so is postoperative rehabilitation. The medical team, social workers, physical therapists, occupational therapists, nursing staff, and social workers compose a team that can facilitate the return of a patient to prefracture function and to a prefracture living situation.[42,43]

Rehabilitation may be adversely affected by the existence of nutritional and strength deficiencies, as well as by depression and the fear of falling that often occurs following a fracture in a geriatric patient.[12] Therefore, the rehabilitation programs should include treatment that focuses not only on physical function, but also on psychological and metabolic well-being. Fracture prevention and osteoporosis treatment should also be incorporated into the rehabilitation process.[44]

Summary

The study of hip fracture care provides most of the data that are available on optimal care of older fracture patients and serves as the model for this care. A well-considered, multidisciplinary approach to the patient's preoperative assessment and medical management, including expeditious timing of surgery and postoperative management, including DVT prophylaxis, pain control, and rehabilitation, can lead to a decrease in complications and mortality.

Annotated References

1. Richmond J, Aharonoff GB, Zuckerman JD, Koval KJ: Mortality risk after hip fracture. *J Orthop Trauma* 2003;17(1):53-56.

2. Strauss EJ, Egol KA: The management of ankle fractures in the elderly. *Injury* 2007;38(suppl 3):S2-S9.

   This is a review comparing the surgical and nonsurgical management of ankle fractures in geriatric patients. Data supporting surgery for displaced ankle fractures in this population are provided.

3. Strauss EJ, Alaia M, Egol KA: Management of distal humeral fractures in the elderly. *Injury* 2007;38(Suppl 3): S10-S16.

   This is a review of the surgical management of distal humerus fractures in geriatric patients. Data on open reduction and internal fixation compared with arthroplasty are outlined. Both techniques have been shown to produce good functional outcome.

4. Beaupre LA, Cinats JG, Senthilselvan A, et al: Reduced morbidity for elderly patients with a hip fracture after implementation of a perioperative evidence-based clinical pathway. *Qual Saf Health Care* 2006;15(5):375-379.

   This review of two separate sequential cohorts of hip fracture patients (each more than 650 patients) describes decreased complications in the cohort in which a standardized clinical pathway was used.

5. Pedersen SJ, Borgbjerg FM, Schousboe B, et al; Hip Fracture Group of Bispebjerg Hospital: A comprehensive hip fracture program reduces complication rates and mortality. *J Am Geriatr Soc* 2008;56(10):1831-1838.

   This retrospective chart review of 535 hip fracture patients compares mortality and morbidity in patients treated by a multidisciplinary team and with hip fracture pathways to those treated without such. In-hospital complications and 1-year mortality were decreased.

6. Heyburn G, Beringer T, Elliott J, Marsh D: Orthogeriatric care in patients with fractures of the proximal femur. *Clin Orthop Relat Res* 2004;425:35-43.

   This review describes a multidisciplinary geriatric fracture care program and some of its important aspects.

7. Friedman SM, Mendelson DA, Kates SL, McCann RM: Geriatric co-management of proximal femur fractures: Total quality management and protocol-driven care result in better outcomes for a frail patient population. *J Am Geriatr Soc* 2008;56(7):1349-1356.

6: Geriatric and Pediatric Trauma

This article describes a geriatric fracture comanagement program, based on treatment algorithms and early discharge planning.

8. Adunsky A, Lusky A, Arad M, Heruti RJ: A comparative study of rehabilitation outcomes of elderly hip fracture patients: The advantage of a comprehensive orthogeriatric approach. *J Gerontol A Biol Sci Med Sci* 2003; 58(6):542-547.

9. Penrod JD, Litke A, Hawkes WG, et al: The association of race, gender, and comorbidity with mortality and function after hip fracture. *J Gerontol A Biol Sci Med Sci* 2008;63(8):867-872.

    This study of three hip fracture cohorts (2,692 patients) followed for 6 months demonstrates higher mortality and worse mobility for nonwhite patients.

10. Sexson SB, Lehner JT: Factors affecting hip fracture mortality. *J Orthop Trauma* 1987;1(4):298-305.

11. Jiang HX, Majumdar SR, Dick DA, et al: Development and initial validation of a risk score for predicting in-hospital and 1-year mortality in patients with hip fractures. *J Bone Miner Res* 2005;20(3):494-500.

    A population-based cohort of 3,981 hip fracture patients was studied. A risk score for predicting in-hospital and 1-year mortality was created. Primary determinants of mortality are older age, male sex, and prefracture comorbidities.

12. Fiatarone Singh MA, Singh NA, Hansen RD, et al: Methodology and baseline characteristics for the Sarcopenia and Hip Fracture study: A 5-year prospective study. *J Gerontol A Biol Sci Med Sci* 2009;64(5):568-574.

    This 5-year prospective cohort study evaluates 193 hip fracture patients for sarcopenia (71%), vitamin D deficiency (55%), and undernourishment (58%). These and other factors consistent with sedentary activity predicted hospital length of stay.

13. Radcliff TA, Henderson WG, Stoner TJ, Khuri SF, Dohm M, Hutt E: Patient risk factors, operative care, and outcomes among older community-dwelling male veterans with hip fracture. *J Bone Joint Surg Am* 2008; 90(1):34-42.

    This study of 5,683 hip fracture patients treated in the Veterans Health Administration system describes poorer 30-day outcomes in patients whose surgery was delayed 4 days or longer and who had a higher ASA score. Regional anesthesia was associated with lower in-hospital mortality.

14. McLaughlin MA, Orosz GM, Magaziner J, et al: Preoperative status and risk of complications in patients with hip fracture. *J Gen Intern Med* 2006;21(3):219-225.

    This prospective cohort study of 571 hip fracture patients identifies potentially modifiable preoperative major abnormalities that increased the risk of postoperative complications. Those abnormalities that should be addressed preoperatively are noted.

15. Marcantonio ER, Flacker JM, Wright RJ, Resnick NM: Reducing delirium after hip fracture: A randomized trial. *J Am Geriatr Soc* 2001;49(5):516-522.

16. Zuckerman JD, Skovron ML, Koval KJ, Aharonoff G, Frankel VH: Postoperative complications and mortality associated with operative delay in older patients who have a fracture of the hip. *J Bone Joint Surg Am* 1995; 77(10):1551-1556.

17. Al-Ani AN, Samuelsson B, Tidermark J, et al: Early operation on patients with a hip fracture improved the ability to return to independent living. A prospective study of 850 patients. *J Bone Joint Surg Am* 2008; 90(7):1436-1442.

    Early operation on patients with a hip fracture improved the ability to return to independent living. This is a prospective study of 850 patients admitted in Sweden during the course of 1 year showed that surgical repair of a hip fracture more than 48 hours after admission resulted in a decrease in independent living, an increase in the development of pressure sores, and an increase in hospital stay.

18. Orosz GM, Magaziner J, Hannan EL, et al: Association of timing of surgery for hip fracture and patient outcomes. *JAMA* 2004;291(14):1738-1743.

    This prospective cohort study evaluated 1,206 hip fractures for outcomes relative to surgery timing. Early surgery was associated with decreased pain and shorter length of stay. Improved function and increased mortality were not noted, however.

19. Powers PJ, Gent M, Jay RM, et al: A randomized trial of less intense postoperative warfarin or aspirin therapy in the prevention of venous thromboembolism after surgery for fractured hip. *Arch Intern Med* 1989;149(4): 771-774.

20. Snook GA, Chrisman OD, Wilson TC: Thromboembolism after surgical treatment of hip fractures. *Clin Orthop Relat Res* 1981;155:21-24.

21. Todd CJ, Freeman CJ, Camilleri-Ferrante C, et al: Differences in mortality after fracture of hip: The east Anglian audit. *BMJ* 1995;310(6984):904-908.

22. Geerts WH, Bergqvist D, Pineo GF, et al; American College of Chest Physicians: Prevention of venous thromboembolism: American College of Chest Physicians Evidence-Based Clinical Practice Guidelines (8th edition). *Chest* 2008;133(6, suppl):381S-453S.

    This is the eighth edition of evidence-based clinical practice guidelines provided by the American College of Chest Physicians. Fondaparinux, warfarin, and low-dose fractionated heparin are recommended for use in the hip fracture population.

23. Brown GA: Venous thromboembolism prophylaxis after major orthopaedic surgery: A pooled analysis of randomized controlled trials. *J Arthroplasty* 2009;24(6, suppl):77-83.

The author of this study hypothesized that when used for VTE prophylaxis after major orthopaedic surgery, aspirin will decrease the rate of surgical site bleeding without an increase in thromboembolic events. A pooled analysis of randomized controlled trials supports aspirin use in this manner.

24. Eriksson BI, Bauer KA, Lassen MR, Turpie AG; Steering Committee of the Pentasaccharide in Hip-Fracture Surgery Study: Fondaparinux compared with enoxaparin for the prevention of venous thromboembolism after hip-fracture surgery. *N Engl J Med* 2001;345(18):1298-1304.

25. Comp P, Happe LE, Sarnes M, Farrelly E: Venous thromboembolism clinically detected after hip fracture surgery with prophylaxis in a clinical practice setting. *Am J Orthop* 2008;37(9):470-475.

    This retrospective cohort study of more than 49,000 hip fracture patients compares thromboembolism rates following the use of dalteparin, enoxaparin, and unfractionated heparin with fondaparinux. Fondaparinux was found to result in fewer DVTs.

26. Patil S, Gandhi J, Curzon I, Hui AC: Incidence of deep-vein thrombosis in patients with fractures of the ankle treated in a plaster cast. *J Bone Joint Surg Br* 2007;89(10):1340-1343.

    One hundred patients treated with casting for ankle fracture were evaluated by duplex Doppler ultrasound for DVT. Five nonclinical DVTs were detected.

27. Willis AA, Warren RF, Craig EV, et al: Deep vein thrombosis after reconstructive shoulder arthroplasty: A prospective observational study. *J Shoulder Elbow Surg* 2009;18(1):100-106.

    One hundred shoulder arthroplasty patients were evaluated for DVT postoperatively. Prevalence of DVT was 13% and PE prevalence was 3% (one fatal). No DVT prophylaxis was used.

28. Lin JT, Lane JM: Rehabilitation of the older adult with an osteoporosis-related fracture. *Clin Geriatr Med* 2006;22(2):435-447, x.

    This review of rehabilitation of the geriatric orthopaedic trauma patient focuses on osteoporosis prevention and treatment.

29. Parker MJ, Handol HH, et al: Anesthesia for hip fracture surgery in adults. *Cochrane Database Syst Rev* 2004;18(4):CD000521.

    This is a meta-analysis of regional compared with general anesthesia in hip fracture patients. The results of 22 trials were pooled. There was insufficient evidence to draw conclusions regarding mortality or other outcomes. There was, however, a tendency toward decreased postoperative confusion in the regional anesthesia patients.

30. Scalea TM, Maltz S, Yelon J, Trooskin SZ, Duncan AO, Sclafani SJ: Resuscitation of multiple trauma and head injury: Role of crystalloid fluids and inotropes. *Crit Care Med* 1994;22(10):1610-1615.

31. Lewis MC, Abouelenin K, Paniagua M: Geriatric trauma: Special considerations in the anesthetic management of the injured elderly patient. *Anesthesiol Clin* 2007;25(1):75-90.

    This article reviews anesthetic management in the geriatric trauma patient.

32. Callaway DW, Wolfe R: Geriatric trauma. *Emerg Med Clin North Am* 2007;25(3):837-860.

    This review of care of the geriatric trauma patient focuses on thorough evaluation and aggressive resuscitation.

33. Liu LL, Wiener-Kronish JP: Perioperative anesthesia issues in the elderly. *Crit Care Clin* 2003;19(4):641-656.

    This review outlines optimal anesthesia recommendations in the geriatric patient.

34. Morrison RS, Magaziner J, Gilbert M, et al: Relationship between pain and opioid analgesics on the development of delirium following hip fracture. *J Gerontol A Biol Sci Med Sci* 2003;58(1):76-81.

35. Gruson KI, Aharonoff GB, Egol KA, Zuckerman JD, Koval KJ: The relationship between admission hemoglobin level and outcome after hip fracture. *J Orthop Trauma* 2002;16(1):39-44.

36. Foss NB, Kehlet H: Hidden blood loss after surgery for hip fracture. *J Bone Joint Surg Br* 2006;88(8):1053-1059.

    This study of 546 hip fracture patients evaluates intraoperative and total in-hospital blood loss. Type of surgery, aspirin use, intraoperative hypotension, and gastrointestinal bleeding were independent predictors of blood loss.

37. Halm EA, Wang JJ, Boockvar K, et al: The effect of perioperative anemia on clinical and functional outcomes in patients with hip fracture. *J Orthop Trauma* 2004;18(6):369-374.

    This prospective observational cohort study of 550 hip fracture patients determines that higher preoperative hemoglobin is associated with shorter hospital stay and lower mortality and readmission within 60 days of discharge. Higher postoperative hemoglobin is associated with shorter length of stay and lower 60-day readmission as well.

38. Foss NB, Kristensen MT, Jensen PS, Palm H, Krasheninnikoff M, Kehlet H: The effects of liberal versus restrictive transfusion thresholds on ambulation after hip fracture surgery. *Transfusion* 2009;49(2):227-234.

    This randomized controlled trial of 120 cognitively intact hip fracture patients shows that more liberal transfusion criteria (10 g/dL compared with 8 g/dL) did not result in improved function postoperatively. However, fewer patients who were transfused with 10 g/dL had cardiovascular complications (2% versus 10%, $p = 0.05$) and the mortality rate was lower (0% versus 8%; $P = 0.02$).

6: Geriatric and Pediatric Trauma

39. Koval KJ, Sala DA, Kummer FJ, Zuckerman JD: Post-operative weight-bearing after a fracture of the femoral neck or an intertrochanteric fracture. *J Bone Joint Surg Am* 1998;80(3):352-356.

40. Moseley AM, Sherrington C, Lord SR, Barraclough E, St George RJ, Cameron ID: Mobility training after hip fracture: A randomised controlled trial. *Age Ageing* 2009;38(1):74-80.

    This is a randomized controlled trial of 150 hip fracture patients. Eighty patients underwent higher intensity rehabilitation and 80 underwent less intense rehabilitation. No difference in strength or walking speed was noted, although those with sound cognition did better with more intense rehabilitation.

41. Egol KA, Koval KJ, Zuckerman JD: Functional recovery following hip fracture in the elderly. *J Orthop Trauma* 1997;11(8):594-599.

42. Wells JL, Seabrook JA, Stolee P, Borrie MJ, Knoefel F: State of the art in geriatric rehabilitation. Part I: Review of frailty and comprehensive geriatric assessment. *Arch Phys Med Rehabil* 2003;84(6):890-897.

43. Wells JL, Seabrook JA, Stolee P, Borrie MJ, Knoefel F: State of the art in geriatric rehabilitation. Part II: Clinical challenges. *Arch Phys Med Rehabil* 2003;84(6): 898-903.

44. Sander B, Elliot-Gibson V, Beaton DE, Bogoch ER, Maetzel A: A coordinator program in post-fracture osteoporosis management improves outcomes and saves costs. *J Bone Joint Surg Am* 2008;90(6):1197-1205.

    This deterministic cost-effectiveness analysis describes the need for the treatment of 350 hip fracture patients to offset the cost of a postfracture osteoporosis treatment coordinator.

6: Geriatric and Pediatric Trauma

Chapter 41

Hip Fractures in the Geriatric Population

Christopher E. Mutty, MD   Lawrence B. Bone, MD

Introduction

Hip fractures in the geriatric population are a common event and carry serious consequences in terms of morbidity, mortality, and societal burden. There were approximately 250,000 hip fractures in the United States in 1990,[1] and 340,000 in 1996.[2] Recent literature suggests that the overall incidence of hip fractures in the United States may be declining, yet the numbers remain large, with an annual incidence of 794 per 100,000 women and 369 per 100,000 men in 2005.[3] More than 90% of these fractures occur in individuals older than 65 years.[4] On a global scale, approximately 1.6 million hip fractures occur annually, and that rate is expected to climb to 6.3 million per year by 2050.[5] Approximately 25% of hip fracture patients who were previously independent will require long-term care after injury; only 50% of hip fracture patients regain prefracture mobility.[4] One-year mortality rates after hip fracture range from 14% to 36%.[2] Although some improvements in short-term mortality rates have been recently reported,[6] overall mortality rates have not changed and may even be increasing as the geriatric population increases.[7,8] The economic burden of hip fracture care in the United States is substantial, with lifetime direct and indirect costs exceeding $20 billion for all hip fractures in 1997 and a current average direct cost of $40,000 per patient in the first year after a hip fracture.[3,4,9]

The most common mechanism of injury in the geriatric patient is a fall from a standing position, which happens to approximately 33% of individuals older than 65 years and 50% of those older than 80 years. Ten percent of these individuals who fall will sustain a fracture, with hip fracture the second most frequent type (following wrist fractures).[10] Femoral neck fractures and intertrochanteric fractures occur with equal

Dr. Bone or an immediate family member has received royalties from DePuy; and research or institutional support from Zimmer. Neither Dr. Mutty nor any immediate family member has received anything of value from or owns stock in a commercial company or institution related directly or indirectly to the subject of this article.

frequency in geriatric patients,[1] and the female-male ratio of fracture has been reported to be from 2:1 to 8:1.[11] A fall from standing height has enough potential energy to result in a proximal femoral fracture even in young individuals, but hip fracture is rare in this population. Four reasons that simple falls more commonly result in hip fractures in older individual have been proposed.[1,12] First, because ambulatory speed is diminished, the elderly tend to fall to the side rather than forward, with the resultant impact on the lateral aspect of the hip. Second, protective responses are diminished. Third, reduced muscle mass about the hip prevents effective energy dissipation. Fourth, decreased bone strength secondary to osteopenia or frank osteoporosis reduces the amount of energy needed to produce a fracture.

Femoral Neck Fractures

Femoral neck fractures are intracapsular proximal femoral fractures that occur in a bimodal age distribution, with most occurring in older individuals.[2] Several classification schemes have evolved to describe these fractures; from a practical standpoint, these fractures should be recognized as displaced or nondisplaced; this is the most critical feature in determining treatment. The Garden classification system is the most widely accepted for these injuries[13] (**Figure 1**). In clinical practice, Garden stage I and II fractures tend to be grouped together as nondisplaced fractures amenable to internal fixation, whereas displaced Garden stage III and IV fractures are generally considered an indication for some form of prosthetic replacement in geriatric patients. Another classification scheme developed by Pauwels and first described in 1935 categorizes femoral neck fractures by the angle of the fracture plane as seen on an AP radiograph[14] (**Figure 2**). Fractures in a low (more horizontal) plane are nearly perpendicular to the compressive force of body weight through the hip. As the fracture plane becomes more vertical, a shearing component becomes more dominant. As the fracture plane becomes more vertical, it more closely approximates the joint reaction force acting on the hip (typically directed downward and 30° lateral in the vertical

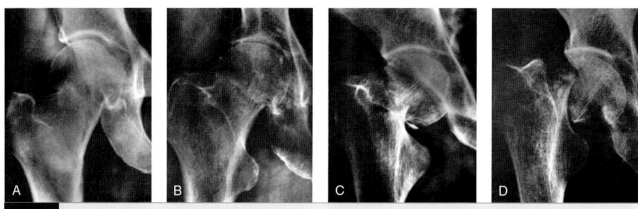

Figure 1 Garden's original classification of femoral neck fractures. **A,** Stage I, incomplete fracture. **B,** Stage II, complete fracture without displacement. **C,** Stage III, complete fracture with partial displacement. **D,** Stage IV, complete fracture with full displacement. (Reproduced with permission from Garden RS: Stability and union in subcapital fractures of the femur. *J Bone Joint Surg Am* 1964;46:630-647.)

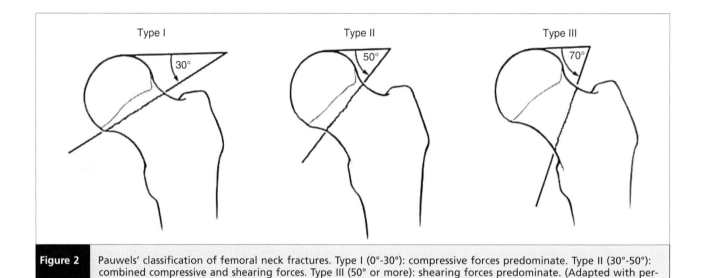

Figure 2 Pauwels' classification of femoral neck fractures. Type I (0°-30°): compressive forces predominate. Type II (30°-50°): combined compressive and shearing forces. Type III (50° or more): shearing forces predominate. (Adapted with permission from Bartonicek J: Pauwels' classification of femoral neck fractures: Correct interpretation of the original. *J Orthop Trauma* 2001;15:358-360.)

plane). The more parallel the fracture line is to the joint rotation force, the more likely the fracture is to displace under typical loading scenarios such as walking. Consideration of the fracture plane becomes important when deciding on fixation technique, as more vertical fractures have been shown to have improved results when treated with sliding hip screw devices versus multiple screws.[15]

There is general acceptance that the risks of nonsurgical treatment (prolonged bed rest/immobility) of geriatric lower extremity fractures outweigh the risks of surgical treatment in most cases. No level I studies compare surgical and nonsurgical treatment of nondisplaced or valgus-impacted femoral neck fractures. An intervention review published through the Cochrane collaboration in 2008 analyzed five randomized trials involving 428 geriatric patients with these fractures.[16] The overall conclusion of this review was that although most of these fractures were treated surgically, there

was insufficient evidence to determine if surgery resulted in better outcomes than bed rest and traction for patients with nondisplaced intracapsular fractures. The authors concluded that nonsurgical treatment avoids the complications of surgery at the cost of slower rehabilitation and increased limb deformity (secondary to fracture displacement). Reviews of this type need to be considered critically in light of current practice trends and earlier comparative studies that showed unacceptable rates of late displacement. More than 98% of Medicare patients with a hip fracture (intracapsular or extracapsular) were treated surgically in 1996 and 1997,[17] highlighting the reduced role of nonsurgical treatment in current practice. This practice trend is supported by the fact that mortality rates in surgically treated patients are lower than those of patients treated nonsurgically at 30 days (7% versus 17%) and 1 year (25% versus 39%).[17,18] In addition, historical studies

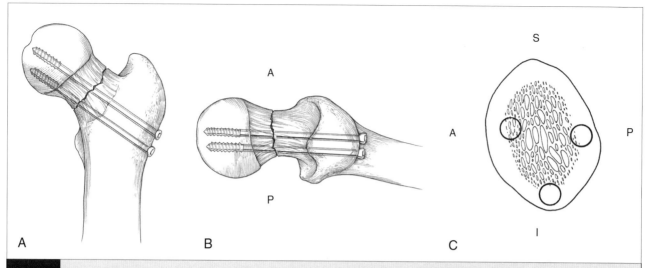

Figure 3 Schematic drawings of the femoral neck. AP (**A**) and lateral (**B**) views showing correct inferior and posterior screw placement for fixation of a subcapital or transcervical fracture. C, Cross-sectional view showing correct placement in three-screw fixation. A = anterior, I = inferior, P = posterior, S = superior. (Reproduced from Probe R, Ward R: Internal fixation of femoral neck fractures. *J Am Acad Orthop Surg* 2006;14:567.)

have shown higher union rates in surgically treated patients and displacement rates as high as 16% for impacted fractures treated nonsurgically.[19] Nondisplaced fractures have no inherent stability and are at high risk for displacement if internal fixation is not used. Nonsurgical management should be reserved only for those patients who are completely nonambulatory and demonstrate minimal discomfort and those with severe medical comorbidities that place them at high risk for anesthesia and surgery-related complications.

Multiple percutaneously placed screws are often used during surgical treatment of nondisplaced fractures. A variety of screw configurations exist; a triangular configuration of three screws either with an inverted or upright pattern is most common. Although the best particular configuration is a topic of debate, a basic principle of screw fixation in the femoral neck is peripheral placement of the screws against the endosteal cortex to enhance support[20] (**Figure 3**). Geriatric patients typically cannot comply with weight-bearing restrictions and this should be taken into consideration when screws are placed. A screw placed along the inferior cortex of the femoral neck will best resist inferior and varus displacement and should be part of any screw configuration. Vertically oriented fracture patterns may benefit from fixation with a sliding hip screw construct, with care taken to avoid proximal fragment rotation during lag screw insertion.[15]

Displaced femoral neck fractures in geriatric patients are typically treated with some form of hemiarthroplasty, given the fact that rates of nonunion and osteonecrosis following internal fixation have been reported at 10% to 30% and 15% to 33%, respectively.[21] However, an increasing proportion of geriatric patients who remain very active, and internal fixation, or conversely, total hip arthroplasty, may be considered

for them. This choice remains a controversial topic. With regard to internal fixation, several studies in the literature have compared various screw types and configurations along with sliding hip screw constructs for displaced femoral neck fractures.[22-27] No single construct has emerged as clearly advantageous in terms of rate of union or risk of displacement. What is clear, however, is that the success of internal fixation of displaced femoral neck fractures is directly related to the accuracy of reduction and that open reduction should be undertaken if an anatomic reduction cannot be achieved through closed or percutaneous means.

Management of displaced femoral neck fractures is a complex and often-debated issue. A survey underscoring this fact demonstrated that there is a lack of consensus regarding the ideal management of these injuries.[28] When making the decision whether to fix a displaced femoral neck fracture or perform arthroplasty, consideration must be given to the risks of fixation (including osteonecrosis, nonunion, and need for revision surgery) versus the risks of replacement (including the potential for longer surgical time, greater blood loss, and dislocation). When reviewing the literature on this subject it is important to note that many studies do not stratify their results based on patient age. However, the mean age of patients in these studies is almost always 65 years or older, making the results of these studies applicable to the geriatric population. A review of 17 trials (10 of which were done after 2000) found that internal fixation led to a decrease in surgical time, less blood loss, and a decreased need for transfusion.[29] Nonunion and osteonecrosis occurred in 28.5% and 9.8%, respectively, of those in the fixation group. Dislocations occurred in 4.3% of those treated with hemiarthroplasty and 13.2% of those treated with total hip arthroplasty. The rate of reoperation was significantly lower in the arthroplasty group over the fixation group. There was no statistically significant difference in either early (less than 6 months after surgery) or late (12 months or greater) mortality between the groups. Pain and mobility scores were inconclusive regarding which treatment had better outcomes. In a 2007 study, hemiarthroplasty was compared with fixation using two screws; functional outcomes were better in the hemiarthroplasty group, with similar mortality rates.[30] Published literature to date supports the fact that internal fixation of displaced fractures has higher rates of complications than arthroplasty and that arthroplasty is not associated with higher mortality.[2]

Additional dilemmas exist within the arthroplasty treatment arm, including the decision to use a cemented rather than a cementless implant when performing a hemiarthroplasty. Several studies have examined the issue of cemented versus cementless hemiarthroplasty for hip fracture.[31,32] The results of these studies favor a cemented design over a cementless design, with the patients receiving cemented prostheses demonstrating decreased postoperative pain and better mobility. However, none of the literature compares a modern, porous-coated prosthesis to a cemented prosthesis. At least one study has shown higher perioperative mortality with a cemented prosthesis.[33] Given this fact, coupled with the increased difficulty of revising a cemented stem in cases of infection and loosening, a reasonable approach includes preparing the canal for a modern ingrowth cementless stem. If excellent rotational and axial stability cannot be achieved, a cemented system should be available as an alternative approach. Future studies comparing results of porous-coated stems against cemented stems will help resolve this debate.

Two types of hemiarthroplasty components currently in common use are unipolar and bipolar designs. In the unipolar design, a stem with a tapered neck is implanted, and a large metal head that matches the size of the native femoral head is placed. A bipolar prosthesis has two articulations—a large metal head that articulates with the acetabulum and a smaller head affixed to the neck that articulates with the larger head through a captured polyethylene liner. In theory, the dual articulation of the bipolar design should result in less acetabular erosion and less stress on the stem-bone interface, at the expense of polyethylene wear as a potential complication. Multiple studies have been conducted to determine if there is any advantage of either design. To date the theoretical advantage of the bipolar design has yet to be demonstrated. The next consideration when deciding on treatment is whether to perform a hemiarthroplasty or a total hip arthroplasty (THA). Indications for THA in patients with a displaced femoral neck fracture have typically centered on the presence of preexisting degenerative joint disease. More recently, there has been interest in performing THA primarily for management of displaced femoral neck fractures in active patients. This interest has arisen in part because painful acetabular erosion can develop

in hemiarthroplasty patients, particularly in those who are active as a result of the metal-on-cartilage articulation. A 2006 randomized trial compared THA and hemiarthroplasty in mobile, independent patients with femoral neck fractures.[34] THA patients demonstrated higher function than their hemiarthroplasty counterparts at a mean 3-year follow-up. There were no dislocations in the hemiarthroplasty group, whereas 3 of 40 THA patients (7.5%) sustained a dislocation. A similar trial was conducted in 2008.[35] THA patients had similar functional results at 6 months, but improved results at 12 and 24 months in comparison with those undergoing hemiarthroplasty. There were no dislocations in the hemiarthroplasty group, compared to 1 of 17 patients (5.8%) in the THA group. Although debate over THA as primary treatment of displaced femoral neck fractures remains, level I and II data support this treatment method for healthy ambulatory patients without dementia.

Intertrochanteric Fractures

Intertrochanteric hip fractures are extracapsular injuries with a portion of the fracture line extending into the area of the femur between the greater and lesser trochanters. Fractures that extend below the lesser trochanter are described as having a subtrochanteric component, and those fractures in which the major fracture plane runs from superomedial to inferolateral are called reverse obliquity fractures. A key differentiating feature separating these injuries from femoral neck fractures is the rich blood supply of the intertrochanteric metaphyseal region, which likely accounts for the improved rates of healing of intertrochanteric fractures. Although most classification systems for intertrochanteric fractures have poor reproducibility, the system most commonly referred to is that originally described in 1949 and published in 1951[36] (**Figure 4**). The most important feature of this early classification is the integrity of the posteromedial cortex. Fractures in which the posteromedial cortex is compromised are unstable, as are those fractures with subtrochanteric extension or a reverse obliquity pattern. Recent research indicates that fractures that compromise the lateral cortex or include extension into the femoral neck are also unstable injuries.[37-39] As a loose rule, any fracture in the AO-OTA classification scheme that is a type 31-A2.2 or above can be considered potentially unstable. The ability of the treating surgeon to distinguish between stable and unstable fracture patterns is important and integral to the selection of surgical approach and choice of fixation methods.

A recent evidence-based review of the literature regarding the management of these injuries included discussion of many of the key issues to be considered.[40] The most basic initial question is whether to use surgical or nonsurgical management. As with femoral neck fractures, most patients with intertrochanteric fractures

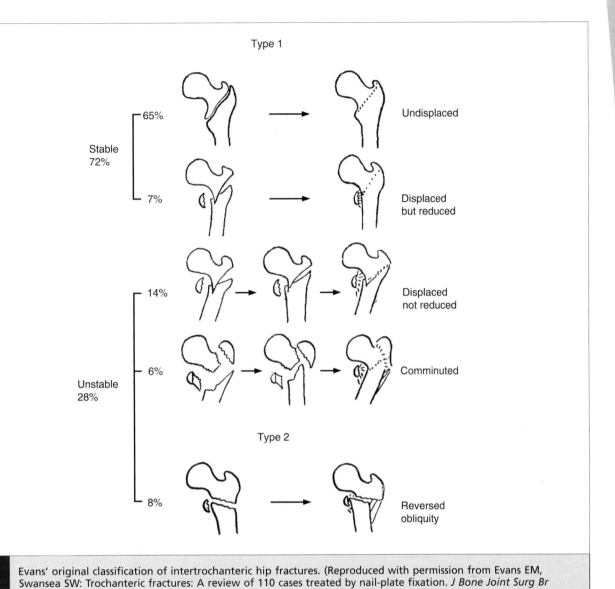

Figure 4 Evans' original classification of intertrochanteric hip fractures. (Reproduced with permission from Evans EM, Swansea SW: Trochanteric fractures: A review of 110 cases treated by nail-plate fixation. *J Bone Joint Surg Br* 1951;33:192-204.)

are treated with surgery, reserving nonsurgical management for those patients with severe medical comorbidities that raise perioperative risk to an unacceptably high level. However, unlike patients with femoral neck fractures, patients with intertrochanteric fractures have been shown to demonstrate excellent results with nonsurgical management including early bed-to-chair mobility and meticulous nursing care.[41-43] Although nonsurgical treatment can result in an excellent outcome, it has been associated with a greater loss of independence at 6 months[31] and a higher rate of mortality at 30 days[43] and should remain a second-line option for patients whose medical conditions can be sufficiently optimized to permit reasonably safe surgical intervention.

The choice of fixation method for intertrochanteric fractures has emerged as a flashpoint in current orthopaedic practice, and intense research has focused on intramedullary and extramedullary fixation devices. The basic premise of both types of fixation is the same: to allow controlled compression of the fracture to a stable position during the healing process, thereby avoiding the problems common to fixed-angle devices such as uncontrolled collapse and either penetration of hardware into the joint or hardware failure. Intramedullary devices consist of either a short or long intramedullary nail inserted through the greater trochanter, through which a sliding lag screw is inserted through the lateral cortex and into the femoral head. Extramedullary sliding hip screw devices consist of a sideplate and barrel through which a sliding lag screw is inserted into the femoral head. The theoretical advantages of intramedullary fixation include the ability of the nail to serve as a buttress against fracture collapse (which provides stability regardless of lateral wall integrity, because the nail serves as a more medial surrogate for the lateral wall) and the potential for insertion through smaller in-

6: Geriatric and Pediatric Trauma

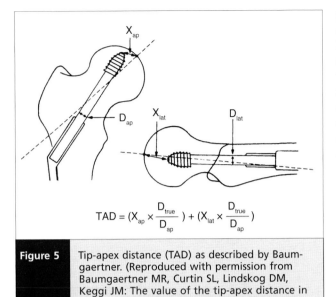

$$TAD = (X_{ap} \times \frac{D_{true}}{D_{ap}}) + (X_{lat} \times \frac{D_{true}}{D_{ap}})$$

Figure 5   Tip-apex distance (TAD) as described by Baumgaertner. (Reproduced with permission from Baumgaertner MR, Curtin SL, Lindskog DM, Keggi JM: The value of the tip-apex distance in predicting failure of fixation of peritrochanteric fractures of the hip. *J Bone Joint Surg Am* 1995; 77:1058-1064.)

cisions with less dissection at the fracture site, minimizing surgical trauma. For generations of orthopaedic surgeons, the sliding hip screw has been the implant of choice for fixation of these fractures. However, recent studies have shown that there now exists significant geographic variation in the use of sliding hip screws in comparison with intramedullary devices in the United States.[44] Also, practice patterns in the United States have begun to shift, with more young surgeons using intramedullary devices.[45] Published results have been contradictory, and relatively recent intramedullary device design changes make correct interpretation of the literature difficult. Despite these difficulties, several important issues can be sorted out when reviewing the data available.

Stable intertrochanteric fractures are well managed with either type of device. A recurrent finding in studies including a review of stable fracture fixation is that there is no difference in surgical indices or postoperative complications between fractures fixed with a sliding hip screw or those fixed with an intramedullary device.[46-53] The most recent Cochrane review[54] on this topic concludes that the sliding hip screw device is superior given the lower rate of complications seen with the sliding hip screw than with the intramedullary devices. However, many of the studies included in this review compared "first generation" imtramedullary devices with the sliding hip screw. These earlier intramedullary designs were short canal-filling nails, frequently impacted with a mallet, had large distal locking screws, and had an increased lateral bend—all factors that contributed to a higher rate of iatrogenic femoral fracture. Newer intramedullary designs and current technique have taken into account the problems seen with earlier versions, and the results of studies using the first-

generation devices probably cannot be extrapolated to devices currently in use. In terms of cost, intramedullary devices are more expensive than the sliding hip screw. A sound conclusion based on current literature is that a well-executed reduction and fixation of a stable intertrochanteric fracture with either a sliding hip screw or intramedullary device can be expected to produce a good result and issues unrelated to implant mechanics, such as surgeon preference, implant availability, and cost, should drive the choice of implant type.

Unstable intertrochanteric fractures are better managed with intramedullary devices. For fractures with an incompetent posteromedial component or lateral trochanteric wall, excessive collapse can occur. When the lag screw in a sliding hip screw device collapses to the point where the threads make contact with the barrel, no further shortening can occur, and the risk of cutout increases. In reverse obliquity patterns, the plane of the fracture is parallel to the plane of motion of the lag screw, and a sideplate is unable to serve as a buttress against displacement. Therefore, lag screw sliding results in progressive fracture displacement and shaft medialization, rather than fracture compression. Sideplate modifications have been developed (such as the Medoff plate, which allows axial compression and a lateral buttress plate that can be added to a sliding hip screw construct) to combat these problems, but these add unnecessary complexity, given the advantages inherent in intramedullary devices for these fracture patterns. Multiple studies have included a review of both sliding hip screw and intramedullary fixation of intertrochanteric fractures that did not specifically focus on a stable versus unstable fracture pattern.[46-53] Although not uniform, in general these studies found no meaningful difference in surgical time, blood loss, revision rates, or postoperative complications between the devices. There is a suggestion that faster recovery time and improved postoperative ambulation may be associated with intramedullary device use. More recent work has specifically addressed the issue of fixation of unstable fracture patterns.[37-39] These studies have provided convincing evidence that a sliding hip screw should not be used to treat these fractures.

Regardless of the type of implant chosen it is important that an accurate reduction be achieved and hardware placed appropriately to maximize the likelihood of a successful outcome. Lag screw placement is a critical part of intertrochanteric fracture fixation. The importance of screw tip placement as a predictor of lag screw cutout has been demonstrated[55] (**Figure 5**). When a sliding hip screw device is used, a key step in the procedure is accurate placement of a guidewire with appropriate version and inclination through the femoral neck to allow for lag screw placement deep in the femoral head to the level of subchondral bone and centered in the head in both AP and lateral planes. Provided guidewire placement is done correctly, the neck-shaft angle in the AP plane will be dictated by the sideplate-barrel angle selected. The surgical technique is different

Table 1

Intertrochanteric Fractures: 10 Tips to Improve Results

1. Aim for a tip-apex distance of less than 20 mm on combined AP and lateral radiograph.

2. Use an intramedullary device if the lateral cortex is compromised.

3. Recognize an unstable fracture and treat with an intramedullary device.

4. Beware of a bow mismatch between the implant and the femur. If a mismatch is identified, either a short nail or alternative fixation should be considered.

5. When using a trochanteric entry nail, start slightly medial to the exact tip of the greater trochanter.

6. Do not ream an unreduced fracture.

7. Be cautious about the nail trajectory, and do not use a hammer to seat the nail.

8. Avoid varus angulation of the proximal fragment: use the relationship between the tip of the trochanter and the center of the femoral head.

9. When nailing, lock the nail distally if the fracture is axially or rotationally unstable.

10. Avoid fracture distraction when nailing.

(Adapted with permission from Haidukewych GJ: Intertrochanteric fractures: Ten tips to improve results. *J Bone Joint Surg Am* 2009;91:712-719.)

when intramedullary devices are used, but the goals are the same. The key principle to keep in mind is that the nail will not reduce the fracture when placed, and acceptable reduction must be achieved before placement of the device. If a closed reduction cannot be achieved, percutaneous pins, clamps, or ball-spike pushers can aid in aligning the fracture.[1] A deformity frequently seen in the lateral fluoroscopic projection is flexion and external rotation of the proximal fragment. This is particularly true when the lesser trochanter remains attached to the proximal fragment. A useful technique to reduce this deformity is to place a Cobb elevator along the anterior femoral neck and then lever the proximal fragment into a reduced position. Only after reduction is achieved is placement of the guidepin for the nail initiated. Ten tips to improving results in intertrochanteric fracture fixation were presented in a recent study[56] (Table 1). These tips should be viewed as basic principles in intertrochanteric fracture fixation; when followed, a successful result will be the rule.

Patient outcomes following intertrochanteric fracture are most dependent on preinjury function and patient age.[57-59] Patients with poor preinjury functional status and older patients can be expected to have poorer outcomes after hip fracture. There is evidence that patients with unstable intertrochanteric fractures experience decreased function at 2 months compared to those treated for stable fractures, but this difference disappears at 6 months.[57] Mortality rates at 1 year par-

allel those of patients with hip fracture in general (14% to 36%).

Ambulatory patients with intertrochanteric fractures who have preexisting symptomatic degenerative hip disease may be considered for prosthetic replacement. Studies have shown good results for this select subset of patients.[60,61] Replacement is also an effective salvage procedure for failed internal fixation of intertrochanteric fractures.[62] However, reconstruction will be more complex than that done in the primary setting because the abductor insertion is usually involved in the fracture and will require supplemental fixation, and the calcar region is often incompetent. Familiarity with revision hip arthroplasty is strongly recommended for surgeons considering prosthetic replacement in these patients.

Patient Management

Older patients with a hip fracture are typically evaluated in the emergency department by both geriatric (medical) and orthopaedic services. The question often arises as to which service should admit and lead the management of the patient. This issue was examined in a recent study; patients admitted to a dedicated hip fracture service led by a geriatrician had a shorter length of stay, decreased time to the operating room, and a reduction in total costs.[63] This work is supported by additional studies demonstrating the advantages and improved outcomes that result from comprehensive management of geriatric hip fracture patients.[4,64]

Surgical Timing

The interval between diagnosis of a hip fracture and definitive surgical management has been scrutinized in terms of its relationship to patient outcomes. Multiple recent studies have demonstrated that surgery performed within 48 hours of admission was associated with lower short- and long-term mortality, an improved ability to return to independent living, and a shortened hospital stay.[65-69] An important factor in surgical timing is the preoperative medical evaluation that sometimes includes cardiac testing in the hip fracture population, discussed in a 2007 study.[70] Patients undergoing elective surgery benefit from the information gained from preoperative testing, and the benefits of these tests far outweigh any risk of delaying surgery. On the other hand, delaying emergent life- or limb-saving surgery for extensive preoperative testing is irrational. Urgent hip fracture surgery falls between these surgical extremes, and the extent of preoperative medical testing that is appropriate and reasonable is not well established. The 2007 study demonstrated that the addition of cardiac testing did not lead to changes in the orthopaedic or medical management of geriatric patients with hip fractures, including those patients with newly diagnosed

6: Geriatric and Pediatric Trauma

cardiac abnormalities and those with known cardiac disease. However, the cardiac workup did contribute significantly to a delay to surgery. Although preoperative evaluation should be tailored to individual patients to identify those medically unstable patients for whom perioperative risk is simply too high, it is important to have in place efficient, established medical protocols to allow for early decision making and prompt surgical intervention in most patients. An additional issue that is becoming more common is the question of surgical delay for those patients on platelet modifiers such as clopidogrel. A recent study demonstrated that there is a complete lack of consensus in the orthopaedic community on this issue.[71] This study was a computer-based survey that was administered to the program directors of academic orthopaedic surgery programs. Seventy-three percent of the respondents indicated that waiting 3 days or less for urgent but nonemergent surgical interventions is acceptable; 23% thought that no delay is necessary.

Summary

Femoral neck and intertrochanteric fractures are common injuries in the geriatric population, and the absolute number of these injuries will continue to rise as the population ages. The ability to manage these fractures remains a fundamental orthopaedic skill. Understanding the basic principles behind internal fixation and prosthetic replacement allows for appropriate surgical approaches and implant selection to maximize patient outcomes from the standpoint of surgeon-controlled variables. Surgeons must be familiar with the outcomes of hip fractures in terms of mortality and function and must be able to communicate effectively with the patient and his or her family so that expectations are established appropriately and early. Comprehensive patient management from emergency department presentation through rehabilitation is important to diminish unnecessary delays to definitive management and provide appropriate support through the recovery period.

Annotated References

1. Lindskog DM, Baumgaertner MR: Unstable intertrochanteric hip fractures in the elderly. *J Am Acad Orthop Surg* 2004;12(3):179-190.

   The authors present a review of the techniques and pitfalls in the management of unstable intertrochanteric hip fractures.

2. Miyamoto RG, Kaplan KM, Levine BR, Egol KA, Zuckerman JD: Surgical management of hip fractures: An evidence-based review of the literature. I: Femoral neck fractures. *J Am Acad Orthop Surg* 2008;16(10): 596-607.

   This thorough and up-to-date review of femoral neck

fracture management incorporates the latest, most pertinent evidence-based articles.

3. Brauer CA, Coca-Perraillon M, Cutler DM, Rosen AB: Incidence and mortality of hip fractures in the United States. *JAMA* 2009;302:1573-1579.

   A current review of the overall statistics for hip fractures in the United States and the trends in these figures from 1985 to 2005 are presented.

4. Friedman SM, Mendelson DA, Kates SL, McCann RM: Geriatric co-management of proximal femur fractures: Total quality management and protocol-driven care result in better outcomes for a frail patient population. *J Am Geriatr Soc* 2008;56(7):1349-1356.

   The authors discuss their geriatric fracture center and demonstrate that improved outcomes are possible for patients with proximal femur fractures when a comanagement approach is used.

5. Ruecker AH, Rupprecht M, Gruber M, et al: The treatment of intertrochanteric fractures: Results using an intramedullary nail with integrated cephalocervical screws and linear compression. *J Orthop Trauma* 2009;23(1): 22-30.

   The authors present a case series in which 100 consecutive patients underwent treatment of an intertrochanteric fracture with a cephalomedullary device that uses two integrated cephalocervical screws.

6. McGinn T, Conte JG, Jarrett MP, ElSayegh D: Decreasing mortality for patients undergoing hip fracture repair surgery. *Jt Comm J Qual Patient Saf* 2005;31(6):304-307.

   Following death after anesthesia induction in a hip fracture patient, a root cause analysis was performed and a recommendation for improved preoperative assessment and communication was made. The authors show reduced mortality after the implementation of a preoperative protocol.

7. Vestergaard P, Rejnmark L, Mosekilde L: Has mortality after a hip fracture increased? *J Am Geriatr Soc* 2007; 55(11):1720-1726.

   A register-based cohort study in which Danish hip fracture patients are compared with age- and sex-matched controls over a 20-year period is presented.

8. Holt G, Smith R, Duncan K, Hutchison JD, Gregori A: Outcome after surgery for the treatment of hip fracture in the extremely elderly. *J Bone Joint Surg Am* 2008; 90(9):1899-1905.

   An outcome study was conducted in Scotland in which hip fracture patients older than 95 years were examined and compared to a control group composed of individuals age 75 to 89 years. Level of evidence: I.

9. Braithewaite RS, Col NF, Wong JB: Estimating hip fracture morbidity, mortality, and costs. *J Am Geriatr Soc* 2003;51:364-370.

   The authors present a computer cohort simulation using estimates from published literature with costs based on Medicare reimbursement rates.

10. Stone ME Jr, Barbaro C, Bhamidipati C, Cucuzzo J, Simon R: Elderly hip fracture patients admitted to the trauma service: Does it impact patient outcome? *J Trauma* 2007;63(6):1348-1352.

    The authors discuss a retrospective chart review of 255 patients (age 65 years or older) who presented to their institution with a hip fracture over a 5-year period and discussed the merits of admitting these patients to a trauma service.

11. Koval KJ, Zuckerman JD: Hip fractures: II. Evaluation and treatment of intertrochanteric fractures. *J Am Acad Orthop Surg* 1994;2(3):150-156.

12. Cummings SR, Nevitt MC: A hypothesis: The causes of hip fractures. *J Gerontol* 1989;44(4):M107-M111.

13. Garden RS: Stability and union in subcapital fractures of the femur. *J Bone Joint Surg Br* 1964;46(4):630-647.

14. Bartoníček J: Pauwels' classification of femoral neck fractures: Correct interpretation of the original. *J Orthop Trauma* 2001;15(5):358-360.

15. Goldstein C, Petrisor BA, Ferguson T, Bhandari M: Evidence-based medicine: Implants for fixation of femoral neck fractures. *Tech Orthop* 2008;23(4):301-308.

    In this article, the authors critically examine the various fixation methods for femoral neck fractures with a focus on cannulated screws, a sliding hip screw, and an intramedullary hip screw device.

16. Handoll HH, Parker MJ: Conservative versus operative treatment for hip fractures in adults. *Cochrane Database Syst Rev* 2008;3(3):CD000337.

    The authors present a review of the literature through 2008 on surgical versus nonsurgical management of both intracapsular (one study reviewed) and extracapsular (four studies reviewed) hip fractures.

17. Sporer SM, Weinstein JN, Koval KJ: The geographic incidence and treatment variation of common fractures of elderly patients. *J Am Acad Orthop Surg* 2006;14(4):246-255.

    The authors examine regional differences in the treatment of common fractures (including hip fractures) in the United States using Medicare data as the source.

18. Weinstein JN, Birkmeyer JD (eds): *The Dartmouth Atlas of Musculoskeletal Health Care*. Chicago, IL: American Hospital Publishing, 2000.

19. Bentley G: Treatment of nondisplaced fractures of the femoral neck. *Clin Orthop Relat Res* 1980;152:93-101.

20. Probe R, Ward R: Internal fixation of femoral neck fractures. *J Am Acad Orthop Surg* 2006;14(9):565-571.

    The authors present a surgical techniques article reviewing the principles of femoral neck fixation.

21. Koval KJ, Zuckerman JD: Hip Fractures: I. Overview and evaluation and treatment of femoral-neck fractures. *J Am Acad Orthop Surg* 1994;2(3):141-149.

22. Parker MJ, Stockton G, Gurusamy KS: Internal fixation implants for intracapsular proximal femoral fractures in adults. *Cochrane Database Syst Rev* 2001;4(4):CD001467.

23. Benterud JG, Husby T, Nordsletten L, Alho A: Fixation of displaced femoral neck fractures with a sliding screw plate and a cancellous screw or two Olmed screws: A prospective, randomized study of 225 elderly patients with a 3-year follow-up. *Ann Chir Gynaecol* 1997;86(4):338-342.

24. Madsen F, Linde F, Andersen E, Birke H, Hvass I, Poulsen TD: Fixation of displaced femoral neck fractures: A comparison between sliding screw plate and four cancellous bone screws. *Acta Orthop Scand* 1987;58(3):212-216.

25. Paus A, Gjengedal E, Hareide A, Jørgensen JJ: Dislocated fractures of the femoral neck treated with von Bahr screws or hip compression screw: Results of a prospective, randomized study. *J Oslo City Hosp* 1986;36(5-6):55-61.

26. Kuokkanen H, Korkala O, Antti-Poika I, Tolonen J, Lehtimäki MY, Silvennoinen T: Three cancellous bone screws versus a screw-angle plate in the treatment of Garden I and II fractures of the femoral neck. *Acta Orthop Belg* 1991;57(1):53-57.

27. Parker MJ, Blundell C: Choice of implant for internal fixation of femoral neck fractures: Meta-analysis of 25 randomised trials including 4,925 patients. *Acta Orthop Scand* 1998;69(2):138-143.

28. Kakar S, Tornetta P III, Schemitsch EH, et al; International Hip Fracture Research Collaborative: Technical considerations in the operative management of femoral neck fractures in elderly patients. A multinational survey. *J Trauma* 2007;63(3):641-646.

    The authors present the results of a survey of 298 Orthopaedic Trauma Association members and AO-affiliated surgeons regarding preferences in specific aspects of the surgical technique for internal fixation as well as arthroplasty for femoral neck fractures.

29. Parker MJ, Gurusamy KS: Internal fixation versus arthroplasty for intracapsular proximal femoral fractures in adults. *Cochrane Database Syst Rev* 2006;4(4):CD001708.

    The authors present a review of the evidence-based literature through 2006 regarding internal fixation versus arthroplasty for femoral neck fractures. Seventeen trials involving 2,694 patients were included.

30. Frihagen F, Nordsletten L, Madsen JE: Hemiarthroplasty or internal fixation for intracapsular displaced femoral neck fractures: Randomised controlled trial. *BMJ* 2007;335(7632):1251-1254.

6: Geriatric and Pediatric Trauma

The authors present the results of a trial comparing 110 patients with femoral neck fractures who underwent hemiarthroplasty to 112 patients who underwent internal fixation for similar fractures. Their primary conclusion is that hemiarthroplasty is associated with better functional outcomes.

31. Parker MJ, Gurusamy KS: Arthroplasties (with and without bone cement) for proximal femoral fractures in adults. *Cochrane Database Syst Rev* 2006;3:CD001706.

    The authors present a review of 19 trials involving 2,115 patients comparing cemented with uncemented arthroplasty for hip fractures. Their primary conclusion is that cemented prostheses may reduce postoperative pain and lead to better mobility.

32. Khan RJ, MacDowell A, Crossman P, Keene GS: Cemented or uncemented hemiarthroplasty for displaced intracapsular fractures of the hip: A systematic review. *Injury* 2002;33(1):13-17.

33. Lennox IA, McLauchlan J: Comparing the mortality and morbidity of cemented and uncemented hemiarthroplasties. *Injury* 1993;24(3):185-186.

34. Baker RP, Squires B, Gargan MF, Bannister GC: Total hip arthroplasty and hemiarthroplasty in mobile, independent patients with a displaced intracapsular fracture of the femoral neck: A randomized, controlled trial. *J Bone Joint Surg Am* 2006;88(12):2583-2589.

    The authors present a British trial comparing total hip arthroplasty (40 patients) with hemiarthroplasty (41 patients) for displaced femoral neck fractures. Their main conclusion is that total hip arthroplasty resulted in superior short-term clinical results and fewer complications.

35. Macaulay W, Nellans KW, Garvin KL; DFACTO Consortium: Prospective randomized clinical trial comparing hemiarthroplasty to total hip arthroplasty in the treatment of displaced femoral neck fractures: *J Arthroplasty* 2008;23(6, suppl 1):2-8.

    The authors present the results of a randomized trial involving 40 patients with displaced femoral neck fractures; 17 received a total hip arthroplasty while 23 received a hemiarthroplasty. The authors conclude that THA is a valuable treatment option.

36. Evans EM, Swansea SW: Trochanteric fractures: A review of 110 cases treated by nail-plate fixation. *J Bone Joint Surg Br* 1951;33(2):192-204.

37. Palm H, Jacobsen S, Sonne-Holm S, Gebuhr P: Integrity of the lateral wall in intertrochanteric hip fractures: An important predictor of a reoperation. *J Bone Joint Surg Am* 2007;89:470-475.

    The authors present a 6-month follow-up study of 214 consecutive patients with an intertrochanteric fracture treated with a sliding hip screw device between 2002 and 2004. Five of 168 patients with an intact lateral wall postoperatively underwent reoperation within 6 months while 10 of 46 patients with an incompetent lateral wall required reoperation within the same period.

38. Gotfried Y: The lateral trochanteric wall: A key element in the reconstruction of unstable pertrochanteric hip fractures. *Clin Orthop Relat Res* 2004;425:82-86.

    In a retrospective study, 24 patients whose hip fractures were treated with a sliding hip screw device were seen in a follow-up clinic over a 12-month period.

39. Kyle RF, Ellis TJ, Templeman DC: Surgical treatment of intertrochanteric hip fractures with associated femoral neck fractures using a sliding hip screw. *J Orthop Trauma* 2005;19:1-4.

    In a retrospective study, 20 fractures were treated at a single institution over a 10-year period; radiographic failure occurred in 5 of 20 fractures.

40. Kaplan K, Miyamoto R, Levine BR, Egol KA, Zuckerman JD: Surgical management of hip fractures: An evidence-based review of the literature. II: Intertrochanteric fractures. *J Am Acad Orthop Surg* 2008;16(11):665-673.

    The authors present a thorough and up-to-date review of intertrochanteric fracture management incorporating the latest, most pertinent evidence-based articles.

41. Hornby R, Evans JG, Vardon V: Operative or conservative treatment for trochanteric fractures of the femur: A randomised epidemiological trial in elderly patients. *J Bone Joint Surg Br* 1989;71(4):619-623.

42. Bong SC, Lau HK, Leong JC, Fang D, Lau MT: The treatment of unstable intertrochanteric fractures of the hip: A prospective trial of 150 cases. *Injury* 1981;13(2):139-146.

43. Jain R, Basinski A, Kreder HJ: Nonoperative treatment of hip fractures. *Int Orthop* 2003;27(1):11-17.

44. Forte ML, Virnig BA, Kane RL, et al: Geographic variation in device use for intertrochanteric hip fractures. *J Bone Joint Surg Am* 2008;90(4):691-699.

    The authors examined national Medicare data for variance in the choice of device used in the treatment of intertrochanteric fractures. Substantial geographic variation was demonstrated.

45. Anglen JO, Weinstein JN; American Board of Orthopaedic Surgery Research Committee: Nail or plate fixation of intertrochanteric hip fractures: Changing pattern of practice. A review of the American Board of Orthopaedic Surgery Database. *J Bone Joint Surg Am* 2008;90(4):700-707.

    The authors reviewed the case lists submitted for Part II of the American Board of Orthopaedic Surgery examination from 1999 through 2006. Over this time period, they found that the use of intramedullary nails had increased dramatically.

46. Adams CI, Robinson CM, Court-Brown CM, McQueen MM: Prospective randomized controlled trial of an intramedullary nail versus dynamic screw and plate for intertrochanteric fractures of the femur. *J Orthop Trauma* 2001;15(6):394-400.

47. Ahrengart L, Törnkvist H, Fornander P, et al: A randomized study of the compression hip screw and gamma nail in 426 fractures. *Clin Orthop Relat Res* 2002;401:209-222.

48. Obrien P, Meek RN, Blachut PA, Broekhuyse HM, Sabharwal S: Intertrochanteric hip fracture fixation: Gamma nail versus dynamic hip screw. A randomized, propspective, study. *J Orthop Trauma* 1993;7(2):193.

49. Utrilla AL, Reig JS, Muñoz FM, Tufanisco CB: Trochanteric gamma nail and compression hip screw for trochanteric fractures: A randomized, prospective, comparative study in 210 elderly patients with a new design of the gamma nail. *J Orthop Trauma* 2005;19(4): 229-233.

The authors present the results of 104 patients treated with a cephalomedullary nail and 106 patients treated with a compression hip screw. Overall there was no difference in functional outcome, nor was there a difference in intraoperative or postoperative complications.

50. Pajarinen J, Lindahl J, Michelsson O, Savolainen V, Hirvensalo E: Pertrochanteric femoral fractures treated with a dynamic hip screw or a proximal femoral nail: A randomised study comparing post-operative rehabilitation. *J Bone Joint Surg Br* 2005;87(1):76-81.

The authors compared 42 patients treated with a proximal femoral nail to 41 patients treated with a dynamic hip screw. Healing and complication rates did not differ. A proximal femoral nail may allow a faster postoperative restoration of walking ability.

51. Baumgaertner MR, Curtin SL, Lindskog DM: Intramedullary versus extramedullary fixation for the treatment of intertrochanteric hip fractures. *Clin Orthop Relat Res* 1998;348:87-94.

52. Sadowski C, Lübbeke A, Saudan M, Riand N, Stern R, Hoffmeyer P: Treatment of reverse oblique and transverse intertrochanteric fractures with use of an intramedullary nail or a 95 degrees screw-plate: A prospective, randomized study. *J Bone Joint Surg Am* 2002; 84(3):372-381.

53. Papasimos S, Koutsojannis CM, Panagopoulos A, Megas P, Lambiris E: A randomised comparison of AMBI, TGN and PFN for treatment of unstable trochanteric fractures. *Arch Orthop Trauma Surg* 2005;125(7): 462-468.

The authors present the results of a Greek study comparing 120 unstable intertrochanteric fractures treated with a dynamic hip screw, a trochanteric nail, or a proximal femoral nail. A higher complication rate was noted in the proximal femoral nail group.

54. Parker MJ, Handoll HH: Gamma and other cephalocondylic intramedullary nails versus extramedullary implants for extracapsular hip fractures in adults. *Cochrane Database Syst Rev* 2008;3(3):CD000093.

The authors review 22 trials (involving 3,871 patients) comparing the gamma nail with the sliding hip screw. They conclude that the gamma nail is associated with an increased risk of intraoperative and postoperative femur fracture.

55. Baumgaertner MR, Curtin SL, Lindskog DM, Keggi JM: The value of the tip-apex distance in predicting failure of fixation of peritrochanteric fractures of the hip. *J Bone Joint Surg Am* 1995;77(7):1058-1064.

56. Haidukewych GJ: Intertrochanteric fractures: Ten tips to improve results. *J Bone Joint Surg Am* 2009;91(3): 712-719.

The author discussed the treatment of intertrochanteric fractures, summarized in 10 key points.

57. Cornwall R, Gilbert MS, Koval KJ, Strauss E, Siu A: Functional outcomes and mortality vary among different types of hip fractures: A function of patient characteristics. *Clin Orthop Relat Res* 2004;425:64-71.

Prospective collected data is reviewed on 537 patients with hip fractures treated in 4 hospitals in New York City. Multivariate analysis identified only preinjury function as an independent predictor of mortality.

58. Lin PC, Chang SY: Functional recovery among elderly people one year after hip fracture surgery. *J Nurs Res* 2004;12:72-78.

One hundred three patients from Taipei with hip fractures and who were older than 65 years were studied from 2000 to 2001. The most important predictor of postinjury function was the preinjury ability to walk outdoors.

59. Paksima N, Koval KJ, Aharanoff G, et al: Predictors of mortality after hip fracture: A 10 year prospective study. *Bull NYU Hosp Joint Dis* 2008;66:111-117.

The role of medical, social, and functional covariates on mortality after hip fracture was studied in 1,109 patients acquired in a prospective database over a 16-year period. Predictors of mortality included advanced age, male gender, high American Society of Anesthesiologists classification, and ambulation with an assistive device.

60. Kim SY, Kim YG, Hwang JK: Cementless calcar-replacement hemiarthroplasty compared with intramedullary fixation of unstable intertrochanteric fractures: A prospective, randomized study. *J Bone Joint Surg Am* 2005;87(10):2186-2192.

The authors present the results of a Korean trial comparing calcar-replacement hemiarthroplasty (29 patients) with a proximal femoral nail (29 patients) in the treatment of unstable intertrochanteric fractures. The authors conclude that the nail provides improved clinical outcome (with similar functional outcome).

61. Stappaerts KH, Deldycke J, Broos PL, Staes FF, Rommens PM, Claes P: Treatment of unstable peritrochanteric fractures in elderly patients with a compression hip screw or with the Vandeputte (VDP) endoprosthesis: A prospective randomized study. *J Orthop Trauma* 1995; 9(4):292-297.

62. Haidukewych GJ, Berry DJ: Salvage of failed treatment of hip fractures. *J Am Acad Orthop Surg* 2005;13(2): 101-109.

6: Geriatric and Pediatric Trauma

Methods and techniques for the treatment of patients with failed fixation of both femoral neck and intertrochanteric hip fractures are discussed.

63. Miura LN, DiPiero AR, Homer LD: Effects of a geriatrician-led hip fracture program: Improvements in clinical and economic outcomes. *J Am Geriatr Soc* 2009;57(1):159-167.

    The authors present a comparison of 91 patients admitted to a dedicated hip fracture service to 72 historical control patients. The authors showed a reduced length of stay, reduced time in the operating room, and reduction in costs in those patients admitted to the hip fracture service.

64. Pedersen SJ, Borgbjerg FM, Schousboe B, et al; Hip Fracture Group of Bispebjerg Hospital: A comprehensive hip fracture program reduces complication rates and mortality. *J Am Geriatr Soc* 2008;56(10):1831-1838.

    The authors present the results of this Danish study in which 178 consecutive hip fracture patients (94% older than 60 years) who were admitted through a comprehensive hip fracture program were compared to 357 historical control patients. The authors conclude that an optimized hip fracture program reduced the rate of in-hospital postoperative complications and mortality.

65. Novack V, Jotkowitz A, Etzion O, Porath A: Does delay in surgery after hip fracture lead to worse outcomes? A multicenter survey. *Int J Qual Health Care* 2007;19(3):170-176.

    The authors present the results of an Israeli study in which data from seven hospitals (involving 4,633 patients) were reviewed. The authors conclude that delays in surgery for hip fracture are associated with significant increase in short-term and 1-year mortality.

66. Shiga T, Wajima Z, Ohe Y: Is operative delay associated with increased mortality of hip fracture patients? Systematic review, meta-analysis, and meta-regression. *Can J Anaesth* 2008;55(3):146-154.

    The authors of this Japanese study reviewed the English language literature from which 16 studies addressing surgical timing and mortality in hip fracture patients were identified. The authors concluded that delay beyond 48 hours was associated with an increase in both 30-day and 1-year all-cause mortality.

67. Verbeek DO, Ponsen KJ, Goslings JC, Heetveld MJ: Effect of surgical delay on outcome in hip fracture patients: A retrospective multivariate analysis of 192 patients. *Int Orthop* 2008;32(1):13-18.

The authors present the results of a retrospective study from The Netherlands examining the outcomes of 192 hip fracture patients. The study results showed a trend toward fewer postoperative complications and shorter length of stay in those patients operated on with a delay of less than 1 day.

68. Al-Ani AN, Samuelsson B, Tidermark J, et al: Early operation on patients with a hip fracture improved the ability to return to independent living: A prospective study of 850 patients. *J Bone Joint Surg Am* 2008;90(7):1436-1442.

    The authors of the Swedish study prospectively examined 850 patients presenting with a hip fracture. Patients were divided into those taken to surgery after 24 hours, after 36 hours, and after 48 hours. The authors conclude that early treatment is associated with an improved ability to return to independent living, lower risk of pressure ulcers, and a shortened hospital stay.

69. Sircar P, Godkar D, Mahgerefteh S, Chambers K, Niranjan S, Cucco R: Morbidity and mortality among patients with hip fractures surgically repaired within and after 48 hours. *Am J Ther* 2007;14(6):508-513.

    The authors present the results of a records review of 49 patients, including 34 who had surgery within 48 hours and 15 who had surgery after 48 hours. They conclude that surgery within the first 48 hours was associated with better health outcomes.

70. Ricci WM, Della Rocca GJ, Combs C, Borrelli J: The medical and economic impact of preoperative cardiac testing in elderly patients with hip fractures. *Injury* 2007;38(Suppl 3):S49-S52.

    The authors present the results of a review of 235 consecutive patients older than 60 years who were admitted with a hip fracture. Thirty-five of these patients (15%) underwent cardiac testing before surgery. The authors conclude that preoperative cardiac testing did not lead to changes in perioperative orthopaedic or medical management.

71. Lavelle WF, Demers-Lavelle EA, Uhl R: Operative delay for orthopedic patients on clopidogrel (Plavix): A complete lack of consensus. *J Trauma* 2008;64:996-1000.

    A computer-based survey was administered to the program directors of academic orthopaedic surgery programs. Seventy three percent of the respondents indicated that waiting 3 days or less for urgent but nonemergent surgical interventions is acceptable; 23% thought that no delay is necessary.

Chapter 42
Osteoporosis and Pathologic Bone

Michael J. Gardner, MD   Jonathan M. Gross, MD, MPH   George J. Haidukewych, MD

Osteoporosis

Overview of Osteoporosis

Osteoporosis is an asymptomatic disease that results in decreased structural bone quality and bone mass, and subsequently predisposes patients to low-energy fractures. Currently in the United States, 10 million people have osteoporosis, confirmed by a T-score on dual energy x-ray absorptiometry (DEXA) scan of -2.5 standard deviation or lower, or the presence of a fragility fracture. An additional 34 million have osteopenia, confirmed by a T-score between -1.0 SD and -2.5 SD, placing them at risk for fractures. Osteoporosis accounts for more than 1.5 million fractures annually in the United States.[1] Although 70% of patients with osteoporosis are women, many men are also affected. Typical osteoporotic fractures include intertrochanteric and femoral neck fractures, vertebral body fractures, and distal radius fractures. However, many other fractures occur as a result of low-energy traumatic mechanisms in elderly patients, including fractures of the proximal humerus, subtrochanteric femur, distal femur, tibial plateau, and ankle. These "fragility fractures," which occur after a fall from a standing height or lower, are increasing in frequency.

Normal bone requires tightly regulated homeostasis to maintain its structural properties. This is based on coordinated bone tissue resorption by osteoclasts and formation by osteoblasts. A key cytokine involved in bone homeostasis is receptor activator of nuclear factor-kappa B ligand (RANK-L), which is mainly produced by osteoblasts and bone marrow stromal cells. Its receptor, RANK, is expressed on osteoclast precursors. The activity of this system is a main mediator of osteoblast-osteoclast coupling and bone turnover.[2]

Pathophysiologically, osteoporosis is caused by dysregulation of the osteoblast-osteoclast interaction, resulting in either a relative increase in bone resorption or a relative decrease in bone formation. Primary (idiopathic) osteoporosis has been divided into two broad categories. Type 1, or postmenopausal osteoporosis (high turnover), is associated with estrogen deficiency. Type 2, or senile, osteoporosis (low turnover) is primarily age-related, and equally affects men and women older than 70 years. Secondary osteoporosis occurs from an identifiable etiology, such as use of certain medications, endocrinopathies, chronic diseases, or nutritional deficiencies.

Alterations in bone turnover dynamics result in altered bone mass and structural properties.[3] Because cancellous bone is more metabolically active than cortical bone, cancellous bone structure is generally affected first.[4,5] Finally, cortical thinning occurs in osteoporosis, which has a dramatic impact on bone strength (**Figure 1**).

Role of the Orthopaedist

Undertreatment of patients with osteoporosis, particularly those with an osteoporotic fracture, has been well documented.[6,7] Typically, patients with an osteoporotic fracture are treated primarily by an orthopaedic surgeon in either an inpatient or outpatient setting. After initial fracture treatment, orthopaedic follow-up includes assessment of fracture healing, maintenance of reduction, and rehabilitation. When the fracture heals and rehabilitation is concluded, the patient is typically discharged from the orthopaedist's care. The patient usually returns to their primary care physician at some point afterward for ongoing care, but this physician is often not aware of the nature of the fracture and osteoporosis evaluation and treatment are never initiated.

Because osteoporosis is an asymptomatic disease, occurrence of a fragility fracture is often its initial manifestation. For this reason, it is incumbent upon any orthopaedic surgeon who treats patients with fragility fractures to be aware of the correlation between low-energy fractures and clinical osteoporosis, and to initiate appropriate work-up and treatment. National Os-

Dr. Gardner or a member of his immediate family serves as a paid consultant to or is an employee of Synthes, DGIMed, and Amgen; and has received research or institutional support from AO, Synthes, Smith & Nephew, Wright Medical Technologies, and Foundation for Orthopaedic Trauma. Dr. Haidukewych or a member of his immediate family serves as a board member, owner, officer, or committee member of Orthopaedic Trauma Association, and American Academy of Orthopaedic Surgeons; has received royalties from DePuy; is a member of a speakers' bureau or has made paid presentations on behalf of DePuy; serves as a paid consultant to or is an employee of DePuy; and has stock or stock options held in Surmodics and Orthopediatrics. Neither Dr. Gross nor a member of his immediate family has received anything of value from or owns stock in a commercial company or institution related directly or indirectly to the subject of this article.

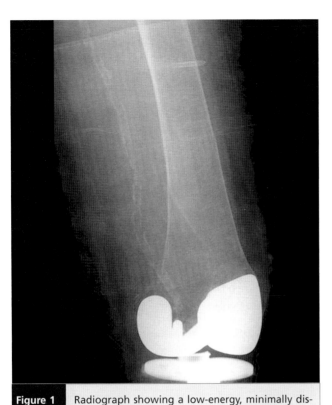

Figure 1 Radiograph showing a low-energy, minimally displaced periprosthetic supracondylar femur fracture in a 91-year-old woman. The marked osteopenia and cortical thinning are evident.

teoporosis Foundation guidelines specify that patients with a low-energy hip or vertebral fracture be considered for medical osteoporotic treatment.[8]

Reasons for the extremely low rate of osteoporosis treatment following a fragility fracture, despite the conclusive evidence-based guidelines for treatment, are not entirely clear, but several theories have been postulated. First, it has been recommended that any patient who sustains an osteoporotic fracture undergo DEXA scanning. DEXA scanning is a better predictor of survival than either blood pressure or cholesterol level.[9] Furthermore, initial DEXA is useful before pharmacologic treatment as a baseline to monitor the effects of therapy. However, it is often logistically difficult to obtain inpatient DEXA scanning, because of difficulties in mobilizing acutely injured patients, technical issues with the test itself, and systematic problems such as the remote location of the DEXA machine and even hospital billing and consultative practices.[10] Even if a DEXA scan is not obtained, National Osteoporosis Foundation guidelines indicate that active antiresorptive medication should be considered.[8] A clinical diagnosis of osteoporosis can be made on the basis of a fragility fracture, without determination of the bone density.[11] Recent surveys have indicated that many orthopaedic surgeons believe it is the responsibility of the primary care physician to diagnose and treat osteoporosis.[12,13] Additionally, many physicians have expressed doubt at the efficacy of antiresorptive medications, and thought

that education regarding their use and adverse effects was inadequate.[12,14] Finally, and perhaps most significantly, patient-related barriers can be a substantial impediment to treatment.[15]

With increasing knowledge of the barriers to osteoporosis treatment following fragility fracture, specific targeted interventions can be instituted. An important prerequisite for any intervention to be effective is that the orthopaedist assumes an active role. Perhaps the most substantial effect can be achieved with patient education. The National Osteoporosis Foundation guidelines are an excellent resource (www.nof.org). More than half of women with fragility fractures are unaware of osteoporosis, or are not psychologically prepared to accept the disease and its treatment.[15] One study provided education to patients newly diagnosed with osteoporosis and gave them a letter to bring to their primary care physician, and found significant improvements in diagnosis and treatment.[16] Also during the inpatient stay, patients should undergo assessment of serum 25-hydroxyvitamin D and calcium levels. Perhaps the most comprehensive and reliable method of improving treatment are systematic changes that designate a specific person or persons who are responsible for coordinating osteoporosis care. Because patients may have difficulty remembering to follow up, standing discharge orders can also improve postfracture treatment.[17]

General Principles of Osteoporotic Fracture Treatment

Many fragility fractures occur in elderly patients with limited physiologic reserves, and fracture treatment should be geared toward this fact. These patients often have significant cardiovascular and pulmonary comorbidities, and are at risk for perioperative morbidity and mortality.[18] Thus, a rational perioperative multidisciplinary management plan should be devised. Optimizing the patient's medical status and providing efficient surgical treatment are equally important. Preoperative considerations include ensuring adequate hydration, correcting electrolyte imbalance, and performing cardiac testing for risk stratification.[19] Recent data indicate that cardiac testing delays hip fracture treatment more than 1 day on average, is costly, and rarely affects perioperative cardiac or orthopaedic management.[20,21] The drawbacks of prolonged surgical delay include an increased risk of infectious complications, including urinary tract infections and pneumonia, thromboembolic disease, decubitus ulcers, and mortality.[22-24] Specifically, the perioperative development of pneumonia or a decubitus ulcer is associated with a 70% increase in mortality among nursing home patients.[25]

Orthopaedic surgical principles must be specifically tailored to the patient with an osteoporotic fracture. In general, obtaining stable fracture fixation is often less predictable due to both decreased bone strength with impaired implant anchorage, and the impaired healing response of the pathologic bone.[26] Comminuted periarticular fractures around the shoulder, elbow, hip, and knee may be considered for arthroplasty replacement. When internal fixation is indicated, proposed procedures should focus on minimizing blood loss and periosteal stripping to avoid excessive biologic insult.

Biomechanical Considerations

Fixation of osteoporotic fractures presents challenges to traditional surgical techniques and expected implant stability. Adherence to sound orthopaedic biomechanical principles maximizes healing rates and patient recovery. Fixation should be planned to allow immediate weight bearing when possible, because many elderly patients are unable to effectively abide by weight-bearing restrictions.[27] These constructs may be different from those selected for similar fracture patterns in younger patients. For this reason, facilitating bone healing and improving the longevity of an implant is imperative.

There are several main categories of implants that are most frequently used for osteoporotic fracture treatment. Besides arthroplasty, these include conventional plate and screw constructs, locked plating constructs, and intramedullary devices. Each device has specific advantages and disadvantages in certain situations.

Plate and Screw Constructs

The ability of a screw to resist load is directly related to its pullout strength and the amount of torque generated during insertion. The pullout strength is derived from the holding power between the screw threads and the material into which the screw is placed. Although pullout strength has classically been defined by the total thread surface area, as the density of the material into which the screw is placed diminishes, thread diameter and number become progressively less important.[28,29] Cortical screw fixation generally is superior to cancellous fixation in osteoporotic bone.[30]

Fixation stability of fractures with unlocked plates relies on the holding strength of the screws in bone, the friction generated between the plate and bone, and the fatigue strength of the plate. The screw holding strength, and consequently the friction generated between the plate and bone, are reduced in osteoporosis. In general, standard plates should be avoided in weaker, predominantly cancellous bone in metaphyseal fractures.[31,32]

When fracture fragments are reduced and stabilized with restoration of bony contact, a more stable mechanical environment is established, and the implant becomes more of a load-sharing device, which may minimize the risk of fixation failure. In osteoporotic fractures, shortening and impaction of the fracture may be desirable in regions such as the distal femur and proximal humerus for increasing bone contact and stability.[33]

The distribution of the screws within the plate can also be optimized to increase the longevity of a plate construct. The working length of a plate is defined by the distance between points of fixation on either side of a fracture. As the working length increases, the focal strain within the plate segment spanning the fracture decreases. In comminuted fractures, the working length typically increases. The overall plate strain decreases as the length of the plate increases and as the points of fixation become more widely spread out.[34] The optimal construct may require more points of fixation on either side of the fracture than is required in normal bone.

In certain anatomic locations, plate orientation can be altered to improve the fixation strength. In the osteoporotic distal fibula, an antiglide nonlocking plate provides more stable fixation than a lateral locked plate.[35]

The strength of unlocked plate and screw constructs can be augmented by increasing the number of implants. Clinical series of nonunions and biomechanical data indicate that fixation stability can be increased with additional plates, placed orthogonal or on the far cortex relative to the primary plate. However, while potentially mechanically favorable, this choice should be used cautiously. The dissection required to place a second orthogonal plate may threaten the viability of the soft-tissue envelope supporting the fracture fragments.

Locked Plates

Locked plates provide additional options for obtaining stable fracture fixation. Locked plates can function as internal external fixators. All of the elements that affect fracture stability with external fixators apply to locked plates, such as the distribution and diameter of screws, the fixed angle nature of the screws, and the plate offset from bone. The improved rigidity of locked plates also affects the failure mode. Because each screw in the plate is secured to the plate, the constructs typically fail catastrophically with either simultaneous screw cutout or plate breakage. Increasing the points of fixation may improve the fatigue strength of the screws, but also decreases the working length of the plate, which increases the plate strain. Longer plates with widely spaced screws may be ideal in osteoporotic bone. Because locked plates can behave as internal external fixators, they are a preferable choice when spanning, or "bridging" comminuted osteoporotic fractures.[36] In these circumstances, healing occurs through endochondral ossification with callus formation.

Minimally invasive insertion and anatomic plate contouring can improve healing by avoiding disruption of the fracture hematoma. Locked plates are amenable to minimally invasive insertion, as targeting arms can be affixed to the plate through the locked holes. Anatomically contoured plates potentially sit closer to the bone than standard plates and this intimate fit can optimize periarticular screw placement and minimize soft-tissue irritation.

In comminuted osteoporotic periarticular fractures, the use of plates that allow both locked and unlocked screws is preferable. Articular reductions can be compressed and rigidly stabilized with multiple lag screws

6: Geriatric and Pediatric Trauma

through the plate, and metaphyseal comminution can be spanned with the same plate. Unlocked screws or indirect reduction tools can be used to indirectly restore mechanical alignment without disrupting the soft-tissue envelope. In osteoporotic fractures, the degree of comminution is often underestimated by plain radiographs, and bridging locked plates can improve fixation in these circumstances. With hybrid fixation, locked screws are placed that flank an unlocked screw on one side of the fracture after reduction has been achieved. The use of hybrid constructs in osteoporotic bone may confer the benefits of both nonlocking and locking plates.[37,38]

Intramedullary Nails

Intramedullary nail fixation is the preferred method of treatment of diaphyseal femoral and tibial fractures in osteoporotic patients. Appropriately sized nails fill broad areas of the intramedullary canal, which allows load-sharing if cortical contact is achieved, and often provide fixation secure enough to accept early weight bearing. Intramedullary nails typically have greater bending strength than plates. They reside closer to the mechanical limb axis, so they are subjected to smaller deforming forces. This mechanical advantage requires that the nail extend past the isthmus of the femur or tibia to minimize toggle. These advantages are most commonly used in subtrochanteric femur fractures and intertrochanteric femur fractures, where the lateral cortex is violated, and where the bending forces are even more significant in patients who cannot abide by weight bearing restrictions.[33]

Improved interlocking technology has broadened the indications of intramedullary devices. Metadiaphyseal distal femur fractures can be treated with intramedullary implants. The weak point in modern nails is the interlocking screw, as the strength of screw fixation is dependent on the quality of the bone in which it is engaged. Interlocking screws in osteoporotic metaphyseal bone of distal femurs are prone to loosening. Newer nail constructs with broader interlocking blade fixation, multidirectional screw orientation, and even locking screws attempt to mitigate the effect of poor bone quality. Extending fixation as distally as possible to achieve interlocking screw fixation closer to denser subchondral bone is also important.

Augmentation of Stability

In an effort to address the limitations of internal fixation in osteoporotic bone, several techniques for augmenting fixation are available. One of the mainstays is using polymethylmethacrylate (PMMA) cement. First used to augment fixation of unlocked condylar buttress plate fixation of supracondylar femur fractures, it has also been used in proximal femur fractures and other fracture locations. Although the material can significantly improve the fixation holding strength, the considerable heat generated during PMMA polymerization may be harmful to the surrounding tissues. Additionally, as a nonresorbable material it can impair healing if it intercalates between viable ends of a fracture, and it can act as third-body wear particle if it is placed intra-articularly. Despite these drawbacks, PMMA augmentation may still be useful when fixation is compromised.

In an effort to address some of the limitations of PMMA, several formulations of calcium phosphate and calcium sulfate have been developed to augment fixation in osteoporotic bone. Calcium phosphate formulations tend to resorb much more slowly than calcium sulfate formulations, which may be an advantage in osteoporotic bone that heals at a slower rate than younger, nonosteoporotic bone. The persistence of the material, however, may share the same disadvantage of PMMA. The primary advantage of the calcium phosphate cement is its ability to resist axial compression. This material is less resistant to bending or torsion forces, and may fragment when a drill is inserted. Calcium phosphate is thus a better augment to support articular fracture fragments that have been elevated from positions of impaction, such as seen in tibial plateau fractures, than to assist with screw fixation. All biologic cements are strongest initially, and progressively weaken with time.

Allograft material can also be used to supplement fixation in osteoporotic fractures. Cortical strut grafts are a mainstay of periprosthetic fracture fixation augmentation at some centers. Although strut grafts incorporate into the host bone slowly, they improve fixation by providing a surface into which screws can be drilled or around which cerclage wires can be securely placed. Strut grafts have also been used to augment intramedullary fixation in the distal femur and have been shown a promising adjunct as an intramedullary augment to locked plate fixation of proximal humerus fractures.[39] In severely osteoporotic or comminuted proximal humerus fractures, an intramedullary fibular strut graft reconstitutes the mechanical integrity of the medial calcar, supports the humeral head fragment, provides additional fixation points for screws, and is relatively inexpensive.

Allograft cancellous chips are an option to augment healing and stabilization of osteoporotic fractures. Although cancellous allograft has been used to buttress reduced articular fracture fragments, their ability to resist compressive loads is less than that of calcium phosphate cement and may allow greater fracture subsidence.[40] Because of its porosity, however, cancellous allograft incorporates more fully than cortical allograft. Cancellous allograft may best be used as a graft expander, by adding it to autograft to effectively increase the volume. The immunogenicity of freeze-dried preparations is relatively low and the material is less expensive than most calcium phosphate and sulfate preparations.

Augmentation of Healing

The historic gold standard for biologic stimulation of bone healing is cancellous autograft. Autograft is osteoconductive, osteoinductive, and a source of pluripotent osteoprogenitor cells. When treating osteoporotic patients, the surgeon must be aware that there is an age-related decline in the number of pluripotent osteoprogenitor cells available in iliac crest autografts. The osteogenic potential is further negatively affected by systemic disease, gender, and environmental factors, such as smoking. Additionally, the same microarchitectural changes that lead to fragility fractures exist in autograft bone. Cancellous autograft harvested from a young, healthy individual has very different structural properties than graft obtained from an older patient with osteoporosis.

Including the bone morphogenetic proteins (BMPs), there are more than 20 families and subfamilies of polypeptide growth factors associated with bone healing. No study has shown that BMP improves fracture healing in osteoporotic bone, and although its routine use is currently not recommended, it might be useful for expediting fracture healing of bones whose fixation is compromised by its altered microarchitecture.

Recombinant parathyroid hormone (PTH, teriparatide) improves bone mineral density in patients with osteoporosis, and may be effective for inducing union in pelvic insufficiency fracture nonunions. Like BMP, routine use of PTH to facilitate fracture union in osteoporotic patients is not presently approved or recommended, but may theoretically have benefit.

Demineralized bone matrix (DBM) contains growth factors, noncollagenous proteins, and collagen. It is a potent inducer of fracture healing and can improve spinal fusion in humans. The osteoinductive effect of DBM, however, is limited by the source of bone from which the material has been derived and the carrier substance with which it is mixed. There is little consistency in the effect, as comparative studies have suggested the osteoinductive effects are highly variable.[41] Nonetheless, DBM may have a role as an adjunct to osteoporotic fracture healing, particularly when large bone deficits are encountered.

Optimizing bone health by correcting vitamin D deficits and ensuring appropriate calcium intake may be as important for osteoporotic bone healing as biologic fracture augmentation. Vitamin D deficiency is endemic to environments with limited sun exposure, people with restrictive diets, and the elderly, who often have subclinical malabsorption syndromes. Similarly, calcium intake requirements are often not met in the elderly. Calcium carbonate is poorly absorbed in the hypochlorhydric or achlorhydric gastrointestinal systems of the elderly, but this formulation is more commonly prescribed, because the pill size required to deliver the same amount of calcium is smaller than the more easily absorbed calcium citrate formulations. Calcium citrate is absorbed without gastric acid, but because the citrate is a larger molecule than the carbonate, the pill tends to be larger for each unit of calcium.

A subset of osteoporotic patients sustains diaphyseal fractures while on bisphosphonate therapy. These fractures have the appearance of chronic stress fractures, typically in the subtrochanteric femur, that may be due to bone turnover suppression from chronic bisphosphonate. In these patients, cessation of bisphosphonate therapy, at least during the initial phases of fracture healing, is theoretically prudent, although bisphosphonates have a half-life of approximately 10 years. Prevention of subsequent fractures may require biologic healing augmentation.

Arthroplasty

Although modern techniques of internal fixation are effective for treating most unstable fractures in patients with osteopenic bone, there are several situations where arthroplasty may be a better choice. Commonly encountered clinical examples include fragility fractures of the proximal humerus, the distal humerus, and the femoral neck. Shoulder, elbow, and hip arthroplasty in these settings may provide more predictable and earlier return to function in this elderly cohort, in whom internal fixation is more likely to fail. This patient population often cannot comply with or tolerate prolonged periods of restricted weight bearing often necessary to achieve fracture union, and immobility of a limb can lead to loss of functional independence.

Perhaps the most common scenario of arthroplasty for acute fractures in osteopenic bone is the displaced femoral neck fracture in the elderly patient. Despite advances in implants and techniques for internal fixation, the fixation failure rate of approximately 40% has not changed over the past 7 decades. This fact has led many surgeons to routinely treat these fractures with some form of hip arthroplasty. Recent prospective randomized studies have demonstrated a significantly lower reoperation rate and better functional outcomes with total hip arthroplasty for displaced femoral neck fractures.[42] Arthroplasty is also cost-effective despite higher implant costs, especially when the costs of salvaging failed internal fixation are compared. Typically, full weight bearing can commence immediately after arthroplasty. Modern cementless and traditional cemented fixation techniques can be effective, and component fixation decisions should be based on bone quality. A more detailed discussion of treatment choices for displaced femoral neck fractures can be found in other chapters of this book.

Other clinical scenarios where arthroplasty may be preferred to internal fixation include selected fractures of the distal femur, acetabulum, and pathologic fractures due to neoplasm in cognitively intact patients. For example, an acetabular fracture in an otherwise healthy octogenarian with femoral head and acetabular articular impaction is likely to result in a poor outcome if treated with internal fixation alone. Combined internal fixation of the acetabulum and total hip arthroplasty in this setting may provide more predictable functional improvement, but is a technically demanding procedure (**Figure 2**). Selected distal femur fractures, for example, extremely distal periprosthetic fractures above a loose total knee arthroplasty in an elderly patient, may be

6: Geriatric and Pediatric Trauma

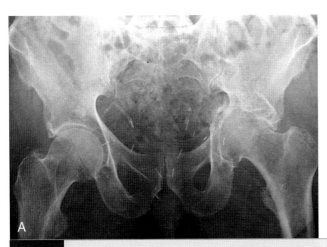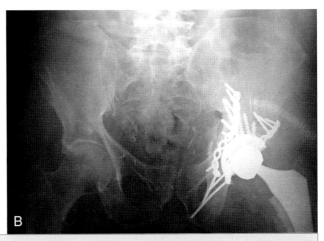

Figure 2 In elderly patients with acetabular fractures with osteoporosis and substantial comminution and/or and associated dome impaction (left panel), consideration may be given to acute ORIF and concomitant total hip arthroplasty (right panel). (Courtesy of A. Sems, MD).

more predictably managed with distal femoral replacement with a so-called "megaprosthesis." It is important to note, however, that most acetabular and distal femoral fractures in elderly patients heal reliably with contemporary and well-executed open reduction and internal fixation (ORIF), and that arthroplasty should be reserved for selected cases.

Arthroplasty for selected acute osteoporotic fragility fractures can provide a predictable alternative to internal fixation, especially in fractures with documented high failure rates with ORIF, and in clinical settings where ORIF is very likely to fail. The surgeon must individualize indications and techniques for the particular patient and fracture pattern. Careful attention to detail is important to minimize complications.

Pathologic Bone

Introduction

Because cancer remains one of the leading causes of death in the United States, it is likely that the orthopaedic surgeon will encounter pathologic bone lesions in his or her practice. Although primary bone malignancies are exceedingly rare, any solitary lesion without a known primary lesion should be considered a primary malignancy until proven otherwise. More commonly, the orthopaedist will encounter multiple bony lesions in a patient with known metastatic disease or multiple myeloma, and will be required to manage impending or completed pathologic fractures. Bone is the third most common site for metastatic disease after the lung and liver. Breast, prostate, lung, thyroid, and kidney cancers commonly metastasize to bone.

Evaluation of Bone Lesions

The evaluation should begin with a thorough history and physical examination. Imaging should include plain radiographs (skeletal surveys), as well as CT for cortical detail, and MRI of the entire bone to evaluate marrow involvement and skip lesions. Bone scan should also be considered to evaluate for distant lesions. CT of the chest, abdomen, and pelvis, mammography, serum electrophoresis, and tumor-specific markers (such as prostate-specific antigen) may be helpful in specific cases. If there is any concern regarding the diagnosis, biopsy may be performed. Recent data have suggested that new osseous lesions in a patient with a known primary carcinoma, especially breast or prostate, should be biopsied and not automatically assumed to be metastatic.[43] It is important that the biopsy be performed by surgeons experienced with the principles of tumor biopsy.

Treatment Considerations and Surgical Indications

The treatment of metastatic cancerous bone lesions is multidisciplinary and may require chemotherapy, radiotherapy, hormonal therapies, bisphosphonates, and surgical stabilization. The size of the lesion and its anatomic location influence the risk of pathologic fracture, and thus guide the surgical indications for prophylactic stabilization of impending pathologic fractures. One of the most commonly used methods for predicting the risk of fracture is the method of Mirels.[44] This system assigns points to tumor characteristics (lytic or blastic), size (cortical loss), presence of pain, and anatomic location. It is important to note that functional pain (for example, hip pain with ambulation) is highly predictive of fracture, and prophylactic intervention is warranted. It is important, therefore, to inquire whether the patient has any other anatomic areas of bony pain. The ideal method of stabilization varies based on the anatomic location of the lesion and the lesion size, among other factors. Life expectancy should be estimated with the input of consultation services, and the risks and benefits for quality of life improvement should be considered and discussed with the pa-

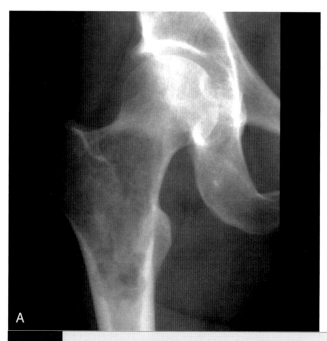
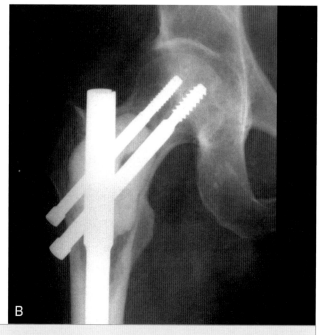

Figure 3 **A,** Radiograph of the hip of a patient with a proximal femoral metastatic lesion and a Mirels score of 12. **B,** Radiograph after treatment prophylactic reconstruction nail stabilization and PMMA augmentation. In this case, after curettage of the lesion, PMMA cement was hand-packed into the cavitary defect just prior to nail insertion.

tient. Typically, most patients with a life expectancy of greater than 3 months are considered for surgical treatment.

Implant Considerations

The appropriate choice of implant will vary based on the anatomic location of the lesion; however, several general principles exist. The fixation should be robust, because it will function in a load-bearing capacity due to the pathologic cortical destruction. Therefore, intramedullary strategies are typically preferred. Prophylactic fixation of diaphyseal lesions generally requires some form of intramedullary fixation to benefit from long and durable fixation constructs, making intramedullary nailing the optimal treatment. Spanning the entire length of the bone with the fixation is generally recommended; for example, cephalomedullary fixation with a long nail is typically selected for a subtrochanteric metastatic lesion. Lesions in the metaphyseal region can be treated with intramedullary fixation or some form of plating, with or without cement augmentation. Epiphyseal lesions are generally treated with resection and prosthetic replacement, typically with some form of megaprosthesis.[45] Acetabular lesions can be managed with antiprotrusio cages and/or internal fixation with cement augmentation if the defects are large. A full discussion of the various reconstructive options can be found in the literature.[46]

Cement Augmentation

The pathologic nature and decreased quantity of bone at the site of a pathologic fracture can substantially in-

hibit stable implant fixation. Because surgical treatment of pathologic extremity fractures is rarely aimed at altering the disease process, but rather at allowing immediate mobilization and pain control, secure fixation is a top priority. Pathologic fractures that occur in a periarticular location, particularly those in the lower extremity, are often treated with arthroplasty. However, in diaphyseal fractures, or in the proximal femoral or humeral metaphysis, cement augmentation can add significant strength to the construct.[47] There is no evidence to suggest that cement augmentation interferes with subsequent radiation therapy. Some studies have recommended that PMMA cement be used for mechanical augmentation to internal fixation whenever possible.[48,49]

PMMA can be used concomitantly with an intramedullary nail or a plate.[50] Lesions are typically treated with open curettage. ORIF can then be performed, and the site of the lesion packed with cement in a viscous state around the implant (**Figure 3**). Alternatively, the cement may be inserted before implant placement. Drill holes for screws can be carefully placed in hardened PMMA, taking care to avoid fragmentation. However, an intramedullary nail should not be placed through a hardened cement mantle.

Failure rates of proximal femoral pathologic fractures treated with internal fixation have been high.[48] In the presence of a large or rapidly expanding lesion, the cortical contact and load sharing ability of the bone progressively declines. Adding cement around the threads of a compression hip screw device can also be considered for potentially increasing the holding strength of the screw, but if the lesion extends into the femoral neck and head, arthroplasty is advisable.

Radiation Therapy

Radiation therapy is a useful adjunct to the management of pathologic fractures. In resected tumors, it is used primarily to minimize local recurrence. For impending fractures, it can be used to reduce the tumor burden. Irradiated healthy bone and soft tissue in the region of the lesion are affected as well as the tumor. Bone may become permanently metabolically hypoactive and osteoporotic. The risk of a late pathologic fracture due to irradiation is relative to the cumulative dose of radiation administered. Typically, adjunctive radiotherapy is administered at least 2 weeks after surgical stabilization, once the surgical wounds have healed. This usually consists of 3,000 to 3,500 Gy of external beam radiation delivered over several fractions. One recent report suggested that as the fracture healed or as the tumor burden diminished, pain and quality of life improved.[51] It may be prudent to irradiate the entire length of a long bone after intramedullary fixation, as tumor cells may have been seeded down the canal during the procedure.[52]

Excessive radiation predisposes patients to osteonecrosis and late fractures and impairs soft-tissue healing, and therefore should be avoided.

Chemotherapy

In the treatment of pathologic fractures, chemotherapy is used to systemically stop or slow down the growth of cancer at the fracture site. This effect helps the musculoskeletal system repair structural damage through bone's inherent ability to regenerate. However, the suppression of the cancer also retards the local progression of the disease, which can further destabilize the skeletal system. In general, the net effects of chemotherapy typically improve the patient's response to surgical management of pathologic fractures. Survival and quality of life improve when pathologic fractures are managed with judicious use of surgery, chemotherapy, and radiation therapy.

Metastatic prostate cancer is usually blastic in nature, but may also be lytic or mixed. Suppression of androgen formation impedes the progression of disease. However, androgens are also instrumental in maintaining osteoblast populations. Androgen suppression therapy is often used as a palliative adjunct in advanced cancers, but results in significant bone mineral density loss, making fracture fixation all the more difficult and predisposing the patient to fragility fractures independent of metastatic disease. Metastatic breast cancer, which is typically lytic, is also often estrogen sensitive. Selective estrogen receptor modulators, such as tamoxifen, can inhibit the progression of metastatic breast cancer, but estrogens are necessary for osteoblast and osteoclast homeostasis. These estrogen analogs can disrupt the normal link between osteoclasts and osteoblasts and have been shown to potentiate osteoporosis

in premenopausal women receiving them for cancer treatment.[51]

In an effort to mitigate the negative effects of chemotherapy, patients are often treated with concomitant bisphosphonates, which interfere with osteoclastic bone resorption. In patients with metastatic breast cancer, intravenous bisphosphonate therapy decreases the risk of skeletal complications. However, the reparative process of diaphyseal fractures may be impaired by its prolonged use.

A major component of chemotherapy for hematopoietic-based malignancies is long-term and high-dose glucocorticoids. Steroids are used as a pain adjuvant, a palliative agent, an antiemetic, and as part of the treatment to reduce inappropriate bone formation. These effects improve function and quality of life. Although the benefits of this chemotherapeutic agent are clear, the detrimental effects on wound and fracture healing, as well as systemic osteoporosis, are also apparent. Prolonged exposure to corticosteroids is the third leading cause of osteoporosis, after menopause and advanced age. Approximately half of people on steroids develop osteoporosis, and fracture risk increases 50% to 100% over the base population. There is essentially a dose- and duration-dependent effect on bone loss and corticosteroid use.[51] Because of the deleterious effect of glucocorticoids on calcium metabolism, all patients on steroids should be initiated on supplemental calcium.

Summary

Osteoporosis is an extremely common disorder caused by dysregulation of bone turnover, whose hallmark is altered structural and mechanical properties of bone. Women are more affected in the sixth decade, but in elderly populations, men are also affected. Prompt diagnosis and treatment are essential, as antiresorptive medications (such as bisphosphonates) are effective in preventing fragility fractures. Historically, rates of diagnosis have been extremely poor following fragility fracture.

Fractures occurring in pathologic bone pose unique difficulties to the orthopaedic surgeon, and the incidence of these fractures continues to increase. Pathologic fractures arise in patients with osteoporosis, whether formally diagnosed or not, or in those with malignancies that have arisen in or metastasized to bone. Management approaches differ in each situation due to the potential for focal disease progression and decreased life expectancy with malignancy. Intramedullary, load sharing fixation of the entire bone is frequently preferable in both instances. Multiple molecular mediators are being tested and refined for biologic augmentation of osteoporotic fractures, and biologic intervention holds promise as the future of pathologic fracture repair.

Annotated References

1. Riggs BL, Melton LJ III: The worldwide problem of osteoporosis: Insights afforded by epidemiology. *Bone* 1995;17(suppl, 5):S505-S511.

2. Rauner M, Sipos W, Pietschmann P: Osteoimmunology. *Int Arch Allergy Immunol* 2007;143(1):31-48.

   An overview of "osteoimmunology," which examines the interactions of inflammatory mediators on bone remodeling, is presented.

3. Kennedy OD, Brennan O, Mahony NJ, et al: Effects of high bone turnover on the biomechanical properties of the L3 vertebra in an ovine model of early stage osteoporosis. *Spine* 2008;33(23):2518-2523.

   In this study of ovarectomized sheep, early bone turnover and mechanical properties of bone were decreased despite retained normal microarchitecture and BMP.

4. Chao EY, Inoue N, Koo TK, Kim YH: Biomechanical considerations of fracture treatment and bone quality maintenance in elderly patients and patients with osteoporosis. *Clin Orthop Relat Res* 2004;425:12-25.

   The authors review important aspects of osteoporotic bone biomechanics and subsequent fracture treatment.

5. Ding M, Odgaard A, Linde F, Hvid I: Age-related variations in the microstructure of human tibial cancellous bone. *J Orthop Res* 2002;20(3):615-621.

6. Feldstein AC, Nichols GA, Elmer PJ, Smith DH, Aickin M, Herson M: Older women with fractures: Patients falling through the cracks of guideline-recommended osteoporosis screening and treatment. *J Bone Joint Surg Am* 2003;85(12):2294-2302.

7. Freedman KB, Kaplan FS, Bilker WB, Strom BL, Lowe RA: Treatment of osteoporosis: are physicians missing an opportunity? *J Bone Joint Surg Am* 2000;82(8):1063-1070.

8. National Osteoporosis Foundation: *Physician's Guide to Prevention and Treatment of Osteoporosis.* Washington, DC: National Osteoporosis Foundation, 2008.

   Comprehensive guidelines for osteoporosis treatment are presented.

9. Johansson C, Black D, Johnell O, Odén A, Mellström D: Bone mineral density is a predictor of survival. *Calcif Tissue Int* 1998;63(3):190-196.

10. Collinge C, LeBus G, Gardner MJ, Gehrig L: Osteoporosis in orthopaedic trauma patients: A diagnosis and treatment protocol. *J Orthop Trauma* 2008;22(8):541-547.

    This study found that using canceal ultrasound, nearly one third of all orthopaedic trauma patients were at high risk for osteoporosis.

11. Simonelli C, Killeen K, Mehle S, Swanson L: Barriers to osteoporosis identification and treatment among primary care physicians and orthopedic surgeons. *Mayo Clin Proc* 2002;77(4):334-338.

12. Taylor JC, Sterkel B, Utley M, et al: Opinions and experiences in general practice on osteoporosis prevention, diagnosis and management. *Osteoporos Int* 2001;12(10):844-848.

13. Skedros JG, Holyoak JD, Pitts TC: Knowledge and opinions of orthopaedic surgeons concerning medical evaluation and treatment of patients with osteoporotic fracture. *J Bone Joint Surg Am* 2006;88(1):18-24.

    According to results from a survey study, many orthopaedic surgeons do not initiate osteoporosis treatment following fragility fracture treatment because they believe it is the role of primary care physicians.

14. Cuddihy MT: Barriers to postfracture osteoporosis care in postmenopausal women. *J Gen Intern Med* 2003;18(1):70-71.

15. Mauck KF, Cuddihy MT, Trousdale RT, Pond GR, Pankratz VS, Melton LJ III: The decision to accept treatment for osteoporosis following hip fracture: Exploring the woman's perspective using a stage-of-change model. *Osteoporos Int* 2002;13(7):560-564.

16. Gardner MJ, Brophy RH, Demetrakopoulos D, et al: Interventions to improve osteoporosis treatment following hip fracture: A prospective, randomized trial. *J Bone Joint Surg Am* 2005;87(1):3-7.

    This prospective, randomized trial identified the effectiveness of providing hip fracture patients with education and a list of questions to bring to their primary care physician after discharge. This significantly increased osteoporosis treatment.

17. Skedros JG: The orthopaedic surgeon's role in diagnosing and treating patients with osteoporotic fractures: Standing discharge orders may be the solution for timely medical care. *Osteoporos Int* 2004;15(5):405-410.

    Following fragility fractures, letters were sent from the orthopaedic surgeon to the patients' primary care physician requesting an appointment. This process was generally ineffective because of noncompliance and inconsistency.

18. Roche JJ, Wenn RT, Sahota O, Moran CG: Effect of comorbidities and postoperative complications on mortality after hip fracture in elderly people: Prospective observational cohort study. *BMJ* 2005;331(7529):1374.

    In patients with hip fractures, the presence of three or more medical comorbidities was the strongest predictor of increased mortality risk.

19. McLaughlin MA, Orosz GM, Magaziner J, et al: Preoperative status and risk of complications in patients with hip fracture. *J Gen Intern Med* 2006;21(3):219-225.

    In elderly hip fracture patients, major correctable electrolyte or physical examination abnormalities should be corrected before surgery to minimize morbidity risk.

6: Geriatric and Pediatric Trauma

20. Ricci WM, Della Rocca GJ, Combs C, Borrelli J: The medical and economic impact of preoperative cardiac testing in elderly patients with hip fractures. *Injury* 2007;38(Suppl 3):S49-S52.

    In a study of 235 hip fracture patients, preoperative cardiac testing was costly and did not alter perioperative management in any case.

21. Boersma E, Poldermans D, Bax JJ, et al; DECREASE Study Group (Dutch Echocardiographic Cardiac Risk Evaluation Applying Stress Echocardiography): Predictors of cardiac events after major vascular surgery: Role of clinical characteristics, dobutamine echocardiography, and beta-blocker therapy. *JAMA* 2001;285(14): 1865-1873.

22. Verbeek DO, Ponsen KJ, Goslings JC, Heetveld MJ: Effect of surgical delay on outcome in hip fracture patients: A retrospective multivariate analysis of 192 patients. *Int Orthop* 2008;32(1):13-18.

    In a cohort of hip fracture patients, surgical delay of greater than 1 day led to greater infectious complications, and a trend toward longer hospital stay.

23. Grimes JP, Gregory PM, Noveck H, Butler MS, Carson JL: The effects of time-to-surgery on mortality and morbidity in patients following hip fracture. *Am J Med* 2002;112(9):702-709.

24. Al-Ani AN, Samuelsson B, Tidermark J, et al: Early operation on patients with a hip fracture improved the ability to return to independent living: A prospective study of 850 patients. *J Bone Joint Surg Am* 2008; 90(7):1436-1442.

    A prospective study of 850 hip fracture patients found that early surgery led to earlier return to independent living, decreased pressure ulcers, and a shorter hospital stay.

25. Berry SD, Samelson EJ, Bordes M, Broe K, Kiel DP: Survival of aged nursing home residents with hip fracture. *J Gerontol A Biol Sci Med Sci* 2009;64(7):771-777.

    The authors of this study examined hip fracture patients who resided in nursing homes, and found a high morbidity associated with potentially avoidable complications such as pressure ulcers and pneumonia.

26. Giannoudis P, Tzioupis C, Almalki T, Buckley R: Fracture healing in osteoporotic fractures: Is it really different? A basic science perspective. *Injury* 2007;38 (suppl 1):S90-S99.

    A review of fracture healing in osteoporotic bone is presented. Although scant, recent data indicate that osteoporotic bone healing may be altered.

27. Koval KJ, Sala DA, Kummer FJ, Zuckerman JD: Postoperative weight-bearing after a fracture of the femoral neck or an intertrochanteric fracture. *J Bone Joint Surg Am* 1998;80(3):352-356.

28. Strømsøe K, Kok WL, Høiseth A, Alho A: Holding power of the 4.5 mm AO/ASIF cortex screw in cortical bone in relation to bone mineral. *Injury* 1993;24(10): 656-659.

29. Asnis SE, Ernberg JJ, Bostrom MP, et al: Cancellous bone screw thread design and holding power. *J Orthop Trauma* 1996;10(7):462-469.

30. Seebeck J, Goldhahn J, Morlock MM, Schneider E: Mechanical behavior of screws in normal and osteoporotic bone. *Osteoporos Int* 2005;16(suppl 2):S107-S111.

    According to a biomechanical study comparing cortical thickness and metaphysis and diaphysis of the tibia to pullout strength of screws, it was suggested that with a cortical thickness of less than 1.5 mm, cancellous density determines pullout strength.

31. Seide K, Triebe J, Faschingbauer M, et al: Locked vs. unlocked plate osteosynthesis of the proximal humerus: A biomechanical study. *Clin Biomech* 2007;22(2): 176-182.

    A biomechanical study of bone density matched cadaveric humeri compared locked and unlocked 4.5-mm, limited contact dynamic compression plates. The study showed significantly greater fatigue strength for locked plates.

32. Strauss EJ, Schwarzkopf R, Kummer F, Egol KA: The current status of locked plating: The good, the bad, and the ugly. *J Orthop Trauma* 2008;22(7):479-486.

    The authors review the current state of biomechanics of locked plating.

33. Cornell CN: Internal fracture fixation in patients with osteoporosis. *J Am Acad Orthop Surg* 2003;11(2):109-119.

34. Sanders R, Haidukewych GJ, Milne T, Dennis J, Latta LL: Minimal versus maximal plate fixation techniques of the ulna: The biomechanical effect of number of screws and plate length. *J Orthop Trauma* 2002;16(3): 166-171.

35. Minihane KP, Lee C, Ahn C, Zhang LQ, Merk BR: Comparison of lateral locking plate and antiglide plate for fixation of distal fibular fractures in osteoporotic bone: A biomechanical study. *J Orthop Trauma* 2006; 20(8):562-566.

    A biomechanical study of matched human cadaveric fibula short oblique osteotomies demonstrated that torque to failure was better with posterolateral convention plate fixation compared with straight lateral locked plate fixation.

36. Smith WR, Ziran BH, Anglen JO, Stahel PF: Locking plates: Tips and tricks. *J Bone Joint Surg Am* 2007; 89(10):2298-2307.

    The authors present a basic review of locked plating along with its indications, uses, and mechanics.

37. Gardner MJ, Griffith MH, Demetrakopoulos D, et al: Hybrid locked plating of osteoporotic fractures of the humerus. *J Bone Joint Surg Am* 2006;88(9):1962-1967.

    In the first biomechanical study comparing locked, unlocked, and hybrid fixation constructs in a synthetic osteoporotic bone model, it was suggested that hybrid screw fixation did not deleteriously affect the strength of the construct.

38. Fitzpatrick DC, Doornink J, Madey SM, Bottlang M: Relative stability of conventional and locked plating fixation in a model of the osteoporotic femoral diaphysis. *Clin Biomech* 2009;24(2):203-209.

   The authors present a biomechanical study using synthetic ostoporotic bone model that compared locked bridge plate to conventional plate stiffness and strength. The study suggested that axial strength may be better with bicortical locked screws, but not bending and torsional strength.

39. Gardner MJ, Boraiah S, Helfet DL, Lorich DG: Indirect medial reduction and strut support of proximal humerus fractures using an endosteal implant. *J Orthop Trauma* 2008;22(3):195-200.

   A clinical series and technique of osteoporotic proximal humerus fractures treated with locked plating and fibular allograft augmentation are presented.

40. Bajammal SS, Zlowodzki M, Lelwica A, et al: The use of calcium phosphate bone cement in fracture treatment: A meta-analysis of randomized trials. *J Bone Joint Surg Am* 2008;90(6):1186-1196.

   A meta-analysis of randomized studies using calcium phosphate to augment fracture healing suggested that patients had less pain and better maintained reductions when augmentation was used.

41. Bae HW, Zhao L, Kanim LE, et al: Intervariability and intravariability of bone morphogenetic proteins in commercially available demineralized bone matrix products. *Spine* 2006;31:1299-1306.

   This molecular biologic study demonstrates more variability between lots than between manufacturers in the concentration BMPs-2, -4, and -7 extricated from commercially available DBM formulations.

42. Baker RP, Squires B, Gargan MF, Bannister GC: Total hip arthroplasty and hemiarthroplasty in mobile, independent patients with a displaced intracapsular fracture of the femoral neck: A randomized, controlled trial. *J Bone Joint Surg Am* 2006;88:2583-2589.

   When compared with hemiarthroplasty, total hip arthoplasty yielded superior short-term clinical results and fewer complications in mobile, independent patients with a displaced fracture of the femoral neck.

43. Clayer M, Duncan W: Importance of biopsy of new bone lesions in patients with previous carcinoma. *Clin Orthop Relat Res* 2006;451:208-211.

   A prospective study of 50 patients is presented that demonstrated assuming a bone lesion is metastatic in patients with known carcinoma can lead to errors in treatment.

44. Mirels H: Metastatic disease in long bones. A proposed scoring system for diagnosing impending pathologic fractures. *Clin Orthop Relat Res* 1989;249:256-264.

45. Chandrasekar CR, Grimer RJ, Carter SR, Tillman RM, Abudu A, Buckley L: Modular endoprosthetic replacement for tumours of the proximal femur. *J Bone Joint Surg Br* 2009;91(1):108-112.

   In this series of pathologic proximal femoral lesions in 100 patients, endoprosthetic replacement led to a 5-year survival rate of 91% and a low complication rate.

46. Damron TA, Sim FH: Surgical treatment for metastatic disease of the pelvis and the proximal end of the femur. *Instr Course Lect* 2000;49:461-470.

47. Miller GJ, Vander Griend RA, Blake WP, Springfield DS: Performance evaluation of a cement-augmented intramedullary fixation system for pathologic lesions of the femoral shaft. *Clin Orthop Relat Res* 1987; 221:246-254.

48. Yazawa Y, Frassica FJ, Chao EY, Pritchard DJ, Sim FH, Shives TC: Metastatic bone disease: A study of the surgical treatment of 166 pathologic humeral and femoral fractures. *Clin Orthop Relat Res* 1990;251:213-219.

49. Gruber G, Zacherl M, Leithner A, et al: Surgical treatment of pathologic fractures of the humerus and femur. *Orthopade* 2009;38(4):324-334, 326-328, 330-334.

   A clinical series on surgical treatment of metastatic bone lesions, in which the authors recommended intralesional curettage and cement augmentation for diaphyseal pathologic fractures is presented.

50. Harrington KD, Sim FH, Enis JE, Johnston JO, Diok HM, Gristina AG: Methylmethacrylate as an adjunct in internal fixation of pathological fractures: Experience with three hundred and seventy-five cases. *J Bone Joint Surg Am* 1976;58(8):1047-1055.

51. Stava CJ, Jimenez C, Hu MI, Vassilopoulou-Sellin R: Skeletal sequelae of cancer and cancer treatment. *J Cancer Surviv* 2009;3(2):75-88.

   A review of the skeletal consequences of chemotherapy is presented. The authors review by class the clinical evidence of the effects of chemotherapeutic agents on skeletal metabolism.

52. Weber KL, Randall RL, Grossman S, Parvizi J: Management of lower-extremity bone metastasis. *J Bone Joint Surg Am* 2006;88(suppl 4):11-19.

   Clinical series of surgically managed metastatic lesions in lower extremities derived from multiple centers provides an algorithm for treatment with useful additional information on management.

6: Geriatric and Pediatric Trauma

Chapter 43

Periprosthetic Fractures

Thomas J. Ellis, MD   Raymond R. White, MD   David W. Lhowe, MD

Upper Extremity Periprosthetic Fractures

Periprosthetic fractures of the upper extremity remain relatively infrequent compared to those of the lower extremity. The reasons for this discrepancy include the relative infrequency of shoulder and elbow arthroplasty in comparison with hip and knee replacement surgeries as well as the decreased mechanical loads placed on the upper extremity. However, with the growing rate of shoulder and elbow replacement surgeries, lengthening life spans, and the high prevalence of osteoporosis, periprosthetic fractures in the upper extremity are an increasing source of concern. The most common fracture site is the proximal humerus involving the humeral component of a shoulder arthroplasty, followed by the distal humerus in association with a total elbow arthroplasty. Periprosthetic ulnar fractures have been described and treatment principles proposed, but case series are lacking because of the relative infrequency of this fracture. Periprosthetic glenoid fractures are exceedingly rare.

As in the evaluation of lower extremity periprosthetic fractures, the following factors are assessed: (1) fracture location and stability, (2) fixation of the implant, and (3) quality of the surrounding bone. Minimally displaced fractures in good-quality bone and associated with well-fixed implants represent the most stable injuries and can be considered for nonsurgical management. At the other end of the spectrum, comminuted unstable fracture patterns in the presence of osteolysis and grossly loose implants require surgical management that is technically difficult and accompanied by higher rates of complication and nonunion. In addition to characteristics of the local bone quality, fracture pattern, and implant status, host factors such

Dr. Ellis or an immediate family member has received royalties from Acumed and is a member of a speakers' bureau or has made paid presentations on behalf of Stryker. Dr. White or an immediate family member serves as a board member, owner, officer, or committee member of the Orthopaedic Associates of Portland; serves as a paid consultant to or is an employee of Zimmer; and has received nonincome support (such as equipment or services), commercially derived honoraria, or other non–research-related funding (such as paid travel) from Synthes. Neither Dr. Lhowe nor any immediate family member has received anything of value from or owns stock in a commercial company or institution related directly or indirectly to the subject of this chapter.

as the presence of local or systemic infection and the ability to safely endure potentially long-lasting general anesthesia must be weighed in devising an approach for these fractures.

Periprosthetic Humerus Fractures Associated With Shoulder Arthroplasty

Periprosthetic proximal humerus fractures occur both during and after shoulder arthroplasty. A recent report from the Mayo Clinic documents an overall 1.5% rate of intraoperative fracture (1.2% in primary surgeries and 3.3% in revision surgeries) from 1980 to 2002.[1] A retrospective review from the same institution found only 19 postoperative fractures in 3,091 patients treated with shoulder arthroplasty between 1976 and 2001.[2] The 0.6% prevalence of postoperative fracture suggested by these numbers may underestimate the actual prevalence, which has been reported at 1.6% and 2.4% in other series.

Intraoperative Fractures

Intraoperative fracture of the humerus during shoulder arthroplasty is most likely when reaming or inserting the stem, removing a previously placed humeral component, retracting the humerus to facilitate glenoid exposure, and dislocating or reducing the glenohumeral joint. Fracture is best avoided by hand reaming the humeral canal and using an appropriate extensile exposure and soft-tissue releases. The use of cortical windows to facilitate stem extraction is advisable in revision cases. Fractured tuberosities should be addressed by suture repair to both the implant and proximal humerus.[3] Metaphyseal fractures are best treated with autologous bone grafting and cerclage cabling, when appropriate. Diaphyseal fractures require a long-stem implant and cerclage fixation, augmented with cortical strut grafting if necessary. Most long stems will not achieve adequate rotational stability with press fitting, and cement fixation is typically necessary. Plate and screw constructs, although frequently successful in the femur, are less advisable in the humerus, where the cortex is much thinner and less likely to provide adequate fixation of cortical screws.

Postoperative Fractures

In a retrospective review,[2] most fractures occurred as the result of a fall; the remainder resulted from a vari-

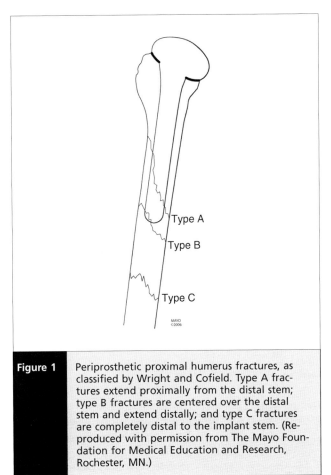

Figure 1 Periprosthetic proximal humerus fractures, as classified by Wright and Cofield. Type A fractures extend proximally from the distal stem; type B fractures are centered over the distal stem and extend distally; and type C fractures are completely distal to the implant stem. (Reproduced with permission from The Mayo Foundation for Medical Education and Research, Rochester, MN.)

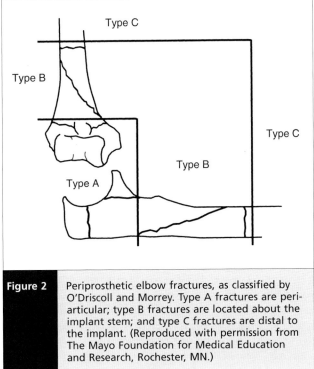

Figure 2 Periprosthetic elbow fractures, as classified by O'Driscoll and Morrey. Type A fractures are periarticular; type B fractures are located about the implant stem; and type C fractures are distal to the implant. (Reproduced with permission from The Mayo Foundation for Medical Education and Research, Rochester, MN.)

ety of other mechanisms, including one fracture that occurred during a shoulder manipulation under anesthesia. Classification is based on fracture location (**Figure 1**), with type A fractures extending proximally from the distal stem, type B fractures centered over the distal stem and extending distally, and type C fractures located completely distal to the implant stem. One third of patients underwent immediate surgical repair and another third healed with nonsurgical treatment. The remaining patients required surgical repair after failure of closed treatment. Treatment recommendations vary somewhat from those for intraoperative fractures.

Surgical repair is recommended for type A fractures in the presence of a loose humeral component, with revision to a cemented long-stem component augmented with iliac crest bone graft. Nonsurgical treatment is considered for type B fractures if the fracture is well aligned and the implant well fixed; however, given the high rate of closed treatment failures, surgical treatment is recommended for fractures that are not united at 3 months. Compression plate–cerclage fixation or allograft cortical strut grafts augmented with autogenous bone graft are recommended. Implant loosening discovered at surgery should be treated by revision to a cemented long-stem component. There are insufficient data to support an adjunctive plate-strut graft fixation

in these revision procedures. Type C fractures with well-fixed stems can be treated nonsurgically if an acceptable alignment is obtained. Failure to unite at 3 months is an indication to proceed with surgical repair.

Periprosthetic Fractures Associated With Elbow Arthroplasty

The available literature on periprosthetic elbow fractures is limited to expert opinion, and even limited case series are lacking. The classification system most often used is that of O'Driscoll and Morrey[4] (**Figure 2**), which is based on their collective experience with 1,000 total elbow arthroplasties. Fracture location, implant fixation, and bone quality are cited as the main factors to guide prognosis and treatment.

Distal Humerus Fractures

Periarticular/condyle fractures (type A) that occur intraoperatively should be treated by suture repair of the common flexor or extensor origin. This treatment is preferable to attempted bone fixation because bone in this area usually is quite osteoporotic and is further compromised by the resection for implant placement. Fractures that are noted postoperatively should be managed without surgery because they typically achieve an asymptomatic fibrous union and rarely result in pain or functional limitations.

Shaft fractures near the tip of the implant (type B) noted during surgery should be immediately repaired with cerclage wiring and possibly with onlay cortical struts or plates. Fractures occurring postoperatively should be repaired if the stem remains well fixed and should be revised to a long-stem prosthesis with bone grafting in the presence of loosening or significant osteolysis. Additional fixation with a plate or strut graft could be considered if fixation was inadequate. Shaft fractures beyond the tip of the stem (type C) should be treated nonsurgically when satisfactory alignment can be obtained.

Proximal Ulna Fractures

Periarticular/olecranon fractures (type A) should be managed nonsurgically unless the fragment is large and significantly displaced. Stable fibrous unions should be anticipated with a good functional outcome in most patients.

Shaft fractures at the tip of the stem (type B) can be managed nonsurgically, if nondisplaced. Otherwise, open reduction and internal fixation with plate and screws should be undertaken. A loose stem or significant osteolysis is an indication for implant revision, possibly augmented with plates or cortical strut grafts.

Shaft fractures beyond the tip of the stem (type C) should be treated with open reduction and internal fixation unless displacement is minimal.

Lower Extremity Periprosthetic Fractures

Periprosthetic fractures of the lower extremity most commonly involve the acetabulum, femur, and proximal tibia. There is substantial published literature on periprosthetic femoral fractures adjacent to both total hip and total knee replacements. There are fewer published studies on periprosthetic acetabular and tibial fractures because these fractures are less common.

Periprosthetic Acetabular Fractures

Periprosthetic acetabular fracture can be challenging to treat. As with other periprosthetic fractures, osteolysis and osteoporosis are common risk factors. Patients will present with persistent groin or pelvic pain. These fractures can occur intraoperatively as a result of over-reaming of the acetabular columns or postoperatively as a result of high- or low-energy trauma.

Evaluation

The initial evaluation should include a patient history to identify (1) when the hip replacement(s) was performed, (2) any history of implant loosening or infection, and (3) how well the hip functioned before the fracture. Groin pain with initial stance, active hip flexion, and the ability to walk only limited distances are signs of possible acetabular implant loosening. If surgery is planned, specific implant information should be obtained. In addition, AP and Judet radiographs should be obtained to determine the integrity of the acetabular columns. In some instances, particularly in patients with severe osteopenia or osteolysis, a CT scan will provide additional information on the location and amount of remaining periacetabular bone. In patients

with severe protrusion or vertical displacement of the acetabulum, skin or skeletal traction can be applied to the limb for comfort and to prevent preoperative muscle contracture.

Treatment

The approach to treating periprosthetic acetabular fractures is the same as for any other periprosthetic fracture: if the implant is stable, leave the implant and treat the fracture. If the implant is loose, then revise the implant and fix the fracture. Periprosthetic acetabular fractures in the setting of a stable implant are usually caused by trauma. As in standard pelvic trauma, surgery is typically only indicated if the pelvis is unstable (for example, vertically unstable iliac fracture) or if the patient is having severe pain that prevents mobilization. If the pelvis is stable (for example, rami fracture), nonsurgical treatment is typically indicated. Periprosthetic acetabular fractures with loose implants may occur either intraoperatively or postoperatively. Intraoperatively, they may result from excessive reaming of the acetabular columns or walls as well as from over-aggressive impaction of the acetabular implant. Postoperative fractures result from either excessive osteolysis or trauma. A loose acetabular implant is usually an indication for surgery.

The basic treatment concept is to restore the integrity of the acetabular columns, with particular focus on the posterior column between the anterosuperior acetabulum and the ischium. If an implant can be wedged between the anterosuperior acetabular rim and the ischium, then a cementless cup with screws can be used. Cementless acetabular implants allow the placement of a larger femoral head; this improves hip stability and avoids cement intrusion into the fracture site, which could delay fracture healing. In patients with a posterior wall fracture or a low anterior wall fracture, this interval is maintained and a cementless acetabular implant can be used. In patients with pelvic discontinuity, this interval is disrupted and its restoration can be accomplished either by plate fixation, acetabular reconstruction ring, or both. In most instances, fixation of the pelvic discontinuity is achieved by plating the posterior column alone. In other situations, insertion of an anterior plate via an ilioinguinal approach is also necessary. This latter approach is indicated when the fracture extends to the iliac wing or when stable reconstruction of the anterosuperior acetabular-ischial segment cannot be restored via a posterior approach alone. Methylmethacrylate can be used to enhance screw purchase because most of these patients have poor bone quality. If stable fixation of the pelvic discontinuity is achieved with plate fixation alone, a cementless implant with screws can be used. After reconstruction of the acetabular columns, bone grafting of residual, contained defects can be done, or trabecular metal augments can be used. If stable fixation of the columns cannot be achieved because of poor bone quality or bone loss, an acetabular reconstruction ring

6: Geriatric and Pediatric Trauma

Table 1

Vancouver Classification of Periprosthetic Femoral Fractures Around Total Hip Implants

Type and Subtype	Location and Characteristics
Type A	
A_G	Greater trochanter
A_L	Lesser trochanter
Type B	
B1	Around stem or stem tip; stem well fixed
B2	Around stem or stem tip; stem loose
B3	Around stem; stem loose; poor proximal bone stock
Type C	Distal to stem

(Reproduced with permission from Springer BD, Berry DJ, Lewallen DG: Treatment of periprosthetic femoral fractures following total hip arthroplasty with femoral component revision. *J Bone Joint Surg Am* 2003;85:2156-2162.)

with or without plate fixation is indicated. If possible, it is preferable to use a hemispherical cup rather than a reconstruction ring because of the head size limitations and impingement issues that can occur with a reconstruction ring.

Postoperative Care

Postoperatively, weight bearing is limited for 6 to 8 weeks to allow for fracture consolidation and implant ongrowth. Radiographs are obtained at 6 weeks and 3 months to confirm the stability of the construct.

Periprosthetic Proximal Femur Fractures

Periprosthetic proximal femur fractures occur in up to 2% of total hip replacements and in 4% of revision surgeries. The most commonly used classification system is the Vancouver classification (**Table 1**), which identifies the location of the fracture and the stability of the implant.[5] This classification system is simple, reliable, and reproducible, and guides treatment.[6] Regardless of the classification system used, the treatment principles applicable to all periprosthetic fractures should be observed: (1) if the implant is stable, treat the fracture; and (2) if the implant is loose, revise the implant and fix the fracture if necessary.

Calcar and Trochanteric Fractures

Intraoperative periprosthetic fractures usually involve the calcar and the greater trochanter. Calcar fractures can occur when broaching or inserting the implant. If identified intraoperatively, a cerclage cable should be placed around the fracture before inserting the implant, especially in cases where proximal fixation is necessary to achieve implant stability. If stable fixation of the fracture cannot be obtained, a stem that achieves stabil-

ity through distal fixation must be used. Fractures of the greater trochanter occur because of excessive lateral pressure on the greater trochanter during retraction, broaching, or implant insertion. Osteolytic lesions or bone defects secondary to previously placed hip screws increase the risk of fracture. If these fractures are identified intraoperatively, they should be fixed with either cerclage wires or cables or with trochanteric claws or plates. Protected weight bearing should be instituted for 6 to 8 weeks. Greater trochanter fractures that occur postoperatively do not always require surgery. Fractures displaced less than 2 cm can be treated successfully with protected weight bearing; in many instances a fibrous union will occur. In fractures with greater displacement, internal fixation is usually indicated because displacement of the hip abductors can lead to hip instability and abductor muscle dysfunction.

Femoral Neck Fractures

Periprosthetic femoral neck fractures are an infrequent complication of hip resurfacing, but if one occurs, femoral revision is necessary. The fracture is typically vertically oriented, resulting in a fracture spike extending distally toward the lesser trochanter. A primary femoral stem may be used at the time of revision surgery, but placement of a cerclage above the lesser trochanter will prevent distal propagation of the fracture during implant insertion.

Treatment

Treatment of periprosthetic femoral fractures around an existing hip replacement depends on the stability of the implant. If the implant is stable (a type B1 fracture), then the implant is retained and the fracture is fixed. Fixation methods depend on both the fracture pattern and the quality of bone. Plates with screws (unicortical or bicortical) or cerclage cables, allograft struts, or a combination can be used.[7-9] In general, bicortical screw fixation is better than unicortical screw fixation (locked or nonlocked) or cerclage cables. Nonlocking screws can often be directed around the implant to achieve this fixation. Locked plating is not advantageous in fractures with good bone stock. Standard nonlocked plating with an anterior allograft strut confers the most stability in type B1 fractures.[10] However, if adequate fixation can be achieved, lateral plating alone may be desirable because of the potential for vascular preservation.[11] The application of allograft struts should be considered when significant osteolytic, deficient cortical bone stock is present.

If the stem is loose (a type B2 fracture), it should be replaced with a cementless, long-stem prosthesis that spans the fracture.[12] The stem is essentially an intramedullary rod that stabilizes the fracture. It may be distally coated or have a fluted stem to achieve distal stability. Placing a cerclage wire around the most proximal aspect of the distal diaphyseal segment before stem insertion will help prevent the development of a longitudinal split in the femur when the femoral com-

Table 2

Lewis and Rorabeck Classification of Periprosthetic Supracondylar Fractures

Type	Characteristics
I	Nondisplaced; prosthesis stable
II	Displaced; prosthesis stable
III	Displaced (IIA) or nondisplaced (IIIB); prosthesis loose or failing

(Adapted from Lewis PL, Rorabeck CH, Angliss RD: Fractures of the femur, tibia, and patella after total knee arthroplasty: Decision making and principles of management. *Instr Course Lect* 1998;47:449-460.)

ponent is inserted. A modular revision prosthesis will help ensure appropriate femoral anteversion and leg lengths in these cases. The construct can be augmented with a lateral plate, allograft strut, or both. In patients with severe proximal femoral bone loss (a type B3 fracture), the use of a proximal femoral replacement or impaction grafting technique is a viable option.[13,14]

In fractures that are distal to a well-fixed hip replacement (a type C fracture), fixation with a lateral plate with unicortical/bicortical screws and proximal cerclage wires if necessary achieves predictable union rates.[15,16] If possible, the use of 90-90 plating and allograft fixation should be avoided because this results in significant soft-tissue and vascular disruption to the fracture site. Allograft fixation alone for the fractures is not indicated. Postoperatively, weight bearing is protected until fracture healing is seen.

Periprosthetic Fractures Above Total Knee Implants

The rate of fractures above total knee arthroplasties is increasing. Patients with knee implants are younger, more active, and are living longer lives. The incidence of these fractures appears to be approximately 2%.[17] This fracture was initially believed to be associated with notching of the femur, but a large 2005 study found no correlation.[18]

Evaluation and Classification

Evaluating a patient with a periprosthetic fracture above a knee implant should include an evaluation of the fracture and an assessment of the whole patient. The patient often has medical comorbidities such as osteoporosis, rheumatoid arthritis, diabetes, and/or cancer. These diseases and their treatments can directly affect fracture healing.

The evaluation includes both AP and lateral radiographs. Oblique views are often necessary to evaluate the size of the distal fragment and loosening. Additional studies are rarely necessary. Careful questioning of the patient regarding preinjury function of the prosthesis helps in determining if the prosthesis was loose before the injury. It is also helpful to identify the exact type of implant, particularly if it is a posterior stabilizing implant with a closed box that would make intramedullary nailing more difficult. Prefracture radiographs are also useful in determining the position of the implants with regard to flexion-extension and varus-valgus alignment of the knee.

Periprosthetic fractures above total knee arthroplasties are most commonly classified by the Lewis and Rorabeck classification[19] (Table 2). There are three fracture types, with the last divided into two subtypes: type I, nondisplaced; type II, displaced; and type III, displaced (IIIA) or nondisplaced (IIIB) with a loose femoral component.

Surgical Indications

Surgical indications depend on the patient's needs and the fracture type. For some patients, surgery is not a safe option because of existing medical conditions. Some patients with severe dementia are poor surgical candidates because of their inability to comply with the postoperative regimen. In patients whose activity level is minimal, nondisplaced fractures can be treated nonsurgically, provided the leg can be controlled with a long leg cast or a brace.

Surgical treatment is indicated for independent and active patients and for most patients with displaced fractures. Surgically treated patients can begin range-of-motion exercises immediately, and they can also be mobilized earlier to avoid the complications associated with bed rest. Displaced fractures generally require surgical fixation to improve limb alignment, ensure proper function, and decrease stress on the implants. Loose implants should be revised using either a long-stem femoral component that stabilizes the fracture or a tumor-type prosthesis.

Technical Considerations

For patients with nondisplaced and stable fractures, the initial treatment can be either a long leg splint or a long knee immobilizer. A long leg cast can be applied when the swelling has subsided. When enough healing has taken place, usually at 4 weeks, the cast can be changed to a hinged cast to allow knee motion. Weight bearing is immediately started at 20 lb. Progressive weight bearing is started at 4 to 6 weeks with the goal of full weight bearing by 8 to 10 weeks. An alternative to casting is the use of a long adjustable hinged knee brace that can be applied early and kept locked straight initially. A gradual increase in motion may be started as soon as it can be tolerated by the patient. Radiographic evaluation at 6 and 12 weeks should show progressive callus formation.

Open reduction and internal fixation allows the surgeon to obtain an accurate reduction and maintain it until the fracture heals. The challenge presented by a periprosthetic fracture above the knee is much the same as that of any supracondylar femoral fracture in a geriatric patient. The surgeon must work with a small and fragile periarticular segment of bone in a patient with

6: Geriatric and Pediatric Trauma

multiple medical comorbidities. In addition, the replacement knee will limit the choice and placement of fixation implants. With posterior stabilized knee implants, positioning the blade into the proper position is usually not possible.

Both nonlocking plates and fixed-angled devices can be used to treat this type of fracture. Nonlocking plates provide multiple points of fixation, but do not resist the varus collapse that is common in comminuted supracondylar femur fractures. Angled blade plates will resist varus collapse, but it can be difficult to achieve adequate fixation when treating fractures that occur around posterior stabilized implants, as well as very distal fractures.[20] Locking periarticular plates offer the advantages of both devices. These implants have multiple points of fixation that lock into the plate, thereby creating a fixed angle. Newer polyaxial locking implants allow screws to be directed into the best bone and then locked to the plate.[21] This is especially useful in periprosthetic fractures, when the femoral component may block placement of conventional fixed-angle locking screws. In addition, most newer locking implants may be placed either percutaneously or with a limited open technique. This minimizes the soft-tissue exposure and stripping around the fracture site.

Surgery is performed with the patient supine on a table that is radiolucent from the hip to the ankle. A small bump is placed under the affected buttock to prevent external rotation of the leg. A sterile tourniquet is applied and used to minimize blood loss, but may need to be removed after reduction and placement of distal screws to allow for placement of proximal screws. A large (10-inch) rolled blanket or radiolucent triangle is placed under the knee to bolster it and facilitate both reduction and exposure. A lateral approach is used and any dissection of the lateralis muscle is done along the posterior intermuscular septum. The periosteum is left intact.

The fracture is reduced with traction and manipulation of the distal fragment to the proximal fragment. The bone is generally osteoporotic, and any reduction clamps must be used judiciously to avoid damaging the distal segment. If necessary, a femoral distractor can be used to gain length by placing one pin in the femoral shaft and another in the tibial shaft, allowing controlled distraction with minimal force on the distal segment. The varus-valgus position can be adjusted by moving the lower leg, and the flexion-extension can be adjusted by moving the bolster under the knee either proximally or distally. If an anatomic reduction is not possible because of severe comminution or impaction, the reduction can be based on the anatomic axis of the knee. The varus-valgus alignment can be determined by using the plane of the distal part of the component, or the surgeon can establish the correct long axis of the entire leg with use of the cautery cord.

In the lateral projection, the anterior aspect of the femoral component should be in line and parallel to the anterior shaft of the femur. In this way the overall axis of the limb is restored.

Once reduction is achieved, provisional fixation may be necessary and can be done with Kirschner wires or a carefully placed pointed reduction forceps. The plate is then applied and its position checked with the image intensifier to verify correct alignment. Verification of correct alignment should be done, especially if the plate is placed percutaneously or submuscularly, because it is important to have the proximal end of the plate centered on the shaft on the lateral view. The plate may need to be moved proximally or distally to allow placement of the distal screws. It may then be applied per the manufacturer's guidelines.

Intramedullary nailing can be used for periprosthetic fractures, provided there is enough bone in the distal segment for placement of interlocking screws.[22,23] It is best to have an open femoral component (cruciate-retaining implant), rather than one with an intramedullary stem. Although some surgeons will cut a hole in the implant to allow for nail placement, this adds an unnecessary level of complexity and risk to the treatment of this fracture.

Intramedullary nailing is done with the patient supine on a table that allows imaging of the entire leg. The position is similar to that for open reduction and internal fixation. A closed technique is generally used and the nail is inserted via an arthrotomy. As with all nailing, the starting point is of utmost importance. In this situation, the presence of the femoral component causes the nail starting point to be more posterior than normal, often resulting in some hyperextension at the fracture site. Reduction techniques are similar to the open reduction and internal fixation techniques. The nail must be inserted deep enough so as not to interfere with the patella, and a minimum of two distal interlocking screws should be used. If there is an option to lock the most distal screw with the end cap device, it should be used.

Revision Arthroplasty

With improvements in plates and the ability to gain purchase in even very small distal fragments, revision arthroplasty is indicated only for loose femoral components or very distal fractures. Even fractures associated with worn polyethylene can be treated with polyethylene exchange and internal fixation. Especially in young patients, every effort should be made to fix the fracture and avoid revision and its associated challenges.

Loose femoral components should be revised. If the patient is physiologically young, revision is done in conjunction with fixation of the fracture to maintain bone stock. Alternatively, in less active patients, the femoral component and the distal bone block can be removed and the knee revised with a distal femoral replacement. This type of constrained prosthesis is not well suited for the young, active patient.

Postoperative Care

With respect to early mobility and functional care, these fractures should be treated in the same manner as any periarticular fracture. If stable fixation is achieved, then early motion is initiated immediately, sometimes even using continuous passive motion. Limited weight bearing is begun, beginning with touchdown weight bearing involving the weight of the lower leg (about 20 lb). At 6 weeks, progressive weight bearing is begun with the goal of full weight bearing by 10 to 12 weeks after surgery. Weight bearing is always limited to that which the patient can tolerate without pain.

Radiographs are obtained at 2, 6, and 10 weeks after surgery. It is often necessary to obtain oblique views to see the anterior and posterior cortex well.

Outcomes

Both open reduction and intramedullary nailing can be used successfully to treat supracondylar femoral fractures.[24,25] However, recent series have shown a lower incidence of malunion with locked plating compared with intramedullary nailing or nonlocked plating, although there are limited numbers in these series.[8,26]

Periprosthetic Fractures Below Total Knee Implants

Fractures of the tibia below total knee implants are unusual and there are no large studies dealing with this fracture or its care. Treatment depends on the fracture pattern and location, the patient's medical and functional status, and the status of the implant. There are no large studies demonstrating the outcomes of these fractures.

Proximal Tibia Fractures

Revision is not necessary for fractures associated with a stable tibial prosthesis. Nondisplaced fractures can be treated with casts or long leg braces, but knee motion should be allowed as quickly as possible to avoid stiffness. Displaced fractures are best treated with internal fixation to restore the correct anatomic axis. This treatment method will allow the limb and the arthroplasty implants to function correctly and last longer. Fixation is limited to plates and screws. Locking periarticular plates offer the benefit of the buttress effect of nonlocking plates, with the added advantage of locking the screws into the plate. Locking the screws into the plate provides better fixation in osteoporotic bone, which is almost always seen in metaphyseal periprosthetic fractures.

The chosen implant can be applied either in a minimally invasive fashion through a separate incision or using the midline incision used for the arthroplasty and extending as necessary. The incision needs to be long enough to see and reduce the fracture. The dissection should be extraperiosteal. The plates should be applied in the buttress mode, meaning that the plate is placed on the side to take advantage of this function: if the fracture is in valgus, then the L-shaped plate is placed laterally to support under the lateral side of the implant. Conversely, if the fracture is in varus, then the medial side must be supported and a T-shaped buttress

plate should be used. The plate should be long enough to support the fracture. It is better to use a longer rather than shorter plate; the distal screws can be placed percutaneously without the need to make a long incision.

If the tibial implant is loose, revision will be necessary. If the fracture is close to the implant, revision with a long tibial stem may address both the loose prosthesis and the fracture. Medial or lateral augments for the tibial baseplate may be necessary if there is metaphyseal fracture comminution or bone loss. If the fracture is distal to the tibial implant, the fracture can be treated to union according to the surgeon's preference, and the tibial revision can be performed at a later date. Alternatively, a revision arthroplasty may be performed in conjunction with plate fixation for the fracture to allow recovery from both conditions simultaneously.

Distal Tibia Fractures

Distal tibia fractures below tibial implants are generally treated with casting or plate fixation. Minimally displaced or nondisplaced fractures can be treated with functional casting. Displaced or severely angulated fractures can be treated with traditional open reduction and internal fixation using either standard plating systems or long distal periarticular plates, depending on the distal extent of the fracture. If the fracture is distal to a long-stem prosthesis, every effort should be made to place bicortical screws around the stem. If this is not possible, then cerclage wire fixation can be used.

Summary

Although upper extremity periprosthetic fractures occur relatively less frequently than those in the lower extremity, both fracture types present similar challenges for the orthopaedic surgeon. Treatment is based on fracture location, implant fixation, and local bone quality. Upper extremity periprosthetic fractures are unlike lower exremity fractures in that successful outcomes may be achieved in certain patients without surgery; however, surgical treatment is usually required in the presenece of a loosened implant or displaced humeral tuberosities. The incidence of periprosthetic fractures will continue to increase as the number of primary total joint replacements increases. The common principle in treating these fractures is to identify whether the implant is loose or stable. If the implant is stable, the component is retained and the fracture is stabilized. If the implant is loose, the implant is revised. Fracture stability is achieved with either the revision implant or accessory plate fixation.

Annotated References

1. Athwal GS, Sperling JW, Rispoli DM, Cofield RH: Periprosthetic humeral fractures during shoulder arthro-

plasty. *J Bone Joint Surg Am* 2009;91(3):594-603.

A case series of 45 intraoperative humeral fractures from the Mayo Clinic (1980-2002) is presented with analysis of risk factors and minimum 2-year follow-up. Level of evidence: IV.

2. Kumar S, Sperling JW, Haidukewych GH, Cofield RH: Periprosthetic humeral fractures after shoulder arthroplasty. *J Bone Joint Surg Am* 2004;86(4):680-689.

This case series of 16 patients with periprosthetic humeral fractures summarizes a 25-year experience at the Mayo Clinic. Treatment recommendations are included. Level of evidence: IV.

3. Campbell JT, Moore RS, Iannotti JP, Norris TR, Williams GR: Periprosthetic humeral fractures: Mechanisms of fracture and treatment options. *J Shoulder Elbow Surg* 1998;7(4):406-413.

4. O'Driscoll SW, Morrey BF: Periprosthetic fractures about the elbow. *Orthop Clin North Am* 1999;30(2):319-325.

5. Duncan CP, Masri BA: Fractures of the femur after hip replacement. *Instr Course Lect* 1995;44:293-304.

6. Rayan F, Dodd M, Haddad FS: European validation of the Vancouver classification of periprosthetic proximal femoral fractures. *J Bone Joint Surg Br* 2008;90(12):1576-1579.

Consultants, trainees, and medical students reviewed 30 cases on two separate occasions. Interobserver agreement was 0.72 and 0.74 for consultants, 0.68 and 0.70 for trainees, and 0.61 for medical students, confirming the reliability and reproducibility of the Vancouver classification system.

7. Bryant GK, Morshed S, Agel J, et al: Isolated locked compression plating for Vancouver Type B1 periprosthetic femoral fractures. *Injury* 2009;40(11):1180-1186.

Ten patients with type B1 periprosthetic femur fractures were treated with locked lateral plating. All fractures healed at an average of 17 weeks, and there were no hardware failures or changes in fracture alignment.

8. Kobbe P, Klemm R, Reilmann H, Hockertz TJ: Less invasive stabilisation system (LISS) for the treatment of periprosthetic femoral fractures: A 3-year follow-up. *Injury* 2008;39(4):472-479.

Sixteen patients with Vancouver types B and C fractures were treated with a locked lateral plate. Proximal screw pullout occurred in two patients.

9. Ebraheim NA, Gomez C, Ramineni SK, Liu J: Fixation of periprosthetic femoral shaft fractures adjacent to a well-fixed femoral stem with reversed distal femoral locking plate. *J Trauma* 2009;66(4):1152-1157.

Vancouver type B1 periprosthetic femoral fractures were stabilized with a reversed distal femoral locking plate in 13 consecutive patients. All fractures healed at an average of 14 weeks after fixation. There were no hardware failures or nonunions.

10. Zdero R, Walker R, Waddell JP, Schemitsch EH: Biomechanical evaluation of periprosthetic femoral fracture fixation. *J Bone Joint Surg Am* 2008;90(5):1068-1077.

This biomechanical study using synthetic bones and cables with allograft struts found that a combination of a lateral nonlocking plate augmented with an anterior allograft strut resulted in the highest stiffness in Vancouver type C fractures.

11. Ricci WM, Bolhofner BR, Loftus T, Cox C, Mitchell S, Borrelli J Jr: Indirect reduction and plate fixation, without grafting, for periprosthetic femoral shaft fractures about a stable intramedullary implant: Surgical Technique. *J Bone Joint Surg Am* 2006;88(suppl 1, pt 2):275-282.

Forty-one patients with a Vancouver type B1 fracture were treated with open reduction and internal fixation using a single lateral plate without structural allografting or other bone grafting. All fractures healed and 31 patients returned to their preinjury ambulatory status.

12. O'Shea K, Quinlan JF, Kutty S, Mulcahy D, Brady OH: The use of uncemented extensively porous-coated femoral components in the management of Vancouver B2 and B3 periprosthetic femoral fractures. *J Bone Joint Surg Br* 2005;87(12):1617-1621.

Twenty-two type B2 and type B3 fractures were treated with an extensively coated revision femoral component. At 33 months, 19 were stable, 2 were loose, and 1 was revised for deep infection.

13. Klein GR, Parvizi J, Rapuri V, et al: Proximal femoral replacement for the treatment of periprosthetic fractures. *J Bone Joint Surg Am* 2005;87(8):1777-1781.

Twenty-one patients with a Vancouver type B3 fracture were treated with a cemented proximal femoral replacement. At a mean of 3.2 years, 20 patients could walk with minimal or no pain. Complications included two dislocations, one femoral fracture, and two infections.

14. Tsiridis E, Narvani AA, Haddad FS, Timperley JA, Gie GA: Impaction femoral allografting and cemented revision for periprosthetic femoral fractures. *J Bone Joint Surg Br* 2004;86(8):1124-1132.

A retrospective review of 106 patients with periprosthetic femoral fractures showed that fractures treated with impaction grafting and long stems were more than five times more likely to unite than those treated by impaction grafting and a short stem.

15. Ricci WM, Borrelli J Jr: Operative management of periprosthetic femur fractures in the elderly using biological fracture reduction and fixation techniques. *Injury* 2007;38(Suppl 3):S53-S58.

Fifty-nine patients (average age, 74 years) with either a fracture of the periprosthetic femoral shaft about an arthroplasty stem or a supracondylar fracture above a total knee arthroplasty were treated with biologic open reduction and internal fixation techniques, but no bone grafts or bone graft substitutes. Forty-nine of 59 patients returned to their baseline level of function, suggesting that adjuvant bone graft may not be routinely necessary in these cases.

16. Chakravarthy J, Bansal R, Cooper J: Locking plate osteosynthesis for Vancouver Type B1 and Type C periprosthetic fractures of femur: A report on 12 patients. *Injury* 2007;38(6):725-733.

    Eleven patients with Vancouver type B1 or type C fractures were treated with a lateral locking plate. Ten fractures healed.

17. Berry DJ: Epidemiology: Hip and knee. *Orthop Clin North Am* 1999;30(2):183-190.

18. Ritter MA, Thong AE, Keating EM, et al: The effect of femoral notching during total knee arthroplasty on the prevalence of postoperative femoral fractures and on clinical outcome. *J Bone Joint Surg Am* 2005;87(11):2411-2414.

    Femoral notching occurred in 29.8% of consecutive total knee replacements (325 of 1,089). At 5.1 years, only two supracondylar fractures occurred, both in total knee replacement without femoral notching.

19. Rorabeck CH, Angliss RD, Lewis PL: Fractures of the femur, tibia, and patella after total knee arthroplasty: Decision making and principles of management. *Instr Course Lect* 1998;47:449-458.

20. Healy WL, Siliski JM, Incavo SJ: Operative treatment of distal femoral fractures proximal to total knee replacements. *J Bone Joint Surg Am* 1993;75(1):27-34.

21. Wilkens KJ, Curtiss S, Lee MA: Polyaxial locking plate fixation in distal femur fractures: A biomechanical comparison. *J Orthop Trauma* 2008;22(9):624-628.

    A polyaxial distal femoral locking plate had greater stiffness when compared with a uniaxial locking plate in a biomechanical testing model. The clinical significance of these data are not known.

22. McLaren AC, Dupont JA, Schroeber DC: Open reduction internal fixation of supracondylar fractures above total knee arthroplasties using the intramedullary supracondylar rod. *Clin Orthop Relat Res* 1994;302:194-198.

23. Jabczenski FF, Crawford M: Retrograde intramedullary nailing of supracondylar femur fractures above total knee arthroplasty: A preliminary report of four cases. *J Arthroplasty* 1995;10(1):95-101.

24. Haidukewych GJ: Periprosthetic distal femur fracture: Plate versus nail fixation. *J Orthop Trauma* 2007;21(3):219-220.

    In this opinion article, the author argues for the superiority of percutaneously applied locked plates over nail fixation for treating periprosthetic distal femoral fractures.

25. Gliatis J: Periprosthetic distal femur fracture: Plate versus nail fixation. *J Orthop Trauma* 2007;21(3):220-221.

    In this opinion article, the author argues for the superiority of nail fixation over percutaneously applied locked plates for treating periprosthetic distal femoral fractures.

26. Large TM, Kellam JF, Bosse MJ, et al: Locked plating of supracondylar periprosthetic femur fractures. *J Arthroplasty* 2008;23(6, suppl 1):115-120.

    Twenty-five patients were treated with a locked distal femoral plate and 19 with a nonlocked distal femoral plate or intramedullary nail. There were significantly fewer nonunions and malunions in the locked-plate group.

Chapter 44

Problematic Pediatric Fractures

David S. Weisman, MD   Steven L. Frick, MD

Pediatric Trauma: General Considerations

Trauma is the leading cause of death and disability in childhood. Infants and children have important physiologic, biomechanical and psychologic differences from adults that should be considered by clinicians caring for injured youth (Table 1).

Pelvic Fractures

Several classifications of pediatric pelvic fractures exist; the most commonly used for the pelvic ring is that of Torode and Zeig, who classified pediatric pelvic fractures into four groups: avulsion fracture, iliac wing fracture, stable pelvic ring fracture, and unstable pelvic ring disruption. Watts classified pediatric acetabular fractures into small fragments associated with a dislocation; nondisplaced fractures associated with stable pelvic fractures; unstable intra-articular fractures; and central fracture-dislocations. The differing fracture patterns are due in large part to the open triradiate cartilage and the plasticity of the bone in children. More commonly the Letournel system is used when describing the fracture patterns.

Avulsion fractures of the pelvis can occur at the anterior-superior iliac spine (sartorius), anterior-inferior iliac spine (rectus femoris, direct head), ischial tuberosity (hamstring), and iliac crest (external oblique). The lesser trochanter can be avulsed by the iliopsoas. All require protected weight bearing during healing. A full return of function can be expected by 6 weeks.

Fractures of the iliac wing and simple ring fractures and most bony ring disruptions (bilateral rami, straddle fractures) are treated nonsurgically because most are mechanically stable with excellent healing potential. Pe-

Dr. Frick or an immediate family member serves as a board member, owner, officer, or committee member of the American Orthopaedic Association, J. Robert Gladden Society, Pediatric Orthopaedic Society of North America, and American Academy of Orthopaedic Surgeons; and has received research or institutional support from Biomet. Neither Dr. Weisman nor an immediate family member has received anything of value from or owns stock in a commercial company or institution related directly or indirectly to the subject of this chapter.

diatric acetabular fracture treatment follows the same principles as in the adult. According to a recent study, surgical treatment of unstable pediatric pelvic and acetabular fractures demonstrated improved results compared to those of historical control subjects.[1] The displaced acetabular fracture needs to be reduced to maintain joint congruity. Nondisplaced fractures can be treated with no weight bearing in the cooperative patient or a spica cast in the younger child. Injuries to the triradiate cartilage before closure have the added risk of growth arrest producing delayed joint incongruity and dysplasia. In a 2005 study, the authors demonstrated that malreduced unstable pelvic fractures at the time of healing have minimal ability to remodel and will result in pelvic asymmetry.[2] They found that pelvic asymmetry greater than 1 cm increased the risk of a worse functional and clinical outcome.

Hip dislocations are surgical emergencies requiring reduction as soon as possible to limit the risk of osteonecrosis. General anesthesia with paralysis and fluoroscopic visualization should be used to avoid possible fracture of the capital femoral epiphysis during reduction. A post-reduction pelvic radiograph is required to assess the congruity of the reduction. When there is a lack of concentricity, a CT scan helps assess for incarcerated fracture fragments. An MRI may be necessary to assess purely cartilaginous fragments. Most isolated dislocations are stable after reduction and require ambulation without weight bearing for the cooperative patient and spica casting for the young or noncompliant patient.

Femoral Neck Fractures

Fractures of the proximal femur have been classified into four groups: type 1, transepiphyseal (A-without dislocation of the proximal fragment, B-with dislocation of the proximal fragment); type 2, transcervical; type 3, cervicotrochanteric; and type 4, intertrochanteric. These are typically high-energy injuries that require rapid treatment with anatomic realignment to minimize the complications of osteonecrosis, growth arrest, malunion, and nonunion.

An immediate reduction of the fracture is strongly recommended. According to a recent study, the quality and timing of the reduction influence the risk of osteonecrosis.[3] Nondisplaced fractures in children younger than 2 years may be treated with spica casting;

Table 1

Important Pediatric Differences for Trauma Management

Characteristic Difference From Adults	Relevance in Trauma Care
Infants are obligatory nasal breathers	Clear nasal and oral pharynx for airway
Large head:body ratio	Predisposes to upper cervical spine injury Large occiput will flex neck when supine; cervical spine at risk and airway access difficult Scalp laceration bleeding may be significant
Total blood volume smaller (80 mL/kg)	Small-volume blood loss proportionately higher
Large surface area to body volume	Higher risk of hypothermia
Pliable rib cage, higher costal margin, smaller and lower pelvis	Less protection to underlying internal organs. Can have severe injury without fractures
Increased physiologic reserve / higher baseline metabolic rate	Hemodynamic response to trauma may be minimal; hypotension is a late sign of shock in children
Rapid intravenous access often difficult	Consider intraosseous infusion
Communication barriers: age/maturity	Remember possible nonaccidental trauma as a cause of injuries; injury identification and pain management more difficult; psychological effects of trauma (may need counseling).

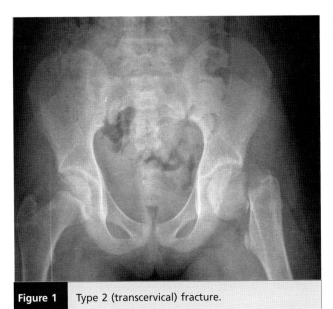

Figure 1   Type 2 (transcervical) fracture.

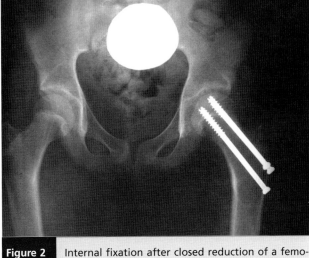

Figure 2   Internal fixation after closed reduction of a femoral neck fracture.

close follow-up is necessary to watch for late displacement. If rigid fixation is required for proximal fractures the growth plate may be crossed. The child older than 2 years should undergo internal fixation to maintain the reduction of the femoral neck regardless of displacement (**Figures 1** and **2**).

The most common complication of a proximal femoral fracture is osteonecrosis. This risk diminishes as the fracture location becomes more distal. The following rates of osteonecrosis have been reported according to type of fracture: type 1, 38%, type 2, 28%, type 3, 18%, and type 4, 5%, with an overall rate of 21%.[4] Coxa vara as a result of malunion is the second most common complication. Premature physeal closure may

ensue and in the younger patient can cause coxa valga or less commonly coxa vara as well as a limb-length discrepancy Nonunion is more common in malreduced fractures or those treated without internal fixation.

The role of capsular decompression in minimizing osteonecrosis risk has not been established. No relationship between capsular decompression and osteonecrosis has been established.[3] According to one study, fracture type and age were the only significant predictors of osteonecrosis.[4]

Femoral Shaft Fractures

Several factors must be considered during the decision-making process for the treatment of a pediatric femoral shaft fracture, the most important of which are patient age, location of the fracture, fracture pattern, and associated injuries. Another important factor may be the weight of the patient. Nonsurgical treatment using spica casting remains the primary treatment of the child younger than 5 years. In children in this age group, femur fractures are typically well maintained in the cast with a greater degree of acceptable deformity. The cast can be either a single-leg or a one and one-half spica cast to control rotation. The exception would be the case of a distal femoral buckle fracture, which is inherently stable and simply requires a long leg cast.

Surgical fixation has been increasingly advocated for femur fractures in children older than 5 years, when the fracture patterns become less stable and the remodeling potential is diminished. This transition is supported by reports of low morbidity and improved social outcomes following surgical compared to nonsurgical management in this age group.

External fixation remains an option for the treatment of femoral fractures, but when used as a definitive treatment, the complication rates remain high in comparison with other techniques. External fixation and intramedullary nails (rigid and flexible) in open femur fractures were compared in patients with an average age of 15 years in a recent study.[5] Complications were five times more likely in the external fixation group (2.7 times if pin tract infections are excluded). Refracture, associated with varus malunion, only occurred in the external fixation group. Thus, external fixation has fallen out of favor for treating pediatric femur fractures. Perhaps its best use is in an unstable patient before definitive treatment.

Flexible nailing with either titanium or stainless steel implants from supracondylar entry points proximal to the growth plate is used for diaphyseal fractures with length-stable fracture patterns.[6] The stainless steel nail may provide more rigidity in fixation but also may increase the risk of fracture comminution during nail passage. A proximal entry point may also be used with c-shaped and s-shaped nails. The need for a cast following flexible nailing is dependent on the stability of the fixation, although it is not typically required. In a recent study of 94 fractures, the complication rate was 17%, and complications were more likely in patients older than 10 years.[7] Complications related to the insertion site are most common. In this series there was one nonunion, one refracture, and one case of limb-length discrepancy requiring epiphysiodesis. In a comparison of titanium and stainless steel flexible intramedullary nails, malunion rates were higher in the titanium group.[8] The authors found that risk of malunion did not correlate with age, weight, fracture stability (comminution), or nail diameter. Using the authors' nail sizing recommendations, if the nail needs to be undersized based on patient requirements, a more rigid nail (for example, stainless steel) may be superior. The more rigid nail does increase the risk of comminution of the fracture site as it passes through. In a situation where the fracture site does not stabilize with the

flexible nails alone, short-term adjuvant buttressing, such as a spica cast or external fixator, may be necessary.

Femoral fracture plating has been advocated in subtrochanteric fractures as well as distal diaphyseal or metadiaphyseal fractures, especially those within 5 cm of the flexible nail insertion site. Both of these fracture patterns are outside of the diaphysis and, therefore, are more difficult to control with flexible nails. High-grade comminution (greater than 50%) can interfere with stability with the flexible nails. Submuscular plating has become a common method of treating these fractures. In a recent review of 32 patients (average age, 11 years) with locking plate fixation, the most common indication for plating was comminution followed by nonmalignant pathologic fractures, extradiaphyseal fractures, and osteopenia.[9] One patient healed in radiographic valgus of no clinical significance. Seven of 32 patients underwent plate removal.

Rigid antegrade nailing as the child reaches skeletal maturity is another treatment option. A lateral trochanteric approach may mitigate the risk of osteonecrosis of the femoral head associated with a piriformis nail entry point. Associated injuries from high-energy trauma often mandate more aggressive surgical management of pediatric femur fractures. In a systematic review of 2,422 pediatric femoral cases of all types and using evidence-based results,[10] the authors concluded that the available literature supports the following statements: (1) early spica casting leads to fewer adverse events and fewer hospital days than traction and later casting, (2) external fixation results in a lower malunion rate than spica casting, (3) flexible intramedullary nail treatment results in a lower malunion rate than traction and casting or external fixation, and (4) surgical treatment results in fewer adverse events and lower malunion rates.

Tibial Spine Fractures

The treatment of tibial spine (intercondylar eminence) fractures is based on the amount of displacement and the ability to reduce the fragment back into its bed. A good relative indication of an adequate reduction is the ability to fully extend the knee, with an inability to achieve extension indicative of a block to reduction. Reduction attempts may be aided by aspiration and administration of a local anesthetic.

Tibial spine avulsions have been classified into three types: type 1, nondisplaced; type 2, posterior hinged; and type 3, complete displacement. The reduction maneuver consists of extending the knee to at least 20° short of full extension. In addition to a bony block to reduction, entrapped meniscus or intermeniscal ligament may also be present. It is also important to consider that throughout all ranges of knee motion, tension is placed on the fracture fragment by some fibers of the anterior cruciate ligament, further contributing to the inability to obtain a reduction. Closed reduction is more commonly successful in types 1 and 2, less so in

6: Geriatric and Pediatric Trauma

type 3. Failure of the fragment to reduce or a block to extension necessitates either open or arthroscopic management. Complications include knee laxity, arthrofibrosis, nonunion, and growth disturbances.

In a 2009 study, 43 patients were treated with aspiration (91%) and extension casting.[11] Only one patient with a type 3 lesion developed delayed union that required surgery. No cases of meniscal entrapment were noted.

Tibial Tubercle Fractures

The treatment of displaced tibial tubercle fractures typically requires surgical fixation to control the force of the extensor mechanism on the fragment. Watson-Jones classified the fracture into three types: type 1, transverse through the apophysis; type 2, in the area between the apophysis and the proximal tibial epiphysis (between the primary and secondary ossification centers of the proximal tibia); and type 3, coronal fracture through the epiphysis. Two additional types have been described: type 4, coronal then transverse through the proximal tibial epiphysis, and type 5, sleeve fracture avulsion from the anterior surface of the tubercle.

One must be aware of the possibility of a coexistent vascular injury in a patient with a proximal tibial physeal fracture. The vascular injury likely results from direct trauma to the popliteal artery as it passes over the displaced distal metaphyseal fragment. A compartment syndrome can be associated with a displaced proximal tibial physeal fracture.

Tibial tubercle screw fixation is acceptable in the older child whose apophysis does not significantly contribute to growth. If the child is more than 3 years from skeletal maturity, smooth pins would be the fixation of choice with a significant risk of recurvatum as the most common growth disturbance. One study found that in type 3 displaced fractures, closed reduction and internal fixation provided a satisfactory result;[12] closed reduction should be attempted before proceeding to an open reduction.

Proximal Tibial Metaphyseal Fractures

Proximal tibial metaphyseal fractures are more common in the younger age groups (3 to 6 years old) and result most commonly from a valgus force at the knee that creates an incomplete fracture of the proximal tibia. Less commonly the fracture is complete or involves the fibula. The injury commonly occurs when a child goes down a slide in an adult lap with the leg extended.

The most common complication associated with a proximal tibial metaphyseal fracture is tibia valgum. The etiology has been ascribed to many factors, including incomplete reduction, concomitant injury to the proximal tibial physis, infolded periosteum, and injury to the insertion of the pes anserine with the subsequent loss of a proximal tibial physeal tether leading to asymmetric physeal growth. Treatment of proximal tibial fractures mandates an anatomic reduction or slight varus overcorrection. If an anatomic reduction cannot be obtained, an open reduction is recommended to remove the interposed tissue. It is also important to place the extremity in a cast in nearly full extension with a varus mold. The extension in the cast makes it simpler to obtain true AP radiographs of the entire tibia to assess maintenance of reduction.

Should a valgus deformity occur, observation until spontaneous recovery is achieved is recommended. Osteotomies are associated with significant complications, including compartment syndromes and recurrence. A less invasive treatment option would be transient hemi-epiphysiodesis (with a staple or plate) to gradually guide remodeling.

Distal Tibial Physeal Fractures

Fractures of the distal tibia can occur as a result of multiple mechanisms: supination-inversion, supination–plantar flexion, supination-external rotation, or pronation–eversion–external rotation creating Salter-Harris type I and II fracture patterns. Most Salter-Harris type III and IV fractures, with the exception of Tillaux and triplane fractures, require supination-inversion to occur. Variables such as degree of physeal closure at the time of injury also affect fracture patterns.

Treatment consists of cast immobilization for healing of the nondisplaced fractures. One study found that for displaced fractures, a residual physeal gap greater than 3 mm is unacceptable because the risk of premature physeal closure increases dramatically.[13] In addition, the number of closed reduction attempts should be limited (maximum of two attempts) in all children. Closed reduction of the extra-articular (physeal-metaphyseal) component of the fracture in the younger patient who has the ability to remodel is unnecessary, and in the older patient runs the risk of further physeal injury. It is not clear if removing interposed periosteum is necessary to avoid a growth arrest or prevent a permanent angular deformity. A 2009 study found that of the three main factors that potentially contribute to early physeal closure, number of reductions, residual gap, and initial displacement, the latter correlated highest with early physeal closure.[14] The number of reductions also has an effect but not to the same degree. The literature in this area is conflicted, and with small numbers of patients in these studies, assessing causation with multiple variables is prone to error. It is likely that all of these variables will have an influence on premature physeal closure. These findings likely indicate the true etiology is multifactorial.

Salter-Harris type III and IV fractures are intra-articular and share the basic tenets that apply to all intra-articular fractures. Inadequate reduction creates articular incongruity that can lead to posttraumatic arthritis. Salter-Harris type IV fractures of the medial malleolus require anatomic restoration of the physis to lessen the risk of a peripheral growth arrest during fracture healing. Nondisplaced fractures should be treated in a long leg cast for the rotational injuries.

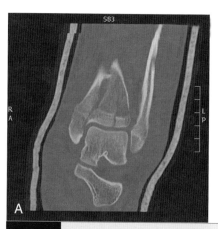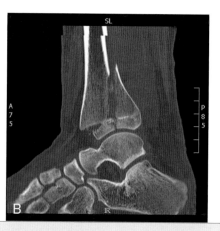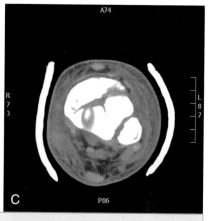

Figure 3 | A through C, Imaging studies showing a four-part triplane fracture.

Following reduction of displaced fractures, a CT scan may be necessary to assess residual intra-articular gap. Screw fixation is the most common method of surgical treatment. When an immature physis is involved, transepiphyseal fixation is used. In the older child (with less than 2 years of growth remaining), transphyseal fixation may be used.

Transitional Fractures of the Distal Tibia
Triplane Fractures/Tillaux Fractures
Transitional fractures (juvenile Tillaux and triplane) occur in the distal tibial physis as it begins to close. The variability in the fracture patterns occurs as a result of the progression of physeal closure. The order of physeal closure of the distal tibial physis is central-posterior-medial-lateral. The mechanism of injury is external rotation except for the medial triplane, which is likely adduction.

The triplane fracture pattern occurs in three planes: sagittal through the epiphysis, transverse through the physis, and coronal through the metaphysis. The fracture is most commonly in two, three, or four parts (**Figure 3**), and the fracture is described as lateral (most common) or medial triplane. An intramalleolar triplane variant has been described where the epiphyseal fracture exits through the medial malleolus. The variance of the fracture patterns is caused by the extent of physeal closure at the time of injury.

The juvenile Tillaux fracture is an avulsion injury of the anterolateral corner of the epiphysis at the insertion of the anteroinferior tibiofibular ligament. This fracture pattern is more common in children nearing the end of growth relative to the triplane fracture, as the anterior lateral corner is the last to fuse.

Treatment is based on the degree of intra-articular displacement. A fracture with greater than 2 mm of articular displacement requires closed or open reduction. A closed reduction is attempted by internally rotating the foot/ankle for Tillaux and lateral triplane fractures and everting the foot for medial triplane fracture. A long leg cast is used because of the rotational nature of the injury. If the fracture gap cannot be closed down to 2 mm or less as typically confirmed on postreduction CT scan, open reduction is indicated. Given that these transitional fractures occur as patients approach skeletal maturity, a transphyseal screw may be used. Uniformly good results were reported in a study of 10 juvenile Tillaux fractures surgically treated and followed long term.[15]

Upper Extremity Fractures

Most pediatric upper extremity fractures are easily treated with nonsurgical methods, with predictable bone union and rapid return to full function. Some of these injuries can be problematic, either because of difficulties in diagnosis or treatment or because surgeons unfamiliar with the healing and recovery potential of skeletally immature patients may believe more aggressive surgical intervention is needed.

Injuries to the Sternoclavicular Joint and Medial Clavicle
The sternoclavicular joint is the connection of the upper extremity to the axial skeleton and as such is susceptible to injury by direct blow or by lateral force applied to the clavicle, acromion, or shoulder. The medial clavicle ossification center appears in the later teenage years, and the physis is the last to close, between the ages of 20 and 25 years. As a result, in teenagers and young adults injuries in the sternoclavicular region are often physeal injuries that mimic dislocations. The main treatment difficulty with injuries in this region is delay in diagnosis, as physical examination and plain radiography are often unreliable in assessing presence of fracture and degree of displacement. Axial CT is recommended in patients with pain and swelling near the sternoclavicular joint to assess for dislocations and physeal injuries and to clarify the direction and magnitude of displacement. Injuries with anterior instability are usually treated nonsurgically, as the functional re-

6: Geriatric and Pediatric Trauma

sults of nonoperative treatment are good. Posteriorly displaced fractures or dislocations can cause injury or compression to the great vessels, trachea, and esophagus, and are usually treated with closed or open reduction to restore anatomic alignment. Because of the structures at risk posterior to the sternum, the lack of data on long-term outcomes of nonsurgically treated patients, the small numbers of patients with these injuries, and the historical recommedations to treat posteriorly displaced sternoclavicular joint injuries with reduction, most surgeons recommend reduction of posteriorly displaced injuries, even in asymptomatic patients. Studies have indicated that medial physeal injuries have remodeling potential and can be treated nonsurgically, but others[16,17] have noted a high frequency of persistent instability after reduction and recommend open reduction and stabilization with suture or wires. Pin fixation in this region is contraindicated because of the risk of pin migration and injury to vital structures. Most authors recommend that a vascular or cardiothoracic surgeon be notified and available at the time of reduction because of the potential for catastrophic hemorrhage at the time of reduction.

For posteriorly displaced dislocations or fractures diagnosed early, closed reduction can usually be accomplished easily, with a bump placed under the ipsilateral scapula toward the midline, with traction on the arm in abduction and extension. Sometimes grasping the midclavicle using fingers or a clamp is needed to pull it anteriorly. If the reduction is believed to be stable, CT should be repeated to document maintenance of reduction. If the reduction is unstable, open reduction with stabilization using suture or wire from the medial clavicle to the sternum or medial epiphysis is recommended. Open reduction is recommended with circumferential subperiosteal dissection around the clavicle beginning at the junction of the medial and middle thirds and progressing medially until the most medial aspect is seen; a clamp can then be used to grasp the clavicle and carefully pull it anteriorly to reduce it.[16,17] After surgery, patients are protected in a sling and swathe for 4 weeks. For injuries treated after a few weeks, attempted closed reduction is not recommended because the medial clavicle may be adherent to vascular structures in the mediastinum.

Proximal Humerus Fractures

Because of the growth and remodeling potential of the proximal humeral physis (contributes 80% of humeral length) and the range of motion of the shoulder joint, most proximal humerus fractures in children and adolescents can be treated nonsurgically with excellent functional results. The problematic fracture is the severely displaced proximal humerus fracture in the patient approaching skeletal maturity. These are typically Salter-Harris type II fracture patterns, with anterior displacement of the distal shaft fragment through the thinner anterior periosteal sleeve. With severe displacement, the concern is that remodeling potential will be

inadequate in patients with only a few years of growth remaining to correct angular deformity that would limit forward elevation and abduction. Despite this concern, most studies report excellent functional outcomes with no advantage of surgical over nonsurgical management, even in patients older than 15 years, approaching skeletal maturity. One study showed that after closed reduction attempts did not improve the position of the fracture, there was no justification for surgical reduction based on the long-term results of older patients in their series.[18] Complications of surgical treatment reported in early studies led some to condemn surgical management for these injuries, but more recent studies demonstrate that surgical reduction and stabilization can be done safely and effectively in adolescents with severely displaced proximal humerus fractures.[19] The Neer-Horowitz classification is used most commonly: grade I – minimally displaced, grade II – one-third width of shaft displaced, grade III – less than two-thirds width of shaft displaced, and grade IV – more than two-thirds width of shaft displaced. The classification can be useful in determining the adequacy of reduction, with a goal for older adolescents being fracture healing in a position with grade II or less displacement.

In adolescents within 2 years of skeletal maturity, fractures with greater than grade II displacement or more than 45° of angulation should undergo closed reduction using adequate analgesia and/or anesthesia, often in the emergency department. Fluoroscopy is very helpful to assess the fracture position and reduction, and the reduction maneuver typically involves flexion, abduction, and external rotation of the arm to realign the distal fragment with the humeral head. Impacting or axially loading the fracture as the arm is brought to the side may help maintain the reduction and allow immobilization in a safe comfortable position in a sling and swathe. If an acceptable reduction is achieved, repeat radiographs should be taken within a few days to document maintenance of acceptable position. If the fracture cannot be reduced to an acceptable position, or if it is unstable and easily displaces after reduction, then a decision about the risks and benefits of surgical intervention should take place. Factors to consider include the age and physiologic maturity of the patient, direction and magnitude of displacement of the fracture, activity level of the patient, and any associated injuries or health problems.

If surgical treatment is chosen, repeat closed reduction is attempted under fluoroscopy. If acceptable position is obtained, the fracture is stabilized with either percutaneous wires or screws. Because of the risks of pin migration around the shoulder girdle, many surgeons use terminally threaded pins and often leave the pins outside the skin with a large bend. Some surgeons bury the pins under the skin in an attempt to lower the incidence of skin problems; the benefits of one approach over the other have not been demonstrated. If an acceptable reduction cannot be obtained, there may be soft-tissue interposition blocking the reduction (biceps tendon or infolded periosteum), and open reduction using a deltopectoral approach is recommended.[19]

Nerve and vascular injuries are uncommonly seen in association with proximal humerus fractures. One series noted associated nerve injuries in only 0.4% of proximal humerus fractures,[20] and all were seen in fractures with valgus displacement (shaft is medial). The four reported nerve deficits resolved by 9 months without treatment. There are no reports of iatrogenic nerve injuries with percutaneous pinning of the proximal humerus, but the axillary nerve is near the common pin locations.

Supracondylar Humerus Fractures

Extension-type supracondylar humerus fractures are the most common childhood elbow fracture. Malunion is common after cast treatment of displaced supracondylar humerus fractures, but malunion rates are now very low with the widespread acceptance of reduction and pin stabilization for displaced fractures. A problematic fracture if not recognized is the Gartland type II fracture (incomplete fracture with posterior angulation) that also has associated collapse or buckling of the medial column.[21] Recognition of this fracture pattern and reduction of the varus in the coronal plane is important to prevent the classic gunstock deformity. Assessing the Baumann angle on injury films and postreduction radiographs can minimize the risk of varus malunion. Comparison radiographs are not usually necessary, unless the patient's uninjured elbow has abnormal alignment.

Traditionally viewed as surgical emergencies, several studies and the experiences of many pediatric trauma centers have demonstrated that closed supracondylar humerus fractures without vascular compromise, severe soft-tissue swelling, or pressure on skin can be managed as surgical "urgencies."[22,23] Many centers have developed protocols where the fracture is splinted in 30° to 40° of elbow flexion and admitted for observation, with closed reduction and pinning performed when the patient has an empty stomach and an expert surgical team is available. Concerns regarding "waiting for the expert" are that swelling may lead to vascular compromise or compartment syndrome or result in greater difficulty in achieving an acceptable closed reduction. The difficulty in assessing the latter argument is that the decision of when to convert from closed to open reduction is highly subjective and not amenable to retrospective analysis. "Next day" treatment has not been found to lead to greater difficulty in obtaining an acceptable reduction. Regarding the risk of compartment syndrome, 11 patients with low-energy fractures developed compartment syndrome after presenting with no signs of vascular compromise.[24] The average time from injury to surgical reduction was 22 hours. As nonemergent treatment of these fractures is slowly becoming more common, the authors recommend early surgical treatment of patients with any of these "red-flag" warning signs: severe elbow swelling, ecchymosis, dimpling or puckered skin, neurologic deficit, and/or a diminished or absent radial pulse. Patients with an ipsilateral forearm or wrist fracture have also been recognized as being at higher risk for the development of compartment syndrome[25] and should be carefully monitored.

Ecchymosis in the anterior distal arm, soft-tissue puckering or skin dimpling, and a palpable subcutaneous proximal fragment constitute components of the brachialis sign, indicating that the proximal fragment has buttonholed through the brachialis muscle. This indicates a more serious injury, with a higher likelihood of arterial injury, skin necrosis, significant swelling, and a more difficult closed reduction. The milking maneuver has been described to reduce the proximal fragment back into the brachialis muscle and allow a closed reduction and is an important technique to master for surgeons caring for these fractures.[26]

The pinning techniques for supracondylar fractures initially described were for medial and lateral entry pins that crossed, but recent studies have advocated lateral-entry–only pinning to diminish the risk of iatrogenic injury to ulnar nerve. The reported risk of injury with crossed pinning ranges from 0 to 4%.[27,28]

The important technical points for fixation with lateral-entry pins are (1) maximize separation of the pins at the fracture site, (2) engage the medial and lateral columns proximal to the fracture, (3) engage sufficient bone in both the proximal segment and the distal fragment, and (4) maintain a low threshold for use of a third lateral-entry pin if there is concern about fracture stability or the location of the first two pins.[27] Stability testing under fluoroscopy has also been recommended, with addition of another lateral-entry pin or a medial-entry pin if the fracture is not stable.[29,30] Stability is assessed by flexing and extending the elbow during lateral fluoroscopy and by anteroposterior fluoroscopic views as the elbow is rotated from outward to inward rotation. The risk of injury to the ulnar nerve with medial-entry pins can be lessened by putting the pin in with the elbow in an extended position, as some children have subluxation of the ulnar nerve over the medial epicondyle with flexion past 90°. Using this technique for medial pinning and a small medial incision, a recent prospective randomized trial comparing lateral-entry pins with medial- and lateral-entry pins found no difference in effectiveness or complications.[28]

Recently, a modification of the Gartland classification introduced a type IV fracture that is unstable in both extension and flexion.[31] This fracture is typically identified after attempted closed reduction when the fluoroscopic lateral view shows that the distal fragment has moved from posterior to anterior relative to the proximal shaft. Tips for obtaining a closed reduction are the use of two parallel lateral-entry pins in only the distal fragment initially to use as joysticks, and rotating the fluoroscopy unit and not the patient's arm to see the lateral view. After fracture reduction, the pins are advanced to engage bone in the proximal fragment, and then a third lateral-entry pin is added.

Management of supracondylar fractures with associated vascular injury follows protocols established by several retrospective studies. Patients with absent radial and ulnar pulses are grouped into those with adequate distal perfusion (pink hand) and those without (white hand). Those with a white hand often have a ruptured brachial artery with inadequate collateral circulation, and the surgical team should be prepared to explore and repair/reconstruct the brachial artery after reducing and pinning the fracture.[32] Arteriography is not indicated in isolated injuries. Patients with a pink hand should undergo closed reduction and pinning. A near-anatomic reduction (no gap) should be obtained; a persistent gap at the fracture may indicate that the artery is entrapped in the fracture or tethered by soft tissues that are pulled into the fracture.

In patients with absent pulses and an irreducible fracture, an anterior approach for open reduction should be used to visualize the artery and reduce the fracture. If the pulse returns after closed reduction, the patient is admitted for observation. If the pulse does not return, there is disagreement about the best management strategy. Many recommend arterial exploration, but if there is a Doppler signal at the wrist and the hand remains well perfused, the patient can be admitted to the hospital for observation and perfusion, swelling, and active finger motion carefully monitored. If a patient with an intact pulse preoperatively loses the pulse after closed reduction and pinning, open reduction is indicated in most cases to assess the artery.

A safe position for immobilization is a concern after supracondylar humerus fractures, and limiting elbow flexion to less than 90° seems to be safest. Studies in supracondylar humerus fracture patients evaluating the radial pulse have shown ablation of the pulse with excessive flexion and pronation, as well as elevated compartment pressure in the deep volar compartment of the forearm with flexion greater than 90°.[33]

Flexion-type fractures are commonly caused by shear mechanism, are usually oblique in orientation, and thus are more unstable than extension-type fractures. Flexion-type supracondylar humerus fractures are much less common, representing less than 5% of supracondylar fractures. The ulnar nerve is the most commonly injured nerve with this injury pattern, and closed reduction is often more difficult.[34,35] There is a higher incidence of open reduction for flexion-type fractures when compared to extension injuries.[34,35]

If open reduction is needed, an anteromedial approach is typically used, although anterolateral and posterior approaches have also been used with good results. Open reduction allows removal of obstacles to reduction (periosteum, muscle) and removal of any entrapped nerves or the brachial artery. Pin placement is percutaneous after reduction with the same techniques used following closed reduction.

Lateral Condyle Fractures

A new classification system has been developed to guide treatment decisions.[36] Nondisplaced or minimally displaced (less than 2 mm) lateral condyle fractures are treated with immobilization and radiographic surveillance to make sure the fracture heals in good position.[37] Oblique radiographs that make the lateral column of the distal humerus visible are helpful to assess the displacement. When the amount of displacement of the joint surface is uncertain because of incomplete or absent epiphyseal ossification, arthrography via injection posteriorly into the olecranon fossa can allow visualization of the articular surface.[36] MRI can be used, but often requires another anesthetic, and arthrography can supply the same information and also allows dynamic assessment. If the fracture is hinged with the articular surface intact, a closed reduction and percutaneous pinning is indicated. Displaced lateral condyle fractures are treated with open reduction and internal fixation to anatomically align the joint surface.[36,37] The risk of nonunion is lessened by surgical technique that preserves soft-tissue attachments to the lateral condyle fragment and provides stable internal fixation. Wire fixation with maximal spread at the fracture level is recommended, unless there is a large metaphyseal fragment that permits screw fixation. Additional stabilization is provided by 3 to 6 weeks of immobilization in an above-elbow cast.

Monteggia Fracture-Dislocations

Late recognition of Monteggia fracture-dislocations still occurs and leads to difficult reconstructive procedures. Assessing the radiocapitellar line on every lateral radiograph of the elbow (a line down the radial shaft should pass through the center of the capitellar ossification center) will prevent missing the diagnosis. Usually closed reduction of the ulnar shaft deformity will result in reduction of the dislocated radial head. If closed reduction is not possible, open reduction through a lateral approach is indicated, with preservation or repair of the annular ligament. In older patients (age 10 years or older) with length-unstable ulnar fractures, plate fixation may be indicated to maintain length and reduction of the radiocapitellar joint. Late reconstruction of missed Monteggia injuries is considered when the radial head retains its concave structure, and typically involves osteotomy of the ulna to correct angular and length deformity, with or without annular ligament reconstruction.[38] Some studies on late reconstruction report excellent results in most patients,[38] but others caution about the significant potential for complications.

Displaced and Angulated Radial Neck Fractures

The management of radial neck fractures with less than 30° angulation and less than 3 to 5 mm of translation is brief immobilization and then graduated return to function. The troublesome fractures are those with greater degrees of angulation and displacement. Healing in this position can result in a cam effect that will block rotation of the radius and limit forearm supination and pronation. Open reduction of displaced radial neck fractures is associated with several complications, including stiffness and osteonecrosis. These risks encourage attempts at closed reduction, percutaneous pin reduction, intramedullary pin reduction, or manipulation of the distal radial neck with a curved elevator – all attempted without opening the fracture or radiocapitellar joint to reduce the fracture to an acceptable position. Multiple methods of closed manipulation are described, and all can be attempted before more invasive methods are used. A stout pin placed distal and posterior to the fracture can be introduced into the fracture and used to lever the radial head back onto the neck, or the pin can be used to directly push on the radial head. If any of these reduction methods is successful, stability is tested with supination and pronation under fluoroscopy, and if needed the fracture is stabilized with obliquely directed wires. Alternatively, excellent success and functional results are reported using a retrograde intramedullary rod, which is driven proximally to the fracture and then rotated and driven into the radial neck/head fragment. Rotation of a curved rod can assist in reducing the fracture, and also provides internal fixation.[39]

If the above techniques fail, a formal open reduction is done with a lateral approach to the radiocapitellar joint. Usually the radial head fragment is displaced laterally and distally, and in exposing it care is taken to avoid injury to the deep branch of the radial nerve and preserve any intact soft-tissue attachments, as they may provide vascularity to the fragment. The annular ligament should be evaluated and may need to be divided and repaired later to replace the radial head in anatomic position in the joint. Obliquely placed wires, small screws, or an intramedullary rod is used for fixation.

Fractures of the Radial and Ulnar Shafts

Most diaphyseal fractures of the radius and ulna can be treated with closed reduction and casting in skeletally immature patients, even in adolescents.[40,41] For those patients who have unacceptable angulation (greater than 10° or 15° in patients older than 10 years), surgical stabilization with flexible intramedullary nails has been shown to be effective.[42-44] Plate and screw fixation is also reliable and effective, and may be favored for length-unstable fractures in patients with less than 2 years of growth remaining. The larger surgical exposure needed for plate fixation, coupled with the more difficult removal of internal fixation, leads most to favor intramedullary nail stabilization in skeletally immature patients. Surgical treatments have higher complication rates than nonsurgical treatment.[45] Reported surgical complications include prominent internal fixation, loss of fixation, delayed union and nonunion, infections, carpal tunnel syndrome, synostosis, nerve injury, and compartment syndrome. Multiple attempts to

pass an intramedullary nail without opening the fracture may be associated with increased swelling and risk of compartment syndrome;[46] thus, if reduction and passage of the rod is not easily accomplished in two or three passes, the fracture should be opened to allow direct visualization and passage of the rod. Refractures are more common in midshaft and proximal fractures and in fractures with delayed healing.[47] For fractures that occur in the distal third of the forearm, two level I studies have found that well-molded below-elbow immobilization is as effective as above-elbow immobilization at maintaining reduction.[48,49]

Summary

Most pediatric patients with fractures can be treated nonsurgically and have good results. As noted previously, certain fractures are treated surgically to preserve growth potential and a smooth articular surface, to improve the functional result compared to nonsurgical treatment, or to minimize the potential for complications. The enhanced healing potential in children, along with the stability of simple fracture patterns and the thicker periosteum, often allow for less rigid fixation than is typically used for adult patients. Modern series of surgical pediatric fracture care generally report excellent outcomes with low complication rates, demonstrating the progress in pediatric fracture care over the past few decades.

Annotated References

1. Karunakar MA, Goulet JA, Mueller KL, Bedi A, Le TT: Operative treatment of unstable pediatric pelvis and acetabular fractures. *J Pediatr Orthop* 2005;25(1):34-38.

   The purpose of this study was to evaluate the results of surgical stabilization of unstable pelvic and acetabular fractures in children and adolescents. Eighteen patients younger than 16 years of age treated over a 7-year period were reviewed. All fractures healed by 10 weeks. No wound complications, infections, or growth arrests were noted with an average follow-up of 30 months. Favorable clinical results can be achieved with a low incidence of complications.

2. Smith W, Shurnas P, Morgan S, et al: Clinical outcomes of unstable pelvic fractures in skeletally immature patients. *J Bone Joint Surg Am* 2005;87:2423-2431.

   The authors studied influences on clinical and functional outcomes in unstable pelvic fractures in skeletally immature patients in a retrospective review.

3. Shrader MW, Jacofsky DJ, Stans AA, Shaughnessy WJ, Haidukewych GJ: Femoral neck fractures in pediatric patients: 30 years experience at a level 1 trauma center. *Clin Orthop Relat Res* 2007;454:169-173.

   The goal of this study was to identify what factors contribute to osteonecrosis in skeletally immature patients with femoral neck fractures. Twenty patients, average age 11 years, comprised the study group. Two of the 20 patients developed osteonecrosis. Five of the patients were treated more than 48 hours after injury including the two with osteonecrosis. Mean time to fixation for the other patients was 12 hours. There was no relationship between capsular decompression and osteonecrosis. Quality of reduction and timing to surgery influenced the risk of osteonecrosis.

4. Moon ES, Mehlman CT: Risk factors for avascular necrosis after femoral neck fractures in children: 25 Cincinnati cases and meta-analysis of 360 cases. *J Orthop Trauma* 2006;20(5):323-329.

The purpose was to identify risk factors for osteonecrosis in pediatric femoral neck fractures. The study reviewed 25 femoral neck fractures, average patient age 8 years, and 300 additional cases from the literature. They found fracture type and age as the only significant predictors of osteonecrosis.

5. Ramseier LE, Bhaskar AR, Cole WG, Howard AW: Treatment of open femur fractures in children: Comparison between external fixator and intramedullary nailing. *J Pediatr Orthop* 2007;27(7):748-750.

The goal of this study was to compare external fixation to intramedullary devices in the treatment of open pediatric femur fractures. Complications were five times more likely in the external fixation group (2.7 times if pin tract infections are excluded). Refracture, associated with varus malunion, only occurred in the external fixation group.

6. Sink EL, Gralla J, Repine M: Complications of pediatric femur fractures treated with titanium elastic nails: A comparison of fracture types. *J Pediatr Orthop* 2005; 25(5):577-580.

The purpose of the study was to analyze complications in femur fractures stabilized with flexible titanium nails comparing their use in stable and unstable fracture patterns. Length-unstable fracture patterns had the highest risk of unplanned follow-up surgery.

7. Ho CA, Skaggs DL, Tang CW, Kay RM: Use of flexible intramedullary nails in pediatric femur fractures. *J Pediatr Orthop* 2006;26(4):497-504.

This study focuses on outcomes of flexible intramedullary nailing. In a review of 94 fractures, an overall complication rate of 17% was found. The complication rate was significantly higher for patients aged 10 years and older (34%) compared to those age 9 years or younger (9%).

8. Wall EJ, Jain V, Vora V, Mehlman CT, Crawford AH: Complications of titanium and stainless steel elastic nail fixation of pediatric femoral fractures. *J Bone Joint Surg Am* 2008;90(6):1305-1313.

This study investigated the outcomes of titanium versus stainless steel flexible nail fixation of pediatric femur fractures. A higher malunion rate was found in the titanium nail group. The malunion rate did not correlate with age, weight, fracture stability or nail diameter using the authors' nail sizing recommendations.

9. Hedequist D, Bishop J, Hresko T: Locking plate fixation for pediatric femur fractures. *J Pediatr Orthop* 2008;28(1):6-9.

The purpose of this study was to assess locking plate fixation for pediatric femur fractures. Thirty-two patients with an average age of 11 years were reviewed. The indications for the use of a locking plate were comminution, nonmalignant pathologic fractures, fracture location, and osteopenia. All patients but one healed in near-anatomic alignment.

10. Poolman RW, Kocher MS, Bhandari M: Pediatric femoral fractures: A systematic review of 2422 cases. *J Orthop Trauma* 2006;20(9):648-654.

This study was a systematic review to determine the effect different treatment options have on complications and outcomes after femoral shaft fractures in children.

11. Wilfinger C, Castellani C, Raith J, Pilhatsch A, Höllwarth ME, Weinberg AM: Nonoperative treatment of tibial spine fractures in children: 38 patients with a minimum follow-up of 1 year. *J Orthop Trauma* 2009; 23(7):519-524.

The purpose of this study was to determine if nonsurgical treatment of tibial spine fractures in children is the treatment of choice. Forty-three patients were treated with aspiration and extension casting. Only one patient required surgery. No cases of meniscal entrapment were noted.

12. Pesl T, Havranek P: Acute tibial tubercle avulsion fractures in children: Selective use of the closed reduction and internal fixation method. *J Child Orthop* 2008; 2(5):353-356.

This study evaluated the selective use of closed reduction and internal fixation in tibial tubercle fractures. They found that for displaced intra-articular fractures, closed reduction with percutaneous fixation was a successful treatment.

13. Barmada A, Gaynor T, Mubarak SJ: Premature physeal closure following distal tibia physeal fractures: A new radiographic predictor. *J Pediatr Orthop* 2003;23(6): 733-739.

14. Leary JT, Handling M, Talerico M, Yong L, Bowe JA: Physeal fractures of the distal tibia: Predictive factors of premature physeal closure and growth arrest. *J Pediatr Orthop* 2009;29(4):356-361.

This study investigated the incidence and predictors of premature physeal closure. Fifteen fractures with premature closure were identified. They found only initial displacement—not residual gap or number of reductions—correlated highest with early physeal closure.

15. Kaya A, Altay T, Ozturk H, Karapinar L: Open reduction and internal fixation in displaced juvenile Tillaux fractures. *Injury* 2007;38(2):201-205.

This study reviewed 10 patients with surgically managed juvenile Tillaux fractures. The results indicate uniformly good results at average follow-up of 54 months.

16. Goldfarb CA, Bassett GS, Sullivan S, Gordon JE: Retrosternal displacement after physeal fracture of the medial clavicle in children: treatment by open reduction and internal fixation. *J Bone Joint Surg Br* 2001;83(8):1168-1172.

17. Waters PM, Bae DS, Kadiyala RK. Short-term outcomes after surgical treatment of traumatic posterior sternoclavicular fracture-dislocations in children and adolescents. *J Pediatr Orthop* 2003;23(4):464-469.

18. Beringer DC, Weiner DS, Noble JS, Bell RH: Severely displaced proximal humeral epiphyseal fractures: A follow-up study. *J Pediatr Orthop* 1998;18(1):31-37.

19. Dobbs MB, Luhmann SL, Gordon JE, Strecker WB, Schoenecker PL: Severely displaced proximal humeral epiphyseal fractures. *J Pediatr Orthop* 2003;23(2):208-215.

20. Hwang RW, Bae DS, Waters PM: Brachial plexus palsy following proximal humerus fracture in patients who are skeletally immature. *J Orthop Trauma* 2008;22(4):286-290.

Neurologic injuries after proximal humerus fracture in children are rare. Valgus displacement places the brachial plexus at greater risk.

21. De Boeck H, De Smet P, Penders W, De Rydt D: Supracondylar elbow fractures with impaction of the medial condyle in children. *J Pediatr Orthop* 1995;15(4):444-448.

22. Mehlman CT, Strub WM, Roy DR, Wall EJ, Crawford AH: The effect of surgical timing on the perioperative complications of treatment of supracondylar humeral fractures in children. *J Bone Joint Surg Am* 2001;83(3):323-327.

23. Gupta N, Kay RM, Leitch K, Femino JD, Tolo VT, Skaggs DL: Effect of surgical delay on perioperative complications and need for open reduction in supracondylar humerus fractures in children. *J Pediatr Orthop* 2004;24(3):245-248.

There were no significant differences between the early and delayed treatment groups in perioperative complication rates, the need to perform an open reduction, neurologic or vascular damage, or pin site infection.

24. Ramachandran M, Skaggs DL, Crawford HA, et al: Delaying treatment of supracondylar fractures in children: Has the pendulum swung too far? *J Bone Joint Surg Br* 2008;90(9):1228-1233.

Patients from multiple centers around the world over a 10-year period who developed compartment syndrome after delayed treatment of supracondylar humerus fractures were identified. All 11 patients presented with low-energy fractures with an intact radial pulse. The mean delay was 22 hours (range, 6 to 64 hours).

25. Blakemore LC, Cooperman DR, Thompson GH, Wathey C, Ballock RT: Compartment syndrome in ipsilateral humerus and forearm fractures in children. *Clin Orthop Relat Res* 2000;376:32-38.

26. Archibeck MJ, Scott SM, Peters CL: Brachialis muscle entrapment in displaced supracondylar humerus fractures: A technique of closed reduction and report of initial results. *J Pediatr Orthop* 1997;17(3):298-302.

27. Skaggs DL, Cluck MW, Mostofi A, Flynn JM, Kay RM: Lateral-entry pin fixation in the management of supracondylar fractures in children. *J Bone Joint Surg Am* 2004;86(4):702-707.

The authors concluded that the use of lateral-entry pins alone was effective for even the most unstable supracondylar humeral fractures. There were no iatrogenic ulnar nerve injuries, and no reduction was lost.

28. Kocher MS, Kasser JR, Waters PM, et al: Lateral entry compared with medial and lateral entry pin fixation for completely displaced supracondylar humeral fractures in children: A randomized clinical trial. *J Bone Joint Surg Am* 2007;89(4):706-712.

The authors did not find significant differences in clinical or radiographic outcomes, or complications, for type III extension supracondylar humerus fractures treated with either lateral-entry pins or medial- and lateral-entry pins. Level of evidence: I.

29. Sankar WN, Hebela NM, Skaggs DL, Flynn JM: Loss of pin fixation in displaced supracondylar humeral fractures in children: Causes and prevention. *J Bone Joint Surg Am* 2007;89(4):713-717.

Eight of 279 supracondylar fractures had postoperative loss of pin fixation. In all cases, technical errors in pin placement were noted.

30. Zenios M, Ramachandran M, Milne B, Little D, Smith N: Intraoperative stability testing of lateral-entry pin fixation of pediatric supracondylar humeral fractures. *J Pediatr Orthop* 2007;27(6):695-702.

A comparison of lateral intraoperative fluoroscopic views in internal and external rotation was used to assess stability, and an additional lateral-entry wire or medial-entry wire was placed if the fracture was not stable. Only 26% of fractures were stable after two lateral-entry wires. After institution of the stability testing protocol, no patient had a return to the operating room for loss of reduction.

31. Leitch KK, Kay RM, Femino JD, Tolo VT, Storer SK, Skaggs DL: Treatment of multidirectionally unstable supracondylar humeral fractures in children: A modified Gartland type-IV fracture. *J Bone Joint Surg Am* 2006;88(5):980-985.

The authors propose a type IV fracture to add to the Gartland classification; this is a very unstable fracture that will displace from an extended to a flexed position secondary to disruption of the soft-tissue envelope on both sides. A method of closed reduction and pinning is described.

32. Choi PD, Melikian R, Skaggs DL: Risk factors for vascular repair and compartment syndrome in the pulseless

supracondylar humerus fracture in children. *J Pediatr Orthop* 2010;30:50-56.

In a large series, 2.6% of patients with supracondylar humerus fractures presented without distal pulses. Of the 33 patients, 24 were well perfused and 9 were poorly perfused at presentation; 4 of the 9 poorly perfused patients had an arerial injury that was repaired. Two of these patients later developed compartment syndrome. None of the 24 well-perfused patients had vascular repair, and none developed compartment syndrome.

33. Battaglia TC, Armstrong DG, Schwend RM: Factors affecting forearm compartment pressures in children with supracondylar fractures of the humerus. *J Pediatr Orthop* 2002;22(4):431-439.

34. Mahan ST, May CD, Kocher MS: Operative management of displaced flexion supracondylar humerus fractures in children. *J Pediatr Orthop* 2007;27(5):551-556.

Flexion-type fractures are more likely to undergo open reduction and have a higher incidence of ulnar nerve injury than extension-type fractures.

35. Steinman S, Bastrom TP, Newton PO, Mubarak SJ: Beware of ulnar nerve entrapment in flexion-type supracondylar humerus fractures. *J Child Orthop* 2007;1(3): 177-180.

Flexion-type fractures were noted to have a higher incidence of open treatment than extension-type fractures, and entrapment of the ulnar nerve in the fracture site medially was noted in three patients.

36. Weiss JM, Graves S, Yang S, Mendelsohn E, Kay RM, Skaggs DL: A new classification system predictive of complications in surgically treated pediatric humeral lateral condyle fractures. *J Pediatr Orthop* 2009;29(6): 602-605.

The authors classified fractures based on amount of displacement and integrity of articular surface. Type I has less than 2 mm displacement, type II has 2 mm or greater displacement with intact articular surface by arthrogram, and type III 2 mm or greater displacement and articular surface disrupted. Type II and III fractures were treated surgically, and type III fractures had a higher complication risk. All type III fractures had displacement of 4 mm or greater.

37. Launay F, Leet AI, Jacopin S, Jouve JL, Bollini G, Sponseller PD: Lateral humeral condyle fractures in children: A comparison of two approaches to treatment. *J Pediatr Orthop* 2004;24(4):385-391.

Nondisplaced fractures treated nonsurgically are at high risk for displacement and should be followed closely. Surgical treatment is indicated for fractures with greater than 2 mm of displacement. Nonunion did not occur after surgical treatment. The authors note the risk of infection with percutaneous pins, and if there are concerns about patient compliance with follow-up the authors believe leaving the pins subcutaneous may reduce this risk, although it will necessitate a second surgery to remove them.

38. Nakamura K, Hirachi K, Uchiyama S, et al: Long-term clinical and radiographic outcomes after open reduction for missed Monteggia fracture-dislocations in children. *J Bone Joint Surg Am* 2009;91(6):1394-1404.

Excellent long-term outcomes are reported in 16 of 22 patients after surgical treatment of missed Monteggia injuries in children younger than 12 years of age and diagnosed within 3 years of injury. At final follow-up 17 patients had a reduced radial head, and 5 had subluxation. Treatment involved open reduction, ulnar osteotomy, and annular ligament reconstruction.

39. Schmittenbecher PP, Haevernick B, Herold A, Knorr P, Schmid E: Treatment decision, method of osteosynthesis, and outcome in radial neck fractures in children: A multicenter study. *J Pediatr Orthop* 2005;25(1):45-50.

A prospective multicenter study of 66 cases from 12 departments found 74% of displaced fractures treated with closed or open reduction had good/excellent results. Fractures that required open reduction had worse results.

40. Jones K, Weiner DS: The management of forearm fractures in children: A plea for conservatism. *J Pediatr Orthop* 1999;19(6):811-815.

41. Zionts LE, Zalavras CG, Gerhardt MB: Closed treatment of displaced diaphyseal both-bone forearm fractures in older children and adolescents. *J Pediatr Orthop* 2005;25(4):507-512.

Closed treatment of displaced diaphyseal forearm fractures in children ages 8 to 15 years resulted in union in all cases and satisfactory functional outcomes.

42. Schmittenbecher PP, Fitze G, Gödeke J, Kraus R, Schneidmüller D: Delayed healing of forearm shaft fractures in children after intramedullary nailing. *J Pediatr Orthop* 2008;28(3):303-306.

In a retrospective review of 532 cases of elastic stable intramedullary nailing of displaced unstable forearm fractures in children (mean age, 12.3 years), only 1.9% showed delayed healing. Ulna fractures, open fractures, and fractures treated with open reduction were more common in the delayed healing group.

43. Rabinovich A, Adili A, Mah J: Outcomes of intramedullary nail fixation through the olecranon apophysis in skeletally immature forearm fractures. *J Pediatr Orthop* 2005;25(5):565-569.

Radiographic and functional measures showed healing and few limitations in 19 patients treated with intramedullary nail fixation through the olecranon apophysis. No significant growth abnormalities were noted in the olecranon.

44. Jubel A, Andermahr J, Isenberg J, Issavand A, Prokop A, Rehm KE: Outcomes and complications of elastic stable intramedullary nailing for forearm fractures in children. *J Pediatr Orthop B* 2005;14(5):375-380.

In a prospective study of 51 children treated with elastic stable intramedullary nailing for displaced diaphyseal forearm fractures, 43 had excellent or good results at 38-month follow-up.

45. Smith VA, Goodman HJ, Strongwater A, Smith B: Treatment of pediatric both-bone forearm fractures: A comparison of operative techniques. *J Pediatr Orthop* 2005;25(3):309-313.

In a retrospective case control study of closed treatment, open reduction and internal fixation with plates and intramedullary rodding showed significantly higher complications in the surgically treated fractures. Intramedullary rodding had a higher incidence of complication, although most were minor, and open reduction and internal fixation with plates had a higher percentage of major complications.

46. Yuan PS, Pring ME, Gaynor TP, Mubarak SJ, Newton PO: Compartment syndrome following intramedullary fixation of pediatric forearm fractures. *J Pediatr Orthop* 2004;24(4):370-375.

Two hundred five of 235 closed fractures were treated with closed reduction and casting, and none developed compartment syndrome. Thirty were treated with closed reduction and intramedullary fixation, and there was a 10% incidence of compartment syndrome. Fifty patients with open fractures were treated with débridement and intramedullary nail fixation, and 6% developed compartment syndrome. Longer surgical times were associated with an increased risk of compartment syndrome. The authors caution against multiple attempts to pass the intramedullary device and recommend open reduction if the fracture is not easily reduced and pinned.

47. Baitner AC, Perry A, Lalonde FD, Bastrom TP, Pawelek J, Newton PO: The healing forearm fracture: A matched comparison of forearm refractures. *J Pediatr Orthop* 2007;27(7):743-747.

Proximal and middle-third forearm fractures were at higher risk for refracture. The time to refracture averaged 10 months. Incomplete healing was noted more frequently in those with refractures.

48. Webb GR, Galpin RD, Armstrong DG: Comparison of short and long arm plaster casts for displaced fractures in the distal third of the forearm in children. *J Bone Joint Surg Am* 2006;88(1):9-17.

A prospective randomized trial of 113 patients with 8-month follow-up is presented. Well-molded short arm casts are as effective as a long arm cast to treat fractures of the distal third of the forearm in children age 4 years and older.

49. Bohm ER, Bubbar V, Yong Hing K, Dzus A: Above and below-the-elbow plaster casts for distal forearm fractures in children: A randomized controlled trial. *J Bone Joint Surg Am* 2006;88(1):1-8.

The authors present a prospective, randomized, blinded trial of 102 children, mean age 8.6 years. Below-elbow casts performed as well as above-elbow casts in maintaining reduction of distal third forearm fractures, and complications were similar.

6: Geriatric and Pediatric Trauma

Index

Blade plating vs. locked plating, 83

Blast injuries, 103–105, 174, 491

Bleeding, gastrointestinal, 540

Blunt injuries
brachial plexus injuries, 193
cervical spine injuries, 357
head injuries, 104
in pelvic injuries, 281
penetrating injuries vs., 61, 174, 176
pulmonary function and, 125
thoracolumbar trauma as, 375

BMPs. *See* Bone morphogenetic proteins

Bohler angle, 521, 524

Bone. *See also* Osteopenic bone;
Pathologic bone
cancellous vs. cortical, 557
defects in
forearm fractures and, 244
grafting for (*See* Bone grafting)
loss of, 62
reaming of, 85

Bone grafting
fracture healing (*See* Bone healing)
for fractures
distal femur, 447, 448
distal radius, 247, 251
femoral neck, 412f
tibial shaft, 491
in lower extremity injuries, 66
for nonunions
aseptic, 455
atrophic, 152
femoral shaft fracture, 439
forearm, 244, 255
scaphoid, 266–267
osteomyelitis and, 166, 167
in osteotomies, 149
in posterior glenohumeral joint
dislocations, 192–193
staged treatment issues, 153
types of
allogenic bone, 149, 152
allograft bone (*See* Allograft bone)
autogenous bone graft, 136–137,
152–153
autogenous bone marrow, 133, 136t,
137
autograft bone (*See* Autograft bone)
autologous bone, 149, 152, 569
iliac crest, 137, 138, 362

Bone graft substitutes, 167
for acetabular fracture fixation, 326
for atrophic nonunions, 152
bone morphogenetic proteins as, 138
calcium phosphates as, 137
calcium sulfates as, 137–138
demineralized bone matrix as, 138
for distal femur fractures, 447
for distal radius fractures, 251
nanotechnology for, 85
platelet concentrates as, 138
systemic agents as, 139

for tibial plateau fracture fixation, 479

Bone healing
critical components of, 133–134
diabetes and, 507
enhancement of, 139–141
in osteoporotic context, 560–561
phases of, 134–135

Bone hooks, 42, 424. *See also* Shoulder
hooks

Bone impactors for plate removal, 46f

Bone marrow regeneration, 342

Bone morphogenetic proteins (BMPs)
for atrophic nonunions, 153
benefits of, 138
for bone defects, 134, 138
as bone graft substitute, 138
bone healing with, 561
for distal femur fractures, 447
limitations of, 138
recommendation grade, 136t, 138
role in electrical stimulation, 138
role in osteoinduction, 133
for tibial shaft fractures, 493

Bone scans, 164f, 404, 562

Bone stimulation, 493

Bone tunnel placement, 31

Bother index. *See* Short Musculoskeletal
Function Assessment (SMFA)

Bowel dysfunction/injuries, 317, 540

Boyd classification system, 417

Brachial plexus injuries
associated nerve injuries, 193
characteristics of, 193
glenohumeral joint dislocations and,
191
with humeral shaft fractures, 209
scapulothoracic dissociation and, 186
treatment of, 193–194

Bracing
for burst fractures, 379
for low lumbar fractures, 388
functional, 209, 210
role of, 373–374
for sacral fractures, 394
for tibial shaft fractures, 489

Brain injuries, 311

Bridge plating
application of, 45–46
benefits of, 135
for humeral diaphyseal fractures, 43
internal, 251
for pilon fractures, 44–45

Bridging external fixation. *See* External
fixation

Burst fractures
as C1 fracture, 349
as flexion-distraction injuries, 380
imaging for, 365f, 378f

low lumbar fractures, 387–388, 388t,
389t, 390
minimally invasive techniques for, 390

osteoporosis and, 379
without neurologic deficits, 378–379

C

Calcaneal fractures
calcium phosphates for, 137
classification of, 522
complications in, 523–524
evaluation of, 521–522
imaging for, 88
locked plating for, 83–84
negative pressure wound therapy for, 87
outcomes, 524, 526
surgical approach, 522–523

Calcaneus, 520–521, 521f

Calcium deficiency, 145, 558, 561

Calcium phosphates
benefits of, 137
as bone graft substitute, 137
as fracture cement, 133, 135f, 251, 255
limitations of, 137
in osteoconduction, 133
for osteoporotic bone fixation, 560
recommendation grade, 136t, 137

Calcium sulfates, 136t, 137–138, 560

Canadian C-Spine Rule (CCR), 358, 358f,
360f

Canadian Orthopaedic Trauma Society,
188

Canale classification system, 519

Cancellous croutons, 251

Cancer, 536, 539, 562, 564

Capacitive coupling. *See* Electrical
stimulation

Capitellum fractures, 8

Capping, of an amputated extremity, 76

Capsular decompression, 580

Cardiovascular risk, 432, 537t

Career development, 19, 20t, 26. *See also*
Practice management

Carpal tunnel syndrome, 245, 257, 266,
587

Cartilage, 87–88

Castile soap, 52, 166

Cauda equina syndrome, 300, 374t,
387–388, 393

C-clamp, 282, 287–288, 288f

Celiotomy, 109

Cell necrosis, 52

Cellular apoptosis, 341

Center of rotation of angulation (CORA),
149, 151f

Centers for Disease Control and
Prevention (CDC), 19, 104

Central cord syndrome, 365–366

Central venous catheterization, 539

Cephalomedullary nailing, 418, 419,
424, 425. *See also* Intramedullary (IM)
nailing

Cephalosporin, 52, 164, 165t

Cerclage techniques

Index

forearm, 243–244, 244f
metacarpal, 269f
odontoid, 350, 351
olecranon, 226–227
patellar, 465–466
pelvic, 286–288, 286f, 288f
periprosthetic, 569–570, 571–573, 574
radial head, 229–230, 229f
tibial plateau, 478f, 479f
fractures caused by, 46
fragment-specific fixation, 250–251
iliosacral screws (*See* Iliosacral screw placement)
implant considerations, 563
importance of imaging for, 42
inadequate, 293, 301–302
infections and, 43, 44
for injuries
ankle syndesmosis, 501, 502
cervical spine, 354, 357, 367
head injuries, 126
injury physiology and, 117
locking screws for, 41
lumbopelvic, 300, 394
malunion in, 42
navigation systems for, 42
osteoporosis issues, 43, 83, 558–559
outcomes for, 83–84
of pelvic ring, 393
for perilunate dislocations, 267
thin wire, 481, 482
timing of, 174, 311
trauma effects, 118
Flail chest, 125
Flap coverage
for bilateral lower extremity injuries, 72f
definitive closure, 74
limb length preservation, 71
for lower extremity injuries, 67
for soft-tissue injuries, 52–53, 176
for transtibial amputation, 72–73
for upper extremity amputation, 73
Flash burns, 104
Flat back, 388
Flexion-distraction injuries, 379–381
Floating elbow injuries, 214f
Floating knee injuries, 436–437, 489
Fluoroscopy
applications of, 31
for classifying nonunions, 147
for dislocations, 462, 579
in fixation
clavicle, 188, 189f
of fractures (general), 41, 42, 43
iliosacral screw placement, 32, 38
pedicle screw placement guidance, 36
pelvic, 287, 288
percutaneous fracture, 32–33
PIP joint, 271
tibial shaft, 492, 493
volar locked plating, 250

for fractures
acetabular, 35–36, 323
distal femur, 451, 452
distal radius, 251, 255f
forearm, 244
odontoid, 36
proximal humeral, 584
supracondylar humerus, 585
tibial plateau, 480
guidewire placement, 33, 33f
for injuries
ankle syndesmosis, 500, 503f
cervical spine, 358
in minimally invasive surgery, 45
for obese patients, 438
pelvic ring disruptions. visualization of, 34
radiation limits for, 37
registration of, 31
sacroiliac joint techniques, 32
three-dimensional, 88
Focused Assessment With Sonography for Trauma (FAST), 282
Fondaparinux, 127, 539
Forearm
anatomy of, 241
fractures of, 241–244, 258, 263, 535
(*See also specific arm fractures*)
Fracture-dislocations. *See also*
Dislocations; Fractures
of cervical spine, 357, 360–361, 363
of elbow (*See under* Elbow)
of femoral head, 401
flexion-distraction injuries vs., 380
of glenohumeral joint, 190
of knee, 475
Lisfranc, 524–525
lumbosacral, 394
Monteggia, 242–243, 586
Monteggia-variant, 234, 234f
of pelvic ring, 295
of PIP joint, 270–271
posteromedial, 235, 235f
posteromedial varus, 231, 235
sacral, 393
of sacroiliac (SI) joint, 112
tibial plateau fractures as, 475
transolecranon, 233–234, 233f
Fractures
acetabular, 34-36, 309-318, 324-329, 399, 401, 402, 561, 571-572, 579
achieving union, 151
anterior impression, 192
avulsion, 112, 279, 350, 363, 521
Barton, 258
bicondylar tibial plateau, 82
bilateral femoral shaft, 124, 435, 436
biology of healing, 133, 492–493
bone grafting for, 136–137
burst, 349, 365, 379-380, 387-390
C1, 348-350

calcaneal, 83-84, 87-88, 137, 521-524, 526
calcar, 572
carpal, 263
classifying, 6–9, 63
clavicle, 83, 181, 186-188, 187f, 188f, 184f, 193
compression-burst, 363
coracoid fractures, 184
coronal plane, 8, 446, 454
coronoid, 225, 226, 228, 232-235
cuboid, 524
dancers, 526
deformity assessment, 146–147
diaphyseal, 31, 36, 37, 42-44, 46, 148, 244, 561, 569
displaced, 191, 201, 207–208
distal femur, 41, 44, 83, 154f, 431, 445-457, 560-562
distal humerus, 8, 215-219, 538-539, 561
distal radius, 83, 84, 137, 245-258, 535
distal tibial, 41, 575, 583
electronic templating for, 88–89
energy determination, study by University of Iowa, 8
evolution of care, 41–42
fixation of (*See* Fixation)
flap coverage for, 53
Galeazzi, 241-242
greater trochanter, 420
greater tuberosity, 191, 192, 202
hangman's, 352-354
healing components, 133–134, 134f
healing enhancement, 139–141
HFS-97 scale, 64
Hoffa, 446, 449, 454, 454f
iliac wing, 112, 279, 296, 571, 579
infection incidence, 159
intercondylar, 82
low lumbar, 378-388, 388t, 390, 394
malleolar, 499, 502, 504-506
minimally displaced, 204
minimally invasive care, 41–47
nightstick, 241
nutcracker (cuboid), 524
olecranon, 225, 226, 228
operating room access, 24
phases of healing, 134–135
pilon, 44-45, 82, 87
rib, 181, 193
role of bracing for, 373–374
Smith, 258
Snowboarder's, 520
stability of
benefits/risks of early stabilization, 171
degrees of, 134–135
locked plate systems, 81–82, 83
mechanical, 133, 134f
open fractures, 12
pelvic fractures, 112

Index

Hip replacement. *See* Total hip arthroplasty (THA)

HIV, 145

Hoffa fracture, 446, 449, 454, 454*f*

Holland nail, 419–420

Holstein-Lewis fracture pattern, 213

Homeostasis, 159, 338, 557

Homologous tissue destruction, 118

Hoop stress, 434

Hospital for Special Surgery Knee Score, 457, 482

Hospitals. *See also* Trauma centers
  community trauma systems, 14
  compensation issues, 22
  contractural deliverables for employed physicians, 21*t*
  disaster preparedness phases, 98–101
  emergency care in, 11
  financial issues, 25–26
  institutional review board approvals, 13
  operational issues, 24–25
  patient care and transfer, 13, 15
  planning for disaster response, 101–102, 105
  practice management issues, 19
  resource allocation, 24
  stakeholders, 101*t*
  system planning and improvement in, 16
  trauma care/facilities in, 12, 19
  trauma center infrastructure, 22

Humerus
  classification of fractures, 8
  distal humerus fractures
    anatomy of, 215–216
    biomechanics of, 218
    classification of, 8, 216, 216*f*
    complications with, 219
    elbow arthroplasty and, 570–571
    evaluation of, 216
    in geriatric population, 538–539
    osteoporosis and, 561
    rehabilitation after, 219
    treatment for, 216–218
  extra-articular distal third fractures, 215
  fracture-dislocation, 206*f*
  humeral diaphyseal fractures (*See also* Diaphyseal fractures)
  minimally invasive care for, 43
  nonunion of, 209
  segmental, 208*f*
  surgical treatment for, 209–210
  humeral shaft fractures, 208–213
  hypertrophic nonunion, 148*f*
  lateral condyle fractures, 586
  periprosthetic humeral fractures, 569–570, 572*t*
  proximal humeral fractures
    anatomy of, 201–202, 202*f*
    approach for, 41
    brachial plexus injuries with, 193
    classification of, 203–204, 203*f*, 204*f*, 570*f*

displaced, 204, 207–208
epidemiology, 201
evaluation of, 202–203, 203*f*
in geriatric patients, 535
glenohumeral dislocations with, 191
locked plating for, 83, 84, 560
minimally invasive care for, 43
osteoporosis and, 557, 559, 561
pediatric considerations, 584–585
periprosthetic fractures, 569–570
treatment for, 204–208
radial nerve injuries with (*See* Radial nerve palsy (RNP))
supracondylar fractures, 585–586

Humpback deformity, 266

Hybrid fixation, 560. *See also* Fixation

Hydroxyapatite, 84–85

Hyperbaric oxygen, 166

Hypercapnia, 125

Hyperglycemia, 119, 160

Hyperinflammation, 117, 118, 122–124

Hyperparathyroidism, 467

Hypertension, uncontrolled, 537*t*

Hypertrophic nonunions. *See* Nonunions

Hypertrophy, 338

Hypogonadism, 145

Hypoperfusion, 113, 120*f*, 122, 124

Hypotension
  after major trauma, 119
  anemia and, 540
  fractures and, 171
  head injuries and, 126
  intraoperative hypotension, 172
  in lower extremity injuries, 63
  mortality and, 110
  in spinal injuries, 339

Hypothermia
  after major trauma, 119
  infections and, 160
  in lower extremity injuries, 63
  patient stability, 125*t*
  with pelvic fractures, 301
  pulmonary function and, 125
  in spinal injuries, 341
  in systemic inflammatory response, 121

Hypoventilation, 125

Hypovolemia, 63, 539

Hypovolemic shock. *See* Shock

Hypoxemia
  after major trauma, 119
  head injuries and, 126
  in lung injuries, 110
  pulmonary function and, 125, 125*t*

Hypoxia, 171, 172

I

Iatrogenic comminution, 434. *See also* Comminuted fractures

Iatrogenic cutaneous nerve, 188, 210, 212–213

ICD-9, orthopaedic coding issues, 25

Ileus, 300

Iliac wing fractures
  in children, 579
  ORIF for, 296*f*
  in pelvic fractures, 279
  periprosthetic fractures, 571
  stability of, 112
  treatment for, 296

Ilioinguinal exposure, 325, 326, 328

Ilioischial line, 316

Iliosacral screw placement
  computer-assisted, 32–33, 32*f*, 33*f*
  need for, 296, 296*f*
  technical considerations, 297–300, 297*f*, 298*f*

Image-guided orthopaedic surgery. *See* Computer-assisted orthopaedic surgery (CAOS)

Imaging. *See also specific imaging techniques*
  cartilage imaging, 87–88
  computer-assisted navigation, 31
  digital, 25
  importance of, in fracture fixation, 42
  for musculoskeletal infection, 163, 163*f*, 164*f*
  T1-rho mapping, 88
  T2 mapping, 87–88
  three-dimensional fluoroscopy, 88
  for triplane fractures, 583, 583*f*
  for upper extremity nerve injuries, 193

Immune response
  genetic components of, 122
  injury physiology, 117–119
  surgery and, 171
  surgical timing, 119*f*

Immunocompromise, 522

Immunologic dysfunction, 117, 118*f*, 119

Immunoscintigraphy, 163

Immunosuppression
  infections and, 159, 161, 162
  metabolic changes, 119
  surgical window for, 124
  trauma and, 117

Implants
  cost containment, 26
  electronic templating for, 89
  fixation issues, 563
  infections and, 165
  nanotechnology effects, 85
  pathologic bone and, 563

Incident Command System (ICS)
  function of, 96
  in hospitals, 102, 103*f*
  organizational structure of, 96, 97*f*

Incontinence, 303

Indium 111, 163

Indomethacin, 328, 329*f*

Infections. *See also* Nosocomial infections; Osteomyelitis
  in acromioclavicular joint repair, 190
  from amputation, 75

Index